THE ROUTLEDGE HANDBOOK OF YOUTH PHYSICAL ACTIVITY

Over the past three decades the study of pediatric physical inactivity has become a public health concern. The decreases in physical activity have been associated with obesity and numerous hypokinetic diseases. In accordance with this public health concern, the study of pediatric physical activity has become a central part of research in the health and exercise science fields.

The Routledge Handbook of Youth Physical Activity is the first book to survey the full depth and breadth of the issues facing this field. Bringing together many of the world's experts and practitioners, the book helps to develop an understanding of the underlying issues related to pediatric physical activity as well as the role physical activity plays on cognitive, psychomotor, and social aspects of childhood. The book addresses issues with physical activity measurement and discusses wide-ranging aspects of physical activity interventions.

With more emphasis than ever on physical activity, this book makes an important contribution to the scholars and practitioners working in the youth physical activity field.

This is the first single text on the state of current knowledge related to pediatric physical activity which offers a comprehensive guide to students and academics on these subjects. *The Routledge Handbook of Youth Physical Activity* is key reading for all advanced students, researchers, practitioners, and policy-makers with an interest in physical activity, youth sport, public health matters, sport studies, or physical education.

Timothy A. Brusseau, Ph.D. is Associate Professor and Director of Health and Kinesiology at the University of Utah, Salt Lake City, UT, USA. He is also the Director of the Physical Activity Research Laboratory.

Stuart J. Fairclough, Ph.D. is Professor of Physical Activity Education at Edge Hill University, UK. He is also a member of the UK Chief Medical Officers' Physical Activity Guidelines for Children and Young People Expert Group.

David R. Lubans is Professor and National Health and Medical Research Council Fellow in the Priority Research Centre for Physical Activity and Nutrition at the University of Newcastle, Australia.

THE ROUTLEDGE HANDBOOK OF YOUTH PHYSICAL ACTIVITY

Edited by
Timothy A. Brusseau, Stuart J. Fairclough, and
David R. Lubans

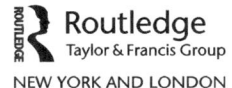

Routledge
Taylor & Francis Group

NEW YORK AND LONDON

First published 2020
by Routledge
605 Third Avenue, New York, NY 10017

and by Routledge
2 Park Square, Milton Park, Abingdon, Oxon, OX14 4RN

First issued in paperback 2022

Routledge is an imprint of the Taylor & Francis Group, an informa business

© 2020 Taylor & Francis

The right of Timothy A. Brusseau, Stuart J. Fairclough, and David R. Lubans to be identified as the authors of the editorial material, and of the authors for their individual chapters, has been asserted in accordance with sections 77 and 78 of the Copyright, Designs and Patents Act 1988.

Publisher's Note
The publisher has gone to great lengths to ensure the quality of this reprint but points out that some imperfections in the original copies may be apparent.

Library of Congress Cataloging-in-Publication Data
A catalog record for this title has been requested

ISBN 13: 978-1-03-240015-0 (pbk)
ISBN 13: 978-1-138-33154-9 (hbk)
ISBN 13: 978-1-003-02642-6 (ebk)

DOI: 10.4324/9781003026426

Typeset in Bembo
by codeMantra

CONTENTS

FIGURES

TABLES

BOXES

CONTRIBUTORS

Salomé Aubert, Children's Hospital of Eastern Ontario Research Institute, Canada.

Lisa M. Barnett, Deakin University, Australia.

Mark R. Beauchamp, University of British Columbia, Canada.

Aaron Beighle, University of Kentucky, USA.

Sarahjane Belton, Dublin City University, Ireland.

David Berrigan, National Cancer Institute, USA.

Stuart J. H. Biddle, University of Southern Queensland, Australia.

Maria Cristina Bisi, University of Bologna, Italy.

Lynne M. Boddy, Liverpool John Moores University, UK.

Amy Bohnert, Loyola University Chicago, USA.

Timothy A Brusseau, University of Utah, USA

Ryan D. Burns, University of Utah, USA.

John Cairney, University of Toronto, Canada.

Lorraine A. Cale, Loughborough University, UK.

Valerie Carson, University of Alberta, Canada.

Anna E. Chalkley, Loughborough University, UK.

Wai Chan, The Chinese University of Hong Kong, Hong Kong.

Cain C. T. Clark, Coventry University, UK.

Ana María Contardo Ayala, Deakin University, Australia.

Kirsten Corder, University of Cambridge, UK.

Sarah A. Costigan, Deakin University, Australia.

Sam G. M. Crossley, Swansea University, UK.

Benedicte Deforche, University of Ghent, Belgium.

Eric S. Drollette, University of North Carolina-Greensboro, USA.

Dean Dudley, Macquarie University, Australia.

Scott Duncan, Auckland University of Technology, New Zealand.

Narelle Eather, University of Newcastle, Australia.

Heather Erwin, University of Kentucky, USA.

Dale W. Esliger, Loughborough University, UK.

Stuart J. Fairclough, Edge Hill University, UK.

Lawrence Foweather, Liverpool John Moores University, UK.

Silvia A. González, Children's Hospital of Eastern Ontario Research Institute, Canada.

Trish Gorely, University of the Highlands and Islands, UK.

Amy S. Ha, Chinese University of Hong Kong, Hong Kong.

Allie Hardin, University of Texas, USA.

Nigel Harris, Auckland University of Technology, New Zealand.

Toni A. Hilland, RMIT University, Australia.

Charles H. Hillman, Northeastern University, USA.

Ryan M. Hulteen, University of British Columbia, Canada.

Stephen Hunter, University of Alberta, Canada.

Erika Ikeda, Auckland University of Technology, New Zealand.

Xanne Janssen, University of Strathclyde, UK.

Rachel A. Jones, University of Wollongong, Australia.

Sarah G. Kennedy, University of Newcastle, Australia.

Andrew P. Kingsnorth, Loughborough University, UK.

Sonja Klingberg, University of Cambridge, UK.

Natalie Lander, Deakin University, Australia.

Justin J. Lang, Public Health Agency of Canada, Canada.

Angus Leahy, University of Newcastle, Australia.

Venurs Loh, Deakin University, Australia.

Monica A. F. Lounsbery, Long Beach State University, USA.

Adam Loveday, Loughborough University, UK.

David R. Lubans, University of Newcastle, Australia.

Kelly A. Mackintosh, Swansea University, UK.

Sandra Mandic, University of Otago, New Zealand.

Taru Manyanga, Children's Hospital of Eastern Ontario Research Institute, Canada.

Anne Martin, University of Glasgow, UK.

Charles E. Matthews, National Cancer Institute, USA.

Emiliano Mazzoli, Deakin University, Australia.

Paul McCrorie, University of Glasgow, UK.

Tara N. McGoey, Canadore College, Canada.

Heather A. McKay, University of British Columbia, Canada.

Thomas L. McKenzie, San Diego State University, USA.

Melitta A. McNarry, Swansea University, UK.

Jennette P. Moreno, Baylor College of Medicine, USA.

Philip J. Morgan, University of Newcastle, Australia.

Kenneth Murfay, University of Kentucky, USA.

Patti Jean Naylor, University of Victoria, Canada.

Johan Y. Y. Ng, The Chinese University of Hong Kong, Hong Kong.

Robert J. Noonan, University of Liverpool, UK.

Wesley O'Brien, University College Cork, Ireland.

Anthony D. Okely, University of Wollongong, Australia.

Anne-Maree Parrish, University of Wollongong, Australia

Michele Peden, University of Wollongong, Australia.

Emma Pollock, University of Newcastle, Australia.

Elizabeth M. Rea, Loyola University Chicago, USA.

Nicola D. Ridgers, Deakin University, Australia.

Nicola D. Ridgers, Loughborough University, UK.

Kate Ridley, Flinders University, Australia.

Alex V. Rowlands, University of Leicester, UK.

James Rudd, Liverpool John Moores University, UK.

Geralyn R. Ruissen, University of British Columbia, Canada.

Ryan S. Sacko, The Citadel, USA.

Shannon Sahlqvist, Deakin University, Australia.

Pedro F. Saint-Maurice, National Cancer Institute, USA.

Jo Salmon, Deakin University, Australia.

Lee Schaefer, McGill University, Canada

Matthew J. Schweickle, University of Wollongong, Australia.

Joseph J. Scott, Edith Cowan University, Australia.

Lauren B. Sherar, Loughborough University, UK.

Cindy H. P. Sit, Chinese University of Hong Kong, Hong Kong.

Jordan J. Smith, University of Newcastle, Australia.

Melody Smith, University of Auckland, New Zealand.

Nicole J. Smith, California State University, USA.

Sonia Sousa, University of Minho, Portugal.

Eduarda Sousa-Sá, University of Wollongong, Australia.

Rita Stagni, University of Bologna, Italy.

Tom Stewart, Auckland University of Technology, New Zealand.

David F. Stodden, University of South Carolina, USA.

Gareth Stratton, Swansea University, UK.

Anna Timperio, Deakin University, Australia.

Grant R. Tomkinson, University of North Dakota, USA.

Mark S. Tremblay, Children's Hospital of Eastern Ontario Research Institute, Canada.

Hans van der Mars, Arizona State University, USA.

Esther van Sluijs, University of Cambridge, UK.

Jenny Veitch, Deakin University, Australia.

Stewart A. Vella, University of Wollongong, Australia.

Ineke Vergeer, University of Southern Queensland, Australia.

Katrina J. Waldhauser, University of British Columbia, Canada.

Gregory Welk, Iowa State University, USA.

Myles D. Young, University of Newcastle, Australia.

Joni H. Zhang, The Chinese University of Hong Kong, Hong Kong.

PREFACE

Physical activity in children and youth is associated with physiological, physical, and mental health benefits with research suggesting that the more physical activity one accumulates, the greater the health benefits (Janssen & LeBlanc, 2010). Physical activity in children and youth is impacted by a variety of psychosocial, environmental, and biological factors (Bauman et al., 2012). Moreover, physical activity peaks in primary school, decreases with age (Farooq et al., 2019), and tracks from childhood through adolescence and into adulthood (Tammelin et al., 2014). Physical activity levels of children and youth are a concern worldwide (Aubert et al., 2018). This lack of physical activity worldwide has been labeled as a global physical inactivity pandemic, with physical inactivity recognized as the fourth leading cause of death worldwide (Andersen, Mota, & Di Pietra, 2016). The high levels of inactivity and the associated risks make it a public health priority, while the direct and indirect economic costs of physical inactivity are extremely burdensome on societies and health care systems (Ding et al., 2016). Thus, physical activity as a public health issue has led to an explosion in research related to causes and barriers, assessment/measurement, and programs/interventions.

This research has been embraced by students, academics, practitioners, educators, and policy-makers to inform knowledge, understanding, practice, programming, and funding decisions. However, navigating through the wealth of research evidence covering these important topics can be challenging. *The Routledge Handbook of Youth Physical Activity* is intended to help with this challenge, and our hope is that it will serve as a comprehensive guide for students, practitioners, and academics, and other research users on the state of current knowledge related to youth physical activity, the current and emerging issues, as well as recommendations for the future.

This text is organized into nine unique parts with 38 chapters in total. Each chapter provides a balanced overview of current knowledge, identifying issues, and discussing relevant debates. Part 1 "Introduction to Physical Activity" includes four chapters addressing the various physical activity domains (Chapter 1), global surveillance of physical activity (Chapter 2), and health-related fitness (Chapter 3), as well as physical activity guidelines and recommendations (Chapter 4). Part 2 highlights the physiological (Chapter 5), psychological (Chapter 6), and cognitive and academic (Chapter 7) benefits of physical activity for youth. Part 3 examines the various correlates of physical activity in youth. Specifically, these chapters focus on the psychological (Chapter 8), interpersonal (Chapter 9), physical environments (Chapter 10), and policy (Chapter 11) factors associated with youth physical activity. Part 4 examines the measurement of physical activity through six chapters addressing various measurement modalities and considerations associated with them. Chapter 12 provides an overall introduction to physical activity measurement and is followed by chapters addressing report-based measures (Chapter 13), direct observation (Chapter 14), pedometers (Chapter 15), accelerometers (Chapter 16), and emerging technologies (Chapter 17). These chapters explore measurement issues when working with youth and offer numerous recommendations for their use. Part 5 looks at the assessment of health-related fitness (Chapter 18) and motor proficiency (Chapter 19). Part 6 explores physical activity programming and interventions focusing on design (Chapter 20), implementation and scale-up (Chapter 21), and evaluation (Chapter 22). Part 7 discusses school-based interventions and includes chapters focused specifically on physical education (Chapter 23), recess (Chapter 24), classroom (Chapter 25), school running programs (Chapter 26), and multicomponent interventions (Chapter 27). This part also has chapters focused on preschool and childcare interventions (Chapter 28) as well as programs designed specifically for children with disabilities (Chapter 29). Part 9 is centered on family and community-based interventions with specific reference to mother/family (Chapter 30) and father-based interventions (Chapter 31). Chapters 32 (before-school and after-school), 33 (summertime), 34 (active commuting), and 35 (technology-based) all explore programming while youth are outside traditional school hours. The final part focuses on movement skill (Chapter 36), exercise (Chapter 37), and sport (Chapter 38) programming.

References

Andersen, L. B., Mota, J., & Di Pietro, L. (2016). Update on the global pandemic of physical inactivity. *Lancet (London, England), 388*(10051), 1255–1256.

Aubert, S., Barnes, J. D., Abdeta, C., Abi Nader, P., Adeniyi, A. F., Aguilar-Farias, N., . . . Chang, C. K. (2018). Global matrix 3.0 physical activity report card grades for children and youth: results and analysis from 49 countries. *Journal of Physical Activity and Health, 15*(Supplement 2), S251–S273.

Bauman, A. E., Reis, R. S., Sallis, J. F., Wells, J. C., Loos, R. J., Martin, B. W., & Lancet Physical Activity Series Working Group. (2012). Correlates of physical activity: Why are some people physically active and others not? *The Lancet, 380*(9838), 258–271.

Ding, D., Lawson, K. D., Kolbe-Alexander, T. L., Finkelstein, E. A., Katzmarzyk, P. T., Van Mechelen, W., . . . Lancet Physical Activity Series 2 Executive Committee. (2016). The economic burden of physical inactivity: A global analysis of major non-communicable diseases. *The Lancet, 388*(10051), 1311–1324.

Farooq, A., Martin, A., Janssen, X., Wilson, M. G., Gibson, A. M., Hughes, A., & Reilly, J. J. (2019). Longitudinal changes in moderate-to-vigorous-intensity physical activity in children and adolescents: A systematic review and meta-analysis. *Obesity Reviews.* doi:10.1111/obr.12953

Janssen, I., & LeBlanc, A. G. (2010). Systematic review of the health benefits of physical activity and fitness in school-aged children and youth. *International Journal of Behavioral Nutrition and Physical Activity, 7*(1), 7–40.

Tammelin, R., Yang, X., Leskinen, E., Kankaanpaa, A., Hirvensalo, M., Tammelin, T., & Raitakari, O. T. (2014). Tracking of physical activity from early childhood through youth into adulthood. *Medicine and Science in Sports Exercise, 46*(5), 955–962.

PART 1

Introduction to Physical Activity

1

PHYSICAL ACTIVITY DOMAINS

Valerie Carson and Stephen Hunter

Introduction

Physical activity is a complex health behavior that has a wide range of health benefits for youth (defined in this book as 3–17 years) (Carson, Lee et al., 2017; Poitras et al., 2016). Physical activity is broadly defined as "any bodily movement produced by skeletal muscles that results in energy expenditure" (Caspersen, Powell, & Christenson, 1985, p 126). Physical activity encompasses a range of activities that occur in a variety of settings (e.g., home, child care, school, community, neighborhood) and that are influenced by many sources (e.g., attitudes, parents and peers, environment, policies) (Sallis et al., 2006). These activities, settings, and sources of influence are dynamic (Spence & Lee, 2003), interact with each other, and can vary by age group (Sallis & Owen, 2015). This chapter on physical activity domains will provide an overview of this complex behavior, including defining common physical activity domains in youth, such as active play and leisure activities, active transportation, organized sport participation, and physical education (ParticipACTION, 2018). This chapter will also highlight key and emerging issues and provide recommendations for research and practice.

Overview of the Literature

Four Components of Physical Activity

Physical activity is often classified and prescribed with the F.I.T.T (frequency, intensity, time, and type) principle.

Frequency

The number of times or how often physical activity is performed (American College of Sports Medicine, 2018; Canadian Society for Exercise Physiology, 2017). For example, the number of times physical activity is performed per week, per day, or per hour.

Intensity

The effort or work of the physical activity performed (American College of Sports Medicine, 2018). Physical activity is usually categorized into three main intensities: light, moderate, and vigorous.

Research in youth often combines moderate and vigorous intensities into one category called moderate- to vigorous-intensity physical activity (MVPA). These different intensities of physical activity are typically defined in terms of energy cost using a metabolic equivalent of task (MET) value, with 1 MET equaling the energy required at rest (Butte et al., 2018). Please see Chapter 5 for more information on intensities of physical activity.

Time

The duration or how long physical activity is performed (American College of Sports Medicine, 2018; Canadian Society for Exercise Physiology, 2017). Most physical activity bouts among younger youth are short and sporadic (Bailey et al., 1995), whereas older youth can engage in physical activity bouts that are longer in duration (Malina, Bouchard, & Bar-Or, 2004). For example, younger youth may take more frequent rest periods during physical activities compared to older youth. Regardless, the accumulation of all bouts of physical activity in youth can contribute to meeting physical activity recommendations.

Type

The kind of physical activity performed (American College of Sports Medicine, 2018). Common types of physical activity included in public health guidelines, in particular for those aged 5–17 years, include aerobic (heart strengthening) and resistance (muscle and bone strengthening) activities (World Health Organization, 2010). Finally, type can also refer to the domains of physical activity, or specific physical activities such as swimming or basketball.

Domains of Physical Activity

In 2006, Sallis and colleagues introduced an ecological model that focused on four mutually exclusive domains of active living that span adult's total physical activity (Sallis et al., 2006). The four domains include active recreation, often referred to as leisure-time activities, active transport, occupation activities, and household activities (Sallis et al., 2006). Each domain has specific behavior settings where physical activity occurs (Sallis et al., 2006). These four domains are commonly used in the adult literature but may not be as applicable for youth, especially younger youth. The domains of physical activity examined in youth vary across studies. For example, some studies and reviews published from 2016 onward have used two to five domains encompassing different combinations of the following: active transportation, school physical activity, school activities outside of physical education, class and recess time, physical education, leisure-time or outside of school activities, organized sport or sport clubs, outdoor play, non-organized physical activity, domestic activity, or chores (Dearth-Wesley, Howard, Wang, Zhang, & Popkin, 2017; Dias et al., 2018; Kemp, Cliff, Chong, & Parrish, 2018; Reimers et al., 2019; Smith, Berdel, Nowak, Heinrich, & Schulz, 2016; Sprengeler, Wirsik, Hebestreit, Herrmann, & Ahrens, 2017; Tsiros, Samaras, Coates, & Olds, 2017; White et al., 2018).

The 2018 ParticipACTION Report Card on Physical Activity for Children and Youth highlighted four main domains of total physical activity that span the entire age group of youth. These included active play and leisure activities, active transportation, organized sport participation, and physical education (ParticipACTION, 2018). These domains are defined below and represented in Figure 1.1.

- *Active play and leisure activities* is generally referred to as unstructured physical activity that is volitional, spontaneous, self-directed, and fun (Barnes et al., 2013). It may be performed alone or with others and may include symbolic play or games with self-made rules

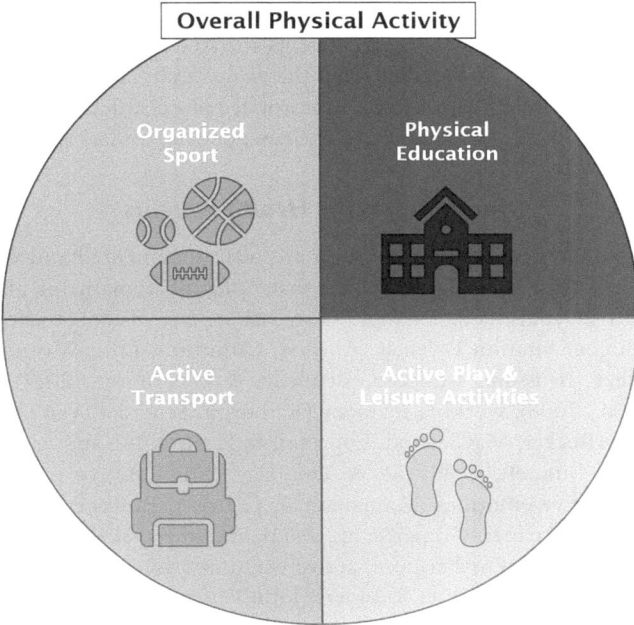

Figure 1.1 Overall physical activity broken into four domains (organized sport, active transport, active play & leisure activities, physical education)

(Brockman, Fox, & Jago, 2011). Active play and leisure activities can occur in different settings, including home, neighborhood, or school/child care settings (e.g., recess, lunch). Active play is often a term more commonly used with younger youth, compared to leisure activities, which may be more relevant for older youth. In younger age groups, active play has been defined as "a form of gross motor or total body movement in which young children exert energy in a freely chosen, fun, and unstructured manner" (Truelove, Vanderloo, & Tucker, 2017). Examples of active play among younger youth include child-directed games like hide-and-go seek and tag or outdoor activities like playing in a pile of leaves, climbing a tree, or sledding down a hill. Examples of leisure activities among older youth include playing basketball with friends, playing catch, or lifting weights (non-competitive) at home, school, or a gym.

- *Active transportation* is physical activity performed to get to and from places (e.g., school, park, friend's house, shopping center) (Tremblay et al., 2016). Main modes of active transportation include walking and cycling (Janssen, 2014). Among younger youth, active transportation is typically performed in the presence of others (e.g., parents, siblings, friends), whereas among older youth, it may occur in the presence of others or independently. See Chapter 34 for more information on active transportation.
- *Organized sport participation* is physical activity in individual or team sports or physical activity programs. It can occur in school or community settings. Unlike active play, organized sports typically have rules, coaching, and specialized equipment (American Academy of Pediatrics & Committee on Sports Medicine and Fitness and Committee on School Health, 2001). Examples include, but are not limited to, swimming, gymnastics, dance, track and field, basketball, soccer/football, hockey, and rugby. See Chapter 38 for more information on organized sport.

- *Physical education* is a curricular subject within the school setting designed for students to develop motor skills, movement-related concepts and strategies, personal and social responsibility, personal fitness, and knowledge about the value of physical activity (SHAPE America, 2013). In youth that are not yet in school, educator-led physical activity opportunities in child care settings could also be encompassed in the category of physical education.

Domain-Specific Health Benefits

The health benefits of physical activity in youth are well documented and will be discussed in detail in Chapters 5–7. It should also be noted that different domains of physical activity can have certain benefits in youth. For example, associations have been observed between active play outdoors and higher vitamin D levels (Absoud, Cummins, Lim, Wassmer, & Shaw, 2011), lower depressed affect (Brussoni, Ishikawa, Brunelle, & Herrington, 2017), better vision (Jin et al., 2015; Rose et al., 2008), working memory (Verburgh, Scherder, Van Lange, & Oosterlaan, 2016), self-regulation (Becker, McClelland, Loprinzi, & Trost, 2014), and relationships with peers (Larouche, Garriguet, Gunnell, Goldfield, & Tremblay, 2016). Active transportation has been linked with higher positive emotions (Ramanathan, O'Brien, Faulkner, & Stone, 2014), better cognitive performance (Martínez-Gómez et al., 2011), and lower likelihood of depressive symptoms (Sun, Liu, & Tao, 2015). Furthermore, active transportation via cycling has been linked to better cardiovascular fitness (Larouche, Saunders, John Faulkner, Colley, & Tremblay, 2014). In terms of organized sport, associations have been observed with better neurocognitive functioning (Verburgh et al., 2016), quality of life (Tsiros et al., 2017), self-esteem and social skills (Eime, Young, Harvey, Charity, & Payne, 2013), school performance (Badura et al., 2016), higher confidence and competence, and fewer depressive symptoms (Eime et al., 2013). Finally, there is evidence suggesting physical education may be associated with better academic performance (Simms, Bock, & Hackett, 2014; Telford et al., 2012; Tremarche, Robinson, & Graham, 2007), cognitive skills (Rasberry et al., 2011), and higher fitness (Burner, Bopp, Papalia, Weimer, & Bopp, 2019), though this appears dependent on the quality of physical education received (Dargavel, Robertson-Wilson, & Bryden, 2017).

Domain-Specific Correlates and Determinants

The ecological model with four domains of active living introduced by Sallis and colleagues highlighted that correlates or determinants of physical activity are domain specific and can span multiple levels from individual factors to policy (Sallis et al., 2006). This model built on the concepts of behavior and context specificity introduced in 2005 in the area of environmental correlates of physical activity (Giles-Corti, Timperio, Bull, & Pikora, 2005). The concept of behavior and context specificity highlights the importance of matching correlates with behavioral domains (e.g., active play, organized sport), settings (e.g., home, school), personal characteristics (e.g., age, sex, ethnicity), and times (e.g., after-school vs weekend) to improve the predictive power of ecological models and the success of physical activity interventions (Atkin, van Sluijs, Dollman, Taylor, & Stanley, 2016; Giles-Corti et al., 2005). Previous research has identified domain-specific and/or context-specific correlates of physical activity in youth. For example, systematic review evidence indicates that distance, household income, and car ownership are consistent negative correlates of active transportation (Pont, Ziviani, Wadley, Bennett, & Abbott, 2009). In another systematic review, perceived encouragement from peers, parents, and/or teachers, portable play equipment, and number of facilities available were consistent positive correlates of physical activity during recess (Ridgers, Salmon, Parrish, Stanley, & Okely, 2012). This evidence can help inform interventions targeting specific domains and/or settings.

Key Issues

A Broadening Perspective on Intensity

All the different domains of physical activity defined earlier in this chapter make important contributions to both light-intensity physical activity (LPA) and MVPA participation among youth. Traditionally, the primary focus of research and promotion of physical activity among youth has been on MVPA (Chaput, Carson, Gray, & Tremblay, 2014). This focus can partly be explained by measurement challenges. Historically, subjective measures of physical activity have been commonly used in physical activity research, but these measures lack the precision to accurately capture LPA (Adamo, Prince, Tricco, Connor-Gorber, & Tremblay, 2009; Kohl, Fulton, & Caspersen, 2000). As measurement has evolved with technological advances, the focus on MVPA has remained steady, given evidence generally supports that the higher the intensity of activity, the stronger the health benefits (Poitras et al., 2016). However, there has also been an increasing focus on LPA (Poitras et al., 2016). There are a couple main reasons for this new focus. First, large proportions of youth populations are not meeting recommended amounts of MVPA (Colley et al., 2017; Fakhouri, 2014; Roman-Vinas et al., 2016). Therefore, targeting LPA as a stepping stone to increasing MVPA may be a more feasible approach for increasing physical activity in inactive youth. Second, even among youth who are meeting MVPA recommendations, MVPA only makes up a small portion of the day (Chaput et al., 2014). Thus, opportunities to increase daily LPA are much larger compared to MVPA.

A systematic review published in 2016 on the associations between objectively measured physical activity and health indicators in 5–17-year-olds highlighted a dearth of evidence and mixed findings for the health impacts of LPA (Poitras et al., 2016). However, two observational studies indicated that the intensity of LPA may be important (Carson et al., 2013; Kwon, Janz, Burns, & Levy, 2011). Specifically, LPA at the higher end of the spectrum, which represents more dynamic activities (e.g., slow walking), may be more important for health than LPA at the lower end, which represents more static activities (e.g., standing) (Carson et al., 2013). Overall, experimental evidence for the health benefits of LPA is lacking (Poitras et al., 2016).

Generational Differences in Active Play

Of the different domains of physical activity, the active play domain has received considerable attention as of late. In several countries, it has been reported that active play has declined over time (Bassett, John, Conger, Fitzhugh, & Coe, 2015; Gray, 2011). The biggest declines are thought to have occurred in outdoor active play (Gray, 2011). For example, in a large sample of 6–12-year-olds from the United States, outdoor activities decreased 37% from 1997 to 2003 (Hofferth, 2009). Additionally, parents have reported that youth today play outside less compared to previous generations (Clements, 2004). The type of outdoor play has also changed with less risky play and more structured, adult-led play (Brussoni et al., 2015). Cultural changes, in particular around parent practices and norms and technology, are thought to be two of the main reasons for the decline in active play (Pynn et al., 2018; Veitch, Bagley, Ball, & Salmon, 2006). Specifically, parents' fears for youth's safety, including stranger danger, traffic danger, and injuries, are considered the biggest barriers to active outdoor play (Clements, 2004; Gray, 2011; Lee et al., 2015; Veitch et al., 2006). Consequently, youth face more rules and restrictions, and are more closely monitored by parents than previous generations (Pynn et al., 2018). Furthermore, allowing youth to play outside unsupervised is now considered as bad parenting or neglectful in some parts of the world, despite it being the norm in previous generations (Lee et al., 2015; Pynn et al., 2018; Veitch et al., 2006). Additionally, the explosion and allure of electronic devices, including smartphones and tablets, are thought to be replacing active play (Gray, 2011; Veitch et al., 2006). Increasing active play could increase the percentage of youth meeting physical activity recommendations and have important health implications as discussed earlier in the chapter. Additionally, it is estimated that for every hour/day that youth spend in active play instead of screen time, energy expenditure would increase 49 calories/day (Janssen, 2014).

Emerging Issues

First 2,000 Days

Research on physical activity domains of youth has typically focused on those who are school-aged (5–17 years), with young children under 5 years largely being neglected (Pate et al., 2013; Timmons, Naylor, & Pfeiffer, 2007). This focus is partly explained by the general assumption that young children are naturally and sufficiently active (Pate et al., 2013; Timmons et al., 2007). However, with the growing knowledge of the importance of the first 2,000 days of life (Thompson, 2001) and the growing concerns that over 41 million children under the age of 5 are overweight (Busch, Manders, & de Leeuw, 2013), research on physical activity in young children has increased. This is particularly true for preschool-aged children (3–4 or 3–5 years), but there is also limited but growing research on physical activity in infant (<1 year) and toddler (1–2 years) age groups (Cliff, Reilly, & Okely, 2009; Worobey, 2014). Given the rapid development that occurs in the first years of life (Thompson, 2001), unique considerations need to be given to the domains of physical activity for young children.

Young children do not have the capacity to maintain intense activity for extended periods of time (Zwiren, 1989) so they frequently engage in short bouts of higher intensity activity intermixed with periods of lower intensity activity and sedentary behavior (Bailey et al., 1995; Cliff et al., 2009). Additionally, all intensities of physical activity, including LPA, have been identified as important for young children (Carson, Lee et al., 2017; Tremblay, Chaput et al., 2017). This is in contrast to school-aged youth where traditionally the focus has been on MVPA. Furthermore, active play is the dominant domain of physical activity in young children but encompasses different activities at different stages of development (Cliff et al., 2009). For infants, active play typically involves floor-based activities and tummy time, which includes arm, leg, and neck movements (Cliff et al., 2009). Active play then progresses to crawling and pulling up on objects to standing and walking unassisted (Cliff et al., 2009; Worobey, 2014). Active play for toddlers typically involves activities that develop and improve locomotor skills (e.g., running, jumping, galloping) and object-control skills (e.g., throwing, catching, kicking) (Cliff et al., 2009). This book focuses on youth 3–17 years of age where the vast majority of the scientific evidence exists for physical activity. Future physical activity research is clearly warranted in children under 3 years.

Objective Measures of Physical Activity Domains

Objective measures of physical activity, such as accelerometers, are typically used to capture frequency, intensity, and duration of physical activity. However, traditionally these monitors have not been able to capture contextual information, such as where physical activity is occurring or the setting (e.g., home, school, neighborhood), the domain (e.g., active play, organized sport) (Dollman et al., 2009), or the specific activity being performed (e.g., basketball, cycling, swimming). However, novel approaches and technological advances have been developed to objectively capture contextual information regarding children's physical activity. First, some activity monitors have specific features that capture contextual information. For example, some accelerometer models include an ambient light sensor that can be used to estimate whether a child is engaging in physical activity indoors or outdoors (Flynn et al., 2014). Second, novel data processing approaches have been used to estimate contextual information. For example, machine learning techniques have been used to determine specific activities being performed (de Vries, Engels, & Garre, 2011; Hagenbuchner, Cliff, Trost, Van Tuc, & Peoples, 2015; Trost, Wong, Pfeiffer, & Zheng, 2012). Finally, multiple objective devices have been combined to provide further contextual information on physical activity. For example, accelerometers have previously been combined with global positioning systems (GPS) devices to determine where physical activity is being performed (Carlson et al., 2016; Cerin et al., 2016). Additionally, algorithms and specific procedures have been developed using accelerometers, GPS devices, and child activity logs to predict time spent in different physical activity domains, including outdoor active play, active transportation, organized sport participation, and physical education (Borghese & Janssen, 2018).

An Integrated Approach

Another recent development in regard to physical activity domains that is applicable across different age groups is taking an integrated approach for researching and promoting movement (Chaput et al., 2014). This approach is in contrast to the segregated approach, which focuses on physical activity in isolation (Chaput et al., 2014). Physical activity, sedentary behavior, and sleep have been identified as three co-dependent, interacting behaviors that make up the full range of movement intensity in a 24-hour period. Sedentary behavior is defined as "any waking behavior characterized by an energy expenditure ≤ 1.5 metabolic equivalents (METs), while in a sitting, reclining or lying posture" (Tremblay, Aubert et al., 2017). Common domains or types of sedentary behavior in youth include screen time (while sitting, reclining, or lying), sitting in school, and passive transport (Tremblay, Aubert et al., 2017). Sleep can be defined as "a naturally recurring state of body and mind characterized by altered consciousness, relatively inhibited sensory activity, inhibition of nearly all voluntary muscles and reduced interactions with surroundings" (Chaput, Saunders, & Carson, 2017, p. 8). Sleep can occur during the day time (e.g., nap) or at night and also has different domains or states, including rapid eye movement (REM) and non-rapid eye movement (NREM) (National Sleep Foundation, 2019). Sedentary behavior and sleep both fall on the lower end of the movement intensity continuum (See Figure 1.2).

Sedentary behavior research among youth has exploded over the past 5–10 years (Carson, Hunter et al., 2016). It is only recently that sleep has been considered in relation to physical activity and sedentary behavior. This is because physical activity, sedentary behavior, and sleep are time-constrained by a 24-hour period, meaning if time in one of these behaviors increases, time in another behavior has to decrease (Chastin, Palarea-Albaladejo, Dontje, & Skelton, 2015). Additionally, physical activity, sedentary behavior, and sleep naturally interact to have synergistic effects on health (Carson, Chaput, Janssen, & Tremblay, 2017; Carson, Tremblay, Chaput, & Chastin, 2016; Saunders et al., 2016). For example, if a youth stays up late on a school night to

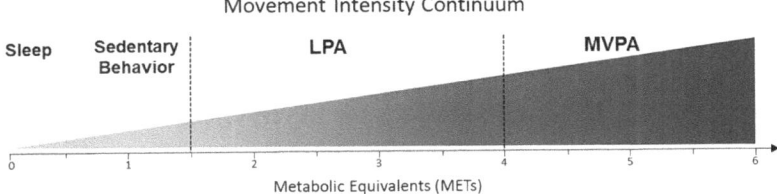

Figure 1.2   Movement intensity continuum for sleep, sedentary behavior, light-intensity physical activity (LPA), and moderate-to vigorous–intensity physical activity (MVPA)

watch TV this results in less sleep, which may lead to a lack of energy to engage in physical education class the next day. In recognizing the importance of this integrated approach for health, several countries and organizations have developed 24-hour movement guidelines, which integrate physical activity, sedentary behavior, and sleep. See Chapter 4 to learn more about the guidelines.

As part of the growing interest and evidence on the integrative nature of physical activity, sedentary behavior, and sleep, novel analytical approaches have started to emerge. These approaches are thought to be superior to standard multiple regression analyses that have typically been used when examining associations with behaviors in isolation because they overcome mathematical challenges of co-dependent data (Chastin et al., 2015; Dumuid, Stanford et al., 2017). Common examples of these novel analytical approaches that have previously been used with samples of youth for physical activity, sedentary behavior, and sleep data include cluster and latent class analysis (Carson, Faulkner, Sabiston, Tremblay, & Leatherdale, 2015; Ferrar, Olds, Maher, & Maddison, 2013), isotemporal substitution modeling (Huang, Wong, He, & Salmon, 2016), and compositional data analysis (Carson, Tremblay et al., 2016; Carson, Tremblay, & Chastin, 2017; Dumuid, Maher et al., 2018; Dumuid, Stanford et al., 2018; Talarico & Janssen, 2018).

Cluster and latent class analyses are two different approaches but both identify mutually exclusive subgroups of participants based on their physical activity, sedentary behavior, and sleep data, and often include specific domains of these behaviors (Beets & Foley, 2010; Ferrar, Chang, Li, & Olds, 2013; Lanza, Collins, Lemmon, & Schafer, 2007; Leech, McNaughton, & Timperio, 2014). Associations between group membership can be explored with correlates and health indicators (Carson et al., 2015; Ferrar, Olds et al., 2013; Lanza et al., 2007). Isotemporal substitution modeling determines the implications of allocating time from one behavior to another while holding time in other behaviors constant (Buman et al., 2014; Mekary, Willett, Hu, & Ding, 2009). Compositional data analysis has been used to examine the collective effects of physical activity, sedentary behavior, and sleep, and the effect of each behavior relative to time spent in other behaviors (Chastin et al., 2015; Dumuid, Stanford et al., 2017). Compositional data analysis has also been used in combination with cluster analysis (Dumuid, Olds et al., 2017, 2018), isotemporal substitution (Carson, Tremblay et al., 2016; Dumuid, Pedisic et al., 2017; Dumuid, Stanford et al., 2018), and when examining the correlates of behaviors among youth (Ezeugwu et al., (submitted)). Researchers are increasingly using 24-hour monitoring study protocols with devices such as accelerometers and/or time use-dairies that capture physical activity, sedentary behavior, and sleep data, and in some cases different domains of these behaviors. Consequently, opportunities to utilize these novel analytical approaches to improve our understanding of these integrated behaviors are also increasing.

Recommendations for Researchers and Practitioners

It is well known that physical activity is an important health behavior for youth of all ages. Collaboration is required across home, child care or school, neighborhood, and community settings to ensure youth are getting ample daily opportunities of physical activity through different domains, such as active play and leisure activities, active transportation, organized sport, and physical education, where relevant. This chapter has highlighted some future directions for research and practice for physical activity domains.

Recommendations for Researchers

1 Research examining domain- and context-specific correlates of physical activity is needed to inform future intervention work.
2 Since all domains of physical activity can include both LPA and MVPA, future research is needed to better understand the role of LPA in health promotion among youth.

3   Future research is needed to understand how to effectively increase active play, in particular outdoor active play, and active transportation (see Chapter 34) within current cultural norms.
4   Given important and unique development occurs during the first 3 years of life, additional physical activity research is needed in this age group.
5   Future research should consider novel measurement and data processing approaches to objectively measure physical activity domains.
6   Research capturing 24-hour data with novel analytical techniques is needed to better understand the health implications and correlates of movement compositions.

Recommendations for Practitioners

1   Consider multiple domains when promoting youth physical activity.
2   Collaborate with stakeholders across settings to promote youth physical activity.
3   Take action to challenge cultural norms that are reducing youth's active outdoor play and active transportation.
4   Adopt an integrated approach to health promotion by considering the inter-relationships between physical activity, sedentary behavior, and sleep domains.

References

Absoud, M., Cummins, C., Lim, M. J., Wassmer, E., & Shaw, N. J. P. O. (2011). Prevalence and predictors of Vitamin D insufficiency in children: A Great Britain population based study. *PloS One, 6*(7), e22179.

Adamo, K. B., Prince, S. A., Tricco, A. C., Connor-Gorber, S., & Tremblay, M. (2009). A comparison of indirect versus direct measures for assessing physical activity in the pediatric population: A systematic review. *International Journal of Pediatric Obesity, 4*(1), 2–27.

American Academy of Pediatrics & Committee on Sports Medicine and Fitness and Committee on School Health. (2001). Organized sports for children and preadolescents. *Pediatrics, 107*(6), 1459–1462.

American College of Sports Medicine. (2018). *ACSM's guidelines for exercise testing and prescription* (Tenth ed.). Philadelphia, PA: Wolters Kluwer.

Atkin, A. J., van Sluijs, E. M. F., Dollman, J., Taylor, W. C., & Stanley, R. M. (2016). Identifying correlates and determinants of physical activity in youth: How can we advance the field? *Preventive Medicine, 87*, 167–169.

Badura, P., Sigmund, E., Geckova, A. M., Sigmundova, D., Sirucek, J., van Dijk, J. P., & Reijneveld, S. A. (2016). Is participation in organized leisure-time activities associated with school performance in adolescence? *PLoS One, 11*(4), e0153276.

Bailey, R. C., Olson, J., Pepper, S. L., Porszasz, J., Barstow, T. J., & Cooper, D. M. (1995). The level and tempo of children's physical activities: An observational study. *Medicine & Science in Sports & Exercise, 27*(7), 1033–1041.

Barnes, J. D., Colley, R. C., Borghese, M., Janson, K., Fink, A., & Tremblay, M. S. (2013). Results from the active healthy kids Canada 2012 report card on physical activity for children and youth. *Paediatrics & Child Health, 18*(6), 301–304.

Bassett, D. R., John, D., Conger, S. A., Fitzhugh, E. C., & Coe, D. P. (2015). Trends in physical activity and sedentary behaviors of United States youth. *Journal of Physical Activity and Health, 12*(8), 1102–1111.

Becker, D. R., McClelland, M. M., Loprinzi, P., & Trost, S. G. (2014). Physical activity, self-regulation, and early academic achievement in preschool children. *Early Education & Development, 25*(1), 56–70.

Beets, M. W., & Foley, J. T. (2010). Comparison of 3 different analytic approaches for determining risk-related active and sedentary behavioral patterns in adolescents. *Journal of Physical Activity and Health, 7*(3), 381–392.

Borghese, M. M., & Janssen, I. (2018). Development of a measurement approach to assess time children participate in organized sport, active travel, outdoor active play, and curriculum-based physical activity. *BMC Public Health, 18*(1), 396.

Brockman, R., Fox, K. R., & Jago, R. (2011). What is the meaning and nature of active play for today's children in the UK?. *International Journal of Behavioral Nutrition and Physical Activity, 8*(1), 15.

Brussoni, M., Gibbons, R., Gray, C., Ishikawa, T., Sandseter, E. B., Bienenstock, A., . . . Tremblay, M. S. (2015). What is the relationship between risky outdoor play and health in children? A systematic review. *International Journal of Environmental Research and Public Health, 12*(6), 6423–6454.

Brussoni, M., Ishikawa, T., Brunelle, S., & Herrington, S. (2017). Landscapes for play: Effects of an intervention to promote nature-based risky play in early childhood centres. *Journal of Environmental Psychology, 54*, 139–150.

Buman, M. P., Winkler, E. A., Kurka, J. M., Hekler, E. B., Baldwin, C. M., Owen, N., . . . Gardiner, P. A. (2014). Reallocating time to sleep, sedentary behaviors, or active behaviors: Associations with cardiovascular disease risk biomarkers, NHANES 2005–2006. *American Journal of Epidemiology, 179*(3), 323–334.

Burner, A., Bopp, M., Papalia, Z., Weimer, A., & Bopp, C. M. (2019). Examining the Relationship between high school physical education and fitness outcomes in college students. *Physical Educator, 76*(1), 285–300.

Busch, V., Manders, L. A., & de Leeuw, J. R. (2013). Screen time associated with health behaviors and outcomes in adolescents. *American Journal of Health Behavior, 37*(6), 819–830.

Butte, N. F., Watson, K. B., Ridley, K., Zakeri, I. F., McMurray, R. G., Pfeiffer, K. A., . . . Berhane, Z. (2018). A youth compendium of physical activities: Activity codes and metabolic intensities. *Medicine and Science in Sports and Exercise, 50*(2), 246–256.

Canadian Society for Exercise Physiology. (2017). Canadian 24-hour movement guidelines: Glossary of terms. Retrieved from http://www.csep.ca/CMFiles/Guidelines/24hrGlines/24HourGuidelinesGlossary_2017.pdf

Carlson, J. A., Schipperijn, J., Kerr, J., Saelens, B. E., Natarajan, L., Frank, L. D., . . . Sallis, J. F. (2016). Locations of physical activity as assessed by GPS in young adolescents. *Pediatrics, 137*(1), e20152430.

Carson, V., Chaput, J. P., Janssen, I., & Tremblay, M. S. (2017). Health associations with meeting new 24-hour movement guidelines for Canadian children and youth. *Preventive Medicine, 95*, 7–13.

Carson, V., Faulkner, G., Sabiston, C. M., Tremblay, M. S., & Leatherdale, S. T. (2015). Patterns of movement behaviors and their association with overweight and obesity in youth. *International Journal of Public Health, 60*(5), 551–559.

Carson, V., Hunter, S., Kuzik, N., Gray, C. E., Poitras, V. J., Chaput, J. P., . . . Tremblay, M. S. (2016). Systematic review of sedentary behaviour and health indicators in school-aged children and youth: An update. *Applied Physiology Nutrition and Metabolism, 41*(6 Suppl 3), S240–S265.

Carson, V., Lee, E. Y., Hewitt, L., Jennings, C., Hunter, S., Kuzik, N., . . . Tremblay, M. S. (2017). Systematic review of the relationships between physical activity and health indicators in the early years (0–4 years). *BMC Public Health, 17*(Suppl 5), 854.

Carson, V., Ridgers, N. D., Howard, B. J., Winkler, E. A., Healy, G. N., Owen, N., . . . Salmon, J. (2013). Light-intensity physical activity and cardiometabolic biomarkers in US adolescents. *PLoS One, 8*(8) e71417.

Carson, V., Tremblay, M. S., Chaput, J. P., & Chastin, S. F. (2016). Associations between sleep duration, sedentary time, physical activity, and health indicators among Canadian children and youth using compositional analyses. *Applied Physiology Nutrition and Metabolism, 41*(6 Suppl 3) S294–S302.

Carson, V., Tremblay, M. S., & Chastin, S. F. M. (2017). Cross-sectional associations between sleep duration, sedentary time, physical activity, and adiposity indicators among Canadian preschool-aged children using compositional analyses. *BMC Public Health, 17*(Suppl 5), 848.

Caspersen, C. J., Powell, K. E., & Christenson, G. M. (1985). Physical activity, exercise, and physical fitness: Definitions and distinctions for health-related research. *Public Health Reports, 100*(2), 126–131.

Cerin, E., Baranowski, T., Barnett, A., Butte, N., Hughes, S., Lee, R. E., . . . O'Connor, T. M. (2016). Places where preschoolers are (in)active: An observational study on Latino preschoolers and their parents using objective measures. *International Journal of Behavioral Nutrition and Physical Activity, 13*, 29.

Chaput, J.-P., Carson, V., Gray, C. E., & Tremblay, M. S. (2014). Importance of all movement behaviors in a 24 hour period for overall health. *International Journal of Environmental Research and Public Health, 11*(12), 12575–12581.

Chaput, J.-P., Saunders, T. J., & Carson, V. (2017). Interactions between sleep, movement and other non-movement behaviours in the pathogenesis of childhood obesity. *Obesity Reviews, 18*(Suppl 1), 7–14.

Chastin, S. F., Palarea-Albaladejo, J., Dontje, M. L., & Skelton, D. A. (2015). Combined effects of time spent in physical activity, sedentary behaviors and sleep on obesity and cardio-metabolic health markers: A novel compositional data analysis approach. *PLoS One, 10*(10), e0139984.

Clements, R. (2004). An investigation of the status of outdoor play. *Contemporary Issues in Early Childhood, 5*(1), 68–80.

Cliff, D. P., Reilly, J. J., & Okely, A. D. (2009). Methodological considerations in using accelerometers to assess habitual physical activity in children aged 0–5 years. *Journal of Science and Medicine in Sport, 12*(5), 557–567.

Colley, R. C., Carson, V., Garriguet, D., Janssen, I., Roberts, K. C., & Tremblay, M. S. (2017). Physical activity of Canadian children and youth, 2007 to 2015. *Health Reports, 28*(10), 8–16.

Dargavel, M., Robertson-Wilson, J., & Bryden, P. J. (2017). The relationship between secondary school physical education and postsecondary physical activity. *Physical Educator, 74*(3), 551–569.

de Vries, S. I., Engels, M., & Garre, F. G. (2011). Identification of children's activity type with accelerometer-based neural networks. *Medicine and Science in Sports and Exercise, 43*(10), 1994–1999.

Dearth-Wesley, T., Howard, A. G., Wang, H., Zhang, B., & Popkin, B. M. (2017). Trends in domain-specific physical activity and sedentary behaviors among Chinese school children, 2004–2011. *International Journal of Behavioral Nutrition and Physical Activity, 14*(1), 141.

Dias, A. F., Brand, C., Lemes, V. B., Stocchero, C. M. A., Agostinis-Sobrinho, C., Duncan, M. J., . . . Gaya, A. C. A. (2018). Differences in physical activity levels of school domains between high-and low-active adolescents. *Motriz: Revista de Educação Física, 24*(4), 1–5, e101800.

Dollman, J., Okely, A. D., Hardy, L., Timperio, A., Salmon, J., & Hills, A. P. (2009). A Hitchhiker's guide to assessing young people's physical activity: Deciding what method to use. *Journal of Science and Medicine in Sport, 12*(5), 518–525.

Dumuid, D., Maher, C., Lewis, L. K., Stanford, T. E., Martin Fernandez, J. A., Ratcliffe, J., . . . Olds, T. (2018). Human development index, children's health-related quality of life and movement behaviors: A compositional data analysis. *Quality of Life Research, 27*(6), 1473–1482.

Dumuid, D., Olds, T., Lewis, L. K., Martin-Fernández, J. A., Katzmarzyk, P. T., Barreira, T., . . . & Kuriyan, R. (2017). Health-related quality of life and lifestyle behavior clusters in school-aged children from 12 countries. *The Journal of Pediatrics, 183*, 178–183.

Dumuid, D., Olds, T., Lewis, L. K., Martin-Fernández, J. A., Barreira, T., Broyles, S., . . . Kurpad, A. (2018). The adiposity of children is associated with their lifestyle behaviours: A cluster analysis of school-aged children from 12 nations. *Pediatric Obesity, 13*(2), 111–119.

Dumuid, D., Pedisic, Z., Stanford, T. E., Martin-Fernandez, J. A., Hron, K., Maher, C. A., ... Olds, T. (2017). The compositional isotemporal substitution model: A method for estimating changes in a health outcome for reallocation of time between sleep, physical activity and sedentary behaviour. *Statistical Methods in Medical Research, 28*(3), 846–857.

Dumuid, D., Stanford, T. E., Martin-Fernandez, J. A., Pedisic, Z., Maher, C. A., Lewis, L. K., . . . Olds, T. (2017). Compositional data analysis for physical activity, sedentary time and sleep research. *Statistical Methods in Medical Research, 27*(12), 3726–3738.

Dumuid, D., Stanford, T. E., Pedisic, Z., Maher, C., Lewis, L. K., Martin-Fernandez, J. A., . . . Olds, T. (2018). Adiposity and the isotemporal substitution of physical activity, sedentary time and sleep among school-aged children: A compositional data analysis approach. *BMC Public Health, 18*(1), 311.

Eime, R. M., Young, J. A., Harvey, J. T., Charity, M. J., & Payne, W. R. (2013). A systematic review of the psychological and social benefits of participation in sport for children and adolescents: informing development of a conceptual model of health through sport. *International Journal of Behavioral Nutrition and Physical Activity, 10*, 98.

Ezeugwu, V. E., Carson, V., Brook, J., Tamana, S. K., Hunter, S., Chikuma, J., . . . Mandhane, P. J. (submitted). Influence of neighborhood characteristics and weather on movement behaviors at age three and five years in a longitudinal birth cohort.

Fakhouri, T. H., Burt, V. L., Song, M., Fulton, J. E., & Ogden. C. L. (2014). Physical activity in U.S. youth aged 12–15 years, 2012. *NCHS Data Brief, 141*, 1–8.

Ferrar, K., Chang, C., Li, M., & Olds, T. S. (2013). Adolescent time use clusters: A systematic review. *Journal of Adolescent Health, 52*(3), 259–270.

Ferrar, K., Olds, T., Maher, C., & Maddison, R. (2013). Time use clusters of New Zealand adolescents are associated with weight status, diet and ethnicity. *Australian and New Zealand Journal of Public Health, 37*(1), 39–46.

Flynn, J. I., Coe, D. P., Larsen, C. A., Rider, B. C., Conger, S. A., & Bassett, D. R. (2014). Detecting indoor and outdoor environments using the ActiGraph GT3X+ light sensor in children. *Medicine and Science in Sports and Exercise, 46*(1), 201–206.

Giles-Corti, B., Timperio, A., Bull, F., & Pikora, T. (2005). Understanding physical activity environmental correlates: Increased specificity for ecological models. *Exercise and Sport Sciences Review, 33*(4), 175–181.

Gray, P. (2011). The decline of play and the rise of psychopathology in children and adolescents. *American Journal of Play, 3*(4), 443–463.

Hagenbuchner, M., Cliff, D. P., Trost, S. G., Van Tuc, N., & Peoples, G. E. (2015). Prediction of activity type in preschool children using machine learning techniques. *Journal of Science and Medicine in Sport, 18*(4), 426–431.

Hofferth, S. L. (2009). Changes in American children's time – 1997 to 2003. *The Electronic International Journal of Time Use Research, 6*(1), 26–47.

Huang, W. Y., Wong, S. H., He, G., & Salmon, J. O. (2016). Isotemporal substitution analysis for sedentary behavior and body mass index. *Medicine and Science in Sports and Exercise, 48*(11), 2135–2141.

Janssen, I. (2014). Active play: An important physical activity strategy in the fight against childhood obesity. *Canadian Journal of Public Health, 105*(1), e22–e27.

Jin, J.-X., Hua, W.-J., Jiang, X., Wu, X.-Y., Yang, J.-W., Gao, G.-P., . . . Zhang, J.-Z. (2015). Effect of outdoor activity on myopia onset and progression in school-aged children in Northeast China: The Sujiatun eye care study. *BMC Ophthalmology, 15*, 73.

Kemp, B. J., Cliff, D. P., Chong, K. H., & Parrish, A.-M. (2018). Longitudinal changes in domains of physical activity during childhood and adolescence: A systematic review. *Journal of Science and Medicine in Sport, 22*(6), 695–701

Kohl, H. W., Fulton, J. E., & Caspersen, C. J. (2000). Assessment of physical activity among children and adolescents: A review and synthesis. *Preventive Medicine, 31*(2), S54–S76.

Kwon, S., Janz, K. F., Burns, T. L., & Levy, S. M. (2011). Association between light-intensity physical activity and adiposity in childhood. *Pediatric Exercise Science, 23*(2), 218–229.

Lanza, S. T., Collins, L. M., Lemmon, D. R., & Schafer, J. L. (2007). PROC LCA: A SAS procedure for latent class analysis. *Structural Equation Modeling, 14*(4), 671–694.

Larouche, R., Garriguet, D., Gunnell, K. E., Goldfield, G. S., & Tremblay, M. S. (2016). *Outdoor time, physical activity, sedentary time, and health indicators at ages 7 to 14: 2012/2013 Canadian health measures survey.* Health Reports, 27(9), 3–13.

Larouche, R., Saunders, T. J., John Faulkner, G. E., Colley, R., & Tremblay, M. (2014). Associations between active school transport and physical activity, body composition, and cardiovascular fitness: A systematic review of 68 studies. *Journal of Physical Activity and Health, 11*(1) 206–227.

Lee, H., Tamminen, K. A., Clark, A. M., Slater, L., Spence, J. C., & Holt, N. L. (2015). A meta-study of qualitative research examining determinants of children's independent active free play. *International Journal of Behavioral Nutrition and Physical Activity, 12*, 5.

Leech, R. M., McNaughton, S. A., & Timperio, A. (2014). The clustering of diet, physical activity and sedentary behavior in children and adolescents: A review. *International Journal of Behavioral Nutrition and Physical Activity, 11*, 4.

Malina, R. M., Bouchard, C., & Bar-Or, O. (2004). *Growth, maturation, and physical activity* (second ed.). Champaign, IL: Human Kinetics.

Martínez-Gómez, D., Ruiz, J. R., Gómez-Martínez, S., Chillón, P., Rey-López, J. P., Díaz, L. E., . . . Marcos, A. (2011). Active commuting to school and cognitive performance in adolescents: The AVENA study. *Archives of Pediatrics & Adolescent Medicine, 165*(4), 300–305.

Mekary, R. A., Willett, W. C., Hu, F. B., & Ding, E. L. (2009). Isotemporal substitution paradigm for physical activity epidemiology and weight change. *American Journal of Epidemiology, 170*(4), 519–527.

National Sleep Foundation. (2019). What happens when you sleep? Retrieved from https://www.sleepfoundation.org/articles/what-happens-when-you-sleep

ParticipACTION. (2018). *The brain + body equation: Canadian kids need active bodies to build their best brains.* Toronto, Canada: ParticipACTION.

Pate, R. R., O'Neill, J. R., Brown, W. H., McIver, K. L., Howie, E. K., & Dowda, M. (2013). Top 10 research questions related to physical activity in preschool children. *Research Quarterly for Exercise and Sport, 84*(4), 448–455.

Poitras, V. J., Gray, C. E., Borghese, M. M., Carson, V., Chaput, J. P., Janssen, I., . . . Tremblay, M. S. (2016). Systematic review of the relationships between objectively measured physical activity and health indicators in school-aged children and youth. *Applied Physiology Nutrition and Metabolism, 41* (6 Suppl 3) S197–S239.

Pont, K., Ziviani, J., Wadley, D., Bennett, S., & Abbott, R. (2009). Environmental correlates of children's active transportation: A systematic literature review. *Health & Place, 15*(3), 827–840.

Pynn, S. R., Neely, K. C., Ingstrup, M. S., Spence, J. C., Carson, V., Robinson, Z., & Holt, N. L. (2018). An intergenerational qualitative study of the good parenting ideal and active free play during middle childhood. *Children's Geographies, 17*(3), 266–277.

Ramanathan, S., O'Brien, C., Faulkner, G., & Stone, M. (2014). Happiness in motion: Emotions, well-being, and active school travel. *Journal of School Health, 84*(8), 516–523.

Rasberry, C. N., Lee, S. M., Robin, L., Laris, B., Russell, L. A., Coyle, K. K., & Nihiser, A. J. (2011). The association between school-based physical activity, including physical education, and academic performance: A systematic review of the literature. *Preventive Medicine, 52*(Suppl 1) S10–S20.

Reimers, A. K., Brzoska, P., Niessner, C., Schmidt, S. C., Worth, A., & Woll, A. (2019). Are there disparities in different domains of physical activity between school-aged migrant and non-migrant children and adolescents? Insights from Germany. *PLoS One, 14*(3), e0214022.

Ridgers, N. D., Salmon, J., Parrish, A. M., Stanley, R. M., & Okely, A. D. (2012). Physical activity during school recess: A systematic review. *American Journal of Preventive Medicine, 43*(3), 320–328.

Roman-Vinas, B., Chaput, J. P., Katzmarzyk, P. T., Fogelholm, M., Lambert, E. V., Maher, C., . . . Group, I. R. (2016). Proportion of children meeting recommendations for 24-hour movement guidelines and associations with adiposity in a 12-country study. *International Journal of Behavioral Nutrition and Physical Activity, 13*(1), 123.

Rose, K. A., Morgan, I. G., Ip, J., Kifley, A., Huynh, S., Smith, W., & Mitchell, P. (2008). Outdoor activity reduces the prevalence of myopia in children. *Ophthalmology, 115*(8), 1279–1285.

Sallis, J. F., Cervero, R. B., Ascher, W., Henderson, K. A., Kraft, M. K., & Kerr, J. (2006). An ecological approach to creating active living communities. *Annual Review of Public Health, 27*, 297–322.

Sallis, J. F., & Owen, N. (2015). Ecological models of health behavior. In K. Glanz, B. K. Rimer, & K. Viswanath (Eds.), *Health behavior: Theory, research, and practice* (Fifth ed., pp. 43–64). San Francisco, CA: Jossey-Bass.

Saunders, T. J., Gray, C. E., Poitras, V. J., Chaput, J. P., Janssen, I., Katzmarzyk, P. T., . . . Carson, V. (2016). Combinations of physical activity, sedentary behaviour and sleep: Relationships with health indicators in school-aged children and youth. *Applied Physiology Nutrition and Metabolism, 41* (6 Suppl 3) S283–S293.

SHAPE America. (2013). *Grade-level outcomes for K-12 physical education.* Reston, VA: Author.

Simms, K., Bock, S., & Hackett, L. (2014). Do the duration and frequency of physical education predict academic achievement, self-concept, social skills, food consumption, and body mass index? *Health Education Journal, 73*(2), 166–178.

Smith, M. P., Berdel, D., Nowak, D., Heinrich, J., & Schulz, H. (2016). Physical activity levels and domains assessed by accelerometry in German adolescents from GINIplus and LISAplus. *PLoS One, 11*(3), e0152217.

Spence, J. C., & Lee, R. L. (2003). Toward a comprehensive model of physical activity. *Psychology of Sport & Exercise, 1*(4), 7–24.

Sprengeler, O., Wirsik, N., Hebestreit, A., Herrmann, D., & Ahrens, W. (2017). Domain-specific self-reported and objectively measured physical activity in children. *International Journal of Environmental Research and Public Health, 14*(3), 242.

Sun, Y., Liu, Y., & Tao, F.-B. (2015). Associations between active commuting to school, body fat, and mental well-being: Population-based, cross-sectional study in China. *Journal of Adolescent Health, 57*(6), 679–685.

Talarico, R., & Janssen, I. (2018). Compositional associations of time spent in sleep, sedentary behavior and physical activity with obesity measures in children. *International Journal of Obesity (London), 42*(8), 1508–1514.

Telford, R. D., Cunningham, R. B., Fitzgerald, R., Olive, L. S., Prosser, L., Jiang, X., & Telford, R. M. (2012). Physical education, obesity, and academic achievement: A 2-year longitudinal investigation of Australian elementary school children. *American Journal of Public Health, 102*(2), 368–374.

Thompson, R. A. (2001). Development in the first years of life. *Future Child, 11*(1), 20–33.

Timmons, B. W., Naylor, P. J., & Pfeiffer, K. A. (2007). Physical activity for preschool children – How much and how? *Canadian Journal of Public Health, 98*(Suppl 2), S122–S134.

Tremarche, P. V., Robinson, E. M., & Graham, L. B. (2007). Physical education and its effect on elementary testing results. *Physical Educator, 64*, 58–64.

Tremblay, M. S., Aubert, S., Barnes, J. D., Saunders, T. J., Carson, V., Latimer-Cheung, A. E., . . . Participants, S. T. C. P. (2017). Sedentary behavior research network (SBRN) – Terminology consensus project process and outcome. *International Journal of Behavioral Nutrition and Physical Activity, 14*, 75.

Tremblay, M. S., Barnes, J. D., Gonzalez, S. A., Katzmarzyk, P. T., Onywera, V. O., Reilly, J. J., . . . Global Matrix 2.0 Research, T. (2016). Global Matrix 2.0: Report card grades on the physical activity of children and youth comparing 38 countries. *Journal of Physical Activity and Health, 13* (11 Suppl 2), S343–S366.

Tremblay, M. S., Chaput, J. P., Adamo, K. B., Aubert, S., Barnes, J. D., Choquette, L., . . . Carson, V. (2017). Canadian 24-hour movement guidelines for the early years (0–4 years): An integration of physical activity, sedentary behaviour, and sleep. *BMC Public Health, 17*(Suppl 5), 874.

Trost, S. G., Wong, W.-K., Pfeiffer, K. A., & Zheng, Y. (2012). Artificial neural networks to predict activity type and energy expenditure in youth. *Medicine and Science in Sports and Exercise, 44*(9), 1801–1809.

Truelove, S., Vanderloo, L. M., & Tucker, P. (2017). Defining and measuring active play among young children: A systematic review. *Journal of Physical Activity and Health, 14*(2), 155–166.

Tsiros, M. D., Samaras, M. G., Coates, A. M., & Olds, T. (2017). Use-of-time and health-related quality of life in 10-to 13-year-old children: Not all screen time or physical activity minutes are the same. *Quality of Life Research, 26*(11), 3119–3129.

Veitch, J., Bagley, S., Ball, K., & Salmon, J. (2006). Where do children usually play? A qualitative study of parents' perceptions of influences on children's active free-play. *Health Place, 12*(4), 383–393.

Verburgh, L., Scherder, E. J., Van Lange, P. A., & Oosterlaan, J. (2016). Do elite and amateur soccer players outperform non-athletes on neurocognitive functioning? A study among 8–12 year old children. *PLoS One, 11*(12), e0165741.

White, R. L., Parker, P. D., Lubans, D. R., MacMillan, F., Olson, R., Astell-Burt, T., & Lonsdale, C. (2018). Domain-specific physical activity and affective wellbeing among adolescents: An observational study of the moderating roles of autonomous and controlled motivation. *International Journal of Behavioral Nutrition and Physical Activity, 15*, 87.

World Health Organization. (2010). *Global recommendations on physical activity for health.* Geneva, Switzerland: World Health Organization Press.

Worobey, J. (2014). Physical activity in infancy: Developmental aspects, measurement, and importance. *The American Journal of Clinical Nutrition, 99*(3), 729S–733S.

Zwiren, L. D. (1989). Anaerobic and aerobic capacities of children. *Pediatric Exercise Science, 1*, 31–44.

2

GLOBAL SURVEILLANCE OF PHYSICAL ACTIVITY OF CHILDREN AND YOUTH

*Salomé Aubert, Silvia A. González, Taru Manyanga,
and Mark S. Tremblay*

Overview

Concepts and Key Terms

The benefits of physical activity for the health of individuals of all ages and for the health of the societies are now well recognized by the international scientific community. Physical inactivity is identified as the fourth leading risk factor for global mortality (World Health Organization, 2009). Consequently, surveillance of physical activity/inactivity is important for understanding the scope and distribution of the public health impact, and informing and assessing future strategies and interventions.

Taking into account the benefits of physical activity in the global context of increasing rates of non-communicable diseases (NCDs) (World Health Organization, 2018e), estimating what proportion of the population is active (i.e., meeting the recommended amount of physical activity) is of obvious importance. This is achieved through physical activity surveillance. In public health, surveillance is defined as the "ongoing, systematic collection, analysis, and interpretation of outcome-specific data for use in the planning, implementation, and evaluation of public health practice" (Thacker & Berkelman, 1988). Based on this definition, the surveillance of physical activity encompasses the collection, analysis, and interpretation of physical activity data, including the complexities of this behavior, in order to assess the physical activity status of populations, identify trends in the levels of physical activity, evaluate policies and interventions, define priorities in physical activity promotion, and identify potential areas of further investigation. Therefore, the objective of the global surveillance of physical activity of children and youth is to estimate the prevalence of (in)active children and youth worldwide.

Physical Activity Measurement Methods

Physical activity surveillance relies on objective (directly measured) and subjective (reported) measurement methods for the assessment of physical activity among children and youth. Objective methods of assessing physical activity include measures based on energy expenditure or oxygen uptake (Schutz, Weinsier, & Hunter, 2001), heart rate monitoring (Schutz et al., 2001), and motion sensors using accelerometry (Schutz et al., 2001), or pedometers measuring step counts (Lubans et al., 2015). Despite providing more accurate measures of movement, motion sensors, like accelerometers, have several limitations: (1) Accelerometry data do not provide information about the type of activity or the context in which it is performed (Fulton & Carlson, 2012); (2) The different available cut-points to estimate the intensity of physical activity measured with accelerometers produce different conclusions about the proportion of individuals meeting physical activity guidelines, and there is a lack of consensus on cut-points selection (Migueles et al., 2018); (3) Objective monitoring of physical activity at the population level may not be a feasible approach for several low- and middle-income countries (LMICs) because of the associated costs, logistic challenges, and expertise required (Lee & Shiroma, 2014).

Subjective measurement of physical activity involves quantitative, qualitative, and/or descriptive recall of active behaviors through the use of interviews, questionnaires or surveys, and diaries or logs. With these methods, the physical activities of a past period of time (e.g., previous week) are reported by children and youth, or by a proxy (e.g., parent, teacher, coach). While objective methods provide a more valid estimation of the physical activity of individuals but are costly, time consuming, and more invasive, subjective methods are less valid, and tend to provide an overestimation of physical activity levels, but they enable collection of physical activity data among large study samples at low cost and provide details characterizing the activity (Sallis & Saelens, 2000; Sylvia, Bernstein, Hubbard, Keating, & Anderson, 2014). The surveillance of the physical activity of children and youth at the population level is challenged by this trade-off between accuracy and feasibility. Questionnaires are today the most commonly used tools to evaluate physical activity at the population level (Ainsworth, Cahalin, Buman, & Ross, 2015).

A thorough presentation and discussion of physical activity measurement procedures and techniques is provided in Part 4, Chapters 14–19.

International Calls for Action and the Need for Surveillance

Over the past few decades, insufficient levels of physical activity have been observed internationally among children and youth (Booth, Rowlands, & Dollman, 2015; Brodersen et al., 2007; Dollman, Norton, & Norton, 2005; Guthold, Stevens, Riley, & Bull, 2018; Kalman et al., 2015), raising concerns for their general health and for the future prevalence of NCDs. In response to this concerning global public health situation, in 2010, the Global Advocacy for Physical Activity (Titze & Oja, 2013), Council of the International Society of Physical Activity and Health (ISPAH), developed the *Toronto Charter for Physical Activity* (Bull et al., 2010). The *Toronto Charter* is a global call to strive for greater political and social commitment to support health-enhancing physical activity for all countries, regions, and communities, and an advocacy tool that outlines four actions based upon nine guiding principles for a population-based approach to support health-enhancing physical activity for all (Bull et al., 2010). The concerted actions for successful population change include implementing a national policy and action plan, introducing policies that support physical activity, and reorienting services and funding to prioritize physical activity and develop partnerships for action. The *Charter* specifically encourages countries and organizations to build capacity and support physical activity surveillance processes.

One year later, the United Nations (UN) hosted a high-level meeting of the General Assembly to discuss the prevention and management of NCDs. In their declaration, the UN acknowledged that the global burden of NCDs is a major threat to the global economy and leads to increasing social inequalities, so is a major threat to global development (United Nations, 2012). The UN stated that it is the responsibility of governments and the international community to promote focused efforts and to engage all sectors of society to address the common risk factors of NCDs including physical inactivity. The UN underlined the importance for Member States to continue addressing common risk factors for NCDs through the implementation of the *World Health Organization (WHO)'s 2008–2013 Action Plan for the Global Strategy for the Prevention and Control of NCDs* and to monitor and report on progress (World Health Organization, 2008).

The *Action Plan for the Global Strategy for the Prevention and Control of NCDs* was re-edited by the WHO with new goals and targets for 2013–2020 (World Health Organization, 2013). The new action plan has six main objectives: raise the priority for prevention and control of NCDs; strengthen national capacity, leadership, governance, multi-sectoral action, and partnerships; reduce modifiable risk factors and underlying social determinants; promote and support high-quality research and development; monitor trends and determinants of NCDs; and evaluate progress. Additionally, this action plan has nine main targets to achieve by 2020, which include a global relative reduction of 10% in the prevalence of insufficient physical activity levels.

During the historic UN Summit on September 25, 2015, in New York (USA), world leaders adopted a set of *Sustainable Development Goals* (SDGs) to end all forms of poverty, fight inequalities, and tackle climate change, while ensuring that no one is left behind as part of a new global sustainable development agenda. The 17 SDGs, which are divided into 169 specific targets, are aimed to be achieved over the next 15 years (United Nations, 2015), the progress of which requires valid and reliable surveillance.

Building on those SDGs, the *Bangkok Declaration on Physical Activity for Global Health and Sustainable Development* was launched in Bangkok at the 2016 ISPAH Congress (ISPAH, 2016). The *Bangkok Declaration* was developed by delegates, ISPAH members, and Congress co-hosts, and provides a new position statement on the importance of physical activity for global health, the prevention of NCDs, and how the co-benefits of population-based actions on physical activity can contribute to achieving 8 of the 17 SDGs. The *Bangkok Declaration* calls upon governments, policy makers, donors, and stakeholders including the WHO, UN, and all relevant non-governmental organizations to contribute to the achievement of these targets by following the guiding principles and recommendations. This requires appropriate surveillance.

The *Report of the Commission on Ending Childhood Obesity* was also built on the UN SDGs. The *Commission on Ending Childhood Obesity* was created in 2014 by the WHO in order to better inform and fashion a comprehensive response to childhood obesity. The Commission published a report in 2016, including a set of recommendations to successfully tackle childhood and adolescent obesity in different contexts around the world, after consultation with over 100 WHO Member States and comments by nearly 180 online reviewers. One of the six main recommendations is to "implement comprehensive programmes that promote physical activity and reduce sedentary behaviors in children and adolescents" (World Health Organization, 2016).

In response to the 17 UN SDGs and the *Bangkok Declaration on Physical Activity for Global Health and Sustainable Development*, the WHO published in 2018 a *Global Action Plan on Physical Activity 2018–2030* (World Health Organization, 2018a). This *Action Plan* is designed to provide guidance to support the implementation of national multi-sectoral physical activity actions that leverage the links and benefits to sectors beyond health, to national economic and sustainable development. Four strategic objectives (1. creating an active society, 2. creating active environments, 3. creating active lives, and 4. creating active systems) and a specific target of a 15% relative reduction in the global prevalence of physical inactivity in adults and adolescents using a baseline of 2016 were formulated in this *Action Plan*. Enhancing data systems and capabilities at national levels to support regular population surveillance of physical activity, across all ages and multiple domains, was identified as one of the strategic actions to reach these objectives.

Within this rich tapestry of international calls for action, the global surveillance of physical activity plays a crucial role. Besides being one of the priority actions for most of these documents, it provides evidence to inform the assessment of the achievement of goals and objectives.

Current State of Surveillance

Global Physical Activity Guidelines for Children and Youth

The WHO recommends that children and youth aged 5–17 years should accumulate at least 60 minutes of moderate- to vigorous-intensity physical activity (MVPA) daily, consisting mostly of aerobic physical activity, and including vigorous-intensity activities, and activities that strengthen muscle and bone at least three times per week (World Health Organization, 2010).

Furthermore, the WHO physical activity guidelines for the early years (0–4 years) (World Health Organization, 2019) state that:

- Infants (less than 1 year) should be physically active several times a day in a variety of ways, particularly through interactive floor-based play; more is better. For those not yet mobile, this includes at least 30 minutes in prone position (tummy time) spread throughout the day while awake;
- Children 1–2 years of age should spend at least 180 minutes in a variety of types of physical activities at any intensity, including MVPA, spread throughout the day; more is better;
- Children 3–4 years of age should spend at least 180 minutes in a variety of types of physical activities at any intensity, of which at least 60 minutes is MVPA, spread throughout the day; more is better.

A thorough presentation and discussion of physical activity recommendations and guidelines is provided in Chapter 5.

Available International Surveillance Surveys and Studies

Implementing and effectively monitoring progress toward benchmarks set out in the various global calls to action requires systematic and standardized surveillance systems. To this end, frameworks such as the WHO STEPwise approach to NCD risk factor surveillance (World Health Organization, 2017) have helped to track the prevalence of physical activity among children and youth worldwide. The use of standardized surveys such as the Modified International Physical Activity Questionnaire for Adolescents (IPAQ-A) (Hagströmer et al., 2008), the Global school-based Student Health Survey (GSHS) (World Health Organization, 2018c), and Health Behaviour in School-Aged Children (HBSC) (Roberts et al., 2009) can facilitate international comparisons. Although standardized surveillance of physical activity among children and youth has substantially increased in the recent past, gaps exist especially in LMICs and physical activity trend data are scarce (Hallal et al., 2012). Table 2.1 presents results from a scoping review that identified 14 international surveillance systems or studies. These international surveillance systems collected physical activity data using standardized methods across three or more countries over the past 20 years.

To the best of our knowledge, most of the international data on the physical activity of children and youth come from specific studies rather than a given physical activity surveillance system. The GSHS, developed by and part of the WHO STEPwise framework, is the most widely adopted surveillance system, with a total of 98 countries having physical activity data available, obtained in a standardized manner (World Health Organization, 2018c). Six international surveys only focus on European and North American countries (Ahrens et al., 2011; Garaulet et al., 2011; McMahon et al., 2017; Riddoch et al., 2005; Roberts et al., 2009; van Stralen et al., 2011), and six others have more geographically distributed study sites across the world (Anderson et al., 2017; International Physical Activity and the Environment Network, 2017; Katzmarzyk et al., 2013; Strachan,

Table 2.1 International studies and surveillance systems of physical activity in children and youth

Name	Location	Target population[a]	Frequency	Description
EuropeaN Energy balance Research to prevent excessive weight Gain among Youth (ENERGY) project	Seven European countries (Belgium, Greece, Hungary, the Netherlands, Norway, Slovenia, and Spain)	Pupils in the final years of primary education (aged 10–12 years)	No established frequency, data were collected once in 2010	The ENERGY project was a school-based cross-sectional survey aiming to provide prevalence of measured overweight, obesity, engagement in energy balance-related behaviors, and blood-sample biomarkers of metabolic function, and to identify personal, family-environmental and school-environmental correlates of these energy balance-related behaviors. Physical activity was assessed by self-report questionnaire measuring the dose (frequency and duration) of active transportation and organized sport, and accelerometers in a subsample (van Stralen et al., 2011)
European Youth Heart Study (EYHS)	Denmark (Odense), Estonia (Tartu), Norway (Oslo), and Portugal (Madeira)	9- and 15-year-old children and youth	No established frequency, data were collected once in 2010	The EYHS was an international multi-center cross-sectional survey focusing on the issue of cardiovascular disease risk factors in children. It investigated a wide range of factors that might influence the progression of CVD risk factors in children. Physical activity was measured objectively using accelerometers worn for four consecutive days, including 2 weekdays and 2 weekend days (Riddoch et al., 2005)
Global School-based Student Health Survey (GSHS)	Datasets currently available for 98 countries from Africa (17), Eastern Mediterranean Region (19), Europe (2), Latin America and the Caribbean (30), South East Asia (9), and Western Pacific Region (21) (World Health Organization, 2018d)	13–17-year-old students	No established frequency, participating countries are encouraged to collect data as often as resources allow them	The GSHS is a relatively low-cost school-based survey using a self-administered questionnaire to evaluate young people's health behavior and protective factors related to the leading causes of morbidity and mortality among children and adults worldwide. Physical activity is measured by three items evaluating the frequency of physical activity, active transportation, and physical education (World Health Organization, 2018c)
Health Behaviour in School-Aged Children (HBSC) Survey	48 countries and regions across Europe and North America (HBSC, 2018)	11-, 13-, and 15-year-old school students	Every 4 years since 1982	HBSC is a school-based survey existing for over 30 years, where data are collected through self-completion questionnaires administered in the classroom. Physical activity is measured using one item evaluating the frequency of moderate-to-vigorous physical activity and two items evaluating the frequency of vigorous physical activity (Roberts et al., 2009)

(Continued)

Name	Location	Target population[a]	Frequency	Description
Health Behaviour and Lifestyle of Pacific Youth (HBLPY) surveys	Vanuatu, Tonga, and Pohnpei (an island of the Federated States of Micronesia)	11-, 13-, and 15-year-old school students	No established frequency, data were collected in 2000–2001	The aim of the study was to collect population-based data on a range of health-related practices, lifestyles, and physical and social environments among school-age students and out-of-school youth. Physical activity was measured using the 2000 version of the HBSC questionnaire (Phongsavan et al., 2005)
Healthy Lifestyle in Europe by Nutrition in Adolescence (HELENA)	Ten European cities in Austria, Belgium, France, Germany, Greece, Hungary, Italy, Spain, and Sweden	12.5–17.5-year-old adolescents	No established frequency, assessment occurred between 2006 and 2008	The HELENA study is a cross-sectional survey that aimed to evaluate the nutritional and health status in European adolescents. Physical activity was assessed by both objective (accelerometers worn for 7 consecutive days) and self-reported methods (using the International Physical Activity Questionnaire for Adolescents) (Garaulet et al., 2011)
Identification and prevention of Dietary- and lifestyle-induced health EFfects In Children and infantS (IDEFICS)	Eight European countries (Sweden, Germany, Hungary, Italy, Cyprus, Spain, Belgium, and Estonia)	2–9-year-old children	Baseline survey at T0 (between September 2007 and May 2008), follow-up survey 2 years later at T1 (September 2009 to May 2010); evaluation of the sustainability of the intervention at T2 (September 2010 to November 2010)	IDEFICS is a cohort study that started in 2006 and ended in 2012. It focused on exploring the risks for overweight and obesity in children as well as associated long-term consequences. Physical activity was objectively monitored over 3 days using accelerometers (Ahrens et al., 2011)
International Physical Activity and the Environment Network (IPEN)	In 2014, data collection was completed in eight countries, under completion in six countries, and under planning in two countries (International Physical Activity and the Environment Network, 2015)	12–17-year-old secondary school students	No established frequency, participating countries are encouraged to collect data as often as resources allow them	The primary aim of IPEN is to estimate strengths of association between detailed measures of the neighborhood-built environment with leisure physical activity, active transportation, and Body Mass Index in all participants, based on self-report survey data collected according to a common protocol. Physical activity is measured by self-completed surveys using 17 items rated on a 4-point Likert scale and accelerometry monitoring over 7 days, including 2 weekend days (Cerin et al., 2017; International Physical Activity and the Environment Network, 2017)

Study		Age group	Frequency	Description
International Study of Asthma and Allergies in Childhood (ISAAC) study phase three	Complete physical activity data available from 73 centers in 32 countries across 6 continents and from 122 centers in 53 countries across 6 continents	6–7-year-old children and 13–14-year-old adolescents	No established frequency, data were collected in each study site between 2001 and 2003	The ISAAC study was a multinational multicenter study, established in 1991, and designed to measure time trends in the prevalence, severity, and risk factors, and the development of asthma and allergies. Data on heights, weights, and physical activity were collected among children and youth during its phase 3. Physical activity was evaluated using parent-reported (for the 6–7-year-olds) and self-reported (for the 13–14-year-olds) frequency of vigorous physical activity (Braithwaite et al., 2017). ISAAC datasets have now been deposited in an openly accessible data archive (Strachan et al., 2017)
International Study of Childhood Obesity, Lifestyle and the Environment (ISCOLE)	12 countries from 5 major geographic regions of the world (Europe, Africa, the Americas, Southeast Asia, and the Western Pacific)	10-year-old children	No established frequency, data were collected in each study site between 2011 and 2013	ISCOLE aimed to determine the relationships between lifestyle behaviors and obesity, and to study the influence of additional characteristics such as behavioral settings, physical, social, and policy environments, on the observed relationships. Physical activity of participants was measured using accelerometers worn for at least 7 days and self-reported daily physical activity, outdoor time, physical education, active transport to school (Katzmarzyk et al., 2013)
Latin American Study of Nutrition and Health (ELANS)	Eight Latin American countries (Argentina, Brazil, Chile, Colombia, Costa Rica, Ecuador, Perú, and Venezuela)	15–18-year-old adolescents	No established frequency, data were collected once in each study site between 2014 and 2015	The ELANS is a multicenter cross-sectional nutrition and health surveillance study evaluating the nutritional intakes, physical activity levels, and anthropometric measurements of nationally representative samples of 15–65 years olds. Physical activity was measured using the Mexican (Spanish) version of the International Physical Activity Questionnaire (IPAQ)–long version, which was adapted for all countries of ELANS. Only the sections leisure–time and transport physical activity were included. In addition, physical activity was also objectively monitored using accelerometers for 7 days in 40% of the samples (Fisberg et al., 2015)
Saving and Empowering Young Lives in Europe (SEYLE) study	Ten European countries (Austria, Estonia, France, Germany, Hungary, Ireland, Italy, Romania, Slovenia, and Spain)	14- and 16-year-old adolescents	No established frequency, data collection took place in 2009–2012	This study explored the prevalence of risk behaviors, and their association with psychopathology and self-destructive behaviors, in adolescents recruited in randomly selected schools across ten European countries. Physical activity was assessed using a modified version of the PACE+ (Patient-Centred Assessment and Counselling for Exercise Plus Nutrition) adolescent physical activity measure. This survey has three items measuring reported frequency of 60 minutes of physical activity over the past 2 weeks, and the regular participation in sport(s) over the past 6 months (McMahon et al., 2017)

(Continued)

Name	Location	Target population[a]	Frequency	Description
SUNRISE International Surveillance Study of 24-hour movement behaviors in the Early Years	36 countries have expressed interest in participating in the SUNRISE Study: five of these are low-income, 11 lower-middle, 8 upper-middle, and 12 high-income countries	4-year-old children	No established frequency yet, pilot testing is underway in 21 countries	The SUNRISE study aims to estimate what proportion of 4-year-old children sampled in participating countries meet the WHO Global 24-hour movement guidelines for the early years and to determine if these proportions differ by sex, socioeconomic status, or urban/rural location between different levels of human and economic development. This study was still at its pilot stage in 2019. Physical activity will be monitored objectively using accelerometers thigh- or hip-worn over 3 days, as well as through parental report (University of Wollongong, 2019)
Global TEENS study	219 centers worldwide over 20 countries in 5 continents	School-aged 8–12-year-old children; 13–18-year-old adolescents	No established frequency, data collection took place in 2012–2013	The TEENs study was a global, observational, cross-sectional study of youth and young adults with type 1 diabetes launched across 5 continents in 20 countries in 2012. The primary aim of this study was to characterize diabetes-specific quality of life and glycemic control of a global sample of patients in predetermined age groups. Physical activity was assessed with self-reported number of days per week spent doing at least 30 minutes of any physical activities or exercise (Anderson et al., 2017)

a Even if some of the surveys have various sample age groups, the characteristics presented here only focus on the pediatric part (0–18) of their study population.

Pearce, Garcia-Marcos, & Asher, 2017; University of Wollongong, 2019; World Health Organization, 2018c). Of the two remaining surveys, one focuses on Latin American countries (Fisberg et al., 2015), and the other one on three South Pacific countries (Phongsavan et al., 2005). A large majority of these international surveys (n = 12/14) collected physical activity data on children and youth aged between 10 and 18 years, while 3 surveys included 6–9-year-old children, and only 2 included children below 5 years old. Only one of these surveys (HBSC) has an officially established frequency of data collection (every 4 years) (Roberts et al., 2009), and data collection in two other international surveys (GSHS and IPEN) is resource dependent (Centers for Disease Control and Prevention, 2016; International Physical Activity and the Environment Network, 2015). The majority of these international surveys are cross-sectional, designed for respondents to answer specific questions at a given time and without any longitudinal follow-up. Finally, self- or proxy-reported physical activity data were collected among seven international surveys (Anderson et al., 2017; McMahon et al., 2017; Phongsavan et al., 2005; Roberts et al., 2009; Strachan et al., 2017; van Stralen et al., 2011; World Health Organization, 2018c), objectively measured data using accelerometers were collected in the samples or subsamples of three of these surveys (Ahrens et al., 2011; Riddoch et al., 2005; University of Wollongong, 2019), and five collected both objective and subjective (reported) data (Fisberg et al., 2015; Garaulet et al., 2011; International Physical Activity and the Environment Network, 2017; Katzmarzyk et al., 2013; University of Wollongong, 2019).

National Surveys and Surveillance Systems

In some countries, physical activity monitoring has been a priority and has been successfully implemented in regular surveillance systems. In the following paragraphs we describe a few examples of good quality surveillance systems that have provided not only national data, but also have been recommended as a reference for other countries to model their own surveys.

Youth Risk Behavior Surveillance System

Developed in 1990 and implemented since 1991, the Youth Risk Behavior Surveillance System (YRBSS) is a nationally representative school-based surveillance system for the United States (Fulton & Carlson, 2012; U.S. Centers for Disease Control and Prevention, 2018a). Informed by multiple sources of data, such as ongoing surveys conducted every 2 years, one-time national surveys, special population surveys, and methods studies, the main objective of YRBSS is to determine the national prevalence and trends of key health risk behaviors among high-school students (grades 9 to 12) (Centers for Disease Control and Prevention, 2013). The surveys are conducted by the Centers for Disease Control and Prevention (CDC) and by education and health agencies. The system monitors six categories of health behaviors associated with the leading causes of morbidity and mortality in youth and young adults from the United States, one of which is physical inactivity (U.S. Centers for Disease Control and Prevention, 2018a). This standardized survey provides comparable data at the national, state, territorial tribal, and local levels (Fulton & Carlson, 2012) and is used to monitor the progress toward achieving national health-related goals, like the Healthy People Objectives (US Department of Health and Human Services, n.d.). The questionnaires used in the YRBSS were developed by a steering committee that included scientific experts from federal agencies, academic institutions, and survey experts from the CDC (Centers for Disease Control and Prevention, 2013). Questionnaires have marginally evolved over time to include adjustments in wording and design to provide better data according to the surveillance priorities. The specific component on physical activity currently includes questions that assess the following: (a) the frequency of engagement in minimum 60 minutes of MVPA in the last 7 days; (b) frequency of engagement in muscle strengthening in the last 7 days; (c) participation in Physical Education classes; (d) involvement in sports teams in the last year; and (e) frequency of concussions from playing sports or being active in the last year (U.S. Centers for Disease Control and Prevention, 2018b). In order to ensure the harmonization of the surveys, a handbook and technical assistance are provided by the CDC to each of the study sites (Centers for Disease Control and Prevention, 2013). Besides the contribution to the US surveillance of physical activity, YRBSS instruments have been adapted and widely used by several countries for the assessment of physical activity (Aubert, Barnes, Abdeta et al., 2018; González, Barnes, Abi Nader et al., 2018).

Canadian Health Measures Survey

This survey was developed in response to the lack of comprehensive population-representative health measures in Canada, and to the need for surveillance of public health indicators to follow-up program and policy initiatives (Tremblay, Wolfson, & Connor Gorber, 2007). Statistics Canada, in partnership with Health Canada and the Public Health Agency of Canada, and in consultation with a team of experts from multiple sectors, spent 3.5 years in the design of this nationally representative survey, with the aim to contribute direct physical measures to advance the Health Information Roadmap Initiative in the country (Canadian Institute for Health Information, 2000). Conducted in 2-year cycles, since 2007, the Canadian Health Measures Survey (CHMS) has several objectives, among those, the most relevant for the topic of this chapter is to estimate the prevalence, distribution, and trends of certain health-related conditions, like physical activity. The survey comprises a household questionnaire and objective measurements at a mobile examination center and includes a nationally representative sample of Canadian people between 6 and 79 years old. The physical activity component for children and youth includes physical activity questions (self-reported for ages ≥12 years or reported by the parents for <12 years) and objective measures with accelerometry. A standardized accelerometry protocol was implemented for the monitoring of physical activity for 7 days, using *Actical* accelerometers, on the right hip. The physical activity variables assessed in CHMS include: (a) adherence to physical activity recommendations; (b) average minutes of MVPA per day; (c) adherence to the Canadian 24-hour movement guidelines for Children and Youth (Tremblay, Carson et al., 2016); (d) amount of hours of physical activity at the school environment; (e) sports participation in the last year; (f) active play participation per week; and (g) active travel participation and time in the last 7 days (Roberts et al., 2017).

National Adolescent School-Based Health Survey from Brazil

Developed since 2004 as part of the Brazilian Surveillance of Risk and Protective Factors for Chronic Diseases, National Adolescent School-Based Health Survey (PeNSE) is a nationally representative school-based survey. The design was led by the Secretary of Health Surveillance of the Ministry of Health, and brought together a group of experts from different academic institutions (Oliveira et al., 2017). This survey has been conducted every 3 years since 2009, by the Ministry of Health and the Brazilian Institute of Geography and Statistics, with support of the Ministry of Education from Brazil and currently is already part of the national surveillance agenda (Oliveira et al., 2017). Since 2015, PeNSE includes the school-enrolled population between 13 and 17 years, from public and private schools, in the morning and afternoon shifts, and from urban and rural areas. In the previous versions only ninth grade students were involved. This change in the sampling was implemented in order to improve the comparability of data at the international level (Oliveira et al., 2017). The objective of PeNSE is to monitor risk and protective factors related to the health of Brazilian adolescents, and it is one of the main sources of information to track public policies targeted at this population. The data from this survey are representative of the 13–17-year-old students in the 26 state capitals of the 5 Brazilian macro-regions and Brazil (Oliveira et al., 2017). The survey comprises two components: one questionnaire about the school environment administered to the school principal, and the other questionnaire to student. Each of these has a specific component of physical activity. The school questionnaire assesses the available infrastructure for physical activity, and the student's questionnaire assesses the practice of physical activity in the previous 7 days and the attendance to Physical Education classes at least twice per week in the previous 7 days. The questionnaires were adapted from the GSHS (World Health Organization, 2018c) and the YRBSS (U.S. Centers for Disease Control and Prevention, 2018b). In order to ensure the quality and comparability of data, standardized training and supervision to the local teams are regularly conducted during the data collection (Oliveira et al., 2017).

Global Initiatives

In response to the global physical inactivity pandemic (Kohl III et al., 2012), research experts, policy makers, and other stakeholders with an interest in promoting physical activity have been mobilizing and establishing initiatives that are designed to systematically compile and synthesize the best available evidence on the levels of physical activity. These initiatives are helping to further our collective understanding of the extent of global physical inactivity, expose data gaps, and identify the most urgent research, interventions, or policy needs. The initiatives include, but are not limited to, the Global Matrix on Physical Activity of Children and Youth (Aubert, Barnes, Abdeta et al., 2018; Tremblay, Carson et al., 2016; Tremblay et al., 2014), WHO Global Health Observatory (GHO) (World Health Organization, 2018b), physical activity factsheets (World Health Organization, 2018f), and the Dedicated Diet and Physical Activity Knowledge Hub (DEDIPAC Determinants of Diet & Physical Activity, 2016b). Details about each of these initiatives are presented in Table 2.2. These initiatives necessarily involve partnerships, enlist experts from multiple jurisdictions, and follow harmonized protocols. The initiatives' particular strength is their adherence to harmonized protocols, reliance on similar appraisal of data either from standalone studies or national surveys, and the collective critical evaluation and interpretation of these data by teams of experts. The involvement of local experts (Active Healthy Kids Global Alliance, 2018; ISPAH, 2019) in collating and appraising the best available evidence, including unpublished data, theses, and reports, bypasses the academic purity and 'gatekeeping' of relying on mostly peer-reviewed literature, and doing so without compromising the quality of the reported findings. This is arguably an innovative approach because it can potentially reduce the publication bias that might arise from the high rejection of articles from LMICs which would have relied on limited and less robust data. Furthermore, the consensus building and consultations among teams of experts during the appraisal and interpretation of data enable them to be thorough, thus formulating recommendations and producing reports that could paint a more complete picture of the status of physical activity in each of the involved countries.

Global Prevalence of Physical (In)activity among Children and Youth

Major relevant findings publicly available from the international surveys and global initiatives previously presented are summarized by categories of interest in this section. When necessary, the presented information was completed with results from specific countries.

Table 2.2 Global Initiatives compiling evidence on physical activity of children and youth

Name	Location	Target population[a]	Frequency	Description
Determinants of Diet and Physical Activity Knowledge Hub – DEDIPAC study	Every country with objective or subjective physical activity data	3–12-year-old children and 13–18-year-old adolescents	No established frequency, the DEDIPAC Knowledge Hub occurred from 2013 to 2016	The DEDIPAC Knowledge Hub was a multidisciplinary consortium of scientists from 46 research centers working on three thematic areas: Assessment and harmonization of methods for future research, surveillance and monitoring, and evaluation of interventions and policies; Determinants of dietary, physical activity, and sedentary behaviors across the life course and in vulnerable groups; Evaluation and benchmarking of public health and policy interventions aimed at improving dietary, physical activity, and sedentary behaviors. This project is now complete, it ended in 2016 (DEDIPAC Determinants of Diet & Physical Activity, 2016b). One of the outputs of this international collaboration was the creation of a Compendium of Datasets on Physical Activity openly available online (DEDIPAC Determinants of Diet & Physical Activity, 2016a)
Global Matrix on physical activity of children and youth	49 countries from 6 continents in 2018	5–17-year-old children and youth	Every 2/3 years since 2014	The Global Matrix initiative, led by the Active Healthy Kids Global Alliance (Active Healthy Kids Global Alliance, 2018), brings together working groups for countries across the world who follow harmonized procedures to develop their Report Cards on Physical Activity for Children and Youth by grading ten common indicators using the best available data (Aubert, Barnes, Abdeta et al., 2018)
International Children's Accelerometry Database (ICAD)	Australia, Brazil, Belgium, Denmark, England, Estonia, Norway, Portugal, Switzerland, and the United States	3–18-year-old children and youth	No established frequency, this initiative only occurred once in 2008–2010	The ICAD was established to pool data on objectively measured physical activity from studies using the same type of accelerometer (Actigraph) worldwide. Investigators from 20 studies with a sample size >400 agreed to participate and shared their raw accelerometry files, and standardized analysis was performed on the pooled datasets (Sherar et al., 2011)

Physical Activity Factsheets	28 European Union Member States of the WHO European Region	0–18-year-old children and youth	First published in 2015, renewed in 2018	The country physical activity factsheets were developed by a partnership between the European Union and WHO. They summarize physical activity monitoring and surveillance-related indicators (including the proportion of children and adolescents reaching the minimum levels of physical activity for health recommended by WHO or another cut-off), as well as policies and action in the area of health-enhancing physical activity promotion, for the European Union Member States of the WHO European Region. National physical activity experts from the noted countries were responsible to report the aforementioned information (World Health Organization, 2018f)
World Health Organization (WHO) Global Health Observatory (GHO)	194 WHO Member States	11–17-year-old adolescents	This first round was performed in 2015 updates over the next 15 years are expected	The GHO is a WHO initiative compiling health-related statistics for more than 1,000 indicators. Concerning physical activity, the WHO GHO compiled surveys that presented sex- and age-specific prevalence with sample sizes (minimum: n = 50), using the definition of not meeting the WHO recommendations on physical activity for health, or a similar definition (less than 60 minutes of activity on less than 5 days per week). Data had to come from a random sample of the adolescent population, with clearly indicated survey methods (World Health Organization, 2018b)

a Even though some of the initiatives cover various sample age groups, the characteristics presented here only focus on the pediatric part (0–18) of their study population.

Early Years (0–4 Years)

- IDEFICS (Identification and prevention of Dietary- and lifestyle-induced health EFfects In Children and infantS) study: Objective data from eight European countries collected in 2007–2010 show that on average, 2.0–2.9-year-olds (boys and girls) engaged in 24 minutes of MVPA per day, 3.0–3.9-year olds engaged in 27 (girls) to 34 (boys) minutes of MVPA per day, and 4.0–4.9-year-olds engaged in 33 (girls) to 42 (boys) minutes of MVPA per day (Konstabel et al., 2014).
- ICAD (International Children's Accelerometry Database) study: The physical activity level of the 3–4-year-old children included in the objective accelerometry data pooled from 11 countries in 2008–2010 was not clearly reported (Cooper et al., 2015).
- Physical activity factsheets: In 2015, only 4 of the 28 European Union countries reported physical activity prevalence data on children aged under 5 years. Their data were not able to estimate intercountry comparisons as the country studies used different methods (World Health Organization Regional Office for Europe, 2015).
- International standardized data on the physical activity of the children younger than 5 years are lacking. It is, however, encouraging that a new international physical activity surveillance system targeting specifically this population, and involving objective measurement of physical activity, the SUNRISE study, is currently under development.

Children and Youth (5–17 Years)

- HELENA (Healthy Lifestyle in Europe by Nutrition in Adolescence) study: In a ten-European country sample (n = 2,200; 1,184 girls), objectively measured data in 2006–2008 indicated that 41.0% of 12.5–17.5-year-old adolescents met the recommended 60 minutes of MVPA daily (Ruiz et al., 2011).
- SEYLE (Saving and Empowering Young Lives in Europe) study: In a ten-European country sample (n = 11,072), self-reported physical activity data collected in 2009–2012 indicated that 13.6% of 14- and 16-year-olds were engaging in 60 minutes of physical activity everyday (McMahon et al., 2017).
- WHO GHO: Globally in 2010, more than 80% of school-going adolescents aged 11–17 years were estimated to be insufficiently physically active (World Health Organization, 2018b).
- Global Matrix 3.0: In 2018, the average grade for the Overall Physical Activity indicator in 49 countries from 6 continents was a "D", which corresponds to an estimation of 27%–33% of children and youth meeting the physical activity guidelines (Aubert, Barnes, Abdeta et al., 2018).

The estimated prevalence of children and youth meeting the WHO physical activity guidelines (World Health Organization, 2019) varies depending on the source of data; however, the proportion of children and youth sufficiently active is consistently low across international data.

Sex/Gender Differences

- HBLPY (Health Behaviour and Lifestyle of Pacific Youth) surveys: Data collected in Pohnpei, Tonga, and Vanuatu in 2000–2001 indicated that among 13-year-old children, 50.5% (Vanuatu) to 71.7% (Tonga) of boys and 29.8% (Vanuatu) to 44.2% (Tonga) of girls declared exercising at least two times per week outside school hours, and 27.4% (Vanuatu) to 33.5% (Pohnpei) of boys and 16.4% (Vanuatu) to 20.3% (Tonga) of girls declared exercising at least 2 hours per week outside school hours (Phongsavan et al., 2005). Similarly, the same data indicated that among 15-year-old children, 58.2% (Vanuatu) to 69.2% (Tonga) of boys and 32.9% (Pohnpei) to 37.5%

(Vanuatu) of girls declared exercising at least two times per week outside school hours, and 33.5% (Pohnpei) to 40.6% (Tonga) of boys and 17.3% (Pohnpei) to 23.6% of girls (Vanuatu) declared exercising at least 2 hours per week outside school hours (Phongsavan et al., 2005).

- HBSC: In physical activity data from 32 participating countries, 23.1% of boys and 14.0% of girls reported at least 60 minutes of MVPA daily (odds ratio/95% confidence interval: 0.546/0.537–0.554) (Kalman et al., 2015). Gender differences were significant in most countries across all age groups (Kalman et al., 2015).
- HELENA study: In Europe, objectively measured data in 2006–2008 indicated that 56.8% of boys vs. 27.5% of girls met the recommended 60 minutes of MVPA daily (p < 0.001) (Ruiz et al., 2011).
- ICAD study: Objective accelerometery data pooled from 11 countries in 2008–2010 indicated that among 5–17-year-olds, 9.0% of boys and 1.9% of girls achieved the WHO physical activity recommendations; that is, on average, activity levels among boys were 0.45 standard deviations higher than in girls at age 9–10 years and 0.66 standard deviations higher at age 12–13 years. There was no country in which this difference was not significant (Cooper et al., 2015).
- IDEFICS study: Objective data from eight European countries collected in 2007–2010 among 2–9-year-old children showed that 2.0% (Cyprus) to 14.7% (Sweden) of girls, and 9.5% (Italy) to 34.1% (Belgium) of boys were meeting the recommended 60 minutes of MVPA daily (Konstabel et al., 2014).
- SEYLE study: In a ten-European country sample (n = 11,072), self-reported physical activity data collected in 2009–2012 indicated that 17.9% (boys) and 10.7% (girls) of 14- and 16-year-olds reported engaging in 60 minutes of physical activity everyday (McMahon et al., 2017).
- WHO GHO: Globally, in 2010, among 11–17-year-old children and youth, it was estimated that the prevalence of adolescents meeting the minimum WHO-recommended activity levels was higher for boys (ranging from 9.0% to 35.4%) than for girls (from 7.4% to 20.4%) (World Health Organization, 2014).

An alarming difference between girls and boys is consistently observed among 5–17-year-old children around the world.

Age Differences

- ICAD study: Every year increase in age was associated with a relative reduction in mean vigorous-intensity physical activity of 6.9% (95% confidence interval [6.2%, 7.5%]) and in mean moderate-intensity physical activity of 6.0% (95% confidence interval [5.6%, 6.4%]) (Corder et al., 2016). The age-related difference in vigorous-intensity physical activity was substantially attenuated, but remained significant, when adjusted for moderate-intensity physical activity (Corder et al., 2016).
- EYHS (European Youth Heart Study): Objectively measured physical activity data from three European countries (Denmark, Estonia, Portugal) among 9-year-old (n = 1,008) and 15-year-old (n = 738) children and youth show that 15-year-old adolescents spent a significantly lower amount of time engaging in low (p < 0.001) and moderate (p < 0.001) physical activity (the time engaging in vigorous physical activity was stable between the two age groups) (Ekelund et al., 2007).
- HBSC surveys: Self-reported physical activity data from 2013 to 2014 were analyzed from 15 countries (n = 61,329) and indicated that more 11- (25.2%; 95% confidence interval [24.5%, 25.8%]) and 13-year-olds (19.8%; 95% confidence interval [19.3%, 20.3%]) met the WHO's physical activity guidelines than 15-year-olds (14.8%; 95% confidence interval [14.3%, 15.3%]) (Ng et al., 2017).

- CHMS survey: Accelerometry data collected on a nationally representative sample of the Canadian population aged 6–19 years showed that the amount of MVPA and average steps per day were decreasing as age category increased (Colley et al., 2011).

Temporal Trends

- HBSC: Overall, in countries and regions across Europe and North America, a small increase in the proportion of boys and girls aged 11–15 years who met the current physical activity recommendations was observed between 2002 and 2010 but these positive trends were not consistent in all countries (Kalman et al., 2015). Many countries reported increasing (n = 16) or stable levels (n = 7) of physical activity; however, the proportion of adolescents achieving the WHO's physical activity guidelines decreased in nine countries (Kalman et al., 2015).
- According to objectively measured data from European countries, there is evidence of little or no significant change in overall physical activity among children and adolescents. Pedometer-derived data from Sweden comparing the number of steps per day between 2000 and 2008 did not find any changes over time. Similarly, a comparison of accelerometer data from Denmark (EYHS study) between 1997–1998 and 2003–2004 did not find apparent changes in the average counts per minute of boys and girls. A study from Czech Republic, comparing the proportion of adolescents achieving the recommended 11,000 steps per day in 1998 and 2010, found a decline among boys (68%–55%), but no changes were observed among girls (75%–74%) (Booth et al., 2015).
- Canadian Report Card: Temporal trend analysis of the Canadian Report Card's physical activity indicators over 12 years (2005–2016) indicated that most physical activity behaviors (overall physical activity, active transportation, sedentary behaviors) among children and youth have not improved since 2005 (Barnes & Tremblay, 2017).

Geographic Variation

- HBSC: Self-reported data from 32 countries in Europe and North America indicate that 23.4% of children were active in 2010. However, there was some variability between countries indicating higher proportions of children meeting the guidelines in Ireland (34.4%), the United States (32.6%), Austria (30.5%), Spain (29.9%), and Finland (29.7%), and the lowest proportions in Italy (10.7%), Denmark (14.3%), Sweden (15.6%), Russia (16.1%), and Estonia (16.6%) (Kalman et al., 2015).
- ICAD study: Results obtained with accelerometry indicate a low proportion of children meet physical activity guidelines in all the involved countries. However, the highest proportions of children meeting the guidelines were found in Norway and Estonia, and the lowest were from the United States and the East of England (Cooper et al., 2015).
- ISCOLE (International Study of Childhood Obesity, Lifestyle and the Environment) study: Objectively measured data of 10-year-old children from 12 countries found that the average MVPA per day varied from 45 minutes per day in China to 71 minutes per day in Kenya and Finland (Katzmarzyk et al., 2015).
- Global Matrix: In 2018, most of the working groups from Asia, Europe North and South America, and Oceania reported "D" or "F" grades (which corresponds to 0%–39% of children and youth meeting the WHO's physical activity guidelines) for the Overall Physical Activity indicator, while the majority of the working groups from Africa assigned "C" grades (which corresponds to 40%–59% of children and youth meeting the WHO's physical activity guidelines) (Aubert, Barnes, Abdeta et al., 2018). These results, presented in Figure 2.1, are consistent with the previous Global Matrices published in 2014 and 2016 (Tremblay, Carson et al., 2016; Tremblay et al., 2014).

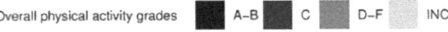

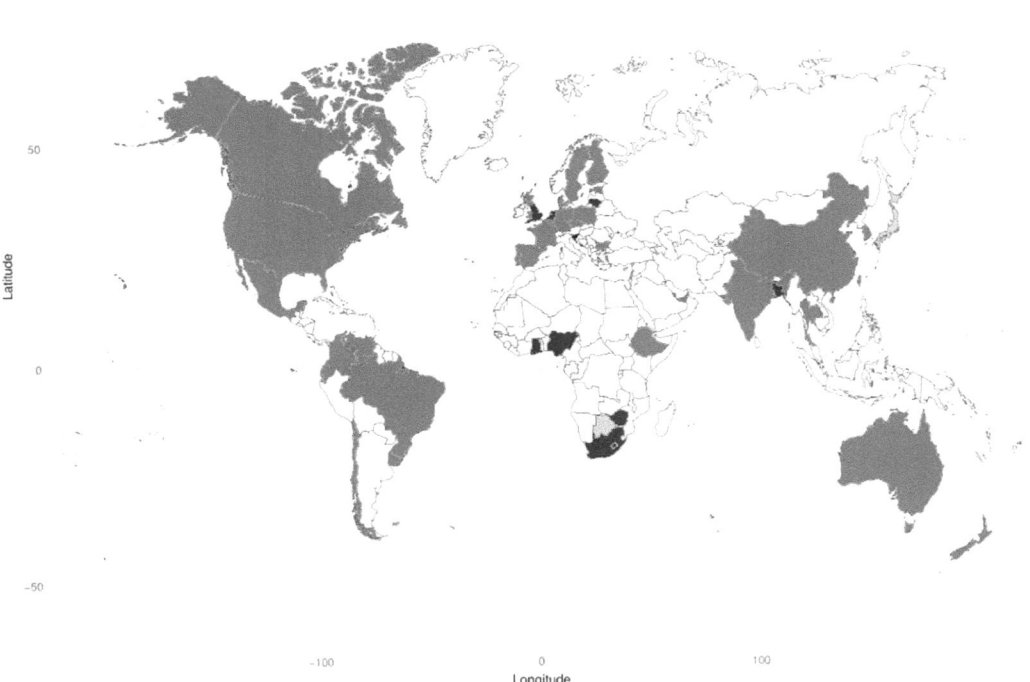

Figure 2.1 Distribution of the grades ("A-B", "C", "D-F", or "INC" grades) for the Overall Physical Activity indicator in the 49 countries that participated in the Global Matrix 3.0 initiative of the Active Healthy Kids Global Alliance

Different patterns are observed between studies, and this could be attributed to the different approaches used to measure physical activity. Several international studies and initiatives including both objectively and subjectively measured physical activity data indicate that children and youth are more active in countries from Africa and Northern/Eastern Europe, while they are less active in North America, the United Kingdom, China, and India; however, the opposite was observed in the HBSC surveys.

Socioeconomic Variation

- HBSC: Across all European and North American countries combined, children with higher Family Affluence Scale scores were more likely to meet the physical activity recommendations than children with low-Family Affluence Scale scores (Kalman et al., 2015).
- Global Matrix 3.0: Distinct letter grade differences were observed for the Overall Physical Activity indicator between the low- and medium-Human Development Index (HDI) countries and the two other HDI groupings. The average grade for the low- and medium-HDI countries was "C-", whereas both the high- and very-high-HDI countries obtained an

average of "D-", which could represent a difference of 14%–26% of children and youth meeting the physical activity guidelines (Aubert, Barnes, Abdeta et al., 2018). In addition, a significant low negative correlation was observed between the Overall Physical Activity indicator and several sociodemographic indicators including the HDI ($r = -0.30$, $P < 0.05$) and the growth national income per capita ($r = -0.33$, $P < 0.05$) (Aubert, Barnes, Abdeta et al., 2018).

- ISCOLE study: Objectively measured physical activity data from 9- to 11-year-old children (n = 4,752) and self-reported parental education level data collected in 12 countries around the world indicated that relationships between maternal and paternal education and child physical activity appear to be related to the developmental stage of different countries. Significant negative associations between parental education and child physical activity were observed in lower economic status countries, and positive non-significant associations between parental education and child physical activity were observed in high-income countries (HICs) (Muthuri et al., 2016).

The presented findings from these international physical activity data align with the recognized influence of the socioeconomic factors on the physical activity of children and youth. More research is needed to explore this relationship; however, available evidence shows that economic factors influence the physical activity of children and youth at two levels – national and individual. Overall, the observed children and youth physical activity levels are higher in low-income countries (LICs). Within LMICs, individual socioeconomic indicators seem to be negatively associated with physical activity behaviors, while the opposite is observed within HICs.

Special Population Data/Issues

- TEENS study: In 2012–2013, 67% of 8–12-year-old children diagnosed with type 1 diabetes spent at least 30 minutes doing any physical activities or exercise 3–7 times per week (against 33% who did 30 minutes of exercise 0–2 times per week) (Anderson et al., 2017). In 2012–2013, 62% of 13–18-year-old children diagnosed with type 1 diabetes spent at least 30 minutes doing any physical activities or exercise per week 3–7 times per week while 38% did 30 minutes of exercise 0–2 times per week (Anderson et al., 2017).
- YRBSS: Self-reported data collected in 2011 among ≤12-, 13-, 14-, 15-, 16-, 17-, and ≥18-year-old students (n = 9,775) indicated that youth with a disability (n =1,986) were less likely to participate in 60 minutes of physical activity at least 5 out of 7 days/week (prevalence = 38% vs. 52%, respectively; odds ratio = 0.5; 95% confidence interval: [0.4–0.6]) (Papas, Trabulsi, Axe, & Rimmer, 2016).
- HBSC surveys: Self-reported physical activity data were analyzed from 15 countries that included the same questions on long-term illnesses or disabilities (LTID) in their 2013/2014 surveys (n = 61,329). Overall, boys with LTID (23.4% meeting the physical activity guidelines) were significantly less likely (odds ratio = 0.89, 95% confidence interval = [0.81–0.98]) to meet the recommendations than boys without LTID (24.6% meeting the physical activity guidelines). The difference among girls with LTID (16.6% meeting the physical activity guidelines) and without LTID (15.4% meeting the physical activity guidelines) was not significant (Ng et al., 2017).
- HBSC surveys: Self-reported physical activity data collected in Finland during 2002, 2006, 2010, and 2014 showed that among adolescents with LTID, the proportion of those physically active in 2014 was higher than in 2002 for girls (15.6% vs. 8.7%) and boys (26.6% vs. 13.0%) (Ng et al., 2016).

- Global Matrix: The Netherlands developed a 2017 Report Card focusing on physical activity indicators for children and youth with disabilities or chronic diseases. In 2017, only 26% of the Dutch youth with a chronic disease or disability met the current national physical activity guidelines (Burghard, de Jong, Vlieger, & Takken, 2018).

The evaluation of physical activity levels of specific populations, including children and youth with disabilities or chronic diseases, aboriginal children and youth, and immigrant children and youth, is lacking globally.

Key/Emerging Issues for the Future

Lack of Standardization and Validation of Measurement of Physical Activity

Despite the global attention on the need for the promotion of physical activity and systematic surveillance, levels of physical inactivity remain high (Guthold et al., 2018). While there is general consensus for making physical activity surveillance a global priority (World Health Organization, 2008), several challenges need to be addressed for current and future initiatives to be successful. Policies, action plans, proposals, and interventions must be anchored in the cultural and contextual realities of each region, and acknowledge the complexities and the myriad of factors that may threaten progress. The lack of standardized and validated global surveillance tools for physical activity creates a predicament for accurate comparisons but also presents an opportunity for the development, trial, and implementation of universal surveillance mechanisms. Without standardized surveillance systems, the existing and urgent research gaps, including the lack of accurate global prevalence estimates of physical activity, will be difficult to fill. At present, although data for younger children may exist in some HICs (Kalman et al., 2015), where country-specific surveys are used, most progress in the global surveillance of physical activity levels has been made for older children and adolescents (11–17 years old) because of data obtained from the GSHS and/or the HBSC surveys (Hallal et al., 2012). Without assessing their universal validity and reliability, the country-specific surveys that are used to obtain data for younger children cannot be adopted in other regions or countries where contexts and cultures may be different. Moreover, a systematic review published in 2010 that evaluated measurement properties of most available questionnaires for children found none that had both acceptable reliability and validity, and therefore proposed to improve and evaluate those with the most promise in multiple high-quality studies (Chinapaw, Mokkink, van Poppel, van Mechelen, & Terwee, 2010).

Despite the reported increase in physical activity surveillance in middle- but not LICs, there still is lack of policy implementation and an absence of meaningful increases in the trends in global physical activity (Sallis et al., 2016). In many LMICs, the dearth of surveillance data can partly be attributable to the lack of validated surveillance tools, infrastructure, resources, and technical capacity. Also, for some countries that have joined international surveillance systems, like the WHO GSHS, the samples studied are not nationally representative. The concern about inadequate physical activity surveillance and a lack of standardized surveillance systems that are adapted to national contexts was recently reiterated as an urgent global necessity (Aubert, Barnes, Abdeta et al., 2018). Furthermore, there is significant heterogeneity in the definitions of key indicators that are relevant for the accurate surveillance of physical activity. For example, there is lack of consensus on how to assess key indicators of physical activity among children and youth such as active transportation, physical education attendance, and active play (Aubert, Barnes, Abdeta et al., 2018); Kohl III et al., 2012; Tremblay, Barnes, et al., 2016; Tremblay et al., 2014). Efforts for consensus and standardization in the approach to assess these indicators can lead to better comparisons and could increase the opportunities to learn from the experiences of countries that are succeeding in the promotion of physical activity in different domains. Currently, most of the physical activity interventions involve different sectors and actions at multiple levels. Consequently, global surveillance systems should incorporate a socioecological framework that monitors indicators at the individual, family/social, school, community, and policy levels (Ding, 2018; Fulton & Carlson, 2012; Kohl III et al., 2012). The resulting data from this comprehensive approach could greatly contribute to the design and improvement of programs and interventions.

Research Gaps

Trends Data

Systematic surveillance of the physical activity of children and youth is still emerging or at very early stages in many countries. It is only recently that it has been prioritized, explaining the absence of continuous surveillance systems (Hallal et al., 2012; Kohl III et al., 2012), particularly in LMICs in sub-Saharan Africa and other resource-limited parts of Latin America and Central Asia (Kohl III et al., 2012). The absence of continuous surveillance of physical activity levels for children and youth explains why there is such a lack of trend data to monitor the progress in physical activity promotion. In fact, the most recent estimates of global trends of physical activity in LICs were based on data from only one country (Benin) (Guthold et al., 2018). In addition, existing surveillance initiatives designed for the assessment of trends in health behaviors, such as the GSHS, have not been regularly administered in some countries due to a combination of insufficient funds, staff turnover, or other in-country barriers (Centers for Disease Control and Prevention, 2016).

Physical Activity in Children under 10 Years

Despite the importance of physical activity in the early years, surveillance of physical activity for younger children, particularly those in LICs, is limited (Sallis et al., 2016; Tremblay et al., 2014). This absence could be due to a lack of valid and reliable questionnaires (Chinapaw et al., 2010). Additionally, it has been reported that less progress has been made in the population-level assessment of physical activity in young people because few countries have surveillance systems covering ages 5–18 years (Bull, Goenka, Lambert, & Pratt, 2017). As part of the surveillance in the early years, future research should incorporate a 24-hour movement behaviors approach in order to better understand the health-related movement behaviors in this age group, and to guide the promotion of healthy development and growth (Tremblay, Carson et al., 2016).

Surveillance of Physical Activity in Vulnerable Groups

There is an absence of global surveillance data on the physical activity levels and opportunities for being active for children belonging to vulnerable groups, like children and youth with disabilities, immigrants and refugees, and children from rural communities and ethnic minorities. To the best of our knowledge, these particularly vulnerable groups have not been specifically included or prioritized in global surveillance initiatives (Aubert, Barnes, Abdeta et al., 2018; Tremblay, Carson et al., 2016; Tremblay et al., 2014). Considering the benefits of physical activity for these populations, it is essential to include and accommodate them in the global surveillance agenda. A good example of the assessment of physical activity levels and opportunities for children with disabilities is the

2017 Dutch Report Card+ on Physical Activity, which is focused on the youth population living with a chronic disease or disability (Burghard et al., 2018). This initiative could guide efforts at the global level to provide a better understanding of the physical activity status of this population.

Characteristics of Specific Behavioral Indicators

As recognized in the Global Matrix initiative and the Report Cards on Physical Activity (Aubert, Barnes, Abdeta et al., 2018); Tremblay, Carson et al., 2016; Tremblay et al., 2014), organized sport and physical activity, active play, and active transport are behaviors that contribute to the overall physical activity levels of children and youth. Certain progress on the assessment of these indicators has been made along the three versions of the Global Matrix initiative (Aubert, Barnes, Abdeta et al., 2018); Tremblay, Carson et al., 2016; Tremblay et al., 2014). However, further research and standardization of the following elements is desirable to improve the comparability of data and provide a better perspective of the current situation of physical activity among children at the global level: (1) Details of the frequency, duration, and intensity of physical activity associated with the practice of sports or organized physical activities (Aubert, Barnes, Abdeta et al., 2018); Tremblay, Carson et al., 2016); (2) Contextual information about the provision of sports and organized physical activity opportunities (i.e., equitable access, private clubs vs. public programs) (Aubert, Barnes, Abdeta et al., 2018); Tremblay, Carson et al., 2016); (3) Definition development as well as valid and reliable measurements to assess active play (Aubert, Barnes, Abdeta et al., 2018); Tremblay, Carson et al., 2016); (4) Dose and characteristics of the engagement in active transportation (Aubert, Barnes, Abdeta et al., 2018); (5) Variation of the dose of active behaviors in and out of school, on school days versus non-school days, and over the four seasons of the year; (6) Variation of the dose of active behaviors in relation to individual characteristics (level of income, education level of parents, religion, ethnicity).

Standardized Surveillance on Multiple-Level Sources of Influence

As suggested by the socioecological framework of active living, there are multiple levels of influence on physical activity (Sallis et al., 2006). While there is broad evidence that supports the importance of family and peers, school, community, built environment, and policy environment on the physical activity of children and youth, there is a lack of standardization on practical and informative indicators to assess these influences (Aubert, Barnes, Abdeta et al., 2018); Tremblay, Barnes, et al., 2016; Tremblay et al., 2014). There is also a lack of multi-sectoral approaches to surveillance, and limited national data on key macro-level indicators among the sources of influence, such as government support, infrastructure, impact evaluation, and implementation monitoring of current policies and programs (Aubert, Barnes, Abdeta et al., 2018); Ding, 2018; Tremblay, Carson et al., 2016).

Lack of Data in LMICs

The lack of infrastructure and paucity of data in LMICs are research gaps that have been universally identified as urgent issues for accurate global estimates of physical activity and promotion, but progress to fulfill this need has been slow (Hallal et al., 2012; Sallis et al., 2016). As part of the Lancet series on physical activity, Sallis et al. reported an improvement from their 2012 data, noting an increase in the overall number of countries with data, a wider range in age groups of adolescents covered, and a larger proportion of the adolescent population covered (Sallis et al., 2016). The fact that systematic surveillance of physical activity has been steadily improving is encouraging. However, it is important to note that although the proportion of countries contributing surveillance data from adolescents increased in most world regions, this was not the case in Africa and Southeast Asia (Sallis et al., 2016). Therefore, despite the improvement in availability of data overall, LICs contributed the least (Sallis et al., 2016). Moreover, assessment methods in LMICs are reported to be weak, not tailored to local contexts, and most of the countries lack clear plans for resource mobilization to enable scaling up of interventions (Sallis et al., 2016). A synthesis of surveillance data for physical activity levels among children and youth from nine LMICs (Manyanga et al., 2018) revealed a glaring lack of data on most of the key indicators in these countries. The limited available data from these countries were mostly self-reported, from small samples and often non-representative samples. The findings showing lack of data from the nine LMICs (Manyanga et al., 2018) are in line with the observation made by Sallis and associates in the Lancet series (Sallis et al., 2016). Without data, accurate estimates and comparisons across regions are difficult to make. In addition, lack of comparable data makes global intervention initiatives difficult to plan, implement, and monitor.

Research Devoted to Surveillance Improvement

There is need for research that can help improve global and national surveillance of physical activity across all ages, and abilities, including testing of new technologies and wearable devices, and methodologies for harmonization of data (World Health Organization, 2018a).

Reporting, Knowledge Translation, and Accountability

There is need for globally accepted and standardized reporting and accountability protocols that countries can follow in order to have meaningful progress in the global surveillance and promotion of physical activity among children and youth. However, reaching consensus and standardizing these reporting and accountability protocols may be challenging. Potential points of contention could range from the common indicators to monitor and regularly report on acceptable quality of data to be used, reporting schedules, and methods of reporting. An additional challenge may be the availability of funding for reporting and the capacity for effective knowledge translation. To facilitate accountability and regular reporting of progress, individual countries could develop and implement national surveillance systems and policy evaluation protocols that conform to established global frameworks and initiatives such as the WHO STEPwise approach (World Health Organization, 2017), the Global Action Plan on Physical Activity or GAPPA (World Health Organization, 2018a), and the Global Matrix initiatives (Aubert, Barnes, Abdeta et al., 2018); Tremblay, Carson et al., 2016; Tremblay et al., 2014). Individual countries could design and concurrently disseminate physical activity promotion plans such as those proposed by global agencies. For example, countries that have limited or no data to inform key indicators of physical activity among children and youth and participate in the Global Matrix initiative could develop and implement complete surveys to inform grades for their Report Cards as was done in Thailand (Amornsriwatanakul et al., 2016). These surveys could be adapted from already existing instruments.

National dissemination and promotion activities should be provided in simple and accessible language, deliberately designed to have a wide reach. For promotional activities, countries could adapt media tool kits from global initiatives such as the Global Matrix (Aubert, Barnes, Abdeta et al., 2018), GAPPA (World Health Organization, 2018a), and other media campaign strategies covering print, audio-visual media, as well as social media.

Issues of Competing Priorities

The combination of limited resources and lack of political will, as well as competing needs, are challenges that are omnipresent and often cited as reasons for lack of dedicated resource allocation to physical activity promotion in most LMICs. Due to lifestyle transitions that have been accelerated by rapid urbanization and industrialization, many LMICs face the dual burden of communicable and NCDs. LMICs, especially those in sub-Saharan Africa, still face a huge disease burden from infectious and other enteral diseases (Agyepong et al., 2018). In these countries, allocating the already limited resources to programs that promote physical activity in priority over communicable diseases or other needs will likely attract criticism, which policy makers may not be willing to accept. Moreover, given that the mortality, morbidity, and healthcare costs associated with physical inactivity do not manifest immediately, it makes for an even harder sell to prioritize. For example, despite evidence of huge direct and indirect healthcare costs of physical inactivity including loss of productivity and a decrease in life expectancy (Ding et al., 2016), governments and policy makers in LMICs have not demonstrated a commitment to prioritizing systematic surveillance of physical activity and interventions. This is especially important given the evidence showing that although HICs bear the largest proportion of the economic burden caused by NCDs, LMICs have a larger proportion of the disease burden (Ding et al., 2016). The disproportionate burden of disease caused by NCDs affecting LMICs, the lack of political will, and the seeming ambivalence by policy makers to urgently prioritize physical activity surveillance including resource allocation may alienate potential allies with whom reliable and enduring partnerships could be established. Furthermore, there is limited capacity development in some LMICs, thus a lack expertise in physical activity research. Without experts who can develop robust surveillance systems and confidently argue for more resource allocation using empirical evidence, physical activity surveillance will continue to lag behind.

Recommendations for Research and Practice

Need for Consensus in the Surveillance Methods

A possible way to address the lack of standardized instruments may involve an approach similar to the one used in the development of 24-hour movement behavior guidelines (Tremblay, Carson et al., 2016). Such an approach could involve combinations of a Delphi process and systematic reviews to gather evidence on all existing surveillance instruments. Once synthesized, common items from each of the instruments could be combined, adding some new items that are adapted to be context and culturally specific. The new instrument would then be pilot-tested, revised, and implemented. Comprehensive global surveillance instruments must have items that assess all domains (e.g., occupational/school-based, leisure, household, travel) and not just leisure-time physical activity. In addition, the following characteristics recommended in the Guidelines for Evaluating Surveillance Systems by the Centers for Disease Control and Prevention (Centers for Disease Control (CDC), 1988) should be taken into account, and consensus about the balance of these attributes should be reached (Fulton & Carlson, 2012).

- Simplicity: Surveillance systems should be as simple as possible in their structure and ease of operation.
- Flexibility: Ability to adapt to changes in the information needs, for example, changes in the definition of cut-points to define active populations. It is desirable that the surveillance instruments allow to re-calculate and adjust estimates as needed.
- Acceptability: It reflects the willingness of individuals to participate in the surveillance system.
- Sensitivity: Ability of the system to accurately measure the outcome of interest.
- Representativeness: Ability of the system to accurately reflect the characteristics of the outcome of interest over time and its distribution in the population.

- Timeliness: It reflects the desired time interval for the availability of the information under surveillance.
- Cost: Resources required to operate the surveillance system.

There is need to exploit the momentum and focused global attention created by the several and repeated global calls for action. To this end, it is critically important to develop partnerships and coalitions of willing entities such as those identified by Kohl and others (Kohl III et al., 2012). These partnerships can serve as the basis to establish cohesive leadership which can organize the various regional physical activity networks, and focus all surveillance research, policy, and practices.

Suggestions for Surveillance across a Range of Resource Availability Contexts

In order to advance in the goal of having comparable estimates of physical activity levels and determinants at a global level, the following recommendations can be useful to guide emerging surveillance initiatives in diverse contexts:

- Whenever possible, physical activity should be approached as a standalone priority in the surveillance agenda. A surveillance system specifically devoted to physical activity could contribute to assess behaviors and determinants in a more comprehensive way. In countries where physical activity is still not a priority for the surveillance agenda, a first step can be to include key indicators, like the proportion of children meeting physical activity guidelines, in other public health surveillance systems. Also, it is important to make visible the lack of data and the importance of its availability to make governments and surveillance-related stakeholders aware of the importance of having effective surveillance systems.
- In countries where physical activity surveillance is emerging and data are still limited, secondary data could help to inform environmental and policy indicators that can be relevant for the study of physical activity determinants. Examples of secondary data that could be used for global surveillance is the Worldwide Survey of School Physical Education conducted by UNESCO (United Nations Educational Scientific and Cultural Organization-UNESCO, 2014), the Multiple Indicator Cluster Survey from UNICEF (United Nations Children's Fund UNICEF, 2019), or environmental data collected with Geographic Information Systems at the global level (Fulton & Carlson, 2012).
- While new and standardized tools are developed, countries can adopt surveillance tools that are being used in similar contexts. Multi-country studies that assess physical activity with multiple measurements, like ISCOLE (Katzmarzyk et al., 2013), represent an opportunity for LMICs to conduct ancillary validity and reliability studies about the instruments used.
- To help fill the data gaps, it is imperative for LMICs to identify and support local researchers who can champion and advocate for the systematic surveillance of physical activity from within their countries. Networking with leaders from countries with more experience in surveillance could lead to fruitful partnerships and opportunities to optimize resources (e.g., workshops for capacity building and agreements between institutions for accelerometer or other devices lending libraries).

Summary

The glaring physical inactivity crisis among children and youth and the global calls to action implore us to prioritize systematic surveillance of physical activity. Given the concerning levels of inactivity among children and youth, the importance of dependable and durable global surveillance systems cannot be overemphasized. Global surveillance systems should carefully balance feasibility and validity. This chapter presents some of the available global surveillance systems and highlights the needs for improvement of the physical activity surveillance systems which mostly focus on older children and adolescents, lack standardization, and are not conducted regularly. Surveillance data are especially scarce for physical activity trends over time in vulnerable populations and in resource-limited LMICs.

References

Active Healthy Kids Global Alliance. (2018). *About – Active healthy kids global alliance*. Retrieved January 31, 2019, from https://www.activehealthykids.org/about/

Agyepong, I. A., Sewankambo, N., Binagwaho, A., Coll-Seck, A. M., Corrah, T., Ezeh, A., . . . Piot, P. (2018). The path to longer and healthier lives for all Africans by 2030: The Lancet commission on the future of health in sub-Saharan Africa. *Lancet (London, England), 390*(10114), 2803–2859. doi:10.1016/S0140-6736(17)31509-X

Ahrens, W., Bammann, K., Siani, A., Buchecker, K., De Henauw, S., Iacoviello, L., . . . Pigeot, I. (2011). The IDEFICS cohort: Design, characteristics and participation in the baseline survey. *International Journal of Obesity, 35*(S1), S3–S15. doi:10.1038/ijo.2011.30

Ainsworth, B., Cahalin, L., Buman, M., & Ross, R. (2015). The current state of physical activity assessment tools. *Progress in Cardiovascular Diseases, 57*(4), 387–395. doi:10.1016/J.PCAD.2014.10.005

Amornsriwatanakul, A., Nakornkhet, K., Katewongsa, P., Choosakul, C., Kaewmanee, T., Konharn, K., . . . Bull, F. C. (2016). Results from Thailand's 2016 report card on physical activity for children and youth. *Journal of Physical Activity and Health, 13*(11 Suppl 2), S291–S298. doi:10.1123/jpah.2016-0316

Anderson, B. J., Laffel, L. M., Domenger, C., Danne, T., Phillip, M., Mazza, C., . . . Mathieu, C. (2017). Factors associated with diabetes-specific health-related quality of life in youth with Type 1 diabetes: The global TEENs study. *Diabetes Care, 40*(8), 1002–1009. doi:10.2337/DC16-1990

Aubert, S., Barnes, J. D., Abdeta, C., Abi Nader, P., Adeniyi, A. F., Aguilar-Farias, N., . . . Tremblay, M. S. (2018). Global Matrix 3.0 physical activity report card grades for children and youth: Results and analysis from 49 countries. *Journal of Physical Activity and Health, 15*(S2), S251–S273. doi:10.1123/jpah.2018-0472

Aubert, S., Barnes, J. D., Aguilar-Farias, N., Cardon, G., Chang, C.-K., Delisle Nyström, C., … Tremblay, M. S. (2018). Report Card Grades on the Physical Activity of Children and Youth Comparing 30 Very High Human Development Index Countries. *Journal of Physical Activity and Health, 15*(S2), S298–S314. doi:10.1123/jpah.2018-0431.

Barnes, J. D., & Tremblay, M. S. (2017). Changes in indicators of child and youth physical activity in Canada, 2005–2016. *Canadian Journal of Public Health, 107*(6), 586. doi:10.17269/cjph.107.5645

Booth, V. M., Rowlands, A. V, & Dollman, J. (2015). Physical activity temporal trends among children and adolescents. *Journal of Science and Medicine in Sport, 18*(4), 418–425. doi:10.1016/j.jsams.2014.06.002

Braithwaite, I. E., Stewart, A. W., Hancox, R. J., Murphy, R., Wall, C. R., Beasley, R., & Mitchell, E. A. (2017). Body mass index and vigorous physical activity in children and adolescents: An international cross-sectional study. *Acta Paediatrica, 106*(8), 1323–1330. doi:10.1111/apa.13903

Brodersen, N. H., Steptoe, A., Boniface, D. R., & Wardle, J. (2007). Trends in physical activity and sedentary behaviour in adolescence: Ethnic and socioeconomic differences. *British Journal of Sports Medicine, 41*(3), 140–144. doi:10.1136/bjsm.2006.031138

Bull, F. C., Gauvin, L., Bauman, A., Shilton, T., Kohl, H. W., & Salmon, A. (2010). The Toronto charter for physical activity: A global call for action. *Journal of Physical Activity and Health, 7*, 421–422. Retrieved from https://pdfs.semanticscholar.org/4b34/24f9139dbf473ac035737ca53ac94c633639.pdf

Bull, F., Goenka, S., Lambert, V., & Pratt, M. (2017). *Physical activity for the prevention of cardiometabolic disease. Cardiovascular, respiratory, and related disorders*. The International Bank for Reconstruction and Development/The World Bank. doi:10.1596/978-1-4648-0518-9/CH5

Burghard, M., de Jong, N. B., Vlieger, S., & Takken, T. (2018). 2017 Dutch report card+: Results from the first physical activity report card plus for Dutch youth with a chronic disease or disability. *Frontiers in Pediatrics, 6*, 122. doi:10.3389/fped.2018.00122

Canadian Institute for Health Information. (2000). *Roadmap initiative… Launching the process*. Ottawa, Canada. Retrieved from https://www.cihi.ca/en/profile_roadmap_launch_pdf_en.pdf

Centers for Disease Control (CDC). (1988). Guidelines for evaluating surveillance systems. *MMWR Supplements, 37*(5), 1–18.

Centers for Disease Control and Prevention. (2013). *Methodology of the youth risk behavior surveillance system–2013. MMWR. Recommendations and reports: Morbidity and mortality weekly report. Recommendations and reports.* Washington, DC: Centers for Disease Control and Prevention.

Centers for Disease Control and Prevention. (2016). Global school-based student health survey. Retrieved May 28, 2019, from https://www.cdc.gov/gshs/background/index.htm

Cerin, E., Sit, C. H. P., Barnett, A., Huang, W. Y. J., Gao, G. Y., Wong, S. H. S., & Sallis, J. F. (2017). Reliability of self-report measures of correlates of obesity-related behaviours in Hong Kong adolescents for the iHealt(H) and IPEN adolescent studies. *Archives of Public Health, 75*(1), 38. doi:10.1186/s13690-017-0209-5

Chinapaw, M. J. M., Mokkink, L. B., van Poppel, M. N. M., van Mechelen, W., & Terwee, C. B. (2010). Physical activity questionnaires for youth: A systematic review of measurement properties. *Sports Medicine, 40*(7), 539–563. doi:10.2165/11530770-000000000-00000

Colley, R. C., Garriguet, D., Janssen, I., Craig, C. L., Clarke, J., & Tremblay, M. S. (2011). Physical activity of Canadian children and youth: Accelerometer results from the 2007 to 2009 Canadian health measures survey. *Statistics Canada, 22*(1). Retrieved from https://www.researchgate.net/profile/Ian_Janssen/publication/51067924_Physical_activity_of_Canadian_children_and_youth_Accelerometer_results_from_the_2007_to_2009_Canadian_Health_Measures_Survey/links/0fcfd4fbd76fb0d3ae000000/Physical-activity-of-Canadian

Cooper, A. R., Goodman, A., Page, A. S., Sherar, L. B., Esliger, D. W., van Sluijs, E. M., . . . Ekelund, U. (2015). Objectively measured physical activity and sedentary time in youth: The international children's accelerometry database (ICAD). *International Journal of Behavioral Nutrition and Physical Activity, 12*(1), 113. doi:10.1186/s12966-015-0274-5

Corder, K., Sharp, S. J., Atkin, A. J., Andersen, L. B., Cardon, G., Page, A., . . . van Sluijs, E. M. F. (2016). Age-related patterns of vigorous-intensity physical activity in youth: The international children's accelerometry database. *Preventive Medicine Reports, 4*, 17–22. doi:10.1016/J.PMEDR.2016.05.006

DEDIPAC Determinants of Diet & Physical Activity. (2016a). Compendium of datasets. Retrieved January 31, 2019, from https://www.dedipac.eu/compendium

DEDIPAC Determinants of Diet & Physical Activity. (2016b). Project – General. Retrieved January 31, 2019, from https://www.dedipac.eu/project

Ding, D. (2018). Surveillance of global physical activity: Progress, evidence, and future directions. *The Lancet Global Health, 6*(10), e1046–e1047. doi:10.1016/S2214-109X(18)30381-4

Ding, D., Lawson, K. D., Kolbe-Alexander, T. L., Finkelstein, E. A., Katzmarzyk, P. T., van Mechelen, W., & Pratt, M. (2016). The economic burden of physical inactivity: A global analysis of major noncommunicable diseases. *The Lancet, 388*(10051), 1311–1324. doi:10.1016/S0140-6736(16)30383-X

Dollman, J., Norton, K., & Norton, L. (2005). Evidence for secular trends in children's physical activity behaviour. *British Journal of Sports Medicine, 39*(12), 892–897; discussion 897. doi:10.1136/bjsm.2004.016675

Ekelund, U., Anderssen, S. A., Froberg, K., Sardinha, L. B., Andersen, L. B., Brage, S., & Group, E. Y. H. S. (2007). Independent associations of physical activity and cardiorespiratory fitness with metabolic risk factors in children: The European youth heart study. *Diabetologia, 50*(9), 1832–1840. doi:10.1007/s00125-007-0762-5

Fisberg, M., Kovalskys, I., Gómez, G., Rigotti, A., Cortés, L. Y., Herrera-Cuenca, M., . . . Tucker, K. L. (2015). Latin American study of nutrition and health (ELANS): Rationale and study design. *BMC Public Health, 16*(1), 93. doi:10.1186/s12889-016-2765-y

Fulton, J. E., & Carlson, S. A. (2012). Surveillance of physical activity. In B. E. Ainsworth & C. A. Macera (Eds.), *Physical activity and public health practice.* Boca Raton, FL: CRC Press.

Garaulet, M., Ortega, F. B., Ruiz, J. R., Rey-López, J. P., Béghin, L., Manios, Y., . . . Moreno, L. A. (2011). Short sleep duration is associated with increased obesity markers in European adolescents: Effect of physical activity and dietary habits. The HELENA study. *International Journal of Obesity, 35*(10), 1308–1317. doi:10.1038/ijo.2011.149

González, S. A., Barnes, J. D., Nader, P. A., Tenesaca, D. S. A., Brazo-Sayavera, J., Galaviz, K. I., . . . & Tremblay, M.S. (2018). Report card grades on the physical activity of children and youth from 10 countries with high human development index: Global Matrix 3.0. *Journal of Physical Activity and Health, 15*(s2), S284–S297.

Guthold, R., Stevens, G. A., Riley, L. M., & Bull, F. C. (2018). Worldwide trends in insufficient physical activity from 2001 to 2016: A pooled analysis of 358 population-based surveys with 1·9 million participants. *The Lancet Global Health, 6*(10), e1077–e1086. doi:10.1016/S2214-109X(18)30357-7

Hagströmer, M., Bergman, P., De Bourdeaudhuij, I., Ortega, F. B., Ruiz, J. R., Manios, Y., . . . Sjöström, M. (2008). Concurrent validity of a modified version of the international physical activity questionnaire

(IPAQ-A) in European adolescents: The HELENA study. *International Journal of Obesity, 32*(S5), S42–S48. doi:10.1038/ijo.2008.182

Hallal, P. C., Andersen, L. B., Bull, F. C., Guthold, R., Haskell, W., & Ekelund, U. (2012). Global physical activity levels: Surveillance progress, pitfalls, and prospects. *The Lancet, 380*(9838), 247–257. doi:10.1016/S0140-6736(12)60646-1

HBSC. (2018). HBSC. Retrieved January 22, 2019, from http://www.hbsc.org/

International Physical Activity and the Environment Network. (2015). IPEN newsletter 2014 edition. Retrieved from https://www.ipenproject.org/

International Physical Activity and the Environment Network. (2017). IPEN. Retrieved January 26, 2019, from https://www.ipenproject.org/

ISPAH. (2016). *The Bangkok declaration on physical aactivity for global health and sustainable development.* Bangkok, Thailand: ISPAH. Retrieved from http://api.ning.com/files/V0BiFi-tkRtNBOh-2povpLXSGLAazPB-z8KItEppPYDz4TzYQ7jUGub6GuuiAdXPIdA6lbCgjeugQswM4vqlpAhOji36u5xE9/BKK_Declaration_Final_2016.pdf

ISPAH. (2019). Global observatory for physical activity. Retrieved January 31, 2019, from http://www.globalphysicalactivityobservatory.com/

Kalman, M., Inchley, J., Sigmundova, D., Iannotti, R. J., Tynjala, J. A., Hamrik, Z., . . . Bucksch, J. (2015). Secular trends in moderate-to-vigorous physical activity in 32 countries from 2002 to 2010: A cross-national perspective. *The European Journal of Public Health, 25*(Suppl 2), 37–40. doi:10.1093/eurpub/ckv024

Katzmarzyk, P. T., Barreira, T. V, Broyles, S. T., Champagne, C. M., Chaput, J.-P., Fogelholm, M., . . . Church, T. S. (2013). The international study of childhood obesity, lifestyle and the environment (ISCOLE): Design and methods. *BMC Public Health, 13*(1), 900. doi:10.1186/1471-2458-13-900

Katzmarzyk, P. T., Barreira, T. V, Broyles, S. T., Champagne, C. M., Chaput, J.-P., Fogelholm, M., . . . Church, T. S. (2015). Physical activity, sedentary time, and obesity in an international sample of children. *Medicine & Science in Sports & Exercise,* (22), 2062–2069. doi:10.1249/MSS.0000000000000649

Kohl III, H. W., Craig, C. L., Lambert, E. V, Inoue, S., Alkandari, J. R., Leetongin, G., & Kahlmeier, S. (2012). The pandemic of physical inactivity: Global action for public health. *Lancet, 380*(1474–547X (Electronic)), 294–305.

Konstabel, K., Veidebaum, T., Verbestel, V., Moreno, L. A., Bammann, K., Tornaritis, M., . . . Pitsiladis, Y. (2014). Objectively measured physical activity in European children: The IDEFICS study. *International Journal of Obesity, 38*(S2), S135–S143. doi:10.1038/ijo.2014.144

Lee, I.-M., & Shiroma, E. J. (2014). Using accelerometers to measure physical activity in large-scale epidemiological studies: Issues and challenges. *British Journal of Sports Medicine, 48*(3), 197–201. doi:10.1136/bjsports-2013-093154

Lubans, D. R., Plotnikoff, R. C., Miller, A., Scott, J. J., Thompson, D., & Tudor-Locke, C. (2015). Using pedometers for measuring and increasing physical activity in children and adolescents. *American Journal of Lifestyle Medicine, 9*(6), 418–427. doi:10.1177/1559827614537774

Manyanga, T., Barnes, J. D., Abdeta, C., Adeniyi, A. F., Bhawra, J., Draper, C. E., . . . Tremblay, M. S. (2018). Indicators of physical activity among children and youth in 9 countries with low to medium human development indices: A Global Matrix 3.0 paper. *Journal of Physical Activity and Health, 15*(S2), S274–S283. doi:10.1123/jpah.2018-0370

McMahon, E. M., Corcoran, P., O'Regan, G., Keeley, H., Cannon, M., Carli, V., . . . Wasserman, D. (2017). Physical activity in European adolescents and associations with anxiety, depression and well-being. *European Child & Adolescent Psychiatry, 26*(1), 111–122. doi:10.1007/s00787-016-0875-9

Migueles, J. H., Cadenas-Sanchez, C., Tudor-Locke, C., Löf, M., Esteban-Cornejo, I., Molina-Garcia, P., . . . Ortega, F. B. (2018). Comparability of published cut-points for the assessment of physical activity: Implications for data harmonization. *Scandinavian Journal of Medicine & Science in Sports.* doi:10.1111/sms.13356

Muthuri, S. K., Onywera, V. O., Tremblay, M. S., Broyles, S. T., Chaput, J.-P., Fogelholm, M., . . . Group, I. R. (2016). Relationships between parental education and overweight with childhood overweight and physical activity in 9–11 year old children: Results from a 12-country study. *PLOS One, 11*(8), e0147746. doi:10.1371/journal.pone.0147746

Ng, K., Rintala, P., Tynjälä, J., Välimaa, R., Villberg, J., Kokko, S., & Kannas, L. (2016). Physical activity trends of finnish adolescents with long-term illnesses or disabilities from 2002–2014. *Journal of Physical Activity and Health, 13*(8), 816–821. doi:10.1123/jpah.2015-0539

Ng, K., Tynjälä, J., Sigmundová, D., Augustine, L., Sentenac, M., Rintala, P., & Inchley, J. (2017). Physical activity among adolescents with long-term illnesses or disabilities in 15 European countries. *Adapted Physical Activity Quarterly, 34*(4), 456–465. doi:10.1123/apaq.2016-0138

Oliveira, M. M., de, Campos, M. O., Andreazzi, M. A. R., de, Malta, D. C., Oliveira, M. M. de, Campos, M. O., . . . Malta, D. C. (2017). Characteristics of the national adolescent school-based health survey – PeNSE, Brazil. *Epidemiologia e Serviços de Saúde, 26*(3), 605–616. doi:10.5123/S1679-49742017000300017

Papas, M. A., Trabulsi, J. C., Axe, M., & Rimmer, J. H. (2016). Predictors of obesity in a US sample of high school adolescents with and without disabilities. *The Journal of School Health, 86*(11), 803–812. doi:10.1111/josh.12436

Phongsavan, P., Olatunbosun-Alakija, A., Havea, D., Bauman, A., Smith, B. J., Galea, G., & Chen, J. (2005). Health behaviour and lifestyle of Pacific youth surveys: A resource for capacity building. *Health Promotion International, 20*(3), 238–248. doi:10.1093/heapro/dah612

Riddoch, C., Edwards, D., Page, A., Froberg, K., Anderssen, S. A., Wedderkopp, N., . . . Team, T. E. Y. H. S. (2005). The European youth heart study – Cardiovascular disease risk factors in children: Rationale, aims, study design, and validation of methods. *Journal of Physical Activity and Health, 2*(1), 115–129. doi:10.1123/jpah.2.1.115

Roberts, C., Freeman, J., Samdal, O., Schnohr, C. W., de Looze, M. E., Nic Gabhainn, S., . . . International HBSC Study Group. (2009). The health behaviour in school-aged children (HBSC) study: Methodological developments and current tensions. *International Journal of Public Health, 54*(Suppl 2), 140–150. doi:10.1007/s00038-009-5405-9

Roberts, K. C., Butler, G., Branchard, B., Rao, D. P., Otterman, V., Thompson, W., & Jayaraman, G. (2017). The physical activity, sedentary behaviour and sleep (PASS) indicator framework. *Health Promotion and Chronic Disease Prevention in Canada, 37*(8), 252–256. doi:10.24095/hpcdp.37.8.04

Ruiz, J. R., Ortega, F. B., Martinez-Gomez, D., Labayen, I., Moreno, L. A., De Bourdeaudhuij, I., . . . Sjostrom, M. (2011). Objectively measured physical activity and sedentary time in European adolescents: The HELENA study. *American Journal of Epidemiology, 174*(2), 173–184. doi:10.1093/aje/kwr068

Sallis, J. F., Bull, F., Guthold, R., Heath, G. W., Inoue, S., Kelly, P., . . . Hallal, P. C. (2016). Progress in physical activity over the olympic quadrennium. *The Lancet, 388*(10051), 1325–1336. doi:10.1016/S0140-6736(16)30581-5

Sallis, J. F., Cervero, R. B., Ascher, W., Henderson, K. A., Kraft, M. K., & Kerr, J. (2006). An ecological approach to creating active living communities. *Annual Review of Public Health, 27*, 297–322. doi:10.1146/annurev.publhealth.27.021405.102100

Sallis, J. F., & Saelens, B. E. (2000). Assessment of physical activity by self-report: Status, limitations, and future directions. *Research Quarterly for Exercise and Sport, 71*(Suppl 2), 1–14. doi:10.1080/02701367.2000.11082780

Schutz, Y., Weinsier, R. L., & Hunter, G. R. (2001). Assessment of Free-living physical activity in humans: An overview of currently available and proposed new measures. *Obesity Research, 9*(6), 368–379. doi:10.1038/oby.2001.48

Sherar, L. B., Griew, P., Esliger, D. W., Cooper, A. R., Ekelund, U., Judge, K., & Riddoch, C. (2011). International children's accelerometry database (ICAD): Design and methods. *BMC Public Health, 11*(1), 485. doi:10.1186/1471-2458-11-485

Strachan, D., Pearce, N., Garcia-Marcos, L., & Asher, I. (2017). International study of asthma and allergies in childhood, 1992–2005 [Data collection]. *UK Data Service, SN: 8131*. doi:10.5255/UKDA-SN-8131-1

Sylvia, L. G., Bernstein, E. E., Hubbard, J. L., Keating, L., & Anderson, E. J. (2014). Practical guide to measuring physical activity. *Journal of the Academy of Nutrition and Dietetics, 114*(2), 199–208. doi:10.1016/j.jand.2013.09.018

Thacker, S. B., & Berkelman, R. L. (1988). Public health surveillance in the United States. *Epidemiologic Reviews, 10*, 164–190.

Titze, S., & Oja, P. (2013). Global advocacy for physical activity. *Public Health Forum, 21*(2), 34–36. doi:10.1016/j.phf.2013.03.018

Tremblay MS, Barnes JD, González SA, Katzmarzyk PT, Onywera VO, Reilly JJ, Tomkinson GR, and the Global Matrix 2.0 Research Team (Aguilar-Farias N, Akinroye KK, Al-Kuwari MG, Amornsriwatanakul A, Aubert S★, Belton S, Gołdys A, Herrera-Cuenca M, Jeon JY, Jürimäe J, Katapally TR, Lambert EV, Larsen LR, Liu Y, Löf M, Loney T, López y Taylor JR, Maddison R, Manyanga T★, Morrison SA, Mota J, Murphy MH, Nardo Junior N, Ocansey RT-A, Prista A, Roman-Viñas B, Schranz NK, Seghers J, Sharif R, Standage M, Stratton G, Takken T, Tammelin TH, Tanaka C, Tang Y, Wong SH). Global Matrix 2.0: Report Card Grades on the Physical Activity of Children and Youth Comparing 38 Countries. *Journal of Physical Activity and Health, 13*(Suppl 2), S343–S366, 2016.

Tremblay, M. S., Carson, V., Chaput, J.-P., Connor Gorber, S., Dinh, T., Duggan, M., . . . Zehr, L. (2016). Canadian 24-hour movement guidelines for children and youth: An integration of physical activity, sedentary behaviour, and sleep. *Applied Physiology, Nutrition, and Metabolism, 41*(6 Suppl 3), S311–S327. doi:10.1139/apnm-2016-0151

Tremblay, M. S., Gray, C. E., Akinroye, K., Harrington, D. M., Katzmarzyk, P. T., Lambert, E. V., . . . Tomkinson, G. (2014). Physical activity of children: A global matrix of grades comparing 15 countries. *Journal of Physical Activity and Health, 11*(s1), S113–S125. doi:10.1123/jpah.2014-0177

Tremblay, M., Wolfson, M., & Connor Gorber, S. (2007). Canadian health measures survey: Rationale, background and overview. *Health Reports, 18*(Suppl), 7–20.

United Nations. (2012). *Political declaration of the UN high-level meeting on the prevention and control of noncommunicable diseases (NCDs): Key points background.* New York, NY. Retrieved from https://ncdalliance.org/sites/default/files/rfiles/Key Points of Political Declaration.pdf

United Nations. (2015). *Transforming our world: The 2030 agenda for sustainable development: Sustainable development knowledge platform.* New York, NY. Retrieved from https://sustainabledevelopment.un.org/post2015/transformingourworld

United Nations Children's Fund UNICEF. (2019). Multiple indicators cluster survey. Retrieved from https://mics.unicef.org/

United Nations Educational Scientific and Cultural Organization-UNESCO. (2014). *World-wide survey of school physical education.* Paris, France: United Nations Educational Scientific and Cultural Organization-UNESCO.

University of Wollongong. (2019). *SUNRISE pilot study phase 2.* Retrieved from https://esri.uow.edu.au/index.html

U.S. Centers for Disease Control and Prevention. (2018a). Youth risk behavior surveillance system (YRBSS). Retrieved from https://www.cdc.gov/healthyyouth/data/yrbs/index.htm

U.S. Centers for Disease Control and Prevention. (2018b). YRBSS questionnaire content 1991–2019. Retrieved from https://www.cdc.gov/healthyyouth/data/yrbs/pdf/2019/YRBS_questionnaire_content_1991-2019.pdf

US Department of Health and Human Services. (2000). *Healthy people 2010.* Office of Disease Prevention and Health Promotion, US Department of Health and Human Services.

van Stralen, M. M., te Velde, S. J., Singh, A. S., De Bourdeaudhuij, I., Martens, M. K., van der Sluis, M., . . . Brug, J. (2011). European energy balance research to prevent excessive weight gain among youth (ENERGY) project: Design and methodology of the ENERGY cross-sectional survey. *BMC Public Health, 11*, 65. doi:10.1186/1471-2458-11-65

World Health Organization. (2008). *2008–2013 Action plan for the global strategy for the prevention and control of noncommunicable diseases.* Geneva, Switzerland. Retrieved from http://apps.who.int/iris/bitstream/handle/10665/44009/9789241597418_eng.pdf;jsessionid=C6F16B3BCF4397A9FA986D5AB37EA6EA?sequence=1

World Health Organization. (2009). *Mortality and burden of disease attributable to selected major risks.* Geneva, Switzerland: WHO. Retrieved from https://www.who.int/healthinfo/global_burden_disease/GlobalHealthRisks_report_full.pdf

World Health Organization. (2010). *Global recommendation on physical activity for health.* Retrieved January 11, 2018, from http://www.who.int/dietphysicalactivity/factsheet_recommendations/en/

World Health Organization. (2013). *Global action plan for the prevention and control of noncommunicable diseases: 2013–2020.* Geneva, Switzerland. Retrieved from http://apps.who.int/iris/bitstream/handle/10665/94384/9789241506236_eng.pdf?sequence=1

World Health Organization. (2014). *Global status report on noncommunicable diseases 2014.* Geneva, Switzerland. Retrieved from http://apps.who.int/iris/bitstream/handle/10665/148114/9789241564854_eng.pdf;jsessionid=F3ECBFD4BB4BA72D42823D9D6B270E06?sequence=1

World Health Organization. (2016). *Report of the commission on ending childhood obesity.* Genava, Switzerland. Retrieved from http://apps.who.int/iris/bitstream/handle/10665/204176/9789241510066_eng.pdf?sequence=1

World Health Organization. (2017). *WHO STEPS surveillance manual – The WHO STEPwise approach to noncommunicable disease risk factor surveillance.* Geneva, Switzerland. Retrieved from https://www.who.int/ncds/surveillance/steps/STEPS_Manual.pdf?ua=1

World Health Organization. (2018a). *Global action plan on physical activity 2018–2030.* Geneva, Switzerland. Retrieved from http://apps.who.int/iris/bitstream/handle/10665/272722/9789241514187-eng.pdf?ua=1

World Health Organization. (2018b). *Global health observatory (GHO) data.* Retrieved January 30, 2019, from https://www.who.int/gho/en/

World Health Organization. (2018c). *Global school-based student health survey (GSHS).* Retrieved January 25, 2019, from https://www.who.int/ncds/surveillance/gshs/en/

World Health Organization. (2018d). *Global school-based student health survey (GSHS) – Datasets.* Retrieved January 25, 2019, from https://www.who.int/ncds/surveillance/gshs/datasets/en/

World Health Organization. (2018e). *Noncommunicable diseases progress monitor 2017.* Geneva, Switzerland: World Health Organization. Retrieved from https://www.who.int/nmh/publications/ncd-progress-monitor-2017/en/

World Health Organization. (2018f). *Physical activity factsheets for the 28 European union member states of the WHO European region.* Copenhagen, Denmark. Retrieved from http://www.euro.who.int/pubrequest

World Health Organization. (2019). *Guidelines on physical activity, sedentary behaviour and sleep for children under 5 years of age.* Geneva, Switzerland: WHO.

World Health Organization Regional Office for Europe. (2015). *Factsheets on health-enhancing physical activity in the 28 European Union member states of the WHO European region.* Retrieved from http://www.euro.who.int/pubrequest

3

GLOBAL SURVEILLANCE OF CARDIORESPIRATORY AND MUSCULOSKELETAL FITNESS

Justin J. Lang, Jordan J. Smith, and Grant R. Tomkinson

Population health surveillance is described as the "systematic, ongoing collection, management, analysis, and interpretation of data followed by the dissemination of these data to public health programs to stimulate [population] health action" (Thacker, Qualters, Lee, & Centers for Disease Control and Prevention, 2012, p. 3). Effective population health surveillance is vital not only to help understand the general health of a population, but also to help inform healthy public policy. For instance, surveillance data can serve two purposes with regard to healthy public policy: (1) it can help guide policy efforts by identifying subpopulations that are outliers (i.e., healthy or unhealthy) through comparing surveillance data across geographic regions, and (2) it can be used to evaluate the effectiveness and monitor the progress of implemented policy efforts through an analysis of temporal trends (Hallal et al., 2012). Among children and adolescents (collectively referred to hereafter as youth), identifying robust surveillance indicators that are strongly related to health is difficult, as youth are generally healthy and without chronic diseases. To date, the primary population health surveillance indicators for youth have been self-reported physical activity levels and body mass index (BMI). The addition of objective measures of physical fitness could help complement current efforts by building a better understanding of population health among youth.

More recently, there has been a growth of interest in using field-based physical fitness measures for population health surveillance (Lang, 2018a), with a particular focus on cardiorespiratory fitness (CRF) and musculoskeletal fitness (MF), as these measures reflect the capacity of underlying systems that relate to the body's ability to perform physical activity. These types of measures could be effective for surveillance purposes because they are meaningfully associated with health (i.e., cardiovascular and/or metabolic health) in youth (Lang et al., 2018b; Ortega, Ruiz, Castillo, & Sjöström, 2008; Smith et al., 2014). In some cases there is evidence to suggest that fitness, particularly CRF, in youth can help predict future health outcomes in adulthood (Mintjens et al., 2018; Ruiz et al., 2009a). This is particularly important for population health planning and adapting to future needs, and therefore bolsters the rationale for surveillance efforts that enable early detection of low fitness and intergenerational trends. There is also evidence to suggest these measures are scalable, especially in the school environment. Domone, Mann, Sandercock, Wade, and Beedie (2016) described the scalability of field-based fitness measures as the ability for a measure to attain six criteria (summarized in Table 3.1): (1) delivery, (2) evidence of operating at scale, (3) effectiveness, (4) cost, (5) resource requirements, and (6) practical implications.

The objective of this chapter is to review the CRF and MF literature that pertains to population health surveillance, with a focus on identifying scalable measures that are favorably associated

Table 3.1 Six criteria for identifying scalable field-based fitness measures

	Criteria	Description
1	Delivery	Feasible testing context, test duration, suitability for longitudinal research, and non-technical delivery staff
2	Evidence of operating at scale	Appropriate for population testing, and are schools likely to accept the test
3	Effectiveness	Validity, reliability, level of participation, and a high completion rate
4	Cost	Is the test cost-effective
5	Resource requirements	Minimal equipment, space, skills, competence, and workforce requirements
6	Practical implication issues	Can the test be implemented and scored with ease

Note: Adapted from Domone et al., (2016).

with health among youth. We will also focus on describing current fitness surveillance efforts worldwide, including trends and cross-country comparisons in specific fitness test measures. Last, we will describe several key emerging issues and areas of future research that could help advance this field of study.

Overview of the Literature

Cardiorespiratory Fitness

CRF is the ability of the body to deliver oxygen to the muscles to support energy production during physical activity (Armstrong, Tomkinson, & Ekelund, 2011; Institute of Medicine, 2012). Although lab-based measures of CRF with indirect calorimetry (measured peak oxygen uptake [$\dot{V}O_{2peak}$]) are considered the gold standard, these types of tests are not feasible for population health surveillance. As a result, field-based measures of CRF are typically used in surveillance as an indication of exercise capacity, while providing an estimate of $\dot{V}O_{2peak}$ values. Among youth, CRF is meaningfully associated with a variety of cardiovascular risk factors: adiposity (e.g., waist circumference, sum of five skinfolds, BMI), systolic and diastolic blood pressure, resting heart rate, total cholesterol, high-density lipoprotein cholesterol, C-reactive protein, and blood glucose levels (Lang, Larouche, & Tremblay, 2019a). There is evidence to suggest that high CRF levels are associated with better academic achievement and cognition among youth (Marques, Santos, Hillman, & Sardinha, 2018). Furthermore, there is strong evidence to support CRF levels in youth being inversely associated with metabolic health and cardiovascular profile in adulthood (Mintjens et al., 2018; Ruiz et al., 2009). In light of this evidence, there is support for CRF as a health indicator for surveillance among youth (Lang et al., 2018c). Among adults, CRF is a strong and independent predictor of cardiovascular diseases, certain cancers, and all-cause mortality (Harber et al., 2017; Ross et al., 2016). More importantly, CRF among adults has been shown to be a stronger predictor of mortality than other well-established risk factors (i.e., smoking, hypertension, high cholesterol) (Ross et al., 2016). It has also been proposed as an important clinical vital sign because of the improved cardiovascular disease mortality risk classification (e.g., net reclassification improvement), when added to traditional risk scores (e.g., Framingham and European risk scores) (Ross et al., 2016). Field-based measures of CRF exist, many of which are scalable and are currently being used in national and international surveillance. Further details on field-based fitness assessments for CRF are provided in Chapter 18. Below, we highlight the most well-established measures of CRF along with a description of their scalability for surveillance purposes.

20-m Shuttle Run Test

The 20-m shuttle run test (20mSRT) (also known as the Progressive Aerobic Cardiovascular Endurance Run [PACER], beep test, bleep test), first described in the 1980s by Professor Luc Léger (Léger, Lambert, Goulet, Rowan, & Dinelle 1984; Léger, Mercier, Gadoury, & Lambert, 1988), is now the most widely used field-based assessment of youth CRF. The 20mSRT has previously been described as potentially the most scalable field-based measure of CRF in youth (#1 Delivery) (Domone et al., 2016). The 20mSRT has been used in large population studies (Tomkinson et al., 2017) (#2 Operating at scale). It has moderate criterion validity and high reliability (Artero et al., 2011a; Mayorga-Vega, Aguilar-Soto, & Viciana, 2015; Ruiz, Silva et al., 2009b), only a small number of youth are unable to complete the first stage of the test (España-Romero, Artero et al., 2010a), and youth appear to enjoy the 20mSRT over other field-based CRF assessments (Zhu, 2013) (#3 Effectiveness). There is no literature describing the cost-effectiveness of the 20mSRT, but it is likely high due to the low cost of equipment needed to conduct the test (#4 Cost) and the lack of training needed for test administrators (e.g., school teachers) (#5 Resource requirements). With the given evidence it appears as though the 20mSRT can be implemented and scored with relative ease (#6 Practical implications).

In recent years there has been considerable effort to pool 20mSRT data to help describe and inform the surveillance of population health among youth. In 2017, Tomkinson et al. provided a systematic analysis of over 1.1 million 20mSRT scores for youth aged 9–17 years from 50 countries (Tomkinson et al., 2017). This dataset helped describe global patterns of 20mSRT performance where youth from Northern Europe and sub-Saharan Africa were identified as being the best performers and those from South America were generally the worst performers (Lang et al., 2018d) (Figure 3.1). Temporal trends indicated a substantial decline in 20mSRT performance since 1981 in high-income countries, with diminishing and stabilizing changes occurring since 2000 (Tomkinson, Lang, & Tremblay, 2019). There are also well-established international normative- and criterion-referenced standards to help with interpreting 20mSRT performance results (Tomkinson et al., 2017; Ruiz et al., 2016; Lang et al., 2019b), an approach that is described in detail in Chapter 18. These types of studies further support the 20mSRT as a scalable measure for population health surveillance.

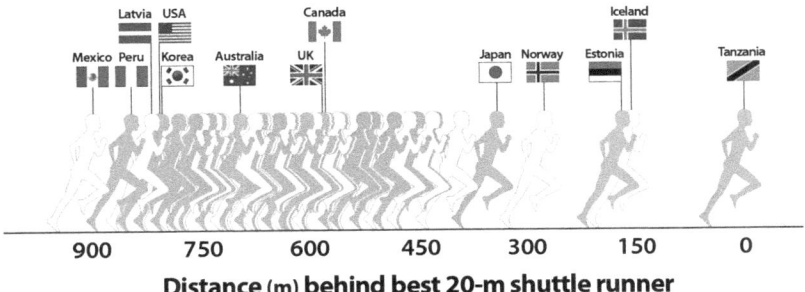

Figure 3.1 International 20mSRT performance among 12-year-old girls from 50 countries. Data available from Lang et al. (2018d)

Distance and Timed Run Tests

Various distance/timed running tests have long been used in large national surveys of youth across the globe (Catley & Tomkinson, 2013; Tomkinson et al., 2012) (#2 Operating at scale). They have low to moderate criterion validity, with the 1.5-mile and the 12-minute walk/run tests having higher validity than other running tests (albeit similar validity to the 20mSRT) (Mayorga-Vega, Bocanegra-Parrilla, Ornelas, & Viciana, 2016), and high reliability (Artero et al., 2011a; Safrit, 1990). Youth with low CRF and/or high BMI appear to better engage in the 1-mile run than other field-based CRF tests (Zhu, 2013) (#3 Effectiveness). There is no literature describing the cost-effectiveness of distance/timed running tests, but it is likely high due to the low cost of equipment needed to conduct the test (#4 Cost; #5 Resource requirements). While distance/timed running tests can be implemented and scored with relative ease, some implementation issues exist. For example, distance runs are preferred over timed runs, because the time taken to complete a known distance can be measured more easily than the distance covered in a fixed time period (Cooper & Storer, 2001); psychosocial factors such as motivation and pacing ability can significantly affect test results (e.g., 1-mile run times can improve by 7%–8% over three trials in the space of 2 weeks [Watkins & Moore, 1983, 1996]) highlighting the need for test familiarization; and it is possible that differences in the test name (e.g., run vs. run/walk) could affect results (#6 Practical implications).

Distance/timed running tests have long been used to describe and inform the surveillance of population health across the lifespan, especially among youth. Unfortunately, there is no universally accepted distance/running test, with different tests used between and within countries over time, making it difficult to pool test results internationally (Tomkinson & Olds, 2007b, 2008). Nonetheless, age- and sex-specific norm-referenced and health-related criterion-referenced standards are available for various distance/timed running tests (e.g., the 1-mile run [Catley & Tomkinson, 2013; The Cooper Institute, 2017]). Cross-country comparisons in distance running test performance have been made within Asia at least, with East Asian youth (Japan, Korea, Hong Kong, and Taiwan) typically outperforming their age- and sex-matched southeast Asian peers (Philippines, Thailand, and Vietnam) (Macfarlane & Tomkinson, 2007). Temporal trends in the distance/timed run performance of >25 million youth from 27 countries (representing 5 continents) have been described and indicate a substantial decline (~4%–5% per decade) since the mid-1970s (Tomkinson et al., 2012; Tomkinson & Olds, 2007). As with the 20mSRT, these data support the potential use of distance/timed running tests as scalable measures for population health surveillance.

Measuring CRF in Preschool Children

The assessment of CRF in preschool children aged 3–5 years is a fairly new and developing area of research. To date, the 20mSRT, the ½-mile run/walk, and the 3-minute run seem to be the dominant field-based measures of CRF in preschool children (Ortega et al., 2015). Of these, the 20mSRT is likely the most practical because it removes the cognitive aspect of pacing, which is a difficult task for some preschool children, and requires considerably less space (Ortega et al., 2015). An adapted version of the 20mSRT that begins at a running speed of 6.5 km/h and increases by 0.5 km/h at every consecutive minute was developed for the PREFIT (Assessing FITness in PREschool children) test battery (Cadenas-Sanchez et al., 2014). It is also recommended that two testers concurrently run with a small group of children during the test to assist with pacing. This is considered a feasible alternative to the original 20mSRT version, which starts at a running speed (8.5 km/h) and may be too quick for preschool-age children to induce a maximum aerobic effort (Cadenas-Sanchez et al., 2016). There is a need for future research to evaluate the validity of the PREFIT 20mSRT, and to further explore the associations between performance and health markers in preschool-age children.

Summary of CRF Surveillance

Evidence supporting the national and international surveillance of CRF as an indicator of population health among youth continues to grow (Lang et al., 2018c). The surveillance of CRF may complement current efforts to understand youth health across jurisdictions and over time to help guide public health policy efforts. Although distance/timed run tests have been used for generations, recent evidence suggests that the 20mSRT is meaningfully associated with a variety of health markers in youth (Lang et al., 2018b), whereas this may not be the case for distance/timed runs tests (Stodden, Sacko, & Nesbitt, 2017). For these reasons, researchers and decision-makers should try to implement CRF surveillance using the 20mSRT over distance/timed run tests, if possible. When reporting 20mSRT results, researchers should follow the Tomkinson recommendations by reporting, at the very least, running speed (km/h) at the last completed stage (Tomkinson et al., 2017). There is also a need to collect more youth CRF data in low-income countries, as this remains a large data gap (Tomkinson, 2019).

There are some important considerations when implementing CRF surveillance efforts. CRF testing using the suggested protocols is generally meant for able-bodied, ambulatory youth, and may not be suitable for those with physical impairment. The 20mSRT and other distance/timed run tests are meant to require a near-maximal effort that may pose an increased risk to sedentary youth or those at risk of cardiovascular and/or musculoskeletal complications. Efforts should be made to appropriately screen individuals before conducting near-maximal CRF testing and any adverse events (or lack thereof) reported (Longmuir, Colley, Wherley, & Tremblay, 2014). While data on adverse events in children performing maximal exercise are rare, no adverse events have been recorded in the two largest UK-based fitness studies (Liverpool SportsLinx and East of England Healthy Hearts Study) in which 20mSRT assessments were made on ~80,000 youth aged 9–16 years (Barker, Williams, Tolfrey, Fawkner, & Sandercock, 2013).

Musculoskeletal Fitness

MF is a multidimensional construct that is made up of three components: *muscular strength*, the ability of a muscle or group of muscles to generate force; *endurance*, the ability of a muscle or a group of muscles to produce force repeatedly; and *power*, the ability of a muscle or a group of muscles to produce force quickly (Caspersen, Powell, & Christenson, 1985). See Chapter 18 for a detailed description of MF field-based assessments. Although tests of MF have been described in the literature for some time, misuse of terms remains commonplace (e.g., referring to 'strength' when describing a test of muscular endurance). The measurement of MF is difficult because there is no single measure that provides an indication of total MF levels. Moreover, MF is site-specific, meaning that a test result obtained at one part of the body (e.g., handgrip strength) does not necessarily reflect MF at another part of the body (e.g., leg strength). As a result, in health surveillance, we often rely on a very small subset of the larger MF picture. For instance, handgrip strength and standing broad jump (SBJ) are widely used measures of MF that provide an indication of upper body isometric strength and lower-body power (or "explosive" strength), respectively. Despite these nuances, MF is considered an important aspect of health-related fitness (Ortega et al., 2008). In 2014, Smith et al. systematically reviewed the literature and found significant negative associations between MF (mainly operationalized as the SBJ) and adiposity (pooled effect size [95% confidence interval]: $r = -0.29$ [−0.44, −0.12]). There was consistent evidence for positive associations between handgrip strength and adiposity, although the direction of association changed if MF was expressed in relative terms (i.e., relative to body size) (Smith et al., 2014). Furthermore, the systematic review highlighted strong evidence supporting positive associations between MF and bone health and self-esteem/self-perceptions, and negative associations between MF and cardiovascular disease and metabolic risk factors (i.e., insulin resistance [Artero et al., 2011b; Benson, Torode, & Singh, 2006] and inflammatory biomarkers [Artero et al., 2014; Steene-Johannessen, Kolle, Andersen, & Anderssen, 2013]). The majority of these associations are low to moderate, and for some health outcomes at least there is evidence that associations may be independent of CRF levels (Artero et al., 2011b). From a health promotion standpoint, analyses that control for CRF are important given CRF and MF tend to be positively correlated in youth (Laurson, Saint-Maurice, Welk, & Eisenmann, 2017). Of note, MF (e.g., handgrip strength) may also provide a stronger indication of cardiometabolic risk among girls, in comparison with boys (Rioux et al., 2017).

In addition to cross-sectional associations, MF levels in childhood and adolescence may provide an indication of population health in adulthood. For instance, in a cohort of more than 1 million Swedish male youth (aged 16–19 years), high levels of muscular strength were associated with a 20%–35% lower risk of all-cause mortality in adulthood over a period of 24 years, independent of BMI and blood pressure (Ortega, Silventoinen, Tynelius, & Rasmussen, 2012). Using the same cohort, it was also identified that high MF in adolescence was associated with a lower risk of disability in adulthood (Henriksson, Henriksson, Tynelius, & Ortega, 2019). Furthermore, in a 2009 systematic review it was identified that changes in MF during childhood and adolescence were negatively associated with changes in overall adiposity in adulthood (Ruiz et al., 2009a). There was inconclusive evidence for associations between changes in MF and changes in cardiovascular disease risk factors in adulthood (Ruiz et al., 2009a). However, more recent evidence has shown strength in late adolescence is significantly and independently (of CRF and adiposity) associated with risk of heart failure in later life (Crump, Sundquist, Winkleby, & Sundquist, 2017). In addition, changes in SBJ, but not handgrip strength, have shown significant longitudinal relationships with clustered metabolic risk over short time periods (i.e., 2 years) (Fraser et al., 2018; García-Hermoso, Ramírez-Campillo, & Izquierdo, 2019; Zaqout et al., 2016). Below, we describe specific measures of MF, including temporal trends in specific measures that are further described in Table 3.2.

Handgrip Strength

Handgrip strength is a test of maximal isometric upper body strength. It takes approximately 2 minutes to assess a person's handgrip strength, and it can be measured by an administrator with little testing experience (#1 Delivery). The test has been conducted in over 200,000 youth in Europe between 1988 and 2016 (Tomkinson et al., 2018), demonstrating its acceptability for population-based testing. It is also recommended by the National Academy of Medicine (formally the Institute of Medicine) as an acceptable measure for school-based testing (Institute of Medicine, 2012) (#2 Operating at scale). Handgrip strength has strong to very strong test-retest reliability in youth (Artero et al., 2011a), and strong construct validity when compared with 1-repetition maximum chest press (Milliken, Faigenbaum, Loud, & Westcott, 2008). Differences in hand size, optimal grip size adjustment, elbow angle, and device calibration are important for valid testing (España-Romero et al., 2008, España-Romero et al., 2010b; Ruiz et al., 2006). To our knowledge, completion rates for the handgrip strength test have never been reported, but they are likely near perfect as the test is short and little motivation on the part of the participant is required (#3 Effectiveness). There are no studies available that have assessed the cost-effectiveness of the handgrip strength test (#4 Cost). The cost of equipment is likely the largest barrier to implementing health surveillance with this measure as the cost for a handgrip dynamometer ranges from US$200 to US$400 (#5 Resource requirements). The results from the test are easily interpretable and scored (#6 Practical implications).

Table 3.2 International secular trends in the MF test performance of children and adolescents

Country	Citation(s)	HG	SU/CU	FAH/BAH	SBJ
Australia	Hardy et al. (2018), Fraser et al. (2019)				↓ (1985–2015)
Belgium	Matton et al. (2007)			↓ (1969–2005)	≈ (1969–2005)
Canada	Tremblay et al., (2010)	↓ (1981–2009)			
China	Mcfarlane and Tomkinson (2007)				↓ (1995–2000)
Czechia	Kopecký and Přidalová (2008)				↓ (1966–2002)
England	Sandercock and Cohen (2019)	↓ (1998–2014)	↓ (1998–2014)	↓ (1998–2014)	↓ (1998–2014)
Estonia	Jürimäe et al. (2007)		≈ (1992–2002)	↓ (1992–2002)	↓ (1992–2002)
Finland	Huatori et al., (2010)				≈ (1976–2001)
France	Jürimäe et al. (2007)				↓ (1985–1998)
Greece	Smpokos, Linardakis, Papadaki, Lionis, and Kafatos (2012)		↑ (1992–2007)		↑ (1992–2007)
Iceland	Jürimäe et al. (2007)				↓ (1986–1999)
Italy	Jürimäe et al. (2007)				↑ (1993–1998)
Japan	Mcfarlane and Tomkinson (2007)				↓ (1929–1969)
Korea	Mcfarlane and Tomkinson (2007)				↓ (1988–1995)
Lithuania	Venckunas et al. (2016)	? (1992–2012)	? (1992–2012)	↓ (1992–2012)	↓ (1992–2012)
Mexico	Malina et al. (2010)	? (1968–2000)			
Mozambique	Dos Santos et al. (2015)	? (1992–2012)			
Netherlands	Runhaar et al. (2010)			↓ (1980–2006)	
New Zealand	Albon, Hamlin, and Ross (2010)		↑ (1991–2003)		
Poland	Ignasiak et al. (2016), Przeweda and Dobosz (2003)	↑ (2001–2011)	↓ (2001–2011)		↓ (2001–2011)
Portugal	Costa et al. (2017)	↓ (2001–2007)	↑ (1993–2013)		≈ (1993–2013)
Spain	Jürimäe et al. (2007), Moliner-Urdiales et al. (2010)			≈ (2001–2007)	↓ (1985–2007)
Sweden	Ekblom, Oddsson, and Ekblom (2004)		↓ (1987–2001)	↓ (1987–2001)	
Thailand	Mcfarlane and Tomkinson (2007)				↓ (1990–2003)
Turkey	Haslofça et al. (2017)	↓ (1983–2013)			↓ (1983–2013)
United States	Silverman (2015)	≈ (1966–2009)			

Note: HG, handgrip strength; SU/CU, sit-ups/curls-ups; FAH/BAH, flexed arm hang/bent arm hang; SBJ, standing broad jump. ↑ = *increasing performance*; ↓ = *decreasing performance*; ≈ = *no change in performance*; ? = *mixed findings (e.g., between age and sex subgroups)*.

A comprehensive review of global changes in young peoples' handgrip strength was recently published in Sports Medicine (Dooley et al, 2020). The available data suggest mixed findings for secular trends in the handgrip strength of youth around the world. A summary of global trends in common field-based measures of muscular fitness can be seen in Table 3.2. With regard to handgrip strength, there appears to have been declines among 7–19-year-olds from Canada (Tremblay et al., 2010), 10-year-olds from England (Sandercock & Cohen, 2019), 12–17-year-old from Spain (Moliner-Urdiales et al., 2010), and 11–12-year-olds from Turkey (Haslofça, Kutlay, & Haslofça, 2017). Conversely, there have been mixed findings between boys and girls from Mexico (Malina, Reyes, Tan, & Little, 2010) and Mozambique (Dos Santos et al., 2015), and no change in the United States (Silverman, 2015).

Cross-country comparisons are largely absent in the literature (Jürimäe, Volbekiene, Jürimäe, & Tomkinson, 2007; Tomkinson, Olds, & Borms, 2007c), making it challenging to determine which nations' youth have the best and worst handgrip strength. When collapsing children, adolescents, and adults together, there is evidence that countries from developed regions perform substantially better than those from developing regions (Dodds et al., 2016). The highest quality international comparison, however, comes from Europe with Tomkinson et al. (2007c), comparing data from >1.1 million youth aged 7–18 years from 23 countries. According to their trends analysis of the handgrip strength of 173,359 youth from 18 European countries, youth from Slovakia, the Netherlands, and Hungary were top-ranked, while youth from France, Italy, and Albania were bottom-ranked (Tomkinson et al., 2007c). The 2013 Asia-fit study, a cross-cultural comparison of 12,590 youth aged 12–15 years from eight Southeast and East Asian metropolitan cities (Hong Kong, Shanghai, Tokyo, Seoul, Kuala Lumpur, Taipei, Singapore, and Bangkok), showed that youth from Tokyo, Shanghai, and Bangkok had the best handgrip strength (Hui et al., 2015).

Standing Broad Jump

The SBJ is a common field-based fitness test used to assess lower-body muscular power (Bianco et al., 2015). Administering the SBJ test should take approximately 5 minutes per participant, including rest time and practice jumps. The test has been used widely in longitudinal research. For example, the SBJ has been used for decades to assess temporal trends (Jürimäe et al., 2007; Tomkinson, 2007a). The test is also easily administered by individuals who do not have a background in fitness testing (#1 Delivery). Between 1981 and 2016 a total of 464,900 European SBJ test scores have been published across 29 countries (Tomkinson et al., 2018). In addition, this test is recommended for school-based testing (Institute of Medicine, 2012) (#2 Operating at Scale). The construct validity of the SBJ ranges from $r = 0.35$ (1 RM chest press) (Holm, Fredriksen, Fosdahl, & Vøllestad, 2008) to $R^2 = 0.83–0.86$ for lower-body muscular strength (Castro-Piñero et al., 2010). SBJ also correlates strongly ($r = 0.70–0.91$) with other lower- and upper-body field-based explosive strength tests (e.g., vertical jump, countermovement vertical jump, explosive basketball throw) in 6–17-year-olds, controlling for age, sex, body mass, and/or BMI (Castro-Piñero et al., 2010; Holm et al., 2008; Larson, 1974; Reid, & Fielding, 2012;). The test-retest reliability is strong to near perfect in youth, with reliability coefficients improving with age (Docherty, 1996). To the authors' knowledge, the completion rate for the SBJ has not been reported, but it is likely to be nearly perfect (#3 Effectiveness). The cost-effectiveness of the SBJ has also not yet been reported (#4 Cost). However, due to low cost equipment, minimal space, and limited training and personnel requirements (#5 Resource Requirements), this test is often described as being cost-effective (Hardy, Merom, Thomas, & Peralta, 2018). Last, the SBJ can be implemented and scored with ease (#6 Practical Implications).

Given the simplicity of test administration and its subsequent widespread use around the world, global trend data for the SBJ is more complete than it is for handgrip strength. Indeed, Tomkinson's (2007a) meta-analysis of 'anaerobic' performance from 1958 to 2003 included jumping test results for 20.9 million youth, of which 18.5 million were on the SBJ test specifically.

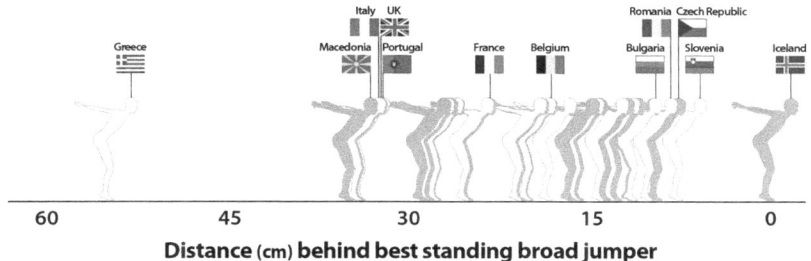

Distance (cm) behind best standing broad jumper

Figure 3.2 International SBJ performance among 12-year-old boys from 22 European countries. Data available from Tomkinson et al. (2007c)

Interestingly, Tomkinson (2007a) concluded global jumping performance had remained relatively stable overall during this period (i.e., mean change = 0.03% p.a.), albeit with substantial variability across countries (range = −0.8% p.a. to 1.2% p.a.). However, it should be noted these trends were based on four separate single jump tests, including but not limited to the SBJ, and the analysis also indicated a downward trajectory in more recent decades with consistent declines observed from approximately 1985 onward (Tomkinson, 2007a). These more recent changes correspond with the majority of findings in the contemporary literature. For example, recent evidence from Australia shows jump distance declined by 4.6–11 cm in 9–15-year-olds (Hardy et al., 2018) and by 16.4 cm (~11%) in 11–12-year-olds (Fraser et al., 2019) between 1985 and 2015. While improvements have been reported, for example, among Italian youth (Jürimäe et al., 2007), declines in SBJ performance have typically been reported in recent decades, including in European youth from Belgium (Lefèvre, Bouckaert, & Duquet, 1998), girls (but not boys) from the Czech Republic (Kopecký, 2006; Kopecký, & Přidalová, 2008), England (Sandercock & Cohen, 2019a), Estonia (Jürimäe et al., 2007), France (Jürimäe et al., 2007), Iceland (Jürimäe et al., 2007), Lithuania (Venckunas, Emeljanovas, Mieziene, & Volbekiene, 2017), Spain (Jürimäe et al., 2007; Moliner-Urdiales et al., 2010), Poland (Ignasiak, Sławińska, & Malina, 2016), and Turkey (Haslofça et al., 2017), as well as among Asian youth from South Korea, China, Thailand, and Japan (Mcfarlane & Tomkinson, 2007). Consequently, there appears to be good support for the view that SBJ performance around the world is generally on the decline. Similar to handgrip strength, high-quality international comparisons in jumping performance are limited. Using SBJ data on 209,674 European youth from 23 countries, Tomkinson et al. (2007c) identified Iceland, Slovenia, and the Czech Republic as the best performing, and Greece, Macedonia, and Italy as the worst performing (see Figure 3.2).

Measures of Local Muscular Endurance

There are many measures of local muscular endurance that are currently used in youth (Bianco et al., 2015). Common tests include partial curl-ups and push-ups to exhaustion or repetitions performed in a set time limit (e.g., 60 seconds), flexed/bent arm hang, isometric knee extension at submaximal intensity, plank test, and maximal pull-ups (Institute of Medicine, 2012; Tomkinson et al., 2018). Chapter 18 provides a detailed description of test protocols for local muscular endurance. Many of these measures are scalable and have been widely used for population-based surveillance (e.g., data have been published on 481,032 and 189,673 youth aged 9–17 years from 23 European countries tested on the sit-ups [n/30 s] and bent arm hang tests, respectively [Tomkinson et al., 2018]). However, while there is some evidence favorably linking abdominal endurance with low-back and neck pain (Mikkelsson et al., 2006; Payne, Gledhill, Katzmarzyk, & Jamnik, 2000), compared to CRF and muscular strength/power measures, there is limited evidence linking muscular endurance measures to health in youth (García-Hermoso et al., 2019). It has previously been shown that popular tests of muscular endurance may be better predictors of body composition than a criterion measure of this MF component (Woods, Pate, & Burgess, 1992). However, low muscular endurance (sit-ups performance) was significantly associated with mortality in Canadian adults (Katzmarzyk, & Craig, 2002) and Japanese men (Fujita et al., 1995) independent of CRF, adiposity, and other covariates. For this reason, there is a need for more research to help identify muscular endurance measures that are strongly linked to health, which would help in selecting a measure for future population health surveillance. Nonetheless, as shown in Table 3.2, there have been mixed findings for secular changes in muscular endurance, with declines reported consistently for the flexed/bent arm hang test (at least within Europe), but both improvements (e.g., in Greece, New Zealand, Portugal) and declines (e.g., in England and Poland) reported for the curl-up/sit-up test.

Measuring MF in Preschool Children

The measurement of MF in preschoolers is a new and developing area of research. A recent systematic review by Ortega et al. (2015) found literature to support the handgrip strength test and the SBJ in preschool children. For handgrip strength, the Lode dynamometer was identified as being more reliable than the Martin vigorimeter (Zuidam, Selles, Stam, & Hovius, 2008). Other authors recommend using the non-digital version of the TKK (model 5001) for its high reliability and validity in older youth (España-Romero et al., 2010b) and its ability to detect values below 5 kg, which is an attainable result in preschoolers. It is important for the hand dynamometer to have an adjustable grip span which seems to optimize reliability when set at 4 cm in youth aged 3–5 years (Sanchez-Delgado et al., 2015). Other than these recommendations, the handgrip strength test should be conducted in preschool children using the same procedures as older youth.

To improve feasibility with the SBJ it is recommended to use additional guidance to help youth understand when to jump. Cadenas-Sanchez et al. (2016) drew footprints at the take-off line to help youth understand when to start their jump. This tactic seemed to improve reliability. Other than this minor modification, the SBJ procedures for preschool children should be conducted following the same procedures described in older youth. Future research should further investigate the validity of MF tests and their associations with health markers in preschool children. There is also a need for more research to identify suitable measures of muscular endurance in young children.

Summary of MF Surveillance

MF during childhood and adolescence is increasingly being viewed as an important marker of current and future health (Ortega et al., 2008; Smith et al., 2014), and should therefore be included in national and international fitness surveillance efforts alongside CRF. The handgrip strength and SBJ tests in particular have demonstrated satisfactory validity and reliability; are relatively fast and simple to administer; require limited resources, personnel, and training; and produce results that are easily interpretable. As such, these tests should form the backbone for population MF surveillance and monitoring in the future. Beyond this, there is a need to identify a suitable test of local muscular endurance that could also be included to give a more complete picture of youth MF. However, the field has yet to determine conclusively that existing field-based measures of local muscular endurance are predictive of health outcomes, independently of confounding factors such as body composition. In addition, future tests would need to demonstrate acceptable feasibility, validity, and reliability, which has yet to be shown in current field-based muscular endurance tests. Consideration should also be given to how MF data are expressed (i.e., absolute value vs. relative to body mass or fat-free mass), as such choices can have substantial impact on the associations between MF and some health outcomes (Plowman, & Meredith, 2014; Smith et al., 2014), and could make the interpretation of population trends in MF challenging. Recommendations for applying scaling methods to MF tests exist in the literature (Jaric, Mirkov, & Markovic, 2005), but are often ignored or used inconsistently by researchers. Finally, there is a clear need to identify health-related criterion-referenced standards for MF tests in youth, as these standards enable us to make meaning of MF test results that can subsequently be used to guide healthy public policy efforts. Such studies are starting to appear in the literature (Castro-Piñero et al., 2019; Saint-Maurice et al., 2018) and should be pursued further.

Examples of Current Fitness Surveillance Efforts

National Health Surveys

National health surveys provide a structured and systematic approach for collecting data on a relatively small sample of participants, using stratified, multistage random sampling, to obtain nationally representative estimates of health using survey weights. Some national health surveys, such as the Canadian Health Measures Survey (CHMS) and the National Health and Nutrition Examination Survey (NHANES) in the United States, include measures of physical fitness. For instance, the CHMS includes CRF using the modified Canadian Aerobic Fitness Test (mCAFT), partial curl-ups (e.g., muscular endurance), and sit-and-reach (e.g., flexibility) in select cycles, and the handgrip strength test in all cycles (2007–2023). Physical fitness measures are also available for certain cycles of the NHANES, including a submaximal/maximal treadmill test for CRF and handgrip strength for MF. In 2012, a National Youth Fitness Survey was conducted jointly with the NHANES to obtain a comprehensive surveillance picture of youth fitness in the United States. This Youth Survey included the core plank test (i.e., muscle endurance), a test of gross motor skill, knee extension strength, handgrip strength, a modified pull-up test (i.e., muscle endurance), and CRF measured using a maximal or submaximal treadmill test (Borrud et al., 2014). Although these types of surveys are costly, they do provide a good national estimate of physical fitness and the ability to develop national normative-referenced standards (Laurson et al., 2017). They are also important for describing the associations between difference physical fitness measures and health outcomes/markers across different age by sex groups, similar to recent work with the CHMS (Lang et al., 2019a).

The school system remains one of the most promising locations to implement national fitness surveillance for youth (Pate, 1989), with several countries conducting national fitness surveillance through schools, including Korea (Tomkinson, Olds, Kang, & Kim, 2007d) and Slovenia (Strel, 2013). For example, Slovenia collects annual national fitness data on school-aged youth through a surveillance initiative called SLOfit (formerly known as the Sport Educational Chart program). SLOfit has been compulsory for all Slovenian primary and secondary school-aged youth since 1987, resulting in >200,000 annual measurements and >7 million in the past 30 years, and a database inclusive of more than half of the Slovenian population (University of Ljubljana, 2019). Individualized feedback is provided, including a comparison of each child's fitness against centile bands to identify expected, better than expected, or worse than expected developmental changes. In response to an analysis of the SLOfit database indicating a decline in youth fitness between 1990 and 2010, Slovenia implemented a national health-promoting physical activity intervention called Healthy Lifestyle in the 2010/2011 school year, offering youth two additional extracurricular hours of physical activity per week. As a result, the fitness and physical activity levels of Slovenian youth have improved (Strel, 2013). Furthermore, in a recent report comparing physical activity levels across 49 countries (representing six continents), Slovenian youth were top-ranked in overall national physical activity levels (Aubert et al., 2018). Slovenia provides an excellent example of how fitness surveillance can be used to monitor and improve population health. Table 3.3 provides more details on the fitness measures included for a select number of national physical fitness surveillance efforts.

Table 3.3 International physical fitness surveillance efforts

Surveillance effort description	Treadmill test	Step test	Distance/timed run test	20-m shuttle run test	Grip strength	Back strength	Lower-body strength	Plank test	Curl-ups	Pull-ups	Push-ups	Bent arm hang	Standing broad jump	Vertical jump
	CRF measures				MF measures									
					Muscular strength				Endurance				Power	
Canadian Health Measures Survey, select cycles, 2007–2023, Canada (Statistics Canada, 2019)		●			●				●					●
National Health and Nutritional Examination Survey, select cycles, 1999–2016, United States (CDC, 2019)	●				●									
National Health and Nutritional Examination Survey National Youth Survey (3–15 years), 2012, United States (CDC, 2016)					●		●	●		●				
Hungarian National Youth Fitness Study (11–19 years), 2013, Hungary (Csányi et al., 2015)	●			●	●								●	
National Surveillance of Physical Fitness (3–6 years), every 5 years, 2000–2015, China (personal communication)				●					●		●		●	
Physical Fitness and Health Surveillance of Chinese Schools (6–19 years), annual, 1985+, China (personal communication)		●	●			●			(girls)	(boys)			●	
Physical Fitness Survey 'Sport Test' (10–17 years), annual, 1964+, Japan (Shingo & Takeo, 2002)			●		●	●				●			●	●
SLOfit National Surveillance System (7–19 years), annual, 1982+, Slovenia (University of Ljubljana, 2019)			●						●			●	●	
Chilean National Physical Education Survey (grade 8), 2011, Chili (Garber, Sajuria, & Lobelo, 2014)				●										●

Physical Fitness Test Batteries

Physical fitness test batteries are comprehensive groupings of field-based tests that are meant to provide an overall understanding of an individual's physical fitness. These types of fitness test batteries have been the focus of youth fitness surveillance since the 1950s with the publication of the American Alliance for Health, Physical Education and Recreation and Dance (AAHPERD) Youth Fitness Test in 1958 (Institute of Medicine, 2012). Worldwide, there are currently more than 15 published physical fitness test batteries (Institute of Medicine, 2012); of these, only three are truly international: FitnessGram, Eurofit, and ALPHA (Table 3.4). FitnessGram has

Table 3.4 Summary of physical fitness test batteries

	PREFIT	*FitnessGram*	*Eurofit*	*ALPHA*
Citation	(Ortega et al., 2015)	(Plowman & Meredith, 2013)	(Council of Europe, Committee for Development of Sport, 1988)	(Ruiz et al., 2011)
Age range	3–5 years	5–18 years	6–18 years	13–17 years
Cardiorespiratory fitness	• Modified 20mSRT	• 20mSRT (PACER) • 1-mile run test[a] • 1-mile walk test[a]	• 20mSRT • PWC170	• 20mSRT
Muscular fitness				
Strength/power	• Handgrip strength • Standing broad jump	• Trunk lift	• Handgrip strength • Standing broad jump	• Handgrip strength • Standing broad jump
Endurance		• 90° push-up • Traditional push-up[a] • Flexed arm hang[a] • Cadence-based curl-up	• Sit-ups in 30 seconds • Bent arm hang	
Flexibility		• Back saver sit-and-reach • Shoulder stretch	• Sit-and-reach	
Agility	• 4 × 10-m shuttle run		• 10 × 5-m shuttle run	• 4 × 10-m shuttle run[a]
Balance	• Standing on one leg test		• Flamingo balance test	
Body composition	• BMI • Waist circumference	• BMI • Skinfold thickness • Bioelectric impedance	• BMI • Skinfold thickness	• BMI • Skinfold thickness[a] • Waist circumference
Other			• Plate tapping (fine motor skills and coordination)	

Note

a indicates optional or alternative tests; PREFIT = Assessing FITness in PREschool children; ALPHA = Assessing Levels of Physical Activity.

been used to describe the prevalence of youth meeting health-related standards across several states in the United States (Bai et al., 2015) and in Hungary (Welk, Saint-Maurice, & Csányi, 2015). The Eurofit test battery has been a core component of youth fitness surveillance, with 30 European countries implementing the test since 1988 (Tomkinson, Lang, & Tremblay, 2019). More recently, the ALPHA (Assessing Levels of Physical Activity) was developed as a rapid health-related fitness test battery that is beginning to gain popularity in Europe (Ruiz et al., 2011). In addition to these, the PREFIT is the first fitness test battery for preschool youth that is currently, widely used in Spain (Cadenas-Sanchez et al., 2019), but could become more international in the near future. Further details on physical fitness test batteries are also provided in Chapter 18.

Web-Based Surveillance of Self-Reported Fitness

Web-based surveillance of physical fitness is a promising avenue to collect large amounts of data worldwide. For instance, between November 2013 and August 2015, Nauman, Tauschek, Kaminsky, Nes, and Wisløff (2017) were able to collect self-reported, estimated CRF for 886,333 (730,432 after data cleaning) adults aged 19–90 years, from 196 counties. This represented the largest effort to date to estimate the CRF levels in individuals, globally. Among youth no such effort has taken place. The International Fitness Scale is a reliable and valid self-report fitness measure for adolescents aged 12–17 years that has been translated into several languages (Ortega et al., 2011). This type of questionnaire could be used to pilot a web-based surveillance effort, similar to efforts conducted in adults. This approach has been described in detail elsewhere (Lang et al., 2018d). There are many strengths of web-based surveillance including its low cost, rapid data collection, and international coverage. Despite these benefits there are some important limitations. First, there is a degree of error involved with self-report measures. Second, voluntary participants that take part in web-based surveillance represent a subset of the population who are generally interested in their fitness. Last, these efforts should not be interpreted as producing nationally or internationally representative results, regardless of the sample size. For these reasons, web-based surveillance should not replace surveillance efforts that use objective measures; instead, web-based surveillance should be seen as a way to complement objective measurement efforts.

Key Issues

Standardized Protocols and Reporting

The accurate use and reporting on protocols and performance results are persisting key issues in physical fitness testing. For instance, there exist three different 20mSRT protocols: Léger (Léger et al., 1984), Eurofit (Council of Europe, Committee for Development of Sport, 1988), and Queens University of Belfast (Riddoch, 1990). The protocol used could have implications when pooling data, especially when the protocol is not accurately reported (Tomkinson et al., 2017; Tomkinson, Léger, Olds, & Cazorla, 2003). The protocol used is particularly important with MF testing as protocol variants could have major implications when comparing performance across countries or studies. For example, having an elbow flexed at 90° during the handgrip strength test can result in a significantly lower score when compared to having a fully extended elbow (España-Romero et al., 2010b). These types of protocol deviations could result in data being unusable during international data pooling and surveillance efforts. It is also important to accurately report performances using a common result metric. Following common reporting standards can help limit data cross-walking (i.e., standardizing data estimates to a common metric) in data pooling efforts, which reduces potential error involved with these procedures. Last, when possible, reporting descriptive means and standard deviations for each physical fitness test by single age and sex groups can also help with international surveillance and data pooling efforts.

A Shared Global Vision on Fitness Surveillance

For the most part, physical fitness surveillance has been conducted in regional or national silos worldwide. It is for this reason that physical fitness surveillance has been largely disjointed internationally, with a variety of fitness tests and protocols being used in some geographic areas but not others. There is certainly a need for a shared global vision on fitness surveillance as these types of measure hold promise for describing health trends and for guiding healthy public policy. In 2018, physical fitness was included as a new indicator in the Global Matrix 3.0 Physical Activity Report Card for Children and Youth (Aubert et al., 2018). Findings from this report indicated that only 22 out of 49 countries were able to identify enough data to produce a meaningful grade, resulting in 27 countries with incomplete grades. It was concluded that there were substantial variability in data (i.e., the type and amount of fitness data, normative values used, age ranges, sample size) making it difficult to compare physical fitness levels across countries (Aubert et al., 2018). These types of findings further reinforce the need for international collaborations in physical fitness surveillance, similar to the Global Matrix 3.0 efforts. International efforts in physical fitness surveillance are encouraged and may help bridge the numerous data gaps worldwide.

Emerging Issues

Using Fitness Surveillance to Evaluate Public Health Interventions

In a 2013 Cochrane systematic review it was identified that there was good evidence that school-based physical activity interventions have a positive impact on CRF, suggesting that CRF measures are sensitive to changes in physical activity levels (Dobbins, Husson, DeCorby, & LaRocca, 2013). This is an important finding that supports the surveillance of scalable CRF measures in schools to help track and understand physical activity levels. In this context, it is important to understand that objective measures of physical activity are time-consuming and costly, and measuring CRF could be a suitable alternative. Moreover, some authors have suggested that researchers should avoid using a dependent variable that is the same as the primary objective of the intervention (e.g., using physical activity as the dependent variable in a physical activity intervention) as a focus on physiological health markers as the dependent variable could provide a better indication of success (Sandercock & Jones, 2019b). In other words, the measurement of CRF could be an important indicator to help understand the impact of school-based physical activity interventions.

Recently, the World Health Organization has launched the Global Action Plan on Physical Activity (GAPPA) with an aim to attain a 15% relative reduction in the global prevalence of insufficient physical activity in youth and adults by 2030 (World Health Organization, 2017). In a recent publication in the Bulletin of the World Health Organization, Lang et al. (2018e) provided a perspective that the measurement of CRF could be used to complement the current GAPPA evaluation efforts which, to date, largely include self-reported physical activity. This emerging development could be a step toward using CRF as a measure to evaluate national and international healthy public policies. There is also a need to explore the possibility of using measures of MF as a way to evaluate the impact of similar policy interventions.

Recommendations for Researchers/Practitioners

The measurement of physical fitness is easy to administer, low in cost, feasible, and scalable in the school environment. Importantly, measures of physical fitness can help describe youth health patterns, and in some cases, may provide valuable information on future population health. Although population surveillance of physical fitness is not common, these measures hold promise and should be used to complement existing population health surveillance efforts among youth. There is a need for integrated international collaboration to help standardize testing protocols to simplify data pooling efforts. These types of efforts would be valuable for guiding healthy public policies and for evaluating public health interventions.

Disclaimer

The content and views expressed in this chapter are those of the authors and do not necessarily reflect those of the Government of Canada.

Conflicts of Interest

All authors declared no conflicts of interest and received no funding for this project.

Contributors

JJL and GRT developed the aims and objectives of the chapter. All authors contributed to writing, editing, and critical reviewing the chapter. All authors approved the final version.

References

Albon, H. M., Hamlin, M. J., & Ross, J. J. (2010). Secular trends and distributional changes in health and fitness performance variables of 10–14-year-old children in New Zealand between 1991 and 2003. *British Journal of Sports Medicine, 44*(4), 263–269.

Armstrong, N., Tomkinson, G., & Ekelund, U. (2011). Aerobic fitness and its relationship to sport, exercise training and habitual physical activity during youth. *British Journal of Sports Medicine, 45*, 849–858.

Artero, E. G., España-Romero, V., Castro-Pinero, J., Ortega, F. B., Suni, J., Castillo-Garzon, M. J., & Ruiz, J. R. (2011a). Reliability of field-based fitness tests in youth. *International Journal of Sports Medicine, 32*(3), 159–169.

Artero, E. G., España-Romero, V., Jiménez-Pavón, D., Martinez-Gómez, D., Warnberg, J., Gómez-Martínez, S., . . . De Henauw, S. (2014). Muscular fitness, fatness and inflammatory biomarkers in adolescents. *Pediatric Obesity, 9*(5), 391–400.

Artero, E. G., Ruiz, J. R., Ortega, F. B., España-Romero, V., Vicente-Rodríguez, G., Molnar, D., . . . Gutiérrez, A. (2011b). Muscular and cardiorespiratory fitness are independently associated with metabolic risk in adolescents: The HELENA study. *Pediatric Diabetes, 12*(8), 704–712.

Aubert, S., Barnes, J. D., Abdeta, C., Nader, P. A., Adeniyi, A. F., Aguilar-Farias, N., . . . Tremblay, M. S. (2018). Global Matrix 3.0 physical activity report card grades for children and youth: Results and analysis form 49 countries. *Journal of Physical Activity and Health, 15*(Suppl 2), S251–S273.

Bai, Y., Saint-Maurice, P. F., Welk, G. J., Allums-Featherston, K., Candelaria, N., & Anderson, K. (2015). Prevalence of youth fitness in the United States: Baseline results from the NFL PLAY 60 FITNESSGRAM partnership project. *The Journal of Pediatrics, 167*(3), 662–668.

Barker, A., Williams, C., Tolfrey, K., Fawkner, S., & Sandercock, G. (2013). *The BASES expert statement on measurement and interpretation of aerobic fitness in young people.* Leeds, UK: British Association of Sport and Exercise Sciences.

Benson, A. C., Torode, M. E., & Singh, M. A. (2006). Muscular strength and cardiorespiratory fitness is associated with higher insulin sensitivity in children and adolescents. *International Journal of Pediatric Obesity, 1*(4), 222–231.

Bianco, A., Jemni, M., Thomas, E., Patti, A., Paoli, A., Roque, J., . . . Tabacchi, G. (2015). A systematic review to determine reliability and usefulness of the field-based test batteries for the assessment of physical fitness in adolescents – The ASSO project. *International Journal of Occupational Medicine and Environmental Health, 28*(3), 445–478.

Borrud, L. G., Chiappa, M., Burt, V., Gahche, J. J., Zipf, G., Dohrmann, S. M., & Johnson, C. L. (2014). *National health and nutrition examination survey: National youth fitness survey plan, operations, and analysis, 2012.* Retrieved from https://stacks.cdc.gov/view/cdc/22313

Cadenas-Sanchez, C., Alcántara-Moral, F., Sanchez-Delgado, G., Mora-Gonzalez, J., Martinez-Tellez, B., Herrador-Colmenero, M., . . . Ortega, F. B. (2014). Assessment of cardiorespiratory fitness in preschool children: Adaptation of the 20 metres shuttle run test [article in Spanish]. *Nutricion Hospitalaria, 30*(6), 1333–1343.

Cadenas-Sanchez, C., Intemann, T., Labayen, I., Peinado, A. B., Vidal-Conti, J., Sanchis-Moysi, J., . . . Martinez-Tellez, B. (2019). Physical fitness reference standards for preschool children: The PREFIT project. *Journal of Science and Medicine in Sport, 22*(4), 430–437.

Cadenas-Sanchez, C., Martinez-Tellez, B., Sanchez-Delgado, G., Mora-Gonzalez, J., Castro-Piñero, J., Löf, M., . . . Ortega, F. B. (2016). Assessing physical fitness in preschool children: Feasibility, reliability and practical recommendations for the PREFIT battery. *Journal of Science and Medicine in Sport, 19*(11), 910–915.

Caspersen, C. J., Powell, K. E., & Christenson, G. M. (1985). Physical activity, exercise, and physical fitness: Definitions and distinctions for health-related research. *Public Health Reports, 100*(2), 126–131.

Castro-Piñero, J., Ortega, F. B., Artero, E. G., Girela-Rejón, M. J., Mora, J., Sjöström, M., & Ruiz, J. R. (2010). Assessing muscular strength in youth: Usefulness of standing long jump as a general index of muscular fitness. *Journal of Strength and Conditioning Research, 24*, 1810–1817.

Castro-Piñero, J., Perez-Bey, A., Cuenca-Garcia, M., Cabanas-Sanchez, V., Gómez-Martínez, S., Veiga, O. L., . . . Nova, E. (2019). Muscle fitness cut points for early assessment of cardiovascular risk in children and adolescents. *The Journal of Pediatrics, 206*, 134–141.

Catley, M, &. J., & Tomkinson, G. R. (2013). Normative health-related fitness values for children: Analysis of 85,374 test results on Australian 9–17 years olds since 1985. *British Journal of Sports Medicine, 47*(2), 98–108.

Center for Disease Control and Prevention. (2016, January 25). *The NHANES national youth fitness survey.* Retrieved from https://www.cdc.gov/nchs/nnyfs/index.htm

Center for Disease Control and Prevention. (2019, July 17). *National health and nutrition examination survey.* Retrieved from https://www.cdc.gov/nchs/nhanes/index.htm

Cooper, C. B., & Storer, T. W. (2001). *Exercise testing and interpretation: A practical approach.* Cambridge, UK: Cambridge University Press.

Costa, A. M., Costa, M. J., Reis, A. A., Ferreira, S., Martins, J., & Pereira, A. (2017). Secular trends in anthropometrics and physical fitness of young Portuguese school-aged children. *Acta medica portuguesa, 30*(2), 108–114.

Council of Europe, Committee for Development of Sport. (1988). *Eurofit: European tests of physical fitness.* Rome, Italy: Edigraf Editoriale Grafica.

Crump, C., Sundquist, J., Winkleby, M. A., & Sundquist, K. (2017). Aerobic fitness, muscular strength and obesity in relation to risk of heart failure. *Heart, 103*(22), 1780–1787.

Csányi, T., Finn, K. J., Welk, G. J., Zhu, W., Karsai, I., Ihász, F., . . . Molnár, L. (2015). Overview of the Hungarian national youth fitness study. *Research Quarterly for Exercise and Sport, 86*(Supp 1), S3–S12.

Dobbins, M., Husson, H., DeCorby, K., & LaRocca, R. L. (2013). School-based physical activity programs for promoting physical activity and fitness in children and adolescents aged 6 to 18. *Cochrane Database of Systematic Reviews, 2*, CD007651.

Docherty, D. (1996). Field tests and test batteries. In D. Docherty (Ed.), *Measurement in pediatric exercise science* (pp. 285–334). Champaign, IL: Human Kinetics.

Dodds, R. M., Syddall, H. E., Cooper, R., Kuh, D., Cooper, C., & Sayer, A. A. (2016). Global variation in grip strength: A systematic review and meta-analysis of normative data. *Age and Ageing, 45*(2), 209–216.

Domone, S., Mann, S., Sandercock, G., Wade, M., & Beedie, C. (2016). A method by which to assess the scalability of field-based fitness tests of cardiorespiratory fitness among schoolchildren. *Sports Medicine, 46*(12), 1819–1831.

Dooley FL, Kaster T, Annandale M, Fitzgerald JS, Walch T, Ferrar K, Lang JJ, Smith JJ, Tomkinson GR. Temporal trends in the handgrip strength of 2,216,589 children and adolescents between 1967 and 2017: a systematic review. *Sports Medicine.* 2020 Feb 6. [Epub ahead of print].

Dos Santos, F. K., Prista, A., Gomes, T. N. Q. F., Daca, T., Madeira, A., Katzmarzyk, P. T., & Maia, J. A. R. (2015). Secular trends in physical fitness of Mozambican school-aged children and adolescents. *American Journal of Human Biology, 27*(2), 201–206.

Ekblom, Ö., Oddsson, K., & Ekblom, B. (2004). Health-related fitness in Swedish adolescents between 1987 and 2001. *Acta Paediatrica, 93*(5), 681–686.

España-Romero, V., Artero, E. G., Jimenez-Pavon, D., Cuenca-Garcia, M., Ortega, F. B., Castro-Pinero, J., . . . Ruiz, J. R. (2010a). Assessing health-related fitness tests in the school setting: Reliability, feasibility and safety; the ALPHA Study. *International Journal of Sports Medicine, 31*(7), 490–497.

España-Romero, V., Artero, E. G., Santaliestra-Pasias, A. M., Gutierrez, A., Castillo, M. J., & Ruiz, J. R. (2008). Hand span influences optimal grip span in boys and girls aged 6 to 12 years. *The Journal of Hand Surgery, 33*(3), 378–384.

España-Romero, V., Ortega, F. B., Vicente-Rodríguez, G., Artero, E. G., Rey, J. P., & Ruiz, J. R. (2010b). Elbow position affects handgrip strength in adolescents: Validity and reliability of Jamar, DynEx, and TKK dynamometers. *Journal of Strength and Conditioning Research, 24*(1), 272–277.

Fraser, B. J., Blizzard, L., Schmidt, M. D., Juonala, M., Dwyer, T., Venn, A. J., & Magnussen, C. G. (2018). Childhood cardiorespiratory fitness, muscular fitness and adult measures of glucose homeostasis. *Journal of Science and Medicine in Sport, 21*, 935–940.

Fraser, B. J., Blizzard, L., Tomkinson, G. R., Lycett, K., Wake, M., Burgner, D., . . . Olds, T. (2019). The great leap backward: Changes in the jumping performance of Australian children aged 11–12-years between 1985 and 2015. *Journal of Sports Sciences, 37*(7), 748–754.

Fujita, Y., Nakamura, Y., Hiraoka, J., Kobayashi, K., Sakata, K., Nagai, M., & Yanagawa, H. (1995). Physical-strength tests and mortality among visitors to health-promotion centers in Japan. *Journal of Clinical Epidemiology, 48*(11), 1349–1359.

Garber, M. D., Sajuria, M., & Lobelo, F. (2014). Geographical variation in health-related physical fitness and body composition among Chilean 8th graders: A nationally representative cross-sectional study. *PLoS One, 9*(9), e108053.

García-Hermoso, A., Ramírez-Campillo, R., & Izquierdo, M. (2019). Is muscular fitness associated with future health benefits in children and adolescents? A systematic review and meta-analysis of longitudinal studies. *Sports Medicine, 49*(7), 1079–1094.

Hallal, P. C., Andersen, L. B., Bull, F. C., Guthold, R., Haskell, W., Ekelund, U., & Lancet Physical Activity Series Working Group. (2012). Global physical activity levels: Surveillance progress, pitfalls, and prospects. *Lancet, 380*(9838), 247–257.

Harber, M. P., Kaminsky, L. A., Arena, R., Blair, S. N., Franklin, B. A., Myers, J., & Ross, R. (2017). Impact of cardiorespiratory fitness on all-cause and disease-specific mortality: Advances since 2009. *Progress in Cardiovascular Diseases, 60*(1), 11–20.

Hardy, L. L., Merom, D., Thomas, M., & Peralta, L. (2018). 30-year changes in Australian children's standing broad jump: 1985–2015. *Journal of Science and Medicine in Sport, 21*(10), 1057–1061.

Haslofça, F., Kutlay, E., & Haslofça, E. (2017). Analysis of three decade changes in physical fitness characteristics of Turkish children aged between 11 and 12. *Spor Hekimligi Dergisi/Turkish Journal of Sports Medicine, 52*(4), 137–145.

Henriksson, H., Henriksson, P., Tynelius, P., & Ortega, F. B. (2019). Muscular weakness in adolescence is associated with disability 30 years later: A population-based cohort study of 1.2 million men. *British Journal of Sports Medicine, 53*(19), 1221–1230.

Holm, I., Fredriksen, P.M., Fosdahl, M., & Vøllestad, N. (2008). A normative sample of isotonic and isokinetic muscle strength measurements in children 7 to 12 years of age. *Acta Paediatrica, 97*, 602–607.

Hui, S. S. C., Suzuki, K., Naito, H., Balasekaran, G., Song, J. K., Park, S. Y., . . . Kijboonchoo, K. (2015). How fit and active in Asian youth? The Asia-fit study: 3412 Board# 173 May 30, 8. *Medicine & Science in Sports & Exercise, 47*(5S), 922.

Huotari, P. R., Nupponen, H., Laakso, L., & Kujala, U. M. (2010). Secular trends in muscular fitness among Finnish adolescents. *Scandinavian Journal of Public Health, 38*(7), 739–747.

Ignasiak, Z., Sławińska, T., & Malina, R. M. (2016). Short term secular change in body size and physical fitness of youth 7–15 years in Southwestern Poland: 2001–2002 and 2010–2011. *Anthropological Review, 79*(3), 311–329.

Institute of Medicine. (2012). *Fitness measures and health outcomes in youth.* Washington, DC: National Academies Press.

Jaric, S., Mirkov, D., & Markovic, G. (2005). Normalizing physical performance tests for body size: A proposal for standardization. *The Journal of Strength & Conditioning Research, 19*(2), 467–474.

Jürimäe, T., Volbekiene, V., Jürimäe, J., & Tomkinson, G. R. (2007). *Changes in Eurofit test performance of Estonian and Lithuanian children and adolescents (1992–2002).* In G. R. Tomkinson & T. S. Olds (Eds.), *Pediatric fitness* (Vol. 50, pp. 129–142). Basel, Switzerland: Karger Publishers.

Katzmarzyk, P. T., & Craig, C. L. (2002). Musculoskeletal fitness and risk of mortality. *Medicine and Science in Sports and Exercise, 34*(5), 740–744.

Kopecký, M. (2006). The secular trends in the somatic development and motoric performance of boys in the Olomouc region within the last 36 years. *Acta Universitatis Palackianae Olomucensis. Gymnica, 36*(3), 55–64.

Kopecký, M., & Přidalová, M. (2008). The secular trend in the somatic development and motor performance of 7–15 year old girls. *Medicina Sportiva, 12*(3), 78–85.

Lang, J. J. (2018a). Exploring the utility of cardiorespiratory fitness as a population health surveillance indicator for children and youth: An international analysis of results from the 20-m shuttle run test. *Applied Physiology, Nutrition, and Metabolism, 43*(2), 211–211.

Lang, J. J., Belanger, K., Poitras, V., Janssen, I., Tomkinson, G. R., & Tremblay, M. S. (2018b). Systematic review of the relationship between 20 m shuttle run performance and health indicators among children and youth. *Journal of Science and Medicine in Sport, 21*(4), 383–397.

Lang, J. J., Larouche, R., & Tremblay, M. S. (2019a). Exploring the relationship between physical fitness and health among Canadian children and youth aged 9 to 17 years. *Health Promotion and Chronic Disease Prevention in Canada, 39*(3), 104–111.

Lang, J. J., Tomkinson, G. R., Janssen, I., Ruiz, J. R., Ortega, F. B., Léger, L., & Tremblay, M. S. (2018c). Making a case for cardiorespiratory fitness surveillance among children and youth. *Exercise and Sport Science Reviews, 46(2)*, 66–75.

Lang, J. J., Tremblay, M. S., Léger, L., Olds, T., & Tomkinson, G. R. (2018d). International variability in 20 m shuttle run performance in children and youth: Who are the fittest from a 50-country comparison? A systematic literature review with pooling of aggregate results. *British Journal of Sports Medicine, 52*(4), 276.

Lang, J. J., Tremblay, M. S., Ortega, F. B., Ruiz, J. R., & Tomkinson, G. R. (2019b). Review of criterion-referenced standards for cardiorespiratory fitness: What percentage of 1 142 026 international children and you are apparently healthy? *British Journal of Sports Medicine, 53*, 953–958.

Lang, J. J., Wolfe Phillips, E., Orpana, H. M., Tremblay, M. S., Ross, R., Ortega, F. B., . . . Tomkinson, G. R. (2018e). Field-based measurement of cardiorespiratory fitness to evaluate physical activity interventions. *Bulletin of the World Health Organization, 96*(11), 794–796.

Larson, L. A. (1974). *Fitness, health, and work capacity: International standards for assessment.* New York, NY: Macmillan.

Laurson, K. R., Saint-Maurice, P. F., Welk, G. J., & Eisenmann, J. C. (2017). Reference curves for field tests of musculoskeletal fitness in US children and adolescents: The 2012 NHANES national youth fitness survey. *The Journal of Strength & Conditioning Research, 31*(8), 2075–2082.

Lefèvre, J., Bouckaert, J., & Duquet, W. (1998). De barometer van de fysieke fitheid van de Vlaamse jeugd 1997: De resultaten. *Sport (Bloso Brussel), 4*, 16–22.

Léger, L. A., Lambert, J., Goulet, A., Rowan, C., & Dinelle, Y. (1984). Aerobic capacity of 6- to 17-year old Quebecoise – 20 metre shuttle run test with 1 minute stages [Article in French]. *Canadian Journal of Applied Sport Sciences, 9*(2), 64–69.

Léger, L. A., Mercier, D., Gadoury, C., & Lambert, J. (1988). The multistage 20 metre shuttle run test for aerobic fitness. *Journal of Sport Sciences, 6*(2), 93–101.

Longmuir, P. E., Colley, R. C., Wherley, V. A., & Tremblay, M. S. (2014). Canadian Society for exercise physiology position stand: Benefit and risk for promoting childhood physical activity. *Applied Physiology, Nutrition, and Metabolism, 39*(11), 1271–1279.

Macfarlane, D. J., & Tomkinson, G. R. (2007). The evolution and variability in fitness test performance of Asian children and adolescents. *Medicine and Sport Science, 50*, 143–167.

Malina, R. M., Reyes, M. E. P., Tan, S. K., & Little, B. B. (2010). Secular change in muscular strength of indigenous rural youth 6–17 years in Oaxaca, southern Mexico: 1968–2000. *Annals of Human Biology, 37*(2), 169–185.

Marques, A., Santos, D. A., Hillman, C. H., & Sardinha, L. B. (2018). How does academic achievement relate to cardiorespiratory fitness, self-reported physical activity and objectively reported physical activity: A systematic review in children and adolescents aged 6–18 years. *British Journal of Sports Medicine, 52*(16), 1039–1039.

Matton, L., Duvigneaud, N., Wijndaele, K., Philippaerts, R., Duquet, W., Beunen, G., . . . Lefevre, J. (2007). Secular trends in anthropometric characteristics, physical fitness, physical activity, and biological maturation in Flemish adolescents between 1969 and 2005. *American Journal of Human Biology, 19*(3), 345–357.

Mayorga-Vega, D., Aguilar-Soto, P., & Viciana, J. (2015). Criterion-related validity of the 20-m shuttle run test for estimating cardiorespiratory fitness: A meta-analysis estimating cardiorespiratory fitness: A meta-analysis. *Journal of Sports Sciences and Medicine, 14*(3), 536–547.

Mayorga-Vega, D., Bocanegra-Parrilla, R., Ornelas, M., & Viciana, J. (2016). Criterion-related validity of the distance- and time-based walk/run field tests for estimating cardiorespiratory fitness: A systematic review and meta-analysis. *PLoS One, 11*(3), e0151671.

Mikkelsson, L. O., Nupponen, H., Kaprio, J., Kautiainen, H., Mikkelsson, M., & Kujala, U. M. (2006). Adolescent flexibility, endurance strength, and physical activity as predictors of adult tension neck, low back pain, and knee injury: A 25 year follow up study. *British Journal of Sports Medicine, 40*(2), 107–113.

Milliken, L. A., Faigenbaum, A. D., Loud, R. L., & Westcott, W. L. (2008). Correlates of upper and lower body muscular strength in children. *Journal of Strength and Conditioning Research, 22*(4), 1339–1346.

Mintjens, S., Menting, M. D., Daams, J. G., van Poppel, M. N., Roseboom, T. J., & Gemke, R. J. (2018). Cardiorespiratory fitness in childhood and adolescence affects future cardiovascular risk factors: A systematic review of longitudinal studies. *Sports Medicine, 48*(11), 2577–2605.

Moliner-Urdiales, D., Ruiz, J. R., Ortega, F. B., Jiménez-Pavón, D., Vicente-Rodriguez, G., Rey-López, J. P., . . . Noriega-Borge, M. J. (2010). Secular trends in health-related physical fitness in Spanish adolescents: The AVENA and HELENA studies. *Journal of Science and Medicine in Sport, 13*(6), 584–588.

Nauman, J., Tauschek, L. C., Kaminsky, L. A., Nes, B. M., & Wisloff, U. (2017). Global fitness levels: Findings from a web-based surveillance report. *Progress in Cardiovascular Diseases, 60*(1), 78–88.

Ortega, F. B., Cadenas-Sánchez, C., Sánchez-Delgado, G., Mora-González, J., Martínez-Téllez, B., Artero, E. G., . . . Ruiz, J. R. (2015). Systematic review and proposal of a field-based physical fitness-test battery in preschool children: The PREFIT battery. *Sports Medicine, 45*(4), 533–555.

Ortega, F. B., Ruiz, M. J., Castillo, M. J., & Sjöström, M. (2008). Physical fitness in childhood and adolescence: A powerful marker of health. *International Journal of Obesity, 32*(1), 1–11.

Ortega, F. B., Ruiz, J. R., Espana-Romero, V., Vicente-Rodriguez, G., Martínez-Gómez, D., Manios, Y., . . . Sjöström, M. (2011). The international fitness scale (IFIS): Usefulness of self-reported fitness in youth. *International Journal of Epidemiology, 40*(3), 701–711.

Ortega, F. B., Silventoinen, K., Tynelius, P., & Rasmussen, F. (2012). Muscular strength in male adolescents and premature death: Cohort study of one million participants. *British Medical Journal, 345*, e7279.

Pate, R. R. (1989). The case for large-scale physical fitness testing in American youth. *Pediatric Exercise Sciences, 1*(4), 290–294.

Payne, N., Gledhill, N., Katzmarzyk, P. T., & Jamnik, V. (2000). Health-related fitness, physical activity, and history of back pain. *Canadian Journal of Applied Physiology, 25*(4), 236–249.

Plowman, S. A., & Meredith, M. D. (Eds.). (2014). *Fitnessgram/activitygram reference guide* (4th ed.). Top 10 research questions related to musculoskeletal physical fitness testing in children and adolescents. *Research Quarterly for Exercise and Sport, 85*(2), 174–187.

Przeweda, R., & Dobosz, J. (2003). Growth and physical fitness of Polish youths in two successive decades. *Journal of Sports Medicine and Physical Fitness, 43*(4), 465–474.

Reid, K. F., & Fielding, R. A. (2012). Skeletal muscle power: A critical determinant of physical functioning in older adults. *Exercise and Sport Sciences Reviews, 40*, 4–12.

Riddoch, C. J. (1990). *The Northern Ireland health and fitness survey – 1989: The fitness, physical activity, attitudes and lifestyles of Northern Ireland post-primary schoolchildren*. Belfast, Northern Island: The Queen's University of Belfast, 1990.

Rioux, B. V., Kuwornu, P., Sharma, A., Tremblay, M. S., McGavock, J. M., & Sénéchal, M. (2017). Association between handgrip muscle strength and cardiometabolic z-score in children 6 to 19 years of age: Results from the Canadian health measures survey. *Metabolic Syndrome and Related Disorders, 15*(7), 379–384.

Ross, R., Blair, S. N., Arena, R., Church, T. S., Després, J. P., Franklin, B. A., . . . Myers, J. (2016). Importance of assessing cardiorespiratory fitness in clinical practice: A case for fitness as a clinical vital sign: A scientific statement from the American Heart Association. *Circulation, 134*(24), e653–e699.

Ruiz, J. R., España-Romero, V., Ortega, F. B., Sjöström, M., Castillo, M. J., & Gutierrez, A. (2006). Hand span influences optimal grip span in male and female teenagers. *The Journal of Hand Surgery, 31*(8), 1367–1372.

Ruiz, J. R., Castro-Piñero, J., Artero, E. G., Ortega, F. B., Sjöström, M., Suni, J., & Castillo, M. J. (2009a). Predictive validity of health-related fitness in youth: A systematic review. *British Journal of Sports Medicine, 43*(12), 909–923.

Ruiz, J. R., Cavero-Redondo, I., Ortega, F. B., Welk, G. J., Andersen, L. B., & Martinez-Vizcaino, V. (2016). Cardiorespiratory fitness cut points to avoid cardiovascular disease risk in children and adolescents: What level of fitness should raise a red flag? A systematic review and meta-analysis. *British Journal of Sports Medicine, 50*(23), 1451–1458.

Ruiz, J. R., España, V. R., Castro, J. P., Artero, E. G., Ortega, F. B., Cuenca, M. G., . . . Gutierrez, A. (2011). ALPHA-fitness test battery: Health-related field-based fitness tests assessment in children and adolescents [Spanish article]. *Nutricion Hospitalaria, 26*(6), 1210–1214.

Ruiz, J. R., Silva, G., Oliveira, N., Ribeiro, J. C., Oliveira, J. F., & Mota, J. (2009b). Criterion-related validity of the 20-m shuttle run test in youths aged 13–19 years. *Journal of Sports Sciences, 27*(9), 899–906.

Runhaar, J., Collard, D., Singh, A., Kemper, H., Van Mechelen, W., & Chinapaw, M. (2010). Motor fitness in Dutch youth: Differences over a 26-year period (1980–2006). *Journal of Science and Medicine in Sport, 13*(3), 323–328.

Safrit, M. J. (1990). The validity and reliability of fitness tests for children: A review. *Pediatric Exercise Science, 2*, 9–28.

Saint-Maurice, P. F., Laurson, K., Welk, G. J., Eisenmann, J., Gracia-Marco, L., Artero, E. G., . . . & Janz, K. F. (2018). Grip strength cutpoints for youth based on a clinically relevant bone health outcome. *Archives of Osteoporosis, 13*(1), 92.

Sanchez-Delgado, G., Cadenas-Sanchez, C., Mora-Gonzalez, J., Martinez-Tellez, B., Chillón, P., Löf, M., . . . Ruiz, J. R. (2015). Assessment of handgrip strength in preschool children aged 3 to 5 years. *Journal of Hand Surgery. European Volume, 40*(9), 966–972.

Sandercock, G. R., & Cohen, D. D. (2019a). Temporal trends in muscular fitness of English 10-year-olds 1998–2014: An allometric approach. *Journal of Science and Medicine in Sport, 22*(2), 201–205. Published Online First: 2018 July 31.

Sandercock, G. R., & Jones, B. (2019b). Is it time to give population health surveillance a late fitness test? *British Journal of Sports Medicine, 53*, 463–464. Published Online First, 02 February 2018.

Shingo, N., & Takeo, M. (2002). The educational experiments of school health promotion for the youth in Japan: Analysis of the 'sport test' over the past 34 years. *Health Promotion International, 17*(2), 147–160.

Silverman, I. W. (2015). Age as a moderator of the secular trend for grip strength in Canada and the United States. *Annals of Human Biology, 42*(3), 201–211.

Smith, J. J., Eather, N., Morgan, P. J., Plotnikoff, R. C., Faigenbaum, A. D., & Lubans, D. R. (2014). The health benefits of muscular fitness for children and adolescents: A systematic review and meta-analysis. *Sports Medicine, 44*(9), 1209–1223.

Smpokos, E. A., Linardakis, M., Papadaki, A., Lionis, C., & Kafatos, A. (2012). Secular trends in fitness, moderate-to-vigorous physical activity, and TV-viewing among first grade school children of Crete, Greece between 1992/93 and 2006/07. *Journal of Science and Medicine in Sport, 15*(2), 129–135.

Statistics Canada. (2019, July 11). *Canadian health measures survey.* Retrieved from https://www.statcan.gc.ca/eng/survey/household/5071

Steene-Johannessen, J., Kolle, E., Andersen, L. B., & Anderssen, S. A. (2013). Adiposity, aerobic fitness, muscle fitness, and markers of inflammation in children. *Medicine and Science in Sports and Exercise, 45*(4), 714–721.

Stodden, D., Sacko, R., & Nesbitt, D. (2017). A review of the promotion of fitness measures and health outcomes in youth. *American Journal of Lifestyle Medicine, 11*(3), 232–242.

Strel, J. (2013). *Analysis of the program healthy lifestyle for the years 2010/11 and 2011/12* [Article in Slovenian]. Ljubljana, Slovenia: Institute for Sport Planica.

Thacker, S. B., Qualters, J. R., Lee, L. M., & Centers for Disease Control and Prevention. (2012). Public health surveillance in the United States: Evolution and challenges. *MMWR Surveillance Summaries, 61*(Suppl), 3–9.

The Cooper Institute. (2017). *FitnessGram administration manual: The journey to MyHealthyZone* (5th ed.). Champaign, IL: Human Kinetics.

Tomkinson, G. R. (2007a). Global changes in anaerobic fitness test performance of children and adolescents (1958–2003). *Scandinavian Journal of Medicine and Science in Sports, 17*(5), 497–507.

Tomkinson, G. R., Carver, K. D., Atkinson, F., Daniell, N. D., Lewis, L., Fitzgerald, . . . Ortega, F. B. (2018). European normative values for physical fitness in children and adolescents aged 9–17 years: Results from 2 779 165 Eurofit performances representing 30 countries. *British Journal of Sports Medicine, 55*(22), 1445–1456.

Tomkinson, G. R., Lang, J. J., & Tremblay, M. S. (2019). Temporal trends in the cardiorespiratory fitness of children and adolescents representing 19 high-income and upper middle-income countries between 1981 and 2014. *British Journal of Sports Medicine, 53*(8), 478–486. Published Online First, 2017 October 30 [Epub ahead of print].

Tomkinson, G. R., Lang, J. J., Tremblay, M. S., Dale, M., LeBlanc, A. G., Belanger, K., . . . Léger, L. (2017). International normative 20 m shuttle run values from 1 142 026 children and youth representing 50 countries. *British Journal of Sports Medicine, 51*(21), 1545–1554.

Tomkinson, G. R., Léger, L. A., Olds, T. S., & Cazorla, G. (2003). Secular trends in the performance of children and adolescents (1980–2000). An analysis of 55 studies of the 20m shuttle run test in 11 countries. *Sports Medicine, 33*(4), 285–300.

Tomkinson, G. R., Macfarlane, D., Noi, S., Kim, D. Y., Wang, Z., & Hong, R. (2012). Temporal changes in long-distance running performance of Asian children between 1964 and 2009. *Sports Medicine, 42*(4), 267–279.

Tomkinson, G. R., & Olds, T. S. (2007b). Secular changes in pediatric aerobic fitness test performance: The global picture. *Medicine and Sport Science, 50,* 46–66.

Tomkinson, G., & Olds, T. S. (2008). Field tests of fitness. In N. Armstrong, & W. Van Mechelen (Eds.), *Paediatric exercise science and medicine* (2nd ed., pp. 109–128). Oxford, UK: Oxford University Press.

Tomkinson, G. R., Olds, T. S., & Borms, J. (2007c). Who are the Eurofittest? In G. R. Tomkinson, & T. S. Old (Eds.), *Pediatric fitness* (Vol. 50, pp. 104–128). Basel, Switzerland: Karger Publishers.

Tomkinson, G. R., Olds, T. S., Kang, S. J., & Kim, D. Y. (2007d). Secular trends in the aerobic fitness test performance and body mass index of Korean children and adolescents (1968–2000). *International Journal of Sports Medicine, 28*(4), 314–320.

Tremblay, M. S., Shields, M., Laviolette, M., Craig, C. L., Janssen, I., & Gorber, S. C. (2010). Fitness of Canadian children and youth: Results from the 2007–2009 Canadian health measures survey. *Health Reports, 21*(1), 7–20.

University of Ljubljana. (2019). *SLOfit.* Retrieved from http://en.slofit.org/

Venckunas, T., Emeljanovas, A., Mieziene, B., & Volbekiene, V. (2017). Secular trends in physical fitness and body size in Lithuanian children and adolescents between 1992 and 2012. *Journal of Epidemiology and Community Health, 71*(2), 181–187.

Watkins, J., & Moore, B. (1983). The performance of Scottish boys in the one mile run test. *Scottish Journal of Physical Education, 11,* 4–10.

Watkins, J., & Moore, B. (1996). The effects of practice on performance in the one mile run test of cardio-respiratory fitness in 12–15 year old girls. *ACHPER Healthy Lifestyles Journal, 43,* 11–14.

Welk, G. J., Saint-Maurice, P. F., & Csányi, T. (2015). Health-related physical fitness in Hungarian youth: Age, sex, and regional profiles. *Research Quarterly for Exercise and Sport, 26*(Suppl 1), S45–S57.

Woods, J. A., Pate, R. R., & Burgess, M. L. (1992). Correlates to performance on field tests of muscular strength. *Pediatric Exercise Science, 4*(4), 302–311.

World Health Organization (WHO). (2017). *More active people for a healthier world. Global action plan on physical activity 2018–2030.* Geneva, Switzerland: World Health Organization.

Zaqout, M., Michels, N., Bammann, K., Ahrens, W., Sprengeler, O., Molnar, D., . . . Jimenez, D. (2016). Influence of physical fitness on cardio-metabolic risk factors in European children. The IDEFICS study. *International Journal of Obesity, 40*(7), 1119–1125.

Zhu, X. (2013). Situational interest and physical activity in fitness testing: A need for pedagogical engineering. *International Journal of Sport and Exercise Psychology, 12,* 76–89.

Zuidam, J. M., Selles, R. W., Stam, H. J., & Hovius, S. E. (2008). Age-specific reliability of two grip-strength dynamometers when used by children. *The Journal of Bone and Joint Surgery. American Edition, 90*(5), 1053–1059.

4

PHYSICAL ACTIVITY GUIDELINES AND RECOMMENDATIONS

Paul McCrorie, Anne Martin, and Xanne Janssen

Introduction

In 1953, the Lancet published two pioneering papers by the late great Professor Jeremiah 'Jerry' Morris that have shaped the field of physical activity (PA) epidemiology as we know it today (Morris, Heady, Raffle, Roberts, & Parks, 1953a, 1953b). The London Transport Workers Study was one of the first to show that the incidence of cardiac events was related to occupational physical (in)activity. Sedentary London Transport Authority bus drivers were at higher risk of coronary heart disease than their more active conductor colleagues. Similar findings were observed between active postal workers and sedentary telephonists. It has been over 65 years since these seminal papers and the body of evidence linking physical inactivity to non-communicable disease have grown in size and strength, including the important recognition of this relationship in children and young people (Carson et al., 2016; Riopel et al., 1986; Strong et al., 2005; Tarp et al., 2018). Chapters 5–7 outline the physical/physiological, mental, and cognitive and academic benefits of PA.

The obvious question is why is this important or even relevant to this particular chapter? Well, linking physical (in)activity to health outcomes is the initial stage of the widely cited behavioral epidemiological framework (Sallis et al., 2006), and the impact of this body of work for guideline development cannot be understated, and its importance undersold. Without it, our ability to understand the role of key PA-related constructs (i.e., frequency, intensity, time, type, and dose) as part of the PA-health relationship would preclude the ability to produce adequate evidence-based guidelines and recommendations. As developers of guideline recommendations for children and young people, we have to consider 'how many times' 'for how long' 'at what level of effort' and 'of what type' is required to observe physical and mental health benefits. You will notice that all of the recommendations within guideline documents are composed of these important constructs; yet without the underlying evidence we are only able to provide recommendations based on expert opinion (See Table 4.1).

What Are PA Recommendations and Why Do We Produce Them?

The main goal of PA (and more recently sedentary behavior) guidelines is to provide a structured and systematic set of evidence-based statements/recommendations that guide the public to improve their health through PA. This includes how much we should do (i.e., PA) and how much is too much (e.g., sedentary behaviors) to "optimise current and future health of all young people" (Cavill, Biddle, & Sallis, 2001, p. 12). PA recommendations are also intended to increase awareness of the health benefits of PA and consequences of sedentary behavior, which in turn can influence positive attitudes toward engaging in PA or reducing time spent in sedentary behavior. Ancillary

Table 4.1 Definition of key terms

Term	Definition
PA guidelines	Piece of non-mandatory advice. Between supporting information (key principles, processes, evidence summary, communication) they provide a set of specific recommendations derived from a systematic review of the scientific literature
PA recommendation(s)	Specific evidence-based advisory statements that incorporate important PA-related constructs that when combined form guidance to population groups of the optimal levels of PA to return the greatest levels of health benefit
PA policy	A course or principle of action adopted or proposed by an organization (e.g., governmental body). Policy includes high-level statements that guide actions and decisions
	Example: The Safe, Affordable, Flexible, Efficient Transportation Equity Act: A Legacy for Users, or SAFETEA-LU (P.L.109-59, 2005) was a 2005–2009 funding and authorization bill that governed US federal surface transportation spending, including cycling and pedestrian infrastructure
PA strategy	The 'bigger picture' that includes the outline of steps to get from point A to B. It is a solution that helps you plan the journey to success
	Examples: 'Get Scotland Walking' (Campbell, Calderwood, Hunter, & Murray, 2018), 'Let's Make Scotland More Active' (PA Task Force, 2003), 'VicHealth's PA Strategy 2018–2023' (VicHealth, 2018)
PA action plan	The who, what, when, why, and how much. Provides detail to the overarching strategy
	Example: Global Action Plan on PA 2018–2030 (GAPPA) – World Health Organization (World Health Organization, 2018)
PA initiatives	Individual examples of programs designed to meet a specific goal that may be the result of/guided by an overarching policy, strategy, and action plan
	Example: Safe Routes to School initiatives

to this is the role guidelines can have on individual level habit formation. Guideline statements should be specific, measurable, achievable/attainable, realistic, and time-bound. For those who are familiar with setting goals, these combine to form the SMART acronym commonly used in goal setting theory (Kirschenbaum, 1997). Guideline statements are produced to allow population groups to work toward, and beyond, the recommended levels of PA. This is only possible through the conscious and explicit structure that they take.

Where population groups can use guideline recommendations to foster habit formation, national governments and international health advocacy agencies and institutions (e.g., the World Health Organization [WHO]) may commission/fund the update of guidelines and recommendations in response to an updated evidence base. They also rely on the specificity of guideline statements – particularly the outcomes – as a set of measurable indicators that can be tracked and surveilled over time; often in response to, or evaluation of, (inter)national strategies/plans/charters to improve population health.

How Have the PA Recommendations Evolved?

PA guidelines and recommendations have matured considerably since the late 1980s when the first 'children and youth' opinion statement from the American College of Sports Medicine (ACSM) was published (American College of Sports Medicine (ACSM), 1988). As the evidence base strengthened, guideline statements were produced initially for adolescents (Sallis & Patrick, 1994), then for children (Cavill et al., 2001); even more recently, we have seen guidelines produced for the 'early years,' including infants (less than 1 year old), toddlers (1–2 years old), and preschoolers (2–4 years old) (Australian Department of Health, 2010). In addition to the evolution of recommendations for specific population groups, there has been a recent development in the understanding of PA as it exists within specific time periods (e.g., a 24-hour cycle). Part of this chapter will present the history of guideline development, and it will become clear how changes in our evidence base have influenced the scientific underpinning of the guideline statements produced for the public.

Chapter Aims and Learning Objectives

As you move through this chapter you will begin to understand how many of the fields within PA research coalesce from basic terminology, to more advanced epidemiology, measurement issues, and policy relevance. PA recommendations have a huge role to play within a larger system of health promotion, and this chapter will demonstrate its importance. The main aim of this chapter is to introduce the concept of PA recommendations and the process in which they are created. By the end of this chapter you will:

- Understand the key constructs that form the basis of PA recommendations and how they vary globally
- Have a clear understanding of how the PA recommendations evolved over time
- Be able to identify how the PA recommendations vary depending on age group
- Have learned about the scientific process underlying the development and creation of PA recommendations
- Know about the key and emerging issues within the field of PA guideline development
- Understand the key research recommendations for future guideline development/updates

Key Issues of PA Guideline Recommendations

Countries all over the world have developed their own PA guidelines, and while differences between these country-specific guidelines exist, many use similar concepts. Therefore, before we start introducing the guidelines and explain the differences and similarities between countries, it is important to understand the key concepts guidelines are based on.

Dose-Response Relationship

All guidelines aim to provide a recommendation around the *dose-response* relationship between PA and/or sedentary behavior and health outcomes. This means that they are based on evidence of how a certain amount of PA (the dose) affects the health outcome of interest (the response). The dose-response relationship can have different forms: for example, a dose-response relationship can be linear, which means that every added unit of something (e.g. 1 minute of extra PA such as jumping, hopping, or skipping) results in a consistent added health benefit. However, often dose-response relationships are not linear, for example, increasing PA by 20 minutes does not necessarily improve a health outcome twice as much as increasing PA by 10 minutes. Instead, the relationship between PA, sedentary behavior, and health outcomes is often *curvilinear*. This means that we see a relative stronger effect of these behaviors on health outcomes at certain points of the curve compared to other points (Figure 4.1). The dose at which we start to see an effect varies between health outcomes and age groups, but in general it has been suggested that greater improvements in health are noticed when increasing PA from lower baseline values (Pate et al., 1995). For example, imagine that an inactive person (high risk of disease) decides to increase their PA by 30 minutes. This change results in a much larger reduction of disease risk compared to an already very active person (low risk of disease) who also increases their PA by 30 minutes

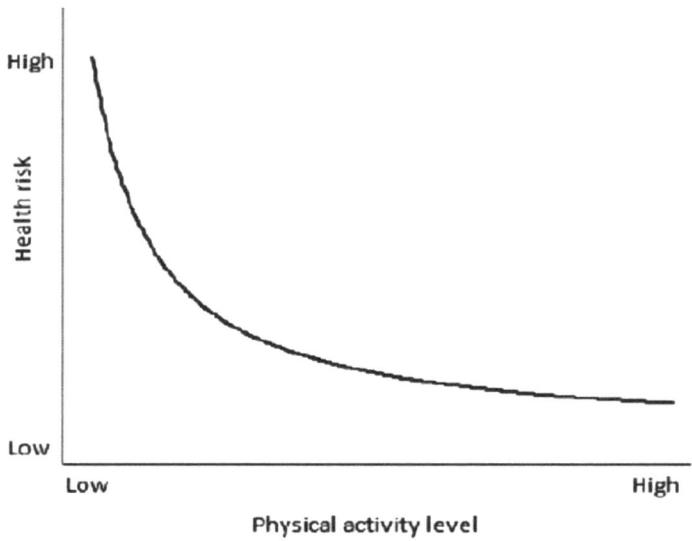

Figure 4.1   Curvilinear dose-response relationship between PA level (x-axis) and health risk (y-axis)

(Figure 4.1). When we move on through this chapter it is important to remember that in addition to differences in dose-response relationships between age groups, movement skills/abilities and behavior patterns also vary with age. Therefore, most guidelines refer to a specific age group. The most commonly used age groups for under 19s are (i) the early years which include infants (0–12 months), toddlers (1–2 years), and preschoolers (3–4 years); (ii) school-aged children 5–11 years; and (iii) young people (12–18 years). However, slight differences between countries exist.

PA and Sedentary Behavior

In the past, guidelines focused purely on PA. However, over the last decade evidence has suggested that high levels of sedentary time can have harmful effects on children's health (Carson et al., 2016; Poitras et al., 2017), and this has led to an increased focus of public health to reduce sedentary time and the inclusion of sedentary behavior in PA guidelines in several countries (e.g. Australian Department of Health, 2014; Pfeifer & Rutten, 2017; Tremblay et al., 2016; UK Department of Health and Social Care, 2019; Weggemans et al., 2018). Sedentary behavior is defined as any waking behavior with an energy expenditure of less than 1.5 metabolic equivalents (METs; 1 MET equals the amount of oxygen consumed while at rest. See Section 'Different intensities of PA' for further explanation) while in a seated or reclined position (Tremblay, Aubert et al., 2017). It is important to acknowledge that sedentary behavior is not physical inactivity. A child is often referred to as physically inactive if they do not meet the PA guidelines. However, an active child (i.e., a child who meets the PA guidelines) can at the same time be a sedentary child; e.g., the child engages in 70 minutes of moderate to vigorous PA per day but spends the rest of the day seated behind his/her computer. Sedentary activities can include but are not limited to reading, sitting in a stroller/buggy, and watching a movie.

Frequency, Intensity, Time, Type of PA

PA guidelines are often based on the FITT principle. FITT stands for Frequency, Intensity, Time, and Type. *Frequency* refers to how often someone should engage in PA and/or sedentary behavior. This can refer to how many times per week or how many sessions per day. The second concept, *intensity*, refers to how hard someone has to work during the activity. Children's and young peoples' PA behavior includes a vast array of different activities, and these all require different amounts of energy. To simplify this, guidelines often classify PA in three different intensities:

- Light PA
- Moderate PA
- Vigorous PA

Whether an activity belongs to the light, moderate, or vigorous category depends on how much energy a child uses when engaging in a certain activity, which we will explain in more detail below. Intensity only applies to PA as there is very little variability in the intensity levels of sedentary behaviors. The third component, *time*, refers to the amount of time someone should engage in PA and/or sedentary behaviors. This can be the amount of time per session, per day, or even per week. The last component *type* refers to what kind of PA and/or sedentary behaviors someone should or should not engage in. Examples of different types of activities are bone- and muscle-strengthening PA, playing a specific sport, reading, etc. We will explain some of these in more detail below.

Different Intensities of PA

The PA intensity of a specific activity can differ between children. The intensity of a specific activity depends on factors such as age and fitness levels. Intensities of PA are classified based on the amount of energy which is used during a specific activity. The MET for a task is a physiological measure which tells us the energy cost of certain activities for an individual person. To establish the MET value of an activity we measure the amount of oxygen used during that activity compared to the amount of oxygen used at rest. This means that if a person is at rest the MET value will be 1, whereas this person will have a much higher MET value during a more intense activity, such as running (e.g., 4 METs). Each intensity has its own MET threshold. It is important to remember that during growth resting energy expenditures of children vary widely, e.g. resting energy expenditure for an 8-year-old is 1.8 times compared to that of adults, which means their resting MET value is 1.8. Consequently, the MET value of high intensities of PA is higher. Therefore, when using METs in children it is recommended to use age-adjusted MET values (described in more detail in Chapter 12).

Light PA

Light PA refers to any activity with an energy expenditure between 1.5 and 3 METs (Pate et al., 1995). Light PA results in a minor raise in heart rate, and children should be able to hold a conversation during the activity without being out of breath. Examples of light PA are dressing up in costumes and getting themselves ready for bed (Ainsworth et al., 2000).

Moderate PA

Moderate PA refers to activities with an energy expenditure between 3 and 6 METs (Pate et al., 1995). Children engaging in these types of activities are often slightly out of breath. Examples of moderate physical activities are brisk walks, cycling, skipping, and climbing activities (Ainsworth et al., 2000).

Vigorous PA

Vigorous PA refers to any activity with an energy expenditure >6 METs (Pate et al., 1995). These activities will result in the child breathing hard and sweating. These activities can include fast running, jumping, playing tag, etc. (Ainsworth et al., 2000).

The guidelines for children and young people often refer to *moderate-to-vigorous intensity PA (MVPA)*. MVPA is often the leading component in PA guidelines for school-aged children and youth.

Total PA

Guidelines for the early years often focus on total PA (i.e., a combination of light, moderate, and vigorous PA). This activity can be accumulated by walking to school, getting dressed, playing with friends, etc.

Different Types of PA

PA and sedentary time can be accumulated in many different forms and types of activities. Cardio-respiratory fitness refers to how well your heart and lungs can supply the rest of your body with oxygen/energy for PA. Activities that enhance cardiorespiratory fitness are of moderate-to-vigorous intensity. This type of activity is often the most promoted type of activity in the guidelines, and the majority of national surveillance data will only report on the percentage of children meeting the guidelines based on this type of PA. However, most PA guidelines for school-aged children and young people include three more types of activities, bone-strengthening, muscle-strengthening, and flexibility activities. *Bone-strengthening physical activities* refer to activities which produce a force on the bones that promotes bone growth and strength. Examples include jumping, gymnastics, and running. These types of physical activities are especially important throughout childhood as this is when the skeletal system develops. *Muscle-strengthening activities* refer to activities which increase muscle strength. Examples include climbing trees, monkey swings, using playground equipment, and resistance training. Flexibility refers to the ability to move joints and muscles to their maximum range of motion. *Flexibility activities* are therefore activities which increase the range of movement in the joints and muscles. These activities can include stretching but activities such as playing on climbing equipment and taking part in gymnastics will also increase flexibility. While most PA guidelines include flexibility, and bone and muscle-strengthening components, these are seldom measured and/or reported in national surveillance reports. More recently, a body of evidence has emerged demonstrating the benefits of active play (Janssen, 2014; Pesce et al., 2016; Yogman, Garner, Hutchinson, Hirsh-Pasek, & Golinkoff, 2018). *Active play* is gross motor or total body movements in which young children exert energy in a freely chosen, fun, and unstructured manner (Truelove, Vanderloo, & Tucker, 2017). Active play includes activities such as jumping, kicking, catching, or running, and is a common type of PA during early childhood but becomes slightly less prominent when children grow older.

Infants, toddlers, and preschoolers all engage in different types of movement behaviors and activities. In addition, the age at which a child starts walking differs between children, resulting in different movement behaviors even between children of the same age. Guidelines focusing on the early years therefore use slightly different terms and concepts. Guidelines may make recommendations specifically for infants, toddlers, and preschoolers, or they may differentiate between walkers and non-walkers. In addition, for infants who cannot crawl, the focus is often on *tummy time,* which refers to the time an infant spends in the prone position (lying on their tummy) while awake. Tummy time is considered to be PA for infants and is thought to be beneficial for their health. Early years guidelines will also often include recommendations on *time spent being restraint*. This refers to any time the child is placed in a position in which it cannot move voluntarily (e.g., car seats, strollers/buggies).

As mentioned previously, sedentary behaviors consist of a range of different activities. Differences are also noted between the content children engage in during sedentary behaviors. An activity can be classed as *educational* (e.g., child doing homework on a computer) or *non-educational* (e.g., child watching a cartoon movie). Another important factor is the social setting, in which sedentary behaviors take place. Children can engage in *social* sedentary activities by engaging with others during the activity (e.g., family TV viewing or children Skype with grandparents), or a child can engage in a *non-social* activity, where they have no social interaction while engaging in the activity (e.g., a child watching TV alone). Guidelines that include sedentary behavior recommendations have recently started to acknowledge the importance of these different types of sedentary behaviors and started to include recommendations around these.

24-Hour Movement Behaviors

If we think about a child's day, they are either sleeping, sedentary, or engaging in PA. All these movement behaviors have shown to influence health independently of each other with the strongest effects seen for MVPA. However, even if children were meeting the guidelines this would only account for approximately 60 minutes of their day (i.e., 4% of waking hours). This means it remains unclear as to what should happen during the other 23 hours of a child's day. This appears to be a problem given the recent evidence suggesting that sleep, sedentary behavior, and PA are not acting independently from each other and that the ultimate health effect of a change in one behavior depends on what behavior it is replaced by (Saunders et al., 2016). Therefore, the 24-hour movement behaviors concept was introduced (Chaput, Carson, Gray, & Tremblay, 2014) (Figure 4.2). This concept follows a 'whole day matters' approach, in that it acknowledges that

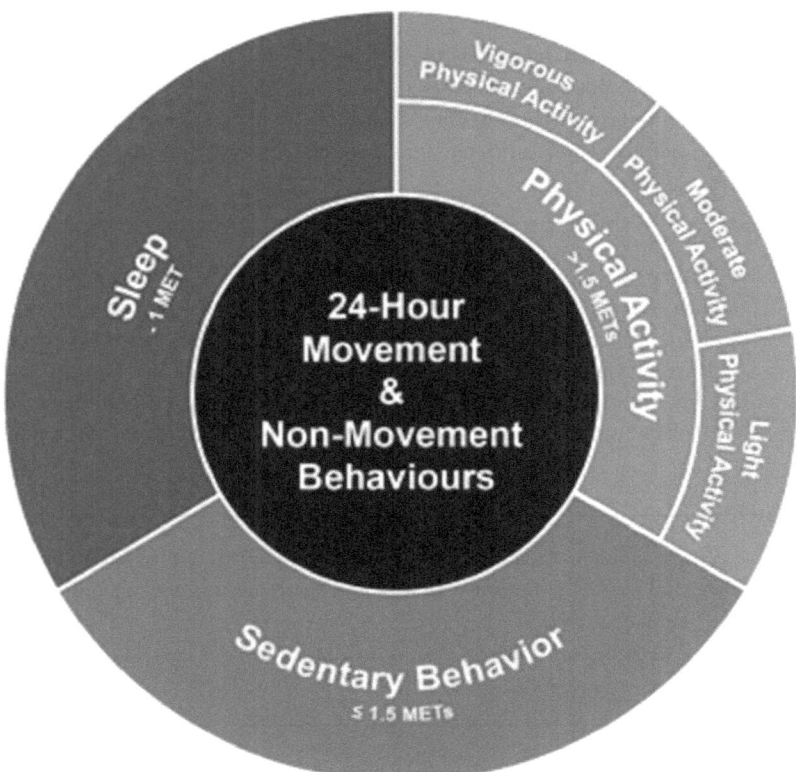

Figure 4.2   24-hour movement concept (Adapted from Tremblay, Aubert et al., 2017, Figure 4.3)

sleep, sedentary behavior, and PA collectively impact health and recommendations for all these behaviors should be made in a 24-hour movement guideline. Several countries (i.e., Canada, Australia, New Zealand, and South Africa) as well as the WHO have developed 24-hour movement behavior guidelines for the early years and/or school-aged children and youth.

Evolution of PA Guidelines for Children and Youth

The Early Days of PA Recommendations

Before national or international PA guidelines were developed, professional and medical organizations published opinion and consensus statements on the amount of PA needed for health benefits in children and youth. For example, the ACSM published an "Opinion statement on physical fitness in children and youth" in 1988 (American College of Sports Medicine, 1988) proposing that children and adolescents should obtain 20–30 minutes of vigorous exercise daily. Scientists were highly critical, acknowledging that the recommendations were based on evidence of the benefits of PA in adults. They concluded that specific guidelines needed to be developed using evidence from the adolescent PA literature (Sallis & Patrick, 1994). In 1992, the International Consensus Conference on PA Guidelines for Adolescents was convened involving scientists and clinicians from North America, Europe, and Australia (Sallis & Patrick, 1994). This conference resulted in two recommendations for youth aged 11–21 years:

1 "All adolescents should be physically active daily, or nearly every day, as part of play, games, sports, work, transportation, recreation, physical education, or planned exercise, in the context of family, school, and community activities.
2 Adolescents should engage in three or more sessions per week of activities that last 20 minutes or more at a time and that require moderate to vigorous levels of exertion" (Sallis & Patrick, 1994, pp. 307–308).

The expert committee acknowledged that the evidence base at that time was not sufficient to provide more definitive recommendations relating to the dose-response relationship of specific types of PA, long-term benefits of PA in adolescence, and effectiveness of individual or community-based PA interventions (Sallis & Patrick, 1994).

In 1997, the UK Health Education Authority began an evidence review and consensus process that resulted in the following international recommendations for children and adolescents aged 5–18 years:

1 "All young people should participate in PA of at least moderate intensity for 1 hour per day.
2 Young people who currently do little activity should participate in PA of at least moderate intensity for at least half an hour per day.
3 At least twice a week, some of these activities should help to enhance and maintain muscular strength and flexibility, and bone health" (Cavill et al., 2001, p. 18).

In 1998, Canada became the first country to produce a national PA guideline with separate recommendations for children and adults. For the first time, a recommendation to reduce sedentary behavior depicting a family with children watching TV was included. Four years later, a new guideline addressing the specific needs of children and youth was developed. In 2002, Canada's PA Guidelines and Guides for children (6–9 years) and youth (10–14 years) recommended (Health Canada and the Canadian Society for Exercise Physiology, 2002a, 2002b):

1	Increase time currently spent on PA, starting with 30 minutes more per day and building up to at least 60 minutes of moderate intensity PA over a 5 months period.
2	Increase time currently spent on PA, starting with 10 minutes of vigorous intensity PA and building up 30 minutes vigorous intensity PA over a 5 months period.
3	Build up physical activities throughout the day in periods of at least 5–10 minutes.
4	Combine three types of activities for best results: endurance activities, flexibility activities, and strength-building activities.
5	Reduce "non-active" time spent on TV, video, computer games, and surfing the internet starting with 30 minutes less per day.

Several other countries followed the Canadian example and developed their own national PA guidelines for children and youth. In 2010, the WHO produced the first global PA guidelines for children and youth aged 5–17 years (World Health Organization, 2010). With a growing body of evidence in the field of child and youth PA over the last two decades, national guidelines have been revised, and updated guidelines have been published. The scientific report of the 2018 PA Guideline for Americans reflected on the change of the evidence used for the first PA guideline for American children and youth back in 2008:

> The evidence has been strengthened by marked increases in the quantity and quality of research on PA and two key health indicators, weight status and/or adiposity and bone health. Further, the evidence has been strengthened by the publication of numerous systematic reviews and meta-analyses on topics related to the impact of PA on health outcomes in children and adolescents.
>
> *(2018 PA Guidelines Advisory Committee, 2018, F7-13)*

How Have PA Guidelines for Children and Young People Changed over Time?

Table 4.2 provides an overview of the key messages of 13 PA guidelines for children and young people aged 5–18 years. The overview shows similarities and differences of guidelines from Canada, Scotland, England, the USA, Australia, the UK, Germany, the Netherlands, and globally (guidelines of the WHO). Table 4.2 also illustrates how the guideline content has changed over time, within and between countries. Table 4.2 does not provide an exhaustive list of all existing PA guidelines; many more countries have their own national PA guideline for children and young people.

In the following paragraphs, we describe the similarities and differences of the recommendations for PA, sedentary behavior, and sleep. In 2016, the 24-hour movement approach was introduced, adding sleep recommendations to PA guidelines for the first time (Tremblay et al., 2016).

Table 4.2 Comparison of PA guidelines for children and youth (5–18 years) between countries over time

Guideline concepts	Canada (2002)	Scotland (2003)	Australia (2004)	England (2004)	USA (2008)	WHO (2010)	Canada (2011)	UK (2011)	Australia (2014)	Germany (2016)	Canada (2016)	The Netherlands (2017)	USA (2018)	Australia (2019)
Light intensity PA	–	–	–	–	–	–	–	–	–	60 minutes/day in everyday activities, e.g. at least 12,000 steps/day (as part of ≥90 minutes/day)	Several hours of a variety of structured and unstructured physical activities	–	–	Several hours of a variety of light physical activities
Moderate intensity PA	Start with ≥30 minutes/day; build up to ≥60 minutes/day	Build up to ≥60minutes on most days of the week	–	–	–	–	–	–	–	–	–	–	–	–
Moderate-to-vigorous intensity PA	–	–	≥60 minutes/day	≥60 minutes/day	≥60 minutes/day (aerobic)	≥60 minutes/day (aerobic)	≥60 minutes/day	≥60 minutes/day	≥60 minutes/day	≥90 minutes/day	≥60 minutes/day	≥60 minutes/day	60 minutes/day (aerobic)	60 minutes/day (mainly aerobic)
Vigorous PA intensity	Start with 10 minutes/day; build up to 30 minutes/day	–	–	≥2 times/week (including muscle- and bone-strengthening activities)	As part of ≥60 minutes/day on ≥3 days/week	As part of ≥60 minutes/day on ≥3 days/week (including muscle- and bone-strengthening activities)	As part of ≥60 minutes/day on ≥3 days/week	≥3 days/week (including muscle- and bone-strengthening activities)	As part of ≥60 minutes/day on ≥3 days/week (including muscle- and bone-strengthening activities)	–	As part of ≥60 minutes/day on ≥3 days/week	–	As part of 60 minutes/day on ≥3 days/week	≥3 days/week (including muscle- and bone-strengthening activities)

Guideline concepts	Canada (2002)	Scotland (2003)	Australia (2004)	England (2004)	USA (2008)	WHO (2010)	Canada (2011)	UK (2011)	Australia (2014)	Germany (2016)	Canada (2016)	The Netherlands (2017)	USA (2018)	Australia (2019)
Muscle- and bone-strengthening PA	–	–	–		As part of ≥60 minutes/day on ≥3 days/week		As part of ≥60 minutes/day on ≥3 days/week			2–3 days/week	As part of ≥60 minutes/day on ≥3 days/week	≥3 times/week	–	
Sedentary behavior	Start with 30 minutes/day less time spent on TV, video, computer games, and surfing the internet; build up to 90 minutes/day less	–	≤2 hours/day using electronic media for entertainment, particularly during daylight hours	–	–	–	–	Minimize the amount of time spent sitting for extended periods	≤2 hours/day using electronic media for entertainment; break up long periods of sitting as often as possible	Avoidable sitting times should be reduced to a minimum. Screen media consumption: ≤60 minutes/day (6–11 years); ≤ 2 hours/day (12–18 years)	≤2 hours/day screen time; Limited sitting for extended periods	Avoid long periods sitting down	–	≤2 hours/day of sedentary recreational screen time; Breaking up long periods of sitting as often as possible
Sleep	–			–	–	–	–	–	–	–	9–11 hours/night (5–13 years); 8–10 hours/night (14–17 years)	–	–	uninterrupted 9–11 hours/per night (5–13 years); 8–10 hours/night (14–17 years); Consistent bed and wake-up times

PA Intensity

- **Light intensity:** Absent from guidelines until 2016 and then included in guidelines from Germany, Canada, and Australia only. The German guideline recommends 60 minutes per day in everyday activities, whereas the Canadian guideline provides a non-specific recommendation of several hours of a variety of structured and unstructured activities.
- **Moderate intensity:** Included in the early guidelines from Canada (2002) and Scotland (2003). Canada provided a specific recommendation of at least 60 minutes per day, whereas Scotland recommended at least 60 minutes on most days.
- **Moderate-to-vigorous intensity:** Part of guidelines of all listed countries from 2004 onward. The duration and frequency are similar between most countries: at least 60 minutes per day.
- **Vigorous intensity:** Introduced first in the Canadian 2002 guideline but not considered in the guidelines from Scotland 2003, Australia 2004, Germany 2016, and the Netherlands 2017. Recommendations varied in duration and frequency in the early 2000 but gained consistency from 2008.

Duration and Frequency of PA

Following the 1997 recommendation of the UK Health Education Authority, nearly all national and global PA guidelines recommended a total of at least 60 minutes of daily PA (of at least moderate intensity). The Canadian 2002 guideline, however, recommended a total of 90 minutes of PA, including 60 minutes of moderate intensity PA and 30 minutes of vigorous intensity PA. This recommendation was revised in 2011 and then aligned with other national and global recommendations. The only country to recommend 90 minutes of daily MVPA has been Germany, as part of their 2016 guideline.

Countries with a specific recommendation for vigorous intensity PA typically recommended that vigorous intensity PA should be done on at least 3 days per week. This recommendation is understood to be part of the total of at least 60 minutes of PA per day. The specific recommendation of daily 30 minutes of vigorous intensity PA in the Canadian 2002 guidelines was not adopted in later guidelines, likely due to a lack of evidence supporting this recommendation which was based on expert opinion at the time. Many guidelines included an additional statement, which encourages to build up the recommended total amount of PA throughout the day in periods of at least 5–10 minutes.

Type of PA

Along with the key recommendation concerning the intensity, duration, and frequency of PA, guidelines also specify the type of physical activities children and young people should do. The recent 2018 PA guideline for children and young people from the USA includes a list of physical activities for each intensity and age group (see Table 3.1 of the American 2018 guideline; US Department of Health and Human Services, 2018). Guidelines typically refer to physical activities that benefit cardiorespiratory fitness, muscle and bone strength, and flexibility.

- **Cardiorespiratory fitness:** To increase and maintain cardiorespiratory fitness, the key recommendation of at least 60 minutes of MVPA daily and vigorous PA on 3 days/week became a fundamental part of PA guidelines. In turn, to achieve this recommendation, guidelines suggested that children and young people should engage in activities such as biking, running, skipping, and jumping. The Germany 2016 and Canada 2016 guidelines recommend walking or stepping as possible types of PA to build cardiorespiratory fitness and so benefit health. In their 2016 guideline, Germany was the only country to recommend a specific daily step count of at least 12,000 steps (Rutten & Pfeifer, 2016).

- **Muscle and bone strength:** Recommendations to combine aerobic physical activities with strength-building activities have been part of PA guidelines as early as the first national PA guideline for children and youth in Canada 2002. However, it took another 6 years for the evidence base to be adequate enough to formulate more specific recommendations, indicating how often children and young people should engage in muscle- and bone-strengthening activities. The American 2008 guideline first introduced that muscle- and bone-strengthening activities should be part of children and youth's daily 60 minutes of MVPA on at least 3 days per week (US Department of Health and Human Services, 2008). Since then, PA guidelines for other nations (Canada 2011, Germany 2016, the Netherlands 2017) also included the same recommendation. Other guidelines differ however; for example, WHO (2010), UK Department of Health and Social Care (2019), and Australian Department of Health (2014) all recommend that 30 minutes of vigorous intensity PA on at least 3 days per week should include muscle- and bone-strengthening activities (Table 4.2).
- **Flexibility:** There is little evidence for the health benefits of flexibility in children and young people. As such, there are no specific recommendations in PA guidelines in terms of duration and frequency of physical activities for improving and maintaining flexibility. However, when providing examples of types of physical activities, some national guidelines include activities that promote flexibility, for example, stretching or yoga.

Sedentary Time

Despite the early recommendation in 1998 to reduce sitting for prolonged periods of time from Canada, the majority of national PA guidelines for children and young people up until 2011 did not contain specific recommendations for reducing time spent in sedentary behavior. Countries, which have included specific sedentary behavior recommendations (Australia, Canada, Germany), suggested limiting time using electronic media for recreational entertainment to a maximum of 2 hours per day. The guidelines from Australia (2014, 2019), Canada (2016), and the Netherlands (2017) also included a recommendation for breaking up extended periods of sitting, but without a specific indication of the duration.

Sleep

In 2016, Canada was the first country to publish the 24-hour movement guidelines, which introduced sleep recommendations in addition to recommendations for PA and sedentary behavior (see Table 4.2). In 2017, New Zealand adopted the Canadian 2016 guidelines, and in 2019 Australia published their own 24-hour movement behavior guidelines for children and young people. None of the other countries that published guidelines in 2017 (The Netherlands), 2018 (USA), and 2019 (UK) have adopted the 24-hour movement guidelines for children and young people.

What about PA Guidelines for Infants, Toddlers, and Preschool Children?

The first nation to mention preschool-aged children in their PA guidelines was Australia in 2004:

> What about pre-school children? PA is important for all children, and infants and toddlers should be given plenty of opportunity to move throughout the day. Children should not be inactive for prolonged periods, except when they're asleep!
>
> (Australian Department of Health and Ageing, 2004, p. 2)

The first mention was an important step and placed research regarding PA for healthy growth and development of young children on the agenda of other nations. In 2005, the Finnish Ministry of Social Affairs and Health published the first PA guidelines for children aged 0–6 years which were part of the National Curriculum Guidelines on Early Childhood Education and Care in Finland recommending:

> A child needs at least two hours of brisk physical activity every day.
>
> Children should be able to train on a daily basis their fundamental motor skills in various settings and in a diversified way.
>
> (Ministry of Social Affairs and Health, 2005, p. 5)

As the evidence base increased, more specific recommendations were developed in 2010 by the Australian Department of Health, and in 2011 by the UK Department of Health and Social Care, stating:

> 1 PA should be encouraged from birth, particularly through floor-based play and water-based activities in safe environments.
> 2 Children of pre-school age who are capable of walking unaided should be physically active daily for at least 180 minutes (3 hours), spread throughout the day.
> 3 All under 5s should minimize the amount of time spent being sedentary (being restrained or sitting) for extended periods (except time spent sleeping).
>
> (UK Department of Health and Social Care, 2019, p. 20)

In 2012, the Canadian guideline expanded the UK 2011 recommendations by providing additional details on what 180 minutes of daily PA for toddlers and preschoolers should look like (Tremblay et al., 2012):

- A variety of activities in different environments
- Activities that develop movement skills
- Progression toward at least 60 minutes of energetic play by 5 years of age

The last point is of particular importance as it considers the transition into the recommendations for children and youth aged 5–18 years. The 2016 German PA guidelines not only included age-specific recommendations for infants, toddlers, and preschoolers – consistent with Australia (2010), UK (2011) and Canada (2012) – but also made specific recommendations for reducing sedentary time in this age group:

> Avoidable sitting times should be reduced to a minimum. In addition to (motorized) transport, e.g. in a baby carrier or child seat, or periods spent inside unnecessarily, this relates in particular to reducing consumption of screen media to a minimum:
>
> - Infants and toddlers: 0 minutes
> - Preschool children: as little as possible, maximum of 30 minutes/day.
>
> (Rutten & Pfeifer, 2016, p. 28)

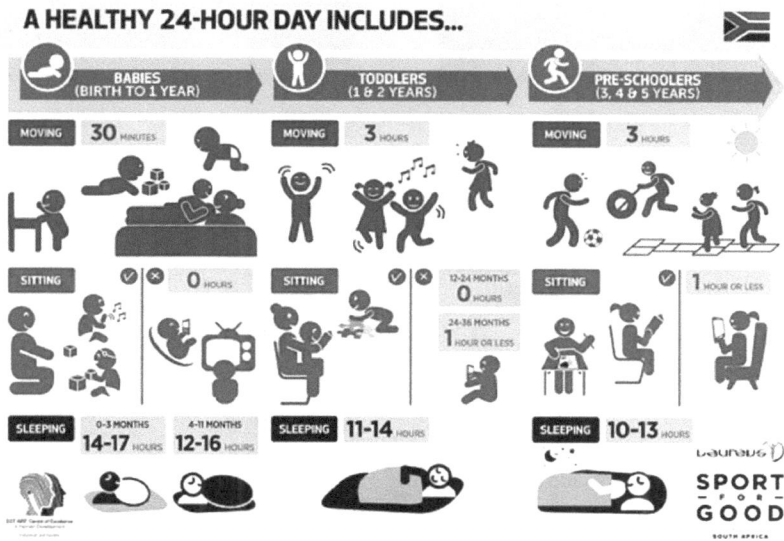

Figure 4.3 South African 24-hour movement guidelines for the early years (birth to five years) 2018 (Reproduced with permission from Laureus Sport for Good Foundation: http://www.laureus.co.za/moving-playing-sleeping-starting-early-with-healthy-habits/)

Updates of PA guidelines for the early years in Canada (2017), Australia (2017), and New Zealand (2017) followed the 'whole day matters' approach leading to the development of the 24-hour movement behavior guidelines (Tremblay, Chaput et al., 2017; Okely et al., 2017). However, the importance of sleep in addition to PA and sedentary behavior was recognized for the first time in the early years guidelines from Finland (2016).

In 2018, the UK, South Africa, and the WHO prepared 24-hour movement behavior guidelines for children under the age of 5 years (Okely, Tremblay, Reilly, Draper, & Bull,, 2018), with the UK guidelines later being ratified as independent behavior guidelines (i.e., non-24 hour). Released in 2018, Figure 4.3 displays the South African 24-hour movement behavior guidelines for children under the age of 5 years.

Despite what appears to be strong available evidence (Carson et al., 2017), international variability exists in its recognition and translation within this age group. For example, the Dutch 2017 PA guideline committee in their review of the literature "found no research that provides a basis for establishing a recommendation for this age group" (Weggemans et al., 2018, p. 7), claiming that "International physical activity guidelines for this age group are based on opinions of experts and experience in practice" (Health Council of the Netherlands, 2017, p. 30). While the 2018 PA Guidelines for Americans did include evidence-based recommendations for children aged 3–5 years, which are consistent with recommendations from other nations, no recommendations for infants and toddlers were developed (US Department of Health and Human Services, 2018). As shown in Figure 4.4, considerable effort has been expended to harmonize PA guidelines for the early years globally. However, there is still some distance to go before there is true international harmonization in the early years: as highlighted above regarding the absence of recommendations for the early years in the Dutch, for infants and toddlers in the US guidelines, and the inconsistency with regard to integrated 24-hour movement behavior guidelines or independent PA guidelines (Figure 4.4).

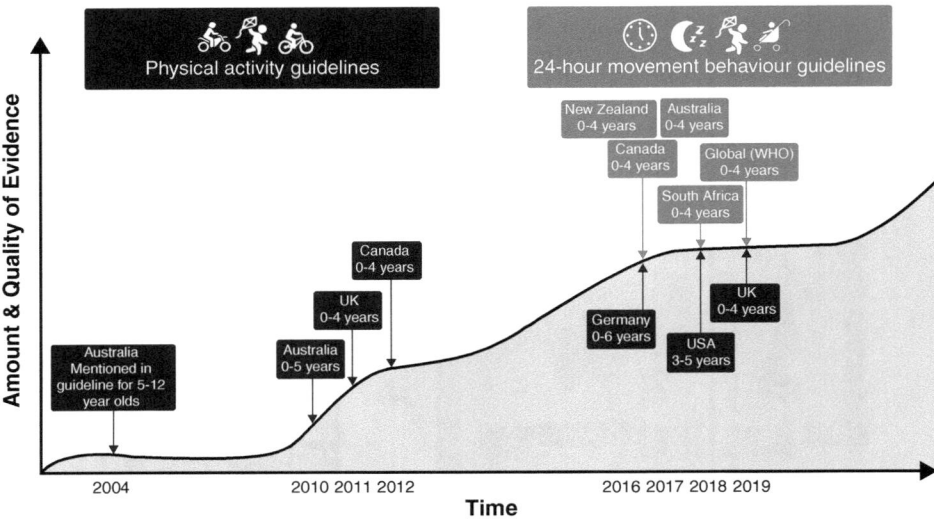

Figure 4.4   Evolution of early years PA guidelines over time (Image created by MRC/CSO Social and Public Health Sciences Unit, University of Glasgow)

The Scientific Process of Creating PA Guidelines

The scientific process for developing PA guidelines was influenced by the processes involved in developing clinical practice guidelines. For example, the updated Canadian PA Guidelines for children and youth in 2011 followed the AGREE (Appraisal of Guidelines, Research and Evaluation) II instrument – a tool typically used for developing clinical practice guidelines (Brouwers et al., 2010; Tremblay et al., 2010). The AGREE II instrument has three purposes: (1) guideline assessment, (2) guidance for guideline reporting, and (3) guidance for guideline development. The AGREE II instrument has 23-items over 6 domains: scope and purpose, stakeholder involvement, rigor of development, clarity of presentation, applicability (concerns implementation of the guideline), and editorial independence (concerns potential bias due to conflicts of interest of guideline developers or funder) (Brouwers et al., 2010).

The AGREE II instrument has not been used universally by all PA guideline developers to guide the process. Nevertheless, the development of PA guidelines shares common steps. It takes about seven steps to get from the idea of creating a PA guideline to the actual recommendations suitable for a variety of population groups. Figure 4.5 summarizes the steps in the scientific process of guideline development in a flow diagram. In the following paragraphs, we describe each step in more detail and outline how the process of developing guidelines changed with a growing body of evidence and existing guidelines globally.

Step 1: Forming Committees

The child and youth PA guideline process typically starts with assembling a leadership and guideline committee. The leadership committee may include the Principal Investigator, representatives from funding organizations, and governmental health departments (Tremblay et al., 2010). The guideline committee comprises leading experts in the field of child and youth PA and guideline development experts. The experts can be scientists or practitioners, who then develop specific questions that need to be answered as part of the guideline development process. In addition to the

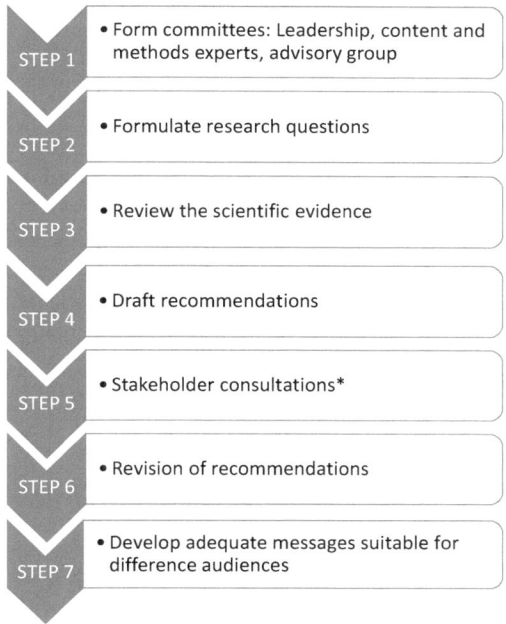

Figure 4.5 Flow diagram of the scientific process of developing PA guidelines

★ Some countries have two rounds of consultations, where they repeat the stakeholder consultation after the first round of revisions of recommendations.

leadership and guideline committee, an external advisory group is formed. The advisory group (or sometimes called steering group) is not actively involved in the guideline development process, but they provide independent feedback on the process and content of the guideline. This ensures that the PA guideline reflects the evidence base correctly and in an unbiased fashion.

Step 2: Formulating Research Questions

Formulating specific research questions is the next step in the process of developing guidelines. Research questions, for the purpose of guideline development, address issues around the health benefits or risks of PA in children and youth, and the characteristics of PA in terms of intensity, type, and duration. In Box 1, we show the research questions that guided the American 2018 PA Guidelines for children and youth (US Department of Health and Human Services, 2018).

Box 4.1: Research Questions to Inform the American 2018 PA Guidelines for Children and Young People

Question 1: In children and adolescents, is PA related to health outcomes?

a   What is the relationship between PA and cardiorespiratory and muscular fitness?
b   What is the relationship between PA and adiposity or weight status? Does PA prevent or reduce the risk of excessive increases in adiposity or weight?
c   What is the relationship between PA and cardiometabolic health?

---

d   What is the relationship between PA and bone health?

e   Are there dose-response relationships? If so, what are the shapes of those relationships?

f   Do the relationships vary by age, sex, race/ethnicity, weight status, or socioeconomic status?

Question 2: In children and adolescents, is sedentary behavior related to health outcomes?

a   What is the relationship between sedentary behavior and cardiometabolic health?

b   What is the relationship between sedentary behavior and adiposity or weight status?

c   What is the relationship between sedentary behavior and bone health?

d   Are there dose-response relationships? If so, what are the shapes of those relationships?

e   Do the relationships vary by age, sex, race/ethnicity, weight status, or socioeconomic status?

Step 3: Reviewing the Scientific Evidence

This step is critical for developing sound and well-informed guidelines. Common to the process of all national and international PA guidelines is that the research questions are answered by reviewing and synthesizing the scientific evidence. Methodologically, the highest quality reviews of evidence are systematic reviews of primary studies or existing evidence reviews. Table 4.3 provides definitions of research designs that inform evidence reviews.

The very first international PA guideline for youth from 1992 was based on seven literature reviews. The purpose of these was to summarize the current body of evidence on the health benefits and risk of PA for the general youth population and high-risk subgroups of youth (Sallis & Patrick, 1994). The guideline committee also produced evidence summaries on the epidemiology of PA in youth and implementation strategies of PA recommendations in primary care.

On some occasions, individual high-quality studies are considered during the guideline development process, specifically if there is no sufficient evidence for conducting a systematic review. What if there is no scientific evidence available to answer a research question? In that case, recommendations are developed based on the scientific opinions of the members of the expert committee as well as experience from child and youth practitioners (for example, pediatricians or teachers). However, expert opinion and practice experience are at the bottom of the evidence hierarchy (Borgerson, 2009). Therefore, they should only be used to develop guidelines when the benefits of having recommendations outweigh the harms of not having. When the likelihood of causing harm by providing certain recommendations is low, the benefits of recommendations based on expert option or practice experience outweigh the risks.

Where possible, experts involved in reviewing the evidence for developing guidelines consult different types of evidence. Evidence can differ as to whether observational or intervention data are being used and which study design has been applied. All types of study designs can be of value for developing PA guidelines depending on the research questions asked. See Tables 4.3 and 4.4 for definitions and summaries of the different study designs/type of research questions.

Knowing the answer to the research questions set out in Step 2 of the guideline process is not enough for formulating guideline recommendations. Step 3 of the process also involves assessing the strength or quality of the evidence. By doing this, we will know how certain we can be that the evidence is likely to be the truth and is unlikely to change when new evidence emerges.

Table 4.3 Research design definitions[a]

Term	Definition
Systematic review	A literature review that summarizes the evidence on a clearly formulated review question according to a predefined protocol, using systematic and explicit methods to identify, select, and appraise relevant studies, and to extract, analyze, collate, and report their findings. It may or may not use statistical techniques, such as meta-analysis to combine results from several similar studies and estimate an overall effect
Randomized control trial (RCT)	A study in which a number of similar people are randomly assigned to two (or more) groups to test a specific drug, treatment, or other intervention. One group (the experimental group) has the intervention being tested (e.g., specific components of the FITT principle), the other (the comparison or control group) has an alternative intervention, a dummy intervention (placebo), or no intervention at all. The groups are followed up to see how effective the experimental intervention was. Outcomes are measured at specific times, and any difference in response between the groups is assessed statistically
Randomization	Assigning people in a research study to different groups without taking any similarities or differences between them into account. For example, it could involve using a random numbers table or a computer-generated random sequence. It means that each individual (or each group in the case of cluster randomization) has the same chance of having each intervention
Effectiveness trials	The performance of an intervention under 'real-world' conditions
Natural experiment	Lacks an exact definition and has many variants. Common thread across most is that exposure to the event or intervention of interest has not been manipulated by the researcher (Craig et al., 2012) – it has occurred naturally
Controlled clinical trial	A clinical study that includes a comparison (control) group. The comparison group receives a placebo, another treatment, or no treatment at all. (National Cancer Institute)
Longitudinal design	A study of the same group of people at different times. This contrasts with a cross-sectional study, which observes a group of people at a point in time
Prospective study	A research study in which the health or other characteristic of patients is monitored (or 'followed up') for a period of time, with events recorded as they happen. This contrasts with retrospective studies
Prospective cohort study	An observational study with two or more groups (cohorts) of people with similar characteristics (e.g., children born in the same year). One group has a treatment, is exposed to a risk factor (e.g. higher levels of PA), or has a particular symptom; the other group does not. The study follows their progress over time and records what happens
Cross-sectional study	A 'snapshot' observation of a group of people at one time point. Contrasts with a longitudinal study that follows a group of people over a period of time
Case control study	A prospective or retrospective study that compares a group of patients who have the disease or condition (cases) with a group of people who do not have it (controls) but are otherwise as similar as possible (in characteristics thought to be unrelated to the causes of the disease or condition)

a Available from https://www.nice.org.uk/Glossary.

The tools are used to assess the strength of the evidence as part of the guideline process has varied between countries. For example, Canada, Australia, the UK (early years only) and the global WHO guidelines have been developed using the framework by the Grading of Recommendations, Assessment, Development and Evaluations (GRADE) working group (Balshem et al., 2011).

Table 4.4 Overview of the different study designs used to answer research questions

Guideline research topic	Study design
Effectiveness of PA for health benefits	Randomized controlled trials, controlled clinical trials, natural experiments
Relationship between PA and health or harm/risk	Prospective or retrospective longitudinal study, cross-sectional study
Long-term benefits of PA	Experimental or observational prospective studies
Dose-response relationship	Cross-sectional, longitudinal, or experimental designs
Physiological mechanisms	Experimental studies, case-control studies

The GRADE approach allows a systematic assessment of the certainty in evidence by evaluating the following factors[1]:

• Risk of bias in the methodology
• Indirectness of evidence
• Imprecision of evidence
• Inconsistency of evidence
• Dose-response relationship
• Magnitude of the effect
• Residual confounding
• Publication bias

Based on these factors, evidence for a particular health outcome can be upgraded or downgraded resulting in four possible quality ratings: high, moderate, low, and very low (Balshem et al., 2011). For developing the 2018 US PA Guidelines, the expert committee adapted the United States Department of Agriculture's (USDA) Nutrition Evidence Library (NEL) Conclusion Statement Evaluation Criteria to evaluate the strength of systematic review evidence. The criteria were applicability, generalizability to the US population, risk of bias and study limitations, quantity and consistency of evidence, and magnitude and precision of effect (2018 PA Guidelines Advisory Committee, 2018). The quality was rated as strong, moderate, limited, or not assignable.

Step 4: Drafting Recommendations

Step 4 of the guideline development process is about translating the reviewed and synthesized evidence into recommendations. This step requires a considerable amount of subjective judgment by the guideline developers, who at times need to balance between science and conservative pragmatism: the direction and strength of a recommendation needs to be established whilst bearing in mind key principles of guideline development for public health. The key principles are as follows:

• Do not change recommendations where new evidence is not compelling enough to support change
• Aim for consistency of recommendations in terms of its content to facilitate international comparison of adherence to guidelines

Determining the strength of a recommendation involves other factors in addition to the quality of the evidence (see Step 3). In Table 4.5, we provide an overview of the factors that determine the strength of recommendations.

Table 4.5 Factors determining the strength of recommendations (adapted from GRADE https://gdt. gradepro.org/app/handbook/)

Factor	Influence on recommendation
Balance between desirable and undesirable outcomes (trade-offs) taking into account: • best estimates of the magnitude of effects on benefits and risks of PA/sedentary behavior/sleep on health • importance of health outcomes (for the public and practitioners)	The larger the differences between the desirable and undesirable consequences, the more likely a strong recommendation is warranted. The smaller the net benefit and the lower certainty for that benefit, the more likely a less strong recommendation is warranted
Confidence in the magnitude of estimates of effect of PA/sedentary behavior/sleep on important outcomes (overall quality of evidence for outcomes)	The higher the quality of evidence, the more likely a strong recommendation is warranted
Confidence in values and preferences of the public (children and youth, parents, practitioners) and the variability of values and preferences	The greater the variability in values and preferences, or uncertainty about typical values and preferences, the more likely a less strong recommendation is warranted
Resource use	The higher the resources consumed of an intervention (increasing PA/reducing sedentary behavior), the less likely a strong recommendation is warranted

The expert committee considers a recommendation as strong following a risk/benefit appraisal: for example, if they are confident that the desirable effects of engaging in MVPA for 60 minutes per day outweigh the risks associated with being physically active. A strong recommendation implies that most or all children and youth will be best served by the recommended course of action (Andrews et al., 2013). In contrast, a less strong or so-called *conditional* recommendation implies that the majority of children and youth will benefit from adhering to the recommendation but also recognizes that many will not, even though the benefits of following the recommendation probably outweigh the risk of not adhering. Expert committees should label recommendations as less strong or conditional if they are not entirely certainty about the benefits. Where the expert committee faces uncertainty, they are advised to consult the intended end user of the guidelines such as youth, parents, and practitioners to ensure that the final decision on the recommendation is consistent with the end users' preferences and values (Andrews et al., 2013). Consultation of the end user and incorporating their feedback into the final recommendation are part of Steps 5–7, described below.

As briefly described earlier in this chapter, some national expert committees opted for not providing PA recommendations for young children under the age of 5 years. In general, there are two reasons for not drafting recommendations:

1 The confidence in evidence is so low that the expert committee feel a recommendation is too speculative.
2 Irrespective of the confidence in evidence, the benefits and risks are so closely balanced, and if the values and preferences of the end user and resource implications are not known or too variable, the expert committee has great difficulty deciding on the direction of a recommendation (Andrews et al., 2013).

However, users of PA guidelines may be frustrated with the lack of guidance when the guideline committees fail to make a recommendation. The frustration of the guideline user is another reason, in addition to providing a measure for surveillance and international comparability, why a guideline committee may devise recommendations based on expert opinion and practice experience.

Steps 5: Stakeholder Consultation

Involvement of stakeholders in the process of developing guidelines is critical to ensuring that the guideline and its recommendations are meaningful, understood, and used widely. For guideline development, stakeholders typically include national and international content experts, health professionals, government and nongovernmental organizations, teachers, and caregivers: in short, the intended users of the guideline.

Stakeholder consultations can take place face-to-face in workshops or conferences, or through online surveys. In face-to-face consultations, the chair of the expert committee presents the draft recommendations to the stakeholders and then they get a chance to express their preferences, values, and concerns regarding the content, language, and implementation of the recommendation. Online consultations also present the draft recommendations, and a set of specific questions allows the stakeholders to provide feedback.

Steps 6–7: Finalizing Recommendations

Steps 6 and 7 refer to revising the recommendations and investing resources in optimizing the messaging of the recommendations to maximize uptake and impact (Figure 4.5). The final recommendations should reflect the feedback given by the intended guideline users obtained from a national or international consultation. The wording of recommendations should offer the guideline user as many indicators as possible for understanding and interpretation (Andrews et al., 2013). Recommendations need to specify for whom the recommendation is intended, and guideline developers should present recommendations in active voice because recommendations in the passive voice lack clarity. Guideline developers collaborate with creative writers and designers to develop different sets of age appropriate messages of the recommendation to be suitable for children and youth as well as parents and practitioners (Sharratt & Hearst, 2007). As part of the development of the Canadian PA Guidelines in 2002, for example, guideline developers obtained feedback from guideline users in a series of workshops, evaluating the graphics and messages of the recommendations (Sharratt & Hearst, 2007). In Figure 4.3, you can see how the recommendations were presented in the recent PA guidelines in South Africa (2018).

New Approaches to PA Guideline Development

A considerable number of countries have established their own national PA guidelines for children and youth. The large number of PA guidelines globally meant that updates of guidelines could draw on already existing guidelines, in addition to conducting systematic reviews of the most recent evidence (Okely et al., 2018). For example, the UK 2011 PA guidelines were developed considering the evidence compiled for the US 2008 and the Canadian 2011 PA guidelines (Bull & the Expert Working Groups, 2010). To update the UK 2011 guidelines for children and young people in 2019, guideline developers consulted national evidence reviews of 15 European countries and an additional 14 systematic reviews and meta-analyses (UK Children and Young People Expert Working Group, 2018).

Table 4.6 Overview of PA guidelines that adopted or adapted existing guidelines using the GRADE-ADOLOPMENT approach

New national guideline	Adopted guideline	Adapted guideline
New Zealand 2017 (Children & Youth)	Canadian 24-hour movement guidelines (2016)	–
New Zealand 2017 (early years)	Canadian 24-hour movement guidelines (2017)	–
Australia 2017 (early years)	Canadian 24-hour movement guidelines (2017; early years)	–
South Africa 2018 (early years)	–	Canadian 24-hour movement guidelines (2017; early years)
United Kingdom 2019 (early years)	–	Canadian 24-hour movement guidelines (2017; early years)
United Kingdom 2019 (Children and Youth)	–	Dutch 2017 PA guidelines
Australia 2019 (Children and Youth)	Canadian 24-hour movement guidelines (2016; Children and Youth)	–
World Health Organization 2019 (early years)	–	Canadian 24-hour movement guidelines (2017; early years)

The process of reviewing and appraising the quality of existing guidelines and developing subsequent recommendations also varies between countries. The German 2016 PA guideline recommendations were developed using quality criteria for existing guidelines. Twenty-eight quality criteria were established through an expert survey and were clustered around four domains: scope and purpose, rigor of development, clarity and comprehensiveness of content, and arrangement and presentation (Geidl & Pfeifer, 2017).

In contrast, for the development of the Australian 2017 24-hour movement behavior guideline for the early years, the AGREE II tool was used to assess the credibility of Canada's 2017 guideline, on which the Australian guideline was based (Okely et al., 2017). Australia's 2017 24-hour movement behavior guidelines followed a novel approach in guideline development, which is called Grading of Recommendations Assessment, Development and Evaluation (GRADE)–Adaptation, Adoption, and De Novo Development (ADOLOPMENT). GRADE-ADOLOPMENT is a model that leads to adoption or adaptation of existing recommendations, or development of new recommendations (Schünemann et al., 2017). As to whether existing guidelines or certain recommendations should be adopted, adapted or newly developed depends on the context in which the existing guidelines were developed and how applicable the context is to the new guideline context, the credibility of existing guidelines, and the available resources needed to develop guidelines. GRADE-ADOLOPMENT has been used by six countries to date, and Table 4.6 highlights which country adapted or adopted existing guidelines.

Emerging Issues

As outlined in earlier sections of the chapter, the Netherlands updated their children and young people PA guidelines in 2017 (Weggemans et al., 2018). Similarly, the USA, the UK, Australia, South Africa, and the WHO also embarked on their own process of updating respective guidelines in 2018/2019. The continuously increasing evidence base means experts have been able to

Table 4.7 Effect of different measurement decisions to evaluate adherence/prevalence estimates

Day	Minutes of MVPA	Meets every day	On average
Monday	60		
Tuesday	61		
Wednesday	60		
Thursday	59		
Friday	60		
Saturday	60		
Sunday	120		
		6 out of 7 days	420/7 = 60 minutes/day

develop more specific and improved guidelines over the years. Expert working groups involved in the guideline development process have identified important gaps in our current knowledge that would be critical for informing the scientific foundation of future guidelines, from both the syntheses of the best available research evidence but also as a result of stakeholder engagement. This section will therefore explain some of the ongoing debates in the PA field and then provide recommendations for future research and practice drawing on the considerations identified in the technical reports of the aforementioned guideline updates.

Measurement of 'Adherence' to the Guideline Recommendations

The majority of the guidelines includes a recommendation around the duration of PA a child needs to engage in per day. In most countries, the recommendation is at least 60 minutes of MVPA for children and youth and 180 minutes of total PA for the early years. However, while there is consistency around the recommendation a key issue is the inconsistency of surveillance studies measuring the adherence to these criteria. Currently, the adherence to these guidelines has been assessed in multiple different ways. Some studies and national surveillance programs examine adherence as an average per week, whereas others follow an everyday approach (i.e., a child has to meet the guidelines every day) (Currie, Zanotti, & Morgan, 2012). This means that a child participating in a total of 420 minutes of MVPA per week (i.e., an average of 60 minutes per day) can meet the guidelines in one surveillance study; however, if the same child misses out on the threshold during one day they may be classed as inactive in another surveillance study (Table 4.7). This discrepancy can lead to significant differences in the reported percentages of children meeting the guidelines (McCrorie, Mitchell, & Ellaway, 2018). Unfortunately, the current evidence base does not provide us with clear results on whether a child needs to be engaging in PA every day, 6 days per week, 5 days a week, etc. Nevertheless, for surveillance purposes, it is recommended that guidelines are specific in their messaging and surveillance studies operationalize adherence to the guidelines following these recommendations.

Durations, Intensities, and Types of PA

Gaps in the evidence base surrounding the PA duration, intensity, and type still exist. Evidence on a dose-response relationship is sparse, and some may question if the recommended 60 minutes is the "magical number". The lack of evidence around a dose-response relationship of PA and health outcomes makes it hard for guideline developers to establish the minimum amount of PA required for good health (i.e., we start to see improvements in health) and the optimum amount of PA required for good health.

Looking at different intensities of PA, it is well established that MVPA has beneficial effects on a child's and future health. However, much less evidence exists around light intensity PA and/or sedentary behavior. Currently, opinions are divided in regard to the effect of increasing light intensity PA and reducing sedentary behavior to improve health outcomes in children. Some say engaging in enough MVPA counteracts any negative effect that sedentary behavior may have on a child's health (Cliff et al., 2016). However, others state that sedentary behavior does affect a child's health independent of their levels of MVPA (Carson et al., 2016). In addition, researchers have started a debate about the health effects of standing still. Standing still would, according to the sedentary behavior definition (Tremblay, Aubert et al., 2017), be classed as light intensity PA. Nevertheless, researchers have questioned as to whether standing still would have the same effect on health as moving around in a light intensity. Research is needed to determine as to whether increasing standing time improves, maintains, or reduces a child's health.

Sedentary behavior can take place in many forms, one of which being screen time. The effect of screen time on health outcomes has been studied frequently in the literature. However, many studies have focused on TV viewing and so the effects of using new types of screens and multiple screens simultaneously are less known. It can be argued that some types of screen time may have benefits, while others may be more harmful to a child's health (e.g., educational versus non-educational; social versus non-social). While this is acknowledged in several guidelines, the evidence to inform guidelines and provide more detailed recommendations is missing. In addition, the current evidence base around screen time is based on self- or parent-reported screen time, which is more likely to introduce bias toward under reporting due to recall bias. Devices to measure screen time and types of screen time are needed to obtain accurate levels of adherence to the guidelines.

24-Hour Movement Behaviors

As previously discussed, certain countries have started to develop 24-hour movement behavior guidelines. While this may be seen as a step forward, this change does not come without challenges. The evidence on the impact of combinations of behaviors is limited, and as described above there is still a debate as to whether or not these "other" behaviors (i.e., sedentary behavior and light PA) are important for health. There is a need for studies to examine the interaction between these behaviors and increase clarity around this subject. In addition, a consistent approach in regard to measuring adherence to the 24-hour movement guidelines internationally should be established and is crucial to enable international comparison.

Measurement of PA and Sedentary Behaviors

Measuring adherence to the guidelines has often been found difficult, and inconsistencies exist in regard to tools and data analysis methods used to measure adherence to the recommendations. Surveillance studies often use self- and/or parent-report measures, whereas more affluent nations and smaller studies may use device-based measures, such as accelerometry. This inconsistency results in different prevalence estimates and makes comparisons between countries and studies very difficult. In addition, even if a similar tool is used, such as accelerometers, data may be processed and analyzed using different methods (e.g., different cut-points, wear time criteria, and epoch settings) which result in significantly different prevalence outcomes (more on this in Chapter 16). The shift to 24-hour movement guidelines has also created another issue around the measurement and analysis of data (e.g., the use of methods such as compositional data analysis). PA, sedentary behavior, and sleep are traditionally measured using different methods. As a 24-hour day includes all three behaviors, there is need to update current surveillance tools. Tools should be able to measure PA accurately, as well as being able to capture sleep, screen time, overall sedentary behavior. To reduce participant burden it would be recommended to measure these behaviors using one or as a maximum, two methods (e.g., accelerometry for duration and intensity, and questionnaire for type of activity (e.g. screen time)).

Messaging, Communication, and Increasing Awareness

The expectation, which comes with the development of new guidelines, is that they will change behaviors population wide. However, guidelines alone do not change behaviors. Developing a messaging and awareness strategy is a crucial part of the guideline development process. However, this is often seen as the most challenging part, and the implementation of appropriate messaging and awareness campaigns is often lacking. To ensure the guidelines are effective in creating awareness around the importance of PA they should cover the what, why, and how (Brawley & Latimer, 2007). Messages should be informative and persuasive and preferably based on theoretical frameworks for behavior change. The development of a messaging campaign takes time and resources, and requires a collaborative approach between researchers and messaging teams. In addition, ensuring that guidelines are rolled out in combination with community-wide and national-wide PA programs plays a key role in the success of the guidelines (Brawley & Latimer, 2007).

Recommendations for Researchers

Overarching, Cross-Cutting Needs

In addition to addressing the key issues highlighted above, across all recent guideline updates, developers have identified a number of overarching areas of investigation, which should be considered for future updates. For all age groups, there is a recognition that the current guidelines have been developed for the general population and there is a pressing need for guidelines to be developed for children and young people with chronic diseases or disability. Additionally, although there is a strong evidence base for the health benefits of PA, greater clarity is required regarding the potential adverse effects, such as injury and harm; popular modern forms of activity such as High Intensity Interval Training (HIIT); poor posture while being active and risk of musculoskeletal problems; and impact of injury (e.g., concussion) in contact sports.

In general, there is a strong call for researchers to conduct more high-quality studies using either prospective (e.g., cohort studies) or randomized control trials (RCT) to address many of the poorly understood gaps in our knowledge. Specific research priorities exist for particular population groups over and above what can be considered as generic recommendations. If systematically developed from the lab to the free-living environment, these types of studies would provide key evidence regarding the associated changes in light intensity and MVPA, and importantly, their impact on health outcomes. Using the most recent US (2018 PA Guidelines Advisory Committee, 2018) and UK technical reports (UK Children and Young People Expert Working Group, 2018; UK Under 5's Expert Working Group, 2018), Figure 4.6 provides an overview of some of the immediate research priorities for the early years, and similarly Figure 4.7 for children and adolescents aged 5–19.

Evidence gap, issue, research need	Specific research questions, designs and decisions
The evidence base surrounding the recent introduction of 24 hour movement guidelines is in its infancy	• A variety of research designs should be employed to answer the following questions: • What are the optimal amounts, intensities (for PA, PA), and frequencies of the behaviors associated with 24-hour movement. • What are the determinants of the movement behaviors? • What is the current prevalence of the population who meet the 24-hour guidelines and how does this vary internationally and by demographic factors (e.g. age, SES, race/ethnicity). • What are the health and developmental consequences of compliance/non compliance with the guidelines ? • Standing as a behavior is poorly understood in the literature and may be misclassified as either light intensity activity or sedentary time, potentially obscuring associations with health outcomes and bias estimates of these behaviors. • How should the 24-hour movement behaviors be quantified? Are there analytical approaches to analysing multiple behaviors other than compositional analysis?
There is a need for more evidence on the health and developmental impact of contemporary screen-technology	• More modern screen-based technology can be interactive (involving social engagement e.g. with family members) and is potentially less harmful than the kinds of sedentary behavior. What are the benefits/harms of modern more interactive/less passive forms of screen time for the Under 5s?
There is a need for high quality studies that investigate the benefits of outdoor play	• Well-controlled RCTs are need to explore the benefits of active outdoor play over active indoor play? Is there evidence that the ratio of children to outdoor and indoor space is related to frequency, duration and level of PA in infants, toddlers, and pre-schoolers?
There is a need to develop valid instruments for measuring PA in the under 5's	• Specific research designs are required to validate PA measurement instruments in the under 5 population. Due to the lack of validated measures in very young children, our knowledge of the relationship between PA/sedentary time and health outcomes between birth and two years in limited.
There is a strong need to develop the evidence base surrounding the sleep (as exposure and outcome), PA/sedentary, health outcome relationship.	• What is the impact of PA on sleep and impact of sleep on PA? • For **infants and toddlers** what are the associations between sleep duration and: growth; motor development; PA; SB; Quality of Life; wellbeing; risk/ harms such as injuries. • For **pre-schoolers** what are the associations between sleep and emotional regulation; motor development; Quality of Life; wellbeing; risks/harms such as injuries. • What is the impact of screen-time on sleep?, and the timing of screen-time exposure before sleeping?

Figure 4.6 Future recommendations for guideline updates in early year's age group

There is a lack of nationally representative PA data which uses device-based measurements of PA for children and young people	• Include objective measurements of PA into nationally representative surveys and in longitudinal cohort studies. The ability to link new surveys to routine data (e.g. health and education) would be particularly advantageous.
The current research on the relationship between sedentary behaviour and health is limited by the lack of device-based measures of time spent in sedentary behaviour	• Longitudinal research designs should be employed to examine specific forms of sedentary behavior (e.g. sitting time, screen time, patterns incuding breaks) and health outcomes. Research is needed to differentiate between the health effects of time spent sedentary and time spent in specific behaviors that typically include sedentary time.
There is a lack of information on the benefits of meeting the 60 minutes MVPA guideline every day vs. an average per day.	• Longitudinal studies that examine the impact of meeting the national guidelines on each day vs. on average are needed in relation to all major health outcomes.
There is a lack of evidence about the benefits of light-intensity PA among children and young people, alone and in combination with MVPA	• Well-controlled RCTs and prospective designs are needed to examine the impact of light-intensity PA on health outcomes using contemporary analysis approaches. Specific information on the impact of displacing sedentary or MVPA time with light-intensity PA on a number of health outcomes is needed.
There is a lack of evidence on the dose-response relationship between PA and mulitple health outcomes, and if these are modified by demographic factors (e.g. age, race/ethnicity.)	• Research is needed to examine the principles of manipulating the FITT principle in relation to health outcomes at different developmental stages. This will necessitate rigorously controlled experimental studies in which the dose of PA is externally managed and confounding variables are controlled.
There is a need for more high quality evidence on the effect of PA on cognitive development and academic attainment.	• Well-controlled RCTs and high quality prospective data are needed to assess the impact of PA on cognitive development and academic attainment.
There is a lack of high quality evidence on the association between PA and mental health in children.	• Well-controlled RCTs and prospective designs are needed to assess the impact of PA on mental health-related outcomes, with additional information specifically warranted on the benefits of different types (e.g. yoga, tai chi, and resistance training) including the quality and quantity of PA. Ideally, these studies would be sufficiently data rich to control for potential confounders.
There is a lack of evidence to identify the optimal age threshold for the adult PA guidelines, or indeed the age for the transition from the early years to children and young people.	• Research is needed to examine whether there should be a fixed transition between the children and young people's and adults' PA guidelines and, if so, what the age threshold should be. Similarly, more evidence is needed on how to manage the transition from the early years guidelines to the children and young people thresholds.
There is a lack of information on the benefits of different strategies to improve motor competence and the effects of those strategies on PA levels across childhood.	• There is a need for RCTs to assess the impact of different types of skill development programmes on fundamental movement skills and motor competency. There is also a need to examine whether increasing these skills has long-term impacts on PA levels.
There is a lack of high quality evidence in relation to the benefits of High-Intensity Interval Training (HIIT) for children and young people.	• High quality RCTs, with standard definitions of HIIT. These should include evaluation of the acceptability (including adverse effects) and sustainability of HIIT-type exercise to identify feasibility of implementing and identify best practice principles for children and young people.

Figure 4.7 Future recommendations for guideline updates in children and young people

Chapter Summary

This chapter had six main goals: (i) to introduce the reader to the concept of PA and sedentary recommendations, and how they vary internationally; (ii) to demonstrate how they have evolved over time in parallel with the advances in our scientific understanding of the relationship between PA, sedentary behaviors, and health; (iii) to identify how the guideline recommendations vary depending on age group; (iv) to make the reader aware of the scientific process that underpins guideline development and updates, and how this has evolved; (v) to introduce the reader to some of the emerging issues and debates related to guideline development; and (vi) to present what may be considered as the key research priorities for future updates of guidelines internationally. Additionally, as an outcome of reading this chapter, you should have a greater understanding of the importance and relevance of our guideline recommendations to other sections and chapters within this handbook. Finally, and most importantly, we hope you use this knowledge and learning to become critical of the guideline process and research evidence in general.

Note

1 https://bestpractice.bmj.com/info/us/toolkit/learn-ebm/what-is-grade/

References

2018 PA Guidelines Advisory Committee. (2018). *2018 PA guidelines advisory committee scientific report*. Washington, DC: US Department of Health and Human Services. Retrieved October 11, 2018 from https://health.gov/paguidelines/second-edition/report/

Ainsworth, B. E., Haskell, W. L., Whitt, M. C., Irwin, M. L., Swartz, A. M., Strath, S. J., . . . Leon, A. S. (2000). Compendium of physical activities: An update of activity codes and MET intensities. *Medicine and Science in Sports Exercise, 32*(9 Suppl), S498–S504.

American College of Sports Medicine (ACSM). (1988). Opinion statement on physical fitness in children and youth ACSM. *Medicine and Science in Sports and Exercise, 20*, 422–423.

Andrews, J. C., Schünemann, H. J., Oxman, A. D., Pottie, K., Meerpohl, J. J., Coello, P. A., . . . Elbarbary, M. (2013). GRADE guidelines: 15. Going from evidence to recommendation – Determinants of a recommendation's direction and strength. *Journal of Clinical Epidemiology, 66*(7), 726–735.

Australian Department of Health. (2010). *Move and play every day. National physical activity recommendations for children 0–5 years*. Commonwealth of Australia, Department of Health and Ageing. Retrieved October 14, 2018 from https://www1.health.gov.au/internet/main/publishing.nsf/content/F01F92328EDADA-5BCA257BF0001E720D/$File/FS%200-5yrs.PDF

Australian Department of Health. (2014). Australia's PA and sedentary behavior guidelines. Retrieved October 14, 2018 from http://www.health.gov.au/internet/main/publishing.nsf/content/health-pubhlth-strateg-phys-act-guidelines

Australian Department of Health and Ageing. (2004). *Australia's physical activity recommendations for 5–12 year olds, Canberra*. Retrieved October 14, 2018 from https://www.walk.com.au/pdfs/DOHA_205465_ParentsCarers.pdf

Balshem, H., Helfand, M., Schünemann, H. J., Oxman, A. D., Kunz, R., Brozek, J., . . . Guyatt, G. H. (2011). GRADE guidelines: 3. Rating the quality of evidence. *Journal of Clinical Epidemiology, 64*(4), 401–406.

Borgerson, K. (2009). Valuing evidence: Bias and the evidence hierarchy of evidence-based medicine. *Perspectives in Biology and Medicine, 52*(2), 218–233.

Brawley, L. R., & Latimer, A. E. (2007). PA guides for Canadians: Messaging strategies, realistic expectations for change, and evaluation. *Canadian Journal of Public Health, 98*(Suppl 2), S170–S184.

Brouwers, M. C., Kho, M. E., Browman, G. P., Burgers, J. S., Cluzeau, F., Feder, G., . . . Littlejohns, P. (2010). AGREE II: Advancing guideline development, reporting and evaluation in health care. *Canadian Medical Association Journal, 182*(18), E839–E842.

Bull, F. C., & the Expert Working Groups. (2010). *Physical activity guidelines in the U.K.: Review and recommendations*. Loughborough, UK: School of Sport, Exercise and Health Sciences, Loughborough University. Retrieved October 8, 2018 from https://assets.publishing.service.gov.uk/government/uploads/system/uploads/attachment_data/file/213743/dh_128255.pdf

Campbell, A., Calderwood, C., Hunter, G., & Murray, A. (2018). PA investments that work – Get Scotland walking: A national walking strategy for Scotland. *British Journal of Sports Medicine, 52*(12), 759–760. doi:10.1136/bjsports-2017-098776

Canadian Society for Exercise Physiology. (2016). *Canadian 24-hour movement guidelines for children and youth.* Ottawa, Canada. Retrieved October 24, 2018 from https://csepguidelines.ca/children-and-youth-5-17/

Carson, V., Hunter, S., Kuzik, N., Gray, C. E., Poitras, V. J., Chaput, J. P., . . . Tremblay, M. S. (2016). Systematic review of sedentary behavior and health indicators in school-aged children and youth: An update. *Applied Physiology Nutrition and Metabolism, 41*(6 Suppl 3), S240–S265. doi:10.1139/apnm-2015-0630

Carson, V., Lee, E. Y., Hewitt, L., Jennings, C., Hunter, S., Kuzik, N., . . . Adamo, K. B. (2017). Systematic review of the relationships between PA and health indicators in the early years (0–4 years). *BMC Public Health, 17*(5), 854.

Cavill, N., Biddle, S. J. H., & Sallis, J. F. (2001). Health enhancing PA for young people: Statement of the United Kingdom expert consensus conference. *Pediatric Exercise Science, 13*(1), 12–25. doi:10.1123/pes.13.1.12

Chaput, J. P., Carson, V., Gray, C. E., & Tremblay, M. S. (2014). Importance of all movement behaviors in a 24 hour period for overall health. *International Journal of Environmental Research and Public Health, 11*(12), 12575–12581. doi:10.3390/ijerph111212575

Cliff, D. P., Hesketh, K. D., Vella, S. A., Hinkley, T., Tsiros, M. D., Ridgers, N. D., . . . Plotnikoff, R. C. (2016). Objectively measured sedentary behavior and health and development in children and adolescents: Systematic review and meta-analysis. *Obesity Reviews, 17*(4), 330–344.

Craig, P., Cooper, C., Gunnell, D., Haw, S., Lawson, K., Macintyre, S., . . . Thompson, S. (2012). Using natural experiments to evaluate population health interventions: New medical research council guidance. *Journal of Epidemiology and Community Health, 66*(12), 1182–1186. doi:10.1136/jech-2011-200375

Currie, C., Zanotti, C., & Morgan, A. (2012). *Social determinants of health and well-being among young people. Health behaviour in school-aged children (HBSC) Study: International report from the 2009/2010 survey.* Copenhagen, Denmark: WHO Regional Office for Europe (Health Policy for Children and Adolescents, No. 6).

Geidl, W., & Pfeifer, K. (2017). Background and methodology of the development of German PA guidelines. *Gesundheitswesen (Bundesverband der Arzte des Offentlichen Gesundheitsdienstes (Germany)), 79*(Suppl 01), S4–S10.

Health Canada and the Canadian Society for Exercise Physiology. (2002a). *Canada's PA guide for youth.* Cat. No. H39-611/2002-1E. Ottawa, Canada: Minister of Public Works and Government Services. Retrieved October 08, 2018 from http://www.sd22.bc.ca/Programs/health/Documents/Appendix-C_Health_Canada_Physical_Fitness_GuideYouth.pdf

Health Canada and the Canadian Society for Exercise Physiology. (2002b). *Canada's PA guide for children.* Cat. No. H39-611/2002-2E. Ottawa, Canada: Minister of Public Works and Government Services. Retrieved October 08, 2018 from http://publications.gc.ca/site/eng/389049/publication.html

Health Council of the Netherlands. (2017). *PA guidelines 2017.* No. 2017/08e. The Hague, The Netherlands. Retrieved November 14, 2018 from https://research.vu.nl/en/publications/the-2017-dutch-physical-activity-guidelines

Janssen, I. (2014). Active play: An important PA strategy in the fight against childhood obesity. *Canadian Journal of Public Health, 105*(1), e22–e27.

Kirschenbaum, D. (1997). *Mind matters: 7 steps to smarter sport performance.* Carmel, IN: Cooper Publishing Group.

McCrorie, P., Mitchell, R., & Ellaway, A. (2018). Comparison of two methods to assess PA prevalence in children: An observational study using a nationally representative sample of Scottish children aged 10–11 years. *BMJ Open, 8*(1), e018369. doi:10.1136/bmjopen-2017-018369

Ministry of Social Affairs and Health. (2005). *Recommendations for physical activity in early childhood education* (p. 15). Finland: Ministry of Social Affairs and Health. Retrieved September 26, 2019 from https://julkaisut.valtioneuvosto.fi/bitstream/handle/10024/72925/URN%3ANBN%3Afi-fe201504225286.pdf?sequence=1

Morris, J. N., Heady, J. A., Raffle, P. A., Roberts, C. G., & Parks, J. W. (1953a). Coronary heart-disease and PA of work. *Lancet, 265*(6796), 1111–1120.

Morris, J. N., Heady, J. A., Raffle, P. A., Roberts, C. G., & Parks, J. W. (1953b). Coronary heart-disease and PA of work. *Lancet, 265*(6795), 1053–1057.

Okely, A. D., Ghersi, D., Hesketh, K. D., Santos, R., Loughran, S. P., Cliff, D. P., . . . Sherring, J. (2017). A collaborative approach to adopting/adapting guidelines – The Australian 24-hour movement guidelines for the early years (birth to 5 years): An integration of PA, sedentary behavior, and sleep. *BMC Public Health, 17*(5), 869.

Okely, A. D., Tremblay, M. S., Reilly, J. J., Draper, C. E., & Bull, F. (2018). PA, sedentary behavior, and sleep: Movement behaviors in early life. *The Lancet Child & Adolescent Health, 2*(4), 233–235.

PA Task Force. (2003). *Let's make Scotland more active: A strategy for PA.* Edinburgh, Scotland: Scottish Executive.

Pate, R. R., Pratt, M., Blair, S. N., Haskell, W. L., Macera, C. A., Bouchard, C., . . . Kriska, A. (1995). PA and public health. A recommendation from the centers for disease control and prevention and the American college of sports medicine. *JAMA, 273*(5), 402–407.

Pesce, C., Masci, I., Marchetti, R., Vazou, S., Saakslahti, A., & Tomporowski, P. D. (2016). Deliberate play and preparation jointly benefit motor and cognitive development: Mediated and moderated effects. *Frontiers in Psychology, 7*, 349. doi:10.3389/fpsyg.2016.00349

Pfeifer, K., & Rutten, A. (2017). National recommendations for PA and PA promotion. *Gesundheitswesen, 79*(Suppl 01), S2–S3. doi:10.1055/s-0042-123346

Poitras, V. J., Gray, C. E., Janssen, X., Aubert, S., Carson, V., Faulkner, G., . . . Tremblay, M. S. (2017). Systematic review of the relationships between sedentary behavior and health indicators in the early years (0–4 years). *BMC Public Health, 17*(Suppl 5), 868. doi:10.1186/s12889-017-4849-8

Riopel, D. A., Boerth, R. C., Coates, T. J., Miller, W. W., Weidman, W. H., & Hennekens, C. H. (1986). Coronary risk factor modification in children: Smoking. A statement for physicians by the committee on atherosclerosis and hypertension in childhood of the council on cardiovascular disease in the young, American Heart Association. *Circulation, 74*(5), 1192A–1194A.

Rutten, A., & Pfeifer, K. (Eds.). (2016). *National recommendations for PA and PA promotion.* Erlangen, Germany: Florida Atlantic University Press. Retrieved October 11, 2018 from https://www.sport.fau.de/files/2015/05/National-Recommendations-for-Physical-Activity-and-Physical-Activity-Promotion.pdf

Sallis, J. F., Cervero, R. B., Ascher, W., Henderson, K. A., Kraft, M. K., & Kerr, J. (2006). An ecological approach to creating active living communities. *Annual Review of Public Health, 27*, 297–322. doi:10.1146/annurev.publhealth.27.021405.102100

Sallis, J. F., & Patrick, K. (1994). PA guidelines for adolescents: Consensus statement. *Pediatric Exercise Science, 6*(4), 302–314. doi:10.1123/pes.6.4.302

Saunders, T. J., Gray, C. E., Poitras, V. J., Chaput, J. P., Janssen, I., Katzmarzyk, P. T., . . . Carson, V. (2016). Combinations of PA, sedentary behavior and sleep: Relationships with health indicators in school-aged children and youth. *Applied Physiology, Nutrition, and Metabolism, 41*(6 Suppl 3), S283–S293. doi:10.1139/apnm-2015-0626

Schünemann, H. J., Wiercioch, W., Brozek, J., Etxeandia-Ikobaltzeta, I., Mustafa, R. A., Manja, V., . . . Santesso, N. (2017). GRADE evidence to decision (EtD) frameworks for adoption, adaptation, and de novo development of trustworthy recommendations: GRADE-ADOLOPMENT. *Journal of Clinical Epidemiology, 81*,101–110.

Sharratt, M. T., & Hearst, W. E. (2007). Canada's PA guides: Background, process, and development. *Applied Physiology, Nutrition, and Metabolism, 32*(S2E), S9–S15.

Strong, W. B., Malina, R. M., Blimkie, C. J., Daniels, S. R., Dishman, R. K., Gutin, B., . . . Trudeau, F. (2005). Evidence based PA for school-age youth. *Journal of Pediatrics, 146*(6), 732–737. doi:10.1016/j.jpeds.2005.01.055

Tarp, J., Child, A., White, T., Westgate, K., Bugge, A., Grontved, A., . . . International Children's Accelerometry Database Collaborators. (2018). PA intensity, bout-duration, and cardiometabolic risk markers in children and adolescents. *International Journal of Obesity (London), 42*(9), 1639–1650. doi:10.1038/s41366-018-0152-8

Tremblay, M. S., Aubert, S., Barnes, J. D., Saunders, T. J., Carson, V., Latimer-Cheung, A., . . . Chinapaw, M. J. M. (2017). Sedentary behavior research network (SBRN) – Terminology consensus project process and outcome. *International Journal of Behavioral Nutrition and PA, 14*(1), 75.

Tremblay, M. S., Carson, V., Chaput, J. P., Connor Gorber, S., Dinh, T., Duggan, M., . . . Zehr, L. (2016). Canadian 24-hour movement guidelines for children and youth: An integration of PA, sedentary behavior, and sleep. *Applied Physiology, Nutrition, and Metabolism, 41*(6 Suppl 3), S311–327. doi:10.1139/apnm-2016-0151

Tremblay, M. S., Chaput, J. P., Adamo, K. B., Aubert, S., Barnes, J. D., Choquette, L., . . . Gruber, R. (2017). Canadian 24-hour movement guidelines for the early years (0–4 years): An integration of PA, sedentary behavior, and sleep. *BMC Public Health, 17*(5), 874.

Tremblay, M. S., LeBlanc, A. G., Carson, V., Choquette, L., Connor Gorber, S., Dillman, C., . . . Kho, M. E. (2012). Canadian PA guidelines for the early years (aged 0–4 years). *Applied Physiology, Nutrition, and Metabolism, 37*(2), 345–356.

Truelove, S., Vanderloo, L. M., & Tucker, P. (2017). Defining and measuring active play among young children: A systematic review. *Journal of Physical Activity and Health, 14*(2), 155–166. doi:10.1123/jpah.2016-0195

UK Under 5's Expert Working Group. (2018). *UK PA guidelines: Draft review and recommendations for the Under 5's.* University of Bristol. Retrieved October 08, 2018 from http://www.bristol.ac.uk/media-library/sites/sps/documents/cmo/under-5s-technical-report.pdf

UK Children and Young People Expert Working Group. (2018). *UK PA guidelines: Draft review and recommendations for children and young people.* University of Bristol. Retrieved October 08, 2018 from http://www.bristol.ac.uk/media-library/sites/sps/documents/cmo/children-young-people-technical-report.pdf

UK Department of Health and Social Care. (2019). UK Chief Medical Officers' physical activity guidelines. London, UK. Retrieved September 08, 2019 from https://assets.publishing.service.gov.uk/government/uploads/system/uploads/attachment_data/file/832868/uk-chief-medical-officers-physical-activity-guidelines.pdf

US Department of Health and Human Services. (2008). *PA guidelines for Americans.* Washington, DC. Retrieved October 08, 2018 from https://health.gov/paguidelines/guidelines

US Department of Health and Human Services. (2018). *PA guidelines for Americans* (2nd ed.). Washington, DC. Retrieved November 16, 2018 from https://health.gov/paguidelines/second-edition/

VicHealth. (2018). *VicHealth's PA strategy 2018–2023.* Victoria, Australia: VicHealth.

Weggemans, R. M., Backx, F. J. G., Borghouts, L., Chinapaw, M., Hopman, M. T. E., Koster, A., . . . de Geus, E. J. C. (2018). The 2017 Dutch PA guidelines. *International Journal of Behavioral Nutrition and Physical Activity, 15*(1), 58. doi:10.1186/s12966-018-0661-9

World Health Organization. (2010). Global recommendations on PA for health. Geneva, Switzerland. Retrieved October 11, 2018 from https://www.who.int/dietphysicalactivity/factsheet_young_people/en/

World Health Organization. (2018). *Global action plan on PA 2018–2030: More active people for a healthier world.* Geneva, Switzerland: World Health Organization.

Yogman, M., Garner, A., Hutchinson, J., Hirsh-Pasek, K., & Golinkoff, R. M. (2018). The power of play: A pediatric role in enhancing development in young children. *Pediatrics, 142*(3). doi:10.1542/peds.2018-2058

PART 2

Benefits of Physical Activity

5

PHYSIOLOGICAL HEALTH BENEFITS OF PHYSICAL ACTIVITY FOR YOUNG PEOPLE

Narelle Eather, Kate Ridley, and Angus Leahy

Introduction

Chapter Overview and Definitions

This chapter focuses on the physiological responses to physical activity and the associated health benefits in children and adolescents. The chapter has a specific focus on the impact of physical activity intensity on health. In the context of physical activity, physiological responses refer to how an individual's cells, tissues, and organs adapt when they are exposed to activity of varying intensity and duration. Physiological responses to physical activity are influenced by factors such as age, sex, physical disability, and environmental conditions (Burton, Stokes, & Hall, 2004; Rivera-Brown & Frontera, 2012). Exercise programs can induce varied physiological responses in individuals when the principles of training are considered and elements such as exercise frequency, intensity, duration, and mode are manipulated (Hoffman, 2002). Changes to heart rate, ventilation rate, skeletal muscle activation and energy metabolism, lactate levels, oxygen uptake, and hormonal and immune responses are typical physiological responses to aerobic and resistance exercise (Rivera-Brown & Frontera, 2012; U.S. Department of Health and Human Services, 1996). The cardiovascular and respiratory systems are primarily responsible for enabling sustained movement over extended periods, with additional and specific physiological adaptations observed in these systems with long-term physical activity participation (Rivera-Brown & Frontera, 2012). The magnitude of these changes is largely contingent on the intensity and duration of the physical activity, the force or load used in training, and an individual's baseline fitness level (Burton et al., 2004; U.S. Department of Health and Human Services, 1996). A reduction or cessation of physical activity or training results in the gradual loss of most physiological adaptations gained.

The earliest evidence linking participation in physical activity with health outcomes was established in adults, and the most commonly reported physical health outcomes are all-cause mortality, cardiovascular disease, metabolic syndrome, overweight and obesity, type 2 diabetes, osteoporosis, and cancer risk (Garber et al., 2011). A curvilinear reduction in disease risk occurs across volume of activity, with the steepest gradient at the lowest end of the activity scale (i.e., some activity is better than none, and more is better than some) (Powell, Paluch, & Blair, 2011).

The physiological mechanisms explaining the relationships between physical activity and health outcomes are complex (a detailed discussion is beyond the scope of this chapter) (Silverman & Deuster, 2014). Research indicates that physical activity exposes an individual to altered hemodynamic and hormonal milieu production, often eliciting substantial structural, functional, and electrical remodeling, and increasing capacities for blood flow and oxygen consumption in many organs of the body (especially the heart and skeletal muscles) (Hamilton, Hamilton, & Zderic, 2004; Heinonen et al., 2014). An active lifestyle also stimulates potent biochemical and molecular processes essential for preventing the impact of inactivity on chronic metabolic diseases. For example, the lipoprotein lipase (LPL: an enzyme assisting in the breakdown of fat) is one of the few proteins studied across the physical activity intensity continuum and data demonstrates a strong and inverse relationship between LPL activity and cardiovascular disease (Hamilton et al., 2004). Furthermore, the anti-inflammatory effects of regular physical activity or exercise have been shown to promote behavioral and metabolic resilience, and protect against various chronic diseases associated with systemic inflammation (Silverman & Deuster, 2014). On the flip side, spending extended periods in sedentary behaviors, such as prolonged sitting, has been shown to have deleterious effects on health, with sedentary individuals at increased risk for all-cause and cardiovascular disease mortality, diabetes, obesity, and risk factors for cardiovascular disease (Powell et al., 2011).

One benefit of engaging in regular physical activity is the development of health-related physical fitness. Indeed, physical activity is central to the development of cardiorespiratory fitness, muscular fitness, and favorable body composition in youth, all of which contribute to overall health (Morrow et al., 2013). Review-level evidence has demonstrated the health-enhancing benefits of attaining sufficient levels of physical fitness (Ortega, Ruiz, Castillo, & Sjostrom, 2008; Smith et al., 2014). Of note, cardiorespiratory fitness has been described as a 'powerful marker of health' (Ortega et al., 2008), and is an important predictor of current and future health. It is worth noting that in adults, children, and adolescents cardiorespiratory fitness is associated with meaningful health outcomes, independent of physical activity levels (Åberg et al., 2015; Lang et al., 2018; Van der Velde, Savelberg, Schaper, & Koster, 2015). There is evidence to suggest a small-to-moderate relationship exists between habitual physical activity and cardiorespiratory fitness; however, the strength of this relationship improves when higher physical activity intensities are examined (Lang et al., 2018). There is clear evidence supporting the inclusion of aerobic physical activities that develop cardiorespiratory fitness within youth physical activity and fitness programs (Ortega et al., 2008; Ruiz et al., 2009). However, recently there has been a growing interest in the utility of promoting resistance-based physical activities to develop components of muscular fitness (Faigenbaum et al., 2009; Lloyd et al., 2014; Wolfe, 2006). The health benefits of developing muscular fitness during youth are extensive (Grøntved et al., 2015; Smith et al., 2014), and muscular fitness has been shown to be a predictor of cardiovascular disease, skeletal health, and psychological health (Catley & Tomkinson, 2013). Clearly, physical fitness is an important predictor of current and future health status (Morrow et al., 2013). For many individuals, modifying the frequency, intensity, duration, or type of physical activity will produce meaningful changes in fitness (Hoffman, 2002); therefore, identifying strategies to engage youth in health-enhancing physical activity should be a public health priority.

Physical Activity Intensity and Physiological Benefits for Children and Adolescents

Physical Activity Intensity Terminology

Physical activity intensity directly relates to energy expenditure, and ranges from activities demanding very low levels of energy expenditure (e.g., sitting quietly) to activities requiring extreme levels of energy expenditure (e.g., professional sports) (Norton, Norton, & Sadgrove, 2010).

Physical activity intensity is commonly expressed as either an absolute measure (such as heart rate, HR; metabolic equivalent task, MET; or oxygen-carrying capacity VO_2 max) or as a relative measure (such as percentage of maximum heart rate). Norton and colleagues (2010) propose five categories spanning the physical activity intensity continuum, these include sedentary, light intensity, moderate intensity, vigorous intensity and high-intensity activities (Norton et al., 2010), although many researchers combine the upper two categories as simply 'vigorous activity' (Pate, O'Neill, & Lobelo, 2008). The categories directly related to the energy demands, physiological stress, and typical metabolic and neuro-humoral responses of individuals participating in physical activities of specific intensity (Norton et al., 2010), and are summarized in Table 5.1. The latest physical activity guidelines published by the U.S. Department of Health and Human Services promote minimum recommended levels of physical activity for children and adolescents and specify the intensity of activity needed for achieving optimal health. Young people (age 6–17 years) are encouraged to participate in a variety of physical activities that are age appropriate and enjoyable for at least 60 minutes each day. It is recommended that the physical activities be of moderate-to-vigorous intensity and include vigorous intensity physical activity on at least three days a week. Furthermore, young people are encouraged to engage in muscle- and bone-strengthening activities at least 3 times per week as part of their 60 minutes or more of daily physical activity (U.S. Department of Health and Human Services, 2018).

Overview of Association between Physical Activity Intensity for Physiological Health Benefits

Observational studies have demonstrated that participating in moderate intensity physical activities leads to many health benefits not achieved through light intensity physical activity (Jansseen & LeBlanc, 2010; Kistler et al., 2011; Saint-Maurice, Troiano, Berrigan, Kraus, & Matthews, 2018). Data also suggest that vigorous intensity activities provide additional health benefits (Jansseen & LeBlanc, 2010; Powell et al., 2011; Tarp et al., 2018). Although the associations are not clear, researchers suggest the increased amount of energy expended and the unique physiological responses exhibited by individuals exposed to acute and chronic bouts of higher intensity physical activities explain the lower incidence of coronary heart disease and more favorable risk factor profiles (Powell et al., 2011). On the other end of the intensity scale, a growing body of evidence supports the independent and unique health risks of prolonged exposure to sedentary activities in adults (Kokkinos, 2012; van der Ploeg, Chey, Korda, Banks, & Bauman, 2012; Zhu & Owen, 2017). Sedentary behavior has a direct influence on metabolism, bone mineral content, and vascular health, with a dose-response relationship observed between time spent in sedentary behaviors (e.g., sitting watching TV, driving a car, or playing computer games) and all-cause and cardiovascular disease mortality, and other important health outcomes (such as diabetes, metabolic syndrome, obesity, cancer, and psychological well-being) (Tremblay, Colley, Saunders, Healy, & Owen, 2010). High-quality investigations exploring the association between various health outcomes and sedentary behaviors in young people are limited, possibly due to the complexity of this research area and the number of possible mediators, moderators, and confounders at play (Biddle, Garcia Bengoechea, & Wiesner, 2017; Biddle, Pearson, & Salmon, 2018; Cliff et al., 2016). However, emerging evidence supports the dose-response relationship between select sedentary behaviors (e.g., screen-time) and some health outcomes (e.g., adiposity, psychological health, health-related quality of life) (Biddle et al., 2017; Wu et al., 2017), with evidence also suggesting that young people who are highly sedentary can minimize the deleterious health effects through high levels of participation in physical activities (Mitchell & Byun, 2014; Wu et al., 2017).

Table 5.1 Categories of physical activity intensity (adapted from Norton et al., 2010)

Category	Description	Activities	Measures
Sedentary	Any waking behavior characterized by minimal energy expenditure, while in a sitting, reclining, or lying posture (Tremblay et al., 2017)	Sitting watching TV, playing non-active video games, computer use, driving, sewing, fishing, and reading	<1.5 METs <40% HR max <20% HRR <20% VO_2 max RPE (C): <8 RPE (C-R): <1 Very, very light
Light	Activities requiring standing up and moving around, either in the home, workplace, or community. The activity does not result in noticeable changes to breathing or heart rate and can be sustained for long periods	Housework (hanging out the washing, ironing, and cooking), walking slowly	Children: 1.5 to 4 METs 40% to 55% HR max. 20% to 40% HRR 2% to 40% VO_2 max. RPE (C): 8–10 RPE (C-R): 1–2 Very light-light
Moderate	Activities requiring some effort but you can still talk while doing them	Brisk walking, recreational swimming, social tennis, leisurely bike ride, heavy cleaning (washing the windows or vacuuming), lawn mowing	Children: 4–6 METs 55% to 70% HR max 40% to 60% HRR 40% to 60% VO_2 max RPE (C): 11–13 RPE (C-R): 3–4 Moderate – Somewhat hard
Vigorous	Activities accelerate the heart rate and cause rapid breathing, or puffing and panting (depending on your fitness) (World Health Organization, 2004). Activity can be sustained for up to about 30 minutes	Aerobics, jogging, competitive sports, resistance training, lifting, carrying and digging, cycling, and playing with children	6–9 METs 70% to 90% HR max 60% to 85% HRR 60% to 85% VO_2 max RPE (C): 14–16 RPE (C-R): 5–6 Hard
High	An activity of intensity that generally cannot be sustained for longer than about 10 minutes	Hard running or sprinting, tackling, periods of team competitive sports	≥ 9 METs ≥90% HR max ≥85% HRR ≥85% VO_2 max RPE (C): ≥17 RPE (C-R): ≥7 Very hard (Welk, Morrow, & Saint-Maurice, 2017)

Notes: One MET is defined as the energy cost of sitting quietly and can be measured in a laboratory by measuring gas exchange varies or predicted using equations based on age, sex, and body characteristics (body mass, height, fat free mass, etc.). In children, one MET is typically equivalent to a caloric consumption of approximately 1.2–1.5 kcal/kg/hour (Herrmann et al., 2017; Honas et al., 2016; Norton et al., 2010; World Health Organization, 2004). As the variability in body composition during growth in childhood influences both resting and activity energy expenditure, the MET cut-point for moderate activity differs between children and adults.; RPE: Borg's Rating of Perceived Exertion (RPE) scale, category scale 0–10 (Borg, 1998); % HRmax: percentage of heart rate maximum (heart rate maximum = 220 − age); %HRR: percentage of heart rate reserve (heart rate reserve = HRmax − resting HR); %VO_2 max: percentage of maximum oxygen uptake.

Physiological Benefits of Physical Activity across the Intensity Spectrum

Overview of Physical Activity for Children and Adolescents

A well-established body of evidence demonstrates the physiological health benefits of children and adolescents who are sufficiently active (Janssen & Leblanc, 2010; Poitras et al., 2016; Reiner, Niermann, Jekauc, & Woll, 2013). Participation in any form of physical activity is beneficial; however, national and international guidelines recommended that children and adolescents should accumulate at least 60 minutes of moderate-to-vigorous physical activity (MVPA) daily, while also engaging in activities that strengthen muscle and bone on at least 3 days per week to accrue the associated benefits (Australian Government, 2014; World Health Organization, 2010).

Light-Intensity Physical Activity

Given that approximately 80% of youth worldwide are currently not meeting physical activity guidelines, improvements in heath are achievable from relatively small increases in regular physical activity. Light physical activity is typically classified as activity performed between 1.6 and 3 metabolic equivalents (METs), and ranges from static (i.e., standing or stationary) to dynamic (i.e., casual walking) activities (Tremblay et al., 2017). It is important to consider that youth engage in activities of light intensity more commonly than MVPA, and therefore, activities of lower intensity may be more attainable and easier to promote to a relatively inactive population (Carson et al., 2013).

Evidence from an observational study in a large sample of adolescents suggests that time spent in light intensity activity was associated with improved cardio-metabolic biomarkers (i.e., lower diastolic blood pressure, and higher high-density lipoprotein [HDL] cholesterol) (Carson et al., 2013). Specifically, each additional hour per day of low light intensity physical activity was associated with a 0.59 mmHG lower diastolic blood pressure. However, it is important to note that greater effects were observed for time spent in activity toward the higher end of the light intensity continuum (i.e., more dynamic activities), with each additional hour per day associated with a 1.67 mmHG lower diastolic blood pressure and 0.04 mmol/L higher HDL cholesterol. There is also evidence to suggest objectively measured light physical activity is associated with cardiorespiratory fitness in adolescents (Ekelund et al., 2007; Martinez-Gomez et al., 2010). However, findings within the literature are not consistent and therefore should be interpreted with caution (Poitras et al., 2016). While there remains a scarcity of research examining the impact of light physical activity in youth (Carson et al., 2013), there is accumulating evidence suggesting that low-intensity activity can have health-enhancing benefits in older populations (Chastin et al., 2018; Fuzeki, Engeroff, & Banzer, 2017; Saint-Maurice, Troiano, Berrigan, Kraus, & Matthews, 2018).

A recent meta-analysis examining acute studies in adults highlighted the benefit of engaging in frequent short bouts of light physical activity on postprandial glucose and insulin levels. Specifically, interrupting sedentary behavior and engaging in light physical activity reduced postprandial glucose by about 17% and insulin by 25% (Chastin et al., 2018). Several chronic studies have also reported improvements in a range of health outcomes. For example, one study reported an improvement in VO_2 max by 5.5% after 6 weeks (Nishida et al., 2011), while another found a 6% reduction in total cholesterol following 12 weeks of mild walking (Okano, Sato, & Murata, 1990). Experimental studies in children and adolescents are lacking, and adult studies have predominantly used physical activities that are not likely to appeal to children and adolescents (e.g., treadmill walking or stationary cycling) (Chastin et al., 2018; Hulteen et al., 2017). As such, innovative intervention designs are warranted. Exergaming appears to be a potentially novel and viable strategy for increasing light physical activity in youth. Several reviews on this topic have highlighted the utility of this approach to motivate and engage youth in physical activity, while providing some evidence of health-enhancing benefits (Gao & Chen, 2014; Lamboglia et al., 2013; Zeng & Gao, 2016). Specifically, one review reported that exergaming has the potential to improve physical activity levels and energy expenditure, and reduce waist circumference (Lamboglia et al., 2013). Although promising, the limited number of experimental trials and low-quality research design requires more research for definitive conclusions to be made on the effects of health-related outcomes (Zeng & Gao, 2016). In summary, there is evidence to support that light physical activity might be a pragmatic approach for producing health benefits, particularly for those individuals engaging in no or minimal physical activity or commencing a physical activity program.

Moderate-Intensity Physical Activity

International guidelines recommend that children and adolescents should aim to accumulate at least 60 minutes of daily activity that is at least moderate intensity (World Health Organization, 2010). A majority of this should comprise activities that are aerobic in nature such as brisk walking, riding a bike or scooter, or mowing the lawn. As part of the recommended 60 minutes, children and adolescents should also include age-appropriate muscle- and bone-strengthening activities on at least three days per week (World Health Organization, 2010). These activities help to develop musculoskeletal fitness and often involve activities such as body weight resistance training (i.e., push-ups, squats), climbing, jumping, and pushing or pulling activities (e.g., tug-o-war). Moderate intensity activities require greater oxygen consumption and effort in comparison to light activities (i.e., noticeably accelerating heart rate and respiratory rate). There is overwhelming evidence demonstrating the health benefits for youth who engage in sufficient doses of moderate physical activity, with greater benefits observed for those who meet or exceed the recommended guidelines (Arundell, Hinkley, Veitch, & Salmon, 2015; Carson, Chaput, Janssen, & Tremblay, 2017; Hoffman, 2002; Janssen & LeBlanc, 2010; Sothern, Loftin, Suskind, Udall, & Blecker, 1999; U.S. Department of Health and Human Services, 2018).

A recent review of key health indicators and physical activity behaviors (including data from over 200,000 children and adolescents from a range of observational and experimental studies) (Poitras et al., 2016) emphasizes that the strongest health benefits are achieved when young people participate in activity of at least moderate intensity and achieve high levels of physical fitness (Janssen & LeBlanc, 2010; Physical Activity Guidelines Advisory Committee, 2018). The risk of premature mortality and chronic diseases decreases by 20%–30% for youth satisfying physical activity intensity guideline recommendations, with greater reductions observed when healthy physical fitness levels are also achieved (Warburton & Bredin, 2017). In addition, higher physical fitness during childhood and adolescence (particularly cardiorespiratory fitness) is associated with a plethora of favorable health outcomes (including lower waist circumference, body fatness, and decreased risk of mortality later in life) (Hogstrom, Nordstrom, & Nordstrom, 2016). Evidence from observational studies suggests a favorable association between moderate intensity activity and aerobic fitness (Gutin, Yin, Humphries, & Barbeau, 2005; Ottevaere et al., 2011); however, these effects appear to be stronger when activity of high intensity (i.e., moderate-to-vigorous, and vigorous intensity activity) is examined independently. It is hard to determine which specific level of physical activity intensity (within the moderate-to-vigorous intensity range) mediates improvements in health outcomes, as very few studies independently examine moderate versus vigorous activity in youth (Owens, Galloway, & Gutin, 2015); higher intensity physical activities (i.e., MVPA and vigorous intensity activity) are more commonly studied (Poitras et al., 2016).

While evidence supports a dose-response relationship for those engaging in greater amounts of MVPA (World Health Organization, 2010), the improvements in health may be attributable to greater amounts of vigorous intensity activity as opposed to moderate intensity activity.

Experimental studies examining the effects of physical activity on cardio-metabolic risk factors suggest that in order for benefits to occur, activities should be aerobic and involve at least moderate intensity (Okely et al., 2012). Moreover, participation in a range of moderate intensity physical activities is sufficient to produce 8%–10% improvements in cardiorespiratory fitness (Baquet, van Praagh, & Berthoin, 2003). For example, the results from two studies involving obese adolescents found that participation in a 12-week moderate intensity interval training program (70%–80% max aerobic speed sessions three times per week) (Racil et al., 2013) or continuous training program (30–60 minutes twice per week) (Corte de Araujo et al., 2012) can significantly improve VO_2 max. Similarly, adolescents participating in a traditional aerobic program (20 minutes of continuous running at 70% of VO_2 max) significantly improved aerobic fitness over a 7-week period (Buchan et al., 2011).

Although the majority of physical activity research in youth has focused on the effects of aerobic exercise, there is also strong and building evidence demonstrating the health benefits of engaging in regular resistance training programs for improving health and fitness levels (Faigenbaum et al., 2009; Lloyd et al., 2014). Recently, the beneficial effects of muscular fitness have been shown to be independent of cardiorespiratory fitness. In addition to the favorable effects on adiposity and bone health, studies have also demonstrated that muscular fitness is important for preventing injury in young people (Smith et al., 2014). Together these findings suggest that in addition to aerobic physical activities, there is strong evidence to support that youth should engage in activities that develop muscular fitness, further supporting the inclusion of muscle- and bone-strengthening activities within the youth physical activity guidelines (World Health Organization, 2010).

Vigorous-Intensity Physical Activity

Recently, international physical activity guidelines were revised and extended to recommend that youth should engage in some vigorous intensity activity. Vigorous physical activity refers to activity that is performed at or above 6 METs, and reflects greater physiological demands than activities of lower intensities. This type of activity elicits more pronounced acute effects such as increased respiration rate, heart rate, and energy consumption (World Health Organisation, 2017). Examples of vigorous physical activities include fast cycling, jogging, and competitive individual/team sports. While participation in any form of physical activity is essential for a range of health outcomes, accumulating evidence suggests that vigorous intensity physical activity is particularly potent for young people's physical health, providing additional benefits to that of lower intensities (Hay et al., 2012; Janssen & LeBlanc, 2010; Swain & Franklin, 2006).

Observational evidence from adult studies has demonstrated the potent health benefits of vigorous physical activity (Gebel et al., 2015; Janssen & Ross, 2012; Lee & Paffenbarger, 2000). These findings are consistent with studies conducted in children and adolescents, with stronger associations observed between favorable health and vigorous physical activity than activities of lower intensity (Andersen et al., 2006; Wittmeier, Mollard, & Kriellaars, 2008). Recently, a cross-sectional study of Canadian youth found that cardio-metabolic risk declined in a dose-response manner with increasing amounts of vigorous physical activity but not with increased light or moderate activity. Specifically, increased vigorous activity produced greater benefits than moderate activity for Body Mass Index (BMI), waist circumference, and cardiorespiratory fitness. Interestingly, health benefits were achieved through only an additional seven minutes/day of vigorous activity (Hay et al., 2012). These findings are in line with a previous cross-sectional study in children which found that vigorous physical activity was the only significant predictor of body fat (as assessed by skinfold thickness and Body Max Index), in comparison to total physical activity, moderate physical activity, and MVPA (Ruiz et al., 2006). Furthermore, greater benefits were observed for those who engaged in higher amounts of vigorous physical activity (i.e., >40 minutes/day) for body fat and cardiorespiratory fitness, which suggests a dose-response relationship (i.e., the more vigorous physical activity, the greater the health benefits). Objectively measured vigorous physical activity was also found to be positively associated with muscular fitness (Smith et al., 2019). Further, similar levels of muscular fitness were observed for adolescents who engaged in greater amounts of vigorous activity and those who engaged in regular resistance training, demonstrating the additional health benefits beyond that of moderate intensity activity (Martinez-Gomez et al., 2011). Overall, it appears that engaging in vigorous physical activity is more beneficial for children and adolescents than moderate physical activity, particularly for adiposity, cardiorespiratory fitness, and bone health (Sacheck, 2017).

To date, a majority of the literature examining the health benefits of vigorous physical activity have been observational, with few experimental studies conducted in youth (Sacheck, 2017). A potentially useful approach for promoting vigorous intensity activity in youth is high-intensity interval training (HIIT). Of note, a recent report compiled by the U.S.' physical activity guidelines review committee recommended that novel approaches to physical activity promotion such as HIIT should be explored (Physical Activity Guidelines Advisory Committee, 2018). Accumulating evidence suggests HIIT can provide health-enhancing benefits, such as improved cardiorespiratory fitness, body composition, and cardiovascular disease biomarker health (Costigan et al., 2015; Eddolls, McNarry, Stratton, Winn, & Mackintosh, 2017; Harris et al., 2017; Leahy et al., 2019; Logan, Harris, Duncan, & Schofield, 2014), and elicit positive affective and psychological responses to exercise in youth (Oliveira, Santos, Kilpatrick, Pires, & Deslandes, 2018). HIIT consists of short, yet intense bouts of activity (>85% of age-predicated maximal heart rate) interspersed with periods of active rest or recovery. While the origins of HIIT can date back to the early 20th century, the utility of HIIT as an exercise modality for the general population has only recently gained traction. The main appeal of this type of training is that it can induce similar physiological benefits to that of moderate intensity continuous training but in a fraction of the time (Engel, Ackermann, Chtourou, & Sperlich, 2018; Milanovic, Sporis, & Weston, 2015), which may help mitigate common barriers to exercise such as lack of time.

The effect to which acute bouts of high-intensity exercise impact health outcomes has been given less attention in comparison to longer study designs. The combined evidence suggests that acute bouts of activity produce a number of health benefits either comparable or superior than prolonged bouts of activity (Bond, Weston, Williams, & Barker, 2017). Evidence from chronic studies also highlights the utility of HIIT for improving body composition and cardio-respiratory fitness (CRF) in adolescents. For example, one study in a large sample of adolescents reported significant improvements in cardio-respiratory fitness following a ten-week program involving only one session per week (Baquet, Berthoin, Gerbeaux, & Van Praagh, 2001). In another study, overweight and obese adolescents who participated in HIIT training twice per week for 3 months significantly improved VO$_2$ max by 9.3% over the study period (Tjonna et al., 2009). In regard to population health, school-based interventions are widely regarded as the most effective way to impact the health of young people. As mentioned previously, a main appeal of HIIT is the time-efficient nature in which it can delivered; therefore, researchers are beginning to design HIIT interventions that can feasibly be embedded into the school day. Though still emerging, there is evidence to support the effectiveness of school-based HIIT programs (Bond et al., 2017; Leahy et al., 2019). Given its relative infancy more research is required; however, preliminary findings are promising and suggest that school-based HIIT programs can positively affect cardiorespiratory fitness, body composition, and blood pressure, and are well received by participants.

Sedentary Behaviors and Physiological Health in Children and Adolescents

Sedentary Behavior Terminology

Compared to the large body of physical activity research generated over decades, sedentary behavior research in children and adolescents is still in its infancy. Sedentary behavior is defined as "any waking behavior characterized by an energy expenditure ≤1.5 metabolic equivalents (METs), while in a sitting, reclining or lying posture" (Tremblay et al., 2017). The definition comprises both a postural (i.e. sitting, reclining, or lying) and an energy expenditure (i.e., ≤1.5 METs) criterion. To be considered sedentary, an activity needs to meet both criteria. For example, sitting while performing a leg press exercise is not considered sedentary as the energy expenditure required to lift the weights would exceed the 1.5 MET sedentary cut-point (Butte et al., 2018). Conversely, an activity such as talking while standing which may require less energy expenditure than 1.5 METs to perform would also not be considered sedentary due to the standing posture. Sedentary behaviors are often further classified by the type of activity performed. Screen-based sedentary behavior includes activities such as watching television, playing video games, and using computer or tablet devices while seated. Non-screen-based sedentary behavior commonly includes activities such as playing board games, reading, and undertaking homework. The way sedentary behavior is accrued across the day is referred to as 'temporal (time) patterning'. Individuals can spend a long time being sedentary in one session, or 'bout' (e.g., while watching a movie), or can accumulate sedentary time in shorter bouts across the day interspersed with other light, moderate, or vigorous activity. While the effects of temporal patterning have been studied more extensively in adults than children to-date, there is evidence that the temporal patterning of sedentary behavior has influence on health outcomes.

Associations between Sedentary Behavior and Physiological Health

The physical health outcomes most commonly researched in relation to sedentary behavior include weight status/body composition, cardio-metabolic health (e.g., blood glucose control and blood lipids), cardiorespiratory fitness, and bone health. The evidence surrounding the associations between overall sedentary time (typically measured objectively) and physical health and development is inconsistent (Cliff et al., 2016). Observational epidemiologic studies show mixed results for body composition, cardio-metabolic risk score, and overall bone health (Carson, Lee et al., 2017). The effect of sedentary behavior on bone health may be most apparent in the lower body, i.e. higher bone mineral density in the femoral neck observed in children who had lower overall sedentary time (Koedijk et al., 2017). Of the physical health outcomes typically investigated, cardiorespiratory fitness has been most consistently associated with total sedentary behavior (van Ekris et al., 2016). Although the effect of overall sedentary time on the physical health of children and adolescents is yet to be determined, different types of sedentary behavior appear to have different associations with health. Of note, screen-time behaviors are more often associated with deleterious health outcomes than non-screen-time behaviors. Time spent watching television is most consistently associated with unfavorable body composition and weight status and cardiorespiratory fitness (Carson, Hunter, et al., 2016), while overall screen-time, encompassing television viewing, computer use, and playing video games, has been associated with lower muscular endurance and strength (Carson, Hunter, et al., 2016).

A number of experimental studies have examined the effect of reducing sedentary behavior on physical health outcomes. Studies conducted in adults have found breaking up prolonged periods of sitting with standing and/or moving at light or moderate intensity assists in controlling blood glucose (Chastin, Egerton, Leask, & Stamatakis, 2015), which plays an important role in the development and management of type 2 diabetes. Experimental laboratory studies in children have involved consuming meals of standardized energy composition followed by different experimental conditions of sedentary behavior to examine the effects on markers of cardio-metabolic risk such as circulating levels of glucose, insulin, and lipids in the blood. In general these experiments have yielded mixed results with some studies reporting no associations with cardio-metabolic risk (Saunders et al., 2013; Verswijveren et al., 2018), and others that find breaking up sitting with MVPA have a positive effect on glucose metabolism specifically (Belcher et al., 2015; Fletcher et al., 2015). Prolonged sitting in children also appears to affect blood vascular function, a significant contributor to cardiovascular disease in later life. Deterioration in vascular function was observed during 3-hour of continuous sitting, but was prevented by interrupting sitting with moderate exercise for 10-minute every hour (McManus et al., 2015). One recent small but novel experimental study attempted to simulate the nature of classroom sitting conditions in a laboratory to examine the short-term physical effects of reducing prolonged bouts of sitting by incorporating breaks of light intensity activity (e.g. standing, stretching) (Penning et al., 2017). Energy intake and MVPA was standardized across the two conditions of a typical school day and reduced sitting with both cognitive function and cardio-metabolic outcomes measured. Significant improvements were observed in apolipoproteins (proteins that play a role in lipid transport) in the reduced sitting condition. The effects for cholesterol profile and cognition didn't reach statistical significance, perhaps influenced by the small sample size, yet medium effect sizes were observed suggesting reducing sitting time in schools for cardio-metabolic and cognitive benefit warrants further experimental investigation.

A small number of experimental studies have examined the effect of reducing sedentary behavior on health outcomes in children. Intervention studies conducted in both home and school environments have attempted to change both screen-based and non-screen sedentary time. Interventions targeting recreational screen-time have used behavior change strategies and have targeted the individual (e.g. goal setting, self-monitoring, and rewards), the social environment (support from peers and family), and the physical environment (electronic television monitoring devices). Many have been successful in achieving small, but significant, reductions in screen-time and positive effects on weight status. Intervention effects have been more pronounced in overweight and obese children (Biddle et al., 2017; Biddle, Petrolini, & Pearson, 2014). Strategies to reduce sedentary behavior in schools have included implementing sit-to-stand desks, taking active breaks from sitting and incorporating physically active lessons. The use of sit-to-stand desks has shown some evidence for increasing overall energy expenditure (Ee et al., 2018), but mixed effects for changes in steps, standing or sitting time (Sherry, Pearson, & Clemes, 2016). Interpreting the evidence from intervention studies can be difficult as interventions often target and report behaviors other than sedentary behaviors, including MVPA and diet, so it is difficult to isolate the effect of reduced sedentary time (Biddle et al., 2017).

Mechanisms Explaining the Associations between Sedentary Behavior and Health

To better understand why sedentary behavior demonstrates associations with physical health independent of MVPA, it is necessary to consider the mechanisms that may be responsible. Three mechanisms that have been proposed to contribute to the observed associations between sedentary time and physical health are displacement of physical activity, concurrent behaviors such as poor diet, and physiological responses to sitting. The displacement hypothesis suggests that sedentary behavior replaces physical activity time leading to increased disease risk. In children and adolescents, the displacement hypothesis is most relevant on weekends and during the daylight after-school period where individuals have more discretion over their activity choices (Arundell et al., 2015). Other behaviors, such as poor diet, that occur while individuals are being sedentary may also have negative effects on health. This concurrent behavior may partially explain the unique associations observed between television viewing and body composition. For example, studies have found increased snacking (Pearson et al., 2017) and consumption of discretionary foods while watching television. However, a systematic review of studies that measured various sedentary behaviors and dietary intake in adolescents found the majority of positive associations between sedentary behavior and adiposity was independent of diet (Fletcher et al., 2015). Finally, the physiological responses to sitting may be different to those observed when participating in MVPA. Laboratory studies of sedentary physiology responses in rats suggest the low level of muscle contraction which is characteristic of sedentary behavior can contribute to cardio-metabolic health (Tremblay et al., 2010). For example, an absence of activity in the muscles of rats resulted in decreased production of the LPL enzyme important in the regulation of fats (i.e., uptake of triglycerides and the production of HDL) (Hamilton et al., 2004).

Chapter Summary

Research studies spanning many decades have investigated the links between physical activity and physical health outcomes and have used a range of cross-sectional, longitudinal, quasi-experimental, and experimental study designs (Strong et al., 2005). These studies have provided strong and consistent evidence supporting an association between physical activity and a range of physical health benefits for children and adolescents, including improved musculoskeletal and cardiovascular health, reduced risk of obesity, and reduced risk of developing metabolic syndrome (Jansseen & LeBlanc, 2010; Strong et al., 2005). Furthermore, data demonstrate a dose-response relationship, whereby greater health benefits are acquired when individuals (all ages) engage in more physical activity (Jansseen & LeBlanc, 2010; Powell et al., 2011; Warburton & Bredin, 2017), and the greatest health benefits are observed when they participate in vigorous physical activities (Jansseen & LeBlanc, 2010; Physical Activity Guidelines Advisory Committee, 2018) and activities that promote aerobic and muscular fitness (Smith et al., 2014). This evidence served to inform the most recent physical activity guidelines for children and adolescents, recommending daily participation in physical activities of moderate-to-vigorous intensity, and regular inclusion of vigorous intensity physical activities and muscle- and bone-strengthening activities (Australian Government, 2014; Weggemans et al., 2018).

Alternatively, evidence relating to benefits of reducing sedentary behavior and increasing light activity is unclear, due to both a lack of studies and equivocal findings. While there is emerging evidence that sedentary behavior (particularly screen-time accrued in long uninterrupted bouts) has negative effects on physical health, and that a dose-response relationship exists between sedentary behavior and physical health outcomes (Carson, Hunter, et al., 2016), it is difficult to isolate the unique effect of sedentary behavior. This is partly due to the nature of how movement behaviors of sleep, sedentary behavior, and physical activity of varying intensities are accrued across a 24-hour day. Unlike other combinations of health behaviors where participation can occur concurrently (e.g. smoking while eating), or be completely absent, an individual can be engaging in only one form of movement behavior at any given time. It is not possible to be engaging in sedentary behavior and vigorous activity at the same time, for example. Consequently, a change in one movement behavior will result in an opposite change, and net equal result, in the other behaviors (Grgic et al., 2018). This means movement behaviors within an individual are highly correlated with each other (e.g., spending less time in sedentary behavior automatically means an individual is spending more time in light, moderate, or vigorous activity). The nature of these relationships has made it difficult for researchers to isolate the effect of one kind of movement behavior, result-ing in difficulty ascertaining associations with health outcomes. More recently, physical activity researchers have started exploring analytical techniques which allow for the compositional nature of movement behavior data by interpreting the health effects of one behavior as a proportion relative to the other behaviors, instead of a behavior being independent of all others (Chastin, Palarea-Albaladejo, Dontje, & Skelton, 2015). While these studies are relatively new and limited in number, results are showing that higher intensity physical activity is particularly important for children and adolescents (Carson, Tremblay, Chaput, & Chastin, 2016; Fairclough et al., 2017), and it is recommended that young people limit their time being sedentary, particularly screen-time, for physical health benefits. These new analytical methods show promise for future research to further elucidate the associations between physical health outcomes and movement behaviors at different intensities. Such research may lead to future public health guidelines adopting a 24-hour day focus and including recommendations for optimal durations of time spent in each of the phys-ical activity intensity categories.

References

Åberg, N. D., Kuhn, H. G., Nyberg, J., Waern, M., Friberg, P., Svensson, J., . . . Nilsson, M. (2015). In-fluence of cardiovascular fitness and muscle strength in early adulthood on long-term risk of stroke in Swedish men. *Stroke, 46*(7), 1769–1776. doi:10.1161/STROKEAHA.115.009008

Andersen, L. B., Harro, M., Sardinha, L. B., Froberg, K., Ekelund, U., Brage, S., & Anderssen, S. A. (2006). Physical activity and clustered cardiovascular risk in children: A cross-sectional study (The European Youth Heart Study). *Lancet, 368*(9532), 299–304. doi:10.1016/S0140-6736(06)69075-2

Arundell, L., Hinkley, T., Veitch, J., & Salmon, J. (2015). Contribution of the after-school period to chil-dren's daily participation in physical activity and sedentary behaviours. *PLoS One, 10*(10), e0140132. doi:10.1371/journal.pone.0140132

Australian Government. (2014). *Australia's physical activity and sedentary behaviour guidelines.* Canberra. Re-trieved from http://www.health.gov.au/internet/main/publishing.nsf/content/health-pubhlth-strateg-phys-act-guidelines#apa1317

Baquet, G., Berthoin, S., Gerbeaux, M., & Van Praagh, E. (2001). High-intensity aerobic training during a 10 week one-hour physical education cycle: Effects on physical fitness of adolescents aged 11 to 16. *Inter-national Journal of Sports Medicine, 22*(4), 295–300. doi:10.1055/s-2001-14343

Baquet, G., van Praagh, E., & Berthoin, S. (2003). Endurance training and aerobic fitness in young people. *Sports Medicine (Auckland, New Zealand), 33*(15), 1127–1143. doi:10.2165/00007256-200333150-00004

Belcher, B. R., Berrigan, D., Papachristopoulou, A., Brady, S. M., Bernstein, S. B., Brychta, R. J., . . . Yanovski, J. A. (2015). Effects of interrupting children's sedentary behaviors with activity on meta-bolic function: A randomized trial. *Journal of Clinical Endocrinology and Metabolism, 100*(10), 3735–3743. doi:10.1210/jc.2015-2803

Biddle, S. J. H., Garcia Bengoechea, E., & Wiesner, G. (2017). Sedentary behaviour and adiposity in youth: A systematic review of reviews and analysis of causality. *International Journal of Behavioral Nutrition and Physical Activity, 14*(1), 43. doi:10.1186/s12966-017-0497-8

Biddle, S. J. H., Pearson, N., & Salmon, J. (2018). Sedentary behaviors and adiposity in young people: Causal-ity and conceptual model. *Exercise Sport Science Review, 46*(1), 18–25. doi:10.1249/jes.0000000000000135

Biddle, S. J. H., Petrolini, I., & Pearson, N. (2014). Interventions designed to reduce sedentary behaviours in young people: A review of reviews. *British Journal of Sports Medicine, 48*(3), 182–186. doi:10.1136/bjsports-2013-093078

Bond, B., Weston, K. L., Williams, C. A., & Barker, A. R. (2017). Perspectives on high-intensity inter-val exercise for health promotion in children and adolescents. *Open Access Journal of Sports Medicine, 8*, 243–265. doi:10.2147/OAJSM.S127395

Borg, G. (1998). *Borg's perceived exertion and pain scales.* Champaign, IL: Human Kinetics.

Buchan, D. S., Ollis, S., Thomas, N. E., Buchanan, N., Cooper, S. M., Malina, R. M., & Baker, J. S. (2011). Physical activity interventions: Effects of duration and intensity. *Scandivanian Journal of Medicinie and Sci-ence in Sports, 21*(6), e341–e350. doi:10.1111/j.1600-0838.2011.01303.x

Burton, D. A., Stokes, K., & Hall, G. M. (2004). Physiological effects of exercise. *Continuing Education in Anaesthesia Critical Care & Pain, 4*(6), 185–188. doi:10.1093/bjaceaccp/mkh050

Butte, N. F., Watson, K. B., Ridley, K., Zakeri, I. F., McMurray, R. G., Pfeiffer, K. A., . . . Fulton, J. E. (2018). A youth compendium of physical activities: Activity codes and metabolic intensities. *Medicine and Science in Sports Exercise, 50*(2), 246–256. doi:10.1249/MSS.0000000000001430

Carson, V., Chaput, J. P., Janssen, I., & Tremblay, M. S. (2017). Health associations with meeting new 24-hour movement guidelines for Canadian children and youth. *Preventive Medicine, 95*, 7–13. doi:10.1016/j.ypmed.2016.12.005

Carson, V., Hunter, S., Kuzik, N., Gray, C. E., Poitras, V. J., Chaput, J. P., . . . Tremblay, M. S. (2016). Systematic review of sedentary behaviour and health indicators in school-aged children and youth: An update. *Applied Physiology, Nutrition, and Metabolism = Physiologie appliquee, nutrition et metabolisme, 41*(6 Suppl 3), S240–S265. doi:10.1139/apnm-2015-0630

Carson, V., Lee, E.-Y., Hewitt, L., Jennings, C., Hunter, S., Kuzik, N., . . . Tremblay, M. S. (2017). Systematic review of the relationships between physical activity and health indicators in the early years (0–4 years). *BMC Public Health, 17*(Suppl 5), 854–854. doi:10.1186/s12889-017-4860-0

Carson, V., Ridgers, N. D., Howard, B. J., Winkler, E. A., Healy, G. N., Owen, N., . . . Salmon, J. (2013). Light-intensity physical activity and cardiometabolic biomarkers in US adolescents. *PLoS One, 8*(8), e71417. doi:10.1371/journal.pone.0071417

Carson, V., Tremblay, M. S., Chaput, J. P., & Chastin, S. F. (2016). Associations between sleep duration, sedentary time, physical activity, and health indicators among Canadian children and youth using compositional analyses. *Applied Physiology, Nutrition, and Metabolism = Physiologie appliquee, nutrition et metabolisme, 41*(6 Suppl 3), S294–S302. doi:10.1139/apnm-2016-0026

Catley, M. J., & Tomkinson, G. R. (2013). Normative health-related fitness values for children: Analysis of 85347 test results on 9–17-year-old Australians since 1985. *British Journal of Sports Medicine, 47*(2), 98–108. doi:10.1136/bjsports-2011-090218

Chastin, S. F., De Craemer, M., De Cocker, K., Powell, L., Van Cauwenberg, J., Dall, P., . . . Stamatakis, E. (2018). How does light-intensity physical activity associate with adult cardiometabolic health and mortality? Systematic review with meta-analysis of experimental and observational studies. *British Journal of Sports Medicine.* Retrieved from http://bjsm.bmj.com/content/early/2018/05/02/bjsports-2017-097563.abstract

Chastin, S. F., Egerton, T., Leask, C., & Stamatakis, E. (2015). Meta-analysis of the relationship between breaks in sedentary behavior and cardiometabolic health. *Obesity (Silver Spring), 23*(9), 1800–1810. doi:10.1002/oby.21180

Chastin, S. F., Palarea-Albaladejo, J., Dontje, M. L., & Skelton, D. A. (2015). Combined effects of time spent in physical activity, sedentary behaviors and sleep on obesity and cardio-metabolic health markers: A novel compositional data analysis approach. *PLoS One, 10*(10), e0139984. doi:10.1371/journal.pone.0139984

Cliff, D. P., Hesketh, K. D., Vella, S. A., Hinkley, T., Tsiros, M. D., Ridgers, N. D., . . . Lubans, D. R. (2016). Objectively measured sedentary behaviour and health and development in children and adolescents: Systematic review and meta-analysis. *Obesity Reviews, 17*(4), 330–344. doi:10.1111/obr.12371

Corte de Araujo, A. C., Roschel, H., Picanco, A. R., do Prado, D. M., Villares, S. M., de Sa Pinto, A. L., & Gualano, B. (2012). Similar health benefits of endurance and high-intensity interval training in obese children. *PLoS One, 7*(8), e42747. doi:10.1371/journal.pone.0042747

Costigan, S. A., Eather, N., Plotnikoff, R. C., Taaffe, D. R., Pollock, E., Kennedy, S. G., & Lubans, D. R. (2015). Preliminary efficacy and feasibility of embedding high intensity interval training into the school day: A pilot randomized controlled trial. *Preventive Medicine Reports, 2*, 973–979. doi:10.1016/j.pmedr.2015.11.001

Eddolls, W. T. B., McNarry, M. A., Stratton, G., Winn, C. O. N., & Mackintosh, K. A. (2017). High-Intensity interval training interventions in children and adolescents: A systematic review. *Sports Medicine.* doi:10.1007/s40279-017-0753-8

Ee, J., Parry, S., IR de Oliveira, B., McVeigh, J. A., Howie, E., & Straker, L. (2018). Does a classroom standing desk intervention modify standing and sitting behaviour and musculoskeletal symptoms during school time and physical activity during waking time? *International Journal of Environmental Research and Public Health, 15*(8), 1668. Retrieved from https://www.mdpi.com/1660-4601/15/8/1668

Ekelund, U., Anderssen, S. A., Froberg, K., Sardinha, L. B., Andersen, L. B., & Brage, S. (2007). Independent associations of physical activity and cardiorespiratory fitness with metabolic risk factors in children: The European youth heart study. *Diabetologia, 50*(9), 1832–1840. doi:10.1007/s00125-007-0762-5

Engel, F. A., Ackermann, A., Chtourou, H., & Sperlich, B. (2018). High-intensity interval training performed by young athletes: A systematic review and meta-analysis. *Frontiers in Physiology, 9*, 1012–1012. doi:10.3389/fphys.2018.01012

Faigenbaum, A. D., Kraemer, W. J., Blimkie, C. J., Jeffreys, I., Micheli, L. J., Nitka, M., & Rowland, T. W. (2009). Youth resistance training: Updated position statement paper from the national strength and conditioning association. *Journal of Strength and Conditioning Research, 23*(5 Suppl), S60–S79. doi:10.1519/JSC.0b013e31819df407

Fairclough, S. J., Dumuid, D., Taylor, S., Curry, W., McGrane, B., Stratton, G., . . . Olds, T. (2017). Fitness, fatness and the reallocation of time between children's daily movement behaviours: An analysis of compositional data. *International Journal of Behavioral Nutrition and Physical Activity, 14*(1), 64. doi:10.1186/s12966-017-0521-z

Fletcher, E., Leech, R., McNaughton, S. A., Dunstan, D. W., Lacy, K. E., & Salmon, J. (2015). Is the relationship between sedentary behaviour and cardiometabolic health in adolescents independent of dietary intake? A systematic review. *Obesity Reviews, 16*(9), 795–805. doi:10.1111/obr.12302

Fuzeki, E., Engeroff, T., & Banzer, W. (2017). Health benefits of light-intensity physical activity: A systematic review of accelerometer data of the national health and nutrition examination survey (NHANES). *Sports Medicine, 47*(9), 1769–1793. doi:10.1007/s40279-017-0724-0

Gao, Z., & Chen, S. (2014). Are field-based exergames useful in preventing childhood obesity? A systematic review. *Obesity Reviews, 15*(8), 676–691. doi:10.1111/obr.12164

Garber, C. E., Blissmer, B., Deschenes, M. R., Franklin, B. A., Lamonte, M. J., Lee, I. M., . . . American College of Sports Medicine. (2011). American college of sports medicine position stand. Quantity and quality of exercise for developing and maintaining cardiorespiratory, musculoskeletal, and neuromotor fitness in apparently healthy adults: Guidance for prescribing exercise. *Medicine and Science in Sports and Exercise, 43*(7), 1334–1359. doi:10.1249/mss.0b013e318213fefb

Gebel, K., Ding, D., Chey, T., Stamatakis, E., Brown, W. J., & Bauman, A. E. (2015). Effect of moderate to vigorous physical activity on all-cause mortality in middle-aged and older Australians. *JAMA Internal Medicine, 175*(6), 970–977. doi:10.1001/jamainternmed.2015.0541

Grgic, J., Dumuid, D., Bengoechea, E. G., Shrestha, N., Bauman, A., Olds, T., & Pedisic, Z. (2018). Health outcomes associated with reallocations of time between sleep, sedentary behaviour, and physical activity: A systematic scoping review of isotemporal substitution studies. *International Journal of Behavioral Nutrition and Physical Activity, 15*(1), 69. doi:10.1186/s12966-018-0691-3

Grøntved, A., Ried-Larsen, M., Møller, N. C., Kristensen, P. L., Froberg, K., Brage, S., & Andersen, L. B. (2015). Muscle strength in youth and cardiovascular risk in young adulthood (the European Youth Heart Study). *British Journal of Sports Medicine, 49*(2), 90. Retrieved from https://bjsm.bmj.com/content/bjsports/49/2/90.full.pdf

Gutin, B., Yin, Z., Humphries, M. C., & Barbeau, P. (2005). Relations of moderate and vigorous physical activity to fitness and fatness in adolescents. *The American Journal of Clinical Nutrition, 81*(4), 746–750. Retrieved from http://ajcn.nutrition.org/content/81/4/746.abstract

Hamilton, M. T., Hamilton, D. G., & Zderic, T. W. (2004). Exercise physiology versus inactivity physiology: An essential concept for understanding lipoprotein lipase regulation. *Exercise and Sport Sciences Reviews, 32*(4), 161–166. Retrieved from http://www.ncbi.nlm.nih.gov/pmc/articles/PMC4312662/

Harris, N. K., Dulson, D. K., Logan, G. R. M., Warbrick, I. B., Merien, F. L. R., & Lubans, D. R. (2017). Acute responses to resistance and high-intensity interval training in early adolescents. *Journal of Strength and Conditioning Research/National Strength & Conditioning Association, 31*(5), 1177–1186. doi:10.1519/JSC.0000000000001590

Hay, J., Maximova, K., Durksen, A., Carson, V., Rinaldi, R. L., Torrance, B., . . . McGavock, J. (2012). Physical activity intensity and cardiometabolic risk in youth. *Archives of Pediatrics & Adolescent Medicine*, 1–8. doi:10.1001/archpediatrics.2012.1028

Heinonen, I., Kalliokoski, K. K., Hannukainen, J. C., Duncker, D. J., Nuutila, P., & Knuuti, J. (2014). Organ-specific physiological responses to acute physical exercise and long-term training in humans. *Physiology, 29*(6), 421–436. doi:10.1152/physiol.00067.2013

Herrmann, S. D., McMurray, R. G., Kim, Y., Willis, E. A., Kang, M., & McCurdy, T. (2017). The influence of physical characteristics on the resting energy expenditure of youth: A meta-analysis. *American Journal of Human Biology, 29*(3), e22944. doi:10.1002/ajhb.22944

Hoffman, J. (2002). *Physiological aspects of sport training and performance* (2nd ed.). Champaign, IL: Human Kinetics.

Hogstrom, G., Nordstrom, A., & Nordstrom, P. (2016). Aerobic fitness in late adolescence and the risk of early death: A prospective cohort study of 1.3 million Swedish men. *International Journal of Epidemiology, 45*(4), 1159–1168. doi:10.1093/ije/dyv321

Honas, J. J., Willis, E. A., Herrmann, S. D., Greene, J. L., Washburn, R. A., & Donnelly, J. E. (2016). Energy expenditure and intensity of classroom physical activity in elementary school children. *Journal of Physical Activity and Health, 13*(6 Suppl 1), S53–S56. doi:10.1123/jpah.2015-0717

Hulteen, R. M., Smith, J. J., Morgan, P. J., Barnett, L. M., Hallal, P. C., Colyvas, K., & Lubans, D. R. (2017). Global participation in sport and leisure-time physical activities: A systematic review and meta-analysis. *Preventive Medicine, 95*, 14–25. doi:10.1016/j.ypmed.2016.11.027

Janssen, I., & LeBlanc, A. G. (2010). Systematic review of the health benefits of physical activity and fitness in school-aged children and youth. *International Journal of Behavioral Nutrition & Physical Activity, 7*(40), 1–49. doi:10.1186/1479-5868-7-40

Janssen, I., & Ross, R. (2012). Vigorous intensity physical activity is related to the metabolic syndrome independent of the physical activity dose. *International Journal of Epidemiology, 41*(4), 1132–1140. doi:10.1093/ije/dys038

Kistler, K. D., Brunt, E. M., Clark, J. M., Diehl, A. M., Sallis, J. F., Schwimmer, J. B., & Group NCR. (2011). Physical activity recommendations, exercise intensity, and histological severity of nonalcoholic fatty liver disease. *American Journal of Gastroenterology, 106*(3), 460–468; quiz 469. doi:10.1038/ajg.2010.488

Koedijk, J. B., van Rijswijk, J., Oranje, W. A., van den Bergh, J. P., Bours, S. P., Savelberg, H. H., & Schaper, N. C. (2017). Sedentary behaviour and bone health in children, adolescents and young adults: A systematic review. *Osteoporosis International: A Journal Established as Result of Cooperation between the European Foundation for Osteoporosis and the National Osteoporosis Foundation of the USA, 28*(9), 2507–2519. doi:10.1007/s00198-017-4076-2

Kokkinos, P. (2012). Physical activity, health benefits, and mortality risk. *ISRN Cardiology, 2012*, 14. doi:10.5402/2012/718789

Lamboglia, C. M., da Silva, V. T., Vasconcelos Filho, J. E., Pinheiro, M. H., Munguba, M. C., Silva Júnior, F., . . . da Silva, C. A. (2013). Exergaming as a strategic tool in the fight against childhood obesity: A systematic review. *Journal of Obesity, 2013*, 8. doi:10.1155/2013/438364

Lang, J. J., Tomkinson, G. R., Janssen, I., Ruiz, J. R., Ortega, F. B., Leger, L., & Tremblay, M. S. (2018). Making a case for cardiorespiratory fitness surveillance among children and youth. *Exercise & Sport Sciences Reviews, 46*(2), 66–75. doi:10.1249/jes.0000000000000138

Leahy, A. A., Eather, N., Smith, J. J., Hillman, C. H., Morgan, P. J., Plotnikoff, R. C., . . . Lubans, D. R. (2019). Feasibility and preliminary efficacy of a teacher-facilitated high-intensity interval training intervention for older adolescents. *Pediatric Exercise Science, 31*(1), 107–117. doi:10.1123/pes.2018-0039

Lee, I. M., & Paffenbarger, R. S., Jr. (2000). Associations of light, moderate, and vigorous intensity physical activity with longevity. The Harvard alumni health study. *American Journal of Epidemiology, 151*(3), 293–299.

Lloyd, R. S., Faigenbaum, A. D., Stone, M. H., Oliver, J. L., Jeffreys, I., Moody, J. A., . . . Myer, G. D. (2014). Position statement on youth resistance training: The 2014 international consensus. *British Journal of Sports Medicine, 48*(7), 498–505. doi:10.1136/bjsports-2013-092952

Logan, G. R., Harris, N., Duncan, S., & Schofield, G. (2014). A review of adolescent high-intensity interval training. *Sports Medicine (Auckland, New Zealand), 44*(8), 1071–1085. doi:10.1007/s40279-014-0187-5

Martinez-Gomez, D., Ruiz, J. R., Ortega, F. B., Casajus, J. A., Veiga, O. L., Widhalm, K., . . . Sjostrom, M. (2010). Recommended levels and intensities of physical activity to avoid low-cardiorespiratory fitness in European adolescents: The HELENA study. *American Journal of Human Biology, 22*(6), 750–756. doi:10.1002/ajhb.21076

Martinez-Gomez, D., Welk, G. J., Puertollano, M. A., Del-Campo, J., Moya, J. M., Marcos, A., & Veiga, O. L. (2011). Associations of physical activity with muscular fitness in adolescents. *Scandivanian Journal of Medicine and Science in Sports, 21*(2), 310–317. doi:10.1111/j.1600-0838.2009.01036.x

McManus, A. M., Ainslie, P. N., Green, D. J., Simair, R. G., Smith, K., & Lewis, N. (2015). Impact of prolonged sitting on vascular function in young girls. *Experimental Physiology, 100*(11), 1379–1387. doi:10.1113/ep085355

Milanovic, Z., Sporis, G., & Weston, M. (2015). Effectiveness of high-intensity interval training (HIT) and continuous endurance training for VO_2 max improvements: A systematic review and meta-analysis of controlled trials. *Sports Medicine (Auckland, New Zealand), 45*(10), 1469–1481. doi:10.1007/s40279-015-0365-0

Mitchell, J., & Byun, W. (2014). Sedentary behavior and health outcomes in children and adolescents. *American Journal of Lifestyle Medicine, 8*(3), 173–199. doi:10.1177/1559827613498700

Morrow, J. R., Tucker, J. S., Jackson, A. W., Martin, S. B., Greenleaf, C. A., & Petrie, T. A. (2013). Meeting physical activity guidelines and health-related fitness in youth. *American Journal of Preventive Medicine, 44*(5), 439–444. doi:10.1016/j.amepre.2013.01.008

Nishida, Y., Iyadomi, M., Higaki, Y., Tanaka, H., Hara, M., & Tanaka, K. (2011). Influence of physical activity intensity and aerobic fitness on the anthropometric index and serum uric acid concentration in people with obesity. *Internal Medicine, 50*(19), 2121–2128. doi:10.2169/internalmedicine.50.5506

Norton, K., Norton, L., & Sadgrove, D. (2010). Position statement on physical activity and exercise intensity terminology. *Journal of Science and Medicine in Sport, 13*(5), 496–502. doi:10.1016/j.jsams.2009.09.008

Okano, G., Sato, Y., & Murata, Y. (1990). Effect of mild walk habit on body composition, blood pressure and serum lipids. *Japanese Journal of Physical Fitness and Sports Medicine, 39*(5), 315–323.

Okely, A. D., Salmon, J., Vella, S. A., Cliff, D., Timperio, A., Tremblay, M. S., . . . Marino, N. (2012). *A systematic review to update the Australian physical activity guidelines for children and young people.* Canberra, Australia: Commonwealth of Australia.

Oliveira, B. R. R., Santos, T. M., Kilpatrick, M., Pires, F. O., & Deslandes, A. C. (2018). Affective and enjoyment responses in high intensity interval training and continuous training: A systematic review and meta-analysis. *PLoS One, 13*(6), e0197124. doi:10.1371/journal.pone.0197124

Ortega, F. B., Ruiz, J. R., Castillo, M. J., & Sjostrom, M. (2008). Physical fitness in childhood and adolescence: A powerful marker of health. *International Journal of Obesity, 32*(1), 1–11. doi:10.1038/sj.ijo.0803774

Ottevaere, C., Huybrechts, I., De Bourdeaudhuij, I., Sjöström, M., Ruiz, J. R., Ortega, F. B., . . . De Henauw, S. (2011). Comparison of the IPAQ-A and actigraph in relation to VO$_2$ max among European adolescents: The HELENA study. *Journal of Science and Medicine in Sport, 14*(4), 317–324. doi:10.1016/j.jsams.2011.02.008

Owens, S., Galloway, R., & Gutin, B. (2015). The case for vigorous physical activity in youth. *American Journal of Lifestyle Medicine, 11*(2), 96–115. doi:10.1177/1559827615594585

Pate, R. R., O'Neill, J. R., & Lobelo, F. (2008). The evolving definition of "sedentary". *Exercise and Sport Sciences Reviews, 36*(4), 173–178. doi:10.1097/JES.0b013e3181877d1a

Pearson, N., Griffiths, P., Biddle, S. J. H., Johnston, J. P., McGeorge, S., & Haycraft, E. (2017). Clustering and correlates of screen-time and eating behaviours among young adolescents. *BMC Public Health, 17*(1), 533. doi:10.1186/s12889-017-4441-2

Penning, A., Okely, A. D., Trost, S. G., Salmon, J., Cliff, D. P., Batterham, M., . . . Parrish, A. M. (2017). Acute effects of reducing sitting time in adolescents: A randomized cross-over study. *BMC Public Health, 17*(1), 657. doi:10.1186/s12889-017-4660-6

Physical Activity Guidelines Advisory Committee. (2018). *2018 Physical activity guidelines advisory committee scientific report.* Retrieved from Washington, DC: https://health.gov/paguidelines/second-edition/report/pdf/PAG_Advisory_Committee_Report.pdf.

Poitras, V. J., Gray, C. E., Borghese, M. M., Carson, V., Chaput, J. P., Janssen, I., . . . Tremblay, M. S. (2016). Systematic review of the relationships between objectively measured physical activity and health indicators in school-aged children and youth. *Applied Physiology, Nutrition and Metabolism, 41*(6 Suppl 3), S197–S239. doi:10.1139/apnm-2015-0663

Powell, K. E., Paluch, A. E., & Blair, S. N. (2011). Physical activity for health: What kind? How much? How intense? On top of what? *Annual Review Public Health, 32*(1), 349–365. doi:10.1146/annurev-publhealth-031210-101151

Racil, G., Ben Ounis, O., Hammouda, O., Kallel, A., Zouhal, H., Chamari, K., & Amri, M. (2013). Effects of high vs. moderate exercise intensity during interval training on lipids and adiponectin levels in obese young females. *European Journal of Applied Physiology, 113*(10), 2531–2540. doi:10.1007/s00421-013-2689-5

Reiner, M., Niermann, C., Jekauc, D., & Woll, A. (2013). Long-term health benefits of physical activity – A systematic review of longitudinal studies. *BMC Public Health, 13*(1), 813. doi:10.1186/1471-2458-13-813

Rivera-Brown, A. M., & Frontera, W. R. (2012). Principles of exercise physiology: Responses to acute exercise and long-term adaptations to training. *PM&R The Journal of Injury, Function and Rehabilitation, 4*(11), 797–804. doi:10.1016/j.pmrj.2012.10.007

Ruiz, J. R., Castro-Piñero, J., Artero, E. G., Ortega, F. B., Sjöström, M., Suni, J., & Castillo, M. J. (2009). Predictive validity of health-related fitness in youth: A systematic review. *British Journal of Sports Medicine, 43*(12), 909. Retrieved from https://bjsm.bmj.com/content/bjsports/43/12/909.full.pdf

Ruiz, J. R., Rizzo, N. S., Hurtig-Wennlof, A., Ortega, F. B., Warnberg, J., & Sjostrom, M. (2006). Relations of total physical activity and intensity to fitness and fatness in children: The European youth heart study. *American Journal of Clinical Nutrition, 84*(2), 299–303. doi:10.1093/ajcn/84.1.299

Sacheck, J. M. (2017). Vigorous physical activity in youth: Just one end of the physical activity spectrum for affecting health? *American Journal of Lifestyle Medicine, 11*(2), 116–118. doi:10.1177/1559827616680565

Saint-Maurice, P. F., Troiano, R. P., Berrigan, D., Kraus, W. E., & Matthews, C. E. (2018). Volume of light versus moderate-to-vigorous physical activity: Similar benefits for all-cause mortality? *Journal of the American Heart Association: Cardiovascular and Cerebrovascular Disease, 7*(7), e008815. doi:10.1161/JAHA.118.008815

Saunders, T. J., Chaput, J. P., Goldfield, G. S., Colley, R. C., Kenny, G. P., Doucet, E., & Tremblay, M. S. (2013). Prolonged sitting and markers of cardiometabolic disease risk in children and youth: A randomized crossover study. *Metabolism: Clinical and Experimental, 62*(10), 1423–1428. doi:10.1016/j.metabol.2013.05.010

Sherry, A. P., Pearson, N., & Clemes, S. A. (2016). The effects of standing desks within the school classroom: A systematic review. *Preventive Medicine Reports, 3*, 338–347. doi:10.1016/j.pmedr.2016.03.016

Silverman, M. N., & Deuster, P. A. (2014). Biological mechanisms underlying the role of physical fitness in health and resilience. *Interface Focus, 4*(5). doi:10.1098/rsfs.2014.0040

Smith, J. J., Eather, N., Morgan, P. J., Plotnikoff, R. C., Faigenbaum, A. D., & Lubans, D. R. (2014). The health benefits of muscular fitness for children and adolescents: A systematic review and meta-analysis. *Sports Medicine (Auckland, New Zealand), 44*(9), 1209–1223. doi:10.1007/s40279-014-0196-4

Smith, J. J., Eather, N., Weaver, R. G., Riley, N., Beets, M. W., & Lubans, D. R. (2019). Behavioral correlates of muscular fitness in children and adolescents: A systematic review. *Sports Medicine.* doi:10.1007/s40279-019-01089-7

Sothern, M. S., Loftin, M., Suskind, R. M., Udall, J. N., & Blecker, U. (1999). The health benefits of physical activity in children and adolescents: Implications for chronic disease prevention. *European Journal of Pediatrics, 158*(4), 271–274.

Strong, W. B., Malina, R. M., Blimkie, C. J. R., Daniels, S. R., Dishman, R. K., Gutin, B., . . . Trudeau, F. (2005). Evidence based physical activity for school-age youth. *Journal of Pediatrics, 146*, 732–737.

Swain, D. P., & Franklin, B. A. (2006). Comparison of cardioprotective benefits of vigorous versus moderate intensity aerobic exercise. *American Journal of Cardiology, 97*(1), 141–147. doi:10.1016/j.amjcard.2005.07.130

Tarp, J., Child, A., White, T., Westgate, K., Bugge, A., Grøntved, A., ... On behalf of the International Children's Accelerometry Database Collaborators. (2018). Physical activity intensity, bout-duration, and cardiometabolic risk markers in children and adolescents. *International Journal of Obesity, 42*(9), 1639–1650. doi:10.1038/s41366-018-0152-8

Tjonna, A. E., Stolen, T. O., Bye, A., Volden, M., Slordahl, S. A., Odegard, R., . . . Wisloff, U. (2009). Aerobic interval training reduces cardiovascular risk factors more than a multitreatment approach in overweight adolescents. *Clinical Science, 116*(4), 317–326. doi:10.1042/CS20080249

Tremblay, M. S., Aubert, S., Barnes, J. D., Saunders, T. J., Carson, V., Latimer-Cheung, A. E., . . . on behalf of SBRN Terminology Consensus Project Participants. (2017). Sedentary behavior research network (SBRN) – Terminology consensus project process and outcome. *International Journal of Behavioral Nutrition and Physical Activity, 14*(1), 75. doi:10.1186/s12966-017-0525-8

Tremblay, M. S., Colley, R. C., Saunders, T. J., Healy, G. N., & Owen, N. (2010). Physiological and health implications of a sedentary lifestyle. *Applied Physiology Nutrition and Metabolism, 35*(6), 725–740. doi:10.1139/H10-079

U.S. Department of Health and Human Services. (1996). *Physical activity and health: A report of the surgeon general.* Retrieved from Atlanta, GA: https://www.cdc.gov/nccdphp/sgr/pdf/prerep.pdf

U.S. Department of Health and Human Services. (2018). *Physical activity guidelines for Americans.* Retrieved from Washington, DC: https://health.gov/paguidelines/second-edition/pdf/Physical_Activity_Guidelines_2nd_edition.pdf

van der Ploeg, H., Chey, T., Korda, R. J., Banks, E., & Bauman, A. (2012). Sitting time and all-cause mortality risk in 222 497 Australian adults. *Archives of Internal Medicine, 172*, 494–500. doi:10.1001/archinternmed.2011.2174

Van der Velde, J., Savelberg, H., Schaper, N., & Koster, A. (2015). Moderate activity and fitness, not sedentary time, are independently associated with cardio-metabolic risk in U.S Adults aged 18–49. *International Journal of Environmental Research and Public Health, 12*, 2330–2343. doi:10.3390/ijerph120302330

van Ekris, E., Altenburg, T. M., Singh, A. S., Proper, K. I., Heymans, M. W., & Chinapaw, M. J. (2016). An evidence-update on the prospective relationship between childhood sedentary behaviour and biomedical health indicators: A systematic review and meta-analysis. *Obesity Reviews, 17*(9), 833–849. doi:10.1111/obr.12426

Verswijveren, S., Lamb, K. E., Bell, L. A., Timperio, A., Salmon, J., & Ridgers, N. D. (2018). Associations between activity patterns and cardio-metabolic risk factors in children and adolescents: A systematic review. *PLoS One, 13*(8), e0201947. doi:10.1371/journal.pone.0201947

Warburton, D. E. R., & Bredin, S. S. D. (2017). Health benefits of physical activity: A systematic review of current systematic reviews. *Current Opinion in Cardiology, 32*(5), 541–556. doi:10.1097/hco.0000000000000437

Weggemans, R. M., Backx, F. J. G., Borghouts, L., Chinapaw, M., Hopman, M. T. E., Koster, A., . . . Committee Dutch Physical Activity Guidelines. (2018). The 2017 Dutch physical activity guidelines. *International Journal of Behavioral Nutrition and Physical Activity, 15*(1), 58. doi:10.1186/s12966-018-0661-9

Welk, G., Morrow, J., & Saint-Maurice, P. (2017). *Measures registry user guide: Individual physical activity.* Retrieved from Washington, DC: http://nccororgms.wpengine.com/tools-mruserguides/wp-content/uploads/sites/2/2017/NCCOR_MR_User_Guide_Individual_PA-FINAL.pdf

Wittmeier, K. D. M., Mollard, R. C., & Kriellaars, D. J. (2008). Physical activity intensity and risk of over-weight and adiposity in children. *Obesity, 16*(2), 415–420. doi:10.1038/oby.2007.73

Wolfe, R. R. (2006). The underappreciated role of muscle in health and disease. *American Journal of Clinical Nutrition, 84*(3), 475–482. doi:10.1093/ajcn/84.3.475

World Health Organization. (2004). *Global strategy on diet, physical activity and health.* Retrieved from Geneva, Switzerland: https://www.who.int/dietphysicalactivity/strategy/eb11344/strategy_english_web.pdf

World Health Organization. (2010). *Global recommendations on physical activity for health.* Geneva, Switzerland: World Health Organization. Retrieved from https://apps.who.int/iris/bitstream/handle/10665/44399/9789241599979_eng.pdf;jsessionid=C24E42398F11DFB89FAF92C89A9715F5?sequence=1

World Health Organization. (2017). *What is moderate-intensity and vigorous-intensity physical activity?* Retrieved from http://www.who.int/dietphysicalactivity/physical_activity_intensity/en/

Wu, X. Y., Han, L. H., Zhang, J. H., Luo, S., Hu, J. W., & Sun, K. (2017). The influence of physical activity, sedentary behavior on health-related quality of life among the general population of children and adolescents: A systematic review. *PLoS One, 12*(11), e0187668. doi:10.1371/journal.pone.0187668

Zeng, N., & Gao, Z. (2016). Exergaming and obesity in youth: Current perspectives. *International Journal of General Medicine, 9*, 275–284. doi:10.2147/ijgm.S99025

Zhu, W., & Owen, N. (2017). *Sedentary behavior and health: Concepts, assessments, and interventions.* Champaign, IL: Human Kinetics.

6

MENTAL HEALTH BENEFITS OF PHYSICAL ACTIVITY FOR YOUNG PEOPLE

Stuart J. H. Biddle and Ineke Vergeer

Introduction

There is a commonly held view that participation in physical activity is good for mental health, and this perception has roots in antiquity. The case for mental health benefits across the lifespan is strong. However, this research field is also complex, and there is uncertainty regarding some issues.

This chapter will consider the links between involvement in physical activity and various mental health outcomes in young people. Given the diversity of psychological and mental health states and conditions that can be experienced, the chapter will focus on the key themes of self-esteem, depression, anxiety, and health-related quality of life (HRQoL). Other important concepts will be discussed, including enjoyment and social outcomes of physical activity. Cognitive functioning is dealt with elsewhere in this book. We will briefly discuss the psychological outcomes of involvement in acute bouts of physical activity, but the main focus will be on involvement over time, the so-called 'chronic' effects of physical activity, such as participation in exercise programs.

It is important to recognize that this field of research is complex. Figure 6.1 highlights a number of key issues, including aspects of physical activity itself (e.g., intensity and type), mental health conditions and outcomes, and characteristics of the individuals, such as their preferences. Even with such a simplified summary shown, Figure 6.1 highlights the potential complexity of the field. Interactions are possible between virtually all elements.

Defining Mental Health

The World Health Organisation states that mental health is more than the absence of mental disorders and is a central component of health. It formally defines mental health as "a state of well-being in which an individual realizes his or her own abilities, can cope with the normal stresses of life, can work productively and is able to make a contribution to his or her community" (see http://www.who.int/features/factfiles/mental_health/en/). This is a broad definition based on positive and effective functioning – it is not centered on poor mental health, illness, or 'deficit'. That said, defining mental health in this way cannot hide the fact that it can be both positive and negative, and that poor mental health is a highly prevalent and serious issue in modern society (see later). As such, mental health organizations (e.g., 'Beyondblue' in Australia) have a focus on reducing depression, anxiety, and suicide (see https://www.beyondblue.org.au/about-us/who-we-are-and-what-we-do).

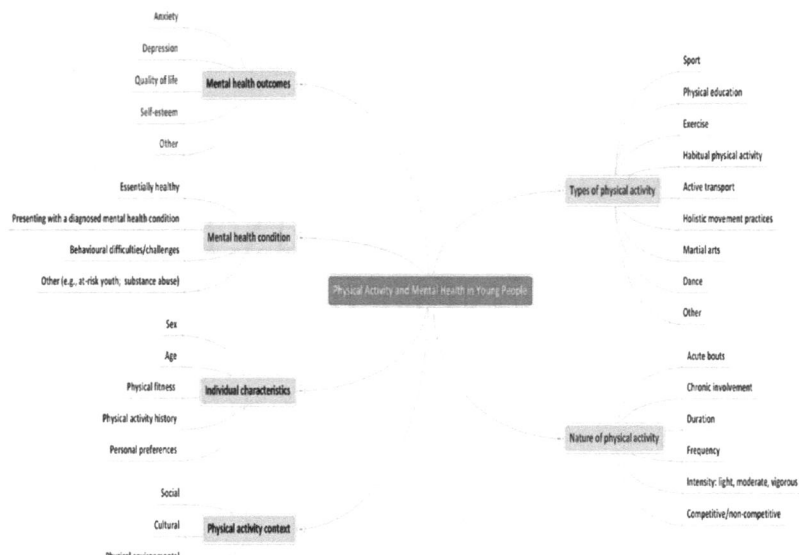

Figure 6.1 Illustration of key issues showing the complexity of the field of physical activity and mental health in young people

For research purposes, mental health has no universal definition; however, key issues include those of self-esteem, depression, anxiety, and HRQoL. Self-esteem, for example, is considered a key indicator of mental health, including emotional stability and subjective well-being, and is often a strong focus for educational programs for young people. The wider concept of HRQoL includes psychological as well physical and functional health components (Bowling, 1997; Rejeski, Brawley, & Shumaker, 1996). Depression and anxiety states and disorders are common, including day-to-day mood changes that may affect functioning.

A useful conceptual model concerning the effects of physical activity on mental health outcomes in children and adolescents is provided by Lubans et al. (2016). They group mental health outcomes into cognitive function, well-being, and ill-being. Well-being includes global self-esteem, subjective and psychological well-being, quality of life, and resilience. Ill-being includes internalizing disorders (e.g., anxiety and depression) and externalizing disorders (e.g., conduct disorder and attention–deficit hyperactivity disorder (ADHD)).

Epidemiology and Prevalence of Mental Health Conditions in Young People

Data suggest that the mental health of many young people is less than optimal. The Mental Health Foundation reported that 20% of those aged 16 years and over in the UK in 2014 had symptoms of anxiety or depression, and this trend appears to be increasing. Moreover, rates are higher among females than males (Mental Health Foundation, 2018). The second National Survey of the Mental Health and Wellbeing of Australian Children and Adolescents, conducted 2013–2014, reported that a mental disorder was experienced by 14% of those aged 4–17 years (equivalent to 560,000 Australian children), including major depressive and anxiety disorders (Lawrence et al., 2015). In the most recent (2017–2018) Australian National Health Survey, 15% of those aged 18–24 years (the youngest age group reported) had distress levels as 'high' or 'very high' (see https://www.abs.gov.au/AUSSTATS).

On a more positive note, a recent large meta-analysis, covering mainly Western countries, has shown that average levels of self-esteem have increased in children from 4 to 11 years of age though remained stable from 11 to 15 years (Orth, Erol, & Luciano, 2018). There will be many potential threats to self-esteem in young people at the individual level, including societal pressures (e.g., appearance), evaluations (e.g., exam performance), and social interactions (e.g., bullying).

Given these data and trends, it is evident that many young people will encounter mental health problems. Moreover, it is widely accepted that as a society we want children and adolescents to live their lives not just free of mental ill-health, but to experience positive growth, high levels of self-esteem, happiness, resilience, psychological well-being, and quality of life. For these reasons, cost-effective solutions to achieve positive mental health – including avoidance of ill-health – are widely sought after. Physical activity is proposed as one such solution.

Historical Context to the Field

Although reference to psychological benefits of physical activity stretch back many centuries, much of this refers to adults rather than young people. One of the earliest research overviews on the topic with adults was authored by Emma McCloy Layman (1960), but it was not until two decades later that research syntheses appeared with a focus on young people (e.g., Brown, 1982). The overview by Brown drew on evidence from student dissertations, other overviews and commentaries, and a few small-scale studies, the earliest dating only to 1977. A clear focus was on self-concept and children with psychological impairment. One of the first meta-analyses in the field was published in 1986 by Gruber, reporting on physical activity and self-concept in young people. Studies only as far back as 1967 were included (Gruber, 1986).

Two important papers were published on physical activity and mental health in young people as part of the first developments of national physical activity guidelines for young people in the US (Calfas & Taylor, 1994) and the UK (Mutrie & Parfitt, 1998). In the latter research review, it was concluded that "some progress" had been made, and that "physical activity is associated with good mental health" (p. 64). But, equally, many questions remained unanswered, including those concerning the mechanisms, or causes, of this link. Overall, therefore, the field concerning physical activity and mental health in young people has quite a short history.

Overview of the Literature

As shown in Figure 6.1, one of the key distinctions to make in considering mental health outcomes is whether the physical activity is taken in single bouts (acute) or over time (chronic). In acute studies, assessments of mental health are usually taken before and after single bouts of exercise with the aim of detecting short-term changes. Chronic studies typically investigate differences or changes over a longer time period, such as before and after involvement in a 12-week physical activity program, or whether there are differences in mental health between those undertaking regular physical activity and those who are inactive.

Acute Affective Responses to Physical Activity

Typically, single session studies will be testing whether physical activity (usually 'exercise') makes you 'feel better'. In practice, this will involve the assessment of changes in 'affect' or 'mood'. 'Affect', sometimes referred to as 'core affect' or 'basic affect', is a generic 'valenced' (good/bad) response. It is considered a basic human response. Russell and Feldman-Barrett (1999) refer to 'core affect' as "the most elementary consciously accessible affective feelings" (p. 806). Mood is a global set of affective (feeling) states we experience on a day-to-day basis and may last hours, days, weeks, or even months. Mood can be conceptualized in terms of distinct mood states, such as vigor and depression. It represents generic feelings rather than a reaction to an event, that is an emotion. The origin of mood states is usually more difficult to specify than the origin of emotions. One can be 'feeling down' for no obvious reason, and hence, moods tend to be 'diffuse' and relatively low in intensity (Ekkekakis, 2013).

An early review of acute affective outcomes of exercise was conducted by Tuson and Sinyor (1993). They concluded that only 'modest' anxiety effects were evident and "no reliable effects were found for any of the other affective states examined" (p. 100). No conclusions could be drawn about young people. However, at the time, assessments of affective states in acute studies used simple 'before and after' measures, typically using multiple-item questionnaires. This precluded the assessment of feelings <u>during</u> exercise, and thus, studies lacked the ability to see how affect changed over the course of an exercise bout.

The assessment of acute mental health effects of physical activity has been debated (Ekkekakis & Petruzzello, 2000), but one framework used mainly with adults is the 'affect circumplex' (Russell, 1980). This model tends to depict affect in terms of the two dimensions of valence (i.e., pleasant–unpleasant) and arousal (i.e., high–low). This allows affective states to be classified into four quadrants, as shown in Figure 6.2. Typically, studies use single item measures of the two dimensions; thus, multiple assessments can be made before, during, and after exercise, allowing for a time-line of affective responses to be plotted. This approach has been used with young people (e.g., Benjamin, Rowlands, & Parfitt, 2012; Malik, Williams, Weston, & Barker, 2018), mainly through the assessment of affective valence, but it remains an understudied population using this method.

Exercise intensity is likely to be an important moderator of the relationship between physical activity and affective reactions. In 2003, Ekkekakis proposed a 'Dual-Mode Model' regarding affective responses, intensity, and temporal aspects of responses (Ekkekakis, 2003). One of his propositions stated that responses that are immediately following what he describes as 'moderately vigorous' exercise (but not 'strenuous') "are almost uniformly positive, regardless of whether the

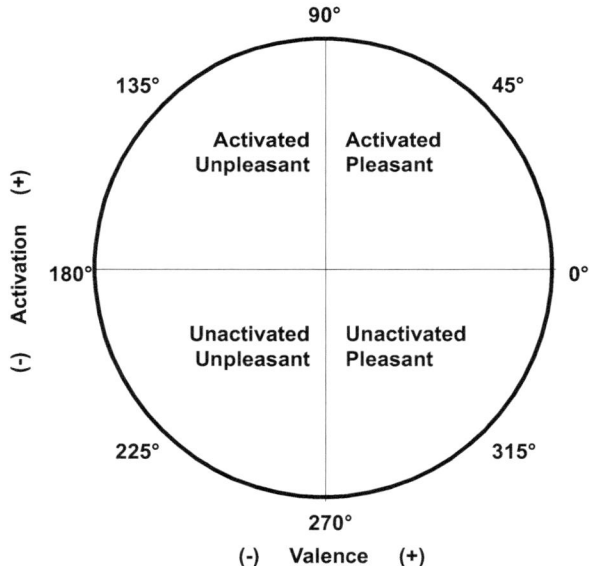

Figure 6.2 A circumplex model of psychological valence and perceived activation

responses during exercise were positive or negative" (p. 221). This is the so-called 'rebound' effect, and Ekkekakis (2003) describes the robustness of this effect as "remarkable" (p. 221). Another proposition states that "affective responses during strenuous exercise unify into a negative trend as the intensity of exercise approaches each individual's functional limits" (p. 222). The ventilatory threshold (VT) has been suggested as one biological marker for when this shift occurs. VT represents a change from the primary use of aerobic metabolism to a significant contribution of anaerobic metabolism, resulting in the accumulation of blood lactate and hyperventilation.

Reed and Ones (2006) conducted a comprehensive meta-analysis of 158 studies investigating acute aerobic exercise and measures reflecting 'positive activated affect' (PAA). This is represented in the circumplex model by high affective valence (feeling 'good') and high arousal/activation (see Figure 6.2). The overall effect size (ES) in the meta-analysis was 0.47, showing a 'moderate' but clear effect. However, while studies were included from all age groups, no analysis was reported testing for the effects of age; thus, we cannot conclude from this meta-analysis if such an effect is evident in young people.

Several studies from Parfitt and colleagues, however, do suggest that this approach is relevant to children and adolescents. In an early study, Sheppard and Parfitt (2008) examined the affective responses of 22 adolescents to each of three exercise conditions on a cycle ergometer. Having determined individual VTs, two exercise intensities were prescribed. The first was considered 'low' intensity and was below the VT, and the second was 'high' intensity and above the VT. For the third condition, the adolescents were able to set a self-selected level of exercise intensity. This was determined by the request to "select an intensity that you would be happy to sustain for 15 minutes and that you would feel happy to do regularly". Affective valence was assessed using the Feeling Scale (Hardy & Rejeski, 1989) which is a single item scale ranging from −5 (feeling 'very bad') through 0, and up to +5 (feeling 'very good'). Results showed that affect was positive throughout the exercise when at the lower intensity or self-selected. Affect declined in the higher intensity condition, but rebounded to more positive responses after exercise. Broadly similar findings have been reported with low-active adolescents (Stych & Parfitt, 2011), younger children (Benjamin et al., 2012), and adolescent girls (Hamlyn-Williams, Freeman, & Parfitt, 2014). Greater declines in affect were also reported by Malik et al. (2018) for high-intensity exercise relative to moderate intensity, although both rebounded to similarly positive values post-exercise.

In conclusion, acute exercise studies with children and adolescents do seem to support the basic tenets of the Dual-Mode Model. Moreover, Parfitt and colleagues have shown that affective responses during exercise seem to be more positive when participants are allowed to choose their own exercise intensity.

Chronic Effects of Physical Activity on Mental Health

It has been more typical to study the effects of chronic (longer term) involvement in physical activity on mental health than it has been to study acute affective reactions to single exercise bouts. Common mental health outcomes that have been studied include self-esteem, depression, and anxiety. All three outcomes have been reviewed by Biddle, Ciaccioni, Thomas, and Vergeer (2019) in an update of a previous review of reviews (Biddle & Asare, 2011), in which evidence linking chronic physical activity to these outcomes was synthesized from published literature reviews.

Self-Esteem and Physical Self-Perceptions

Self-esteem is a term used in daily life, including in general conversations by parents, teachers, and managers at work. It is generally seen as a key indicator of psychological well-being (Fox, 2000). Self-esteem reflects the degree to which individuals appraise and value themselves, and reflects a core sense of self-worth. It is concerned with feelings of 'good' in oneself, however that is perceived. Typically, self-concept <u>describes</u> aspects of the self (e.g., 'I am an exerciser'), whereas self-esteem attaches a <u>value</u> to such descriptors (e.g., 'I feel good about myself because I exercise'). In the research literature, however, the two terms are often used interchangeably.

A commonly used theory of self-esteem involves a hierarchical model proposing that our global view of ourselves ('global self-esteem') – how we feel about ourselves in general – is underpinned by perceptions and feelings of ourselves in specific domains in our lives. These include, among others, social, academic, and physical domains, and each of these is constructed from perceptions in relevant further sub-domains or more focused contexts (Shavelson, Hubner, & Stanton, 1976). This is illustrated in Figure 6.3 with example domains and sub-domains. Constructs lower down the hierarchy, and likely even further beneath those illustrated in Figure 6.3, are more open to change and, consequently, those higher up will require more intensive or prolonged experiences to change.

There is an assumption that physical activity is a positive influence on self-esteem. The potential to enhance self-esteem is frequently used as a rationale for promoting participation and is a common justification for the teaching of physical education (PE) to children. However, it is likely that relationships between self-esteem and physical activity are bi-directional. That is, not only might we expect physical activity to affect self-esteem, but we could hypothesize that those with high or low self-esteem may choose to adopt and maintain behaviors that reflect this. For example, if an adolescent has low perceptions of their physical competence (see Figure 6.3), why would they risk exposing this in a public context, such as PE?

One of the first meta-analyses in the field of physical activity concerned self-esteem and was reported by Gruber (1986). It was centered on play and PE programs for children. From 27 studies, an overall moderate ES was reported for physical activity on self-esteem and over 60% of the studies found positive effects. A more recent meta-analysis examined whether exercise interventions improved global self-esteem among children and young people aged 3–20 years (Ekeland, Heian, & Hagen, 2005; Ekeland, Heian, Hagen, Abbott, & Nordheim, 2004), and also showed a moderate effect for exercise. The authors concluded that exercise can lead to improvements in self-esteem in young people, at least in the short term, and among those considered at-risk. A meta-analysis from 18 randomized controlled trials by Liu, Wu, and Ming (2015) reported an overall small but significant positive effect for physical activity when the intervention was 'physical activity alone'.

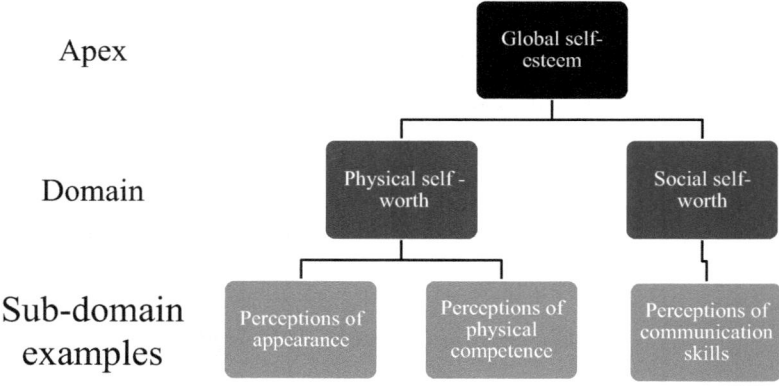

Figure 6.3 A multidimensional and hierarchical model of self-esteem, with example domains of physical and social self-worth

In a recent update of the 2011 review of reviews by Biddle and Asare (2011), Biddle et al. (2019) located ten systematic reviews on physical activity and self-esteem in young people in the 8 years up to the end of 2017, suggesting that the field is expanding quite rapidly. The reviews tended to include healthy samples, with ages ranging from pre-school to late adolescence. Physical activity was broadly defined, including leisure-time physical activity, yoga, recreational dance, and muscle-strengthening exercise. Overall, the reviews were suggestive of positive associations between physical activity and self-esteem, with six reviews concluding positive findings and four reporting inconclusive, mixed, or null results.

Alongside the review of reviews itself, an analysis was conducted to assess whether the association between physical activity and self-esteem could be considered causal according to criteria proposed by Hill (1965). Overall, it was concluded that the association was not causal because the criterion of strength of the association was only partially supported, and there was no support for physical activity preceding, rather than following, self-esteem ('temporal sequencing'), or for a dose-response relationship (Biddle et al., 2019). However, there was evidence from experimental designs. Given that experimental evidence is a cornerstone of scientific enquiry, this does suggest that physical activity may have a causal role in enhancing self-esteem in youth. However, when put alongside other criteria concerning causality, the weight of evidence was not supportive of a causal relationship based on evidence from recent systematic reviews.

In slight contrast to the conclusions regarding causality from the review by Biddle et al. (2019), Lubans et al. (2016) came to the conclusion that a causal link is evident between physical activity and self-esteem in young people. However, they used a different perspective, and their conclusions were arrived at by reviewing the mechanisms linking physical activity and mental health in youth. Specifically, they identified studies where it was possible to test whether physical activity changed potential mechanisms affecting self-esteem – a different analysis to that undertaken by Biddle et al. (2019). Changes in appearance were associated with changes in self-esteem in five of six studies. Physical self-worth (in two of three studies) and perceived competence (in three of four studies) also showed associations with self-esteem.

The work of Lubans et al. does point to the potential importance of studying changes in aspects of <u>physical</u> self-perceptions rather than just global self-esteem. Moreover, this might highlight a key weakness of this field. Why would we expect global self-esteem to change significantly as a result of greater physical activity? It is more likely that perceptions lower in the hierarchy will be amenable to change (see Figure 6.3). Of course, such changes may then filter through and affect global self-esteem, but these changes may be slow and difficult to assess, as well as global self-esteem being affected by other, non-physical, experiences.

Interestingly, a meta-analysis by Babic et al. (2014), concerning the association between <u>physical</u> self-concept/self-worth and physical activity, showed clear, but somewhat moderate, associations across cross-sectional, longitudinal, and intervention designs. As shown in Figure 6.4, general physical self-concept had a small association with physical activity, whereas perceived competence and perceived fitness both had 'moderate' associations. Perceived appearance had only a small association, and this could be expected given that many other factors beyond physical activity could affect such perceptions. Associations tended to be larger for boys than girls for general physical self-concept and perceived fitness. Study design was not a significant moderator for any of the four outcomes.

One issue to consider is the nature of the physical activity undertaken. Although it is often the case that we emphasize moderate-to-vigorous physical activity (typically meant as 'aerobic activity'), national and international guidelines also recommend that children and adolescents take part in activities that strengthen muscle and bone (for Australia, see: http://www.health.gov.au/internet/main/publishing.nsf/content/health-pubhlth-strateg-phys-act-guidelines). These activities might involve resistance exercise (e.g., using body weight or external equipment) and

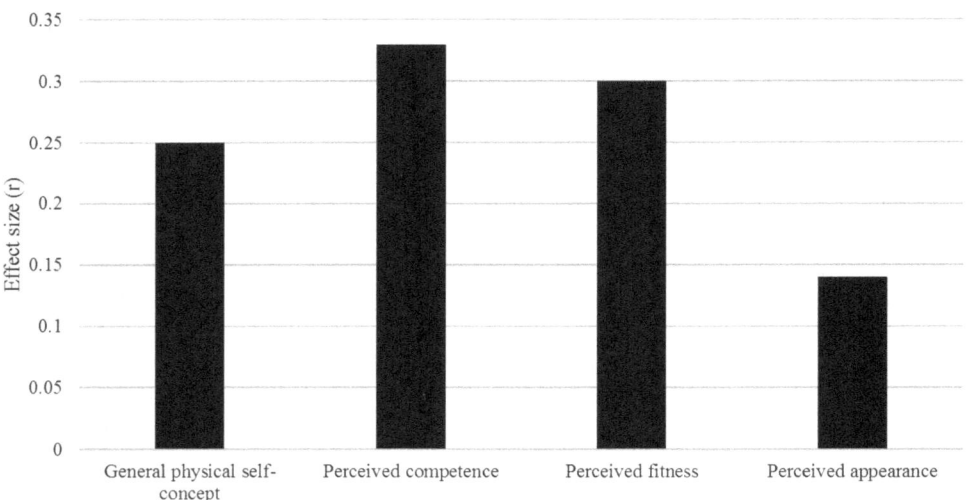

Figure 6.4 Associations from a meta-analysis by Babic et al. (2014) for physical activity with sub-domains of physical self-worth

movement with substantial weight bearing. Such 'muscle strength exercise' has been considered to be the forgotten part of the guidelines (Strain, Fitzsimons, Kelly, & Mutrie, 2016) even though the evidence for health benefits is clearly emerging (Bennie, Lee et al., 2018).

A review of the association between muscle strength exercise and health outcomes in young people by Smith et al. (2014) found a moderate association between muscular fitness and perceptions of sport competence when a meta-analytic synthesis was possible. They also reported positive cross-sectional associations between muscular fitness and physical self-perceptions, including appearance and perceived competence, but no analyses by sex were reported. However, of importance is that the only experimental study included in Smith et al.'s review showed that changes in muscular fitness were not related to changes in any of the measures of physical self-perceptions. Moreover, a large school-based randomized controlled trial in Australia did not show any significant changes in self-esteem from involvement in a resistance exercise program (Smith et al., 2018) but did show changes in resistance training self-efficacy at 6 months follow-up, although this was not sustained at 12 months (Kennedy et al., 2018). These experimental findings suggest that the complexity of this field may still be clouding our view of how physical activity is associated with global self-esteem or its domains.

In conclusion, it might be better to have a re-think about the role of physical activity in the promotion of global self-esteem. Obviously, it is desirable to achieve changes in self-esteem, but equally we should not expect large changes at that level of the hierarchy. We should be more optimistic that positive experiences in physical activity, such as improved fitness and competence, will affect the domain of physical self-worth. This in itself will be positive and should perhaps be the goal of physical activity programs. Moreover, many of the studies in this field are conducted with healthy populations, thus being open to ceiling effects. Further sub-group analyses are needed to test effects for those with impaired levels of self-esteem or challenged in other ways in their mental health.

The relationship between self-esteem and physical activity is complex, and this needs greater recognition. More emphasis is needed on the social-emotional contexts in which physical activity is delivered or takes place. It could be argued that we should look more at the conditions in which physical activity can support more positive and stable self-esteem in young people than testing for simple linear associations.

We have argued that global self-esteem is just one part of the wider view of the self. In addition, other conceptualizations, for example, look at what constitutes vulnerable (Roberts & Monroe, 1994) or contingent self-esteem (Bos, Huijding, Muris, Vogel, & Biesheuvel, 2010). Vulnerable self-esteem means the absence of a stable, inner anchor of self-worth, which makes one overly dependent on external sources of self-worth. These tend to vary according to circumstances and thus make self-esteem temporally unstable and fluctuating. High or low levels of self-esteem will be contingent on the perceived presence or withdrawal of love and appreciation and/or on perceived success or failure. In addition, vulnerable self-esteem is often accompanied by cognitive self-evaluations that include unrealistically high criteria for achievement, and an inability to tolerate even small discrepancies between real and ideal self. Furthermore, feelings of self-worth may rely on a very limited number of sources and/or sources that are difficult to maintain (Roberts & Monroe, 1994).

It is important to consider the sources of self-esteem, and how and why physical activity might affect these. Self-esteem, in the context of physical activity, is dependent on, or influenced by, psychosocial and interpersonal processes, as well as the experience of success and failure. Other influences include social inclusion and stressful life events. How the young person is guided through failure, loss, and rejection experiences in the physical activity context is important. The sport domain, for example, with its proliferation of possibilities for experience of both success and failure, is full of potential opportunities for both enhancing and degrading self-esteem. When failure experiences dominate, this will be a challenge for self-esteem in all children, but particularly so for those with few other positive sources of self-esteem.

Depression

As stated, one of the most frequently encountered mental health problems is depression. Depression can be characterized by the absence of positive affective states, such as enjoyment, as well as persistent low depressive mood. In addition, depression symptoms can be emotional, cognitive, physical, and behavioral. However, over many years physical activity has been seen as a viable strategy for preventing or managing depressive episodes. Despite some inaccurate appraisals of the literature concerning adults (see Ekkekakis, 2015; Ekkekakis, Hartman, & Ladwig, 2018, for critiques), or underestimated effects due to publication bias (Schuch et al., 2016), it has been concluded that "compared to non-active interventions, exercise has a large and significant anti-depressant effect", and that the evidence "confirms and strengthens the case that exercise is an evidence-based treatment for depression" (Schuch et al., 2016, p. 49). However, rather less is known about children and adolescents.

Biddle and Asare (2011) concluded from four systematic reviews that "physical activity over no intervention seems to be potentially beneficial for reduced depression, but the evidence base is limited" (p. 888). When updating this evidence, Biddle et al. (2019) located a further ten systematic reviews.

From reviews of intervention studies, six of seven meta-analytic ESs varied between −0.41 and −0.61, which shows 'moderate' strength. Reviews of depressed participants seemed to show slightly stronger effects than those from mixed or healthy samples. In the review by Carter, Morres, Meade, and Callaghan (2016) concerning treatment effects from physical activity for adolescents, a meta-analysis of eight trials showed a significant overall moderate difference between intervention and controls for depressive symptom reduction. A similar strength of effect was shown in trials that studied only clinical samples. For trials with a higher methodological rating, the ES was also similar but marginally non-significant.

One trial illustrative of the field was reported by Nabkasorn and colleagues (2006). Adolescent females with mild-to-moderate depression were randomized to a group jogging condition for 5 × 50 minutes weekly sessions for 8 weeks or a control group. Not only did depression scores decline in comparison to controls, but neurobiological markers also indicated favorable effects. Two issues should be noted. One is the relatively high volume of exercise. Although the level is below the standard physical activity guideline for young people of 60 minutes/day on most or all days of the week, this may still prove to be a challenge to many. Second, the exercise took place in groups, and any favorable psychological effect could be due to social effects.

Biddle et al. (2019) also conducted an analysis concerning whether physical activity is causally associated with depression in young people (see Table 6.1). It was concluded that only a 'partial' case could be made for causality. Compared to adults, where it has been suggested that physical activity is causally associated with clinical depression (Biddle, Mutrie, & Gorely, 2015; Mutrie, 2000), the evidence appears less convincing for young people for both clinical and non-clinical populations. As indicated in Table 6.1, while the evidence is encouraging from interventions, there is little evidence showing an appropriate temporal sequencing of physical activity preceding changes in depression. Moreover, reverse causality has not been tested whereby those with higher levels of depression become less active. There was also little to suggest that indicators of exercise dose (e.g., intensity or frequency) affected depression. If studies on chronic involvement in physical activity mirror data from acute studies, one might expect highly variable affective responses to 'heavy' exercise, but largely favorable responses to lighter (light and moderate) exercise. 'Severe' (very high) intensity exercise can be associated with negative affective states (Ekkekakis & Dafermos, 2012; Ekkekakis, Vazou, Bixby, & Georgiadis, 2016). However, these issues are in need of further testing in programs of physical activity involvement over time.

The somewhat mixed findings concerning physical activity and depression in young people could be due to several reasons. First, studies show great diversity in the sampling of young people, and have included those apparently 'healthy', those with mild depressive moods, as well as those with clinical levels of depression. In addition, youth with other conditions have also been studied

Table 6.1 Appraisal of evidence, drawn from a review of systematic reviews (2012–2017), for whether the association between physical activity and depression in young people can be considered causal (Biddle et al., 2019)

Criterion proposed by Hill (1965)	*Research question*	*Assessment*	
		Is there evidence for causality?	Comments
Strength of association	How strong is the association between physical activity and depression in young people?	Partial	Interventions show moderate ESs. Observational studies show small to very small negative associations
Temporal sequencing	Does physical inactivity precede the development of depression in young people?	No	Longitudinal studies do not support temporal sequencing, with null to small associations or effects. Reverse causality not tested but plausible
Dose-response relationship	Do higher levels of physical activity show lower levels of depression in young people?	No	Largely null effects for intensity, frequency, and duration as moderators
Experimental evidence	Is there evidence using experimental methods in young people for changes in depression resulting from changes in physical activity?	Yes	Evidence from experimental intervention trials shows moderate ESs

(e.g., ADHD). The identification of the reasons for <u>why</u> physical activity might be beneficial for the reduction of depression in young people remains less well studied. Most commentary on the 'why' question – so called 'mechanisms' – has referred to adults. Psychological mechanisms that have been proposed include the enhancement of self-efficacy, the regulation of affect and mood, and the reinforcement of positive behaviors (Craft, 2013). Neurobiological mechanisms have also been proposed, including the monoamine and neurotrophin hypotheses (see Chen, 2013).

Lubans and colleagues' (2016) conceptual model for the effects of physical activity on mental health in youth includes neurobiological, psychosocial, and behavioral mechanisms. These authors also conducted a systematic review of mechanisms by synthesizing studies that are tested for mediation effects. Rather few studies were available concerning depression. Only one of four studies presented evidence showing a change in a mediator (physical self-concept) and change in depression. No conclusions could be made regarding causality, and, clearly, more is needed using this kind of approach.

Anxiety and Stress

Another frequently encountered mental health problem is anxiety. It is also common to hear anecdotal reports of day-to-day 'stress', such as examinations, concerns about money, and family and social conflicts. These point to the need to find accessible and affordable treatments or coping strategies. Physical activity has long been thought to be suitable for stress relief. This could be immediately following an exercise session (acute effects), or a gradual decline in trait levels of anxiety over time as a result of participation in an exercise program (chronic effects). Moreover, reactions to psychosocial stressors can also be attenuated through physical activity (Crews & Landers, 1987; Utschig, Otto, Powers, & Smits, 2013). For example, the cross-stressor-adaptation (CSA) hypothesis suggests that exposure to physical stress, such as through exercise, will trigger a stress response similar to that of psychosocial stressors. This can lead to positive adaptions to stress which can also generalize to other stressors (Mücke, Ludyga, Colledge, & Gerber, 2018). However, little work on this has been conducted with children and adolescents.

Biddle and Asare (2011) concluded from four systematic reviews that "physical activity interventions for young people have been shown to have a small beneficial effect for reduced anxiety. However, the evidence is limited and in need of development" (pp. 888–889). In their updated review, Biddle et al. (2019) located only three new systematic reviews between 2012 and 2017, suggesting that the field did not progress a great deal over this time period. Overall, results from the updated reviews show anxiety reduction effects from physical activity, with ESs ranging from very small to moderate. The latter was for young people with ADHD. The reviews showed moderate-to-large intervention effects for healthy young people. No evidence was available in the review by Lubans et al. (2016) concerning possible mechanisms for anxiety-reducing effects of physical activity in youth.

With scant attention being paid to young people, it is important to note findings and issues gleaned from research with adults. For example, Utschig et al. (2013) conclude that "physical activity is beneficial for most anxiety, most of the time" (p. 112). Research directions that could equally apply to young people include interventions for people with anxiety disorders, the nature of the dose-response relationship, and self-selected versus prescribed exercise intensities (Utschig et al., 2013). Moreover, there is a need to test bi-directional effects between physical activity and anxiety (Burg et al., 2017). Regarding mechanisms for anxiety reduction effects, Gaudlitz, von Lindenberger, Zschucke, & Strohle (2013) and Mücke et al. (2018) suggest a number of possibilities, including the following:

- Psychological: exposure to internal bodily sensations; anxiety sensitivity; self-efficacy; self-esteem; changes in accessibility or intensity of ruminations, worries, and anxiety; modification of emotional action tendencies; social contact/engagement

- Biological: serotonin, opioids, stress hormone system, atrial natriuretic peptide, brain-derived neurotrophic factor (BDNF), genetics.
- Positive adaptation of the hypothalamic-pituitary-adrenocortical (HPA) axis activity and the sympathoadrenal medullary (SAM) system during exercise.

Despite the importance of anxiety as a mental health construct, the literature regarding physical activity and anxiety reduction in youth seems rather limited in comparison to the other constructs discussed in this chapter.

Health-Related Quality of Life

Perceived quality of life is considered an over-arching concept of importance to well-being and is similar to concepts such as life satisfaction. At this generic level it can include perceptions of health, well-being, personal circumstances, happiness, and even where you live (e.g., 'livability'). In most physical activity studies where quality of life has been assessed, it has usually been as health-related quality of life (HRQoL) (Focht, 2012), including 'subjective well-being'. Rejeski et al. (1996) suggest that it is typical for HRQoL to be defined in terms of participants' perceptions of function, as shown in Table 6.2.

Some have suggested a simple division of HRQoL into functional measures and those assessing quality of life itself (Muldoon, Barger, Flory, & Manuck, 1998). The assessment of quality of life has become increasingly important because health economists use it to quantify the benefits of different approaches to treatment. The unit of 'quality adjusted life year' (QALY) is used to estimate how much it would cost to improve someone's quality of life or extend that person's life with a new treatment.

Given the emphasis in HRQoL measures on functional status, it is not surprising that when this is included in physical activity studies, it has been in the context of special populations. These have included older adults (Elavsky & McAuley, 2013), those with disability or with chronic conditions, including cancer and cardiovascular disease (e.g., Vallance, Culos-Reed, Mackenzie, & Courneya, 2013). Focht (2012) concludes that findings "clearly demonstrate that exercise consistently results in … clinically meaningful improvements in a variety of quality-of-life outcomes …" (p. 110). However, while some evidence exists for young people (e.g., Page et al., 2009), this is considerably less than for adults and more research is needed (Marker, Steele, & Noser, 2018).

In a systematic review by Marker and colleagues (2018), 33 studies were identified concerning physical activity and HRQoL in young people. They found from cross-sectional observational studies that there was a small, positive association when self-reported by the child. However, when the assessments were completed by the parents, the association was smaller. For intervention studies, there was a small effect using reports by the child. This ES was greater when parent reports were used. The authors concluded that physical activity was related to better HRQoL in children

Table 6.2 Dimensions of HRQoL (Rejeski et al., 1996)

Indexes of HRQoL	Include
Global	General life satisfaction and self-esteem
Physical function	Perceptions of function, physical self-perceptions, health-related perceptions
Physical symptoms	Fatigue, energy, sleep
Emotional function	Depression, anxiety, mood, affect
Social function	Social dependency and family/work roles
Cognitive function	Memory, attention, problem-solving

and adolescents. However, they stated that the "magnitude of these effects did not represent a minimal clinically important difference (MCID) in most studies". There also appears to be inconsistency of findings based on whether the data were reported by children or parents.

Possible Moderators of Mental Health Effects from Physical Activity

The association between physical activity and mental health in young people may be moderated by various factors, including sex, age, mental health status of the participants, and type of physical activity. In our analysis of causality of the effects of physical activity on self-esteem and depression (Biddle et al., 2019), we found no consistency in evidence across systematic reviews for differential effects for sex and age. While some studies or reviews have shown sex and age differences, these are not consistent.

An important moderator that has been found is that of the mental health status of participants. It has been a problem in the literature for many years that studies often concern essentially healthy participants. While physical activity could affect daily mood, for example, it is less likely to influence depression or anxiety if such mental health conditions are of a 'normal' or non-clinical level. In our updated review of reviews (Biddle et al., 2019), we found a great deal of diversity in the reviews concerning depression. For example, reviews included studies where the young people were mentally 'healthy', had mild depressive moods, and had clinically assessed depression at least at a 'moderate' level, as well as some studies addressing youth with ADHD. Such diversity is likely to lead to some inconsistency in findings. However, for those diagnosed as depressed, results favored physical activity quite consistently. For self-esteem, the issue may be different as it is possible for physical activity to boost the self-esteem of those with low self-esteem, as well as enhance it to levels higher than 'normal'. Equally, negative physical activity experiences may undermine self-esteem.

Different Types of Physical Activity

It would be naive to expect all types of physical activity to affect mental health in the same way. While results suggest that key indicators of mental health in youth can be positively affected by physical activity, a great deal more needs to be known about how different types of physical activity operate, especially across different contexts. In a systematic review covering all age groups, including adults, White et al. (2017) reported that mental health was weakly and positively associated with participation in leisure-time and work-related physical activity. Household physical activity, as well as school sport and PE, was not significantly associated with better mental health. These findings suggest that greater attention needs to be paid to different domains of physical activity.

Moreover, different types and domains of physical activities can have different qualities, and different contexts could affect mental health outcomes. Key activity domains include school PE, competitive sport, exercise programs, recreational activities (e.g., surfing), incidental/habitual physical activity (e.g., active transport), dance, martial arts, and holistic movement practices (e.g., yoga).

Physical Education

Physical education in schools has the primary aim of educating children about movement and their bodies. It will include some elements of competition and largely unavoidable public display of skills and competencies, which may lead to diverse psychological reactions. It will also include elements of compulsion and thus will not always be a 'free choice' behavior. In a survey of perceptions of their school PE lessons in the US, respondents reported on their 'worst memories'.

Feelings of embarrassment were reported by 34%, lack of enjoyment by 18%, bullying by 17%, and social-physique anxiety by 14% (Ladwig, Vazou, & Ekkekakis, 2018). While 'best memories' included enjoyment of the activities in class (56%; see later) and experiencing feelings of physical competence (37%), 7% expressed their best memory was not having to take PE class any longer or missing the class altogether! It appears that the context of school PE – experienced by nearly all children and adolescents – leads to diverse psychological responses. Any conclusions, therefore, that PE 'boosts self-esteem', for example, are too simplistic.

Sport

Competitive sport is a key physical activity opportunity for young people and tends to be highly valued in many societies. It usually places clear emphasis on competence, skills, and comparative abilities, and outcomes can create negative as well as positive feelings. Equally, it can challenge young people to improve and structure their practice, as well as help them learn about persistence and striving. Such diversity of approaches and outcomes based on outcome- versus self-focused is reflected in a great deal of research concerning achievement goals of youth in physical activity (Keegan, 2019; Roberts & Papaioannou, 2014). This remains an important explanatory framework, alongside other theories such as Self-Determination Theory (Ryan & Deci, 2000b; Standage, Curran, & Rouse, 2019).

Youth sport can also assist in creating strong social bonds (see later) and positive feelings of affiliation and group goal-seeking. However, as shown in seminal research over half a century ago, inter-group competition can create negative as well as positive environments and responses (Sherif, 1958; Sherif, Harvey, White, Hood, & Sherif, 1961).

Exercise

Exercise programs usually have the aim of improving fitness and health. They can involve solo or group exercising but are often structured and repetitive forms of movement (Caspersen, Powell, & Christenson, 1985). Exercise programs are likely to impact body image and physical self-perceptions in positive ways, but also challenge discipline and adherence (Lunt et al., 2014). It is likely that structured exercise training with a personal trainer will reach those from lower socio-economic groups less than those from more affluent sectors (Bennie, Thornton, van Uffelen, Banting, & Biddle, 2016), and personal trainers appear to have only a modest level of interest in training high health-risk groups (Bennie, Thomas et al., 2018). But the appeal of 'traditional' exercise sessions may not be appealing to many young people, although may develop as young people progress from adolescence to young adulthood and thus adopt more adult-like lifestyles. For younger children, 'exercise' will be part of active play, active transport, and sport.

For exercise, as well as PE and sport, an excellent framework to consider for optimizing the experience of physical activity for young people, and enhancing its appeal, is the 'SAAFE' framework, developed by Lubans et al. (2017). SAAFE is an acronym for supportive, active, autonomous, fair, and enjoyable. This is an "an evidence-based framework designed to guide the planning, delivery, and evaluation of organized physical activity sessions in school, after-school, and community sports setting" (p. 2). The SAAFE principles were informed by various motivational theories, including self-determination theory and achievement goal theory.

Recreational Activities

There are a number of active recreational pursuits that might provide a different psychosocial context for young people compared with, say, school PE or sport. This may include activities such as surfing, hiking, and mountain biking. The context may be non-competitive, and is likely to include possibilities not only for being outside in nature, but also providing thrill and adventure-seeking. Mental health benefits could easily accrue from such experiences (Araújo, Brymer, Brito, Withagen, & Davids, 2019; Brymer, Davids, & Mallabon, 2014; Davids, Araujo, & Brymer, 2016). 'Green gym' initiatives, aimed mainly at adults, are examples of combining physical activity with nature-based tasks and environments.

Incidental Physical Activity

What might be termed 'incidental physical activity' – sometimes referred to as 'habitual physical activity' – includes physical activity that is undertaken throughout the day in less structured bouts. This might involve stair climbing, and walking and cycling as forms of transport. It is unclear whether the utilitarian purpose of some of these behaviors will affect mental health, particularly in young people, and may in some cases be seen as unpleasant effort or inconvenient, and less comfortable ways to travel. This needs further research.

Dance

Dance comes in a multitude of forms and types of engagement varying from performance-oriented forms such as ballet, to competitive forms, social dances, as well as creative and free movement forms, delivered both within and outside of school education. Dance forms and contexts can vary greatly in terms of their emphases on what is important, ranging from skill learning, mastery, and technical perfection aimed at performance or competition, to fun and social interaction, and to self-expression, self-knowledge, and sometimes self-transcendence.

Some performance-oriented dance contexts, particularly the ballet environment, can provide strong pressures on young dancers. This may include absorbing a great deal of critical assessment, competition for performance roles, conforming to certain body shapes, and the pressures of performing itself. This environment has been shown to be associated with lower levels of self-esteem, and higher levels of body dissatisfaction and disordered eating in young female dancers (Bettle, Bettle, Neumärker, & Neumärker, 2001; Ravaldi et al., 2006). On the other hand, committed young dancers often thrive on the discipline that is part of this type of dance environment (Bond & Stinson, 2007; Stinson, Blumenfield, & van Dyke, 1990).

There are also dance contexts for children that encourage free movement, self-exploration, and self-expression. Koff (2000) has argued that this type of creative involvement in dance should be the basis of dance education in schools. Research is still limited in terms of what these types of dance engagement can do for young people's mental health. But it has been suggested, for example, that free movement forms of dance could help young people, girls in particular, to experience and appreciate their bodies from the inside out and as a way of improving physical self-esteem (Johansson, 2015). This could act as an antidote to society's objectification of the female body as outlined in Fredrickson and Roberts' (1997) objectification theory. This posits that girls and women are typically acculturated to internalize an observer's perspective on their physical selves, which can lead to shame, anxiety, eating disorders, and low physical self-esteem, rather than a lived and empowered appreciation of one's physicality.

Martial Arts

Traditional martial arts (e.g., judo, karate, taekwondo) can provide structure, predictability, and discipline, in addition to grading systems that reward personal mastery and commitment. A review by Vertonghen and Theeboom (2010) indicated that research on martial arts in youth has shown positive psychosocial benefits, with a number of studies finding beneficial effects for anxiety, self-reliance, cognitive and affective self-regulation, self-acceptance, and personal growth, and decreases in hostility and aggression. However, they also noted some inconsistency in findings, and some studies showed associations with increases in hostility and anti-social behavior. Martial arts have been found to be relatively popular choices for intervention programs targeted at socially vulnerable or 'at risk' youth (Theeboom, De Knop, & Wylleman, 2008).

Holistic Movement Practices

Holistic movement practices (HMPs) are physical practices embedded in philosophies of holistic well-being. The most well known of these in western society are the imported Asian practices of yoga, t'ai chi and qigong. These include a range of internally focused skills, including meditation, breathing, mindful attention, self-acceptance, body awareness, mental and emotional awareness, and sometimes imagery (Park et al., 2018; Wayne & Kaptchuk, 2008). Research on psychological effects of holistic movement practices on children and adolescents is still very limited but these practices have potential for training and improving internal processes related to self-knowledge and self-regulation.

A systematic review of psychosocial and other outcomes of yoga in schools was reported by Ferreira-Vorkapic and colleagues (2015). Results were supportive of the benefits of yoga in some studies, but overall there was uncertainty in findings. A number of problems with the literature were identified, and these might have contributed to this uncertainty. These included inadequate sample sizes, variability in the type of yoga being taught, and failure to measure intervening variables such as mindfulness and body awareness.

In a recent systematic review, Riskowski and Almeheyawi (2017) concluded that there was insufficient evidence to evaluate the effect of t'ai chi and qigong interventions on psychological well-being and behavior of children and adolescents. The authors noted that there was a large variety in type, dose, and duration of the interventions, as well as in the outcome measures studied. Although the slowness and required levels of concentration of t'ai chi/qigong may act as a deterrent to some young people (Riskowski & Almeheyawi, 2017), t'ai chi and qigong's ingredients of slow movements, concentration, mindful awareness, imagery, intention, and body awareness offer potential avenues for relaxation, stress management, and self-regulation when taught with age-appropriate adaptations.

Overall, given their inclusion of internally focused self-regulation skills, the holistic movement practices discussed, and others, may offer particular benefits to young people in whom these skills are impaired.

In conclusion, more research is required concerning the effect of different types and contexts of physical activity for mental health in young people. The belief that all physical activities will automatically be positive for mental health, or operate in similar ways, is unlikely to be true. A more nuanced approach is required that recognizes the complexity of this field.

Emerging Issues and Other Perspectives

In this chapter, we have focused on evidence linking the key mental outcomes of self-esteem, anxiety, and depression with physical activity in young people. However, there are other important concepts and perspectives requiring attention. These include the following:

- Enjoyment as a significant antecedent and outcome of physical activity
- Combining affective and reflective perspectives on physical activity motivation and psychological outcomes
- Social benefits of physical activity

Discussion on enjoyment is included because enjoyment can act as both a mental health-related outcome and an antecedent of physical activity choices and motivation. It is often a misunderstood concept in exercise science and requires some clarification. Similarly, affect can play an important role as both an outcome and antecedent of physical activity.

Enjoyment as a Psychological Outcome

Enjoyment is a rather elusive or 'slippery' concept in physical activity research. It is not easy to define or measure, and it can act as an antecedent as well as a consequence of physical activity. Indeed, it is likely to act in a cyclical fashion, with people choosing activities they expect to enjoy and, if they then 'enjoy' the participation and experience, will come back for more. Equally, other important motives will need to operate to adhere to a program of exercise that is not inherently enjoyable. For example, in the study cited earlier by Ladwig et al. (2018), an online questionnaire was completed by over 1,000 American adults in which they were asked to rate their retrospective enjoyment of school PE, as well other perceptions, including attitudes and intentions for physical activity. In responses concerning their 'best memories', 56% referred to enjoyment of their PE class activities.

The notion of enjoyment being linked to participation might be considered common sense. In Australia, for example, it is recognized in national physical activity guidelines (see http://www.health.gov.au/internet/main/publishing.nsf/content/health-pubhlth-strateg-phys-act-guidelines#apa512). The Australian brochure summarizing guidelines for adolescents suggests to "choose activities you enjoy doing, and you will be more likely to continue doing them". But such statements are not as dominant as those concerning the physical health benefits of physical activity. In the 2018 updated guidelines from the US, a key summary paper in *JAMA*, with 115,736 online 'views' in the 30 days prior to November 22, 2018, has just one mention of the word 'enjoy(ment)', yet uses the word 'health' more than 60 times (Piercy et al., 2018). In the new 'Sport Plan' for Australia (see https://www.sportaus.gov.au/home), which includes wider aspects of physical activity, the word 'enjoy(ment)' is mentioned once in 70 pages and only in the context of swimming.

It was over three decades ago when Dishman, Sallis, and Orenstein (1985) stated, "Knowledge of and belief in the health benefits of physical activity may motivate initial involvement, but feelings of enjoyment and well-being seem to be stronger motives for continued participation" (p. 162). This is likely to be even more important for young people as health consequences of physical activity will not be as highly salient for them.

There are several ways to view enjoyment, including the concept of 'flow', intrinsic motivation, and affective states (Biddle et al., 2015). Csikszentmihalyi (1975) described activities that people invested a great deal of time and energy in as 'autotelic' (meaning 'self-goal' or 'self-purpose'). When asking people in a range of activities (e.g., rock climbers, composers, dancers) why they enjoyed their chosen activity, 'intrinsic' factors were clearly evident. For example, 'enjoyment of the experience and use of skills' was strongly endorsed as a reason for involvement. Csikszentmihalyi concluded that motivation seemed highest when the difficulty of the task (challenge) was matched by the personal abilities and skills of the individual. This matching led to a state of 'flow', or supreme enjoyment and engagement in the task. A mismatch can lead to either boredom (low challenge relative to skills) or anxiety (high challenge relative to skills). This is shown in Figure 6.5.

The concept of flow is one way to view physical activity enjoyment and suggests that greater emphasis is required on the matching of the challenges of the activity with capabilities. Of course, while gains in fitness (and skill) will require increasing the challenge of exercise, large mismatches in this regard will likely lead to anxiety or negative affect, and possible dropout.

Intrinsic motivation is a commonly studied aspect of physical activity psychology. High intrinsic motivation includes feelings of enjoyment as well as high effort, competence, and autonomy

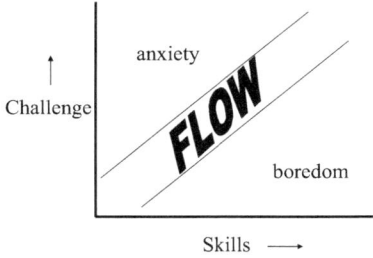

Figure 6.5 Illustration of the concept of 'flow' where high levels of enjoyment are thought to result from a matching of skills and challenge

(self-determination), and low levels of pressure and anxiety (Deci & Ryan, 1985). Intrinsic motivation, enjoyment, and flow are clearly interrelated. However, 'pure' intrinsic enjoyment is likely to be rare in some forms of physical activity, whereas we might be motivated more by what are called states of 'identified' motivation, such as being physically active for the satisfaction of achieving goals or mastering tasks, rather than just 'fun'. For example, in a meta-analysis, the association was assessed between 'affective judgment' and physical activity in young people (Nasuti & Rhodes, 2013). Affective judgment was defined as the "overall pleasure/displeasure, enjoyment, and feeling states expected from enacting an activity or from reflection on past activity" (p. 358). The ES was small (0.2) but significant. In a similar review with young people, it was found that autonomous forms of motivation (i.e., intrinsic motivation and identified regulation) had moderate, positive associations with physical activity, whereas controlled forms of motivation (i.e., introjection and external regulation) had weak, negative associations (Owen, Smith, Lubans, Ng, & Lonsdale, 2014). Therefore, it may not be appropriate to assume a simple relationship between physical activity and enjoyment given that 'intrinsic' states can vary in quality (Ryan & Deci, 2000a).

Returning to the circumplex model of affect discussed earlier, it is logical to expect positive feeling states, accompanied by high activation ('positive activated affect' – PAA (Reed & Ones, 2006)), to be associated with enjoyment during physical activity. Similarly, the positive engagement sub-scale of the Exercise-Induced Feeling Inventory (Gauvin & Rejeski, 1993) is closely associated with enjoyment. However, while enjoyment is a key to motivation, its nature and measurement is still in need of development and refinement. The only specific scale purporting to assess physical activity enjoyment is Kendzierski and DeCarlo's (1991) 18-item Physical Activity Enjoyment Scale (PACES), and this may include too many items for some studies wishing to assess many other constructs. Moreover, the scale contains multiple constructs that may produce differential responses to varied forms of physical activity. Items reflect the diverse feelings of enjoyment, boredom, pleasure, challenge, accomplishment, frustration, gratification, exhilaration, and others.

In summary, enjoyment is a key mental health-related outcome of physical activity, but can also act as an antecedent of decisions regarding physical activity involvement. It is a poorly understood concept and requires more work to clarify exactly what it is and how it can be assessed.

Affective States and Appraisals as Motivation

Similar to enjoyment, affective reactions and mental health outcomes of physical activity can also act as reinforcement for participation and motivation for adherence. However, this approach is rarely considered in the light of the mental health literature for young people. Moreover, the literature on motivation for physical activity in general tends to adopt a cognitive approach that assumes people are rational decision-makers in such matters. Other perspectives, such as dual-process models, provide additional insight (Brand & Ekkekakis, 2018). Essentially, humans will operate two psychological processes that can lead to a behavior. The 'type-2' process involves the typical social-cognitive approach in exercise psychology whereby people think through and plan their actions – that is, it involves 'reflective' evaluations and processes. An example would be where people schedule an exercise session, and plan the time, type, and location (referred to as 'action plans'). Hence, this is seen as a 'slow' route. 'Type-1' processes, on the other hand, involve more 'automatic' and 'gut response' reactions. This might involve a spontaneous decision to walk home from work when the weather is nice (referred to as 'action impulse'). Little conscious thought or planning is involved, and hence, it is a 'fast' processing route. This perspective underpins the 'Affective-Reflective Theory' (ART) of physical inactivity proposed by Brand and Ekkekakis (2018). The ART claims to differ from other approaches by, among other things, focusing on the role of affect and automaticity. Brand and Ekkekakis state that "individuals tend to seek pleasurable experiences and avoid displeasure", and

> hedonistic theories differ significantly from most theories presently used in the study of exercise motivation, which are based on a cognitive core and assert that, once enough information is available … individuals will inevitably make the rational decision to change their behavior and will be motivated to do so more or less regardless of any hardship they have to endure in the process.
>
> *(pp. 50–51)*

The ART provides an additional approach to conventional views by combining affective and reflective constructs in the advancement of knowledge concerning physical activity motivation. The role of affect is important in this but extends the notion of affect simply being a response to an event, such as exercise, as described earlier in the chapter. Moreover, it may be highly relevant to young people because of their propensity for more spontaneous forms of physical activity (e.g., active play). These are important ways to be active, although more research is required on the mental health outcomes of such forms of physical activity, as suggested earlier.

Social Benefits of Participation

The focus of research on physical activity and mental health in young people has tended to adopt a strongly psychological orientation. Outcomes described in this chapter (e.g., depression, self-esteem) are obviously 'psychological'. However, as Carless and Douglas (2010) argue, research should not only investigate the effects of physical activity, but also explore the meaning of physical activity in the context of people's lives, including those with mental ill-health. To do this, a broader perspective is required where the social context of physical activity is accounted for, and social outcomes are also studied.

It is frequently claimed that physical activity can bring about positive social benefits for the individual, as well as society. Moreover, important developmental tasks include developing healthy interpersonal skills, a coherent sense of identity, and the ability to function as a socially and morally responsible member of society.

In a review of psychological and social benefits of sport participation for young people, Eime, Young, Harvey, Charity, and Payne (2013) identified a number of 'social' outcomes. These included relationships with coaches and friends, respect for teachers and neighbors, social functioning, social interactions, social self-concept, social well-being, sportsmanship, and teamwork. Initiatives and research concerning 'positive youth development' and 'sport for development' are examples where participation in physical activity – in this case mainly sport – is structured and delivered with explicit social outcomes in mind. Coalter (2005) states that participation in sport has claimed psychosocial and sociological benefits, for the latter including increased community identity, social coherence, and integration. Whether non-sport physical activity can have similar effects for young people remains to be seen, but future research should avoid narrowly focusing only on psychological outcomes and consider broader outcomes of perceived well-being and social benefits at the individual and community level.

Recommendations for Research and Professional Practice

In this final section, we provide recommendations for research concerning physical activity and mental health in young people, as well for professional practice. The latter include the settings of education, health, community, and family.

Recommendations for Research

Figure 6.1 shows the complexity of this field. An important part of this overall picture is the nature of the mental health outcome itself. In this chapter, we have focused – quite narrowly some might argue – on self-esteem, anxiety, depression, and HRQoL. But there are many psychological outcomes that could be considered, including externalizing disorders (e.g., ADHD and anger), feelings of energy and fatigue, and sleep. In addition, applications to wider contexts are recommended. These might include the role of physical activity in specific conditions, such as schizophrenia, addictions, behavioral difficulties, pain, and mood disorders.

Equally, research needs to continue to address how physical activity operates in different populations. These might include those with physical disabilities, with learning difficulties, presenting with pre-existing mental health problems, from different socio-economic backgrounds, and with different physical activity histories. One avenue to pursue is to see if types or characteristics of activities can be matched to mental health conditions for effective mental health promotion.

Different types of physical activity also require greater research attention. Mental health may be associated with a number of activity types or domains in different ways. For example, the context, interactions, and settings for sport and active transport are quite different, and thus, mental health relationships may not show similar patterns. A priority for future research is to study the mental health effects of different forms of transport for young people, such as comparisons between active and passive forms of transport. It is also worth studying the effects of holistic movement practices, which emphasize internal self-regulation skills, such as yoga and t'ai chi, on young people's mental health.

All studies involving physical activity struggle with measurement. In the present context, this will involve assessment of the exposure (physical activity) and outcome (mental health), both of which provide challenges. While physical activity measurement has advanced a great deal in recent years through the employment of new technology, there are still many unresolved issues. The use of movement-detection wearable technology devices (e.g., pedometers and accelerometers) is often referred to as using 'objective' assessment. However, there are many 'subjective' decisions used in the application of, say, accelerometers. Hence, it is recommended to refer to 'device-based assessment' rather than 'objective assessment'. Conversely, using self-report measures to assess physical activity is not necessarily 'subjective'. A self-report scale can distinguish between types of physical activities very well ('did you go swimming today?"), and, in such cases, the assessment is not 'subjective'. It is recommended to refer to such measures as 'self-reported physical activity'. Of course, deriving accurate values from some self-report measures is difficult, and associations with mental health may be underestimated due to large variability in the data. Equally, accelerometers will not report all activities very well (e.g., cycling) or not be able to distinguish between different types of activity.

As we have suggested in the reviews concerning self-esteem and depression, there is a case to be made for the assessment of whether physical activity is causally associated with mental health. The updated review of reviews by Biddle et al. (2019) used the criteria proposed by Sir Austin Bradford Hill (Hill, 1965), and these are well known in epidemiological research. The key point to note is that many different factors are taken into account, including strength of association, dose-response relationship, and experimental evidence. This 'triangulation' is important for arriving at decisions in research (Munafò & Davey Smith, 2018), and it is recommended that further analyses of this type are undertaken. Moreover, any conclusions reached using these criteria should be updated periodically. Other methods for testing causation are also possible, such as Mendelian randomization (Richmond et al., 2014).

Finally, it is clear from the evidence reviewed that the field is still dominated by quantitative studies. Given the nature of mental health, and the different contexts and experiences of physical activity, it is surprising that there are still rather few qualitative studies in this area. In addition, more mixed-methods studies are recommended where outcomes can be assessed in quantitative terms, but participant views and stories can be gathered through qualitative methods to help enrich and contextualize our understanding of such effects. But let us not fall into the trap of stating that quantitative studies are unable to 'explain' findings and that qualitative studies are 'in-depth' and thus able to provide the 'why' for mental health change. Both methods can operate in-depth or be superficial, and both offer explanations for the study findings in their own way. It will depend on how they were conducted.

Recommendations for Professional Practice

As the evidence accumulates supporting the role of physical activity in the development of positive mental health in youth, and given the national trends showing considerable prevalence of mental ill-being in young people, it is important to promote physical activity – for mental health as well as other positive outcomes – in different settings. Physical activity environments need to be able to support healthy psychological development (see Lubans et al., 2017). This will require pleasant and attractive environments that encourage physical activity, and provide plenty of opportunities for active rather than passive alternatives. Moreover, it is vital to have physically and emotionally safe, non-abusive, well-guided psychosocial environments provided by responsible adults in sport and other physical activity settings.

Perhaps the most obvious setting to consider is the education system. With nearly all children and adolescents attending school, this provides a highly suitable context for not only promoting physical activity, but also for exploring the role of active lifestyles in mental health. For example, schools can continue to offer high-quality PE for all, as well as offer extra-curricular opportunities to be active (e.g., dance, sport, active video games, and holistic physical activities that can foster stress management and emotion regulation skills). In addition, a whole-school approach should be encouraged whereby active living is supported in all aspects of school life, including active travel to and from school, inclusive sport and physical activity opportunities, and active classrooms designed for movement-based subject learning (Hinckson et al., 2015; Routen et al., 2017). Active living initiatives in schools should also have mental health outcomes as goals, and plan activities to boost self-esteem and HRQoL as standard practice.

Physical activity for positive mental health should also be promoted for young people in health and health care settings. Routine encounters with health care professionals should include assessment and advice about active lifestyles and mental well-being. Training of health professionals will be required.

Community facilitation of active living needs greater priority. A key area for this is to promote active forms of transport to and from school, and provide excellent local public transport systems, thus allowing a mix of passive and active forms of transport in favor of car-dependent travel. In addition, provision of 'green space', such as parks and play areas, is essential. Such environmental supports are usually provided at the 'community' level. Therefore, it is important that physical activity experts are involved in early discussions regarding urban planning.

Finally, the family should be considered as an important setting for the promotion of physical activity for the mental health of young people. Linking to issues raised in this section, parents need to be supportive of active opportunities at school, in health care, and in the local community. Where possible, driving children to school should be avoided, and active safe alternatives provided. Within the home, play spaces and equipment should be provided and supported, and young people encouraged to regulate (usually meaning 'reduce') their sitting time, such as at computer games.

Conclusions

This chapter has defined mental health and provided a historical context to contemporary research on physical activity and mental health in young people. We have highlighted that the prevalence of mental ill-being in youth is high. Evidence has been summarized on the key mental health outcomes of self-esteem, anxiety, depression, and HRQoL, and on balance, evidence is supportive of the role of physical activity in mental health promotion. However, many unresolved issues remain, including the role of different types of physical activities and preferences, the different contexts for physical activity, and possible moderators. We have suggested that additional issues should be considered; these include enjoyment, affective and reflective approaches in considering physical activity motivation, and the social benefits of activity. Finally, we summarized key recommendations for research and professional practice.

References

Araújo, D., Brymer, E., Brito, H., Withagen, R., & Davids, K. (2019). The empowering variability of affordances of nature: Why do exercisers feel better after performing the same exercise in natural environments than in indoor environments? *Psychology of Sport and Exercise, 42*, 138–145. doi:10.1016/j.psychsport.2018.12.020

Babic, M. J., Morgan, P. J., Plotnikoff, R. C., Lonsdale, C., White, R. L., & Lubans, D. R. (2014). Physical activity and physical self-concept in youth: Systematic review and meta-analysis. *Sports Medicine, 44*(11), 1589–1601. doi:10.1007/s40279-014-0229-z

Benjamin, C. C., Rowlands, A., & Parfitt, G. (2012). Patterning of affective responses during a graded exercise test in children and adolescents. *Pediatric Exercise Science, 24*, 275–288.

Bennie, J. A., Lee, D.-C., Khan, A., Wiesner, G. H., Bauman, A. E., Stamatakis, E., & Biddle, S. J. H. (2018). Muscle-strengthening exercise participation patterns among 397,423 American adults and associations with adverse health conditions. *American Journal of Preventive Medicine, 55*(6), 864–874. doi:10.1016/j.amepre.2018.07.022

Bennie, J. A., Thomas, G., Wiesner, G. H., Van Uffelen, J. G. Z., Khan, A., Kolbe-Alexander, T., . . . Biddle, S. J. H. (2018). Australian fitness professionals' level of interest in engaging with high health-risk population subgroups: Findings from a national survey. *Public Health, 160*, 108–115. doi:10.1016/j.puhe.2018.03.035

Bennie, J. A., Thornton, L. E., van Uffelen, J. G. Z., Banting, L. K., & Biddle, S. J. H. (2016). Variations in area-level disadvantage of Australian registered fitness trainers usual training locations. *BMC Public Health, 16*(1), 1–7. doi:10.1186/s12889-016-3250-3

Bettle, N., Bettle, O., Neumärker, U., & Neumärker, K. (2001). Body image and self-esteem in adolescent ballet dancers. *Perceptual and Motor Skills, 93*, 297–309. doi:10.2466/pms.2001.93.1.297

Biddle, S. J. H., & Asare, M. (2011). Physical activity and mental health in children and adolescents: A review of reviews. *British Journal of Sports Medicine, 45*, 886–895. doi:10.1136/bjsports-2011-090185

Biddle, S. J. H., Ciaccioni, S., Thomas, G., & Vergeer, I. (2019). Physical activity and mental health in children and adolescents: An updated review of reviews and an analysis of causality. *Psychology of Sport and Exercise, 42*, 146–155. doi:10.1016/j.psychsport.2018.08.011

Biddle, S. J. H., Mutrie, N., & Gorely, T. (2015). *Psychology of physical activity: Determinants, well-being and interventions* (3rd ed.). Abingdon, UK: Routledge.

Bond, K. E., & Stinson, S. W. (2007). 'It's work, work, work, work': Young people's experiences of effort and engagement in dance. *Research in Dance Education, 8*(2), 155–183. doi:10.1080/14647890701706115

Bos, A. E. R., Huijding, J., Muris, P., Vogel, L. R. R., & Biesheuvel, J. (2010). Global, contingent and implicit self-esteem and psychopathological symptoms in adolescents. *Personality and Individual Differences, 48*, 311–316. doi:10.1016/j.paid.2009.10.025

Bowling, A. (1997). *Measuring health: A review of quality of life measurement scales* (2nd ed.). Buckingham, UK: Open University Press.

Brand, R., & Ekkekakis, P. (2018). Affective–reflective theory of physical inactivity and exercise. *German Journal of Exercise and Sport Research, 48*, 48–58. doi:10.1007/s12662-017-0477-9

Brown, R. S. (1982). Exercise and mental health in the pediatric population. *Clinics in Sports Medicine, 1*(3), 515–527.

Brymer, E., Davids, K., & Mallabon, L. (2014). Understanding the psychological health and well-being benefits of physical activity in nature: An ecological dynamics analysis. *Ecopsychology, 6*(3), 189–197. doi:10.1089/eco.2013.0110

Burg, M. M., Schwartz, J. E., Kronish, I. M., Diaz, K. M., Alcantara, C., Duer-Hefele, J., & Davidson, K. W. (2017). Does stress result in you exercising less? Or does exercising result in you being less stressed? Or is it both? Testing the bi-directional stress-exercise association at the group and person (N of 1) level. *Annals of Behavioral Medicine, 51*(6), 799–809. doi:10.1007/s12160-017-9902-4

Calfas, K. J., & Taylor, W. C. (1994). Effects of physical activity on psychological variables in adolescents. *Pediatric Exercise Science, 6*, 406–423.

Carless, D., & Douglas, K. (2010). *Sport and physical activity for mental health.* Chichester, UK: John Wiley.

Carter, T., Morres, I. D., Meade, O., & Callaghan, P. (2016). The effect of exercise on depressive symptoms in adolescents: A systematic review and meta-Analysis. *Journal of the American Academy of Child and Adolescent Psychiatry, 55*(7), 580–590. doi:10.1016/j.jaac.2016.04.016

Caspersen, C. J., Powell, K. E., & Christenson, G. M. (1985). Physical activity, exercise and physical fitness: Definitions and distinctions for health-related research. *Public Health Reports, 100*, 126–131.

Chen, M. J. (2013). The neurobiology of depression and physical exercise. In P. Ekkekakis (Ed.), *Routledge handbook of physical activity and mental health* (pp. 169–183). London, UK: Routledge.

Coalter, F. (2005). Sport, social inclusion, and crime reduction. In G. E. J. Faulkner & A. H. Taylor (Eds.), *Exercise, health and mental health. Emerging relationships* (pp. 190–209). London, UK: Routledge.

Craft, L. L. (2013). Potential psychological mechanisms underlying the exercise and depression relationship In P. Ekkekakis (Ed.), *Routledge handbook of physical activity and mental health* (pp. 161–168). London, UK: Routledge.

Crews, D. J., & Landers, D. M. (1987). A meta-analytic review of aerobic fitness and reactivity to psychosocial stressors. *Medicine and Science in Sports and Exercise, 19*(5 Suppl), S114–S120.

Csikszentmihalyi, M. (1975). *Beyond boredom and anxiety.* San Francisco, CA: Jossey-Bass.

Davids, K., Araujo, D., & Brymer, E. (2016). Designing affordances for health-enhancing physical activity and exercise in sedentary individuals. *Sports Medicine, 46*(7), 933–938. doi:10.1007/s40279-016-0511-3

Deci, E. L., & Ryan, R. M. (1985). *Intrinsic motivation and self-determination in human behavior.* New York, NY: Plenum Press.

Dishman, R. K., Sallis, J. F., & Orenstein, D. (1985). The determinants of physical activity and exercise. *Public Health Reports, 100*, 158–171.

Eime, R. M., Young, J. A., Harvey, J. T., Charity, M. J., & Payne, W. R. (2013). A systematic review of the psychological and social benefits of participation in sport for children and adolescents: Informing development of a conceptual model of health through sport. *International Journal of Behavioral Nutrition and Physical Activity, 10*(1), 98. doi:10.1186/1479-5868-10-98

Ekeland, E., Heian, F., & Hagen, K. B. (2005). Can exercise improve self-esteem in children and young people? A systematic review of randomised controlled trials. *British Journal of Sports Medicine, 39*, 792–798.

Ekeland, E., Heian, F., Hagen, K. B., Abbott, J., & Nordheim, L. V. (2004). Exercise to improve self-esteem in children and young people. *The Cochrane Database of Systematic Reviews*, (1). Article No. CD003683. doi:10.1002/14651858.CD003683.pub2

Ekkekakis, P. (2003). Pleasure and displeasure from the body: Perspectives from exercise. *Cognition and Emotion, 17*, 213–239. doi:10.1080/02699930244000282

Ekkekakis, P. (2013). *The measurement of affect, mood, and emotion: A guide for health-behavioral research.* Cambridge, UK: Cambridge University Press.

Ekkekakis, P. (2015). Honey, I shrunk the pooled SMD! Guide to critical appraisal of systematic reviews and meta-analyses using the Cochrane review on exercise for depression as example. *Mental Health and Physical Activity, 8*, 21–36. doi:10.1016/j.mhpa.2014.12.001

Ekkekakis, P., & Dafermos, M. (2012). Exercise is a many-splendored thing, but for some it does not feel so splendid: Staging a resurgence of hedonistic ideas in the quest to understand exercise behavior. In E. O. Acevedo (Ed.), *The Oxford handbook of exercise psychology* (pp. 295–333). New York, NY: Oxford University Press.

Ekkekakis, P., Hartman, M. E., & Ladwig, M. A. (2018). Mass media representations of the evidence as a possible deterrent to recommending exercise for the treatment of depression: Lessons five years after the extraordinary case of TREAD-UK. *Journal of Sports Sciences, 36*(16), 1860–1871. doi:10.1080/02640414.2018.1423856

Ekkekakis, P., & Petruzzello, S. J. (2000). Analysis of the affect measurement conundrum in exercise psychology: I. Fundamental issues. *Psychology of Sport & Exercise, 1*, 71–88.

Ekkekakis, P., Vazou, S., Bixby, W. R., & Georgiadis, E. (2016). The mysterious case of the public health guideline that is (almost) entirely ignored: Call for a research agenda on the causes of the extreme avoidance of physical activity in obesity. *Obesity Reviews, 17*(4), 313–329. doi:10.1111/obr.12369

Elavsky, S., & McAuley, E. (2013). Role of physical activity in older adults' quality of life. In P. Ekkekakis (Ed.), *Routledge handbook of physical activity and mental health* (pp. 493–504). Abingdon, UK: Routledge.

Ferreira-Vorkapic, C., Feitoza, J. M., Marchioro, M., Simoes, J., Kozasa, E., & Telles, S. (2015). Are there benefits from teaching yoga at schools? A systematic review of randomized control trials of yoga-based interventions. *Evidence Based Complementary and Alternative Medicine, 2015*, 345835. doi:10.1155/2015/345835

Focht, B. C. (2012). Exercise and health-related quality of life. In E. O. Acevedo (Ed.), *The Oxford handbook of exercise psychology* (pp. 97–116). New York, NY: Oxford University Press.

Fox, K. R. (2000). The effects of exercise on self-perceptions and self-esteem. In S. J. H. Biddle, K. R. Fox, & S. H. Boutcher (Eds.), *Physical activity and psychological well-being* (pp. 88–117). London, UK: Routledge.

Fredrickson, B., & Roberts, T. (1997). Objectification theory: Toward understanding women's lived experiences and mental health risks. *Psychology of Women Quarterly, 21*, 173–206. doi:10.1111/j.1471-6402.1997.tb00108.x

Gaudlitz, K., von Lindenberger, B.-L., Zschucke, E., & Strohle, A. (2013). Mechanisms underlying the relationship between physical activity and anxiety: Human data. In P. Ekkekakis (Ed.), *Routledge handbook of physical activity and mental health* (pp. 117–129). Abingdon, UK: Routledge.

Gauvin, L., & Rejeski, W. J. (1993). The exercise-induced feeling inventory: Development and initial validation. *Journal of Sport & Exercise Psychology, 15*, 403–423.

Gruber, J. J. (1986). Physical activity and self-esteem development in children: A meta-analysis. In G. A. Stull & H. M. Eckert (Eds.), *Effects of physical activity on children* (pp. 30–48). Champaign, IL: Human Kinetics.

Hamlyn-Williams, C. C., Freeman, P., & Parfitt, G. (2014). Acute affective responses to prescribed and self-selected exercise sessions in adolescent girls: An observational study. *BMC Sports Science, Medicine, and Rehabilitation, 6*, 35. http://www.biomedcentral.com/2052-1847/6/35

Hardy, C. J., & Rejeski, W. J. (1989). Not what, but how one feels: The measurement of affect during exercise. *Journal of Sport and Exercise Psychology, 11*, 304–317.

Hill, A. B. (1965). The environment and disease: Association or causation? *Proceedings of the Royal Society of Medicine, 58*(5), 295–300.

Hinckson, E., Salmon, J., Benden, M., Clemes, S. A., Sudholz, B., Barber, S. E., . . . Ridgers, N. D. (2015). Standing classrooms: Research and lessons learned from around the world. *Sports Medicine.* Published Online: 01 December 2015. doi:10.1007/s40279-015-0436-2

Johansson, M. (2015). *Holistic movement practices and psychological benefits of embodied self-awareness.* Paper presented at the 14th European Congress of Sport Psychology, Bern, Switzerland.

Keegan, R. J. (2019). Achievement goals in sport and physical activity. In T. S. Horn & A. L. Smith (Eds.), *Advances in sport and exercise psychology* (4th ed., pp. 265–287). Champaign, IL: Human Kinetics.

Kendzierski, D., & DeCarlo, K. J. (1991). Physical activity enjoyment scale: Two validation studies. *Journal of Sport & Exercise Psychology, 13*, 50–64.

Kennedy, S. G., Smith, J. J., Morgan, P. J., Peralta, L. R., Hilland, T. A., Eather, N., . . . Lubans, D. R. (2018). Implementing resistance training in secondary schools: A cluster randomized controlled trial. *Medicine & Science in Sports & Exercise, 50*(1), 62–72. doi:10.1249/mss.0000000000001410

Koff, S. R. (2000). Toward a definition of dance education. *Childhood Education, 77*, 27–32. doi:10.1080/00094056.2000.10522134

Ladwig, M. A., Vazou, S., & Ekkekakis, P. (2018). "My best memory is when I was done with it": PE memories are associated with adult sedentary behavior. *Translational Journal of the American College of Sports Medicine, 3*(16), 119–129. doi:10.1249/tjx.0000000000000067

Lawrence, D., Johnson, S., Hafekost, J., Boterhoven De Haan, K., Sawyer, M., Ainley, J., & Zubrick, S. R. (2015). *The mental health of children and adolescents: Report on the second Australian child and adolescent survey of mental health and wellbeing.* Canberra, Australia: Department of Health.

Layman, E. M. (1960). Contributions of exercise and sports to mental health and social adjustment. In W. R. Johnson (Ed.), *Science and medicine of exercise and sports* (pp. 560–599). New York, NY: Harper.

Liu, M., Wu, L., & Ming, Q. (2015). How does physical activity intervention improve self-esteem and self-concept in children and adolescents? Evidence from a meta-analysis. *PLoS One, 10*(8), e0134804. doi:10.1371/journal.pone.0134804

Lubans, D. R., Lonsdale, C., Cohen, K., Eather, N., Beauchamp, M. R., Morgan, P. J., . . . Smith, J. J. (2017). Framework for the design and delivery of organized physical activity sessions for children and adolescents: Rationale and description of the 'SAAFE' teaching principles. *International Journal of Behavioral Nutrition and Physical Activity, 14*(1), 24. doi:10.1186/s12966-017-0479-x

Lubans, D. R., Richards, J., Hillman, C., Faulkner, G., Beauchamp, M., Nilsson, M., . . . Biddle, S. J. H. (2016). Physical activity for cognitive and mental health in youth: A systematic review of mechanisms. *Pediatrics, 138*(3), e20161642. doi:10.1542/peds.2016-1642

Lunt, H., Draper, N., Marshall, H. C., Logan, F. J., Hamlin, M. J., Shearman, J. P., . . . Frampton, C. M. A. (2014). High intensity interval training in a real world setting: A randomized controlled feasibility study in overweight inactive adults, measuring change in maximal oxygen uptake. *PLoS One, 9*(1), e83256. doi:10.1371/journal.pone.0083256

Malik, A. A., Williams, C. A., Weston, K. L., & Barker, A. R. (2018). Perceptual responses to high- and moderate-intensity interval exercise in adolescents. *Medicine and Science in Sports & Exercise, 50*(5), 1021–1030. doi:10.1249/MSS0000000000001508

Marker, A. M., Steele, R. G., & Noser, A. E. (2018). Physical activity and health-related quality of life in children and adolescents: A systematic review and meta-analysis. *Health Psychology, 37*(10), 893–903. doi:10.1037/hea0000653

Mental Health Foundation. (2018). *Statistics.* Retrieved from https://www.mentalhealth.org.uk/statistics

Mücke, M., Ludyga, S., Colledge, F., & Gerber, M. (2018). Influence of regular physical activity and fitness on stress reactivity as measured with the Trier social stress test protocol: A systematic review. *Sports Medicine, 48*(11), 2607–2622. doi:10.1007/s40279-018-0979-0

Muldoon, M. F., Barger, S. D., Flory, J. D., & Manuck, S. B. (1998). What are the quality of life measurements measuring? *British Medical Journal, 316*, 542–545.

Munafò, M. R., & Davey Smith, G. (2018). Repeating experiments is not enough. *Nature, 553*, 399–401. doi:10.1038/d41586-018-01023-3

Mutrie, N. (2000). The relationship between physical activity and clinically defined depression. In S. J. H. Biddle, K. R. Fox, & S. H. Boutcher (Eds.), *Physical activity and psychological well-being* (pp. 46–62). London, UK: Routledge.

Mutrie, N., & Parfitt, G. (1998). Physical activity and its link with mental, social and moral health in young people. In S. J. H. Biddle, J. F. Sallis, & N. Cavill (Eds.), *Young and active? Young people and health-enhancing physical activity: Evidence and implications* (pp. 49–68). London, UK: Health Education Authority.

Nabkasorn, C., Miyai, N., Sootmongkol, A., Junprasert, S., Yamamoto, H., Arita, M., & Miyashita, K. (2006). Effects of physical exercise on depression, neuroendocrine stress hormones and physiological fitness in adolescent females with depressive symptoms. *European Journal of Public Health, 16*(2), 179–184. doi:10.1093/eurpub/cki159

Nasuti, G., & Rhodes, R. E. (2013). Affective judgment and physical activity in youth: Review and meta-analyses. *Annals of Behavioral Medicine, 45*(3), 357–376. doi:10.1007/s12160-012-9462-6

Orth, U., Erol, R. Y., & Luciano, E. C. (2018). Development of self-esteem from age 4 to 94 years: A meta-analysis of longitudinal studies. *Psychological Bulletin*, Online First Publication, July 16, 2018. doi:10.1037/bul0000161

Owen, K. B., Smith, J., Lubans, D. R., Ng, J. Y. Y., & Lonsdale, C. (2014). Self-determined motivation and physical activity in children and adolescents: A systematic review and meta-analysis. *Preventive Medicine, 67*, 270–279. doi:10.1016/j.ypmed.2014.07.033

Page, R. M., Simonek, J., Ihász, F., Hantiu, I., Uvacsek, M., Kalabiska, I., & Klarova, R. (2009). Self-rated health, psychosocial functioning, and other dimensions of adolescent health in Central and Eastern European adolescents. *European Journal of Psychiatry, 23*(2), 101–114.

Park, C. L., Elwy, A. R., Maiya, M., Sarkin, A. J., Riley, K. E., Eisen, S. V., . . . Groessl, E. J. (2018). The Essential properties of yoga questionnaire (EPYQ): Psychometric properties. *International Journal of Yoga Therapy, 28*, 23–38. doi:10.17761/2018-00016R2

Piercy, K. L., Troiano, R. P., Ballard, R. M., Carlson, S. A., Fulton, J. E., Galuska, D. A., . . . Olson, R. D. (2018). The physical activity guidelines for Americans. *JAMA, 320*(19), 2020–2028. doi:10.1001/jama.2018.14854

Ravaldi, C., Vannacci, A., Bolognesi, E., Mancini, S., Faravelli, C., & Ricca, V. (2006). Gender role, eating disorder symptoms, and body image concern in ballet dancers. *Journal of Psychosomatic Research, 61*, 529–535. doi:10.1016/j.jpsychores.2006.04.016

Reed, J., & Ones, D. S. (2006). The effect of acute aerobic exercise on positive activated affect: A meta-analysis. *Psychology of Sport and Exercise, 7*(5), 477–514.

Rejeski, W. J., Brawley, L. R., & Shumaker, S. A. (1996). Physical activity and health-related quality of life. *Exercise and Sport Sciences Reviews, 24*, 71–108.

Richmond, R. C., Davey Smith, G., Ness, A. R., den Hoed, M., McMahon, G., & Timpson, N. J. (2014). Assessing causality in the association between child adiposity and physical activity levels: A Mendelian randomization analysis. *PLoS Medicine, 11*(3), e1001618. doi:10.1371/journal.pmed.1001618

Riskowski, J. L., & Almeheyawi, R. (2017). Effects of tai chi and qigong in children and adolescents: A systematic review of trials. *Adolescent Research Review.* doi:10.1007/s40894-017-0067-y

Roberts, G. C., & Papaioannou, A. G. (2014). Achievement motivation in sport settings. In A. G. Papaioannou & D. Hackfort (Eds.), *Routledge companion to sport and exercise psychology* (pp. 49–66). London, UK: Routledge.

Roberts, J. E., & Monroe, S. M. (1994). A multidimensional model of self-esteem in depression. *Clinical Psychology Review, 14*(3), 161–181. doi:10.1016/0272-7358(94)90006-X

Routen, A. C., Biddle, S. J. H., Bodicoat, D. H., Cale, L., Clemes, S., Edwardson, C. L., . . . Sherar, L. B. (2017). Protocol for an implementation evaluation of an intervention to reduce and break-up sitting time in the school classroom: The CLASS PAL (physically active learning) project. *BMJ Open, 7*, e019428. doi:10.1136/bmjopen-2017-019428

Russell, J. A. (1980). A circumplex model of affect. *Journal of Personality and Social Psychology, 39*, 1161–1178.

Russell, J. A., & Feldman-Barrett, L. (1999). Core affect, prototypical emotional episodes, and other things called emotion: Dissecting the elephant. *Journal of Personality & Social Psychology, 76*, 805–819.

Ryan, R. M., & Deci, E. L. (2000a). Intrinsic and extrinsic motivations: Classic definitions and new directions. *Contemporary Educational Psychology, 25*, 54–67.

Ryan, R. M., & Deci, E. L. (2000b). Self-determination theory and the facilitation of intrinsic motivation, social development, and well-being. *American Psychologist, 55*, 68–78.

Schuch, F. B., Vancampfort, D., Richards, J., Rosenbaum, S., Ward, P. B., & Stubbs, B. (2016). Exercise as a treatment for depression: A meta-analysis adjusting for publication bias. *Journal of Psychiatric Research, 77.* doi:10.1016/j.jpsychires.2016.02.023

Shavelson, R. J., Hubner, J. J., & Stanton, G. C. (1976). Self-concept: Validation of construct interpretations. *Review of Educational Research, 46*, 407–441.

Sheppard, K. E., & Parfitt, G. (2008). Acute affective responses to prescribed and self-selected exercise intensities in young adolescent boys and girls. *Pediatric Exercise Science, 20*, 129–141.

Sherif, M. (1958). Superordinate goals in the reduction of intergroup conflict. *American Journal of Sociology, 63*, 349–356. doi:10.1086/222258

Sherif, M., Harvey, O. J., White, B. J., Hood, W. R., & Sherif, C. W. (1961). *Intergroup conflict and cooperation: The Robbers Cave experiment* (Vol. 10). Norman, OK: University Book Exchange.

Smith, J. J., Beauchamp, M. R., Faulkner, G., Morgan, P. J., Kennedy, S. G., & Lubans, D. R. (2018). Intervention effects and mediators of well-being in a school-based physical activity program for adolescents: The 'resistance training for teens' cluster RCT. *Mental Health and Physical Activity, 15*, 88–94. doi:10.1016/j.mhpa.2018.08.002

Smith, J. J., Eather, N., Morgan, P. J., Plotnikoff, R. C., Faigenbaum, A. D., & Lubans, D. R. (2014). The health benefits of muscular fitness for children and adolescents: A systematic review and meta-analysis. *Sports Medicine, 44*(9), 1209–1223. doi:10.1007/s40279-014-0196-4

Standage, M., Curran, T., & Rouse, P. C. (2019). Self-determination-based theories of sport, exercise, and physical activity motivation. In T. S. Horn & A. L. Smith (Eds.), *Advances in Sport and Exercise Psychology* (4th ed., pp. 289–311). Champaign, IL: Human Kinetics.

Stinson, S. W., Blumenfield, D., & van Dyke, J. (1990). Voices of young women dance students: An interpretive study of meaning in dance. *Dance Research Journal, 22*(2), 13–22. doi:10.2307/1477780

Strain, T., Fitzsimons, C., Kelly, P., & Mutrie, N. (2016). The forgotten guidelines: Cross-sectional analysis of participation in muscle strengthening and balance & co-ordination activities by adults and older adults in Scotland. *BMC Public Health, 16*(1), 1108. doi:10.1186/s12889-016-3774-6

Stych, K., & Parfitt, G. (2011). Exploring affective responses to different exercise intensities in low-active young adolescents. *Journal of Sport & Exercise Psychology, 33*, 548–568.

Theeboom, M., De Knop, P., & Wylleman, P. (2008). Martial arts and socially vulnerable youth: An analysis of Flemish initiatives. *Sport, Education and Society, 13*(3), 301–318. doi:10.1080/13573320802200677

Tuson, K. M., & Sinyor, D. (1993). On the affective benefits of acute aerobic exercise: Taking stock after twenty years of research. In P. Seraganian (Ed.), *Exercise psychology: The influence of physical exercise on psychological processes* (pp. 80–121). New York, NY: Wiley.

Utschig, A. C., Otto, M. W., Powers, M. B., & Smits, J. A. J. (2013). The relationship between physical activity and anxiety and its disorders. In P. Ekkekakis (Ed.), *Routledge handbook of physical activity and mental health* (pp. 105–116). Abingdon, UK: Routledge.

Vallance, J., Culos-Reed, S. N., Mackenzie, M., & Courneya, K. S. (2013). Physical activity and psychosocial health among cancer survivors. In P. Ekkekakis (Ed.), *Routledge handbook of physical activity and mental health* (pp. 518–529). Abingdon, UK: Routledge.

Vertonghen, J., & Theeboom, M. (2010). The social-psychological outcomes of martial arts practise among youth: A review. *Journal of Sports Science & Medicine, 9*(4), 528–537.

Wayne, P. M., & Kaptchuk, T. J. (2008). Challenges inherent to T'ai Chi research: Part I – T'ai Chi as a complex multicomponent intervention. *The Journal of Alternative and Complementary Medicine, 14*, 95–102. doi:10.1089/acm.2007.7170A

White, R. L., Babic, M. J., Parker, P. D., Lubans, D. R., Astell-Burt, T., & Lonsdale, C. (2017). Domain-specific physical activity and mental health: A meta-analysis. *American Journal of Preventive Medicine, 52*(5), 653–666. doi:10.1016/j.amepre.2016.12.008

7

COGNITIVE AND ACADEMIC BENEFITS OF PHYSICAL ACTIVITY FOR SCHOOL-AGE CHILDREN

Eric S. Drollette and Charles H. Hillman

Introduction

Modern conveniences resulting from advances in technology over the past century have rapidly outpaced our evolved genetic need for a healthy mind and body (Vaynman & Gomez-Pinilla, 2006). Industrialized societies have shifting from a work force of human physical labor to automation, resulting in a reduction in daily occupation-related energy expenditure over recent decades (Church et al., 2011). Consequently, the rising generations are the beneficiaries of our new environment with data revealing that children today fail to meet physical activity recommendations for maintaining and improving not only physical health – including cardiovascular, muscular, metabolic, bone, and cancer-related health – but also mental health (2018 Physical Activity Guidelines Advisory Committee, 2018). As a consequence, children today are more overweight and obese, and less active and fit compared to previous generations (Gahche et al., 2014; Ogden, Carroll, Fryar, & Flegal, 2015). Unfortunately, public schools, who are intimately involved with over 50.7 million U.S. children for nearly two-thirds of waking hours (US Department of Education, National Center for Education Statistics, Common Core of Data, 2017), have further contributed to the declining health in youth by reducing physical activity opportunities during the school day – 16.2% reduction in daily physical education attendance from 1991 to 2015 (Kann, 2016) – in an effort to accommodate academic learning time. However, research over the past two decades demonstrating a positive relationship between increased physical activity and improved cognition, brain health, and academic achievement (Donnelly et al., 2016) suggests that this direction is counter to intended academic goals and represents a reciprocal maladaptive approach (Sallis, 2010). This surgency in scientific evidence provides a new direction for advocates of physical activity to educate administrative representatives regarding the necessity of physical activity opportunities as a significant factor for a healthy developing mind and should be a priority when intended educational goals are to improve academic achievement in developing youth.

This chapter will begin with definitions of key concepts associated with outcome measures of cognition and academic achievement. Next, specific research domains, including acute and chronic physical activity, with an emphasis on novel research derived from neuroimaging techniques will be discussed. The chapter will conclude with future directions with a particular focus on mechanisms that may better inform the design and application of physical activity interventions in school-age children. It should be noted that this chapter is not intended to be a comprehensive review of the extent of the research. Rather, the purpose is to provide an overview of current trends while highlighting general outcomes and practical conclusions that may better inform educators and administrators seeking to understand the current state of the literature.

Overview of the Literature

Defining Cognition and Academic Achievement

Researchers investigating the relation of physical activity to cognition often associate performance on a cognitive task as evidence of potential classroom success (Drollette et al., 2014; Harveson et al., 2016; Hogan et al., 2013; Pirrie & Lodewyk, 2012). However, such a leap may be an oversimplification of the many factors underlying academic achievement. Thus, an understanding of differences and similarities of cognition and academic achievement is necessary. Academic achievement is defined as a measurable performance outcome that reveals the extent to which a person has accomplished specific goals across different domains of learning in an instructional environment (Ramachandran, 2012). These measures, collected within the school system, stem from a prevailing concern among educators and policy makers seeking to identify and promote particular skills that children need in order to assure long-term academic and vocational success (Scott-Little, Lesko, Martella, & Milburn, 2007). Multiple methods have been implemented in school systems for measuring academic success over the past century (i.e., letter grades, and grade point average or GPA) with an increasing emphasis on standardized test batteries that are widely available, and have the advantage of comparing test results regionally, nationally, and globally. The variety of standardized tests are extensive and include Stanford Achievement Tests, National Assessment of Educational Progress (NAEP), and school- and state-level achievement tests. Interestingly, these measures, including standardized tests, have become a 'gate keeper' to future life outcomes with research demonstrating educational differences as a significant factor in social disparities including vocational success, income, and socioeconomic status (SES) (Jimerson, Egeland, & Teo, 1999).

Cognition represents a set of mental processes that contribute to perception, memory, intellect, and action. Cognitive function can be assessed using a variety of techniques including paper-and pencil-based tests, neuropsychological testing, and computerized testing methods. Cognitive functions are largely divided into different domains that capture both the type of process and the brain areas and circuits that control those functions. Furthermore, unlike academic achievement, cognition is not socially constructed and is composed of a collection of underlying mental processes that are utilized in a systematic order to accomplish an intended goal or outcome. These mental processes include (but are not limited to) memory, perception, attention, problem-solving, reasoning, learning, creativity, and language. Today, advances in neuroimaging technology compliment ongoing cognitive research and provide a new avenue for understanding mental operations occurring in the brain with an added benefit for observing mental processing in the absence of overt behavior.

In sum, cognition represents the set of underlying mental operations that are utilized to accomplish academic (as well as other) outcomes. To use an analogy, cognition can be viewed as a collection of tools that a carpenter has available to build a table, and academic achievement can be viewed as the finished table. Completion of the project requires multiple tools administered in an appropriate and particular order for the desired outcome. However, if the table has obvious wood splints around the edges (i.e., academic outcomes) it might be because the carpenter used a dull saw (i.e., underlying cognitive construct). In practical terms, a child might perform poorly on a mathematics exam because they did not pay attention to the lesson and may have poor memory ability to maintain and recall the necessary mathematical principles needed to solve the problem. Although this is an oversimplification of actual mental processing, while also ignoring other extraneous factors that play a critical role in academic success including parental involvement (Jeynes, 2007), personality (Poropat, 2009; Rimfeld, Kovas, Dale, & Plomin, 2016), environment (Hair, Hanson, Wolfe, & Pollak, 2015), and SES (White, 1982), it provides a framework for how these two domains are inter-related yet unique, thus providing a reference for understanding the relation with physical activity. Additionally, such clarification may assist with dispelling the notion that 'physical activity makes you smart', rather, physical activity sharpens the tools, but it does not build the table.

Cognitive Control

Of particular interest in this field of research is the set of cognitive operations known as cognitive control, or executive function, given the moderating link with academic achievement and physical activity. That is, research in children demonstrates that in many cases, physical activity effects are selectively greater for tasks involving cognitive control (Donnelly et al., 2016; Hillman, Kamijo, & Scudder, 2011), the relation of cognitive control to academic achievement is more robust compared to other cognitive domains (Bull & Scerif, 2001; Clair-Thompson & Gathercole, 2006; Swanson & Alloway, 2012), and physical activity is associated with academic achievement outcomes (Álvarez-Bueno et al., 2017) (see Figure 7.1).

Additionally, healthy development of cognitive control during childhood extends beyond these factors and is an important predictor of positive health outcomes during adulthood, including social outcomes, psychological disorders, risk of certain cancers, obesity, and life satisfaction (Gale et al., 2012; Koenen et al., 2009; Martin & Kubzansky, 2005; Moffitt et al., 2011), among other health factors. Together, it appears that cognitive control is the common underlying factor that may be most susceptible to physical activity behavior and may also be implicated in observed improvements in academic achievement. Further, cognitive control plays an important role across multiple domains that are important for healthy life outcomes. Thus, a detailed description is warranted to further elucidate the relation with physical activity and underlying implications for academic achievement.

Cognitive control refers to top-down, goal-directed mental operations that aid with selection, scheduling, maintaining, and coordinating processes that underlie perception, memory, and action (Botvinick, Braver, Barch, Carter, & Cohen, 2001; Norman & Shallice, 1986; Rogers & Monsell, 1995). The core cognitive processes underlying cognitive control include a set of unified yet diverse processes including working memory, inhibitory control, and cognitive flexibility (Miyake & Friedman, 2012; Miyake, Friedman, Emerson, Witzki, & Howerter, 2000). Young

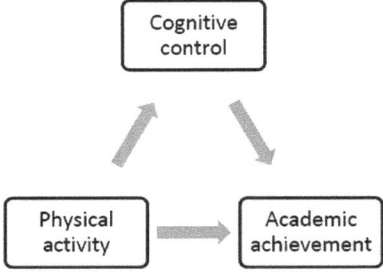

Figure 7.1 Illustration depicting the relation of physical activity to cognitive control and academic achievement

children appear to demonstrate a more unitary operation of cognitive control during early maturation and reveal functionally distinct processes with age. As such, analyses of the dimensionality of cognitive control demonstrate the emergence of inhibitory control earlier in development relative to working memory and cognitive flexibility (Barkley, 1997; Brocki & Bohlin, 2004); the latter two processes are not clearly detected until later in development (Korkman, Kemp, & Kirk, 2001), suggesting that inhibitory control is a robust driving factor of other developing cognitive control operations (Raaijmakers et al., 2008).

Cognitive Control and Brain Function

The interaction of cognitive control processes is dependent on the development and coordinative actions occurring in cortical and subcortical brain structures including the prefrontal cortex (PFC), basal ganglia, superior frontal sulcus, and the anterior cingulate cortex (ACC) (Bunge & Crone, 2009; Bunge, Dudukovic, Thomason, Vaidya, & Gabrieli, 2002; Rueda, Rothbart, McCandliss, Saccomanno, & Posner, 2005). For example, prior investigations demonstrate that patients with PFC lesions perform poorly on select cognitive control tasks compared to healthy controls (Stuss & Levine, 2002). Interestingly, healthy children demonstrate a similar pattern of performance (Bunge et al., 2002), indicating that the PFC follows a protracted development reaching maturation late in adolescence and in adulthood (Diamond, 2002). Therefore, given the delicate and early stages of neural development occurring in regions associated with cognitive control, children represent a critical population for examining physical activity (and other health and lifestyle factors) that potentially alters the developmental trajectory of cognitive control operations and associated brain processes.

Further representation of cognitive control can be assessed via a neuroimaging technique known as event-related potentials (ERPs), which refer to voltage fluctuations measured at the scalp (i.e., summation of postsynaptic potentials) that are time-locked to an event such as a stimulus in the environment or a response to that stimulus (Luck, 2014). These time-locked fluctuations are characterized by positive (P) and negative (N) components identified according to their relative time of occurrence after the event (Hruby & Marsalek, 2003; Luck, 2014). Unlike overt behavior, ERPs provide a continuous millisecond-by-millisecond measure of cognitive processing prior to and following an event, and thus provide high-temporal resolution of cognitive operations as they occur (Luck, 2014).

Cognitive Control and Academic Achievement

Healthy development of cognitive control in children entering preschool and kindergarten reveals notable links with school readiness, literacy, and arithmetic ability (Blair & Razza, 2007; Duncan et al., 2007; McClelland et al., 2007). For example, cognitive control outcomes in elementary age children demonstrate a relationship with language arts, arithmetic, and science (Clair-Thompson & Gathercole, 2006). Additionally, longitudinal data indicate that level of cognitive control upon school entry is a significant predictor of verbal comprehension, understanding directions, and math by first grade (Clark & Woodward, 2007), and higher achievement across various domains by second grade (McClelland, Morrison, & Holmes, 2000). Interestingly, when evaluating individual differences in SES, children from low-income families revealed a significant positive relation of cognitive control with standardized test scores accounting for 40% of the variance (Waber, Gerber, Turcios, Wagner, & Forbes, 2006). Further, cognitive control is also related to behaviors that complement the educational environment. That is, beyond test scores, cognitive control predicts behavior regulation (Cole, Usher, & Cargo, 1993) and classroom disruptive behavior (McGlamery, Ball, Henley, & Besozzi, 2007) in children from preschool to second grade with further longitudinal evidence, demonstrating a relation of cognitive control to teacher-rated classroom behavior from kindergarten to adolescence (Séguin, Nagin, Assaad, & Tremblay, 2004). Some research further suggests that cognitive control deficits in kindergarten were greater predictors of school dropout compared to aggression and defiant or resistant behavior (Vitaro, Brendgen, Larose, & Trembaly, 2005).

Physical Activity, Cognition, Brain Function, and Academic Achievement

Acute Physical Activity

To date, the overall findings following the cessation of an acute bout of physical activity on cognition generally favor improved performance with recent meta-analytical evidence revealing an effect size of 0.52 (Ludyga, Gerber, Brand, Holsboer-Trachsler, & Pühse, 2016). However, the available evidence in children is limited with significant variability in the characteristics of the physical activity bout, thus complicating attempts to delineate unique trends that may inform dose-response relationships. As such, caution is advised regarding the specificity of a prescribed 'dose' of acute physical activity intended to improve cognitive function and academic achievement in children. Rather, a general interpretation may be the best approach until additional research better informs on the dose-response relationship, with a specific emphasis on differences in intensity, duration, timing, and type of the activity bout.

This chapter will briefly discuss overall trends observed across specific cognitive and academic outcomes with a focus on children and adolescence. Findings will be clustered similar to the classification scheme used by Chang and colleagues (Chang, Labban, Gapin, & Etnier, 2012) and adopted by Pontifex et al. (2019), who provided a comprehensive evaluation of the after-effects of acute physical activity on cognition across the lifespan, including a critical evaluation of challenges for future research including discussions of dose-response effects, potential moderators, and underlying mechanisms.

The cognitive and academic outcomes that have received little attention in the literature include selective and sustained attention, information processing, memory, and academic achievement. Specifically, of the nine peer-reviewed articles examining attention (Budde, Voelcker-Rehage, Pietraßyk-Kendziorra, Ribeiro, & Tidow, 2008; Caterino & Polack, 1999; Chen, Yan, Yin, Pan, & Chang, 2014; Fearnbach et al., 2016; Ma, Le Mare, & Gurd, 2015; Metcalfe et al., 2016; Mierau et al., 2014; Raviv & Low, 1990; van den Berg et al., 2016) the majority demonstrate no beneficial effects, with only three revealing improvements following short high-intensity classroom breaks (Ma et al., 2015), coordinative body movement (Budde et al., 2008), and regular physical education instruction (Caterino & Polack, 1999). Research evaluating information processing demonstrates improvements following a variety of physical activity bouts (Gabbard & Barton, 1979; Howie, Schatz, & Pate, 2015; McNaughten & Gabbard, 1993; Samuel et al., 2017), with only one investigation revealing no change in performance (Cooper et al., 2016). Also, memory investigations have revealed selective findings for serial position of memory items (Etnier, Labban, Piepmeier, Davis, & Henning, 2014; Pesce, Crova, Cereatti, Casella, & Bellucci, 2009) and no benefits for successive processing or short-term memory (Di Pietro, 1986; Pirrie & Lodewyk, 2012). Lastly, assessments of academic achievement have revealed positive effects for word reading (Dickinson, Duncan, & Eyre, 2016; Hillman, Pontifex, et al., 2009; Pontifex, Saliba, Raine, Picchietti, & Hillman, 2013), mixed results for arithmetic achievement (Hillman, Pontifex, et al., 2009; Pontifex et al., 2013), and no change in performance for non-verbal matrices (Pirrie & Lodewyk, 2012) and spelling (Dickinson et al., 2016; Hillman, Pontifex, et al., 2009; Pontifex

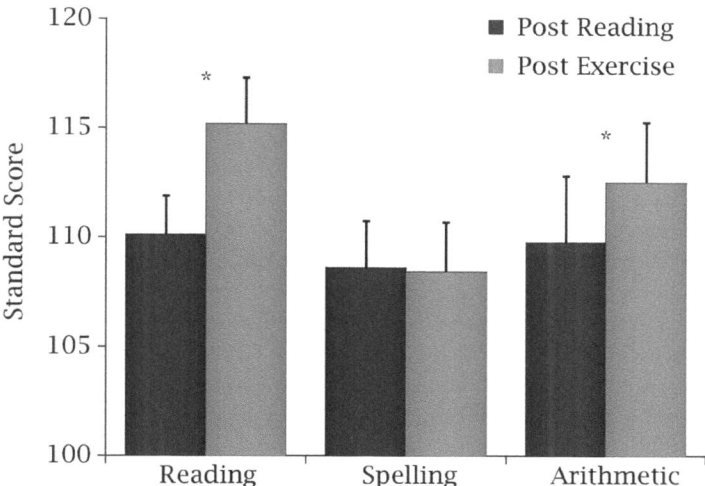

Figure 7.2 Standardized academic achievement scores (WRAT3) following acute exercise or reading (Pontifex et al., 2013)

et al., 2013). However, it should be noted that timing of assessment following the acute bout may be critical to observe beneficial effects for academic achievement following cessation of physical activity. For example, Hillman and colleagues revealed a non-significant trend in arithmetic performance when assessment occurred approximately 58 minutes following cessation of the acute bout of physical activity (Hillman, Pontifex, et al., 2009). Follow-up evaluations shortened the post-physical activity duration by nearly 20 minutes (i.e., 38 minutes) and demonstrated improvements in arithmetic performance while all other parameters of the physical activity bout remained consonant (see Figure 7.2) (Pontifex et al., 2013).

Together, these findings suggest selective improvements for information processing, reading, arithmetic, and memory, while attention and other academic achievement results are not as clear. Indeed, more research is needed in these areas to fully understand how acute bouts of physical activity influence a broad spectrum of cognitive and academic achievement outcomes. Furthermore, as research continues to assess academic achievement, a critical approach will be the practical application, especially with continued efforts to evaluate performance in classroom settings that represent an appropriate ecological environment.

The majority of evidence in this research domain has focused on cognitive control with a significant number of investigations evaluating inhibitory control [41% of all investigations across the lifespan; 48% in children and adolescence (Pontifex et al., 2019)]. Overall, results have generally observed improvements following a wide variety of physical activity modalities (Chen et al., 2014; Chu et al., 2017; Cooper et al., 2016; Drollette et al., 2014; Drollette, Shishido, Pontifex, & Hillman, 2012; Harveson et al., 2016; Hillman, Pontifex, et al., 2009; Hogan et al., 2013; Ishihara, Sugasawa, Matsuda, & Mizuno, 2017; Jäger, Schmidt, Conzelmann, & Roebers, 2014; Piepmeier et al., 2015; Pontifex et al., 2013) while only a few investigations observed no change in performance (Pirrie & Lodewyk, 2012; Soga, Shishido, & Nagatomi, 2015; Stroth et al., 2009). Conversely, the number of investigations evaluating working memory and cognitive flexibility is minimal in comparison to inhibitory control, and has generally yielded mixed results. That is, investigations evaluating working memory have revealed both improvements (Chen et al., 2014;

Cooper et al., 2016; Ishihara et al., 2017; Samuel et al., 2017) and no change in performance (Drollette et al., 2012; Jäger et al., 2014; Soga et al., 2015; van den Berg et al., 2016) with similar trends for cognitive flexibility (Harveson et al., 2016; Howie et al., 2015; Hung, Huang, Tsai, Chang, & Hung, 2016; Ishihara et al., 2017; Piepmeier et al., 2015; Pirrie & Lodewyk, 2012). Together, the abundant evidence for inhibitory control is relatively consistent in suggesting benefits following acute physical activity in a classroom and laboratory setting while the effects on working memory and cognitive flexibility appear less known.

More recently, emerging research has evaluated underlying brain function utilizing various neuroimaging and psychophysiological measures including EEG, ERP, and functional near-infrared spectroscopy. These tools provide insight into psychological processing occurring after a stimulus encounter in the environment and is not limited to a behavior response. The majority of research in children has focused on the P3-ERP component, which is associated with the allocation of attentional resources and timing of stimulus engagement. These investigations have commonly observed enhancements of (i.e., larger) P3 amplitude (Chu et al., 2017; Drollette et al., 2014; Hillman, Pontifex, et al., 2009, 2013), with some demonstrating no change after physical activity (Stroth et al., 2009); however, midline electrode sites were not collected in Stroth et al.'s study which represents a protocol deviation from all other studies in the area. Additionally, research evaluating activation in select brain regions via functional near-infrared spectroscopy has demonstrated that a significant proportion of change in inhibitory control performance following acute physical activity was associated with up-regulation in PFC perfusion and oxygenation (Lambrick, Stoner, Grigg, & Faulkner, 2016). Such neuroimaging findings further suggest that the observed physical activity effects on cognition may be subserved by neural markers associated with distinct brain regions implicated in cognitive control operations. Thus, these investigations provide a window into underlying cortical and subcortical functioning most influenced by single bouts of physical activity.

Overall, this research reveals a potential pattern regarding the beneficial after-effects of acute physical activity on different aspects of cognition and academic achievement, with effects appearing larger for tasks that require greater amounts of inhibitory control. Further, not only does this evidence demonstrate improvements in select cognitive domains, but a robust conclusion points to the evidence that acute bouts of physical activity are not detrimental to cognitive and academic performance, which stands in opposition to recent education practices that have obviated physical activity from the school day. Together with additional evidence in the classroom demonstrating improvements in time on task behavior (Grieco, Jowers, & Bartholomew, 2009; Mahar et al., 2006), and given that multiple repeated bouts of physical activity improve physiological health (i.e., improved fitness, and decreased body mass index or BMI), a practical interpretation of this literature is that, at a minimum, increasing physical activity during the school day will not harm intended educational goals, while promoting positive healthy behaviors in children, and at a maximum may benefit cognitive health and academic performance.

Fitness

This section will focus on cross-sectional investigations with an emphasis on research evaluating cardiorespiratory fitness as a proxy measure of physical activity. Although fitness is linked with physical activity and other extraneous factors – including genetics, physical environment, and morbidity (Bouchard, Shephard, & Stephens, 1994) – it should be noted that fitness represents an objective and accurate physiological measure that, if relations with cognition and brain health are present, supports physical activity interventions aimed at improving fitness (Etnier, Drollette, & Slutsky, 2019). Furthermore, ongoing cross-sectional investigations have consistently demonstrated a positive association of fitness with cognitive operations including cognitive control, memory, language, arithmetic, and learning in children (Berchicci et al., 2015; Buck, Hillman, &

Castelli, 2008; Chaddock, Erickson, Prakash, Kim, et al., 2010; Chaddock, Erickson, Prakash, VanPatter, et al., 2010; Chaddock et al., 2012; Hillman, Buck, Themanson, Pontifex, & Castelli, 2009; Kao, Drollette, et al., 2017; Kao, Westfall, Parks, Pontifex, & Hillman, 2017; Moore, Drollette, Scudder, Bharij, & Hillman, 2014; Pontifex et al., 2011; Pontifex, Scudder, Drollette, & Hillman, 2012; Raine et al., 2013; Scudder, Federmeier, et al., 2014; Scudder, Lambourne, et al., 2014; Voss et al., 2011; Westfall, Kao, Scudder, Pontifex, & Hillman, 2017; Wu et al., 2011), with further evidence demonstrating enhanced brain function (Berchicci et al., 2015; Pontifex et al., 2011), greater cerebral blood flow in subcortical brain regions (Chaddock-Heyman et al., 2016), and increased structural integrity in select cortical and subcortical regions (Chaddock, Erickson, Prakash, Kim, et al., 2010; Chaddock, Erickson, Prakash, VanPatter, et al., 2010; Voss et al., 2011). Such observations are not limited to children as older adults demonstrate similar associations in cognition, brain function, and brain structure (for review see Etnier et al., 2019). Thus, fitness appears robustly related to brain health and cognitive functioning across the lifespan.

Similar to the acute physical activity literature, investigations among children have mainly focused on measures of inhibitory control, which has consistently demonstrated better task performance in higher-fit children compared to their lower-fit peers. In many cases, selectivity is observed such that greater performance differences emerge for trial types or conditions that necessitate greater cognitive control demand (Chaddock, Erickson, Prakash, VanPatter, et al., 2010; Chaddock et al., 2012; Pontifex et al., 2011; Scudder, Lambourne, et al., 2014; Voss et al., 2011); however, it should be noted that some studies have reported more global fitness-related benefits (Hillman, Buck, et al., 2009). These differences are consonant across structural and functional investigations suggesting underlying neural processes that facilitate improved performance. For example, investigations of brain structure have demonstrated unique fitness-related differences in regions associated with cognitive control processing. Specifically, Chaddock and colleagues (2010) demonstrate greater volume in the basal ganglia, a subcortical structure implicated in cognitive control operations, for higher-fit children compared to their lower-fit peers, with further positive associations observed for inhibitory control (Chaddock, Erickson, Prakash, VanPatter, et al., 2010). Additionally, Pontifex and colleagues (2011) incorporated compatible and incompatible response conditions of an inhibitory control task when evaluating individual differences in fitness. Results demonstrated that performance of task conditions requiring lesser amounts of inhibition compared to the condition requiring greater amounts of inhibition was equivalent for higher-fit children, while lower-fit children exhibited reduced accuracy for the condition with greater inhibitory demands. These results were further supported by ERP indices with higher-fit children exhibiting larger P3 amplitude (i.e., greater allocation of attentional resources), shorter P3 latency (i.e., faster cognitive processing speed), and decrease error-related negativity (ERN) amplitude (lower threshold for evaluation of stimulus-response conflict) for the less demanding condition, with greater modulation of ERP components across conditions requiring variable amounts of inhibition (demonstrating greater flexibility in the allocation of neuroelectric resources). Thus, given the unique modulatory patterns observed for behavior and ERP indices between fitness groups, the researchers suggested that higher-fit participants were better able to flexibly adjust inhibitory control processes across conditions to meet the requirements of the task demands (Pontifex et al., 2011).

Further research in the academic domain reveals similar findings such that greater fitness is associated with higher academic scores across a variety of academic topics with the majority focusing on arithmetic and reading achievement (Bass, Brown, Laurson, & Coleman, 2013; Castelli, Hillman, Buck, & Erwin, 2007; Chomitz et al., 2009; Coe, Peterson, Blair, Schutten, & Peddie, 2013; Eveland-Sayers, Farley, Fuller, Morgan, & Caputo, 2009; Grissom, 2005; Rauner, Walters, Avery, & Wanser, 2013). Together with results demonstrating a relation with cognition and brain structure and function, these data demonstrate that fitness is a robust health factor associated with important cognitive, academic, and brain outcomes that are critical for healthy development and functioning in young children. However, to date, these data are mainly cross-sectional and limit causal interpretations with randomized control trials (RCTs) necessary to better understand these effects.

Chronic Physical Activity

Over the past decade there has been a steady increase in the number of RCTs evaluating physical activity effects on cognition and academic achievement in school-age children (Donnelly et al., 2016). Specifically, results across 26 investigations evaluating academic achievement revealed significant benefits following a physical activity intervention for overall composite scores of academic achievements (ES: 0.28) with additional selective benefits for arithmetic (ES: 0.21) and reading ability (ES: 0.13) (Álvarez-Bueno et al., 2017). Additionally, a recent meta-analysis evaluating cognition revealed a small but significant effect (ES: 0.2) of physical activity participation on cognitive control, specifically inhibitory control (Jackson, Davis, Sands, Whittington, & Sun, 2016).

Most of these RCT investigations evaluating cognitive outcomes have utilized neuroimaging tools to evaluate underlying structural and/or functional changes associated with a physical activity intervention (Chaddock-Heyman et al., 2013, 2018; Davis et al., 2011; Drollette et al., 2018; Hillman et al., 2014; Kamijo et al., 2011; Krafft et al., 2014). For example, the FITKids clinical trial (Chaddock-Heyman et al., 2013, 2018; Drollette et al., 2018; Hillman et al., 2014; Kamijo et al., 2011; Monti, Hillman, & Cohen, 2012) had preadolescent children participate every weekday in a 9-month after-school physical activity intervention designed to improve cardiorespiratory fitness. Children were randomized to either a physical activity intervention or a wait-list control. Both groups were administered a cognitive control battery, while brain function (fMRI and ERPs) and structure (MRI) were measured at baseline and following the intervention. Results revealed distinct functional differences between groups including increases in P3 amplitude and shorter P3 latency (Hillman et al., 2014), greater amplitude in contingent negative variation (CNV; greater prefrontal motor task preparation) (Kamijo et al., 2011), stability of the ERN component (suggestive of greater neural efficiency in conflict monitoring across a 9-month span) (Drollette et al., 2018), and reductions in hemodynamic activation in the PFC (Chaddock-Heyman et al., 2013) for the intervention group, while no such effect was observed for the wait-list control group. Together, these findings are broadly similar to other RCT investigations (Krafft et al., 2014) and suggest that participation in a physical activity intervention may facilitate early cortical development, with functional activation similar to more mature neural brain patterns observed in young adults (Chaddock-Heyman et al., 2013).

In addition, a recent publication from the FITKids trial evaluated structural differences in white matter tracts. Specifically, Chaddock-Heyman and colleagues (Chaddock-Heyman et al., 2018) investigated changes in white matter microstructure between baseline and following a 9-month physical activity intervention (or wait-list control). This approach is particularly interesting in children given that healthy development of white matter integrity is important for efficient transmission within neural networks. Results revealed increased white matter microstructure in the corpus callosum selective for children in the intervention, with no changes observed for the wait-list group. This area of the brain is critical for transmitting information across hemispheres and, with underdevelopment, is linked with neurodevelopmental disorders (Paul, 2011). Hence, these data are the first to demonstrate unique modulatory links of regular physical activity participation on structural regions within the developing brain that are critical for effective functioning.

Collectively, these findings from RCTs suggest that participation in a regular physical activity enhances cognition and academic achievement in developing children. Additionally, these enhancements are subserved by structural and functional brain changes that accompany regular physical activity participation. Although additional research is necessary, given that only three large-scale RCTs have been conducted in children evaluating cognitive and brain outcomes, the available evidence provides a foundation for future investigations to more fully elucidate physical activity effects on cognition and academic achievement.

Mechanisms

A recent systematic review by Lubans and colleagues (Lubans et al., 2016) clustered mechanisms associated with physical activity and mental health in children and adolescence into three categories including neurobiological (enhanced cognition via alterations in structure and function of brain networks), psychosocial (enhanced well-being, self-efficacy, perceived competence etc.), and behavioral (altered behavior patterns associated with sleep). The majority of evidence evaluating cognitive outcomes has focused on neurobiological underpinnings with only a few RCTs in children (previously discussed) specifically evaluating changes in brain structure and function. Herein, this chapter will discuss additional evidence from animal models as well as older adult research that provides further support for neurobiological mechanisms that have important implications for healthy maturation of young children.

Much of the evidence of the effects of physical activity on brain growth and development stems from research using non-human animal models (Voss, Vivar, Kramer, & Van Praag, 2013). Such investigations demonstrate physical activity-induced up-regulation of angiogenesis (i.e., growth of new blood vessels) (Black, Isaacs, Anderson, Alcantara, & Greenough, 1990; Creer, Romberg, Saksida, Van Praag, & Bussey, 2010; Isaacs, Anderson, Alcantara, Black, & Greenough, 1992; Swain et al., 2003), neurogenesis (i.e., growth of new neurons) (Aguiar, Speck, Prediger, Kapczinski, & Pinho, 2008; Neeper, 1995; Van Praag, Christie, Sejnowski, & Gage, 1999), and synaptogenesis (i.e., formation of new synapses between neurons) (Eadie, Redila, & Christie, 2005; Hu, Ying, Gomez-Pinilla, & Frautschy, 2009) in select cortical and subcortical regions including cerebellum (Black et al., 1990; Isaacs et al., 1992), primary motor cortex (Kleim, Cooper, & VandenBerg, 2002; Swain et al., 2003), hippocampus (Creer et al., 2010; Van Praag, Shubert, Zhao, & Gage, 2005), basal ganglia (Becker, Kutz, & Voelcker-Rehage, 2016), and PFC (Brockett, LaMarca, & Gould, 2015). These physical activity-induced processes have been observed during the developmental period (Kim, Lee, Kim, Yoo, & Kim, 2007; Lou, Liu, Chang, & Chen, 2008), and are crucial for effective brain health and functioning – especially during the maturation years – by enhancing cell proliferation and providing neuroprotection for developing brain regions. For example, voluntary wheel running in mice has been shown to up-regulate neurogenesis in the hippocampus by increasing the production of brain-derived neurotrophic factor (BDNF) and insulin-like growth factor (IGF-1) (Van Praag et al., 1999). These neurotrophic factors facilitate longevity of synaptic efficacy and neuronal connectivity (McAllister, Katz, & Lo, 1999). Additionally, these exercise-induced changes undergo synaptogenesis such that new neurons are further integrated functionally into the neural network (Eadie et al., 2005; Hu et al., 2009), potentially facilitating healthy communication within these neural cortices.

Together, these exercise-induced processes that facilitate brain health and structural integrity in select cortical regions in animals have significant implications for brain health in children. Furthermore, although such invasive observations are not possible in human participants, advances in neuroimaging techniques provide compelling evidence to corroborate the results from animal models. Specifically, children (previously discussed) and older adult (for review see Etnier et al., 2019) investigations demonstrate that physical activity participation has a positive effect on large-scale brain networks such that improvements in neural connectivity are observed in regions that support the cognitive control network. Collectively, these findings provide evidence for the link between healthy brain infrastructure and physical activity participation, with further implications for functional significance of cognitive processes including cognitive control.

Key Issues

Limitations

Given the developing nature of this field of study, there are multiple limitations facing researchers who aim to grow the field and improve content and impact of future research endeavors. That is, a major challenge worth noting is determining ideal control groups for physical activity interventions. Unlike blinded placebo-controlled methods in other clinical research domains, most participants are aware of the positive physiological outcomes associated with physical activity participation, and therefore, may bias the results either by expectancy effect or by motivation for intended outcome. Additionally, participants who attend a physical activity intervention are exposed to multiple extraneous factors that are difficult to quantify and control including, for example, social interaction, educational information, and/or positive affirmation from adult figures. Some of these factors have also been shown to have a positive effect on psychological well-being, self-efficacy, and academic achievement, and could certainly influence the outcome measures of interest. Hence, establishing the ideal control for physical activity has proven difficult. However, researchers suggest that future methods might consider multiple treatment groups with the intention of isolating the desired characteristics of the intervention that may be critical for intended outcomes (e.g., intensity, duration, and time) while holding all other factors constant (Huffman, Slentz, & Kraus, 2011).

Another limitation of the field is that the majority of investigations of sample children loosely described as preadolescent (age 7 to 10 years). That is, during this stage of the lifespan, development occurs rapidly, and it is naïve to think that children of different ages will perform similarly. In fact, different testing instruments may be necessary to explore similar cognitive functions across different age groups. Hence, a developmental perspective may provide additional insight into the cognitive response to physical activity interventions. Future research would benefit by the inclusion of additional age groups to better characterize physical activity effects on cognition across the developmental spectrum, while accounting for known differences in cognition as a function of age.

Publication bias also presents a limitation due to the tendency for only statistically significant results to be published (Rosenthal, 1979) and/or for research clustering such that when a novel and highly significant effect is published, other researchers pursue the same domain. For example, the majority of published data discussed in this chapter has focused on cognitive control with limited published research available focusing on other aspects of cognition (Pontifex et al., 2019). This trend may have been due to clustering that occurred following seminal research (Kramer et al., 1999), and/or because other avenues of cognition have been explored without observation of statistical effects, yielding difficulty in publishing null effects. Nevertheless, additional research is needed, which focuses on exploring unexplored factors using more rigorous study designs.

Lastly, there remains a disconnect between laboratory-based research and practical implementation of physical activity opportunities in schools and classrooms. Laboratory research should seek to design studies that have the potential for implementation within school systems and are appealing to administrators and teachers. For example, models of acute physical activity research have been accomplished in controlled laboratory environments with children, who walk for 20–30 minutes on a treadmill and then perform academic achievement tests (e.g., Hillman, Pontifex, et al., 2009). However, children rarely maintain a constant walking speed for an extended duration, and such physical activity bouts are not appealing to physical education instructors and teachers to implement in a school setting. Thus, while such models provide proof of concept, they lack external validity, and as such, more research is needed to progress from the laboratory to the school environment in order to make the application appealing.

Emerging Issues

Individual Differences

Collectively, the majority of investigations discussed in this chapter evaluated overall effects of physical activity on cognition and academic achievement, with only a few investigations exploring moderating or mediating factors associated with individual differences. For example, previous research evaluating acute physical activity effects on working memory and inhibitory control parsed groups of children in accordance with baseline cognitive performance, and then evaluated the after-effects of acute physical activity on cognition. Results revealed greater improvements in performance following the physical activity bout selective for those children with poor initial baseline performance compared to higher performers (Budde et al., 2010; Drollette et al., 2014). Although this research focused on performance outcome as the grouping factor, this method may have been efficacious as a 'backend' approach by arbitrarily clustering similar extraneous characteristics that are associated with differences in cognitive ability. Hence, it may be beneficial for future research to incorporate advanced statistical methods to more fully elucidate and identify characteristics that contribute to high and low responders to physical activity effects on cognition and academic achievement. Therefore, this chapter will highlight individual difference factors that demonstrate significant relations with cognition and academic achievement and discuss novel research that has explored such factors.

A wealth of research has demonstrated unique sexual dimorphic differences in cognitive ability across the lifespan (Cahill, 2006; Satterthwaite et al., 2014; Voyer, Postma, Brake, & Imperato-McGinley, 2007; Voyer, Voyer, & Saint-Aubin, 2017). These sex differences have been attributed to various dimorphic developmental trajectories of brain structure and function between male and female children (Allen, Damasio, Grabowski, Bruss, & Zhang, 2003; Filipek, Richelme, Kennedy, & Caviness Jr, 1994; Nopoulos, Flaum, O'Leary, & Andreasen, 2000; Ruigrok et al., 2014), with evidence suggesting unique maturation patterns and early specialization of brain networks selective for females (Christakou et al., 2009; Giedd et al., 1999, 2006; Raznahan et al., 2010). These sexual dimorphic maturation patterns in brain function may share similar pathways with networks associated with physical activity engagement. Interestingly, Drollette and colleagues (Drollette et al., 2016) evaluated the relation of fitness to working memory performance parsed by sex in young prepubescent children. Results across three separate samples of children – evaluating three distinct working memory tasks – revealed the same behavior pattern between males and females. That is, greater fitness in males was associated with greater working memory with no such relation observed for female children. Furthermore, sex differences in working memory were only evident at higher fitness levels, with no difference in performance observed between males and females at lower fitness levels (see Figure 7.3) (Drollette et al., 2016). Similar evidence has been observed with academic achievement demonstrating greater academic achievement with higher fitness for male children (Bass et al., 2013; Kwak et al., 2009). Thus, evaluating sexual dimorphic responses of physical activity to cognition may provide unique insight into common mechanisms most susceptible to physical activity participation.

SES is also a significant modulating factor of cognition, brain function, and academic achievement. Specifically, SES has been shown to be a strong predictor of overall health, psychological well-being, and emotional development across the lifespan (Adler & Rehkopf, 2008; Bradley & Corwyn, 2002; Brooks-Gunn & Duncan, 1997; Conger & Donnellan, 2007; Evans, 2004). Further, children of lower SES face not only economic barriers for success but also have the added disadvantage of greater likelihood of depression, anxiety, attentional disorders, with further evidence demonstrating reductions in prefrontal cortical thickness, attenuated cognitive control processes of neural development, and poorer task performance on measures of cognitive control

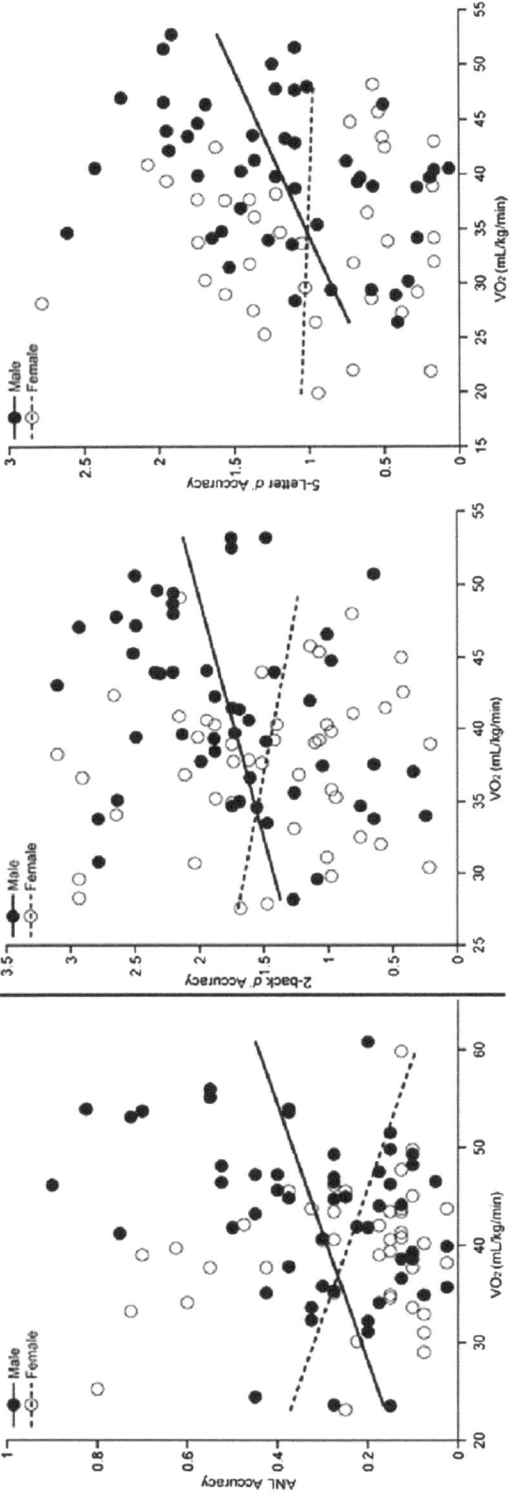

Figure 7.3   Scatter plots representing the sexual dimorphic relation of fitness to working memory across three separate investigations (Drollette et al., 2016)

compared to their higher SES peers (Kishiyama, Boyce, Jimenez, Perry, & Knight, 2009; Lawson, Duda, Avants, Wu, & Farah, 2013; Mezzacappa, 2004, p. 2; Noble, Houston, Kan, & Sowell, 2012; Stevens, Lauinger, & Neville, 2009). Conversely, cognitively stimulating environments have been shown to mediate the deleterious effects of SES on neural development. Specifically, animal models demonstrate that enriched environments facilitate up-regulation in cellular processes associated with healthy neural functioning including IGF-1 and BDNF (Kempermann, Kuhn, & Gage, 1997; Sale, Berardi, & Maffei, 2009; Van Praag, Kempermann, & Gage, 2000) with additional research demonstrating greater functional benefits for mice that were exposed to stressful life factors early in life, simulating low SES (Rampon et al., 2000; Sale et al., 2009). Of interest to the present chapter, such up-regulation processes are also observed following several days of voluntary wheel running in mice and to a greater extent when enriched environments were supplemented with a running wheel (Kobilo et al., 2011). Thus, given that physical activity interventions and enriched environments share a similar underlying neural mechanism, it is apparent that SES factors may be critical to evaluate in future research when assessing physical activity effects on brain health and functioning.

Recommendations for Researchers/Practitioners

Although this chapter addressed a growing body of novel research, there still remains a lack of physical activity interventions in youth with untapped possibilities for isolating underlying mechanisms, dose-response relationships, and individual difference factors that potentially alter brain health, cognition, and academic achievement associated with daily physical activity participation. Further, the extent to which such beneficial effects are observed in other domains of cognition and academic achievement, and across the developmental trajectory remains unknown until further investigations pursue this course of study. Regardless, the present state of the literature provides the beginnings of a growing evidence-base for the utility of physical activity as a means of facilitating cognitive and brain health in youth and provides an opportunity to positively influence the educational setting and the context of learning.

References

2018 Physical Activity Guidelines Advisory Committee. (2018). *2018 Physical activity guidelines advisory committee scientific report*. Washington, DC: U.S. Department of Health and Human Services.

Adler, N. E., & Rehkopf, D. H. (2008). US disparities in health: Descriptions, causes, and mechanisms. *Annual Review of Public Health, 29*, 235–252.

Aguiar, A. S., Speck, A. E., Prediger, R. D., Kapczinski, F., & Pinho, R. A. (2008). Downhill training upregulates mice hippocampal and striatal brain-derived neurotrophic factor levels. *Journal of Neural Transmission, 115*(9), 1251–1255.

Allen, J. S., Damasio, H., Grabowski, T. J., Bruss, J., & Zhang, W. (2003). Sexual dimorphism and asymmetries in the gray–white composition of the human cerebrum. *Neuroimage, 18*(4), 880–894.

Álvarez-Bueno, C., Pesce, C., Cavero-Redondo, I., Sánchez-López, M., Garrido-Miguel, M., & Martínez-Vizcaíno, V. (2017). Academic achievement and physical activity: A meta-analysis. *Pediatrics, 140*(6), e20171498.

Barkley, R. A. (1997). Behavioral inhibition, sustained attention, and executive functions: Constructing a unifying theory of ADHD. *Psychological Bulletin, 121*, 65–94. doi:10.1037/0033-2909.121.1.65

Bass, R. W., Brown, D. D., Laurson, K. R., & Coleman, M. M. (2013). Physical fitness and academic performance in middle school students. *Acta Paediatrica, 102*(8), 832–837. doi:10.1111/apa.12278

Becker, L., Kutz, D., & Voelcker-Rehage, C. (2016). Exercise-induced changes in basal ganglia volume and their relation to cognitive performance. *Journal of Neurology and Neuromedicine, 1*(5), 19–24.

Berchicci, M., Pontifex, M., Drollette, E., Pesce, C., Hillman, C., & Di Russo, F. (2015). From cognitive motor preparation to visual processing: The benefits of childhood fitness to brain health. *Neuroscience, 298*, 211–219.

Black, J. E., Isaacs, K. R., Anderson, B. J., Alcantara, A. A., & Greenough, W. T. (1990). Learning causes synaptogenesis, whereas motor activity causes angiogenesis, in cerebellar cortex of adult rats. *Proceedings of the National Academy of Sciences, 87*, 5568–5572.

Blair, C., & Razza, R. P. (2007). Relating effortful control, executive function, and false belief understanding to emerging math and literacy ability in kindergarten. *Child Development, 78*(2), 647–663.

Botvinick, M. M., Braver, T. S., Barch, D., Carter, C. S., & Cohen, J. D. (2001). Conflict monitoring and cognitive control. *Psychological Review, 108*, 624–652. doi:10.1037/0033-295X.108.3.624

Bouchard, C. E., Shephard, R. J., & Stephens, T. E. (1994). *Physical activity, fitness, and health: International proceedings and consensus statement*. Presented at the International Consensus Symposium on Physical Activity, Fitness, and Health, 2 May 1992, Toronto, ON, Canada.

Bradley, R. H., & Corwyn, R. F. (2002). Socioeconomic status and child development. *Annual Review of Psychology, 53*, 371–399.

Brockett, A. T., LaMarca, E. A., & Gould, E. (2015). Physical exercise enhances cognitive flexibility as well as astrocytic and synaptic markers in the medial prefrontal cortex. *PLoS One, 10*(5), e0124859.

Brocki, K. C., & Bohlin, G. (2004). Executive functions in children aged 6 to 13: A dimensional and developmental study. *Developmental Neuropsychology, 26*, 571–593.

Brooks-Gunn, J., & Duncan, G. J. (1997). The effects of poverty on children. *The Future of Children, 7*, 55–71.

Buck, S. M., Hillman, C. H., & Castelli, D. M. (2008). The relation of aerobic fitness to Stroop task performance in preadolescent children. *Medicine & Science in Sports & Exercise, 40*, 166–172.

Budde, H., Voelcker-Rehage, C., Pietrassyk-Kendziorra, S., Machado, S., Ribeiro, P., & Arafat, A. M. (2010). Steroid hormones in the saliva of adolescents after different exercise intensities and their influence on working memory in a school setting. *Psychoneuroendocrinology, 35*, 382–391.

Budde, H., Voelcker-Rehage, C., Pietraßyk-Kendziorra, S., Ribeiro, P., & Tidow, G. (2008). Acute coordinative exercise improves attentional performance in adolescents. *Neuroscience Letters, 441*(2), 219–223. doi:10.1016/j.neulet.2008.06.024

Bull, R., & Scerif, G. (2001). Executive functioning as a predictor of children's mathematics ability: Inhibition, switching, and working memory. *Developmental Neuropsychology, 19*(3), 273–293. doi:10.1207/S15326942DN1903_3

Bunge, S. A., & Crone, E. A. (2009). Neural correlates of the development of cognitive control. In J. M. Rumsey & M. Ernst (Eds.), *Neuroimaging in developmental clinical neuroscience* (pp. 22–37). New York, NY: Cambridge University Press.

Bunge, S. A., Dudukovic, N. M., Thomason, M. E., Vaidya, C. J., & Gabrieli, J. D. (2002). Immature frontal lobe contributions to cognitive control in children: Evidence from fMRI. *Neuron, 33*(2), 301–311.

Cahill, L. (2006). Why sex matters for neuroscience. *Nature Reviews Neuroscience, 7*(6), 477–484.

Castelli, D. M., Hillman, C. H., Buck, S. M., & Erwin, H. E. (2007). Physical fitness and academic achievement in third- and fifth-grade students. *Journal of Sport & Exercise Psychology, 29*, 239–252.

Caterino, M. C., & Polack, E. D. (1999). Effects of two types of activity on the performance of second-, third-, and fourth-grade students on a test of concentration. *Perceptual and Motor Skills, 89*, 245–248.

Chaddock, L., Erickson, K. I., Prakash, R. S., Kim, J. S., Voss, M. W., VanPatter, M., . . . Kramer, A. F. (2010). A neuroimaging investigation of the association between aerobic fitness, hippocampal volume, and memory performance in preadolescent children. *Brain Research, 1358*, 172–183. doi:10.1016/j.brainres.2010.08.049

Chaddock, L., Erickson, K. I., Prakash, R. S., VanPatter, M., Voss, M. W., Pontifex, M. B., . . . Kramer, A. F. (2010). Basal ganglia volume is associated with aerobic fitness in preadolescent children. *Developmental Neuroscience, 32*(3), 249–256. doi:10.1159/000316648

Chaddock, L., Erickson, K. I., Prakash, R. S., Voss, M. W., VanPatter, M., Pontifex, M. B., . . . Kramer, A. F. (2012). A functional MRI investigation of the association between childhood aerobic fitness and neurocognitive control. *Biological Psychology, 89*(1), 260–268. doi:10.1016/j.biopsycho.2011.10.017

Chaddock-Heyman, L., Erickson, K. I., Chappell, M. A., Johnson, C. L., Kienzler, C., Knecht, A., . . . Kramer, A. F. (2016). Aerobic fitness is associated with greater hippocampal cerebral blood flow in children. *Developmental Cognitive Neuroscience, 20*, 52–58. doi:10.1016/j.dcn.2016.07.001

Chaddock-Heyman, L., Erickson, K. I., Kienzler, C., Drollette, E., Raine, L., Kao, S.-C., . . . Hillman, C. (2018). Physical activity increases white matter microstructure in children. *Frontiers in Neuroscience, 12*(950), 1–11.

Chaddock-Heyman, L., Erickson, K. I., Voss, M., Knecht, A., Pontifex, M. B., Castelli, D., . . . Kramer, A. (2013). The effects of physical activity on functional MRI activation associated with cognitive control in children: A randomized controlled intervention. *Frontiers in Human Neuroscience, 7*, 72–79.

Chang, Y. K., Labban, J. D., Gapin, J. I., & Etnier, J. L. (2012). The effects of acute exercise on cognitive performance: A meta-analysis. *Brain Research, 1453*(Suppl C), 87–101. doi:10.1016/j.brainres.2012.02.068

Chen, A.-G., Yan, J., Yin, H.-C., Pan, C.-Y., & Chang, Y.-K. (2014). Effects of acute aerobic exercise on multiple aspects of executive function in preadolescent children. *Psychology of Sport and Exercise, 15*(6), 627–636. doi:10.1016/j.psychsport.2014.06.004

Chomitz, V. R., Slining, M. M., McGowan, R. J., Mitchell, S. E., Dawson, G. F., & Hacker, K. A. (2009). Is there a relationship between physical fitness and academic achievement? Positive results from public school children in the northeastern United States. *Journal of School Health, 79*, 30–37. doi:10.1111/j.1746-1561.2008.00371.x

Christakou, A., Halari, R., Smith, A. B., Ifkovits, E., Brammer, M., & Rubia, K. (2009). Sex-dependent age modulation of frontostriatal and temporo-parietal activation during cognitive control. *Neuroimage, 48*(1), 223–236.

Chu, C.-H., Kramer, A. F., Song, T.-F., Wu, C.-H., Hung, T.-M., & Chang, Y.-K. (2017). Acute exercise and neurocognitive development in preadolescents and young adults: An ERP study. *Neural Plasticity, 2017*, 13. doi:10.1155/2017/2631909

Church, T. S., Thomas, D. M., Tudor-Locke, C., Katzmarzyk, P. T., Earnest, C. P., Rodarte, R. Q., . . . Bouchard, C. (2011). Trends over 5 decades in US occupation-related physical activity and their associations with obesity. *PloS One, 6*(5), e19657.

Clair-Thompson, H. L. S., & Gathercole, S. E. (2006). Executive functions and achievements in school: Shifting, updating, inhibition, and working memory. *The Quarterly Journal of Experimental Psychology, 59*(4), 745–759. doi:10.1080/17470210500162854

Clark, C., & Woodward, L. (2007). *Preschool executive functioning as a predictor of children's academic achievement at age six years.* Poster presented at the biennial meeting of the Society for Research on Child Development, Boston, MA.

Coe, D. P., Peterson, T., Blair, C., Schutten, M. C., & Peddie, H. (2013). Physical fitness, academic achievement, and socioeconomic status in school-aged youth. *Journal of School Health, 83*(7), 500–507. doi:10.1111/josh.12058

Cole, P. M., Usher, B. A., & Cargo, A. P. (1993). Cognitive risk and its association with risk for disruptive behavior disorder in preschoolers. *Journal of Clinical Child Psychology, 22*(2), 154–164.

Conger, R. D., & Donnellan, M. B. (2007). An interactionist perspective on the socioeconomic context of human development. *Annual Review of Psychology, 58*, 175–199.

Cooper, S. B., Bandelow, S., Nute, M. L., Dring, K. J., Stannard, R. L., Morris, J. G., & Nevill, M. E. (2016). Sprint-based exercise and cognitive function in adolescents. *Preventive Medicine Reports, 4*, 155–161. doi:10.1016/j.pmedr.2016.06.004

Creer, D. J., Romberg, C., Saksida, L. M., Van Praag, H., & Bussey, T. J. (2010). Running enhances spatial pattern separation in mice. *Proceedings of the National Academy of Sciences, 107*(5), 2367–2372. doi:10.1073/pnas.0911725107

Davis, C. L., Tomporowski, P. D., McDowell, J. E., Austin, B. P., Miller, P. H., Yanasak, N. E., . . . Naglieri, J. A. (2011). Exercise improves executive function and achievement and alters brain activation in overweight children: A randomized, controlled trial. *Health Psychology, 30*(1), 91–98. doi:10.1037/a0021766

Di Pietro, J. A. (1986). Effect of physical stimulation on motor inhibition in children. *Perceptual and Motor Skills, 63*(1), 207–214. doi:10.2466/pms.1986.63.1.207

Diamond, A. (2002). Normal development of prefrontal cortex from birth to young adulthood: Cognitive functions, anatomy, and biochemistry. In D. Stuss & R. Knight (Eds.), *Principles of frontal lobe function* (pp. 466–503). New York, NY: Oxford University Press.

Dickinson, B. D., Duncan, M. J., & Eyre, E. L. J. (2016). Exercise and academic achievement in children: Effects of acute class-based circuit training. *Human Movement, 17*, 4–7. doi:10.1515/humo-2016-0007

Donnelly, J. E., Hillman, C. H., Castelli, D., Etnier, J. L., Lee, S., Tomporowski, P., . . . Szabo-Reed, A. N. (2016). Physical activity, fitness, cognitive function, and academic achievement in children: A systematic review. *Medicine and Science in Sports and Exercise, 48*(6), 1223–1224. doi:10.1249/MSS.0000000000000966

Drollette, E. S., Pontifex, M. B., Raine, L. B., Scudder, M. R., Moore, R. D., Kao, S., . . . Castelli, D. M. (2018). Effects of the FITKids physical activity randomized controlled trial on conflict monitoring in youth. *Psychophysiology, 55*(3), e13017.

Drollette, E. S., Scudder, M. R., Raine, L. B., Moore, R. D., Pontifex, M. B., Erickson, K. I., & Hillman, C. H. (2016). The sexual dimorphic association of cardiorespiratory fitness to working memory in children. *Developmental Science, 19*(1), 90–108. doi:10.1111/desc.12291

Drollette, E. S., Scudder, M. R., Raine, L. B., Moore, R. D., Saliba, B. J., Pontifex, M. B., & Hillman, C. H. (2014). Acute exercise facilitates brain function and cognition in children who need it most: An

ERP study of individual differences in inhibitory control capacity. *Developmental Cognitive Neuroscience, 7*, 53–64. doi:10.1016/j.dcn.2013.11.001

Drollette, E. S., Shishido, T., Pontifex, M. B., & Hillman, C. H. (2012). Maintenance of cognitive control during and after walking in preadolescent children. *Medicine and Science in Sports and Exercise, 44*, 2017–2024. doi:10.1249/MSS.0b013e318258bcd5

Duncan, G. J., Dowsett, C. J., Claessens, A., Magnuson, K., Huston, A. C., Klebanov, P., . . . Brooks-Gunn, J. (2007). School readiness and later achievement. *Developmental Psychology, 43*(6), 1428–1446.

Eadie, B. D., Redila, V. A., & Christie, B. R. (2005). Voluntary exercise alters the cytoarchitecture of the adult dentate gyrus by increasing cellular proliferation, dendritic complexity, and spine density. *Journal of Comparative Neurology, 486*(1), 39–47.

Etnier, J. L., Drollette, E. S., & Slutsky, A. (2019). Physical activity and cognition: A narrative review of the evidence for older adults. *Psychology of Sport and Exercise, 42*, 156–166.

Etnier, J. L., Labban, J. D., Piepmeier, A. T., Davis, M. E., & Henning, D. A. (2014). Effects of an acute bout of exercise on memory in 6th grade children. *Pediatric Exercise Science, 26*, 250–258. doi:10.1123/pes.2013-0141

Evans, G. W. (2004). The environment of childhood poverty. *American Psychologist, 59*(2), 77–92.

Eveland-Sayers, B. M., Farley, R. S., Fuller, D. K., Morgan, D. W., & Caputo, J. L. (2009). Physical fitness and academic achievement in elementary school children. *Journal of Physical Activity and Health, 6*(1), 99–104. doi:10.1123/jpah.6.1.99

Fearnbach, S. N., Silvert, L., Keller, K. L., Genin, P. M., Morio, B., Pereira, B., . . . Thivel, D. (2016). Reduced neural response to food cues following exercise is accompanied by decreased energy intake in obese adolescents. *International Journal of Obesity, 40*(1), 77–83.

Filipek, P. A., Richelme, C., Kennedy, D. N., & Caviness, V. S., Jr. (1994). The young adult human brain: An MRI-based morphometric analysis. *Cerebral Cortex, 4*(4), 344–360.

Gabbard, C., & Barton, J. (1979). Effects of physical activity on mathematical computation among young children. *The Journal of Psychology, 103*, 287–288.

Gahche, J., Fakhouri, T., Carroll, D. D., Burt, V. L., Wang, C.-Y., & Fulton, J. E. (2014). *Cardiorespiratory fitness levels among US youth aged 12–15 years: United States, 1999–2004 and 2012. NCHS Data Brief No. 153* (pp. 1–8). Hyattsville, MD: CDC; National Center for Health Statistics.

Gale, C. R., Cooper, R., Craig, L., Elliott, J., Kuh, D., Richards, M., . . . Deary, I. J. (2012). Cognitive function in childhood and lifetime cognitive change in relation to mental wellbeing in four cohorts of older people. *PLoS One, 7*(9), e44860.

Giedd, J. N., Blumenthal, J., Jeffries, N. O., Castellanos, F. X., Liu, H., Zijdenbos, A., . . . Rapoport, J. L. (1999). Brain development during childhood and adolescence: A longitudinal MRI study. *Nature America, 2*, 861–863.

Giedd, J. N, Clasen, L. S., Lenroot, R., Greenstein, D., Wallace, G. L., Ordaz, S., . . . Stayer, C. (2006). Puberty-related influences on brain development. *Molecular and Cellular Endocrinology, 254*, 154–162.

Grieco, L. A., Jowers, E. M., & Bartholomew, J. B. (2009). Physically active academic lessons and time on task: The moderating effect of body mass index. *Medicine & Science in Sports & Exercise, 41*(10), 1921–1926. doi:10.1249/MSS.0b013e3181a61495

Grissom, J. B. (2005). Physical fitness and academic achievement. *Journal of Exercise Physiology, 8*, 11–25.

Hair, N. L., Hanson, J. L., Wolfe, B. L., & Pollak, S. D. (2015). Association of child poverty, brain development, and academic achievement. *JAMA Pediatrics, 169*(9), 822–829.

Harveson, A. T., Hannon, J. C., Brusseau, T. A., Podlog, L., Papadopoulos, C., Durrant, L. H., . . . Kang, K. (2016). Acute effects of 30 minutes resistance and aerobic exercise on cognition in a high school sample. *Research Quarterly for Exercise and Sport, 87*(2), 214–220. doi:10.1080/02701367.2016.1146943

Hillman, C. H., Buck, S. M., Themanson, J. R., Pontifex, M. B., & Castelli, D. M. (2009). Aerobic fitness and cognitive development: Event-related brain potential and task performance indices of executive control in preadolescent children. *Developmental Psychology, 45*(1), 114–129. doi:10.1037/a0014437

Hillman, C. H., Kamijo, K., & Scudder, M. (2011). A review of chronic and acute physical activity participation on neuroelectric measures of brain health and cognition during childhood. *Preventive Medicine, 52*, S21–S28. doi:10.1016/j.ypmed.2011.01.024

Hillman, C. H., Pontifex, M. B., Castelli, D. M., Khan, N. A., Raine, L. B., Scudder, M. R., . . . Kamijo, K. (2014). Effects of the FITKids randomized controlled trial on executive control and brain function. *Pediatrics, 134*(4), e1063–e1071. doi:10.1542/peds.2013-3219

Hillman, C. H., Pontifex, M. B., Raine, L. B., Castelli, D. M., Hall, E. E., & Kramer, A. F. (2009). The effect of acute treadmill walking on cognitive control and academic achievement in preadolescent children. *Neuroscience, 159*(3), 1044–1054. doi:10.1016/j.neuroscience.2009.01.057

Hogan, M., Kiefer, M., Kubesch, S., Collins, P., Kilmartin, L., & Brosnan, M. (2013). The interactive effects of physical fitness and acute aerobic exercise on electrophysiological coherence and cognitive performance in adolescents. *Experimental Brain Research, 229*(1), 85–96. doi:10.1007/s00221-013-3595-0

Howie, E. K., Schatz, J., & Pate, R. R. (2015). Acute effects of classroom exercise breaks on executive function and math performance: A dose-response study. *Research Quarterly for Exercise and Sport, 86*(3), 217–224. doi:10.1080/02701367.2015.1039892

Hruby, T., & Marsalek, P. (2003). Event-related potentials – The P3 wave. *Acta Neurobiologiae Experimentalis, 63*, 55–63.

Hu, S., Ying, Z., Gomez-Pinilla, F., & Frautschy, S. A. (2009). Exercise can increase small heat shock proteins (sHSP) and pre-and post-synaptic proteins in the hippocampus. *Brain Research, 1249*, 191–201.

Huffman, K. M., Slentz, C. A., & Kraus, W. E. (2011). Control arms in exercise training studies: Transitioning from an era of intervention efficacy to one of comparative clinical effectiveness research. *Journal of Applied Physiology, 111*(3), 946–948.

Hung, C.-L., Huang, C.-J., Tsai, Y.-J., Chang, Y.-K., & Hung, T.-M. (2016). Neuroelectric and behavioral effects of acute exercise on task switching in children with attention-deficit/hyperactivity disorder. *Frontiers in Psychology, 7*, 1589. doi:10.3389/fpsyg.2016.01589

Isaacs, K. R., Anderson, B. J., Alcantara, A. A., Black, J. E., & Greenough, W. T. (1992). Exercise and the brain: Angiogenesis in the adult rat cerebellum after vigorous physical activity and motor skill learning. *Journal of Cerebral Blood Flow and Metabolism, 12*, 110–119.

Ishihara, T., Sugasawa, S., Matsuda, Y., & Mizuno, M. (2017). The beneficial effects of game-based exercise using age-appropriate tennis lessons on the executive functions of 6–12-year-old children. *Neuroscience Letters, 642*, 97–101.

Jackson, W. M., Davis, N., Sands, S. A., Whittington, R. A., & Sun, L. S. (2016). Physical activity and cognitive development: A meta-analysis. *Journal of Neurosurgical Anesthesiology, 28*(4), 373–380. doi:10.1097/ANA.0000000000000349

Jäger, K., Schmidt, M., Conzelmann, A., & Roebers, C. M. (2014). Cognitive and physiological effects of an acute physical activity intervention in elementary school children. *Frontiers in Psychology, 5*. doi:10.3389/fpsyg.2014.01473

Jeynes, W. H. (2007). The relationship between parental involvement and urban secondary school student academic achievement: A meta-analysis. *Urban Education, 42*, 82–110.

Jimerson, S., Egeland, B., & Teo, A. (1999). A longitudinal study of achievement trajectories: Factors associated with change. *Journal of Educational Psychology, 91*(1), 116–126.

Kamijo, K., Pontifex, M. B., O'Leary, K. C., Scudder, M. R., Wu, C.-T., Castelli, D. M., & Hillman, C. H. (2011). The effects of an afterschool physical activity program on working memory in preadolescent children. *Developmental Science, 14*(5), 1046–1058. doi:10.1111/j.1467-7687.2011.01054.x

Kann, L. (2016). Youth risk behavior surveillance– United States, 2015. *MMWR. Surveillance Summaries, 65.* doi:10.15585/mmwr.ss6506a1

Kao, S.-C., Drollette, E. S., Scudder, M. R., Raine, L. B., Westfall, D. R., Pontifex, M. B., & Hillman, C. H. (2017). Aerobic fitness is associated with cognitive control strategy in preadolescent children. *Journal of Motor Behavior, 49*(2), 150–162.

Kao, S.-C., Westfall, D. R., Parks, A. C., Pontifex, M. B., & Hillman, C. H. (2017). Muscular and aerobic fitness, working memory, and academic achievement in children. *Medicine and Science in Sports and Exercise, 49*(3), 500–508. doi:10.1249/MSS.0000000000001132

Kempermann, G., Kuhn, H. G., & Gage, F. H. (1997). More hippocampal neurons in adult mice living in an enriched environment. *Nature, 386*(6624), 493–495.

Kim, H., Lee, S. H., Kim, S. S., Yoo, J. H., & Kim, C. J. (2007). The influence of maternal treadmill running during pregnancy on short-term memory and hippocampal cell survival in rat pups. *International Journal of Developmental Neuroscience, 25*, 243–249.

Kishiyama, M. M., Boyce, W. T., Jimenez, A. M., Perry, L. M., & Knight, R. T. (2009). Socioeconomic disparities affect prefrontal function in children. *Journal of Cognitive Neuroscience, 21*(6), 1106–1115.

Kleim, J. A., Cooper, N. R., & VandenBerg, P. M. (2002). Exercise induces angiogenesis but does not alter movement representations within rat motor cortex. *Brain Research, 934*(1), 1–6.

Kobilo, T., Liu, Q.-R., Gandhi, K., Mughal, M., Shaham, Y., & Van Praag, H. (2011). Running is the neurogenic and neurotrophic stimulus in environmental enrichment. *Learning & Memory (Cold Spring Harbor, New York), 18*(9), 605–609. doi:10.1101/lm.2283011

Koenen, K. C., Moffitt, T. E., Roberts, A. L., Martin, L. T., Kubzansky, L., Harrington, H., . . . Caspi, A. (2009). Childhood IQ and adult mental disorders: A test of the cognitive reserve hypothesis. *American Journal of Psychiatry, 166*(1), 50–57.

Korkman, M., Kemp, S. L., & Kirk, U. (2001). Effects of age on neurocognitive measures of children ages 5 to 12: A cross-sectional study on 800 children from the United States. *Developmental Neuropsychology, 20*(1), 331–354.

Krafft, C. E., Pierce, J. E., Schwarz, N. F., Chi, L., Weinberger, A. L., Schaeffer, D. J., . . . McDowell, J. E. (2014). An eight month randomized controlled exercise intervention alters resting state synchrony in overweight children. *Neuroscience, 256*, 445–455. doi:10.1016/j.neuroscience.2013.09.052

Kramer, A. F., Hahn, S., Cohen, N. J., Banich, M. T., McAuley, E. M., Harrison, C. R., . . . Colcombe, A. (1999). Ageing, fitness and neurocognitive function. *Nature, 400*, 418–419. doi:10.1038/22682

Kwak, L., Kremers, S. P. J., Bergman, P., Ruiz, J. R., Rizzo, N. S., & Sjöström, M. (2009). Associations between physical activity, fitness, and academic achievement. *The Journal of Pediatrics, 155*(6), 914–918.e1. doi:10.1016/j.jpeds.2009.06.019

Lambrick, D., Stoner, L., Grigg, R., & Faulkner, J. (2016). Effects of continuous and intermittent exercise on executive function in children aged 8–10 years: Acute exercise and executive function. *Psychophysiology, 53*(9), 1335–1342. doi:10.1111/psyp.12688

Lawson, G. M., Duda, J. T., Avants, B. B., Wu, J., & Farah, M. J. (2013). Associations between children's socioeconomic status and prefrontal cortical thickness. *Developmental Science, 16*(5), 641–652.

Lou, S., Liu, J., Chang, H., & Chen, P. (2008). Hippocampal neurogenesis and gene expression depend on exercise intensity in juvenile rats. *Brain Research, 1210*, 48–55.

Lubans, D., Richards, J., Hillman, C., Faulkner, G., Beauchamp, M., Nilsson, M., . . . Biddle, S. J. H. (2016). Physical activity for cognitive and mental health in youth: A systematic review of mechanisms. *Pediatrics, 138*(3), e20161642.

Luck, S. J. (2014). *An introduction to the event-related potential technique.* Cambridge: MIT Press.

Ludyga, S., Gerber, M., Brand, S., Holsboer-Trachsler, E., & Pühse, U. (2016). Acute effects of moderate aerobic exercise on specific aspects of executive function in different age and fitness groups: A meta-analysis. *Psychophysiology.* doi:10.1111/psyp.12736

Ma, J. K., Le Mare, L., & Gurd, B. J. (2015). Four minutes of in-class high-intensity interval activity improves selective attention in 9- to 11-year olds. *Applied Physiology, Nutrition, and Metabolism = Physiologie Appliquee, Nutrition Et Metabolisme, 40*(3), 238–244. doi:10.1139/apnm-2014-0309

Mahar, M. T., Murphy, S. K., Rowe, D. A., Golden, J., Shields, A. T., & Raedeke, T. D. (2006). Effects of a classroom-based program on physical activity and on-task behavior. *Medicine & Science in Sports & Exercise, 38*, 2086–2094. doi:10.1249/01.mss.0000235359.16685.a3

Martin, L. T., & Kubzansky, L. D. (2005). Childhood cognitive performance and risk of mortality: A prospective cohort study of gifted individuals. *American Journal of Epidemiology, 162*(9), 887–890.

McAllister, A. K., Katz, L. C., & Lo, D. C. (1999). Neurotrophins and synaptic plasticity. *Annual Review of Neuroscience, 22*(1), 295–318.

McClelland, M. M., Cameron, C. E., Connor, C. M., Farris, C. L., Jewkes, A. M., & Morrison, F. J. (2007). Links between behavioral regulation and preschoolers' literacy, vocabulary, and math skills. *Developmental Psychology, 43*(4), 947–959.

McClelland, M. M., Morrison, F. J., & Holmes, D. L. (2000). Children at risk for early academic problems: The role of learning-related social skills. *Early Childhood Research Quarterly, 15*(3), 307–329.

McGlamery, M. E., Ball, S. E., Henley, T. B., & Besozzi, M. (2007). Theory of mind, attention, and executive function in kindergarten boys. *Emotional and Behavioural Difficulties, 12*(1), 29–47.

McNaughten, D., & Gabbard, C. (1993). Physical exertion and the immediate mental performance of sixth-grade children. *Perceptual and Motor Skills, 77*, 1155–1159.

Metcalfe, A. W. S., MacIntosh, B. J., Scavone, A., Ou, X., Korczak, D., & Goldstein, B. I. (2016). Effects of acute aerobic exercise on neural correlates of attention and inhibition in adolescents with bipolar disorder. *Translational Psychiatry, 6*(5), e814. doi:10.1038/tp.2016.85

Mezzacappa, E. (2004). Alerting, orienting, and executive attention: Developmental properties and socio-demographic correlates in an epidemiological sample of young, urban children. *Child Development, 75*, 1373–1386. doi:10.1111/j.1467-8624.2004.00746.x

Mierau, A., Hülsdünker, T., Mierau, J., Hense, A., Hense, J., & Strüder, H. K. (2014). Acute exercise induces cortical inhibition and reduces arousal in response to visual stimulation in young children. *International Journal of Developmental Neuroscience, 34*, 1–8. doi:10.1016/j.ijdevneu.2013.12.009

Miyake, A., & Friedman, N. P. (2012). The nature and organization of individual differences in executive functions: Four general conclusions. *Current Directions in Psychological Science, 21*(1), 8–14.

Miyake, A., Friedman, N. P., Emerson, M. J., Witzki, A. H., & Howerter, A. (2000). The unity and diversity of executive functions and their contributions to complex "frontal lobe" tasks: A latent variable analysis. *Cognitive Psychology, 41*, 49–100. doi:10.1006/cogp.1999.0734

Moffitt, T. E., Arseneault, L., Belsky, D., Dickson, N., Hancox, R. J., Harrington, H., . . . Caspi, A. (2011). A gradient of childhood self-control predicts health, wealth, and public safety. *Proceedings of the National Academy of Sciences, 108*(7), 2693–2698. doi:10.1073/pnas.1010076108

Monti, J. M., Hillman, C. H., & Cohen, N. J. (2012). Aerobic fitness enhances relational memory in preadolescent children: The FITKids randomized control trial. *Hippocampus, 22*, 1876–1882. doi:10.1002/hipo.22023

Moore, R. D., Drollette, E. S., Scudder, M. R., Bharij, A., & Hillman, C. H. (2014). The influence of cardiorespiratory fitness on strategic, behavioral, and electrophysiological indices of arithmetic cognition in preadolescent children. *Frontiers in Human Neuroscience, 8*. doi:10.3389/fnhum.2014.00258

Neeper, S. A. (1995). Exercise and brain neurotrophins. *Nature, 373*, 109.

Noble, K. G., Houston, S. M., Kan, E., & Sowell, E. R. (2012). Neural correlates of socioeconomic status in the developing human brain. *Developmental Science, 15*(4), 516–527.

Nopoulos, P., Flaum, M., O'Leary, D., & Andreasen, N. C. (2000). Sexual dimorphism in the human brain: Evaluation of tissue volume, tissue composition and surface anatomy using magnetic resonance imaging. *Psychiatry Research: Neuroimaging, 98*(1), 1–13.

Norman, D. A., & Shallice, T. (1986). Attention to action: Willed and automatic control of behavior. In R. J. Davidson, G. E. Schwartz, & D. Shapiro (Eds.), *Consciousness and self-regulation: Advances in research and theory* (Vol. 4, pp. 1–18). New York, NY: Plenum.

Ogden, C. L., Carroll, M. D., Fryar, C. D., & Flegal, K. M. (2015). *Prevalence of obesity among adults and youth: United States, 2011–2014*. Washington, DC: US Department of Health and Human Services, Centers for Disease Control and Prevention, National Center for Health Statistics.

Paul, L. K. (2011). Developmental malformation of the corpus callosum: A review of typical callosal development and examples of developmental disorders with callosal involvement. *Journal of Neurodevelopmental Disorders, 3*(1), 3–27.

Pesce, C., Crova, C., Cereatti, L., Casella, R., & Bellucci, M. (2009). Physical activity and mental performance in preadolescents: Effects of acute exercise on free-recall memory. *Mental Health and Physical Activity, 2*(1), 16–22. doi:10.1016/j.mhpa.2009.02.001

Piepmeier, A. T., Shih, C.-H., Whedon, M., Williams, L. M., Davis, M. E., Henning, D. A., . . . Etnier, J. L. (2015). The effect of acute exercise on cognitive performance in children with and without ADHD. *Journal of Sport and Health Science, 4*(1), 97–104.

Pirrie, A. M., & Lodewyk, K. R. (2012). Investigating links between moderate-to-vigorous physical activity and cognitive performance in elementary school students. *Mental Health and Physical Activity, 5*(1), 93–98. doi:10.1016/j.mhpa.2012.04.001

Pontifex, M. B., McGowan, A. L., Chandler, M. C., Gwizdala, K. L., Parks, A. C., Fenn, K., & Kamijo, K. (2019). A primer on investigating the after effects of acute bouts of physical activity on cognition. *Psychology of Sport and Exercise, 40*, 1–22. doi:10.1016/j.psychsport.2018.08.015

Pontifex, M. B., Raine, L. B., Johnson, C. R., Chaddock, L., Voss, M. W., Cohen, N. J., . . . Hillman, C. H. (2011). Cardiorespiratory fitness and the flexible modulation of cognitive control in preadolescent children. *Journal of Cognitive Neuroscience, 23*(6), 1332–1345. doi:10.1162/jocn.2010.21528

Pontifex, M. B., Saliba, B. J., Raine, L. B., Picchietti, D. L., & Hillman, C. H. (2013). Exercise improves behavioral, neurocognitive, and scholastic performance in children with ADHD. *The Journal of Pediatrics, 162*(3), 543–551. doi:10.1016/j.jpeds.2012.08.036

Pontifex, M. B., Scudder, M. R., Drollette, E. S., & Hillman, C. H. (2012). Fit and vigilant: The relationship between poorer aerobic fitness and failures in sustained attention during preadolescence. *Neuropsychology, 26*(4), 407–413. doi:10.1037/a0028795

Poropat, A. E. (2009). A meta-analysis of the five-factor model of personality and academic performance. *Psychological Bulletin, 135*, 322–338.

Raaijmakers, M. A., Smidts, D. P., Sergeant, J. A., Maassen, G. H., Posthumus, J. A., Van Engeland, H., & Matthys, W. (2008). Executive functions in preschool children with aggressive behavior: Impairments in inhibitory control. *Journal of Abnormal Child Psychology, 36*(7), 1097–1107.

Raine, L. B., Lee, H. K., Saliba, B. J., Chaddock-Heyman, L., Hillman, C. H., & Kramer, A. F. (2013). The influence of childhood aerobic fitness on learning and memory. *PLoS One, 8*(9), e72666. doi:10.1371/journal.pone.0072666

Ramachandran, V. S. (2012). Encyclopedia of human behavior. In B. Spinath (Ed.), *Academic achievement* (pp. 1–8). San Diego, CA: Academic Press.

Rampon, C., Tang, Y.-P., Goodhouse, J., Shimizu, E., Kyin, M., & Tsien, J. Z. (2000). Enrichment induces structural changes and recovery from nonspatial memory deficits in CA1 NMDAR1-knockout mice. *Nature Neuroscience, 3*(3), 238–244.

Rauner, R. R., Walters, R. W., Avery, M., & Wanser, T. J. (2013). Evidence that aerobic fitness is more salient than weight status in predicting standardized math and reading outcomes in fourth-through eighth-grade students. *The Journal of Pediatrics, 163*(2), 344–348.

Raviv, S., & Low, M. (1990). Influence of physical activity on concentration among junior high-school students. *Perceptual and Motor Skills, 70*(1), 67–74. doi:10.2466/pms.1990.70.1.67

Raznahan, A., Lee, Y., Stidd, R., Long, R., Greenstein, D., Clasen, L., . . . Giedd, J. N. (2010). Longitudinally mapping the influence of sex and androgen signaling on the dynamics of human cortical maturation in adolescence. *Proceedings of the National Academy of Sciences, 107*(39), 16988–16993.

Rimfeld, K., Kovas, Y., Dale, P. S., & Plomin, R. (2016). True grit and genetics: Predicting academic achievement from personality. *Journal of Personality and Social Psychology, 111*(5), 780–789.

Rogers, R. D., & Monsell, S. (1995). Cost of a predictable switch between simple cognitive tasks. *American Psychological Association, 124*, 207–231.

Rosenthal, R. (1979). The file drawer problem and tolerance for null results. *Psychological Bulletin, 86*(3), 638–641.

Rueda, M. R., Rothbart, M. K., McCandliss, B. D., Saccomanno, L., & Posner, M. I. (2005). Training, maturation, and genetic influences on the development of executive attention. *Proceedings of the National Academy of Sciences of the United States of America, 102*(41), 14931–14936. doi:10.1073/pnas.0506897102

Ruigrok, A. N., Salimi-Khorshidi, G., Lai, M.-C., Baron-Cohen, S., Lombardo, M. V., Tait, R. J., & Suckling, J. (2014). A meta-analysis of sex differences in human brain structure. *Neuroscience & Biobehavioral Reviews, 39*, 34–50.

Sale, A., Berardi, N., & Maffei, L. (2009). Enrich the environment to empower the brain. *Trends in Neurosciences, 32*(4), 233–239.

Sallis, J. F. (2010). We do not have to sacrifice children's health to achieve academic goals. *The Journal of Pediatrics, 156*, 696–697.

Samuel, R. D., Zavdy, O., Levav, M., Reuveny, R., Katz, U., & Dubnov-Raz, G. (2017). The effects of maximal intensity exercise on cognitive performance in children. *Journal of Human Kinetics, 57*, 85–96. doi:10.1515/hukin-2017-0050

Satterthwaite, T. D., Wolf, D. H., Roalf, D. R., Ruparel, K., Erus, G., Vandekar, S., . . . Hakonarson, H. (2014). Linked sex differences in cognition and functional connectivity in youth. *Cerebral Cortex, 25*(9), 2383–2394.

Scott-Little, C., Lesko, J., Martella, J., & Milburn, P. (2007). Early learning standards: Results from a national survey to document trends in state-level policies and practices. *Early Childhood Research & Practice, 9*(1), n1.

Scudder, M. R., Federmeier, K. D., Raine, L. B., Direito, A., Boyd, J. K., & Hillman, C. H. (2014). The association between aerobic fitness and language processing in children: Implications for academic achievement. *Brain and Cognition, 87*, 140–152.

Scudder, M. R., Lambourne, K., Drollette, E. S., Herrmann, S., Washburn, R., Donnelly, J. E., & Hillman, C. H. (2014). Aerobic capacity and cognitive control in elementary school-age children. *Medicine and Science in Sports and Exercise, 46*(5), 1025–1035.

Séguin, J. R., Nagin, D., Assaad, J.-M., & Tremblay, R. E. (2004). Cognitive-neuropsychological function in chronic physical aggression and hyperactivity. *Journal of Abnormal Psychology, 113*(4), 603–613.

Soga, K., Shishido, T., & Nagatomi, R. (2015). Executive function during and after acute moderate aerobic exercise in adolescents. *Psychology of Sport and Exercise, 16*, 7–17.

Stevens, C., Lauinger, B., & Neville, H. (2009). Differences in the neural mechanisms of selective attention in children from different socioeconomic backgrounds: An event-related brain potential study. *Developmental Science, 12*(4), 634–646.

Stroth, S., Kubesch, S., Keiterle, K., Ruchsow, M., Heim, R., & Kiefer, M. (2009). Physical fitness, but not acute exercise modulates event-related potential indices for executive control in healthy adolescents. *Brain Research, 1269*, 114–124.

Stuss, D. T., & Levine, B. (2002). Adult clinical neuropsychology: Lessons from studies of the frontal lobes. *Annual Review of Psychology, 53*(1), 401–433.

Swain, R. A., Harris, A. B., Wiener, E. C., Dutka, M. V., Morris, H. D., Theien, B. E., . . . Greenough, W. T. (2003). Prolonged exercise induces angiogenesis and increases cerebral blood volume in primary motor cortex of the RAT. *Neuroscience, 117*, 1037–1046.

Swanson, H. L., & Alloway, T. P. (2012). Working memory, learning, and academic achievement. In K. R. Harris, S. Graham, T. Urdan, C. McCormick, G. Sinatra, & J. Sweller (Eds.), *APA educated psychology handbook: Theories, constructs, and critical issues* (pp. 327–366). Washington, DC: American Psychological Association.

US Department of Education, National Center for Education Statistics, Common Core of Data. (2017). *State nonfiscal survey of public elementary and secondary education.* Retrieved from https://nces.ed.gov/programs/digest/d17/tables/dt17_105.20.asp?current=yes

van den Berg, V., Saliasi, E., de Groot, R. H. M., Jolles, J., Chinapaw, M. J. M., & Singh, A. S. (2016). Physical activity in the school setting: Cognitive performance is not affected by three different types of acute exercise. *Frontiers in Psychology, 7.* doi:10.3389/fpsyg.2016.00723

Van Praag, H., Christie, B. R., Sejnowski, T. J., & Gage, F. H. (1999). Running enhances neurogenesis, learning, and long-term potentiation in mice. *Proceedings of the National Academy of Sciences, 96*(23), 13427–13431. doi:10.1073/pnas.96.23.13427

Van Praag, H., Kempermann, G., & Gage, F. H. (2000). Neural consequences of environmental enrichment. *Nature Reviews Neuroscience, 1*(3), 191–198.

Van Praag, H., Shubert, T., Zhao, C., & Gage, F. H. (2005). Exercise enhances learning and hippocampal neurogenesis in aged mice. *Journal of Neuroscience, 25*(38), 8680–8685.

Vaynman, S., & Gomez-Pinilla, F. (2006). Revenge of the "sit": How lifestyle impacts neuronal and cognitive health through molecular systems that interface energy metabolism with neuronal plasticity. *Journal of Neuroscience Research, 84*, 699–715. doi:10.1002/jnr.20979

Vitaro, F., Brendgen, M., Larose, S., & Trembaly, R. E. (2005). Kindergarten disruptive behaviors, protective factors, and educational achievement by early adulthood. *Journal of Educational Psychology, 97*(4), 617–629.

Voss, M. W., Chaddock, L., Kim, J. S., VanPatter, M., Pontifex, M. B., Raine, L. B., . . . Kramer, A. F. (2011). Aerobic fitness is associated with greater efficiency of the network underlying cognitive control in preadolescent children. *Neuroscience, 199*, 166–176. doi:10.1016/j.neuroscience.2011.10.009

Voss, M. W., Vivar, C., Kramer, A. F., & Van Praag, H. (2013). Bridging animal and human models of exercise-induced brain plasticity. *Trends in Cognitive Sciences, 17*(10), 525–544. doi:10.1016/j.tics.2013.08.001

Voyer, D., Postma, A., Brake, B., & Imperato-McGinley, J. (2007). Gender differences in object location memory: A meta-analysis. *Psychonomic Bulletin & Review, 14*(1), 23–38.

Voyer, D., Voyer, S. D., & Saint-Aubin, J. (2017). Sex differences in visual-spatial working memory: A meta-analysis. *Psychonomic Bulletin & Review, 24*(2), 307–334.

Waber, D. P., Gerber, E. B., Turcios, V. Y., Wagner, E. R., & Forbes, P. W. (2006). Executive functions and performance on high-stakes testing in children from urban schools. *Developmental Neuropsychology, 29*(3), 459–477.

Westfall, D. R., Kao, S.-C., Scudder, M. R., Pontifex, M. B., & Hillman, C. H. (2017). The association between aerobic fitness and congruency sequence effects in preadolescent children. *Brain and Cognition, 113*, 85–92. doi:10.1016/j.bandc.2016.12.005

White, K. R. (1982). The relation between socioeconomic status and academic achievement. *Psychological Bulletin, 91*, 461–481.

Wu, C.-T., Pontifex, M. B., Raine, L. B., Chaddock, L., Voss, M. W., Kramer, A. F., & Hillman, C. H. (2011). Aerobic fitness and response variability in preadolescent children performing a cognitive control task. *Neuropsychology, 25*(3), 333–341. doi:10.1037/a0022167

PART 3

Factors Associated with Physical Activity

8

PSYCHOLOGICAL FACTORS ASSOCIATED WITH PHYSICAL ACTIVITY IN YOUTH

Katrina J. Waldhauser, Geralyn R. Ruissen, and Mark R. Beauchamp

Physical Inactivity and Sedentary Behavior: Implications for Youth

With the increased popularity of, and reliance on, technology in recent years, it is not surprising that children and adolescents are spending large amounts of time in front of a screen (i.e., computers, mobile devices, and TV) and less time being physically active (Herman, Hopman, & Sabiston, 2015). According to a recent global report, overall physical activity levels for children and adolescents across 49 countries were rated as low/poor (Aubert et al., 2018). The authors of the report suggest the majority of youth across the globe are failing to meet the suggested physical activity guidelines of at least 60 minutes of moderate-to-vigorous intensity physical activity per day (on average). Moreover, children and adolescents failed to limit their average recreational screen time use to less than 2 hours per day, as recommended by Canadian guidelines (Aubert et al., 2018). Those who spend more time in sedentary behavior experience increased health risks, such as cardiovascular disease and obesity (Carson et al., 2016). In addition to these health risks, school-aged children who spend more than 2 hours per day sitting in front of a screen are at greater risk of having poor pro-social behaviors, decreased self-worth and self-concept, as well as experience poorer academic performance (Carson et al., 2016). Moreover, sedentary behavior has also been found to have negative implications for mental health, such as increased risk of depression (Zhai, Zhang, & Zhang, 2015) and anxiety (Teychenne, Costigan, & Parker, 2015).

Balanced against the costs of inactivity and sedentary lifestyles, engaging in regular and sustained physical activity has consistently been associated with an extensive range of physical/physiological and psychological health benefits that extend across the age span. For example, in the general population, regular physical activity is associated with reduced risk of many non-communicable diseases such as breast cancer, colon cancer, diabetes, heart disease, and stroke (Kyu et al., 2016), as well as a reduced risk of mortality (Hupin et al., 2015). In terms of mental health, regular activity is also associated with improvements in psychological well-being (Penedo & Dahn, 2005), reductions in depression (Rebar et al., 2015), and a lower likelihood of experiencing mood disorders (Hearing et al., 2016). For children and adolescents, in particular, additional physiological benefits include improvements in bone and cardiovascular health, as well as a reduced likelihood of obesity (Smith et al., 2014). Psychological benefits for this population include improvements in self-esteem (Biddle & Asare, 2011; Smith et al., 2014), and from a scholastic perspective, when youth are more active they can benefit from enhanced cognitive functioning (Biddle & Asare, 2011; Hillman et al., 2014), as well as improvements in academic performance (Álvarez-Bueno et al., 2017).

Based on the consistent (physical and psychological) benefits associated with involvement of physical activity, an extensive body of research has accumulated to examine some of the personal, social, and environmental factors/antecedents associated with sustained involvement in physical activity among children and adolescents. In this chapter, we focus on psychological factors implicated in the pursuit of health-enhancing physical activity, and in particular those factors associated with physical activity involvement among youth. In light of the fact that the relations between these psychological factors and physical activity are often explained (i.e., mediated) by other intermediary variables, and also moderated by different boundary conditions, we examine the relations between these psychological factors and youth physical activity but also examine the underlying theoretical models that explain these complex relationships. Specifically, in this chapter, we look at some of the most prominent theories, along with recent insights, that have been applied to understand the various psychological factors implicated in predicting and explaining physical activity behavior among youth. In so doing, we also examine the extant empirical evidence (or absence thereof) in support of those theoretical frameworks. We then conclude by mapping out some viable directions for future research.

Prominent Psychological Theories and Frameworks Applied to the Study of Physical Activity

Psychological Factors Embedded within Social Cognitive Theory

Social cognitive theory (SCT) (Bandura, 1986, 2001) represents one of the most widely applied theoretical models to examine how psychological factors coalesce to influence physical activity (Beauchamp, Crawford, & Jackson, 2018). Broadly conceived, SCT describes the way in which personal factors, environmental (or situational) factors, and human behavior influence and are influenced by each other. The theory recognizes that (a) thought processes are shaped by various social determinants, but also that (b) humans can self-regulate their thoughts and behaviors and demonstrate personal control (or agency) over one's actions (Bandura, 1986, 2001). Personal agency represents a core feature of this framework (Bandura, 1997) and is practiced through *intentionality* (acting with intent based on a plan of action), *forethought* (anticipating outcomes of actions and guiding behavior accordingly), *self-reactiveness* (maintaining motivation towards, and regulation of, a chosen action plan), and *self-reflectiveness* (reflecting upon one's motives, values, and meaning behind a chosen action).

The focal variable within SCT corresponds to self-efficacy, which reflects a person's beliefs in their capabilities to perform various tasks (Bandura, 1997). According to Bandura (2004), self-efficacy beliefs causally influence behavioral outcomes such as physical activity, both directly and also via (i.e., mediated by) a number of intermediary psychological processes. These include (a) the outcomes people envision for themselves (i.e., outcome expectations), which can be physical, social, and/or self-evaluative; (b) the goals they set for themselves with more efficacious individuals setting more challenging goals to pursue; and (c) displays of resilience in overcoming various sociocultural and environmental barriers (Bandura, 2004).

Although self-efficacy beliefs begin to form in childhood, they are malleable and can change across the lifespan (Voskuil & Robbins, 2015). Beliefs in one's capabilities are influenced by six primary sources of information (Bandura, 1997; Maddux, 1995). The strongest source of efficacy information corresponds to past mastery attainments, which in the case of a young child playing school sport might include previous successes in playing the relevant sport. Other sources include vicarious observations of others (e.g., watching other school friends performing certain movement skills in sport), imaginal experiences (e.g., visualizing oneself prior to an important sports match), verbal persuasion (e.g., a teacher's encouragement to play a certain sport), and perceptions of one's physiological states (e.g., improved fitness in the lead up to a sports match) and emotional states (e.g., feelings of enjoyment associated with playing a certain sport).

In the context of understanding the psychological determinants of physical activity behavior among youth, two types of self-efficacy belief are particularly pertinent. The first type corresponds to *task* self-efficacy which, in physical activity settings, corresponds to a person's belief in their capabilities to perform the various movement skills involved in an activity (Bandura, 1997). Recent research has highlighted the importance of youth acquiring the (fundamental) movement skills necessary for involvement in physical activities and sports (Logan, Kipling Webster, Getchell, Pfeiffer, & Robinson, 2015). Furthermore, when youth lack the efficacy beliefs to perform those movement/motor skills, then they are less likely to stick with them (Wrotniak, Epstein, Dorn, Jones, & Kondilis, 2006). What this means, by way of understanding the long-term pursuit of active lifestyles, is that if children and adolescents lack confidence to perform these movement skills, they are less likely to get involved in the various activities (e.g., recreational or competitive sports) that require them (Chase, 2001).

The second type of efficacy belief that is particularly pertinent for supporting the sustained involvement in physical activity by youth corresponds to *self-regulatory efficacy* (Bandura, 2004). Self-regulatory efficacy corresponds to the belief a person has in their capabilities to perform volitional behaviors despite the various obstacles and challenges that one might face, such as being active despite inclement weather or against the backdrop of other competing demands (e.g., homework). A recent longitudinal study involving a large multi-ethnic sample of adolescents from the United States highlights the prospective benefits of youth (between the fifth and seventh Grades), displaying high levels of self-regulatory efficacy beliefs (Dishman, Dowda, McIver, Saunders, & Pate, 2017). Specifically, Dishman and colleagues (2017) were interested in whether the declines in physical activity that one tends to observe between childhood and early adolescence can be explained by naturally occurring changes in children's motives and beliefs. What they found was that physical activity tended to decline less in children who displayed lessened declines in self-efficacy for overcoming barriers to physical activity involvement as well as greater parental support. In another study with a large sample of adolescents, Hagger, Chatzisarantis, and Biddle (2001) found that higher levels of self-regulatory efficacy beliefs were associated with stronger intentions to be physically active, even after controlling for past physical activity behavior.

Among physical activity interventions for youth, self-efficacy has been identified as the most commonly assessed and supported mediator variable (Lubans, Foster, & Biddle, 2008). In a recent meta-analysis examining physical activity in adolescents, Plotnikoff, Costigan, Karunamuni, and Lubans (2013) found that SCT-related variables accounted for 24% of the variance in physical activity behavior; however, the theory was found to be less effective in explaining physical activity behavior when compared to other theories (which explained 31%–37%). In this meta-analytic review, the core construct of SCT (self-efficacy) was commonly and significantly associated with physical activity behavior (Plotnikoff et al., 2013). In a separate review of physical activity interventions for adolescent girls, Owen and colleagues noted that SCT was the most common theory used to guide interventions (Owen, Curry, Kerner, Newson, & Fairclough, 2017). However, they found that all interventions (including those guided by SCT) resulted in mixed effectiveness in promoting physical activity and the overall effect of physical activity interventions was very small ($g = 0.07$, $p = 0.05$). In sum, observational and experimental research guided by SCT suggests that beliefs of personal efficacy and goals are important in fostering physical activity behavior among youth. However, in light of the inconsistent effects of physical activity interventions guided by SCT in relation to youth physical activity behavior, further work is clearly warranted to identify exactly which SCT-informed interventions (or combinations of interventions) are most likely to *consistently support* physical activity *behavior change* among children and adolescents.

Intentions and Youth Physical Activity

Another prominent psychological theory that shares some similarities (but also some notable differences) with SCT corresponds to the theory of planned behavior (TPB; Ajzen, 1985, 1991). The precursor to the TPB was the theory of reasoned action (TRA; Fishbein & Ajzen, 1975) which posited that intention is the proximal determinant of behaviors such as physical activity, with intention itself influenced by a person's attitude toward the behavior as well as subjective norms (perceptions of the norms tied to the behavior). Behavior according to the TRA was posited to be 'reasoned' by virtue of the contention that behavior is shaped by rational or reasoned judgments. Despite the early intuitive appeal of the TRA, early critics (Sheppard, Hartwick, & Warshaw, 1988) highlighted limits to a model that did not include a component that accounts for a person's control over the target behavior. With this in mind, the TRA was expanded to become the TPB by incorporating perceptions of behavioral control (Ajzen, 1985, 1991). Within the TPB, perceived behavioral control is theorized to influence behavior both directly and also via (i.e., mediated by) a person's intentions to perform the behavior. In the ensuing decades after its formulation, the TPB became subject to considerable investigation in relation to multiple behaviors including health-enhancing physical activity. With direct relevance to the current chapter, a number of cross-sectional and passive prospective (i.e., non-experimental) studies involving children and adolescents (e.g., Mummery, Spence, & Hudec, 2000; Uijtdewilligen et al., 2011) provided evidence for the theoretical associations linking attitudes, subjective norms, and perceptions of control to intentions and thereafter physical activity behavior.

Interestingly, this body of correlational evidence suggests that attitudes, subjective norms, and perceived control are much better predictors of intention than behavior (Armitage & Conner, 2001). Interestingly, the relationships between intention and behavior tend to be significantly weaker among children and adolescents than they are for adults (Downs & Hausenblas, 2005). That is, even when youth report intending to be active, those intentions often do not result in concomitant behavioral responses among this population. Furthermore, when researchers have used experimental designs, the utility of the TPB has been particularly challenged. For example, the results of a meta-analysis by Rhodes and Dickau (2012) revealed that when intentions are manipulated experimentally, the resultant changes in physical activity behavior tend to be modest. This finding highlights what is now widely recognized as a substantive limitation of the TPB; that is, there tends to exist a notable intention-behavior gap that is not explained by the model (Rhodes & de Bruijn, 2013), whereby a person's intentions often do not readily translate into changes in physical activity behavior. To illustrate, in the context of a randomized experimental study involving youth, Tessier and colleagues presented lectures to inactive high school students on the benefits of physical activity, wherein each group received either an additional message targeting the various belief constructs embedded within the TPB along with intentions, or no message (control; Tessier, Sarrazin, Nicaise, & Dupont, 2015). The intervention was found to positively influence the TPB belief constructs as well as intentions to be physically active, but not actual physical activity behavior.

In light of concerns about the TPB, some researchers have suggested that the theory be 'retired' and cast to the winds of history (Sniehotta, Presseau, & Araújo-Soares, 2014). Others, however, have suggested drawing from the lessons learned from this body of work by developing interventions that specifically focus on turning intentions *into* behaviors (Armitage, 2015), rather than targeting the distal constructs in the model (e.g., attitudes, subjective norms, perceived control). Examples of psychological constructs that may be able to bridge (or reduce) the intention-behavior gap include action planning (Rhodes & Yao, 2015) and implementation intentions (Gollwitzer, 1999). Action planning (Leventhal, Singer, & Jones, 1965) involves specifying when, where, and how the intended behavior will be performed, and has shown to be effective for increasing physical activity behavior change in adults (Norman & Conner, 2005). However, some research with adolescents has indicated that younger people may require more planning support, such as the addition of coping plans to strategically overcome barriers (Araújo-Soares, McIntyre, & Sniehotta, 2009). As a complement to goal setting, implementation intentions represent conditional plans, wherein the individual forms '*if-then*' strategies to support the intended behavior and buffer against anticipated barriers to success (e.g., *if* it is raining, *then* I will play badminton inside). In a meta-analysis on physical activity, implementation intentions were found to be effective in supporting physical activity behavior change (Bélanger-Gravel, Godin, & Amireault, 2013). In children, in particular, the use of implementation intentions (e.g., "if it is playtime, then I will run around as much as possible") has been shown to be effective in influencing physical activity during playtime (Armitage & Sprigg, 2010).

In sum, research on the TPB in physical activity settings (among youth) has highlighted a number of important findings. In particular, research suggests that psychological factors involving attitudes, subjective norms, and perceived control are related to intentions to engage in the target behavior (e.g., physical activity), but that there exists a substantive intention-behavior gap. In light of this 'gap' researchers are continuing to examine what psychological strategies, or interventions, can be best applied to narrow that disconnect between youths' intentions to be active and their actual physical activity behaviors.

Psychological Needs and Motivational Regulation

Both of the major theoretical models described thus far emphasize the importance of believing in one's own capabilities, by way of self-efficacy beliefs (SCT) and perceived behavioral control (TPB), and both highlight to varying degrees the importance of human motivation in shaping behavior. For example, within SCT, Bandura (1977, 2004) emphasizes the role that goal states and the anticipation of successful outcomes play as important predictors of behavior. Similarly, within the TPB, intentions represent a summary conception of one's readiness to perform the behavior. Despite both models identifying the importance of motivation in facilitating behavior, they do not explicate the downstream effects that result from different *types* of motivation. For example, people can engage in physical activity for a slew of reasons, and so the key question is 'are some reasons or motives more powerful in influencing human behaviors than others'?

It is with this question in mind that we turn to self-determination theory (SDT; Deci & Ryan, 1985, 2002) and the psychological processes explicated within that framework, in particular with regard to physical activity behavior in youth. Broadly conceived, SDT is concerned with examining the effects of different types of motivational regulations, in relation to subsequent health- and achievement-striving behaviors. It is also concerned with understanding the nutriments, or sources, of those different types of motivational regulations, which include the multiple personal, contextual, and environmental factors acting upon people in social settings along with the mediating mechanisms that account for those effects.

Specifically, within SDT, Deci and Ryan (2000) posit that people engage in behaviors for multiple reasons that include those that are self-determined as well as those that are shaped by extrinsic reasons. They also recognized that some people (or some people in certain instances) are simply unmotivated (i.e., display a complete lack of intentionality), and such are considered to be amotivated (Deci & Ryan, 2000). Other than amotivation which simply represents an *absence* of motivation, Deci and Ryan (2000) contend that self-determined (or autonomous) and extrinsic (or controlled) forms of motivation should be considered along a continuum, with more self-determined forms typically displaying more adaptive behavioral and emotional responses than extrinsic (or controlled) forms of motivation.

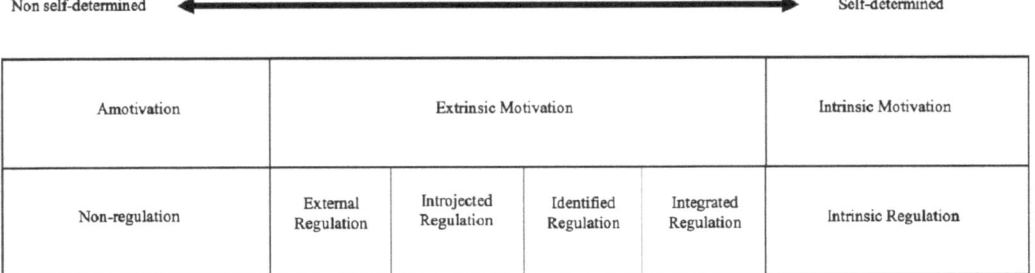

Figure 8.1   Deci and Ryan's continuum of self-determined motivation. Reproduced from Deci., E. L., & Ryan, R. M. (1985). *Intrinsic motivation and self-determination in human behavior.* New York, NY: Plenum Press

The most self-determined 'type' of motivation (see Figure 8.1) corresponds to intrinsic motivation, whereby a behavior is pursued based on personal interest and enjoyment. Extrinsic motivation includes the following: (a) *integrated regulation,* whereby a person pursues a given activity because it aligns, and is integrated with, other important life goals (e.g., a child continuing to participate in sport because they identify as an athlete), (b) *identified regulation*, whereby a person is motivated because the outcome reflects a personal value (e.g., an adolescent who engages in physical activity because they know it is good for their health), (c) *introjected regulation*, whereby a person is motivated by internal self-contingent rewards, such as self-worth or the avoidance of negative affect (e.g., a child who continues to work hard in sport because they experience a sense of pride when they perform well, or because they want to avoid feeling ashamed for not performing well), and (d) *external regulation*, which involves being motivated by external pressure or rewards (e.g., a child who continues to play basketball because they want to please their parents). These four forms of extrinsic motivation each display varying levels of internalization, with integrated regulation representing the most autonomous form of extrinsic motivation, and identified, introjected, and external regulations each displaying decreasing levels of autonomy.

With regard to adolescent involvement in physical activity, Owen and colleagues (2014) conducted a systematic review and found that autonomous motivation demonstrated stronger positive associations with physical activity (pooled effect size (ρ) = 0.27 to 0.38) when compared to controlled motivation (ρ = −0.03 to −0.17). Furthermore, displays of amotivation were negatively correlated with levels of physical activity (ρ = −0.11 to −0.21). Interestingly, displays of self-determined motivation were positively correlated with physical activity during school (i.e., physical education class), as well as during leisure-time (Owen, Smith, Lubans, Ng, & Lonsdale, 2014). In sport, the extent to which self-determined motivation is enhanced has been found to predict reduced drop-out rates and improved participation in adolescents (Calvo, Cervelló, Jiménez, Iglesias, & Murcia, 2010; Ryska, Hohensee, David, Cooley, Dean, Jones, 2002).

According to SDT, the quality of a person's motivation is shaped by the extent to which three basic psychological needs are supported (or actively thwarted). Specifically, the extent to which people feel *competent* (i.e., capable of being successful in one's environment), *autonomous* (i.e., displaying volition), and *related* (i.e., connected to others) enables them to experience more self-determined forms of motivation. When these needs are supported among children and adolescents, they tend to be more physically active (McDavid, Cox, & McDonough, 2014).

Several school-based interventions targeting self-determined motivation have shown to be effective in increasing students' autonomous motivation toward physical activity, often using physical education teachers to bolster students' basic needs (Cheon, Reeve, & Song, 2016; Lonsdale et al., 2013; Tessier, Sarrazin, & Ntoumanis, 2010; Wallhead, Garn, & Vidoni, 2014). Specifically,

SDT-based interventions have successfully increased students' perceived autonomy (Lonsdale et al., 2013), relatedness (Tessier et al., 2010), and competence (Murillo Pardo, Bengoechea, Clemente, & Generelo Lanaspa, 2016), which, in turn, bolsters students' self-determined motivation and physical activity engagement. For example, González-Cutre, Sierra, Beltrán-Carrillo, Peláez-Pérez, and Cervelló (2018) found that when physical education teachers supported students' basic needs, students were more likely to display autonomous motivation and physical activity behavior (González-Cutre et al., 2018). Balanced against these findings, although school-based SDT interventions have been found to be effective at bolstering students' in-class physical activity, they also demonstrate limited effectiveness with regard to changing youth's extracurricular (Wallhead et al., 2014) and long-term (González-Cutre et al., 2018) physical activity behaviors.

How Youth Frame Success and Failure: Does It Matter?

Underpinned initially by research in education, but later extended to the study of achievement-striving in physical activity settings, a considerable body of work has accumulated over the past three decades that has sought to examine the way in which children and adolescents 'frame' conceptions of success and failure and the implications of such framing for sustained involvement in various forms of physical activity (e.g., sports and physical education). This work was largely studied through a cluster of achievement goal theories (Dweck, 1986; Dweck & Sorich, 1999; Nicholls, 1984; Nicholls, Cheung, Lauer, & Patashnick, 1989) which posited that conceptions of success can be considered either in relation to one's own past performances or in relation to the capacity and performances of others. The first conception of achievement came to be known as task involvement, whereby improved personal mastery generates a sense of accomplishment and where success is conceived in relation to one's personal standards (Nicholls, 1984). The latter conception of achievement came to be known as ego involvement, whereby a sense of accomplishment (or success) is only considered by displaying superior performances relative to others within one's social setting (i.e., winning). According to Nicholls (1984) children and youth display a sense of task and/or ego involvement in achievement settings, as a result of a dispositional goal orientation (to be either ego-oriented or task-oriented), which itself emerges through early socialization (i.e., from parents, schooling, culture).

Individuals who tend to approach challenges with a task orientation (otherwise known as 'mastery' orientation) are more likely to persist when experiencing difficulty and maintain high levels of effort over the long term (Dweck, 1986). However, individuals with an ego orientation (also known as a performance orientation) tend to avoid challenges for fear of failure and are more likely to perceive such failure as a direct reflection of their lack of competence (Dweck, 1986). From the perspective of physical activity involvement, children who adopt task goal orientations have been found to be more physically active compared to children with an ego orientation (Ahmed et al., 2017). Interestingly, gender differences suggest that boys are more likely to be ego-oriented and girls more task-oriented (Barić, Vlašić, & Cecić Erpič, 2014; Gråstén & Watt, 2016), a trend that has also been found in adults (D'Lima, Winsler, & Kitsantas, 2014).

The social settings in which physical activities take place, whether in school physical education, competitive sports, or exercise settings, play an important role in shaping youth goal orientations. Early work by Ames and her colleagues (Ames, 1984; Ames & Archer, 1988) contended that motivational climates that promote task involvement (in the form of a mastery climate) or ego involvement (in the form of a performance climate) play an important role in shaping the way youth approach achievement-striving settings or tasks. *Mastery* climates reinforce task goals by focusing on effort and learning. For example, this might involve a coach praising their athletes for working hard during a game, regardless of whether the team won. In contrast, *performance* climates focus on normative outcomes (i.e., winning), such as a coach emphasizing winning rather than focusing on athletic development or enjoyment (Ames, 1992). When children are exposed to and perceive the motivational climate to be mastery-focused this is associated with the greater adoption of a task goal orientation, whereas when children are exposed to and perceive the climate to be performance-focused this tends to be associated with the adoption of an ego orientation (Standage, Duda, & Ntoumanis, 2003). Although much of the work on motivational climates in physical activity settings has been correlational in nature, experimental evidence for the above effects has also been found. For example, in a school-based intervention, when physical education teachers created a mastery climate, students were more likely to perceive a mastery climate and adopt a task goal orientation when compared to students in a regular physical education class (Digelidis, Papaioannou, Laparidis, & Christodoulidis, 2003). From an adolescent engagement perspective, research suggests that when children and youth perceive the prevailing climate to be supportive of mastery involvement this results in a range of adaptive outcomes such as increased intrinsic motivation, enjoyment/interest, and higher levels of after-school physical activity (Ommundsen & Kvalø, 2007). In contrast, when youth perceive the climate to be performance-driven this tends to be associated with a range of negative outcomes, such as lower levels of physical activity during class time (Johnson, Erwin, Kipp, & Beighle, 2017), as well as higher levels of stress, humiliation, shame, anxiety, and negative affect (Hogue, Fry, & Fry, 2017).

The Self-Concept

While goal orientations reflect the way in which people appraise success and failure, people also develop perceptions that reflect their overall sense of self. Self-concept reflects the way in which a person describes him or herself, and is considered a multidimensional construct that includes a range of domain-specific indicators (e.g., social, physical, and emotional domains; Fox, 1997; Marsh, & O'Mara, 2008). Although some researchers have interchangeably used the terms self-esteem and self-concept, Marsh and O'Mara (2008) suggest that the term 'self-esteem' should be used to describe to the global component of self-concept and to further differentiate this global conceptualization from the various subdomains of the self-concept construct (e.g., physical, social, and academic domains).

Over the past few decades, a considerable amount of research has sought to examine the relationships between a person's self-concept (and self-esteem) and physical activity behavior, especially among children and adolescents. The results of a recent meta-analysis revealed that when youth displayed higher levels of physical self-concept, they tended to be more active (Babic et al., 2014). The authors concluded that physical self-concept may act as both a determinant and an outcome of physical activity behavior in youth, with the strength of relations being comparable irrespective of whether physical self-concept and physical activity were operationalized as predictors or criterion measures. In a more recent meta-analysis of randomized and non-randomized controlled experimental studies, Liu, Wu, and Ming (2015) found that physical activity alone is associated with improvements in both self-concept and self-esteem. When taken together, there appears to be strong evidence for relations between physical activity and subsequent self-concept and self-esteem, but with regard to reverse causality (self-concept and self-esteem promoting physical activity behavior) more high-quality experimental evidence is required before firm conclusions can be made.

Affective Factors and Physical Activity

Affect and affect-related constructs are critical psychological factors in understanding the adoption and maintenance of physical activity behavior (e.g., Nasuti & Rhodes, 2013; Rhodes & Kates, 2015). Overall, affect is defined as "an evaluative neurobiological state that manifests in: (1) coordinated patterns of physiological (e.g., release of hormones, increased heart rate) and involuntary behavioral (e.g., facial expression, vocalization) changes, and (2) subjective experiential feelings (e.g., the phenomenal experience of pleasure, anger, embarrassment, etc.)" (Williams, Rhodes, & Conner, 2018, p. 7). In response to the heavy emphasis on rational/cognitive approaches to changing physical activity behavior (e.g., SCT, TPB), recent theoretical efforts have focused on the affective factors that relate to bolstering health-enhancing behavior generally, and physical activity in particular (cf. Williams et al., 2018). Overall, this body of empirical work, examined across diverse theoretical and methodological perspectives, has demonstrated that affect and affect-related constructs are better able to predict and explain physical activity behavior than more rational/instrumental approaches.

Although affect has been conceptualized in a variety of ways by different researchers (for an excellent discussion see Williams et al., 2018), most researchers in the physical activity domain seem to agree that there are several ways in which affect can influence physical activity behavior. Accordingly, distinctions have been made between *different types of affect* in relation to the various ways in which affect can influence physical activity behavior. In line with the preliminary taxonomy proposed by Rhodes, Williams, and Conner (2018) the first distinction that has been made is between *affect proper* and *affect processing* (i.e., cognitions about affect).

Affect proper is an umbrella term encompassing three interrelated concepts: core affect, moods, and emotions (Ekkekakis, 2013; Rhodes, Williams et al., 2018). Core affect is characterized as being "the most elementary consciously accessible affective feeling" (pg. 47) that is continually ebbing and flowing over the course of the day and is further characterized by two orthogonal dimensions: valence (i.e., positive vs. negative) and activation (i.e., high vs. low; Ekkekakis, 2013). Examples of core affect include feelings of pleasure (cf. displeasure) and energy (cf. relaxation). Core affect provides the foundation, or 'building blocks', of moods and emotions. However, while core affect does not involve a cognitive appraisal component, both moods (e.g., feeling irritated, grumpy, cheerful) and emotions (e.g., anger, guilt, sadness, love) do. Specifically, *emotions* are comprised of cognitive appraisals attributed to a specific stimulus (e.g., an event or person), which lead to a change in core affect (i.e., coordinated patterns of physiological and/or behavioral responses and subjective feelings), and can change rapidly in response to an unfolding event and/or reappraisals (Ekkekakis, 2013; Williams et al., 2018). Similarly, *moods* also include cognitive appraisals and changes in core affect; however, unlike emotions, the cause of a mood may not be easily attributed to a specific stimulus and have a longer duration, sometimes persisting for days or weeks (Ekkekakis, 2013; Williams et al., 2018).

One particularly notable theoretical framework through which affect proper is suggested to influence physical activity behavior corresponds to the dual-mode model developed by Ekkekakis and colleagues (Ekkekakis, Hall, & Petruzzello, 2008; Ekkekakis, Parfitt, & Petruzzello, 2011). Specifically, Ekkekakis and colleagues (Ekkekakis et al., 2008, 2011) theorized that an individual's affective response to physical activity becomes unpleasant when he/she reaches his or her ventilatory/lactate thresholds (i.e., the intensity of exercise where breathing becomes labored, and the concentration of lactic acid in the body begins to increase exponentially). Conversely, at sub-threshold intensities, physical activity is associated with pleasant affective responses (Ekkekakis et al., 2011). These pleasant responses to physical activity predict whether an individual will engage in future physical activity efforts. For example, a recent systematic review found that the affective response that individuals had during moderate intensity exercise had a significant and meaningful positive correlation in the medium effect size range with subsequent physical activity behavior (Rhodes & Kates, 2015). However, no relationship was found between post-exercise affect and subsequent physical activity behavior (Rhodes & Kates, 2015).

Recent experimental evidence among children and adolescents has also demonstrated similar relationships between one's affective response to physical activity and subsequent physical activity behavior. For example, among adolescents, it was demonstrated that affective responses *during* moderate intensity physical activity were positively associated with objectively measured physical activity behavior, whereas adolescents' affective response *after* exercise was not (Schneider, Dunn, & Cooper, 2009). Accordingly, based on the dual-mode model of physical activity, children and adolescents should be encouraged to self-select a physical activity intensity that "feels good," as opposed to be imposed by someone else (e.g., a parent, teacher, coach), in order to bolster physical activity adherence. This is particularly pertinent given experimental evidence which demonstrates that when asked to exercise at an intensity that "feels good," adolescents self-selected an intensity that was necessary to achieve the health-enhancing benefits of physical activity (i.e., moderate intensity activity; Schneider & Schmalbach, 2015).

In addition to affect proper, *affect processing* relates to the cognitive processing of previous or anticipated affective responses to physical activity (Williams et al., 2018; Williams & Evans, 2014). There now exists strong meta-analytic evidence that one type of affective processing, known as affective judgment (i.e., evaluations regarding emotions or feelings one associates with being physically active), is better predictor of physical activity behavior than instrumental judgment (i.e., evaluations regarding the utility of a given behavior; Nasuti & Rhodes, 2013; Rhodes, Fiala, & Conner, 2009; Rhodes, Gray, & Husband, 2018). Specifically, among youth, Nasuti and Rhodes (2013) observed a medium-sized relationship between affective judgments and physical activity behavior based on observational research, which was larger than other meta-analytic relationships among youth, such as between parental support and adolescent activity. With respect to experimental evidence, recent meta-analytic evidence, among adults, demonstrated a significant mediation effect, such that targeting affective judgments through intervention, resulted in positive changes in affective judgments, which in turn was associated with increases in physical activity, with a large effect size (Rhodes, Gray et al., 2018). In comparison, the most recent meta-analytic evidence for youth regarding the efficacy of physical activity interventions that targeted affective judgments revealed a small-sized effect with considerable heterogeneity, which may in part be due to the limited number of intervention studies available (Nasuti & Rhodes, 2013). Accordingly, targeting affective judgments through intervention represents a highly promising area for future research among children and adolescents.

Future Research Directions for Understanding Psychological Factors that Underpin Physical Activity Behavior with Youth

The study of psychological processes implicated in the prediction and explanation of physical activity behavior has been extensive in the last few decades, and will likely continue with as much vigor in the next few decades. While there are clearly many worthwhile directions for future research, in the final section of this chapter, we discuss two broad avenues that may be particularly worthwhile for studies with youth that build on some of the earlier work (and frameworks) highlighted above, but also substantively expand on these. The first corresponds to the application of dual-process theories, and the second corresponds to the application and testing of a new theory (Dweck, 2017), which may have particular utility in understanding and intervening to influence physical activity behavior with youth.

Dual-Process Approaches

In recent years, there has been an increased emphasis of *dual-process theories* to understand physical activity behavior (Brand & Ekkekakis, 2018; Ekkekakis & Zenko, 2016; Rhodes, 2017; Schinkoeth & Antoniewicz, 2017; Wiers, Anderson, Van Bockstaele, Salemink, & Hommel, 2018; Zenko, Ekkekakis, & Kavetsos, 2016). The application of dual-process theories in the physical activity domain emerged in response to limitations of previous theories, particularly the expectancy-value tenets of social cognitive models (e.g., SCT, TPB), which assume that individuals act as rational decision-makers who, when provided with complete and accurate information regarding physical activity benefits and guidelines, will logically process this information and change their behavior accordingly (Gibbons, Houlihan, & Gerrard, 2009). However, individuals often do not engage in behaviors that are most adaptive from a cost-benefit perspective (Tversky & Kahneman, 1974). For example, as highlighted above, a prominent criticism of the TPB corresponds to the large discordance between one's intention to be active and their actual engagement in physical activity behavior, known as the "intention-behavior gap" (Rhodes & de Bruijn, 2013). That is, people often do not act upon their own stated intentions (Rhodes, 2017).

To date, there has been a multitude of dual-process theories applied to the study of physical activity behavior. Some of these theories have been derived from social psychology, such as the *associative-propositional evaluation* model (Gawronski & Bodenhausen, 2014), as well as the *reflective-impulsive* model (Strack & Deutsch, 2014). Recent efforts have also sought to create dual-process models specific to physical activity behavior, such as the *multi-process action control* framework (Rhodes, 2017) and the *affective-reflective theory* of physical inactivity and exercise (Brand & Ekkekakis, 2018). Although the definitions vary, generally dual-process models assume that there are two distinct systems operating in the brain: *Type 1* processes, which are generally fast and automatic, require minimal mental effort or processing (also described as *implicit, associative, reflexive, affective,* or *heuristic*), and *Type 2* processes, which are slower, rational, and deliberative (also described as *explicit, reflective*, or *propositional*). Type 1 processes are generally conceived as being more evolutionarily primitive than Type 2 processes and therefore represent the default mode of responding to a situation (Evans & Stanovich, 2013). Further, the influence of Type 1 processes may not be consciously accessible to an individual, therefore potentially exacerbating their biasing powers (Ekkekakis & Zenko, 2016). Accordingly, with respect to physical activity, although an individual may rationally evaluate physical activity as having important health benefits or making them 'feel good' through the slower Type 2 processes, if one's fast and automatic associations regarding physical activity are incongruent (i.e., Type 1 processes evaluate physical activity as unpleasant or unimportant), these may lead an individual to refrain from being active.

To date, the application of dual-process theories to understanding physical activity behavior has primarily been conducted with adult populations (e.g., Antoniewicz & Brand, 2016; Schinkoeth, & Antoniewicz, 2017; Zenko et al., 2016). This, therefore, represents a critical area for future inquiry in youth. Not only would the application for dual-process theories be suitable for youth populations, it has been further suggested that dual-process theories may be even more relevant to youth populations (Gibbons et al., 2009). For example, meta-analytic evidence demonstrates that for health-enhancing behaviors, such as physical activity, age is a salient moderating factor in the intention-behavior gap, such that the discordance between intention and behavior is greater for adolescents than it is for adults (Hagger, Chatzisarantis, & Biddle, 2002). This may be due, in part, to the fact that areas of the brain involved in 'rational decision making' required in traditional social cognitive models are not fully developed until an individual reaches adulthood (Anderson & Briggs, 2016; Wiers et al., 2018). This means that children and adolescents might represent excellent candidates for physical activity interventions that tap into Type 1 processes.

Dweck's (2017) Unified Theory of Motivation, Personality, and Development

Most of the psychological theories and frameworks that have been applied to the study of physical activity behavior propose psychological mechanisms and processes that are invariant across the human lifespan. That is, they tend to propose that the same (or similar) psychological processes apply

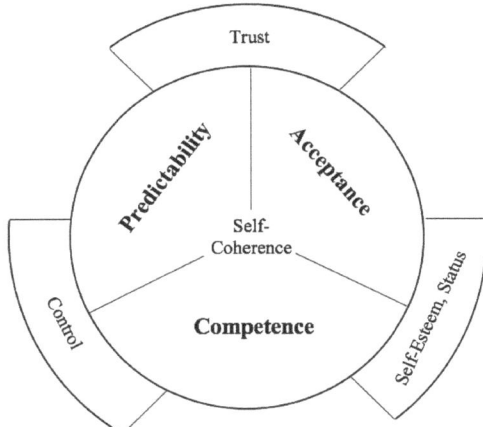

Figure 8.2 Dweck's model of basic needs. Reproduced from Dweck, C. S. (2017). From needs to goals and representations: Foundations for a unified theory of motivation, personality, and development. *Psychological Review, 124*(6), 689–719

to children in the same way that they do for middle-aged and older adults. An exception to this, and a model which may hold particular relevance for understanding and promoting physical activity behavior among youth (and also adults) corresponds to Dweck's (2017) recent unified theory of motivation, personality, and development. This framework draws from the extant personality, social, cultural, evolutionary, motivational, developmental, and clinical psychology literatures (Dweck, 2017). Similar to SDT, Dweck suggests that humans have three basic needs. However, in the case of her model, these correspond to *acceptance* (i.e., supportive social interactions), *predictability* (i.e., being able to understand the world), and *competence* (i.e., having the skills to be successful in the world). Unlike many psychological theories, which consider basic needs in the context of adulthood, Dweck considers basic needs to be fundamental and to begin from infancy. Dweck provides evidence that these basic needs are displayed in early childhood, such as an infant relying on the support of their mother (acceptance), an infant learning from their current environment in an attempt to predict future events (predictability), or an infant turning their reactive actions into intentional ones (competence). It is not until later in childhood, when people begin to recognize their potential for personal agency that additional *compound needs* emerge. These compound needs are derived from an integration of the above three basic needs (see Figure 8.1). This includes the *need for trust* (formed after and from developing the need for acceptance and predictability), the *need for control* (formed from a greater sense of awareness, combining the needs of predictability and competence), and the *need for self-esteem and status* (formed from the ability to compare oneself, combining the need for acceptance and competence) (Figure 8.2).

The essential and central 'hub' of the theory is the need for *self-coherence*, defined as "the sense that the self is intact and firmly rooted" (p. 690), which is comprised of two sub-needs: *identity* ("who am I?") and *meaning* ("how does/should the world work, in ways that are important to me?"). Dweck contended that the fulfillment of the aforementioned three needs supports self-coherence, further leading to enhanced well-being and optimal psychological development. Although this theoretical framework has yet to be applied to the study of physical activity behavior (among youth or adults), it represents a particularly promising model for three main reasons. First, the model has a strong developmental component, which recognizes the importance of tapping into psychological needs that manifest from infancy onward. Second, extensive research in the physical activity domain has examined the predictive utility of some aspects of the model (e.g., competence, control); however, other features of the model remain largely unstudied as predictors of physical activity behavior. For example, although trust has been identified as an important feature in adolescent development (Szcześniak, Colaço, & Rondón, 2012), it has yet to be examined as a psychological 'need,' or targeted as a mechanism for intervention, in physical activity settings. Third, the model provides several testable hypotheses related to the extent to which compound needs develop through the merging of basic psychological needs. Indeed, it would be fascinating to examine the extent to which such compound needs manifest themselves in physical activity settings, as well as the relative predictive validity of these (multiple) psychological needs in supporting the sustained involvement of youth in health-enhancing physical activity.

Conclusion

The overall purpose of this chapter was to provide an overview of the various psychological factors implicated in predicting, understanding, and changing physical activity behavior among children and adolescents. The extant literature to date has provided good support for the prediction of physical activity behaviors, based on longitudinal research, and has also shown that psychological factors represent important and viable targets for intervention. When taken together, that vast majority of research in this area has drawn from deliberative cognitive models, which contend that human behavior is largely guided by rationale forethought. Recent research in the physical activity domain points the importance of other psychological factors such as affective processes, as well as habitual and unconscious psychological mechanisms, that may represent highly viable targets for physical activity promotion and intervention involving youth. In light of these conceptual and empirical advances, the study of psychological factors implicated in physical activity involvement among children and adolescents represents a field of enquiry with considerable potential for advancement.

References

Ahmed, M. D., Ho, W. K. Y., Van Niekerk, R. L., Morris, T., Elayaraja, M., Lee, K. C., & Randles, E. (2017). The self-esteem, goal orientation, and health-related physical fitness of active and inactive adolescent students. *Cogent Psychology, 4*, 1–14. doi:10.1080/23311908.2017.1331602

Ajzen, I. (1985). From intentions to actions: A theory of planned behavior. In J. Kuhl & J. Beckmann (Eds.), *Action control* (pp. 11–39). Berlin, Germany: Springer.

Ajzen, I. (1991). The theory of planned behavior. *Organizational Behavior and Human Decision Processes, 50*, 179–211.

Álvarez-Bueno, C., Pesce, C., Cavero-Redondo, I., Sánchez-López, M., Garrido-Miguel, M., & Martínez-Vizcaíno, V. (2017). Academic achievement and physical activity: A meta-analysis. *Pediatrics, 140*(6), e20171498.

Ames, C. (1984). Achievement attributions and self-instructions under competitive and individualistic goal structures. *Journal of Educational Psychology, 76*(3), 478–487. doi:10.1037/0022-0663.76.3.478

Ames, C. (1992). Classrooms: Goals, structures, and student motivation. *Journal of Educational Psychology, 84*(3), 261–271. Retrieved from http://psycnet.apa.org/journals/edu/84/3/261.html?uid=1993-03487-001

Ames, C., & Archer, J. (1988). Achievement goals in the classroom: Student learning strategies and motivation processes. *Journal of Educational Psychology, 80*(3), 260–267. doi:10.1037/0022-0663.80.3.260

Anderson, K. G., & Briggs, K. E. L. (2016). Self-regulation and decision making. In S. A. Brown & R. A. Zucker (Eds.), *Oxford handbook of adolescent substance abuse*. New York, NY: Oxford University Press.

Antoniewicz, F., & Brand, R. (2016). Learning to like exercising: Evaluative conditioning changes automatic evaluations of exercising and influences subsequent exercising behavior. *Journal of Sport and Exercise Psychology, 38*, 138–148.

Araújo-Soares, V., McIntyre, T., & Sniehotta, F. F. (2009). Predicting changes in physical activity among adolescents: The role of self-efficacy, intention, action planning and coping planning. *Health Education Research, 24*(1), 128–139. doi:10.1093/her/cyn005

Armitage, C. J. (2015). Time to retire the theory of planned behaviour? A commentary on Sniehotta, Presseau and Araújo-Soares. *Health Psychology Review, 9*(2), 151–155. doi:10.1080/17437199.2014.892148

Armitage, C. J., & Conner, M. (2001). Efficacy of the theory of planned behaviour: A meta-analytic review. *British Journal of Social Psychology, 40*, 471–499. doi:10.1348/014466601164939

Armitage, C. J., & Sprigg, C. A. (2010). The roles of behavioral and implementation intentions in changing physical activity in young children with low socioeconomic status. *Journal of Sport and Exercise Psychology, 32*, 359–376.

Aubert, S., Barnes, J. D., Abdeta, C., Nader, P. A., Adeniyi, A. F., Tenesaca, D. S. A., . . . Tremblay, M. S. (2018). Global Matrix 3.0 physical activity report card grades for children and youth: Results and analysis from 49 countries. *Journal of Physical Activity and Health, 15*(2), 251–273.

Babic, M. J., Morgan, P. J., Plotnikoff, R. C., Lonsdale, C., White, R. L., & Lubans, D. R. (2014). Physical activity and physical self-concept in youth: Systematic review and meta-analysis. *Sports Medicine, 44*, 1589–1601.

Bandura, A. (1977). Self-efficacy: Toward a unifying theory of behavioral change. *Psychological Review, 84*(2), 191–215. doi:10.1037/0033-295X.84.2.191

Bandura, A. (1986). *Social foundations of thought and action: A social cognitive theory*. Englewood Cliffs, NJ: Prentice-Hall.

Bandura, A. (1997). *Self-efficacy: The exercise of control*. New York, NY: Freeman.

Bandura, A. (2001). Social cognitive theory: An agentic perspective. *Annual Review of Psychology, 52*, 1–26.

Bandura, A. (2004). Health promotion by social cognitive means. *Health Education and Behavior, 31*(2), 143–164. doi:10.1177/1090198104263660

Barić, R., Vlašić, J., & Cecić Erpič, S. (2014). Goal orientation and intrinsic motivation for physical education: Does perceived competence matter? *Kinesiology, 46*(1), 117–126. doi:10.1080/07303084.2015.1086620

Beauchamp, M. R., Crawford, K. L., & Jackson, B. (2018). Social cognitive theory and physical activity: Mechanisms of behavior change, critique, and legacy. *Psychology of Sport and Exercise*, 1–8. doi:10.1016/j.psychsport.2018.11.009

Bélanger-Gravel, A., Godin, G., & Amireault, S. (2013). A meta-analytic review of the effect of implementation intentions on physical activity. *Health Psychology Review, 7*(1), 23–54. doi:10.1080/17437199.2011.560095

Biddle, S. J. H., & Asare, M. (2011). Physical activity and mental health in children and adolescents: A review of reviews. *British Journal of Sports Medicine, 45*(11), 886–895. doi:10.1136/bjsports-2011-090185

Brand, R., & Ekkekakis, P. (2018). Affective–reflective theory of physical inactivity and exercise. *German Journal of Exercise and Sport Research, 48*, 48–58. doi:10.1007/s12662-017-0477-9

Calvo, T. G., Cervelló, E., Jiménez, R., Iglesias, D., & Murcia, J. A. M. (2010). Using self-determination theory to explain sport persistence and dropout in adolescent athletes. *The Spanish Journal of Psychology, 13*(2), 677–684. doi:10.1017/S1138741600002341

Carson, V., Hunter, S., Kuzik, N., Gray, C. E., Poitras, V. J., Chaput, J.-P., . . . Kho, M. (2016). Systematic review of sedentary behaviour and health indicators in school-aged children and youth: An update. *Applied Physiology, Nutrition, and Metabolism, 41*, 240–265. doi:10.1139/apnm-2015-0630

Chase, M. A. (2001). Children's self-efficacy, motivational intentions, and attributions in physical education and sport. *Research Quarterly for Exercise and Sport, 72*(1), 47–54. doi:10.1080/02701367.2001.10608931

Cheon, S. H., Reeve, J., & Song, Y.-G. (2016). A teacher-focused intervention to decrease PE students' amotivation by increasing need satisfaction and decreasing need frustration. *Journal of Sport and Exercise Psychology, 38*, 217–235. doi:10.1123/jsep.2015-0236

D'Lima, G. M., Winsler, A., & Kitsantas, A. (2014). Ethnic and gender differences in first-year college students' goal orientation, self-efficacy, and extrinsic and intrinsic motivation. *Journal of Educational Research, 107*(5), 341–356. doi:10.1080/00220671.2013.823366

Deci, E. L., & Ryan, R. M. (1985). *Intrinsic motivation and self-determination in human behavior*. New York, NY: Plenum.

Deci, E. L., & Ryan, R. M. (2000). The "what" and "why" of goal pursuits: Human needs and the self-determination of behaviour. *Psychological Inquiry, 11*(4), 227–268. doi:10.1002/maco.19730240806

Deci, E. L., & Ryan, R. M. (2002). An overview of self-determination theory. In E. L. Deci & R. M Ryan (Eds.), *Handbook of self-determination research* (pp. 3–33). Rochester, NY: University of Rochester Press.

Digelidis, N., Papaioannou, A., Laparidis, K., & Christodoulidis, T. (2003). A one-year intervention in 7th grade physical education classes aiming to change motivational climate and attitudes towards exercise. *Psychology of Sport and Exercise, 4*, 195–210. doi:10.1016/s1469-0292(02)00002-x

Dishman, R. K., Dowda, M., McIver, K. L., Saunders, R. P., & Pate, R. R. (2017). Naturally-occurring changes in social-cognitive factors modify change in physical activity during early adolescence. *PLoS One, 12*(2), 1–16. doi:10.1371/journal.pone.0172040

Downs, D. S., & Hausenblas, H. A. (2005). The theories of reasoned action and planned behavior applied to exercise: A meta-analytic update. *Journal of Physical Activity and Health, 2*(1), 76–97. doi:10.1123/jpah.2.1.76

Dweck, C. S. (1986). Motivational processes affecting learning. *American Psychologist, 41*(10), 1040–1048. doi:10.1037/0003-066X.41.10.1040

Dweck, C. S. (2017). From needs to goals and representations: Foundations for a unified theory of motivation, personality, and development. *Psychological Review, 124*(6), 689–719. doi:10.1037/rev0000082

Dweck, C. S., & Sorich, L. A. (1999). Mastery-oriented thinking. In C. R. Snyder (Ed.), *Coping: The psychology of what works* (p. 368). New York, NY: Oxford University Press.

Ekkekakis, P. (2013). *The measurement of affect, mood, and emotion: A guide for health-behavioral research.* New York, NY: Cambridge University Press.

Ekkekakis, P., Parfitt, G., & Petruzzello, S. J. (2011). The pleasure and displeasure people feel when they exercise at different intensities. *Sports Medicine, 41*(8), 641–671. doi:10.2165/11590680-000000000-00000

Ekkekakis P, Hall, E. E., & Petruzzello, S. J. (2008) The relationship between exercise intensity and affective responses demystified: To crack the forty-year-old nut, replace the forty-year-old nutcracker! *Annals of Behavioral Medicine, 35*, 136–149. doi:10.1007/s12160-008-9025-z

Ekkekakis, P., & Zenko, Z. (2016). Escape from cognitivism: Exercise as hedonic experience. In M. Raab, P. S. Wylleman, E. A. Roland, & A. Hatzigeorgiadis (Eds.), *Sport and exercise psychology research: From theory to practice* (pp. 389–414). London, UK: Academic Press. doi:10.1016/B978-0-12-803634-1.00018-2

Evans, J. S. B. T., & Stanovich, K. E. (2013). Dual-process theories of higher cognition: Advancing the debate. *Perspectives on Psychological Science, 8*(3), 223–241. doi:10.1177/1745691612460685

Fishbein, M., & Ajzen, I. (1975). *Belief, attitude, intention and behavior: An introduction to theory and research.* Reading, MA: Addison-Wesley.

Fox, K. R. (1997). *The physical self: From motivation to well-being.* Champaign, IL: Human Kinetics.

Gawronski, B., & Bodenhausen, G. V. (2014). Implicit and explicit evaluation: A brief review of the associative-propositional evaluation model. *Social and Personality Psychology Compass, 8*(8), 448–462. doi:10.1111/spc3.12124

Gibbons, F. X., Houlihan, A. E., & Gerrard, M. (2009). Reason and reaction: The utility of a dual-focus, dual-processing perspective on promotion and prevention of adolescent health risk behaviour. *British Journal of Health Psychology, 14*(2), 231–248. doi:10.1348/135910708X376640

Gollwitzer, P. M. (1999). Implementation intentions: Strong effects of simple plans. *The American Psychologist, 54*, 493–503. doi:10.1103/PhysRevE.87.032905

González-Cutre, D., Sierra, A. C., Beltrán-Carrillo, V. J., Peláez-Pérez, M., & Cervelló, E. (2018). A school-based motivational intervention to promote physical activity from a self-determination theory perspective. *Journal of Educational Research, 111*(3), 320–330. doi:10.1080/00220671.2016.1255871

Gråstén, A., & Watt, A. (2016). Perceptions of motivational climate, goal orientations, and light- to vigorous-intensity physical activity engagement of a sample of Finnish grade 5 to 9 students. *International Journal of Exercise Science, 9*(3), 291–305.

Hagger, M. S., Chatzisarantis, N., & Biddle, S. J. H. (2001). The influence of self-efficacy and past behaviour on the physical activity intentions of young people. *Journal of Sports Sciences, 19*(9), 711–725.

Hagger, M. S., Chatzisarantis, N., & Biddle, S. J. H. (2002). A meta-analytic review of the theories of reasoned action and planned behavior in physical activity: An examination of predictive validity and the contribution of additional variables. *Journal of Sport and Exercise Psychology, 24*(1), 3–32. doi:10.1123/jsep.24.1.3

Hearing, C. M., Chang, W. C., Szuhany, K. L., Deckersbach, T., Nierenberg, A. A., & Sylvia, L. G. (2016). Physical exercise for treatment of mood disorders: A critical review. *Current Behavioral Neuroscience Reports, 3*(4), 350–359. doi:10.1007/s40473-016-0089-y

Herman, K. M., Hopman, W. M., & Sabiston, C. M. (2015). Physical activity, screen time and self-rated health and mental health in Canadian adolescents. *Preventive Medicine, 73*, 112–116. doi:10.1016/j.ypmed.2015.01.030

Hillman, C. H., Pontifex, M. B., Castelli, D. M., Khan, N. A., Raine, L. B., Scudder, M. R., . . . Kamijo, K. (2014). Effects of the FITKids randomized controlled trial on executive control and brain function. *Pediatrics, 134*(4), e1063–e1071. doi:10.1542/peds.2013-3219

Hogue, C. M., Fry, M. D., & Fry, A. C. (2017). The differential impact of motivational climate on adolescents' psychological and physiological stress responses. *Psychology of Sport & Exercise, 30*, 118–127. doi:10.1016/j.psychsport.2017.02.004

Hupin, D., Roche, F., Gremeaux, V., Chatard, J. C., Oriol, M., Gaspoz, J. M., . . . Edouard, P. (2015). Even a low-dose of moderate-to-vigorous physical activity reduces mortality by 22% in adults aged ≥60 years: A systematic review and meta-analysis. *British Journal of Sports Medicine, 49*(19), 1262–1267. doi:10.1136/bjsports-2014-094306

Johnson, C. E., Erwin, H. E., Kipp, L., & Beighle, A. (2017). Student perceived motivational climate, enjoyment, and physical activity in middle school physical education. *Journal of Teaching in Physical Education, 36*(4), 398–408. doi:10.1123/jtpe.2016-0172

Kyu, H. H., Bachman, V. F., Alexander, L. T., Mumford, J. E., Afshin, A., Estep, K., . . . Forouzanfar, M. H. (2016). Physical activity and risk of breast cancer, colon cancer, diabetes, ischemic heart disease, and ischemic stroke events: Systematic review and dose-response meta-analysis for the Global Burden of Disease Study 2013. *British Medical Journal, 354*, 1–10. doi:10.1136/bmj.i3857

Leventhal, H., Singer, R., & Jones, S. (1965). Effects of fear and specificity of recommendation upon attitudes and behavior. *Journal of Personality and Social Psychology, 2*(1), 20–29. doi:10.1037/h0022089

Liu, M., Wu, L., & Ming, Q. (2015). How does physical activity intervention improve self-esteem and self-concept in children and adolescents? Evidence from a meta-analysis. *PLoS One, 10*(8), 1–17. doi:10.1371/journal.pone.0134804

Logan, S. W., Kipling Webster, E., Getchell, N., Pfeiffer, K. A., & Robinson, L. E. (2015). Relationship between fundamental motor skill competence and physical activity during childhood and adolescence: A systematic review. *Kinesiology Review, 4*(4), 416–426. doi:10.1123/kr.2013-0012

Lonsdale, C., Rosenkranz, R. R., Sanders, T., Peralta, L. R., Bennie, A., Jackson, B., . . . Lubans, D. R. (2013). A cluster randomized controlled trial of strategies to increase adolescents' physical activity and motivation in physical education: Results of the motivating active learning in physical education (MALP) trial. *Preventive Medicine, 57*(5), 696–702. doi:10.1016/j.ypmed.2013.09.003

Lubans, D. R., Foster, C., & Biddle, S. J. H. (2008). A review of mediators of behavior in interventions to promote physical activity among children and adolescents. *Preventive Medicine, 47*(5), 463–470. doi:10.1016/j.ypmed.2008.07.011

Maddux, J. E. (1995). *Self-efficacy, adaptation and adjustment.* New York, NY: Plenum Press.

Marsh, H. W., & O'Mara, A. (2008). Reciprocal effects between academic self-concept, self-esteem, achievement, and attainment over seven adolescent years: Unidimensional and multidimentional perspectives of self-concept. *Personality and Social Psychology Bulletin, 34*(4), 542–552.

McDavid, L., Cox, A. E., & McDonough, M. H. (2014). Need fulfillment and motivation in physical education predict trajectories of change in leisure-time physical activity in early adolescence. *Psychology of Sport and Exercise, 15*(5), 471–480. doi:10.1016/j.psychsport.2014.04.006

Mummery, W. K., Spence, J. C., & Hudec, J. C. (2000). Understanding physical activity intention in Canadian school children and youth: An application of the theory of planned behavior. *Research Quarterly for Exercise and Sport, 71*(2), 116–124. doi:10.1080/02701367.2000.10608889

Murillo Pardo, B., Bengoechea, E. G., Clemente, J. A. J., & Generelo Lanaspa, E. (2016). Motivational outcomes and predictors of moderate-to-vigorous physical activity and sedentary time for adolescents in the Sigue La Huella intervention. *International Journal of Behavioral Medicine, 23*, 135–142.

Nasuti, G., & Rhodes, R. E. (2013). Affective judgment and physical activity in youth: Review and meta-analyses. *Annals of Behavioral Medicine, 45*(3), 357–376. doi:10.1007/s12160-012-9462-6

Nicholls, J. G. (1984). Achievement motivation: Conceptions of ability, subjective experience, task choice, and performance. *Psychological Review, 91*(3), 328–346. doi:10.1016/j.cherd.2018.02.018

Nicholls, J. G., Cheung, P. C., Lauer, J., & Patashnick, M. (1989). Individual differences in academic motivation: Perceived ability, goals, beliefs, and values. *Learning and Individual Differences, 1*(1), 63–84. doi:10.1080/0268117X.2001.10555494

Norman, P., & Conner, M. (2005). The theory of planned behavior and exercise: Evidence for the mediating and moderating roles of planning on intention-behavior relationships. *Journal of Sport and Exercise Psychology, 27*, 488–504.

Ommundsen, Y., & Kvalø, S. E. (2007). Autonomy-mastery, supportive or performance focused? Different teacher behaviours and pupils' outcomes in physical education. *Scandinavian Journal of Educational Research, 51*(4), 385–413.

Owen, M. B., Curry, W. B., Kerner, C., Newson, L., & Fairclough, S. J. (2017). The effectiveness of school-based physical activity interventions for adolescent girls: A systematic review and meta-analysis. *Preventive Medicine, 105*, 237–249. doi:10.1016/j.ypmed.2017.09.018

Owen, K., Smith, J., Lubans, D. R., Ng, J. Y., & Lonsdale, C. (2014). Self-determined motivation and physical activity in children and adolescents: A systematic review and meta-analysis. *Preventive Medicine, 67*, 270–279. doi:10.1016/j.ypmed.2014.07.033.

Penedo, F. J., & Dahn, J. R. (2005). Exercise and well-being: A review of mental and physical health benefits associated with physical activity. *Current Opinion in Psychiatry, 18*, 189–193.

Plotnikoff, R. C., Costigan, S. A., Karunamuni, N., & Lubans, D. R. (2013). Social cognitive theories used to explain physical activity behavior in adolescents: A systematic review and meta-analysis. *Preventive Medicine, 56*(5), 245–253. doi:10.1016/j.ypmed.2013.01.013

Rebar, A. L., Stanton, R., Geard, D., Short, C., Duncan, M. J., & Vandelanotte, C. (2015). A meta-meta-analysis of the effect of physical activity on depression and anxiety in non-clinical adult populations. *Health Psychology Review, 9*(3), 366–378. doi:10.1080/17437199.2015.1022901

Rhodes, R. E. (2017). The evolving understanding of physical activity behavior: A multi-process action control approach. In A. J. Elliot (Ed.), *Advances in motivation science* (Vol. 4, pp. 186–195). Cambridge, MA: Academic Press.

Rhodes, R. E., & de Bruijn, G. J. (2013). How big is the physical activity intention-behaviour gap? A meta-analysis using the action control framework. *British Journal of Health Psychology, 18*, 296–309. doi:10.1111/bjhp.12032

Rhodes, R. E., & Dickau, L. (2012). Experimental evidence for the intention-behaviour relationship in the physical activity domain: A meta-analysis. *Health Psychology, 31*(12), 724–727. doi:10.1136/bjsports-2011-090411

Rhodes, R. E., Fiala, B., & Conner, M. (2009). A review and meta-analysis of affective judgments and physical activity in adult populations. *Annals of Behavioral Medicine, 38*(3), 180–204. doi:10.1007/s12160-009-9147-y

Rhodes, R. E., Gray, S. M., & Husband, C. (2018). Experimental manipulation of affective judgments about physical activity: A systematic review and meta-analysis of adults. *Health Psychology Review*, 1–61. doi:10.1080/17437199.2018.1530067

Rhodes, R. E., & Kates, A. (2015). Can the affective response to exercise predict future motives and physical activity behavior? A systematic review of published evidence. *Annals of Behavioral Medicine, 49*(5), 715–731. doi:10.1007/s12160-015-9704-5

Rhodes, R. E., Williams, D. M., & Conner, M. T. (2018). Affective determinants of health behavior: Common themes, future directions, and implications for health behavior change. In D. M. Williams, R. E. Rhodes, & M. T. Conner (Eds.), *Affective determinants of health behavior*. New York, NY: Oxford University Press. doi:10.1093/oso/9780190499037.003.0021

Rhodes, R. E., & Yao, C. A. (2015). Models accounting for intention-behavior discordance in the physical activity domain: A user's guide, content overview, and review of current evidence. *International Journal of Behavioral Nutrition and Physical Activity, 12*(1), 1–14. doi:10.1186/s12966-015-0168-6

Ryska, T. A., Hohensee, D., Cooley, D., & Jones, C. (2002). Participation motives in predicting sport drop-out among Australian youth gymnasts. *North American Journal of Psychology, 4*(2), 199–210.

Schinkoeth, M., & Antoniewicz, F. (2017). Automatic evaluations and exercising: Systematic review and implications for future research. *Frontiers in Psychology, 8*(2103). doi:10.3389/fpsyg.2017.02103

Schneider, M., Dunn, A. L., & Cooper, D. (2009). Affective, exercise and physical activity among healthy adolescents. *Journal of Sport & Exercise Psychology, 31*(6), 706–723. doi:10.1007/978-3-319-96089-0_72

Schneider, M., & Schmalbach, P. (2015). Affective response to exercise and preferred exercise intensity among adolescents. *Journal of Physical Activity and Health, 12*(4), 546–552. doi:10.1123/jpah.2013-0442. Affective

Sheppard, B. H., Hartwick, J., & Warshaw, P. R. (1988). The theory of reasoned action : A meta-analysis of past research with recommendations for modifications and future research. *Journal of Consumer Research, 15*(3), 325–343. doi:10.1086/209170

Smith, J. J., Eather, N., Morgan, P. J., Plotnikoff, R. C., Faigenbaum, A. D., & Lubans, D. R. (2014). The health benefits of muscular fitness for children and adolescents: A systematic review and meta-analysis. *Sports Medicine, 44*(9), 1209–1223. doi:10.1007/s40279-014-0196-4

Sniehotta, F., Presseau, J., & Araújo-Soares, V. (2014). Time to retire the theory of planned behaviour. *Health Psychology Review, 8*(1), 1–7. doi:10.1080/17437199.2013.869710

Standage, M., Duda, J. L., & Ntoumanis, N. (2003). Predicting motivational regulations in physical education: The interplay between dispositional goal orientations, motivational climate and perceived competence. *Journal of Sports Sciences, 21*(8), 631–647. doi:10.1080/0264041031000101962

Strack, F., & Deutsch, R. (2014). The reflective-impulsive model. In J. W. Sherman, B. Gawronski, & Y. Trope (Eds.), *Dual-process theories of the social mind* (pp. 92–104). New York, NY: Guildford Press.

Szcześniak, M., Colaço, M., & Rondón, G. (2012). Development of interpersonal trust among children and adolescents. *Polish Psychological Bulletin, 43*(1), 50–58. doi:10.1016/S0140-6736(02)88363-5

Tessier, D., Sarrazin, P., Nicaise, V., & Dupont, J. P. (2015). The effects of persuasive communication and planning on intentions to be more physically active and on physical activity behaviour among low-active adolescents. *Psychology & Health, 30*(5), 583–604. doi:10.1080/08870446.2014.996564

Tessier, D., Sarrazin, P., & Ntoumanis, N. (2010). The effect of an intervention to improve newly qualified teachers' interpersonal style, students motivation and psychological need satisfaction in sport-based physical education. *Contemporary Educational Psychology, 35*(4), 242–253. doi:10.1016/j.cedpsych.2010.05.005

Teychenne, M., Costigan, S. A., & Parker, K. (2015). The association between sedentary behaviour and risk of anxiety: A systematic review. *BMC Public Health, 15*(513), 1–8. doi:10.1186/s12889-015-1843-x

Tversky, A., & Kahneman, D. (1974). Judgment under uncertainty: Heuristics and biases. *Science, 185*(4157), 1124–1131.

Uijtdewilligen, L., Nauta, J., Singh, A. S., Van Mechelen, W., Twisk, J. W. R., Van Der Horst, K., & Chinapaw, M. J. M. (2011). Determinants of physical activity and sedentary behaviour in young people: A review and quality synthesis of prospective studies. *British Journal of Sports Medicine, 45*(11), 896–905. doi:10.1136/bjsports-2011-090197

Voskuil, V. R., & Robbins, L. B. (2015). Youth physical activity self-efficacy: A concept analysis. *Journal of Advanced Nursing, 71*(9), 2002–2019. doi:10.1111/jan.12658

Wallhead, T. L., Garn, A. C., & Vidoni, C. (2014). Effect of a sport education program on motivation for physical education and leisure-time physical activity. *Research Quarterly for Exercise and Sport.* Taylor & Francis. doi:10.1080/02701367.2014.961051

Wiers, R. W., Anderson, K. G., Van Bockstaele, B., Salemink, E., & Hommel, B. (2018). Affect, dual-processing, developmental psychopathology, and health behaviors. In D. M. Williams, R. E. Rhodes, & C. M. T (Eds.), *Affective determinants of health behavior* (pp. 158–184). Oxford, UK: Oxford University Press.

Williams, D. M., & Evans, D. R. (2014). Current emotion research in health behavior science. *Emotion Review, 6*(3), 277–287. doi:10.1177/1754073914523052

Williams, D. M., Rhodes, R. E., & Conner, M. T. (2018). Overview of affective determinants in health behavior. In D. M. Williams, R. E. Rhodes, & M. T. Conner (Eds.), *Affective determinants of health behavior* (pp. 1–18). New York, NY: Oxford University Press.

Wrotniak, B. H., Epstein, L. H., Dorn, J. M., Jones, K. E., & Kondilis, V. A. (2006). The relationship between motor proficiency and physical activity in children. *Pediatrics, 118*(6), 1758–1765. doi:10.1542/peds.2006-0742

Zenko, Z., Ekkekakis, P., & Kavetsos, G. (2016). Changing minds: Bounded rationality and heuristic processes in exercise-related judgments and choices. *Sport, Exercise, and Performance Psychology, 5*(4), 337–351. doi:10.1037/spy0000069

Zhai, L., Zhang, Y., & Zhang, D. (2015). Sedentary behaviour and the risk of depression: A meta-analysis. *British Journal of Sports Medicine, 49*, 705–709. doi:10.1136/bjsports-2014-093613

9

CHILDREN'S AND ADOLESCENTS' INTERPERSONAL-LEVEL CORRELATES OF PHYSICAL ACTIVITY BEHAVIOR

Toni A. Hilland and Sarah A. Costigan

Introduction

Physical activity behavior is complex, multi-faceted, and multi-dimensional, particularly during the stages of childhood and adolescence (Bauman et al., 2012; Ferreira et al., 2007; Sallis, Prochaska, & Taylor, 2000). Participation in physical activity is influenced by a whole host of factors across multiple domains (e.g., individual, interpersonal, psychosocial, environmental, policy, and global factors). Identifying the variables that influence physical activity behavior is essential for understanding the complexity of behaviors, and contributes to evidence based planning of public health interventions (Bauman et al., 2012). Examining the variables that influence physical activity behavior is typically referred to as the study of correlates or determinants. Correlates are factors associated with physical activity (Bauman et al., 2012), determinants are reproducible associations which are potentially causal (Buckworth & Dishman, 2002), and mediators are intervening causal variables (Bauman, Sallis, Dzewaltowski, & Owen, 2002). This chapter will focus on interpersonal-level correlates of physical activity for youth. Identifying and understanding children's and adolescents' physical activity correlates is of public health significance (Hallal et al., 2012; Tremblay et al., 2014). To design evidence-based interventions and promote physical activity in youth, the factors that influence the acquisition of this behavior must first be understood (Bauman et al., 2012; Ferreira et al., 2007). In this chapter, we will provide an overview of the literature concerning children's and adolescents' correlates of physical activity behavior, a discussion of the key issues, and a summary of recommendations for researchers and practitioners "Why the study of physical activity correlates is important?"

- To understand the factors that directly or indirectly influence or associate with a particular behavior or set of behaviors (e.g. physical activity);
- Programs and interventions can then target factors that influence physical activity, therefore increasing the chance of being effective;
- To understand why some groups are active, while other groups are inactive;
- To identify targets for change in campaigns, interventions, and policy;
- To inform the development of effective intervention strategies for the public or particular population groups;
- To shape the focus and content of programs for particular groups in particular settings;
- Correlates of physical activity are included in theories that explain and predict a behavior and are important in physical activity intervention design.

Theories

Behavioral theories can be applied to help explain why children and adolescents initiate and maintain physical activity behaviors, and can be used to inform intervention design, delivery, and evaluation. Interpersonal-level constructs are featured in a number of models and behavioral change theories, for example the Social Ecological Model (Bronfenbrenner, 1994), Health Belief Model (Hochbaum, Rosenstock, & Kegels, 1952), Theory of Planned Behavior (Ajzen, 1985), and Social Cognitive Theory (Bandura, 1989). These interpersonal models explain health behavior and health behavior change by focusing on social and physical environmental factors. The Social Cognitive Theory (Bandura, 1989) and Social Ecological Model (Bronfenbrenner, 1994) emphasize that behaviors have multiple levels of influence that include intrapersonal, interpersonal, environmental, and policy variables. At an interpersonal level, social support, cultural norms, and practices are key influences on youth physical activity behavior, which were discussed in Chapter 8.

Interpersonal-Level Correlates of Physical Activity for Youth

Interpersonal factors encompass the social relationships and cultural settings within which individuals function and interact (Casper, 2001), which help to shape physical activity behavior. This domain highlights the role of significant others (e.g., parents, peers, teachers, and coaches), and cultural norms and practices as directly and indirectly influencing physical activity behavior (Bauman et al., 2012; Rowe, Raedeke, Wiersma, & Mahar, 2007; Sterdt, Liersch, & Walter, 2014; Welk, 1999). Social-level correlates that have been consistently associated with physical activity in children and adolescents include the influence of family, parents, peers, teachers, and coaches (Beets, Cardinal, & Alderman, 2010; Sallis et al., 2000).

Overview of the Literature

Influence from the social domain on physical activity behavior, specifically in the form of social support, has been the subject of numerous investigations. The term "social support" broadly describes actions which help a person adopt and/or maintain a particular behavior or practice (Beets, Vogel, Forlaw, Pitetti, & Cardinal, 2006). Social support is a multidimensional umbrella term that describes the various resources provided from interactions with significant others (e.g., parents, peers, teachers, coaches) that can influence physical activity behavior (Beets et al., 2010; Langford, Bowsher, Maloney, & Lillis, 1997; Sheridan & Radmacher, 1992). Social support can be provided in a number of different ways:

- Instrumental/direct/logistical support is characterized by the provision or sharing of sports equipment, facilitating transport to local practices, and engaging in the desired behavior together.
- Psychological/emotional is provided via incentives, verbal motivation, encouragement, and praise.
- Instructional/informative support is characterized by acts of orientation, counseling, and talks about the importance and appropriate ways of engaging in the desired behavior (Barr-Anderson, Robinson-O'Brien, Haines, Hannan, & Neumark-Sztainer, 2010; Beets et al., 2006, 2010; Duncan, Duncan, & Strycker, 2005).

Social support is always intended to be helpful, is consciously provided, and is delivered in an interpersonal context of caring, trust, and respect for each person's right to make their own choices (Heaney & Israel, 2008). Social support is recognized as an important correlate of physical activity participation in individuals of all ages. Social-level approaches commonly include strategies which assist in developing or strengthening the social environment, so that physical activity is encouraged or physical activity barriers are overcome.

Interpersonal-level influences of children's and adolescents' physical activity behavior, specifically social support, have been widely researched. The influence of parents, other family members and peers on physical activity behavior appears to have been most comprehensively documented, whereas evidence for social support from teachers and coaches is less conclusive (Duncan et al., 2005; Fitzgerald, Fitzgerald, & Aherne, 2012; Hutchens & Lee, 2018; Xu, Wen, & Rissel, 2015).

Key Issues

Parental Social Support

In the context of physical activity behavior, Beets et al. (2010) define parental social support as "functional characteristics associated with the interactions between a parent and his or her children in the context of intentionally participating in, prompting, discussing, and/or providing activity-related opportunities" (p. 624). Parents are considered to be one of the key influences of their children's health-related behaviors (Perry, Crockett, & Pirie, 1987; Wertlieb, 2003), as they are one of the immediate and primary sources of health information, education, and physical activity opportunities (Hopper, Gruber, Munoz, & Herb, 1992). Parents have been previously described as 'gate-keepers' to physical activity education and opportunities through their provision of social support (Beets et al., 2016; Thompson, Humbert, & Mirwald, 2003). In addition, parents have been identified as a key influencing factor over the physical activity behavioral patterns of their children (Biddle, Atkin, Cavill, & Foster, 2011; Hobbs, 1998; Lindsay, Sussner, Kim, & Gortmaker, 2006; Sallis et al., 2000). This is due to the fact that the majority of young people spend roughly 18 years of their life in close proximity to their parents (Goldscheider, Thornton, & Young-DeMarco, 1993).

Parents serve as models, reinforces, and advocates of physical activity behaviors (Schor, 2003), and participation in physical activity can be encouraged or deterred by the actions of parents (Davison & Birch, 2001). Parents can influence their children's participation in physical activity through a variety of mechanisms (Hutchens & Lee, 2018; Xu et al., 2015). These include modeling, direct involvement, provision of resources, establishment or elimination of barriers, co-participation, and positive reinforcement of physical activity participation (Davidson, Simen-Kapeu, & Veugelers, 2010; Mendonça & Farias Júnior, 2015; Norton, Froelicher, Waters, & Carrieri-Kohlman, 2003). Furthermore, parents can foster positive physical activity behaviors in their children by providing encouragement and facilitating environments conducive to activity (Golan, 2006; Gustafson & Rhodes, 2006). For example, support from family members, such as watching, encouraging, or participating in physical activity, was longitudinally positively related to total and after-school physical activity in adolescents (Morrissey, Janz, Letuchy, Francis, & Levy, 2015) (see Table 9.1).

Review-level evidence suggests parental social support is an important and well-established correlate of physical activity among young people (Biddle et al., 2011; van Sluijs, Kriemler, & McMinn, 2011). Previous research evaluating the effectiveness of physical activity interventions for children highlights the importance of parent involvement (Miller, 2011), and of directly targeting parental supportive behavior (Rhodes et al., 2013) as effective strategies. It is therefore not surprising that parental involvement in physical activity interventions has been previously recommended to enhance children's physical activity participation (Norton et al., 2003; O'Connor, Jago, & Baranowski, 2009). However, most interventions have not effectively targeted fathers (Davison et al., 2018; Morgan et al., 2017; O'Connor et al., 2009) (see Chapter 31). The Social Cognitive Theory (Bronfenbrenner, 1994) and the Youth Physical Activity Promotion Model (Welk, 1999) highlight that the amount of social support and involvement provided by parents is an important component for children and adolescents initiating and maintaining positive physical activity behavior.

Table 9.1 Summary of parental social support correlates

Correlate				Association
Parents	Tangible	Instrumental	Transportation	+
			Payment of fees	+
			Purchasing of equipment	?
			Enrolling in sport/PA programs	+
		Conditional	Parent-child co-activity	+
			Parents watching/supervising	+
	Intangible	Motivational	Encouragement	+
			Praise	?
		Informational	Advice/suggestions/information	?

Note: "+" denotes a positive association; "?" denotes an indeterminate association.

Categories of Parental Support: Direct vs Indirect and Tangible vs Intangible

The various mechanisms of parental social support for children's and adolescents' physical activity behaviors have been previously classified in the literature as 'direct' and 'indirect' support (Beets et al., 2006). Direct support refers to the overt provision of assistance to an individual in creating or providing opportunities to be active, and may include provision of transportation or co-participation in activities (Beets et al., 2006). Indirect support refers to the encouragement to perform activities and praise associated with performance (Beets et al., 2006). However, systematic review evidence summarizing the influence of parental support and youth physical activity behaviors led Beets et al. (2010) to develop a more comprehensive framework that identified four categories of parental social support (instrumental, conditional, motivational, and informational), falling under the two discrete categories of 'tangible' and 'intangible' social support.

Tangible social support is defined as "overt behaviors performed by parents that directly facilitate the involvement in activity" (p. 629), for example providing transportation to places where the child/adolescent can be active (Beets et al., 2010). Tangible support is considered one of the most effective means of social support for youth physical activity (Sallis et al., 1992; Trost et al., 2003), and can be further classified as instrumental or conditional support (Beets et al., 2010). Intangible social support is defined as "verbally encouraging one's child to participate in physical activity and praising them for involvement and effort" (p. 632) and can be categorized as motivational (including encouragement and praise) or informational support (Beets et al., 2010).

Tangible – Instrumental Social Support

Instrumental social support consists of provision of tangible aid and/or services that support physical activity such as transportation to places to be active, purchasing of equipment, payment of fees, and enrolment in activities/sports.

Transportation

Parents providing transportation to places where their child can engage in a variety of physical activity-related behaviors is a key component to children and adolescents accessing these places (Beets et al., 2010, 2016). This may include transporting them to sports, team practices, to play with friends or to play at local community parks and recreation facilities (Davison, Cutting, & Birch, 2003). Cross-sectional analyses indicate that parental provision of transport is linked to greater levels of physical activity in both children and adolescents (Beets et al., 2006; Hoefer, McKenzie, Sallis, Marshall, & Conway, 2001; Sallis, Alcaraz, McKenzie, & Hovell, 1999).

Beets et al. (2010) suggest that younger children are likely in need of some form of transportation to be physically active, given restrictions placed upon them to self-transport. This support maybe even more important considering that nowadays children are less independent and 'freerange' than in previous generations (Pimentel, 2016). In addition, Edwardson, Gorely, Pearson, and Atkin (2013) reported that no differences were found in transportation/logistic support for younger and older adolescents, indicating that throughout adolescence perceptions of logistic support from parents remain stable. These results suggest that even as children reach their teenage years, they may still need to rely upon their parents to transport them to some modes of physical activity (Duncan et al., 2005; Edwardson et al., 2013). It is important to note, however, that these are cross-sectional findings and do not demonstrate change over time but are indicative that forms of support may change as children become older. In contrast, evidence suggests that parental logistic support decreases as children get older (Craggs, Corder, Van Sluijs, & Griffin, 2011; Davison & Jago, 2009).

In Beets et al.'s (2010) systematic review, 17% of the studies reported findings linking transportation social support to youth physical activity levels. In addition, in Mendonça, Cheng, Mélo, and de Farias Júnior (2014) review, ten studies found a significant association between some types of social support from the instrumental/direct dimension (e.g., transportation) and physical activity levels of adolescents. This suggests that these associations are rather robust, with transportation appearing as a predictor of activity levels from both self-report and objective physical activity measures. Pugliese and Tinsley (2007) conducted the only meta-analysis in this area by aggregating associations across 30 studies between parental socialization factors and child or adolescent physical activity. They reported significant but small associations between young people's physical activity and parents transporting the child (Pugliese & Tinsley, 2007).

With regard to parental transportation, social support and gender differences, Sallis et al. (1999) found that over a 20-month period, transportation was the only type of social support related to change in activity for boys and girls, highlighting the importance of transportation for both genders. In contrast, research has concluded that boys were more likely to be transported to sporting events than girls (Hoefer et al., 2001; Sallis et al., 1992), suggesting that boys perceived more transport support than girls. A potential reason for this difference may be due to the significantly higher amount of sport that boys participate in. Therefore, the more sport that a child participates in, the greater the amount of transport support required (Beets et al., 2006).

Payment of Fees, Purchasing of Equipment, Enrolling in Sport and Physical Activity Programs

There are other various instrumental support variables where parents can provide opportunities for their children to be active or facilitate activity involvement. These include the payment of fees, purchasing of equipment and enrolling children in physical activity programs (Eccles, Jacobs, & Harold, 1990). However, these variables are less commonly measured (Davison et al., 2003; Sallis et al., 1999). Within Beets et al.'s (2010) review, only four studies assessed the association between parental payment of fees and purchasing of equipment and physical activity behaviors. Though limited in number, these studies do indicate that payment of fees is associated with higher activity levels of boys during a 20-month period (Sallis et al., 1999). It has also been found that the provision of money may be a fruitful means by which adolescent boys and girls can be more physically active (Wright, Wilson, Griffin, & Evans, 2008).

Furthermore, research has reported that mothers and fathers purchase more equipment for sport-related activity for their sons rather than for their daughters (Fredricks & Eccles, 2005; Sallis et al., 1999). In addition, Fredricks and Eccles (2005) concluded that in homes where mothers bought more athletic equipment, children reported higher competence and beliefs about the benefits of physical activity and sport. However, due to the cross-sectional nature of this study it is not possible to rule out that the direction of causality goes from child to parent, as mothers may respond to their child's interests and competencies by buying them more equipment. In addition, the number of items of exercise equipment available at home has been significantly related to physical activity (Loucaides, Chedzoy, Bennett, & Walshe, 2004; Stuckyropp & DiLorenzo, 1993; Trost, Pate, Ward, Saunders, & Riner, 1999).

Davison (2004) developed and validated a questionnaire to assess maternal, paternal, general familial, peer, and sibling support of physical activity. Confirmatory factor analysis supported the presence of logistic support (e.g., parents enrolling their children in sports and activities) for maternal and paternal support of physical activity (Davison, 2004). This is consistent with Davison, Cutting, and Birch's (2003) conclusions that parental support provided by enrolling their children (girls) in sports and activities was associated with participation in physical activity. In this study, it was found that in comparison to fathers, mothers provided higher levels of logistic support, demonstrating that they were more likely to enroll their daughters in sports (Davison et al., 2003).

Tangible – Conditional Social Support

Parent conditional support for physical activity is defined as parents being directly involved or within proximity of the activity with the child (Duncan et al., 2005; Welk, Wood, & Morss, 2003). Therefore, conditional social support can involve parent's involvement in an activity that the child/adolescent is engaging in (e.g., co-activity) or providing support toward the child/adolescent via watching and/or supervising the activity (Beets et al., 2010; Prochaska, Rodgers, & Sallis, 2002; Raudsepp, 2006). An abundance of studies report conditional support correlates to have positive associations with children's and adolescents' physical activity levels (Adkins, Sherwood, Story, & Davis, 2004; Beets, Vogel, Chapman, Pitetti, & Cardinal, 2007; Heitzler, Martin, Duke, & Huhman, 2006; Loucaides et al., 2004; Prochaska et al., 2002; Sallis et al., 1992; Sallis et al., 1999; Welk et al., 2003).

Parent-Child Co-Activity

One component of tangible conditional social support is parent-child co-activity, such as playing together and active family time (Thompson et al., 2003; Welk et al., 2003). Physical activity co-participation by parents has been reported to positively influence youth physical activity (Edwardson & Gorely, 2010). Specifically, evidence suggests that parent-child co-activity is positively associated with the likelihood of young people meeting recommended physical activity levels (Nelson, Gordon-Larsen, Adair, & Popkin, 2005; Pyper, Harrington, & Manson, 2016). This may suggest that the direct involvement from parents in physical activity with their children and engaging in family physical activities can act to directly and positively reinforce a child's physical activity behavior.

A number of studies have found that supportive parental behavior in the form of co-activity is likely to facilitate youth physical activity (Morgan et al., 2014; Pugliese & Tinsley, 2007; Pyper et al., 2016; Yao & Rhodes, 2015). Similarly, meta-analytic evidence reported that parent-child co-activity was significantly related to physical activity; however, only a small effect size was evident (r = 0.28; 95% CI [confidence interval] 0.03–0.50) (Yao & Rhodes, 2015). While much of the existing evidence is from cross-sectional studies, Yao and Rhodes (2015) also highlight that the effectiveness of social support from parents for young people's physical activity should be examined collectively rather than as separate supportive behaviors.

Parental social support for physical activity in the form of co-activity appears to vary by age. Parents are particularly influential in supporting physical activity behaviors of children under 12 years, when parent-child co-activity is likely to be most prevalent (Yao & Rhodes, 2015). Parental supportive behaviors have been found to correlate closely with physical activity of pre-school and school-aged children (Klesges, Malott, Boschee, & Weber, 1986; Spurrier, Magarey, Golley, Curnow, & Sawyer, 2008). In addition, previous literature emphasizes the promotion of parent-based co-activity interventions during a child's early years of development (Yao & Rhodes, 2015). As children progress into adolescence the influence of parents for supporting physical activity via engagement in co-activity appears to be less influential, with a shift toward support from peer participation in physical activity becoming increasingly influential (Lown & Braunschweig, 2008). This may be explained by children having less volitional control in comparison to adolescents, as adolescents gain increased autonomy over their physical activity behaviors (World Health Organization, 2014).

The provision of social support for physical activity through co-activity also appears to vary according to whether the maternal or paternal parent is participating in the physical activity. Much of the available literature has examined social support for physical activity attributed to 'parental co-activity' as a generic/non-specific term for a child's primary caregiver(s). However, evidence reflecting the differing influence of maternal and paternal figures suggests that mothers and fathers provide different types of support for physical activity under the category of 'co-activity', which effects children's physical activity in different ways. For instance, in Yao et al.'s (2015) meta-analysis, moderation analyses showed that parental gender moderated the relationship between children and parents' activity; however, few studies have included fathers (Morgan et al., 2017) (see Chapter 31).

Furthermore, Beets et al. (2010) reported that the amount of time fathers spent with their kindergarten-aged children throughout the week was a significant predictor of the children's activity levels. A growing body of evidence has demonstrated that fathers are more likely to establish and lead co-activity with their child(ren) in both home and community settings (Lamb, 2010; Zahra, Sebire, & Jago, 2015). Therefore, it is not surprising that children have identified fathers as the main parent responsible for participating in physical activity and sport with them, while mothers were commonly cited as spectators (Noonan, Boddy, Fairclough, & Knowles, 2016). In addition, research examining parental influences on girls' physical activity (Davison et al., 2003) suggests that modeling positive physical activity behaviors (which included parents' own physical activity and being active with their daughters) was associated with higher physical activity among girls, and that fathers were reported as providing higher levels of physical activity support via modeling compared to mothers. The positive influence of fathers' co-activity for their children's physical activity levels may be explained by differences in parenting styles between mothers and fathers. For example, active play time including greater 'physicality' (Lamb, 2010), and opportunities to practice fundamental movement skills (Hardy, King, Espinel, Cosgrove, & Bauman, 2016; Telford, Telford, Olive, Cochrane, & Davey, 2016), commonly begins when children are young and are key characteristics of father's parenting styles. For instance, Morgan et al. (2019) provided the first experimental evidence to suggest that meaningful engagement from fathers can increase physical activity in pre-adolescent girls (e.g., rough and tumble play, fitness and physical activity, sports skills, challenge and adventure) (Morgan et al., 2018).

Maternal involvement in physical activity has been reported as being positively associated with children's physical activity levels; however, the association appears to be different depending on the sex of the child. Previous research suggests mothers have a stronger influence on their daughter's physical activity compared to their sons (Cleland et al., 2011; Hallal et al., 2012), and an additional study reported mothers who are physically active are more likely to have active daughters (Aarnio, Winter, Kujala, & Kaprio, 1997). The differing influence on children's physical activity may be explained by the distinctive maternal bonds observed between females (Gustafson & Rhodes, 2006). Furthermore, it appears that the number of parents providing support for physical activity is an important factor for girls' engagement in physical activity. Davison et al. (2004) found a linear relationship between parental involvement in physical activity and girls' physical activity levels. As such, girls' participation in high levels of physical activity increased as the number of parents providing support for physical activity increased (no parent support: 32%, one supportive parent: 56%, two supportive parents: 70%) (Davison, 2004).

More research is needed in this area considering the diverse nature of families, and therefore the diverse provision of conditional social support, which is given by a range of 'parental figures' (e.g., step-parents, foster parents, and other significant adults providing primary care). Understanding differences in how the provision of conditional social support is provided by parental figures is important for intervention design (Morgan et al., 2018).

Parents Watching/Supervising

Conditional social support from parents also encompasses social support for physical activity provided by parental figures watching and/or supervising their children while engaging in physical activity or sport (Beets et al., 2007). Children whose parents provide support by being present at an activity/sport, without being directly involved in the activity, have been reported to engage in higher physical activity levels (Duncan et al., 2005; Heitzler et al., 2006; Prochaska et al., 2002). However, this area has been less frequently explored in the child/adolescent physical activity literature compared to conditional social support via parent co-activity. For instance, review-level evidence conducted by Beets and colleagues found only 9% of included studies had reported findings examining the effect of parental support for physical activity in the form of watching/supervising children's physical activity (Beets et al., 2010). Interestingly, findings of this review demonstrate differences in perceived support between sex, specifically boys perceived more parental social support in the form of supervising and spectating in comparison with girls (Beets et al., 2010).

Supportive parental behaviors have been found to facilitate youth physical activity, with meta-analytic evidence demonstrating small significant effects on children's physical activity attributed to parental watching/spectating (r = 0.16; 95% CI 0.05–0.27) (Yao & Rhodes, 2015). However, when combining a range of indicators of parental social support (e.g., co-activity, encouragement, praise, watching, transport, equipment, and monitoring), a larger effect size is observed (r = 0.34; 95% CI = 0.30–0.46). Therefore, it may be that the provision of a range of social support strategies by parents is likely to result in positive physical activity messages being regularly reinforced, compared to providing social support exclusively via supervision and watching activities (Yao & Rhodes, 2015). It does not appear that any other specific parental support behavior was as effective for children's physical activity. The small effect sizes observed when examining different types of parental social support for physical activity separately (e.g., co-activity, watching, transport, equipment, and monitoring) may suggest that the provision of multiple parental supportive behaviors is required.

Intangible – Motivational Social Support

Intangible motivational social support is believed to enhance motivation for on-going participation (Prochaska et al., 2002), by providing feedback on current performance, and by contributing to greater levels of perceived competence, which have been shown to lead to higher levels of physical activity (Brustad, 1993). Motivational support includes encouragement and praise for engaging in physical activity (Beets et al., 2010).

Encouragement and Praise

Encouragement is the provision of verbal and non-verbal prompts or suggestions provided by parents to foster the involvement and engagement of their child in physical activity (Beets et al., 2010). Parental encouragement has been cited as having a moderate effect on children's physical activity (Yao & Rhodes, 2015), which can be a precursor or reinforcer of the behavior. In contrast, praise is a motivational response provided by parents that serves to validate their child's performance and/or effort in physical activity. Therefore, unlike encouragement, praise is reserved until after the activity has been performed.

Encouragement is the most extensively studied intangible supportive behavior (Beets et al., 2010). Encouragement has been found to be positively related to the intensity of physical activity (Bauer, Nelson, Boutelle, & Neumark-Sztainer, 2008; King, Tergerson, & Wilson, 2008; Springer, Kelder, & Hoelscher, 2006) and to the amount of physical activity (Alderman, Benham-Deal, & Jenkins, 2010; Anderssen & Wold, 1992; Bauer et al., 2008; Cardon et al., 2005; Mcguire, Hannan, Neumark-Sztainer, Cossrow, & Story, 2002; O'Loughlin, Paradis, Kishchuk, Barnett, & Renaud, 1999). Furthermore, Pugliese and Tinsley's (2007) meta-analysis found that parental encouragement was significantly related to child and adolescent physical activity and confirmed review findings from Sallis et al. (2000). Given the consistent findings in the literature, encouragement appears to be one of the more influential forms of intangible supportive behaviors (Beets et al., 2010).

Pugliese and Tinsley (2007) also found that parental encouragement for physical activity did not vary as a function of age. In contrast, Bauer, Laska, Fulkerson, and Neumark-Sztainer (2011) reported that during the transition from early to middle adolescence, significant decreases were observed in both males' and females' reports of parental encouragement to be physically active. However, as adolescents self-reported their parental encouragement in this study, the results may reflect changes in adolescents' perceptions rather than actual changes in parental behavior. Qualitative evidence suggests youth would like to receive more encouragement from their parents (O'Dea, 2003; Ries, Voorhees, Gittelsohn, Roche, & Astone, 2008; Wright et al., 2008). These findings signify that while encouragement may be present, the amount perceived is insufficient to fully influence activity levels, or the means through which parents are encouraging is not fully adequate.

Within studies investigating social cognitive models, encouragement has been demonstrated to be related to children's competency, behavioral intentions and motivation for on-going participation in physical activity (Biddle & Goudas, 1996; Prochaska et al., 2002). For example, Brustad (1996) reported that the extent to which parents encouraged their children to participate in physical activity was significantly related to their children's level of perceived physical competence, which was predictive of their attraction to physical activity. These findings highlight the importance of the type and amount of encouragement and opportunities parents offer their children to be physically active.

Beets et al. (2006) reported that praise was one of the primary influences of activity, and additional support for praise was found in a sample of Californian youth (Prochaska et al., 2002). Furthermore, it has been found that boys reported receiving greater amounts of praise than girls (Beets et al., 2006), which is likely to influence activity by reinforcing behaviors and validating the effort associated with involvement. However, given the insufficient amount of studies examining these relationships, care must be taken in establishing a connection. Nevertheless, the studies conducted to date indicate that praise may be a potentially important correlate to activity involvement and certainly one that deserves greater research attention.

Intangible – Informational Social Support

Informational social support has been described as the "provision of advice, suggestions, and information to address the behavior of interest" (Beets et al., 2010, p. 633). This functional dimension of intangible supportive behavior includes the provision of information regarding how to perform activities/sports and why one should be physically active (e.g., health benefits) (Duncan et al., 2005; Thompson et al., 2003). These types of social support appear to have been studied less in youth physical activity literature in comparison with other dimensions of social support (Beets et al., 2010).

A limited number of studies have investigated the discrete influence of parents providing informational support for youth physical activity. For example, Mendonça and Farias Júnior (2015) found that for male youth, instructional/informational social support provided by parents via positive comments regarding the activity was positively associated with physical activity. In an additional study examining preschool-aged children, parental support by providing information on physical activity was positively associated with active play (r = 0.16, p = 0.02) (Schary, Cardinal, & Loprinzi, 2012).

When assessed, informational support has been typically included with other support items (e.g., encouragement, transportation, and co-activity) to create an aggregate social support score (Dowda et al., 2011; Loprinzi, Herod, Cardinal, & Noakes, 2013; Loprinzi & Trost, 2010; Williams & Mummery, 2011). This therefore reduces the ability to determine the exclusive influence that parental informational support has on youth physical activity levels. For instance, in Wing and colleagues' study which examined how parents influence their children's physical activity during- and after-school hours, scores for informational, motivational, and role modeling items were averaged to create an overall intangible support score (Wing, Bélanger, & Brunet, 2016). While study findings highlight the importance of targeting a range of intangible parental support behaviors to increase the likelihood of positive physical activity behaviors for youth, the influence of parents providing advice, suggestions, and information regarding the benefits of participating in physical activity to their children remains unknown. Research conducted to date suggests informational support may be an important correlate of youth physical activity; however, further investigation in needed given the scarce number of studies examining these relationships.

Overall, with the exception of parental encouragement/praise which has been cited as having a moderate effect on children's physical activity in meta-analytic reviews (Yao & Rhodes, 2015), it does not appear that any other single parental support behavior was as effective for children's and adolescents' physical activity. The small effect sizes observed when examining numerous types of parental social support for physical activity separately (e.g., co-activity, watching, transport, equipment, and monitoring) suggests parental support should be targeted cumulatively in future interventions (Yao & Rhodes, 2015).

Peer Support

Although a relatively extensive body of research has examined the links between the different dimensions of parental support and physical activity, noticeably less research has examined the influence of peers who are part of the physical activity support network for children and adolescents (Duncan et al., 2005; Sallis et al., 1999). Peers have been defined and referred to in the literature as youth's best and closest friends (Kobus, 2003). Additionally, a peer can be described as a person who is equal to another with respect to certain characteristics such as skills, education level, age, background, and social status (Reber, 2001).

As children move toward adolescence, they spend an increasing amount of time with their peers, compared with parents and family, in such contexts as organized sport, Physical Education (PE), and neighborhood games and activities (Lown & Braunschweig, 2008). This therefore enhances the potential for peers to exert their influence in several domains (Brooks-Gunn & Graber, 1994; Montemayor, 1983): for example, health-enhancing and health-compromising behaviors of youth, including physical activity and inactivity (Perry, Klepp et al., 1987; Sallis & Patrick, 1994). Furthermore, peers may act as powerful role models (Wold & Anderssen, 1992), as they can influence norms and behaviors to shape physical activity levels (Duncan, Duncan, Strycker, & Chaumeton, 2007). Several longitudinal studies have found that the majority of adolescents' physical activity is undertaken with friends (Duncan et al., 2007; Rusby, Westling, Crowley, & Light, 2014). It has also been found that adolescents participate in more vigorous activities when they are with friends compared to when they are alone (Fitzgerald et al., 2012; Salvy et al., 2008).

The support of peers may serve a number of different functions, including social integration, companionship, and direct support (when participating in physical activities together); emotional and motivational support (e.g., encouragement and praise); informational and instrumental support (e.g., sharing equipment or transportation); and observational support (peer modeling of physical activity behavior) (Duncan et al., 2005; Duncan et al., 2007; Fitzgerald et al., 2012). Peers may also provide esteem support or reassurance of worth, which might bolster self-efficacy to participate in physical activity and to overcome perceived barriers (Duncan et al., 2005; Pender, Sallis, Long, & Calfas, 1994). Fitzgerald et al. (2012) categorized six processes through which peers and friends may have an influence on physical activity: peer/friend support, presence of peers/friends, peer norms, friendship quality and acceptance, peer crowds, and peer victimization (see Table 9.2).

The influence from the social domain in peers has been the focus of empirical investigations (Beets et al., 2006). The benefits of social support are substantiated by research that has repeatedly shown that peer support is associated with higher physical activity participation among youth of varying ages (Davison, 2004; Duncan et al., 2007; Gustafson & Rhodes, 2006; Hohepa, Scragg, Schofield, Kolt, & Schaaf, 2009; Pugliese & Tinsley, 2007; Sallis et al., 2000; Voorhees et al., 2005). Duncan et al. (2005) examined the relationship between the sources (parents, siblings, and friends) and types (encourage, do with, watch, talk, and transport) of support for physical activity among youth aged 10–14 years. They concluded that the source of support most highly related to physical activity was friends, and that youth who perceived greater support for physical activity from friends had higher levels of physical activity (Duncan et al., 2005). Likewise, Beets et al. found that peers were the only social support provider related to the physical activity levels of fifth to eighth graders (Beets et al., 2006).

Table 9.2 Summary of peer social support correlates

	Correlate	*Association*
Peers	Peer co-activity	+
	Peer modeling/observing/watching	+
	Sharing transport	?
	Encouragement	?
	Praise	?
	Esteem support/reassurance of worth	?
	Peer norms	?
	Sharing equipment	?
	Advice/suggestions/information	?

Note: "+" denotes a positive association; "?" denotes an indeterminate association.

Furthermore, Sallis et al. (2002) concluded that peer support was the most consistent and crucial correlate of physical activity in young people from grades 1 to 12. In addition, with regard to the intensity of physical activity, Sallis et al. (2002) found that peer support influenced vigorous physical activity among youth and was significant in the youngest groups of boys and girls, suggesting that peer support in physical activity is important for younger children as well as adolescents. In line with this, Salvy et al. (2008) concluded that children were more likely to report more intense physical activity when in the company of peers or close friends, and found that time spent alone is related to lower activity intensity. It therefore appears that social support from peers holds considerable potential as a mechanism for effective activity-based interventions.

Silva and colleagues (2014) found that peer social support had a direct effect on children's moderate to vigorous physical activity. In contrast, Chen, Dai, and Sun (2016) concluded that peer support does not directly influence physical activity. Yet both studies reported the importance of peer social support with regard to self-efficacy and enjoyment of physical activity which has also been reported elsewhere (Duncan, 1993). Silva et al. (2014) found that peer social support significantly influenced levels of enjoyment and self-efficacy, and Chen, Sun, and Dai (2017) concluded that peer support indirectly impacts physical activity through self-efficacy and enjoyment independently. Furthermore, in Fitzgerald et al.'s (2012) systematic review, seven articles demonstrated that friendship quality and acceptance were associated with enjoyment and motivation for physical activity in adolescents. For example, Salvy et al. (2008) found that friendships increased youth's motivation to engage in physical activity (Salvy et al., 2008).

Previous studies have supported the importance of peers as reinforcing factors of physical activity behavior. For example, Duncan and colleagues' (2007) longitudinal study found that the efficacy to overcome barriers, social support from peers, and physically active peers were the main factors in reducing the decline in physical activity typically observed during adolescence. Their results also highlight the importance of friends, as boys and girls with physically active friends were more physically active at age 12. For girls, having physically active friends also played a protective role, in that those with an increase in physically active friends over time also had less of a decline in physical activity from ages 12 to 17. Therefore, findings on the importance of friends' activity and support imply that health promotion programs aimed at increasing youth physical activity might be most effective if they included efforts targeting friends or peers.

Another function of peer social support includes direct support which involves participating in physical activities together. For example, Voorhees et al. (2005) found that co-activity with friends in class or on a sports team, participating in, or having friends ask each other to be active were all positively associated with increased activity. Furthermore, Barkley et al.'s (2014) study was the first to experimentally assess the effect of the presence of a friend on the amount of physical activity in pre- or early-elementary school-age children. They found that children exhibited 54% greater average accelerometer counts during the friend condition than during the solo play condition (≤6 years old) (Barkley et al., 2014). Research has also found that the presence of a friend increased overweight and non-overweight adolescents' physical activity, and that adolescents were more likely to report more intense physical activity when in the company of peers than when alone (Salvy et al., 2007, 2008). These findings are consistent with previous studies (Faith, Leone, Ayers, Heo, & Pietrobelli, 2002; Jurg, Kremers, Candel, Van der Wal, & Meij, 2006; Simon et al., 2004; Storch et al., 2006; Voorhees et al., 2005), suggesting that the presence of peers and friends contributes to increased physical activity behavior in children and adolescents (Salvy, De La Haye, Bowker, & Hermans, 2012).

Watching children takes part in physical activity is considered an emotional and motivational form of support. Reports suggest that friends watching each other participating in physical activity is an important correlate of behavior (United States Department of Health and Human Services, 1996). Further evidence for the importance of emotional types of support was provided by Duncan et al. (2005), who found that children reporting that their friends more frequently watched them engaging in physical activity had higher levels of physical activity (Duncan et al., 2005). Longitudinal, cross-sectional, and review-level evidence suggests the importance of peer support for children and adolescents' physical activity. However, there is a need to measure dimensions of peer social support separately to help target specific types of peer support for interventions.

Sibling Support

Support from family members and peers has been consistently reported as a positive correlate of young people's physical activity (Beets et al., 2010; Sallis et al., 2000; Salvy et al., 2008). While the influence of parents features predominantly in available literature (Barr-Anderson et al., 2010; Beets et al., 2006; Duncan et al., 2005), evidence for social support from siblings as correlates of physical activity appears to be less conclusive, mainly as a result of fewer studies examining such influences (Sallis et al., 2000). Some previous studies examining physical activity correlates for children and adolescents have noted that sibling physical activity may be an important correlate of physical activity particularly for adolescents (Sallis et al., 2000). However, to date it does not appear that the impact of social support for physical activity from siblings has been thoroughly investigated (Duncan et al., 2005). For instance, in one study, adolescents with active siblings receiving greater physical activity support had higher levels of physical activity (Davison, 2004). Furthermore, sex differences appear to exist in regard to the level of perceived support for physical activity attained from an individual's brother or sister (Davison, 2004). While similar levels of physical activity support for boys and girls from brothers were found, girls reported significantly higher levels of physical activity support from a sister. In another study of 372 youth, Duncan et al. (2005) found greater levels of physical activity among children whose siblings regularly watched them participating in physical activity and sport. In this particular study, older children and those from higher-income families also perceived more social support for physical activity from siblings (Duncan et al., 2005). In addition, in a study of 3,471 New Zealand school students, encouragement from siblings (and cousins) was found to be significantly associated with frequency of engaging in after-school physical activity among junior students (Hohepa, Scragg, Schofield, Kolt, & Schaaf, 2007).

Although limited in quantity, the findings of these studies suggest siblings may be important for providing physical activity social support via modeling, watching, and encouragement. These findings also suggest that perceived social support for physical activity may differ by the sex of the sibling, age of child/adolescent, and family income. However, the cross-sectional design of the studies inhibits the ability to identify the direction of the association between sibling social support and physical activity engagement (see Table 9.3). Future research is needed to extend the limited evidence, as most of the evidence is based on self-reported physical activity and therefore, device-based measures of physical activity are necessary (e.g., accelerometery).

Table 9.3 Summary of sibling social support correlates

	Correlate	*Association*
Siblings	Sibling modeling	?
	Sibling observing/watching	?
	Encouragement	?

Note: "+" denotes a positive association; "?" denotes an indeterminate association.

Teacher and Coach Support

A comprehensive body of research has examined the influence of various types of parental and peer support for youth physical activity, while less evidence is available examining the influence of teachers and coaches for physical activity promotion. Schools represent an ideal setting for promoting physical activity for children and adolescent populations (Beets et al., 2010) as young people spend 6–8 hours per day in schools, which have facilities, staff, and curriculum to provide a range of opportunities to be active. Teachers play a significant role in promoting physical activity in the school setting via the provision of quality learning experiences and creating a learning environment that is supportive of movement and physically active (McLeroy, Bibeau, Steckler, & Glanz, 1988; Sallis et al., 2000; Whitehead & Corbin, 1997). Teachers play a key role in reinforcing the importance of being physically active during breaks, in the classroom and in the periods before and after school, by providing a range of supportive behaviors such as provision of opportunities, modeling of behaviors, and encouragement to be active (Donnelly & Lambourne, 2011).

There appears to be great potential for teachers and coaches to provide support for children's and adolescents' physical activity. However, only limited evidence investigating the role of teacher or coach-based social support for physical activity exists. For example, of the six studies included in Sallis' review of physical activity correlates for children and adolescents, no association between teacher social support and adolescent physical activity was found (Sallis et al., 2000). Similarly, meta-analytic evidence investigating the influence of social support for adolescent girls' physical activity reported no association when specifically examining teacher social support and physical activity (Laird, Fawkner, Kelly, McNamee, & Niven, 2016). Additionally, for young people it appears that the influence of social support for physical activity from coaches has been rarely assessed. Of the six studies assessing the influence of coach social support for physical activity included in Sallis' review of correlates for youth (Sallis et al., 2000), four studies found that coach social support was not related to adolescent physical activity; no studies examining children were included in the review.

Furthermore, involvement in physical activity and modeling by PE teachers may be particularly important for children's and adolescents' physical activity motivation. McDavid, Cox, and Amorose (2012) posit that students appear to be influenced by how they perceive teachers to be involved in physical activities and may relate teachers' physical activity behavior to their own behaviors via self-determined motivation (McDavid et al., 2012). Similarly, Zhang, Solmon, and Gu (2012) emphasize the role of teachers' competence and autonomy support for fostering both motivation and achievement in PE lessons (Zhang et al., 2012), and a study conducted by Shen, Li, Sun, and Rukavina (2010) highlights the negative consequences of inadequate teacher social support for physical activity to their students, commonly resulting in students' amotivation (Shen et al., 2010) (see Table 9.4).

Increased encouragement and support from teachers for children and adolescents to engage in physical activities and sports may not directly result in changes to physical activity in the school setting; however, it appears to be important for motivation to be active. More recently, Eather, Morgan, and Lubans (2013) found that social support from teachers mediated physical activity behavior change in children participating in the Fit-4-Fun intervention (Eather et al., 2013),

Table 9.4 Summary of teacher/coach social support correlates

	Correlate	*Association*
Teachers/coaches	Teachers	?
	Physical Education teachers	?
	Coaches	?

Note: "?" denotes an indeterminate association.

suggesting further research in this area is necessary. This is in line with the SAAFE principles which provide a framework for promoting positive experiences in PE and other organized activity settings (Lubans et al., 2017).

Recommendations for Researchers and Practitioners

To improve our understanding of how the social context influences children's and adolescents' physical activity behavior, more research is needed in the area. Future research should build upon the current evidence and examine:

Sample/Participants

- More diverse samples, including marginalized and disadvantaged community groups, particularly ethnic/racial groups, different education levels, rural and remote dwellers, and youth from low- and middle-income countries (Davison, 2004; Davison et al., 2003; Davison & Jago, 2009; Edwardson et al., 2013; Mendonça et al., 2014; O'Connor et al., 2009);
- More diverse families with alternative living situations, for example, postmodern family arrangements such as blended families, binuclear families (an extended family consisting of two separate households formed by the children and subsequent spouses of the partners after a divorce), single-parent families, and children of same-sex parents (Davison et al., 2003; Trost & Loprinzi, 2011);
- Larger and more representative sample sizes (Barr-Anderson et al., 2010);
- More mediation studies as there is a need for identifying the mechanisms of influence in experimental studies.

Measurement of Physical Activity

- Physical activity using previously tested, consistent, reliable, and validated instruments with suitable psychometric properties (Mendonça et al., 2014; Sterdt et al., 2014);
- Physical activity with device-based measures, such as accelerometers (Davison, 2004; Mendonça et al., 2014; Trost & Loprinzi, 2011);
- Physical activity using multiple measures to provide a more complete description of children's and adolescents' activity (Sterdt et al., 2014), for example, employing a combination of objective and self-report measures (Edwardson & Gorely, 2010).

Measurement of Correlates

- Social support using previously tested, reliable, and validated instruments with suitable psychometric properties (Mendonça et al., 2014; Yao & Rhodes, 2015);
- Social support using standardized measures (due to the very high number of possible combinations of types and providers of support identified), so that more informative comparisons can be made (Laird et al., 2016; Mendonça et al., 2014);
- Social support by developing and/or adapting scales in accordance with the physical activity domain under study (Mendonça et al., 2014)
- Social support using multi-methods of assessment (e.g., child and parent report), this would decrease the likelihood of response bias linked with this self-report measure (Davison, 2004);
- Measuring social support dimensions separately, rather than aggregating an overall score would help to target specific types of social support for interventions, as most studies to date use overall measures of social support.

Study Design

- Interpersonal and psychosocial correlates by using longitudinal designs to assess the temporal sequence, and to evaluate the association between social support (parent, family and peer) and children's and adolescents' physical activity at different developmental stages (Davison et al., 2003; Edwardson & Gorely, 2010; Mendonça et al., 2014; Pugliese & Tinsley, 2007; Trost & Loprinzi, 2011);
- Correlates studies that employ prospective designs, both observational and experimental, are required (Barr-Anderson et al., 2010; Gustafson & Rhodes, 2006);
- Correlates studies employing fully powered, well-designed randomized control trials to target physical activity parenting practices (O'Connor et al., 2009);
- Support on physical activity behavior through qualitative exploration (Barr-Anderson et al., 2010).

In addition, future research in this area should:

- Analyze the effect of different types and sources of social support, considering physical activity domains, physical activity intensity, and the organization of activities, by gender and age group (Duncan et al., 2005; Mendonça et al., 2014);
- Be conducted to understand how parents can provide, and adolescents can perceive, high levels of support for physical activity during the transition into young adulthood (Bauer et al., 2011);
- Use different approaches when providing male and female parents and/or guardians with ideas about how they might be physically active with or promote the physical activity of their children, because mothers and fathers influence their child's physical activity levels differently (Beets et al., 2010);
- Investigate and consider the potential negative influences of parents and peers (e.g., modeling of inactive behavior) (Edwardson & Gorely, 2010) and the negative effect of over-competitive parents for boys and girls;
- Increase girls' exposure to multiple types and providers of social support in interventions (Laird et al., 2016).

References

Aarnio, M., Winter, T., Kujala, U., & Kaprio, J. (1997). Familial aggregation of leisure-time physical activity – A three generation study. *International Journal of Sports Medicine, 18*(07), 549–556.

Adkins, S., Sherwood, N. E., Story, M., & Davis, M. (2004). Physical activity among African-American girls: The role of parents and the home environment. *Obesity Research, 12*(S9), 38S–45S.

Ajzen, I. (1985). From intentions to actions: A theory of planned behavior. In J. Kuhl & J. Beckman (Eds.), *Action control: From cognitive to behavior* (pp. 11–39). Heidelberg, Germany: Springer.

Alderman, B. L., Benham-Deal, T. B., & Jenkins, J. M. (2010). Change in parental influence on children's physical activity over time. *Journal of Physical Activity and Health, 7*(1), 60–67.

Anderssen, N., & Wold, B. (1992). Parental and peer influences on leisure-time physical activity in young adolescents. *Research Quarterly for Exercise and Sport, 63*(4), 341–348.

Bandura, A. (1989). Human agency in social cognitive theory. *American Psychologist, 44*(9), 1175–1184.

Barkley, J. E., Salvy, S.-J., Sanders, G. J., Dey, S., Von Carlowitz, K.-P., & Williamson, M. L. (2014). Peer influence and physical activity behavior in young children: An experimental study. *Journal of Physical Activity and Health, 11*(2), 404–409.

Barr-Anderson, D. J., Robinson-O'Brien, R., Haines, J., Hannan, P., & Neumark-Sztainer, D. (2010). Parental report versus child perception of familial support: Which is more associated with child physical activity and television use? *Journal of Physical Activity and Health, 7*(3), 364–368.

Bauer, K. W., Laska, M. N., Fulkerson, J. A., & Neumark-Sztainer, D. (2011). Longitudinal and secular trends in parental encouragement for healthy eating, physical activity, and dieting throughout the adolescent years. *Journal of Adolescent Health, 49*(3), 306–311.

Bauer, K. W., Nelson, M. C., Boutelle, K. N., & Neumark-Sztainer, D. (2008). Parental influences on adolescents' physical activity and sedentary behavior: Longitudinal findings from Project EAT-II. *International Journal of Behavioral Nutrition and Physical Activity, 5*(1), 12.

Bauman, A. E., Reis, R. S., Sallis, J. F., Wells, J. C., Loos, R. J., Martin, B. W., & Lancet Physical Activity Series Working Group. (2012). Correlates of physical activity: Why are some people physically active and others not? *The Lancet, 380*(9838), 258–271.

Bauman, A. E., Sallis, J. F., Dzewaltowski, D. A., & Owen, N. (2002). Toward a better understanding of the influences on physical activity: The role of determinants, correlates, causal variables, mediators, moderators, and confounders. *American Journal of Preventive Medicine, 23*(2), 5–14.

Beets, M. W., Cardinal, B. J., & Alderman, B. L. (2010). Parental social support and the physical activity-related behaviors of youth: A review. *Health Education and Behavior, 37*(5), 621–644.

Beets, M. W., Okely, A., Weaver, R. G., Webster, C., Lubans, D., Brusseau, T., . . . Cliff, D. P. (2016). The theory of expanded, extended, and enhanced opportunities for youth physical activity promotion. *International Journal of Behavioral Nutrition and Physical Activity, 13*(1), 120.

Beets, M. W., Vogel, R., Chapman, S., Pitetti, K. H., & Cardinal, B. J. (2007). Parent's social support for children's outdoor physical activity: Do weekdays and weekends matter? *Sex Roles, 56*(1–2), 125–131.

Beets, M. W., Vogel, R., Forlaw, L., Pitetti, K. H., & Cardinal, B. J. (2006). Social support and youth physical activity: The role of provider and type. *American Journal of Health Behavior, 30*(3), 278–289.

Biddle, S. J. H., Atkin, A. J., Cavill, N., & Foster, C. (2011). Correlates of physical activity in youth: A review of quantitative systematic reviews. *International Review of Sport and Exercise Psychology, 4*(1), 25–49.

Biddle, S. J. H., & Goudas, M. (1996). Analysis of children's physical activity and its association with adult encouragement and social cognitive variables. *Journal of School Health, 66*(2), 75–78.

Bronfenbrenner, U. (1994). Ecological models of human development. *International Encyclopedia of Education, 3*(2), 37–43.

Brooks-Gunn, J., & Graber, J. A. (1994). Puberty as a biological and social event: Implications for research on pharmacology. *Journal of Adolescent Health, 15*(8), 663–671.

Brustad, R. J. (1993). Who will go out and play? Parental and psychological influences on children's attraction to physical activity. *Pediatric Exercise Science, 5*(3), 210–223.

Brustad, R. (1996). Attraction to physical activity in urban schoolchildren: Parental socialization and gender influences. *Research Quarterly for Exercise and Sport, 67*(3), 316–323.

Buckworth, J., & Dishman, R. (2002). Determinants of exercise and physical activity. *Exercise Psychology*, 191–209. Champaign: Human Kinetics.

Cardon, G., Philippaerts, R., Lefevre, J., Matton, L., Wijndaele, K., Balduck, A.-L., & De Bourdeaudhuij, I. (2005). Physical activity levels in 10-to 11-year-olds: Clustering of psychosocial correlates. *Public Health Nutrition, 8*(7), 896–903.

Casper, M. (2001). A definition of "social environment". *American Journal of Public Health, 91*, 465.

Chen, H., Sun, H., & Dai, J. (2017). Peer support and adolescents' physical activity: The mediating roles of self-efficacy and enjoyment. *Journal of Pediatric Psychology, 42*(5), 569–577.

Chen, H., Dai, J., & Sun, H. (2016). Direct and indirect effects of peer support on adolescents' physical activity. *Research Quarterly for Exercise and Sport, 87*(S2), A85.

Cleland, V., Timperio, A., Salmon, J., Hume, C., Telford, A., & Crawford, D. (2011). *A longitudinal study of the family physical activity environment and physical activity among youth.* Los Angeles, CA: SAGE Publications.

Craggs, C., Corder, K., Van Sluijs, E. M., & Griffin, S. J. (2011). Determinants of change in physical activity in children and adolescents: A systematic review. *American Journal of Preventive Medicine, 40*(6), 645–658.

Davidson, Z., Simen-Kapeu, A., & Veugelers, P. (2010). Neighborhood determinants of self-efficacy, physical activity, and body weights among Canadian children. *Health & Place, 16*(3), 567–572.

Davison, K. K. (2004). Activity-related support from parents, peers, and siblings and adolescents' physical activity: Are there gender differences? *Journal of Physical Activity, 1*(4), 363–376.

Davison, K. K., & Birch, L. L. (2001). Childhood overweight: A contextual model and recommendations for future research. *Obesity Reviews, 2*(3), 159–171.

Davison, K. K., Cutting, T. M., & Birch, L. L. (2003). Parents' activity-related parenting practices predict girls' physical activity. *Medicine and Science in Sports and Exercise, 35*(9), 1589–1595.

Davison, K. K., & Jago, R. (2009). Change in parent and peer support across ages 9 to 15 yr and adolescent girls' physical activity. *Medicine and Science in Sports and Exercise, 41*(9), 1816–1825.

Davison, K. K., Kitos, N., Aftosmes-Tobio, A., Ash, T., Agaronov, A., Sepulveda, M., & Haines, J. (2018). The forgotten parent: Fathers' representation in family interventions to prevent childhood obesity. *Preventive Medicine, 111*, 170–176.

Donnelly, J. E., & Lambourne, K. (2011). Classroom-based physical activity, cognition, and academic achievement. *Preventive Medicine, 52*, S36–S42.

Dowda, M., Pfeiffer, K. A., Brown, W. H., Mitchell, J. A., Byun, W., & Pate, R. R. (2011). Parental and environmental correlates of physical activity of children attending preschool. *Archives of Pediatrics & Adolescent Medicine, 165*(10), 939–944.

Duncan, S. C., Duncan, T. E., & Strycker, L. A. (2005). Sources and types of social support in youth physical activity. *Health Psychology, 24*(1), 3–10.

Duncan, S. C., Duncan, T. E., Strycker, L. A., & Chaumeton, N. R. (2007). A cohort-sequential latent growth model of physical activity from ages 12 to 17 years. *Annals of Behavioral Medicine, 33*(1), 80–89.

Eather, N., Morgan, P. J., & Lubans, D. R. (2013). Social support from teachers mediates physical activity behavior change in children participating in the Fit-4-Fun intervention. *International Journal of Behavioral Nutrition and Physical Activity, 10*(1), 68.

Eccles, J. S., Jacobs, J. E., & Harold, R. D. (1990). Gender role stereotypes, expectancy effects, and parents' socialization of gender differences. *Journal of Social Issues, 46*(2), 183–201.

Edwardson, C. L., & Gorely, T. (2010). Activity-related parenting practices and children's objectively measured physical activity. *Pediatric Exercise Science, 22*(1), 105–113.

Edwardson, C. L., Gorely, T., Pearson, N., & Atkin, A. (2013). Sources of activity-related social support and adolescents' objectively measured after-school and weekend physical activity: Gender and age differences. *Journal of Physical Activity and Health, 10*(8), 1153–1158.

Faith, M. S., Leone, M. A., Ayers, T. S., Heo, M., & Pietrobelli, A. (2002). Weight criticism during physical activity, coping skills, and reported physical activity in children. *Pediatrics, 110*(2), e23.

Ferreira, I., Van Der Horst, K., Wendel-Vos, W., Kremers, S., Van Lenthe, F. J., & Brug, J. (2007). Environmental correlates of physical activity in youth – A review and update. *Obesity Reviews, 8*(2), 129–154.

Fitzgerald, A., Fitzgerald, N., & Aherne, C. (2012). Do peers matter? A review of peer and/or friends' influence on physical activity among American adolescents. *Journal of Adolescence, 35*(4), 941–958.

Fredricks, J. A., & Eccles, J. S. (2005). Family socialization, gender, and sport motivation and involvement. *Journal of Sport Exercise Psychology, 27*(1), 3–31.

Golan, M. (2006). Parents as agents of change in childhood obesity – From research to practice. *International Journal of Pediatric Obesity, 1*(2), 66–76.

Goldscheider, F., Thornton, A., & Young-DeMarco, L. (1993). A portrait of the nest-leaving process in early adulthood. *Demography, 30*(4), 683–699.

Gustafson, S. L., & Rhodes, R. E. (2006). Parental correlates of physical activity in children and early adolescents. *Sports Medicine, 36*(1), 79–97.

Hallal, P. C., Andersen, L. B., Bull, F. C., Guthold, R., Haskell, W., Ekelund, U., & Lancet Physical Activity Series Working Group. (2012). Global physical activity levels: Surveillance progress, pitfalls, and prospects. *The Lancet, 380*(9838), 247–257.

Hardy, L., King, L., Espinel, P., Cosgrove, C., & Bauman, A. (2016). *NSW schools physical activity and nutrition survey (SPANS) 2010: Full report 2011.* Sydney, Australia: NSW Ministry of Health Google Scholar.

Heaney, C. A., & Israel, B. A. (2008). Social networks and social support. *Health Behavior and Health Education: Theory, Research, and Practice, 4*, 189–210.

Heitzler, C. D., Martin, S. L., Duke, J., & Huhman, M. (2006). Correlates of physical activity in a national sample of children aged 9–13 years. *Preventive Medicine, 42*(4), 254–260.

Hobbs, K. (1998). Development of physical activity behaviors among children and adolescents. *Pediatrics, 101*(3 Pt 2), 549–554.

Hochbaum, G., Rosenstock, I., & Kegels, S. (1952). *Health belief model.* Washington, DC: United States Public Health Service.

Hoefer, W. R., McKenzie, T. L., Sallis, J. F., Marshall, S. J., & Conway, T. L. (2001). Parental provision of transportation for adolescent physical activity. *American Journal of Preventive Medicine, 21*(1), 48–51.

Hohepa, M., Scragg, R., Schofield, G., Kolt, G. S., & Schaaf, D. (2007). Social support for youth physical activity: Importance of siblings, parents, friends and school support across a segmented school day. *International Journal of Behavioral Nutrition and Physical Activity, 4*(1), 54.

Hohepa, M., Scragg, R., Schofield, G., Kolt, G. S., & Schaaf, D. (2009). Self-reported physical activity levels during a segmented school day in a large multiethnic sample of high school students. *Journal of Science and Medicine in Sport, 12*(2), 284–292.

Hopper, C. A., Gruber, M. B., Munoz, K. D., & Herb, R. A. (1992). Effect of including parents in a school-based exercise and nutrition program for children. *Research Quarterly for Exercise and Sport, 63*(3), 315–321.

Hutchens, A., & Lee, R. E. (2018). Parenting practices and children's physical activity: An integrative review. *The Journal of School Nursing, 34*(1), 68–85.

Jurg, M. E., Kremers, S. P., Candel, M. J., Van der Wal, M. F., & Meij, J. S. D. (2006). A controlled trial of a school-based environmental intervention to improve physical activity in Dutch children: JUMP-in, kids in motion. *Health Promotion International, 21*(4), 320–330.

King, K. A., Tergerson, J. L., & Wilson, B. R. (2008). Effect of social support on adolescents' perceptions of and engagement in physical activity. *Journal of Physical Activity and Health, 5*(3), 374–384.

Klesges, R. C., Malott, J. M., Boschee, P. F., & Weber, J. M. (1986). The effects of parental influences on children's food intake, physical activity, and relative weight. *International Journal of Eating Disorders, 5*(2), 335–345.

Kobus, K. (2003). Peers and adolescent smoking. *Addiction, 98*, 37–55.

Laird, Y., Fawkner, S., Kelly, P., McNamee, L., & Niven, A. (2016). The role of social support on physical activity behaviour in adolescent girls: A systematic review and meta-analysis. *International Journal of Behavioral Nutrition and Physical Activity, 13*(1), 79.

Lamb, M. E. (2010). *The role of the father in child development.* Hoboken, NJ: John Wiley & Sons.

Langford, C. P. H., Bowsher, J., Maloney, J. P., & Lillis, P. P. (1997). Social support: A conceptual analysis. *Journal of Advanced Nursing, 25*(1), 95–100.

Lindsay, A. C., Sussner, K. M., Kim, J., & Gortmaker, S. (2006). The role of parents in preventing childhood obesity. *The Future of Children, 16*, 169–186.

Loprinzi, P. D., Herod, S. M., Cardinal, B. J., & Noakes, T. D. (2013). Physical activity and the brain: A review of this dynamic, bi-directional relationship. *Brain Research, 1539*, 95–104.

Loprinzi, P. D., & Trost, S. G. (2010). Parental influences on physical activity behavior in preschool children. *Preventive Medicine, 50*(3), 129–133.

Loucaides, C. A., Chedzoy, S. M., Bennett, N., & Walshe, K. (2004). Correlates of physical activity in a Cypriot sample of sixth-grade children. *Pediatric Exercise Science, 16*(1), 25–36.

Lown, D. A., & Braunschweig, C. L. (2008). Determinants of physical activity in low-income, overweight African American girls. *American Journal of Health Behavior, 32*(3), 253–259.

Lubans, D. R., Lonsdale, C., Cohen, K., Eather, N., Beauchamp, M. R., Morgan, P. J., . . . Smith, J. J. (2017). Framework for the design and delivery of organized physical activity sessions for children and adolescents: Rationale and description of the 'SAAFE' teaching principles. *International Journal of Behavioral Nutrition and Physical Activity, 14*(1), 24.

McDavid, L., Cox, A. E., & Amorose, A. J. (2012). The relative roles of physical education teachers and parents in adolescents' leisure-time physical activity motivation and behavior. *Psychology of Sport and Exercise, 13*(2), 99–107.

McGuire, M. T., Hannan, P. J., Neumark-Sztainer, D., Cossrow, N. H. F., & Story, M. (2002). Parental correlates of physical activity in a racially/ethnically diverse adolescent sample. *Journal of Adolescent Health, 30*(4), 253–261.

McLeroy, K. R., Bibeau, D., Steckler, A., & Glanz, K. (1988). An ecological perspective on health promotion programs. *Health Education Quarterly, 15*, 351–377.

Mendonça, G., Cheng, L. A., Mélo, E. N., & de Farias Júnior, J. C. (2014). Physical activity and social support in adolescents: A systematic review. *Health Education Research, 29*(5), 822–839.

Mendonça, G., & Farias Júnior, J. C. (2015). Physical activity and social support in adolescents: Analysis of different types and sources of social support. *Journal of Sports and Science, 33*(18), 1942–1951.

Miller, S. C. (2011). Families moving together: Increasing physical activity by targeting parents exclusively versus parents together with children. [Doctoral dissertation, San Marcos, Texas]. Retrieved from https://digital.library.txstate.edu/bitstream/handle/10877/2412/MILLER-DISSERTATION.pdf?sequence=1

Montemayor, R. (1983). Parents and adolescents in conflict: All families some of the time and some families most of the time. *The Journal of Early Adolescence, 3*(1–2), 83–103.

Morgan, P. J., Collins, C. E., Plotnikoff, R. C., Callister, R., Burrows, T., Fletcher, R., . . . Lloyd, A. B. (2014). The 'healthy dads, healthy kids' community randomized controlled trial: A community-based healthy lifestyle program for fathers and their children. *Preventive Medicine, 61*, 90–99.

Morgan, P. J., Young, M. D., Barnes, A. T., Eather, N., Pollock, E. R., & Lubans, D. R. (2018). Engaging fathers to increase physical activity in girls: The "dads and daughters exercising and empowered" (DADEE) randomized controlled trial. *Annals of Behavioral Medicine, 53*(1), 39–52.

Morgan, P. J., Young, M. D., Lloyd, A. B., Wang, M. L., Eather, N., Miller, A., . . . Pagoto, S. L. (2017). Involvement of fathers in pediatric obesity treatment and prevention trials: A systematic review. *Pediatrics, 139*(2), e20162635.

Morrissey, J. L., Janz, K. F., Letuchy, E. M., Francis, S. L., & Levy, S. M. (2015). The effect of family and friend support on physical activity through adolescence: A longitudinal study. *International Journal of Behavioral Nutrition and Physical Activity, 12*(1), 103.

Nelson, M. C., Gordon-Larsen, P., Adair, L. S., & Popkin, B. M. (2005). Adolescent physical activity and sedentary behavior: Patterning and long-term maintenance. *American Journal of Preventive Medicine, 28*(3), 259–266.

Noonan, R. J., Boddy, L. M., Fairclough, S. J., & Knowles, Z. R. (2016). Write, draw, show, and tell: A child-centred dual methodology to explore perceptions of out-of-school physical activity. *BMC Public Health, 16*(1), 326.

Norton, D. E., Froelicher, E. S., Waters, C. M., & Carrieri-Kohlman, V. (2003). Parental influence on models of primary prevention of cardiovascular disease in children. *European Journal of Cardiovascular Nursing, 2*(4), 311–322.

O'Connor, T. M., Jago, R., & Baranowski, T. (2009). Engaging parents to increase youth physical activity: A systematic review. *American Journal of Preventive Medicine, 37*(2), 141–149.

O'Dea, J. A. (2003). Why do kids eat healthful food? Perceived benefits of and barriers to healthful eating and physical activity among children and adolescents. *Journal of the American Dietetic Association, 103*(4), 497–501.

O'Loughlin, J., Paradis, G., Kishchuk, N., Barnett, T., & Renaud, L. (1999). Prevalence and correlates of physical activity behaviors among elementary schoolchildren in multiethnic, low income, inner-city neighborhoods in Montreal, Canada. *Annals of Epidemiology, 9*(7), 397–407.

Pender, N., Sallis, J., Long, B., & Calfas, K. J. (1994). Health care provider counseling to promote physical activity. In R. K. Dishman (Ed.), *Advances in exercise adherence* (pp. 213–236). Champaign, IL: Human Kinetics.

Perry, C. L., Klepp, L. I., Halper, A., Dudovitz, B., Golden, D., Griffin, G., & Smyth, M. (1987). Promoting healthy eating and physical activity patterns among adolescents: A pilot study of 'slice of life'. *Health Education Research, 2*(2), 93–103.

Perry, C. L., Crockett, S. J., & Pirie, P. (1987). Influencing parental health behavior: Implications of community assessments. *Health Education, 18*(5), 68–77.

Pimentel, D. (2016). Protecting the free-range kid: Recalibrating parents' rights and the best interest of the child. *Cardozo Law Review, 38*, 1.

Prochaska, J. J., Rodgers, M. W., & Sallis, J. F. (2002). Association of parent and peer support with adolescent physical activity. *Research Quarterly for Exercise Sport, 73*(2), 206–210.

Pugliese, J., & Tinsley, B. (2007). Parental socialization of child and adolescent physical activity: A meta-analysis. *Journal of Family Psychology, 21*(3), 331–343.

Pyper, E., Harrington, D., & Manson, H. (2016). The impact of different types of parental support behaviours on child physical activity, healthy eating, and screen time: A cross-sectional study. *BMC Public Health, 16*(1), 568.

Raudsepp, L. (2006). The relationship between socio-economic status, parental support and adolescent physical activity. *Journal of Acta Paediatrica, 95*(1), 93–98.

Reber, A. S. (2001). *The Penguin dictionary of psychology*. London, UK: Penguin Press.

Rhodes, R. E., Berry, T., Craig, C. L., Faulkner, G., Latimer-Cheung, A., Spence, J. C., & Tremblay, M. S. (2013). Understanding parental support of child physical activity behavior. *American Journal of Health Behavior, 37*(4), 469–477.

Ries, A. V., Voorhees, C. C., Gittelsohn, J., Roche, K. M., & Astone, N. M. (2008). Adolescents' perceptions of environmental influences on physical activity. *American Journal of Health Behavior, 32*(1), 26–39.

Rowe, D. A., Raedeke, T. D., Wiersma, L. D., & Mahar, M. T. (2007). Investigating the youth physical activity promotion model: Internal structure and external validity evidence for a potential measurement model. *Pediatric Exercise Science, 19*(4), 420–435.

Rusby, J. C., Westling, E., Crowley, R., & Light, J. M. (2014). Psychosocial correlates of physical and sedentary activities of early adolescent youth. *Health Education & Behavior, 41*(1), 42–51.

Sallis, J. F., Alcaraz, J. E., McKenzie, T. L., Hovell, M. F., Kolody, B., & Nader, P. R. (1992). Parental behavior in relation to physical activity and fitness in 9-year-old children. *American Journal of Diseases of Children, 146*(11), 1383–1388.

Sallis, J. F., Alcaraz, J. E., McKenzie, T. L., & Hovell, M. F. (1999). Predictors of change in children's physical activity over 20 months: Variations by gender and level of adiposity. *American Journal of Preventive Medicine, 16*(3), 222–229.

Sallis, J. F., & Patrick, K. (1994). Physical activity guidelines for adolescents: Consensus statement. *Pediatric Exercise Science, 6*(4), 302–314.

Sallis, J. F., Prochaska, J. J., & Taylor, W. C. (2000). A review of correlates of physical activity of children and adolescents. *Medicine Science in Sports Exercise, 32*(5), 963–975.

Salvy, S.-J., Bowker, J. W., Roemmich, J. N., Romero, N., Kieffer, E., Paluch, R., & Epstein, L. H. (2007). Peer influence on children's physical activity: An experience sampling study. *Journal of Pediatric Psychology, 33*(1), 39–49.

Salvy, S.-J., De La Haye, K., Bowker, J. C., & Hermans, R. C. (2012). Influence of peers and friends on children's and adolescents' eating and activity behaviors. *Physiology & Behavior, 106*(3), 369–378.

Salvy, S.-J., Roemmich, J. N., Bowker, J. C., Romero, N. D., Stadler, P. J., & Epstein, L. H. (2008). Effect of peers and friends on youth physical activity and motivation to be physically active. *Journal of Pediatric Psychology, 34*(2), 217–225.

Schary, D. P., Cardinal, B. J., & Loprinzi, P. D. (2012). Parental support exceeds parenting style for promoting active play in preschool children. *Early Child Development and Care, 182*(8), 1057–1069.

Schor, E. L. (2003). Family pediatrics: Report of the task force on the family. *Pediatrics, 111*(6 Pt 2), 1541–1571.

Shen, B., Li, W., Sun, H., & Rukavina, P. B. (2010). The influence of inadequate teacher-to-student social support on a motivation of physical education students. *Journal of Teaching in Physical Education, 29*(4), 417–432.

Sheridan, C. L., & Radmacher, S. A. (1992). *Health psychology: Challenging the biomedical model.* New York, NY: John Wiley & Sons.

Silva, P., Lott, R., Mota, J., & Welk, G. (2014). Direct and indirect effects of social support on youth physical activity behavior. *Pediatric Exercise Science, 26*(1), 86–94.

Simon, C., Wagner, A., DiVita, C., Rauscher, E., Klein-Platat, C., Arveiler, D., . . . Triby, E. (2004). Intervention centred on adolescents' physical activity and sedentary behaviour (ICAPS): Concept and 6-month results. *International Journal of Obesity, 28*(S3), S96–S103.

Springer, A. E., Kelder, S. H., & Hoelscher, D. M. (2006). Social support, physical activity and sedentary behavior among 6th-grade girls: A cross-sectional study. *International Journal of Behavioral Nutrition and Physical Activity, 3*(1), 8–17.

Spurrier, N. J., Magarey, A. A., Golley, R., Curnow, F., & Sawyer, M. G. (2008). Relationships between the home environment and physical activity and dietary patterns of preschool children: A cross-sectional study. *International Journal of Behavioral Nutrition and Physical Activity, 5*(1), 31.

Sterdt, E., Liersch, S., & Walter, U. (2014). Correlates of physical activity of children and adolescents: A systematic review of reviews. *Health Education Journal, 73*(1), 72–89.

Storch, E. A., Milsom, V. A., DeBraganza, N., Lewin, A. B., Geffken, G. R., & Silverstein, J. H. (2006). Peer victimization, psychosocial adjustment, and physical activity in overweight and at-risk-for-overweight youth. *Journal of Pediatric Psychology, 32*(1), 80–89.

Stuckyropp, R. C., & DiLorenzo, T. M. (1993). Determinants of exercise in children. *Preventive Medicine, 22*(6), 880–889.

Telford, R. M., Telford, R. D., Olive, L. S., Cochrane, T., & Davey, R. (2016). Why are girls less physically active than boys? Findings from the LOOK longitudinal study. *PloS One, 11*(3), e0150041.

Thompson, A. M., Humbert, M. L., & Mirwald, R. L. (2003). A longitudinal study of the impact of childhood and adolescent physical activity experiences on adult physical activity perceptions and behaviors. *Qualitative Health Research, 13*(3), 358–377.

Tremblay, M. S., Gray, C. E., Akinroye, K., Harrington, D. M., Katzmarzyk, P. T., Lambert, E. V., . . . Onywera, V. O. (2014). Physical activity of children: A global matrix of grades comparing 15 countries. *Journal of Physical Activity and Health, 11*(s1), S113–S125.

Trost, S. G., & Loprinzi, P. D. (2011). Parental influences on physical activity behavior in children and adolescents: A brief review. *American Journal of Lifestyle Medicine, 5*(2), 171–181.

Trost, S. G., Pate, R. R., Ward, D. S., Saunders, R., & Riner, W. (1999). Correlates of objectively measured physical activity in preadolescent youth. *American Journal of Preventive Medicine, 17*(2), 120–126.

Trost, S. G., Sallis, J. F., Pate, R. R., Freedson, P. S., Taylor, W. C., & Dowda, M. (2003). Evaluating a model of parental influence on youth physical activity. *American Journal of Preventive Medicine, 25*(4), 277–282.

United States Department of Health and Human Services. (1996). *Physical activity and health: A report of the surgeon general.* Retrieved from https://www.cdc.gov/nccdphp/sgr/pdf/sgrfull.pdf

van Sluijs, E. M., Kriemler, S., & McMinn, A. M. (2011). The effect of community and family interventions on young people's physical activity levels: A review of reviews and updated systematic review. *British Journal of Sports Medicine, 45*(11), 914–922.

Voorhees, C. C., Murray, D., Welk, G., Birnbaum, A., Ribisl, K. M., Johnson, C. C., . . . Jobe, J. B. (2005). The role of peer social network factors and physical activity in adolescent girls. *American Journal of Health Behavior, 29*(2), 183–190.

Welk, G. J. (1999). The youth physical activity promotion model: A conceptual bridge between theory and practice. *Quest, 51*(1), 5–23.

Welk, G. J., Wood, K., & Morss, G. (2003). Parental influences on physical activity in children: An exploration of potential mechanisms. *Pediatric Exercise Science, 15*(1), 19–33.

Wertlieb, D. (2003). American academy of pediatrics task force on the family converging trends in family research and pediatrics: Recent findings for the American academy of pediatrics task force on the family. *Pediatrics, 111*(6 Pt 2), 1572–1587.

Whitehead, J. R., & Corbin, C. B. (1997). Self-esteem in children and youth: The role of sport and physical education. In K. R. Fox (Ed.), *The physical self: From motivation to well-being* (pp. 175–203). Champaign, IL: Human Kinetics.

Williams, S. L., & Mummery, W. K. (2011). Links between adolescent physical activity, body mass index, and adolescent and parent characteristics. *Health Education & Behavior, 38*(5), 510–520.

Wing, E. K., Bélanger, M., & Brunet, J. (2016). Linking parental influences and youth participation in physical activity in-and out-of-school: The mediating role of self-efficacy and enjoyment. *American Journal of Health Behavior, 40*(1), 31–37.

Wold, B., & Anderssen, N. (1992). Health promotion aspects of family and peer influences on sport participation. *International Journal of Sport Psychology, 23*(4), 343–359.

World Health Organization. (2014). *Health for the world's adolescents: A second chance in the second decade: Summary.* Retrieved from http://apps.who.int/adolescent/second-decade/

Wright, M. S., Wilson, D. K., Griffin, S., & Evans, A. (2008). A qualitative study of parental modeling and social support for physical activity in underserved adolescents. *Health Education Research, 25*(2), 224–232.

Xu, H., Wen, L. M., & Rissel, C. (2015). Associations of parental influences with physical activity and screen time among young children: A systematic review. *Journal of Obesity.*

Yao, C. A., & Rhodes, R. E. (2015). Parental correlates in child and adolescent physical activity: A meta-analysis. *International Journal of Behavioral Nutrition Physical Activity, 12*(1), 10.

Zahra, J., Sebire, S. J., & Jago, R. (2015). "He's probably more Mr. Sport than me" – A qualitative exploration of mothers' perceptions of fathers' role in their children's physical activity. *BMC Pediatrics, 15*(1), 101.

Zhang, T., Solmon, M. A., & Gu, X. (2012). The role of teachers' support in predicting students' motivation and achievement outcomes in physical education. *Journal of Teaching in Physical Education, 31*(4), 329–343.

10

PHYSICAL ENVIRONMENTAL FACTORS ASSOCIATED WITH PHYSICAL ACTIVITY IN YOUNG PEOPLE

Anna Timperio, Shannon Sahlqvist, Venurs Loh,
Benedicte Deforche, and Jenny Veitch

The physical environment encompasses natural and built environments. The natural environment refers to the geography and climate of a particular area, such as bodies of water, weather, natural landscapes and topography (Australian Institute of Health and Welfare, 2011). The built environment refers to the physical and functional spaces designed and built by people for people, including street networks, public transport systems, land uses, open spaces, recreational amenities and the aesthetic quality of the area (Australian Institute of Health and Welfare, 2011; Transportation Research Board & Institute of Medicine, 2005), as well as public and private buildings and grounds such as schools and residences. Both the natural and built environments have an independent and synergistic capacity to shape behaviors and health (Macintyre, Ellaway, & Cummins, 2002).

The physical environment is an important part of socio-ecological perspectives often used as a theoretical basis to understand and encourage the adoption of a physically active lifestyle (Catalano, 1979; Sallis & Owen, 2015). Socio-ecological models emphasize that health behaviors such as physical activity are influenced by an interplay of factors that operate at multiple levels, and recognize the importance of factors at the social environmental, physical environmental and policy levels, as well as at the intrapersonal level (Sallis et al., 2006). Different levels of determinants are discussed within this book, including the intrapersonal, interpersonal/social environmental, physical environmental (current chapter) and policy levels.

Research on physical activity and the environment to date has most often focused on the built environment. Most of us use and interact with multiple aspects of the built environment daily; however, certain built environments may be more important than others in shaping our behavior, including physical activity (Matthews & Yang, 2013). This chapter focuses on the links between physical activity and the built environment around the home, commonly known as the neighborhood built environment. The impact of other built environments on physical activity will be discussed in Part 7 (School Environment) and Part 8 (Family and Community).

The design of communities or neighborhoods and decisions impacting the built environment involve decision-makers and designers from the public and private sectors. For example, town or urban planners and land developers make decisions about the layout of communities and infrastructure, transport planners determine the road environment and public transport availability, architects can impact the look and feel of a community and governments regulate what can and can't be built in particular locations. Once developed, the design of the built environment and major infrastructure can be expensive and difficult to change, and can have important implications for health and well-being for generations. The built environment can have a long-term and sustainable impact on physical activity at the population level, especially given the number of people repeatedly exposed to it over time (D'Haese, Cardon, & Deforche, 2015; Sallis, Floyd, Rodriguez, & Saelens, 2012). Creating active environments is recognized as a key strategic objective of the World Health Organization's Global Action Plan on Physical Activity 2018–2030, developed to help member states increase population levels of physical activity (World Health Organization, 2018). Such active environments can also have a range of 'co-benefits' in addition to physical activity. For example, a built environment that encourages active transport through pedestrian- and cyclist-friendly design can potentially confer numerous and diverse environmental, economic and social co-benefits, such as less reliance on motor vehicles, reduced vehicle-generated gas emissions and traffic congestion, boost of local micro-economies and fostering of community cohesion (Giles-Corti, Foster, Shilton, & Falconer, 2010; Sallis, Spoon et al., 2015).

The world is becoming more and more urbanized. Globally, 55% of the population currently live in urban areas, a figure projected to increase to 68% by 2050 (United Nations, 2018). As cities become denser, it is important to consider children and adolescents in urban planning and community design to facilitate physical activity and active free play. Time spent outdoors is an important correlate of physical activity among children (Gray et al., 2015). The neighborhood environment provides a setting for walking and cycling for fun or to reach places and for outdoor unstructured play (Carver, Timperio, & Crawford, 2008), both independently and with others, as well as opportunities for structured physical activity. Neighborhood features can support or inhibit movement and use of spaces and contribute to parental perceptions of safety and constraints they place on their child's physical activity (Carver, Timperio, Hesketh, & Crawford, 2010a, 2010b, 2012). Safety concerns, for example, are considered one of the key reasons for rapid declines in active school travel over recent decades in some countries (Carver et al., 2008; Hillman, Adams, & Whitelegg, 1990). With increasing independence during adolescence, it is critical that the local environment supports opportunities to be active at a time when physical activity typically declines rapidly.

Overview of the Literature

Evolution of the Field

Research on the neighborhood physical environment and physical activity among children and youth has evolved rapidly over the past few decades. A seminal study published in 1990 on children's independent mobility on school journeys was among the earliest work to explore the role of the environment in shaping children's physical activity (Hillman et al., 1990). In that study, the top reason parents provided for not allowing their child to return home from school on their own was traffic danger. The same study also documented diminishing rates of walking to school with increasing distance between home and school (Hillman et al., 1990). Between 1970 and 1988, research on environments and physical activity among children and youth focused predominantly on access to neighborhood recreation facilities for physical activity (Sallis, Prochaska, & Taylor, 2000). As the concept of 'walkability' gained prominence outside the transportation field in the 2000s and research on neighborhood environments and physical activity burgeoned (Harris, Lecy, Hipp, Brownson, & Parra, 2013), studies conducted among children and youth began to consider a wider range of neighborhood attributes (Davison & Lawson, 2006; Pont, Ziviani, Wadley, Bennett, & Abbott, 2009). Most research examining the role of the environment in shaping the physical activity of children and youth has been conducted since mid-2000 (Ding, Sallis, Kerr,

Lee, & Rosenberg, 2011). These studies have explored a number of neighborhood environmental attributes; most common among these are urban design elements (encompassing walkability), traffic safety, the presence of walking and cycling infrastructure, the aesthetics of the neighborhood, the availability of recreational facilities and access to parks and public open spaces. Methods used to measure and characterize aspects of the built environment have also evolved rapidly, from survey measures of perceived characteristics to physical audits of streetscapes (both in person and by 'desktop') and sophisticated spatial mapping techniques (Brownson, Hoehner, Day, Forsyth, & Sallis, 2009; Sallis, 2009).

Key Concepts

Measurement Techniques: Subjective Approaches

Environmental attributes can be measured either subjectively (also termed perceived) or objectively. Traditionally, the most common method of measuring the built environment has been via a questionnaire, either interviewer- or self-administered, where individuals (child or parent) report their views of relevant aspects of their neighborhood environment. Surveys gather quantitative data by typically asking individuals to indicate agreement with statements relating to connectivity, residential density, traffic safety, aesthetics, land use mix, proximity to recreational facilities and the presence of walking and cycling infrastructure or features of routes to destinations. The Neighborhood Environment Walkability Scale (NEWS) (Saelens, Sallis, Black, & Chen, 2003) is an example of a commonly used self-report instrument assessing a range of neighborhood features. This instrument has been adapted for use with adolescents (Rosenberg et al., 2009), and several country-specific versions have also been tested (Cerin et al., 2010; Oyeyemi et al., 2016).

Measurement Techniques: Objective Approaches

Audit techniques are typically used to objectively and systematically measure or record features of the physical environment, including features related to community design, streetscapes or routes (Timperio, Veitch, & Sahlqvist, 2018). Historically, such audits were completed in person by direct observation. However, more recently, audits have been conducted using online imagery. Virtual audits of the built environment using Google Street View, for example, have shown good validity against on-site auditing (Badland, Opit, Witten, Kearns, & Mavoa, 2010), and are much quicker to complete as the auditor does not have to physically visit the areas. In addition, there are no restrictions based on weather conditions and the audit can be conducted from any location and at any time of day. Recently, such an audit tool (EGA-Cycling) was developed to assess street characteristics of children's cycling routes to school (Vanwolleghem, Van Dyck, Ducheyne, De Bourdeaudhuij, & Cardon, 2014). The tool can assess macro-environmental features along cycling routes, such as street connectivity, distance to destinations and number of houses. However, the tool should be complemented with direct observations to assess environmental features that may be difficult to capture with imagery, such as traffic and aesthetics.

Spatial mapping techniques, such as Geographic Information Systems (GIS), are another common way of measuring the built environment. GIS is a spatial data management system defined as "digital systems that can integrate, store, adjust, analyze and arrange geographically-referenced information" (Fradelos et al., 2014, p. 403). These systems layer different types of geographically referenced data so that spatial relationships, such as counts of specific attributes or distances between attributes, can be computed. For example, homes can be mapped and features within a user-defined area around the home are analyzed to provide information about the individual's neighborhood.

Measurement Techniques: New methodologies

In recent years, new and novel ways to understand the physical environment have emerged. Photovoice, for example, is a media-based methodology where participants are asked to take photos of perceived environmental supports and barriers for physical activity, which are later discussed with the researcher. This method captures the reality of the participants' environment and has been an effective way to understand environmental exposures (Findholt, Michael, Davis, & Brogoitti, 2010; Heidelberger & Smith, 2016; Hennessy et al., 2010). However, this approach may miss detailed contextual information as children discuss their experiences based on photos rather than from within the photographed environment. To overcome this limitation, 'walk-along' interviews, where individuals walk with a researcher in an environment familiar to them, such as their neighborhood, allow in-situ data collection from participants while they are experiencing the environment (Carpiano, 2009). Although more time-consuming than photovoice, walk-along interviews have been used to capture children's use and perceptions of their neighborhood (Loebach & Gilliland, 2010) and detailed and context-specific information about aspects of public open spaces (e.g. squares, skate parks, parks and sport fields/playgrounds) that may influence physical activity among adolescents (Van Hecke et al., 2016). Similarly, bike-along interviews with children have also been used to capture neighborhood environmental factors (e.g. traffic, urban design, cycling infrastructure, end-of-trip facilities, aesthetics and topography) relevant to cycling for transport (Ghekiere et al., 2014). Photographic images have also been used to study the relative importance of neighborhood features (Veitch et al., 2016), and manipulated photographic images of neighborhood features (e.g. streetscapes and parks) have been used to quantify "virtual" changes in features (Ghekiere, Deforche et al., 2015; Van Cauwenberg et al., 2016; Van Hecke, Ghekiere, Van Cauwenberg et al., 2018).

Study Design Considerations

Children accumulate their daily physical activity in a variety of ways, including via active play, active travel and structured sport. Conceptually, specific features of the physical environment are likely to influence different types of physical activity, a concept called 'behavioral specificity' (Giles-Corti, Timperio, Bull, & Pikora, 2005). For example, urban design elements such as road crossings and footpaths are likely to influence the ways in which young people move around their neighborhood (e.g. active transport), but are less likely to influence participation in organized sport. Likewise, access to parks is most likely to influence active play and leisure-time physical activity. For this reason, associations between specific aspects of the environment and physical activity tend to be stronger when specific physical activity behaviors, as opposed to total physical activity, are the outcome of interest (Ding et al., 2011; Timperio, Reid, & Veitch, 2015). The aspect of the physical environment being studied should be conceptually matched to the type of physical activity of interest.

Studies that rely on self-reported information to characterize both the physical environment and self-reported physical activity are further subject to 'same source bias'. Same source bias may create spurious associations because the physical activity may affect the perception of the built environment (Brownson et al., 2009; Diez-Roux, 2007). For example, those who are less likely to walk within their neighborhood may inaccurately report the availability of built environment features than those who walk. Several studies have shown varying levels of concordance between self-reports and objective measures of the same features among both adolescents and adults (Orstad, McDonough, Stapleton, Altincekic, & Troped, 2017; Prins, Oenema, van der Horst, & Brug, 2009), with better concordance among adults who are most active (Ball et al., 2008; Gebel, Bauman, Sugiyama, & Owen, 2011). This suggests that those who are physically active may have more realistic or accurate perceptions potentially because they spend more time being active (e.g. walking or cycling) in their neighborhood surroundings.

A further consideration is the size of the 'environment' being studied or how the geographic scale of that environment is defined, which can vary considerably from study to study. In studies using GIS, small or large administrative areas, as well as distances from 400 meters to several kilometers from resident addresses have been used (Brownson et al., 2009). Self-report surveys define the neighborhood in different ways as well. The NEWS, for example, defines the neighborhood as within a 10–15-minute walk from the respondent's home (Rosenberg et al., 2009; Saelens, Sallis, Black et al., 2003). This is because environmental features closer to home may be more important influences on some types of physical activity than on others.

Several comprehensive reviews have been conducted (de Vet, de Ridder, & de Wit, 2011; Ding et al., 2011; Giles-Corti, Kelty, Zubrick, & Villanueva, 2009; McGrath, Hopkins, & Hinckson, 2015; Oliveira, Moreira, Abreu, Mota, & Santos, 2014; Panter, Jones, & van Sluijs, 2008; Pont et al., 2009; Timperio et al., 2015): some examining associations with total physical activity (Ding et al., 2011; McGrath et al., 2015; Oliveira et al., 2014) and others exploring associations separately for the domains of physical activity, most commonly active travel (D'Haese, Vanwolleghem et al., 2015; Panter et al., 2008; Pont et al., 2009; Timperio et al., 2015). The evidence to date is overwhelmingly from cross-sectional studies that can only provide information about *associations* between characteristics of the physical environment and a particular physical activity behavior. Cross-sectional studies do not explore temporal relationships and therefore cannot determine *causal* relationships. This is particularly relevant for environmental research as it may be that those who are inclined to engage in active travel, for example, choose to reside in a neighborhood that supports such behaviors. This is termed 'self-selection bias' and may overestimate associations between the built environment and physical activity within cross-sectional studies. Study designs that inform causal inference, such as longitudinal or natural experiment studies, are less common. Natural experiments typically examine the impact of changes in the neighborhood environment where exposure to the change has not been assigned by the researcher (Craig et al., 2012). Randomized controlled trials are generally not possible because the 'change' and the exposure to the change are outside the control of the researcher (Craig et al., 2012; Sallis, Story, & Lou, 2009).

Associations between the Physical Environment and Physical Activity

Urban Design

Much of the evidence exploring the association between the built environment and physical activity has focused on elements of urban design or how areas are arranged, specifically those elements that contribute to 'walkability' including land use mix (diversity of different types of destinations/services/land uses), residential density and street connectivity. Conceptually, in a neighborhood with high 'walkability' these three aspects of urban design can provide residents with short, direct routes to a range of destinations, thereby ensuring that walking and cycling for transport are viable options (Saelens, Sallis, & Frank, 2003). Neighborhood walkability is consistently associated with higher levels of walking and cycling, particularly for transport, among adults (Cerin et al., 2017; Christiansen et al., 2016; McCormack & Shiell, 2011). In youth, however, associations are less clear (D'Haese, Vanwolleghem et al., 2015; Ding et al., 2011; McGrath et al., 2015; Panter et al., 2008; Pont et al., 2009; Timperio et al., 2015).

On balance, it seems that young people who live in more walkable neighborhoods are more likely to engage in active travel, in particular on the journey to school. For example, in their comprehensive review, D'Haese and colleagues explored associations between the neighborhood environment and active travel, distinguishing between both the behavior (i.e., walking, cycling or all active travel) and the context (i.e., active travel to get to and from school and active travel to destinations other than school) (D'Haese, Vanwolleghem et al., 2015). They found convincing evidence that overall walkability was associated with walking to/from school specifically and walking or cycling places more generally, and strong evidence that specific elements of walkability, including residential density, land use mix diversity and accessibility, are associated with walking to school. Although active travel to non-school destinations has been less studied, in their review, findings indicated a possible association between residential density and walking for transport during leisure time. These findings are broadly supported by Ding et al. (2011) among both children and adolescents. In contrast, a review that included more recent studies found inconsistent evidence between residential density, land use mix and walkability with active travel in general and no association with these aspects of urban design and total physical activity (Timperio et al., 2015).

The lack of strong evidence linking walkability with physical activity in young people may indicate that these relationships are complex and nuanced. Street connectivity, for example, is an important influence on adult physical activity but is rarely associated with active travel or overall physical activity in young people, and in some cases is negatively associated (Pont et al., 2009). This may be because well-connected streets may expose children to more traffic, contributing to safety concerns (Pont et al., 2009). This hypothesis has not been widely tested but is supported by findings from a study in Perth, Australia, which found children with both low traffic exposure *and* high street connectivity around their school had higher odds of regularly walking to school (Giles-Corti et al., 2011). In addition, neighborhood streets are an important location for active play in children (Veitch, Salmon, & Ball, 2008, 2010). Cul-de-sacs or dead-end streets are often prominent in areas with low connectivity, but can be conducive to outdoor play among children (Handy, Cao & Mokhtarian, 2008; Veitch, Bagley, Ball, & Salmon, 2006; Veitch et al., 2010). As another example, high residential density reflects smaller residential land size. However, in Australia there is evidence that the home backyard is an important place for young people to be active (Veitch et al., 2008). Therefore, in the absence of easy access to public open space, it is possible that neighborhoods with high residential density may deter active play in children.

Distance to school, an artefact of both planning decisions regarding school siting and school zoning policies, is one of the most widely studied attributes of the built environment. Studies consistently show a strong negative association between distance to school and active travel (Larouche et al., 2015; Panter et al., 2008; Pont et al., 2009; Timperio et al., 2015). For example, a large multi-country study of children aged 9–11 years found that a trip duration longer than 15 minutes was associated with lower odds of school active travel in 8 of the 12 countries (Larouche et al., 2015). One of the few longitudinal studies to be conducted found that among 10-year olds, the odds of taking up school active travel 1 year later were nearly five times higher, and of maintaining active travel almost three times higher, among those living within 1 km of school compared with those living more than 2 km from school (Panter, Corder, Griffin, Jones, & van Sluijs, 2013).

Traffic Safety and Walking and Cycling Infrastructure

Parental concern about traffic and road safety is a frequently cited barrier to young people's physical activity (Carver et al., 2008). The volume and speed of the traffic and the presence of pedestrian safety structures (i.e., safe road crossings) and dedicated walking and cycling infrastructure (e.g. footpaths and cycling lanes) can all affect the ability of children and adolescents to safely walk or cycle from place to place, both in their neighborhood and on their journey to school. While there are some inconsistencies, on balance, the evidence suggests that both pedestrian safety structures and the speed and volume of traffic influences active travel among children (D'Haese, Vanwolleghem et al., 2015; Ding et al., 2011; Oliveira et al., 2014; Timperio et al., 2015). For example, in their review, D'Haese, Vanwolleghem et al. (2015) found evidence of a possible association between general measures of traffic safety (e.g. traffic volume, traffic lights, speed humps and traffic hazards) and school active travel in general, and walking to school and cycling to school specifically. There was no evidence, however, that traffic safety was associated with active travel during leisure time. In their review, Ding et al. (2011) found convincing evidence that the presence of objectively measured pedestrian safety structures was positively associated with active travel to school and playing outdoors, and perceived presence of pedestrian safety structures was positively associated with reported physical activity. Further, objectively measured traffic speed/volume was consistently negatively associated with reported active travel and walking. In adolescents however, there was no evidence that pedestrian safety structures or traffic speed/volume influenced physical activity.

Purpose-built walking and cycling infrastructure, including footpaths, cycle lanes and dedicated off-road walking and cycling paths, separate users from traffic, thereby making journeys safer and more pleasant. Additionally, if this infrastructure is well connected and provides a direct route to destinations, it may make travel on foot and by bike more convenient. There appears to be consistent evidence that walking and cycling facilities are positively associated with walking to school specifically among children (D'Haese, Vanwolleghem et al., 2015; Ding et al., 2011; Oliveira et al., 2014), though not necessarily cycling to school, school active travel in general, or active travel to non-school destinations.

Natural experiment studies provide evidence that changing the safety-related elements of routes to school can result in higher rates of active transport and closing streets to traffic can increase physical activity, most likely through active play. In the US, positive impacts on rates of walking or cycling to school were found in natural experiments evaluating the impact of the installation or widening of bicycle lanes and crossings or upgrading footpaths along routes to school (Boarnet, Anderson, Day, McMillan, & Alfonzo, 2005) and of introducing bicycle parking at school, and signage and traffic calming in addition to these engineering solutions (McDonald et al., 2014). In Belgium, researchers evaluated the impact of *Play Streets*, residential streets that are closed to traffic for several hours for the purpose of providing children with a place to play, on children's physical activity (D'Haese, Van Dyck, De Bourdeaudhuij, Deforche, & Cardon, 2015). During the hours of operation (1,400–1,900), children living in a Play Street increased their physical activity from 27 to 36 minutes, whereas children in the control group experienced a decrease in physical activity.

Aesthetics

In adults, the visual appeal or pleasantness of the neighborhood environment is a common correlate of physical activity (Choi, Lee, Lee, Kang, & Choi, 2017). Among children and adolescents, reviews published before 2010 have indicated a possible positive association between aesthetics of the built environment and physical activity in the small number of studies available (Giles-Corti et al., 2009; Limstrand, 2008). Ding et al. (2011) also found some evidence that the presence of trees on the street (vegetation) was positively associated with reported physical activity in children, but not adolescents. On balance, however, a recent review contradicts these earlier findings, suggesting that there is little to no evidence to support an association between the aesthetics of the neighborhood environment and overall physical activity or active travel specifically (Timperio et al., 2015) among children and youth.

Availability of Facilities

Conceptually, the presence of sport and recreation facilities in the neighborhood can provide young people with opportunities for structured and unstructured physical activity outside the home, thereby increasing their leisure-time physical activity. If these facilities are in close proximity to the home, they may also afford important opportunities for active travel. The findings from re-view papers suggest that access to facilities is likely to be positively associated with overall physical activity in children and youth (D'Haese, Vanwolleghem et al., 2015; Ding et al., 2011; Giles-Corti et al., 2009; Limstrand, 2008; Timperio et al., 2015). For example, Ding and colleagues found objectively measured recreation facilities (access/density/proximity) to be strongly associated with reported leisure-time physical activity in children. In adolescents, this association was present in some but not all studies. A meta-analysis of studies that included objective measures of the en-vironment found small effects of availability of facilities on objectively assessed physical activity, representing a 6% increase in physical activity when one additional facility was present (McGrath et al., 2015). In addition, D'Haese, Vanwolleghem et al. (2015) found some evidence to suggest that access to recreation facilities was positively associated with school active travel, and active travel to non-school destinations (i.e., in leisure time).

Nicosia and Datar (2018) capitalized on the opportunity to measure impact of change in resi-dential neighborhood environment on physical activity levels among adolescents in military fam-ilies when they were re-assigned to a new station in a different neighborhood. In this natural experiment, 12–13-year olds who experienced increased opportunities for physical activity (as measured by the number of fitness and recreation facilities available within 2 miles of home at baseline and follow-up) after moving to a new neighborhood had significantly increased time spent in total and vigorous physical activity compared to non-movers.

Parks, Public Open Space and Natural Environments

Like recreation facilities, public open spaces, parks and urban green spaces are considered import-ant locations where young people can play and participate in sport and more structured recreation (Koohsari et al., 2015). Summarizing data from studies that explored objectively determined access or proximity to parks or density of nearby parks, Ding et al. (2011) found evidence of a positive association with some form of physical activity among children in 42% of results and among adolescents in 38%. Oliveira et al. (2014) also reported a consistent positive association between park and playground proximity and physical activity, particularly walking and cycling trips, among children.

While access to green space appears to be important, empirical evidence also suggests that specific qualities of parks and public open spaces are important to encourage physical activity (Gardsjord, Tveit, & Nordh, 2014). For example, a review of 32 studies conducted with children or youth found that the presence of sports facilities and perceptions of crime safety as well as more specific qualities of parks including lighting, maintenance and aesthetics were positively associated with physical activity (Gardsjord et al., 2014). Extending this work, Van Hecke, Ghekiere, Veitch et al. (2018) reviewed the evidence to understand the specific qualities and characteristics of public open spaces that are associated with both visitation and physical activity among adolescents. They found that the presence of specific sport fields, adventurous playgrounds and trails or walking paths was positively associated with visitation, and to a lesser extent physical activity, among ad-olescents (Van Hecke, Ghekiere, Veitch et al., 2018). They also found some contrasting findings between boys and girls, where the presence of skateboard ramps was associated with more physical activity among boys and less physical activity among girls.

The effect of refurbishing existing parks on visitation and physical activity levels has been evaluated in natural experiment studies, primarily in Australia and the US (Hunter et al., 2015). In Australia, the upgrade of a park to include an all-abilities playground, walking track, BBQ facilities, a dog off-leash park and a fence to protect motor vehicle access to the park, as well as improvements to the landscaping resulted in substantial increases in park visitation among children (2–18 years) relative to the control park (Veitch, Ball, Crawford, Abbott, & Salmon, 2012). Similarly, another Australian study evaluating the impact of the installation of a 'play-scape' in a large park, reported significant increases in the total number of children visiting the park and engaging in park-based physical activity at the intervention park compared with the control park (Veitch et al., 2018). Based on its potential to increase physical activity, that study also found that the play-scape installation was cost-effective (Lal et al., 2019). In contrast, another Australian study found no significant differences between either park visitation or number of children engaging in moderate-to-vigorous physical activity (MVPA) in the intervention and control parks following extensive refurbishment involving the addition of three new children's playgrounds, upgrades to walking paths, landscaping, lighting, amenities and sports fields open for public use (Bohn-Goldbaum et al., 2013). Another US study found that park visitation increased substantially in children following a comprehensive renovation to two parks (including new play equipment as well as landscaping and group surfaces, adult gym equipment and a recreation center in one of the parks), but declined by 51% in adolescents (Cohen et al., 2015). In summary, the findings on the impact of park refurbishment on visitation and physical activity are mixed, and may be context specific. There is little evidence regarding the impact of fitness or parkour equipment in parks or the co-location of these infrastructure with playgrounds designed for younger children. Parks with features that attract people of all ages are desirable. In general, findings indicate that not all park features are attractive to all groups of people.

Urban Development and Renewal

While not common, studies have begun to examine the sum impact of new developments and urban renewal projects on physical activity among children or adolescents, where multiple aspects of the built environment are designed or changed to support more active lifestyles. Smart Growth is an urban planning strategy that designs neighborhoods to ensure compact building design, mixed land use, access to public open space and infrastructure for walking and cycling (Knaap & Talen, 2005). In a small study in California (US), the nature of physical activity among children aged 9–13 years was compared soon after moving to a 'Smart Growth' area relative to children who continued to reside in a conventional low-to-medium density neighborhood. Using ecological momentary assessment, children who had recently moved to the smart growth community were more likely to engage in activity with friends, close to home at venues that they could walk to, compared with children living in the traditional neighborhood. However, after 6 months there were no significant differences in MVPA between the groups (Dunton, Intille, Wolch, & Pentz, 2012). The authors suggest that more time might be needed for the new environment to impact overall physical activity, despite changes in the nature of physical activity (Dunton et al., 2012).

In Copenhagen, Denmark, researchers evaluated the impact of a large-scale urban renewal project on the physical activity levels of adolescents residing in the area (Andersen et al., 2017). The renewal included renovations to public housing and courtyards, the addition of street lights, renovation and establishment of new urban green spaces, playgrounds and sports facilities and the opening of two civic centers. Using data obtained from both accelerometers and Global Positioning System (GPS) receivers, the researchers determined the change in time spent in, and the physical activity done within, the gentrified area among 11–16-year olds in a baseline sample and a sample recruited 2 years later. Compared to baseline, adolescents spent an additional 25 minutes/day in the area. Of that time, there was a small increase in MVPA (4.5 minutes/day). Results were similar among those living within or outside the renewal district.

Key and Emerging Issues

Objective vs. Perceived Measures

As described above, both objective and perceived measures of the environment are commonly used to understand how the physical environment influences physical activity among children and youth. A limitation of self-reported measures of the neighborhood environment is that perceptions are highly subjective, often don't match objectively assessed estimates of the same neighborhood attribute and vary between people (Ball et al., 2008; Gebel et al., 2011; Orstad et al., 2017; Prins et al., 2009). Studies based on objective measures of environmental exposures may better inform policy and practice given exposures are systematically and consistently appraised, and may have less measurement error (Ding et al., 2011), and better alignment with planning metrics and concepts. While it is plausible that a person's perceptions are stronger influences on their behavior or the freedoms they give their child, a systematic review among children and adolescents found that objectively measured built environment attributes were more consistent correlates of physical activity than perceived attributes (Ding et al., 2011). However, some studies (Ding et al., 2011) have found the opposite, with certain features of the perceived environment being stronger correlates of physical activity than objective measures. It is likely that both objective and perceived measures capture distinct constructs that explain unique variances in physical activity.

Interaction between Individual, Social and Environmental Factors

It is important to identify how, for whom and when attributes in the built environment influence physical activity. As highlighted by socio-ecological models, relationships between different levels of influences on physical activity are complex (Rhodes, Saelens, & Sauvage-Mar, 2018) and there is also evidence that different features of the physical environment interact to influence physical activity in different ways. Psychosocial factors such as perceptions of safety from crime, social support and co-participation, and self-efficacy have been examined as potential moderators of associations between the built environment and physical activity among children and adolescents (D'Haese et al., 2016; De Meester, Van Dyck, De Bourdeaudhuij, Deforche, & Cardon, 2013; Deforche, Van Dyck, Verloigne, & De Bourdeaudhuij, 2010; Ghekiere et al., 2016; Wang et al., 2017). These kinds of analyses may help explain inconsistencies in the literature (Sawyer et al., 2017), where the association of a particular environmental attribute on physical activity may depend on another environmental, social or individual factor, and can help inform interventions (Rhodes et al., 2018). Among children in Belgium, no strong interaction was observed between psychosocial factors and walkability on physical activity (D'Haese et al., 2016); however, an Australian study found that parental co-participation in walking or cycling (but not public open space, sport options or population density) moderated associations between street connectivity and walking/cycling trips (Ghekiere et al., 2016). Also in Belgium, a significant interaction was found between walkability and perceived barriers and benefits of physical activity and behavior among adolescents (De Meester et al., 2013). No moderation was found for other psychosocial variables. In the US, Wang et al. (2017) found significant interactions between self-efficacy and walkability and self-efficacy and number of parks/recreation facilities in explaining active transportation among adolescents. Indeed, a recent review among all age groups found, on balance, some support for the premise that social cognitive variables moderated associations between aspects of the built environment and leisure-time physical activity, but not overall or transport-related physical activity (Rhodes et al., 2018).

Parental Fears

Given that children and adolescents are not totally independent and rely on parents to help make decisions, parents perceptions of 'risk' in the neighborhood environment and parental fears may be critical influences on children's activities (Timperio et al., 2015). For example, parental road safety concerns have been associated with more 'constrained behavior' (e.g. preventing their child from engaging in physical activity in certain circumstances or locations, and defensive behaviors such as requiring supervision when playing inside, outdoors or in the neighborhood) among girls, but not boys (Carver et al., 2012). Constrained behaviors such as these are associated with lower levels of physical activity. Importantly, associations between road safety concerns and constrained behavior were 'mediated' by perceived risk (likelihood) of harm to their child (Carver et al., 2012). This suggests that parental fears may explain associations between some aspects of the physical environment and physical activity among youth, especially among girls.

Looking beyond Urban Residential Neighborhood

Most research examining links between the physical environment and physical activity is restricted in focus to the environment within residential neighborhoods in urban locations (Matthews, 2008; Matthews & Yang, 2013), despite it being increasingly recognized that most people spend significant time in places other than their residential neighborhood (Matthews & Yang, 2013). This approach assumes that the relationship between exposure and outcomes is static across places and is termed as 'the local trap' (Cummins, 2007). It is uncommon for researchers to link individuals to multiple places. Physical activity can be carried out at various locations, such as around home, school, as well as the journey between these places, but to date the focus has largely been on neighborhood exposures, with the location of the physical activity not known. Studies that incorporate GPS, GIS and accelerometers may offer opportunities to unpack the complex built environment and physical activity relationship. Studies focused on how the built environment influences physical activity in rural areas are also lacking. It is possible that different features of the built environment are important in rural areas, with unique barriers to physical activity (Hansen, Umstattd Meyer, Lenardson, & Hartley, 2015). In addition, most tools for measuring perceptions of the built environment were developed for urban areas, though several audit tools have been developed to measure aspects of the environment that may relate to physical activity (Hansen et al., 2015).

Use of GPS-enabled devices can be useful for determining locations where individuals engage in physical activity. When participants wear a GPS logger together with a device measuring physical activity (such as an accelerometer), it is possible to identify where the individual engages in physical activity. For example, GPS devices, accelerometers and one-on-one interviews were recently used with adolescents to determine location-specific physical activity, duration of visitation, accompaniment and reasons for using public open spaces (Van Hecke, Verhoeven et al., 2018). About three quarters of the adolescents in the study used a public open space and among those that did, boys accumulated more MVPA in public open space than did girls. Another study utilized both GPS and accelerometers to examine locations where most MVPA occurred among youth and found that most MVPA occurred during the journey between locations through commuting (e.g. between home and school) (Rainham et al., 2012). This finding suggests that the use of specific boundaries such as census tract or buffers within a single residential environment (e.g. home or school) may not either accurately or adequately measure the spatiotemporal realities of daily life.

Natural Experiment Studies

Study designs that are capable of informing causal inference are needed to further the evidence base, but as mentioned earlier, these designs are not common. Natural experiment studies have been identified by experts as the top scoring research priority in this field (Sallis et al., 2009). While natural experiment studies are emerging, very few have examined the impact of changes to the environment on child and youth physical activity (Audrey & Batista-Ferrer, 2015; MacMillan et al., 2018). Part of the reason for the lack of natural experimental evidence is that studies are often opportunistic (i.e., usually identified based on planned changes being implemented by city departments). As such, it is difficult to plan for interventions and the timing of delivery is out of the control of the researcher (Craig et al., 2012; Veitch et al., 2017). Opportunities for natural experiment studies should be selected carefully based on their likely impact on physical activity (Craig et al., 2012). In addition, it is also important to ensure that follow-up assessments allow sufficient time for behaviors to become habitual or for residents to become aware of the change (Dunton et al., 2012; Veitch et al., 2014).

Virtual Experiments

Although more natural experiment studies evaluating real-world changes to the environment are needed, virtual experiments are emerging as a potential cost-effective and less time-consuming alternative to examine the relative importance of environmental characteristics for optimizing physical activity. For example, manipulated photos of micro-environmental street factors (e.g. speed limits, evenness of a cycle path) have been used to examine the perceived supportiveness of street characteristics for transportation cycling among 10–12-year-old children (Ghekiere, Deforche et al., 2015; Ghekiere, Van Cauwenberg et al., 2015) and among adolescents (Verhoeven et al., 2017), and the relative importance of park features among adolescents (Mertens, Van Cauwenberg, Veitch, Deforche, & Van Dyck, 2019; Van Hecke, Ghekiere, Van Cauwenberg et al., 2018) in Belgium. Manipulated photos are a "virtual" experiment, whereby environmental changes are examined without actually making real changes to the environment. As such, virtual experiments are not subject to the risk of negative side-effects that may occur with real-world changes, serving as a first step before conducting a more costly and time-consuming natural experiment. Future research should explore methodologies that can provide participants with exposure to virtual environments, that may provide a sufficiently realistic representation of the environment. For example, emerging technologies such as computer-generated virtual walk through environments provide 3D simulations on which participants can provide feedback on different environmental changes.

Developing Countries

Compared to high-income countries, comparatively few studies have focused on associations between the physical environment and physical activity among children and adolescents in low- or middle-income countries (LMIC) (Day, 2018). Consistent with high-income countries, children in Brazil, China, Kenya, South Africa and Vietnam appear to be more likely to use active transport to school the closer they live to school (Larouche et al., 2015; Trang, Hong, & Dibley, 2012). Among children, walking and cycling infrastructure in Kenya (Muthuri, Wachira, Onywera, & Tremblay, 2016) and pedestrian amenities on streets around home in Mexico (Lee et al., 2016) were associated with higher leisure-time physical activity and outdoor play, respectively. Obstructions on footpaths or sidewalks in the areas around school were shown to impede, and low traffic volume on the most road segments near home was shown to promote, outdoor play in Mexico (Lee et al., 2016). However, parental perceptions that most drivers speed were associated with lower odds of using active transport in Brazil, but higher odds in India (Larouche et al., 2015). In relation to urban design attributes, proximity to destinations is a consistent correlate of higher physical activity among children in LMIC (Sallis et al., 2016). A study in China found that adolescents living in areas with high residential density were less likely to engage in >11 hours/week of recreational physical activity compared to those with the lowest residential density (Xu et al., 2010). It has been suggested that an extremely high level of density may deter physical activity due to perceived overcrowding (Day, 2016), air pollution (Cerin, Chan, Macfarlane, Lee, & Lai, 2011) and/or closer proximity to destinations and public transport than less dense areas (Cerin et al., 2014, 2016). While some findings in LMIC are consistent with those from high-income countries, the limited evidence suggest that there may be some distinct differences.

Air Pollution

Exposure to air pollution is being recognized as a potential barrier to outdoor physical activity, with studies showing negative associations between level of air pollution and physical activity among children and adults (An, Zhang, Ji, & Guan, 2018). Exposure to air pollution increases the risk of mortality, and cardiovascular and respiratory diseases such as stroke and asthma and lung cancer, and can reduce lung function, elevate blood pressure and impair exercise capacity and performance (Cohen et al., 2005; Kurt, Zhang, & Pinkerton, 2016). Due to smaller airways and immature development of the respiratory system, children and youth are more susceptible to the effects of air pollution than adults (Kurt et al., 2016). However, evidence syntheses have found pedestrians to be the least exposed to particulates and car users the most exposed, with cyclists and bus riders having similar exposure, although some disparities between studies were observed (de Nazelle, Bode, & Orjuela, 2017). Among adults, the benefits of physical activity have been shown to outweigh the risk of exposure to air pollution, despite increased exposure to pollution in the majority of settings worldwide (Tainio et al., 2016). More studies are required among children in highly polluted and developing cities (Raza, Forsberg, Johansson, & Sommar, 2018).

There are several ways in which the physical environment can be modified to reduce exposure for pedestrians and cyclists. For example, bicycle lanes next to traffic can draw cyclists to more polluted routes. Solutions may include the provision of dense networks of attractive bike paths and bike boulevards (traffic-calmed streets which provide priority for cyclists) and separation from traffic, especially in locations where rate of respiration is likely to be high (e.g. steep hills) (Bigazzi & Figliozzi, 2014). It is important, however, that low-pollution route alternatives do not lead to excess travel time, which could add to total inhaled pollution dose (Broach & Bigazzi, 2017) or discourage people from walking or cycling. Policies that encourage direct, lower-pollution routes separated from traffic are needed (Bigazzi & Figliozzi, 2014; Broach & Bigazzi, 2017) and should also be considered in regard to routes to school for children. Provision of adequate parks and green space is also important as visiting or being active in parks or traveling through parks may result in less exposure. For example, a recent study among adults (60+ years) showed that walking in a park led to an increase in lung and forced vital capacity; however, these responses were attenuated by walking on a highly polluted street (Sinharay et al., 2018). Perceived personal safety and surveillance on alternative routes is also important to maintain.

The Need for Cross-Government and Strategic Multi-Sectoral Partnerships

The World Health Organization's Global Action Plan on Physical Activity 2018–2030 (World Health Organization, 2018) highlights the need for a co-ordinated and "systems-based" response to ensure effective and successful implementation of changes to the built environment to support physical activity. The physical environment is shaped by decisions, policies and practices within diverse government departments (including planning, transport, parks, and sport and recreation), as well as a range of professionals in the private sector (e.g. developers and landscape architects). As health and physical activity are often not core priorities within these sectors, creating or modifying the built environment to support increased physical activity requires cross-government and strategic multi-sectoral partnerships (Matsudo, 2012; Saelens, Sallis, & Frank, 2003; World Health Organization, 2018) and policies (Giles-Corti et al., 2010). Alignment with broader government objectives, such as the United Nations' Sustainable Development Goals (United Nations, 2018) and other co-benefits (Giles-Corti et al., 2010; Sallis, Spoon et al., 2015), may also help to foster cross-government action.

Recommendations

Recommendations for Research

- Natural experiment studies are needed to inform causal inference on the role of the environment on influencing physical activity. Natural experiment studies evaluating real-world infrastructure changes of different types should ideally incorporate residents of all ages to determine if there are unanticipated impacts on specific groups, or if particular changes yield different results for different groups. Further, in addition to exploring the impact and cost-effectiveness of 'natural experiments' on physical activity, researchers should explore the context in which the changes take place and the mechanisms underpinning the change (or causal pathways). Opportunities should be carefully selected. Guidance on designing natural experiments is available (Craig et al., 2012).
- 'Virtual' methods of studying the potential impact of environmental changes can be explored as a pre-cursor to natural experiments.
- Given the challenges associated with prospectively studying the impact of planned changes to the built environment, opportunities should be sought to retrospectively examine the impact of specific built environment changes within ongoing cohort studies or using existing data sources if degree of exposure can be ascertained. Relocation within cohort studies also offers the opportunity to study the impact of changes in exposure to a range of built environment attributes due to relocation, relative to those who did not relocate (Ding et al., 2018). Longitudinal studies capable of examining within-person changes can provide stronger evidence for causal claims.
- Measurement techniques that extend current methods of obtaining parent and child perceptions of the neighborhood environment should continue to be explored.
- Care should be taken to ensure conceptual specificity within studies of the environment and physical activity. This includes the study of context-specific behaviors (e.g. behaviors likely to occur in the 'neighborhood' when studying the neighborhood environment) as well as behavior-specific environments (e.g. routes to school when studying active transport) (Giles-Corti et al., 2005).
- Conceptual thinking and statistical techniques that explore the complexity of environment-behavior relationships should be applied to determine how, when and for whom environmental attributes influence physical activity. This includes an exploration of inter-relationships with personal, social and family influences on physical activity.
- More studies on the role of the physical environment in shaping physical activity in under-represented areas such as developing countries and rural areas are needed.
- Interdisciplinary collaboration and participatory co-design approaches should be considered. In particular, input from children and youth regarding their perceptions on what features of the built environment are most important to prioritize in interventions or natural experiments could result in larger effects.
- To comprehensively study the impact of the environment on physical activity, environmental contexts beyond the residential neighborhood, such as the environment surrounding schools or other places where children and adolescents spend time, should be studied.

Recommendations for Practice

- Prior to approval of urban planning and renewal projects, an assessment of the likely impact on physical activity for people of all ages, including child pedestrians and cyclists, should be carried out (Timperio et al., 2018). Assessments of likely health, economic and environmental impacts of urban planning policies; infrastructure changes; and other interventions should also be conducted (World Health Organization, 2018).
- The World Health Organization's Global Action Plan on Physical Activity 2018–2030 outlines five key actions for creating active environments to assist in meeting global physical activity targets by 2030 (World Health Organization, 2018). These include the following: integrating urban and transport planning policies to prioritize walking and cycling and use of public transport through compact, mixed use and highly connected streets; improving safety, quality, connectedness and completeness of walking and cycling infrastructure; improving road and personal safety of pedestrians and cyclists; improving access to quality public and green open space, recreational spaces and sports amenities; and strengthening policy, regulatory and design guidelines/frameworks to allow physical activity at and around key neighborhood destinations and access by pedestrians, cyclists and public transport. Safe and equitable access, including for children and youth, is at the heart of each key action.
- Best practice evidence and design guidelines should be used where possible. A number of such resources have been developed (e.g. the Healthy Active by Design website: http://www.healthyactivebydesign.com.au/; Centre for Active Design's *Active Design Guidelines* and checklists: https://centerforactivedesign.org/guidelines/).
- Where possible, examples of best practice, case studies and impacts of changes to the environment should be shared.
- Cross-government and strategic multi-sectoral partnerships and policies to help shape built environments that support active lifestyles for all residents must be fostered.
- Acknowledging the multiple co-benefits of active travel and investing in environmental strategies to shift people from cars (e.g. provision of bicycle highways, shortcuts for walkers and cyclists, cycle and walking paths separated from high traffic streets) should be a priority.
- There is a need for initiatives to encourage children and youth to spend more time outdoors.
- Consider shared use of facilities (e.g. after hours use of school facilities for recreation) and creative options such as closing streets to increase opportunities for active play and leisure-time physical activity.

References

An, R., Zhang, S., Ji, M., & Guan, C. (2018). Impact of ambient air pollution on physical activity among adults: A systematic review and meta-analysis. *Perspectives in Public Health, 138*(2), 111–121.

Andersen, H. B., Christiansen, L. B., Klinker, C. D., Ersbøll, A. K., Troelsen, J., Kerr, J., & Schipperijn, J. (2017). Increases in use and activity due to urban renewal: Effect of a natural experiment. *American Journal of Preventive Medicine, 53*(3), e81–e87.

Audrey, S., & Batista-Ferrer, H. (2015). Healthy urban environments for children and young people: A systematic review of intervention studies. *Health and Place, 36*, 97–117.

Australian Institute of Health and Welfare. (2011). *Health and the environment: A compilation of evidence* (Cat No. PHE 136). Canberra, Australia: Australian Institute of Health and Welfare.

Badland, H. M., Opit, S., Witten, K., Kearns, R. A., & Mavoa, S. (2010). Can virtual streetscape audits reliably replace physical streetscape audits? *Journal of Urban Health, 87*(6), 1007–1016.

Ball, K., Jeffery, R. W., Crawford, D. A., Roberts, R. J., Salmon, J., & Timperio, A. F. (2008). Mismatch between perceived and objective measures of physical activity environments. *Preventive Medicine, 47*(3), 294–298.

Bigazzi, A. Y., & Figliozzi, M. A. (2014). Review of urban bicyclists' intake and uptake of traffic-related air pollution. *Transport Reviews, 34*(2), 221–245.

Boarnet, M. G., Anderson, C. L., Day, K., McMillan, T., & Alfonzo, M. (2005). Evaluation of the California safe routes to school legislation: Urban form changes and children's active transportation to school. *American Journal of Preventive Medicine, 28*(2), 134–140.

Bohn-Goldbaum, E. E., Phongsavan, P., Merom, D., Rogers, K., Kamalesh, V., & Bauman, A. E. (2013). Does playground improvement increase physical activity among children? A quasi-experimental study of a natural experiment. *Journal of Environment and Public Health, 2013*, 109841.

Broach, J., & Bigazzi, A. Y. (2017). Existence and use of low-pollution route options for observed bicycling trips. *Transportation Research Record, 2662*(1), 152–159.

Brownson, R. C., Hoehner, C. M., Day, K., Forsyth, A., & Sallis, J. F. (2009). Measuring the built environment for physical activity: State of the science. *American Journal of Preventive Medicine, 36*(4 Suppl), S99–S123, e112.

Carpiano, R. M. (2009). Come take a walk with me: The "go-along" interview as a novel method for studying the implications of place for health and well-being. *Health and Place, 15*(1), 263–272.

Carver, A., Timperio, A., & Crawford, D. (2008). Playing it safe: The influence of neighborhood safety on children's physical activity. A review. *Health and Place, 14*(2), 217–227.

Carver, A., Timperio, A., Hesketh, K., & Crawford, D. (2010a). Are children and adolescents less active if parents restrict their physical activity and active transport due to perceived risk? *Social Science and Medicine, 70*(11), 1799–1805.

Carver, A., Timperio, A., Hesketh, K., & Crawford, D. (2010b). Are safety-related features of the road environment associated with smaller declines in physical activity among youth? *Journal of Urban Health, 87*(1), 29–43.

Carver, A., Timperio, A., Hesketh, K., & Crawford, D. (2012). How does perceived risk mediate associations between perceived safety and parental restriction of adolescents' physical activity in their neighborhood? *International Journal of Behavioral Nutrition and Physical Activity, 9*, 57.

Catalano, R. (1979). *Health, behavior and the community: An ecological perspective.* New York, NY: Pergamon Press.

Cerin, E., Chan, K. W., Macfarlane, D. J., Lee, K. Y., & Lai, P. C. (2011). Objective assessment of walking environments in ultra-dense cities: Development and reliability of the Environment in Asia Scan Tool–Hong Kong version (EAST-HK). *Health and Place, 17*(4), 937–945.

Cerin, E., Nathan, A., van Cauwenberg, J., Barnett, D. W., Barnett, A., & Council on Environment and Physical Activity (CEPA) – Older Adults Working Group. (2017). The neighborhood physical environment and active travel in older adults: A systematic review and meta-analysis. *International Journal of Behavioral Nutrition and Physical Activity, 14*(1), 15.

Cerin, E., Sit, C. H., Barnett, A., Johnston, J. M., Cheung, M. C., & Chan, W. M. (2014). Ageing in an ultra-dense metropolis: Perceived neighborhood characteristics and utilitarian walking in Hong Kong elders. *Public Health Nutrition, 17*(1), 225–232.

Cerin, E., Sit, C. H., Cheung, M. C., Ho, S. Y., Lee, L. C., & Chan, W. M. (2010). Reliable and valid NEWS for Chinese seniors: Measuring perceived neighborhood attributes related to walking. *International Journal of Behavioral Nutrition and Physical Activity, 7*, 84.

Cerin, E., Zhang, C. J. P., Barnett, A., Sit, C. P. H., Cheung, M. C. M., Johnston, J. M., . . . Lee, R. S. Y. (2016). Associations of objectively-assessed neighborhood characteristics with older adults' total physical activity and sedentary time in an ultra-dense urban environment: Findings from the ALECS study. *Health and Place, 42*, 1–10.

Choi, J., Lee, M., Lee, J. K., Kang, D., & Choi, J. Y. (2017). Correlates associated with participation in physical activity among adults: A systematic review of reviews and update. *BMC Public Health, 17*(1), 356.

Christiansen, L. B., Cerin, E., Badland, H., Kerr, J., Davey, R., Troelsen, J., . . . Sallis, J. F. (2016). International comparisons of the associations between objective measures of the built environment and transport-related walking and cycling: IPEN adult study. *Journal of Transport and Health, 3*(4), 467–478.

Cohen, A. J., Ross Anderson, H., Ostro, B., Pandey, K. D., Krzyzanowski, M., Kunzli, N., . . . Smith, K. (2005). The global burden of disease due to outdoor air pollution. *Journal of Toxicology and Environmental Health A, 68*(13–14), 1301–1307.

Cohen, D. A., Han, B., Isacoff, J., Shulaker, B., Williamson, S., Marsh, T., . . . Bhatia, R. (2015). Impact of park renovations on park use and park-based physical activity. *Journal of Physical Activity and Health, 12*(2), 289–295.

Craig, P., Cooper, C., Gunnell, D., Haw, S., Lawson, K., Macintyre, S., . . . Thompson, S. (2012). Using natural experiments to evaluate population health interventions: New medical research council guidance. *Journal of Epidemiology and Community Health, 66*(12), 1182–1186.

Cummins, S. (2007). Commentary: Investigating neighborhood effects on health – Avoiding the 'local trap'. *International Journal of Epidemiology, 36*(2), 355–357.

Davison, K. K., & Lawson, C. T. (2006). Do attributes in the physical environment influence children's physical activity? A review of the literature. *International Journal of Behavioral Nutrition and Physical Activity, 3*, 19.

Day, K. (2016). Built environmental correlates of physical activity in China: A review. *Preventive Medicine Reports, 3*, 303–316.

Day, K. (2018). Physical environment correlates of physical activity in developing countries: A review. *Journal of Physical Activity and Health, 15*(4), 303–314.

Deforche, B., Van Dyck, D., Verloigne, M., & De Bourdeaudhuij, I. (2010). Perceived social and physical environmental correlates of physical activity in older adolescents and the moderating effect of self-efficacy. *Preventive Medicine, 50*(Suppl 1), S24–S29.

De Meester, F., Van Dyck, D., De Bourdeaudhuij, I., Deforche, B., & Cardon, G. (2013). Do psychosocial factors moderate the association between neighborhood walkability and adolescents' physical activity? *Social Science and Medicine, 81*, 1–9.

de Nazelle, A., Bode, O., & Orjuela, J. P. (2017). Comparison of air pollution exposures in active vs. passive travel modes in European cities: A quantitative review. *Environment International, 99*, 151–160.

de Vet, E., de Ridder, D. T., & de Wit, J. B. (2011). Environmental correlates of physical activity and dietary behaviours among young people: A systematic review of reviews. *Obesity Reviews, 12*(5), e130–e142.

D'Haese, S., Cardon, G., & Deforche, B. (2015). The environment and physical activity. In M. Frelut (Ed.), *The ECOG's eBook on child and adolescent obesity*. Brussels, Belgium: European Childhood Obesity Group (ECOG).

D'Haese, S., Gheysen, F., De Bourdeaudhuij, I., Deforche, B., Van Dyck, D., & Cardon, G. (2016). The moderating effect of psychosocial factors in the relation between neighborhood walkability and children's physical activity. *International Journal of Behavioral Nutrition and Physical Activity, 13*(1), 128.

D'Haese, S., Van Dyck, D., De Bourdeaudhuij, I., Deforche, B., & Cardon, G. (2015). Organizing "Play Streets" during school vacations can increase physical activity and decrease sedentary time in children. *International Journal of Behavioral Nutrition and Physical Activity, 12*, 14.

D'Haese, S., Vanwolleghem, G., Hinckson, E., De Bourdeaudhuij, I., Deforche, B., Van Dyck, D., & Cardon, G. (2015). Cross-continental comparison of the association between the physical environment and active transportation in children: A systematic review. *International Journal of Behavioral Nutrition and Physical Activity, 12*, 145.

Diez-Roux, A. V. (2007). Neighborhoods and health: Where are we and were do we go from here? *Revue d'Epidemiologie et de Sante Publique, 55*(1), 13–21.

Ding, D., Nguyen, B., Learnihan, V., Bauman, A. E., Davey, R., Jalaludin, B., & Gebel, K. (2018). Moving to an active lifestyle? A systematic review of the effects of residential relocation on walking, physical activity and travel behaviour. *British Journal of Sports Medicine, 52*(12), 789–799.

Ding, D., Sallis, J. F., Kerr, J., Lee, S., & Rosenberg, D. E. (2011). Neighborhood environment and physical activity among youth a review. *American Journal of Preventive Medicine, 41*(4), 442–455.

Dunton, G. F., Intille, S. S., Wolch, J., & Pentz, M. A. (2012). Investigating the impact of a smart growth community on the contexts of children's physical activity using ecological momentary assessment. *Health and Place, 18*(1), 76–84.

Findholt, N. E., Michael, Y. L., Davis, M. M., & Brogoitti, V. W. (2010). Environmental influences on children's physical activity and diets in rural Oregon: Results of a youth photovoice project. *Online Journal of Rural Nursing and Health Care, 10*(2), 11–20.

Fradelos, E. C., Papathanasiou, I. V., Mitsi, D., Tsaras, K., Kleisiaris, C. F., & Kourkouta, L. (2014). Health based geographic information systems (GIS) and their applications. *Acta Informatica Medica, 22*(6), 402–405.

Gardsjord, H. S., Tveit, M. S., & Nordh, H. (2014). Promoting youth's physical activity through park design: Linking theory and practice in a public health perspective. *Landscape Research, 39*(1), 70–81.

Gebel, K., Bauman, A. E., Sugiyama, T., & Owen, N. (2011). Mismatch between perceived and objectively assessed neighborhood walkability attributes: Prospective relationships with walking and weight gain. *Health and Place, 17*(2), 519–524.

Ghekiere, A., Carver, A., Veitch, J., Salmon, J., Deforche, B., & Timperio, A. (2016). Does parental accompaniment when walking or cycling moderate the association between physical neighborhood environment and active transport among 10–12 year old? *Journal of Science and Medicine in Sport, 19*(2), 149–153.

Ghekiere, A., Deforche, B., Mertens, L., De Bourdeaudhuij, I., Clarys, P., de Geus, B., . . . Van Cauwenberg, J. (2015). Creating cycling-friendly environments for children: Which micro-scale factors are most important? An experimental study using manipulated photographs. *PLoS One, 10*(12), e0143302.

Ghekiere, A., Van Cauwenberg, J., de Geus, B., Clarys, P., Cardon, G., Salmon, J., . . . Deforche, B. (2014). Critical environmental factors for transportation cycling in children: A qualitative study using bike-along interviews. *PLoS One, 9*(9), e106696.

Ghekiere, A., Van Cauwenberg, J., Mertens, L., Clarys, P., de Geus, B., Cardon, G., . . . Deforche, B. (2015). Assessing cycling-friendly environments for children: Are micro-environmental factors equally import-ant across different street settings? *International Journal of Behavioral Nutrition and Physical Activity, 12*, 54.

Giles-Corti, B., Foster, S., Shilton, T., & Falconer, R. (2010). The co-benefits for health of investing in active transportation. *NSW Public Health Bulletin, 21*(5–6), 122–127.

Giles-Corti, B., Kelty, S. F., Zubrick, S. R., & Villanueva, K. P. (2009). Encouraging walking for transport and physical activity in children and adolescents: How important is the built environment? *Sports Medicine, 39*(12), 995–1009.

Giles-Corti, B., Timperio, A., Bull, F., & Pikora, T. (2005). Understanding physical activity environmental correlates: Increased specificity for ecological models. *Exercise and Sport Science Reviews, 33*(4), 175–181.

Giles-Corti, B., Wood, G., Pikora, T., Learnihan, V., Bulsara, M., Van Niel, K., . . . Villanueva, K. (2011). School site and the potential to walk to school: The impact of street connectivity and traffic exposure in school neighborhoods. *Health and Place, 17*(2), 545–550.

Gray, C., Gibbons, R., Larouche, R., Sandseter, E., Bienenstock, A., Brussoni, M., . . . Tremblay, M. S. (2015). What is the relationship between outdoor time and physical activity, sedentary behaviour, and physical fitness in children? A systematic review. *International Journal of Environmental Research and Public Health, 12*(6), 6455–6474.

Handy, S., Cao, X., & Mokhtarian, P. (2008). Neighborhood design and children's outdoor play: Evidence from Northern California. *Children, Youth and Environments, 18*(2), 160–179.

Hansen, A. Y., Umstattd Meyer, M. R., Lenardson, J. D., & Hartley, D. (2015). Built environments and active living in rural and remote areas: A review of the literature. *Current Obesity Reports, 4*(4), 484–493.

Harris, J. K., Lecy, J., Hipp, J. A., Brownson, R. C., & Parra, D. C. (2013). Mapping the development of research on physical activity and the built environment. *Preventive Medicine, 57*(5), 533–540.

Heidelberger, L., & Smith, C. (2016). Low-income, urban children's perspectives on physical activity: A photovoice project. *Maternal and Child Health Journal, 20*(6), 1124–1132.

Hennessy, E., Kraak, V. I., Hyatt, R. R., Bloom, J., Fenton, M., Wagoner, C., & Economos, C. D. (2010). Active living for rural children community perspectives using PhotoVOICE. *American Journal of Preventive Medicine, 39*(6), 537–545.

Hillman, M., Adams, J., & Whitelegg, J. (1990). *One false move... A study of children's independent mobility.* London, UK: PSI Publishing.

Hunter, R. F., Christian, H., Veitch, J., Astell-Burt, T., Hipp, J. A., & Schipperijn, J. (2015). The impact of interventions to promote physical activity in urban green space: A systematic review and recommenda-tions for future research. *Social Science in Medicine, 124*, 246–256.

Knaap, G., & Talen, E. (2005). New urbanism and smart growth: A few words from the academy. *International Regional Science Review, 28*(2), 107–118.

Koohsari, M. J., Mavoa, S., Villanueva, K., Sugiyama, T., Badland, H., Kaczynski, A. T., . . . Giles-Corti, B. (2015). Public open space, physical activity, urban design and public health: Concepts, methods and research agenda. *Health and Place, 33*, 75–82.

Kurt, O. K., Zhang, J., & Pinkerton, K. E. (2016). Pulmonary health effects of air pollution. *Current Opinion in Pulmonary Medicine, 22*(2), 138–143.

Lal, A., Moodie, M., Abbott, G., Carver, A., Salmon, J., Giles-Corti, B., . . . Veitch, J. (2019). The impact of a park refurbishment in a low socioeconomic area on physical activity: A cost-effectiveness study. *International Journal of Behavioral Nutrition and Physical Activity, 16*(1), 26.

Larouche, R., Sarmiento, O. L., Broyles, S. T., Denstel, K. D., Church, T. S., Barreira, T. V., . . . ISCOLE Research Group. (2015). Are the correlates of active school transport context-specific? *International Journal of Obesity, 5*(Suppl 2), S89–S99.

Lee, R. E., Soltero, E. G., Jauregui, A., Mama, S. K., Barquera, S., Jauregui, E., . . . Levesque, L. (2016). Dis-entangling associations of neighborhood street scale elements with physical activity in Mexican school children. *Environment and Behavior, 48*(1), 150–171.

Limstrand, T. (2008). Environmental characteristics relevant to young people's use of sports facilities: A review. *Scandinavian Journal of Medicine and Science in Sports, 18*(3), 275–287.

Loebach, J., & Gilliland, J. (2010). Child-led tours to uncover childrens' perceptions and use of neighbor-hood environments. *Children, Youth and Environments, 20*(1), 52–90.

Macintyre, S., Ellaway, A., & Cummins, S. (2002). Place effects on health: How can we conceptualise, op-erationalise and measure them? *Social Science and Medicine, 55*(1), 125–139.

MacMillan, F., George, E. S., Feng, X., Merom, D., Bennie, A., Cook, A., . . . Astell-Burt, T. (2018). Do natural experiments of changes in neighborhood built environment impact physical activity and diet? A systematic review. *International Journal of Environmental Research and Public Health, 15*(2), E217.

Matsudo, V. (2012). The role of partnerships in promoting physical activity: The experience of Agita Sao Paulo. *Health and Place, 18*(1), 121–122.

Matthews, S. A. (2008). The salience of neighborhood – Some lessons from sociology. *American Journal of Preventive Medicine, 34*(3), 257–259.

Matthews, S. A., & Yang, T. C. (2013). Spatial polygamy and contextual exposures (SPACEs): Promoting activity space approaches in research on place and health. *American Behavioral Scientist, 57*(8), 1057–1081.

McCormack, G. R., & Shiell, A. (2011). In search of causality: A systematic review of the relationship between the built environment and physical activity among adults. *International Journal of Behavioral Nutrition and Physical Activity, 8*, 125.

McDonald, N. C., Steiner, R. L., Lee, C., Smith, T. R., Zhu, X. M., & Yang, Y. Z. (2014). Impact of the safe routes to school program on walking and bicycling. *Journal of the American Planning Association, 80*(2), 153–167.

McGrath, L. J., Hopkins, W. G., & Hinckson, E. A. (2015). Associations of objectively measured built-environment attributes with youth moderate-vigorous physical activity: A systematic review and meta-analysis. *Sports Medicine, 45*(6), 841–865.

Mertens, L., Van Cauwenberg, J., Veitch, J., Deforche, B., & Van Dyck, D. (2019). Differences in park characteristic preferences for visitation and physical activity among adolescents: A latent class analysis. *PLoS One, 14*(3), e0212920.

Muthuri, S. K., Wachira, L. J., Onywera, V. O., & Tremblay, M. S. (2016). Associations between parental perceptions of the neighborhood environment and childhood physical activity: Results from ISCOLE-Kenya. *Journal of Physical Activity and Health, 13*(3), 333–343.

Nicosia, N., & Datar, A. (2018). Neighborhood environments and physical activity: A longitudinal study of adolescents in a natural experiment. *American Journal of Preventive Medicine, 54*(5), 671–678.

Oliveira, A. F., Moreira, C., Abreu, S., Mota, J., & Santos, R. (2014). Environmental determinants of physical activity in children: A systematic review. *Archives of Exercise in Health and Disease, 4*(2), 254–261.

Orstad, S. L., McDonough, M. H., Stapleton, S., Altincekic, C., & Troped, P. J. (2017). A systematic review of agreement between perceived and objective neighborhood environment measures and associations with physical activity outcomes. *Environment and Behavior, 49*(8), 904–932.

Oyeyemi, A. L., Kasoma, S. S., Onywera, V. O., Assah, F., Adedoyin, R. A., Conway, T. L., . . . Sallis, J. F. (2016). NEWS for Africa: Adaptation and reliability of a built environment questionnaire for physical activity in seven African countries. *International Journal of Behavioral Nutrition and Physical Activity, 13*, 33.

Panter, J., Corder, K., Griffin, S. J., Jones, A. P., & van Sluijs, E. M. (2013). Individual, socio-cultural and environmental predictors of uptake and maintenance of active commuting in children: Longitudinal results from the SPEEDY study. *International Journal of Behavioral Nutrition and Physical Activity, 10*, 83.

Panter, J. R., Jones, A. P., & van Sluijs, E. M. (2008). Environmental determinants of active travel in youth: A review and framework for future research. *International Journal of Behavioral Nutrition and Physical Activity, 5*, 34.

Pont, K., Ziviani, J., Wadley, D., Bennett, S., & Abbott, R. (2009). Environmental correlates of children's active transportation: A systematic literature review. *Health and Place, 15*(3), 827–840.

Prins, R. G., Oenema, A., van der Horst, K., & Brug, J. (2009). Objective and perceived availability of physical activity opportunities: Differences in associations with physical activity behavior among urban adolescents. *International Journal of Behavioral Nutrition and Physical Activity, 6*, 70.

Rainham, D. G., Bates, C. J., Blanchard, C. M., Dummer, T. J., Kirk, S. F., & Shearer, C. L. (2012). Spatial classification of youth physical activity patterns. *American Journal of Preventive Medicine, 42*(5), e87–e96.

Raza, W., Forsberg, B., Johansson, C., & Sommar, J. N. (2018). Air pollution as a risk factor in health impact assessments of a travel mode shift towards cycling. *Global Health Action, 11*(1), 1429081.

Rhodes, R. E., Saelens, B. E., & Sauvage-Mar, C. (2018). Understanding physical activity through interactions between the built environment and social cognition: A systematic review. *Sports Medicine, 48*(8), 1893–1912.

Rosenberg, D., Ding, D., Sallis, J. F., Kerr, J., Norman, G. J., Durant, N., . . . Saelens, B. E. (2009). Neighborhood environment walkability scale for youth (NEWS-Y): Reliability and relationship with physical activity. *Preventive Medicine, 49*(2–3), 213–218.

Saelens, B. E., Sallis, J. F., Black, J. B., & Chen, D. (2003). Neighborhood-based differences in physical activity: An environment scale evaluation. *American Journal of Public Health, 93*(9), 1552–1558.

Saelens, B. E., Sallis, J. F., & Frank, L. D. (2003). Environmental correlates of walking and cycling: Findings from the transportation, urban design, and planning literatures. *Annals of Behavioral Medicine, 25*(2), 80–91.

Sallis, J. F. (2009). Measuring physical activity environments: A brief history. *American Journal of Preventive Medicine, 36*(4 Suppl), S86–92.

Sallis, J. F., Bull, F., Guthold, R., Heath, G. W., Inoue, S., Kelly, P., . . . Lancet Physical Activity Series 2 Executive Committee. (2016). Progress in physical activity over the olympic quadrennium. *Lancet, 388*(10051), 1325–1336.

Sallis, J. F., Cervero, R. B., Ascher, W., Henderson, K. A., Kraft, M. K., & Kerr, J. (2006). An ecological approach to creating active living communities. *Annual Review of Public Health, 27*, 297–322.

Sallis, J. F., Floyd, M. F., Rodriguez, D. A., & Saelens, B. E. (2012). Role of built environments in physical activity, obesity, and cardiovascular disease. *Circulation, 125*(5), 729–737.

Sallis, J. F., & Owen, N. (2015). Ecological models of health behavior. In K. Glanz, B. K. Rimer, & K. "V." Viswanath (Eds.), *Health behavior: Theory, research, and practice* (p. 43–64). San Francisco, USA: Jossey-Bass.

Sallis, J. F., Prochaska, J. J., & Taylor, W. C. (2000). A review of correlates of physical activity of children and adolescents. *Medicine and Science in Sports and Exercise, 32*(5), 963–975.

Sallis, J. F., Spoon, C., Cavill, N., Engelberg, J. K., Gebel, K., Parker, M., . . . Ding, D. (2015). Co-benefits of designing communities for active living: An exploration of literature. *International Journal of Behavioral Nutrition and Physical Activity, 12*, 30.

Sallis, J. F., Story, M., & Lou, D. (2009). Study designs and analytic strategies for environmental and policy research on obesity, physical activity, and diet: Recommendations from a meeting of experts. *American Journal of Preventive Medicine, 36*(2 Suppl), S72–S77.

Sawyer, A. D. M., Jones, R., Ucci, M., Smith, L., Kearns, A., & Fisher, A. (2017). Cross-sectional interactions between quality of the physical and social environment and self-reported physical activity in adults living in income-deprived communities. *PLoS One, 12*(12), e0188962.

Sinharay, R., Gong, J., Barratt, B., Ohman-Strickland, P., Ernst, S., Kelly, F. J., . . . Chung, K. F. (2018). Respiratory and cardiovascular responses to walking down a traffic-polluted road compared with walking in a traffic-free area in participants aged 60 years and older with chronic lung or heart disease and age-matched healthy controls: A randomised, crossover study. *Lancet, 391*(10118), 339–349.

Tainio, M., de Nazelle, A. J., Gotschi, T., Kahlmeier, S., Rojas-Rueda, D., Nieuwenhuijsen, M. J., . . . Woodcock, J. (2016). Can air pollution negate the health benefits of cycling and walking? *Preventive Medicine, 87*, 233–236.

Timperio, A., Reid, J., & Veitch, J. (2015). Playability: Built and social environment features that promote physical activity within children. *Current Obesity Reports, 4*(4), 460–476.

Timperio, A., Veitch, J., & Sahlqvist, S. (2018). Built and physical environment correlates of active transportation. In R. Larouche (Ed.), *Children's active transportation* (pp. 141–153). Amsterdam, Netherlands: Elsevier.

Trang, N. H. H. D., Hong, T. K., & Dibley, M. J. (2012). Active commuting to school among adolescents in Ho Chi Minh City, Vietnam change and predictors in a longitudinal study, 2004 to 2009. *American Journal of Preventive Medicine, 42*(2), 120–128.

Transportation Research Board, & Institute of Medicine. (2005). *Does the built environment influence physical activity?: Examining the evidence–special report 282.* Washington, DC: The National Academies Press.

United Nations, Department of Economic and Social Affairs, Population Division. (2019). *World urbanization prospects: The 2018 revision (ST/ESA/SER.A/420).* New York, NY: United Nations. Retrieved from https://population.un.org/wup/Publications/Files/WUP2018-Report.pdf

Van Cauwenberg, J., De Bourdeaudhuij, I., Clarys, P., Nasar, J., Salmon, J., Goubert, L., & Deforche, B. (2016). Street characteristics preferred for transportation walking among older adults: A choice-based conjoint analysis with manipulated photographs. *International Journal of Behavioral Nutrition and Physical Activity, 13*, 6.

Van Hecke, L., Deforche, B., Van Dyck, D., De Bourdeaudhuij, I., Veitch, J., & Van Cauwenberg, J. (2016). Social and physical environmental factors influencing adolescents' physical activity in urban public open spaces: A qualitative study using walk-along interviews. *PLoS One, 11*(5), e0155686.

Van Hecke, L., Ghekiere, A., Van Cauwenberg, J., Veitch, J., De Bourdeaudhuije, I., Van Dyck, D., . . . Deforche, B. (2018). Park characteristics preferred for adolescent park visitation and physical activity: A choice-based conjoint analysis using manipulated photographs. *Landscape and Urban Planning, 178*, 144–155.

Van Hecke, L., Ghekiere, A., Veitch, J., Van Dyck, D., Van Cauwenberg, J., Clarys, P., & Deforche, B. (2018). Public open space characteristics influencing adolescents' use and physical activity: A systematic literature review of qualitative and quantitative studies. *Health and Place, 51*, 158–173.

Van Hecke, L., Verhoeven, H., Clarys, P., Van Dyck, D., Van de Weghe, N., Baert, T., . . . Van Cauwenberg, J. (2018). Factors related with public open space use among adolescents: A study using GPS and accelerometers. *International Journal of Health Geographics, 17*(1), 3.

Vanwolleghem, G., Van Dyck, D., Ducheyne, F., De Bourdeaudhuij, I., & Cardon, G. (2014). Assessing the environmental characteristics of cycling routes to school: A study on the reliability and validity of a Google Street View-based audit. *International Journal of Health Geographics, 13*, 19.

Veitch, J., Bagley, S., Ball, K., & Salmon, J. (2006). Where do children usually play? A qualitative study of parents' perceptions of influences on children's active free-play. *Health and Place, 12*(4), 383–393.

Veitch, J., Ball, K., Crawford, D., Abbott, G. R., & Salmon, J. (2012). Park improvements and park activity: A natural experiment. *American Journal of Preventive Medicine, 42*(6), 616–619.

Veitch, J., Salmon, J., & Ball, K. (2008). Children's active free play in local neighborhoods: A behavioral mapping study. *Health Education Research, 23*(5), 870–879.

Veitch, J., Salmon, J., & Ball, K. (2010). Individual, social and physical environmental correlates of children's active free-play: A cross-sectional study. *International Journal of Behavioral Nutrition and Physical Activity, 7*, 11.

Veitch, J., Salmon, J., Carver, A., Timperio, A., Crawford, D., Fletcher, E., & Giles-Corti, B. (2014). A natural experiment to examine the impact of park renewal on park-use and park-based physical activity in a disadvantaged neighborhood: The REVAMP study methods. *BMC Public Health, 14*, 600.

Veitch, J., Salmon, J., Crawford, D., Abbott, G., Giles-Corti, B., Carver, A., & Timperio, A. (2018). The REVAMP natural experiment study: The impact of a play-scape installation on park visitation and park-based physical activity. *International Journal of Behavioral Nutrition and Physical Activity, 15*(1), 10.

Veitch, J., Salmon, J., Giles-Corti, B., Crawford, D., Dullaghan, K., Carver, A., & Timperio, A. (2017). Challenges in conducting natural experiments in the built environment – Lessons from the REVAMP study. *International Journal of Behavioral Nutrition and Physical Activity, 14*, 5.

Veitch, J., Salmon, J., Parker, K., Bangay, S., Deforche, B., & Timperio, A. (2016). Adolescents' ratings of features of parks that encourage park visitation and physical activity. *International Journal of Behavioral Nutrition and Physical Activity, 13*, 73.

Verhoeven, H., Ghekiere, A., Van Cauwenberg, J., Van Dyck, D., De Bourdeaudhuij, I., Clarys, P., & Deforche, B. (2017). Which physical and social environmental factors are most important for adolescents' cycling for transport? An experimental study using manipulated photographs. *International Journal of Behavioral Nutrition and Physical Activity, 14*(1), 108.

Wang, X., Conway, T. L., Cain, K. L., Frank, L. D., Saelens, B. E., Geremia, C., . . . Sallis, J. F. (2017). Interactions of psychosocial factors with built environments in explaining adolescents' active transportation. *Preventive Medicine, 100*, 76–83.

World Health Organization. (2018). *Global action plan on physical activity 2018–2030: More active people for a healthier world.* Geneva, Switzerland: WHO.

Xu, F., Li, J., Liang, Y., Wang, Z., Hong, X., Ware, R. S., . . . Owen, N. (2010). Associations of residential density with adolescents' physical activity in a rapidly urbanizing area of Mainland China. *Journal of Urban Health, 87*(1), 44–53.

11

SCHOOL AND COMMUNITY POLICIES

Implications for Youth Physical Activity and Research

Monica A. F. Lounsbery, Thomas L. McKenzie, and Nicole J. Smith

This chapter provides an overview of the nature of school and community policies in relation to youth physical activity and research. To accomplish this, we have divided the chapter into three sections. To begin, we provide an introduction that highlights the complex problem of sedentary living and the need to increase physical activity among youth in school and community environments, and we discuss both school and community sources of physical activity for youth. In the next section, we discuss policy and their implications for increasing youth physical activity. We describe policy, how they are formulated and enacted, and their relationship to practices. Lastly, we provide an overview of physical activity policy research. To accomplish this, we provide a general description of the nature of school policy research and findings, and close with a brief overview of recommended research resources.

Overview of the Literature

As described in Chapters 5–7, physical activity is essential for the growth and development of children and adolescents and to their current and future health (2018 Physical Activity Guidelines Advisory Committee, 2018). Additionally, there is growing evidence of its contributions to academic behavior and achievement (CDC, 2010). Sedentary living remains a public health concern worldwide and in response the World Health Organization (WHO) recently released its *Global Action Plan on Physical Activity for 2018–2030: More Active People for a Healthier World* (WHO, 2018a). This plan calls for children and adolescents aged 5–17 years to engage in at least 60 minutes of moderate to vigorous physical activity (MVPA) daily that includes muscle- and bone-strengthening activities at least three times per week.

Approximately 80% of adolescents do not meet these recommendations (WHO, 2018b), and among the most serious consequences of physical inactivity is increased risk for overweight and obesity. Worldwide rates of these conditions have risen sharply in the past 20 years, and in 2016 an estimated 41 million children under 5 years of age were classified as overweight with the count rising to 340 million when those aged 5–19 were considered (WHO, 2018c).

Physical activity is complex and the accrual of it extends well beyond purposeful exercise and active play – therefore promoting and assessing its occurrence are challenging endeavors. WHO (2011, p. 1), for example, identified that for children and youths, "... physical activity includes play, games, sports, transportation, chores, recreation, physical education (PE), or planned exercise, in the context of family, school, and community activities." Thus, physical activity occurs in numerous locations and in situations where it is influenced via specific contexts – some of which are physical (e.g., structures, equipment, people) and others are sociocultural (e.g., regulations, prompts/reinforcers/punishers for being active).

The complexity of physical activity as part of diverse environments has also been recognized by the Active Healthy Kids Global Alliance, which has supported the development and dissemination of country Report Cards on youth physical activity (Tremblay et al., 2016). These Report Cards use a standardized grading framework (from A = excellent to F = failing) to assess nine separate indicators: Overall Physical Activity, Organized Sport Participation, Active Play, Active Transportation, Sedentary Behavior, Family and Peers, School, Community and the Built Environment, and Government Strategies and Investments. In 2016, 38 countries from 6 continents (representing 60% of the world's population) presented Report Cards at the International Congress on Physical Activity and Public Health in Bangkok, Thailand. The results for each of these countries are available at https://www.activehealthykids.org. While there was substantial variability in indicator grades and across countries, the average grade for physical activity indicators around the world was poor (e.g., a "D" grade). The 2018 Report Cards for 49 countries were recently released by the Active Healthy Kids Global Alliance at the "Global Matrix 3.0" meeting in Adelaide on November 27, 2018. Summaries for the countries and four related papers are available free in a special edition of the *Journal of Physical Activity and Health*.

The need to promote and to subsequently assess changes in child and adolescent physical activity as it occurs in diverse locations is obvious. Studying policies (e.g., laws, rules, regulations) related to physical activity in specific environments is particularly important because policies affect everyone who uses that setting. Investigations using an ecological approach involve considering multiple spheres of influence that include targeting individuals, social environments, physical environments, and policies in order to affect population change (Sallis et al., 2006). Ecological models are particularly well-suited for studying physical activity and public health because they incorporate people's interactions with their physical and sociocultural settings and they specifically include environmental and policy variables (Sallis & Owen, 2015; Stokols, 1992). As a minimum, it is important to identify the times and places of physical activity and to assess the resources and barriers that might hinder or facilitate physical activity there. Once these factors are identified, the environment can be modified to attract people to the location and engage them actively.

Widespread (e.g., national, global) studies using an ecological approach in diverse settings have yet to be conducted. Nonetheless, of the many venues where children and adolescents engage in physical activity, schools settings are studied most often, and Lounsbery (2017) recently provided a thorough discussion of how policies affect physical activity within school environments. Schools are particularly important for promoting physical activity because they reach nearly all children and for extended time periods. All countries have established recommendations for PE programs, and most of these recognize the importance of students engaging in developmentally appropriate MVPA in order to develop physical fitness, motor skills, and related behaviors that will support engagement in lifetime physical activity (UNESCO, 2014; Pühse & Gerber, 2005).

A few global efforts have been initiated to assess PE and other school-based PA opportunities. In addition to the country Report Cards initiated by The Active Healthy Kids Global Alliance (Tremblay et al., 2016), the United Nations Educational, Scientific and Cultural Organization (UNESCO) recently conducted a worldwide survey of PE in 232 countries (UNESCO, 2015). While these efforts demonstrate a widespread commitment to monitoring PE and improving its quality, the data are limited because objective assessment tools have not been widely adopted. Nonetheless, similar to those found in the U.S. (McKenzie & Lounsbery, 2009), there are common barriers that impact the quantity and quality of PE, including limited class schedules, inadequately trained teachers, lack of curricular resources, and insufficient equipment and facilities.

PE is only one school physical activity program, and a whole-of-school approach toward increasing physical activity on school campuses is being advanced. These approaches are frequently referred to as "Comprehensive School Physical Activity Programs" (CSPAP; CDC, 2013; Institute of Medicine, 2013). CSPAPs involve collaborative efforts to promote and provide physical activity within a variety of structured and unstructured school contexts (e.g., PE; recess; before-, during-, and after-school sport; dance; exercise; and play opportunities). The widespread adoption, feasibility, and effectiveness of CSPAPs and their various components are still not well known, and the *School Health Profiles 2016* reported only about 3% of secondary schools in the U.S. had a full CSPAP (Brener et al., 2017). Meanwhile, the National Federation of State High School Associations (NFHS) indicated that nearly 8 million adolescents (4.6 million boys, 3.4 million girls in 2017–2018) participate annually in high school athletic programs in the U.S. alone (NFHS, 2018).

In community settings, organized youth sport has consistently been identified as an important context for physical activity accrual. In addition to school settings, (e.g., after-school programs and summer camps), youth sports programs are often organized as part of public park and recreational offerings, private sports clubs, and faith-based programs (e.g., church sport leagues), and studies have shown that youths engage in substantially more MVPA on "sport" days than on "non-sport" days (Machado-Rodrigues et al., 2012; Wickel & Eisenmann, 2007).

Local park and recreation settings are also important locations for non-sport, leisure time physical activity. In the U.S., for example, 89% of neighborhood parks in a nationally representative study had playgrounds that supported the physical activity of young people, and many adults reported that they came to parks to accompany their children (Cohen et al., 2016). Increasing the variety of playground features (e.g., climbing apparatus) and adding amenities such as restrooms have been shown to have potential for increasing playground use and MVPA. Direct observations of 147 nationally representative playgrounds in 25 U.S. cities, for example, found that most playgrounds had features that promoted swinging, climbing, and sliding, but less than half of them had features that supported spinning, balancing, crawling, and sand or water play. Each additional feature increased playground use substantially, and those with restrooms, spinning equipment, and splashpads attracted more users and generated more on-site MVPA than playgrounds without those features (Cohen et al., 2020). While studies such as these indicate that neighborhood parks are certainly not created equal, they do indicate that local park and recreation settings are rich resources that support child and adolescent physical activity.

Lastly, countries, cities, and communities can promote safe active transportation (e.g., walking and biking to and from school) by designing built environments and enacting policies to support pedestrian needs and improve access to parks and other recreation spaces. Studies on the built environment have identified aspects of the community that have important implications for walking or biking to destinations, and these include residential density, mixed land use, and short distances to destinations (e.g., Frank, Kerr, Chapman, & Sallis, 2007; Gordon-Larsen, Nelson, Page & Popkin, 2006; Saelens & Handy, 2008). Research has also found that parent perceptions of personal safety from traffic and other hazards have important implications for walking and biking and that children who walk or bike to school accumulate more physical activity than their counterparts who are driven (McMillan, 2009).

Key Issues

About Policy

Though school and community settings provide youths with opportunities for physical activity in both structured and unstructured ways, factors within the settings may hinder physical activity accrual. For example, physical activity in PE can be limited when lessons are canceled, delivered in ineffective ways, and/or have inadequate equipment and facilities. Once these hindrances are known, potential policy solutions can be identified, analyzed, and prioritized (CDC, 2017a, 2017b).

From an ecological perspective, physical activity policies are appealing because they have the potential to change guiding principles and procedures within an environment to target specific actions and behaviors (Brownson et al., 2001). Public policy determines what services will be provided, and in school and community settings policies shape the structure of programs (e.g., how much, how often, and who delivers them) as well as their function (e.g., aim, scope, and expected outcomes). Additionally, policies inform community physical environments, including the design and siting locations for homes, schools, parks, and businesses. For interventionists, policies hold wide appeal because once established, they continue as part of the environment and affect behaviors over time.

Public policies are a result of a deliberative process and take the form of laws, constitutions, charters, regulations, ordinances, statutes, resolutions, and administrative actions. These can be local, county, state/provincial, and/or federal in nature. They are formalized in writing and most often are linked to a specific environmental context. For example, schools have numerous contexts (e.g., PE, interscholastic sports), in which specific physical activity policies exist and these guide the prevalence and delivery of programs (commonly referred to as "practices"). Practices include not only the frequency and the duration of programs (e.g., PE; recess; classroom physical activity breaks; and before-, during-, and after-school programs), but also aspects such as program content and how it is delivered and by whom. Practices also relate indirectly to aspects such as staff training; program funding; and the design, use, and maintenance of school facilities. Numerous school-based physical activity studies have been conducted, resulting in the identification of multiple evidence-based school practices for optimizing children's physical activity (McKenzie & Lounsbery, 2009; Sallis et al., 2012) and the development and promotion of school physical activity policy recommendations (e.g., IOM, 2013).

Although communities, through administrative actions, may establish policies that directly impact physical activity (e.g., parks and recreation facility design, hours of operation, types of programing), community policies are typically global and more distal from physical activity itself (e.g., municipal zoning, urban containment, and land use policies). For example, rapid growth and urban sprawl present challenges for communities such as reduced farmland and green space, and increasing traffic, air pollution, and school crowding. As a result, urban sprawl increases distances between salient locations, subsequently requiring time and inactive modes of transportation (e.g., cars, buses) to reach destinations and thus reducing overall time available for leisure and time that could be used for physical activity. Policy responses to alleviate or contain urban sprawl, although not directly aimed at physical activity, might affect it positively (e.g., increase community walkability).

Policy proposals and their enactment and implementation involve many actors, and legislative bodies play a primary role in public policy decisions. In the U.S., legislative bodies exist at both state and local levels of government. A clear description of local policy making is provided by the Municipal Research & Services Center of Washington (1999, p. 11),

> At the local level, city, town, and county councilmembers and county commissioners are legislators. Together they constitute a legislative body which is given authority by the state constitution and state law to make local law. Local legislative authority is generally limited to what the state specifically grants to counties, cities and towns.

Different forms of government exist, and thus, there is variability in how policies are formulated and implemented. In many instances an elected official, such as a mayor, serves as the presiding member of the city council and has a major role in proposing and formulating policies and in implementing them. Authority for policy implementation, however, is typically delegated to heads of city departments who hire and fire employees and perform administrative actions that are consistent within a defined scope of work. In some cases, these administrative actions form practice and policies of their own which could have implications for physical activity, such as neighborhood police patrols, bus routes, traffic abatement, and rules establishing the hours of operation for park and recreation programs.

Relative to school policy making, the vast majority of public education in the U.S. is funded by a state tax base which is often supplemented by local governments through property and other tax forms. States work with local governments to establish local education agencies which are commonly known as school districts. While school siting and zoning policies are typically determined by city councils, policies and procedures related to curricula and graduation requirements are normally established at the state level. Hence, like communities, schools have multiple actors playing roles in formulating policy and these actors are at different levels. At the state level, the state legislature, governor, superintendent, and school board have pivotal roles in policy formulation. At the local level, the school district superintendent, school board, and curriculum directors play roles that are germane to policy formulation and implementation. Additionally, many school districts subscribe to site-based management and this gives local schools substantial authority over their programs which might include funding, facilities, and hiring practices. Thus, state school laws (and their implementation) impact district policy, and this in turn impacts individual school policy and environmental conditions that affect student physical activity (Lounsbery, McKenzie, Morrow Jr, Monnat, & Holt, 2013).

The nature of both school and community and governance structures germane to the formulation and implementation of policies is complex; therefore, the relationship between policies and youth physical activity is also complex. In schools, for example, the interrelationship between policies and practices and the nested nature of classes within schools, schools within districts, and districts within states make assessing children's physical activity relative to policy challenging. Furthermore, even when policies are enacted, there may not be compliance. Even full compliance to a policy does not guarantee changes will be made in physical activity engagement. For example, a school might comply with a state policy of providing 30 minutes of PE daily; however, research indicates that PE is commonly provided in ways that do not fully optimize the accrual of MVPA (McKenzie & Lounsbery, 2009). In the next section, we provide an overview of physical activity policy research including its general nature and sample findings.

Emerging Issues

Physical Activity Policy Research

Research on physical activity policy has been conducted for little over two decades – thus, it is still in its infancy in terms of producing knowledge advancement and generalizable findings. As described previously, the complex nature of policies and the nuances of policy making and implementing it in diverse settings make policy research challenging. Subsequently, near all existing physical activity policy research is descriptive or correlational in nature, and in a broad sense it has focused on assessing the policy prevalence and enactment, policy implementation, and policy associations. As illustration, we use these three broad areas to outline school policy research as community policy research is similarly focused. The information we present is not intended to be exhaustive, but to provide a general understanding of physical activity policy research and shed light on emergent priorities for investigators.

Policy Prevalence and Enactment

Physical activity policy prevalence studies assess the presence of specific policies (e.g., school recess) in specific contexts (e.g., elementary schools). In the U.S., two significant national-level efforts conduct surveillance of physical activity policies in schools. The Division of Adolescent School Health within the Center for Disease Control and Prevention administers the *School Health Policies and Practices Study* (SHPPS; CDC, 2017a). SHPPS assesses school health policies and practices at the state, district, school, and classroom levels and includes physical activity. In addition, the Society of Health and Physical Educators (SHAPE America) conducts periodic assessments of PE policies in U.S. schools and publishes findings in the *Shape of the Nation* report (SHAPE America, 2016).

Unfortunately, the most recent findings from both the SHPPS and *Shape of the Nation* reports highlight that many opportunities for improving physical activity within school environments are being missed. For example, SHPPS (CDC, 2017b) reported only two states were meeting the national recommendations for weekly time in PE at both the elementary and middle school levels, and the 2016 *Shape of the Nation* report found that fewer than ten states required daily recess in elementary schools (SHAPE America, 2016).

Surveillance of physical activity policies is also a priority for international researchers (Ramirez-Varela et al., 2017; Bauman, Nelson, Pratt, Matsudo, & Schoeppe, 2006). The International Society for Physical Activity and Health (ISPAH) Global Observatory for Physical Activity (GoPA!), for example, conducts surveillance of international physical activity policy and research with the goal of increasing global physical activity. Their early findings indicated positive relationships between policy prevalence, policy surveillance, and policy research, suggesting that research and surveillance may play an important role in informing policy (Hallal & Ramirez, 2015).

In addition to large-scale surveillance efforts, other researchers have conducted policy prevalence studies using instrumentation designed specifically for assessing physical activity policies in individual schools and school districts (e.g., S-PAPA; Lounsbery, McKenzie, Morrow Jr, Holt, & Budnar, 2013) and communities (e.g., CHANGE; Lillehoj, Daniel-Ulloa, & Nothwehr, 2016).

While studies of the prevalence of policies are valuable, they are typically limited to only self-reported data (e.g., SHPPS and the *Shape of the Nation* reports). Additional general limitations are that prevalence studies usually fall short of assessing policy strength, implementation fidelity, and level of adoption. In consideration of these limitations, some researchers have broadened the scope of their physical activity policy research to investigate policy enactment.

Policy enactment studies are an extension of prevalence studies, and one of the most significant advances related to policy enactment research was the development of the Physical Education-Related State Policy Classification System (PERSPCS; Masse et al., 2007). PERSPCS was developed by experts based on methods employed by the National Cancer Institute to study tobacco laws, and it is available for researchers via the National Classification of Laws Associated with School Students website (C.L.A.S.S.; National Cancer Institute, 2014). C.L.A.S.S. is a scoring system that evaluates codified state laws that include school PE and nutrition.

Policy enactment studies often aim to understand how policies are formulated, accepted, interpreted, resisted, subverted, or adopted. For example, researchers may try to identify predictors of enactment in order to inform advocacy efforts. One such study reported that bill-level factors were stronger predictors of bill enactment (e.g., having more than one sponsor, bipartisan sponsors, introduction in the state senate) than state-level factors (e.g., duration of legislative session, and party in control) (Boehmer, Luke, Haire-Joshu, Bates, & Brownson 2008).

Policy enactment studies may also evaluate the strength of policies by evaluating the scope, specificity, and strength of the language used in the policies. In these studies, researchers commonly rate policy language from weak to strong (Carlson et al., 2013; Monnat, Lounsbery, & Smith, 2014; Schwartz et al., 2009; Taber et al., 2013). Strong policy language is important because language that is ambiguous or lacking specificity creates opportunities for "loopholes," potentially compromises the general policy aim (Anderson, 2003), and ultimately could limit the impact of a policy on children's accrual of physical activity.

Weakly worded laws are more prevalent than strongly worded ones (Carslon et al., 2013; Taber et al., 2013), and an important finding of physical activity policy enactment studies is that the requirements specified in laws generally fall short of professional recommendations and evidence-based practices. For example, only two U.S. states had laws requiring schools to provide the recommended number of weekly minutes (150 minutes for elementary and 225 for secondary schools), and of 16 states with recess laws, none required the recommended 30 minutes daily (National Cancer Institute, 2014). While only a few physical activity enactment policy studies have been conducted, they are still meaningful. Nonetheless, they are limited, in that they fall short of examining the extent to which policies are disseminated and implemented and they often do not examine the relationships between the implementation of policies and their effect on targeted behaviors/outcomes.

Policy Dissemination and Implementation

Dissemination refers to how policies are communicated and distributed to key constituents (e.g., administrators, teachers) in order to increase awareness of a policy and help ensure it is implemented with fidelity. Few studies have examined policy dissemination (Weatherson, Bradford, Berg, & Sloboda 2016); however, researchers may seek to understand the extent to which policies are adopted or to assess the multiple levels of influence that affect policy adoption. Studies could also examine barriers and facilitators related to policy dissemination, and these have value because what works in one setting may not necessarily work in another.

Strategies are needed to increase the likelihood of widespread dissemination and adoption of policies, and Bauman and colleagues (2006) developed a framework for disseminating international physical activity policies. Their framework suggests that developing evidence-based resources or innovations, defining the target audience, selecting communication channels, engaging decision-makers, and developing evaluation frameworks are all essential components to successful dissemination efforts (Bauman et al., 2006).

Only a few dissemination studies, however, have been conducted since the framework was proposed. In one, a timeline analysis to trace the history of school-based daily physical activity policies in Canada was conducted (Olstad, Campbell, Raine, & Nykiforuk 2015), and Lyn, Sheldon, and Eriksen (2017) conducted a similar analysis in Georgia, U.S. Both studies illustrated (a) the importance of identifying contextual factors that could potentially influence the widespread adoption of policies including the current social and political climate within the organization, and (b) the mobilization of key stakeholders that have a vested interest in the policy agenda. Currently, policy dissemination studies are limited, in that they do not necessarily assess the strength of policy language or the degree to which the policies are implemented.

Implementation refers to the extent to which access, practices, and programs reflect what is espoused within the policy language. It depends on a host of factors and includes, but may not be limited to, the clarity and strength of policy language (e.g., required vs. recommended), dissemination, adequate resources, and accountability measures. Implementation studies are extremely important because they help us to understand the effect of policies and their potential to change practices and ultimately, children's physical activity.

Policy implementation varies substantially from setting to setting, and so the results from individual studies may not generalize well to other settings. To date, researchers have reported that policy implementation plans are lacking (Stylianou & Walker, 2018), and if in place, they typically only include school self-reports of practice (Carlson et al., 2013). Others have examined the role that state organizations can play in monitoring policy implementation and identified opportunities to bolster implementation support particularly as it relates to compliance and impact evaluations (Craddock et al., 2013).

Policy Associations

Policy association studies are a broad category of research that generally aim to assess the associations between policies and outcomes of interest (e.g., access, practices, and programs). They are significant because they have potential to increase understanding about the influence or impact policies have on programs or practices (e.g., MVPA, physical fitness), and they have the potential to generate evidence that is useful for advocacy campaigns.

Researchers commonly view policy associations as an extension of policy prevalence and/or enactment studies. A number of researchers have used C.L.A.S.S. (e.g., PERSPCS) to assess relationships between strong and weak policies and other variables. For example, some studies have aimed to determine the correlates of enactment (e.g., Monnat, Lounsbery, & Smith, 2014), while others have assessed contextual influences on weight status among impoverished adolescents (Oh, Hennessy, McSpadden, & Perna 2015; Taber et al., 2013). Investigations such as these have consistently illustrated the importance of strong policies, as evidenced with disadvantaged populations where strong policies were associated with lower odds of being obese (Oh et al., 2015) and increased PE attendance and physical activity among girls (Taber et al., 2013).

As well, compliance with PE time policies may have important implications for health-fitness outcomes. One study, for example, found that students in school districts that complied with a state policy for PE time had greater odds of meeting the physical fitness standards than districts that did not comply (Sanchez-Vaznaugh et al., 2017). Researchers have also examined the associations between policy and exposure to an evidence-based program or practice (Slater, Nicholson, Chriqui, Turner, & Chaloupka 2012), engagement in MVPA (Kim, 2012), time in PE (Perna et al., 2012), and recess (Turner, Chriqui, & Chaloupka, 2013). The results of these studies have been mixed, but many have shown that state and district policies, even when worded weakly, have important implications for school practices (Slater et al., 2012).

Research Resources

Active Living Research, formerly a national program of the Robert Wood Johnson Foundation (2001–2013), was initiated under the visionary leadership of James F. Sallis, and it continues to play a substantial role in advancing physical activity policy research. Through its more than a decade-long program of competitive grantmaking, carefully designed annual meetings deliberately arranged to foster and support the growth and development of an international community of diverse, multidisciplinary researchers, and its extensive website repletes with research resources (e.g., archived research presentations, published papers, research syntheses, policy briefs, and research instrumentation), Active Living Research continues to be a major resource for researchers and others interested in promoting physical activity.

As we've emphasized throughout this chapter, the nature of physical activity policies is complex, and therefore researching the topic is challenging. As indicated previously, physical activity policies exist at different levels of enactment, including those initiated at the national, state/province, district, city, and local levels (e.g., schools, classes, parks, recreation centers). As well, there are differences in policy language (e.g., strong, such as 'schools will …', and weak, such as 'schools should …'), degrees of implementation (e.g., fully, partially, not at all), and the frequency and level of enforcement (e.g., annual monitoring with substantial penalties for non-compliance).

Nearly two decades ago, Bauman, Sallis, and Owen (2002) provided an overview of relevant measures to assess environmental and policy variables associated with physical activity. They indicated that self-reports, direct observation, existing records, and unobtrusive measures (e.g., electronic and video technology) were important for assessing environments and policies related to physical activity. Nonetheless, self-reports have remained the mainstay, and much of what we know about physical activity policies and practices comes from survey methods. While valuable at the macro level, surveys have limited utility when they are completed only by those distal to the activity sites, such as by officials in state/provincial or central city offices. And even when completed by those directly working in the same environment (e.g., schools), answers to questions may vary depending on respondent status/position (e.g., school principal, PE teacher) (Lounsbery, McKenzie, Holt et al., 2013). Surveys are also subject to potential recall error and social desirability bias, and response rates may be low if the results might cast them or their program in a negative light (Thompson et al., 2018).

Nonetheless, time and resources often limit researchers to self-report methods for collecting policy and practice data. In these cases, we recommend that the appropriate key informants be identified and that whenever possible they respond to items via an interview format. We have designed specific instrumentation and checklists for use with key informants in our own policy-related work. For example, we developed and validated the School Physical Activity Policy Assessment (S-PAPA) tool to assess district and school-level policy relative to physical activity practices at individual school sites (Lounsbery, McKenzie, Holt et al., 2013; Lounsbery, McKenzie, Morrow et al., 2013). S-PAPA uses open-ended, dichotomous, multichotomous, and checklist formatting, and has seven background items and three modules: (a) Physical Education (40 items); (b) Recess (27 items); and (c) Other Before-, During-, and After-School Programs (15 items). It assesses school- and district-level physical activity policy areas and related physical activity policy practices. It also includes background items on respondent's professional role, brief profile of the school and student composition, and the facilities (e.g., gymnasium, multipurpose room, fields) that are available for specific physical activity programs.

We also created PARC (Physical Activity Record for Classes) to generate information on the PA opportunities a school provides to students at the classroom unit level. It is typically completed by classroom teachers who specify opportunities for PA that their homeroom class receives during PE lessons, recess, active lunch recess periods, and PA breaks during the school day. PARC has been used in research studies to assess school PA policies (Lounsbery, McKenzie, Morrow et al., et al., 2013) and as a process measure during the CATCH (Child and Adolescent Trial for Cardiovascular Health) intervention (McKenzie et al., 1994).

Additionally, we created SPAS (Structured Physical Activity Survey) which was designed initially to assess participation in organized school physical activity programs beyond PE and free play sessions (e.g., recess) (Powers, Conway, McKenzie, Sallis, & Marshall, 2002). SPAS has also been used to investigate the shared use of school facilities by community organizations during the school day, on weekends, and over the summer (Carlton et al., 2017; Kanters et al., 2014). The on-site PA leader typically completes SPAS daily by recording the frequency and duration of sessions, how many males and females participated, when programs were offered, who sponsored them, and whether or not there was a participation fee. Total weekly hours are calculated for each program (number of participants x time) as well as overall for the site/school.

The above three tools assess environments and practices that provide opportunities for children and adolescents to accrue physical activity. They can be useful in providing insight into policy compliance, but it is important to emphasize that they do not assess physical activity itself! Assessing physical activity (both directly and indirectly) can be done in many ways, and in our work we have used heart rate monitoring, accelerometry, pedometry, self-reports, and direct observation. Relative to studying policy implementation, systematic observation has advantages over other methods. These include being a direct method that supports the generation of information on setting concurrent physical and social factors that have implications for policy (McKenzie, 2016; McKenzie & van der Mars, 2015). For more information about these methods, see Chapters 13–17.

As a direct method, systematic observation has strong internal (or face) validity, requires little or no participant burden, and can be conducted in locations where other assessment tactics don't work well (e.g., aquatic and martial arts settings). Instructional and assessment videos on the web make observer training readily available and reliable, and apps for electronic recording devices facilitate data entry and file sharing. Nonetheless, there are disadvantages to using direct observation, including the time and costs of training and recalibrating observers and potential participant reactivity.

Considerations for selecting observation instruments and training observers to use them reliably in both structured and unstructured activity settings have recently been described in "Top 10 Research Questions Related to Assessing Physical Activity and Its Contexts" (McKenzie & van der Mars, 2015) and in "Context matters: Systematic observation of place-based physical activity" (McKenzie, 2016). The latter paper emphasizes observational strategies for assessing group-level physical activity, an important consideration in "open" environments where people come and go in a seemingly indiscriminate manner (e.g., in parks and recreation settings). As physical activity is contextual, being able to assess the number of area users and their characteristics (e.g., gender, activity levels) in locations is important for both public health research and for helping practitioners assess their programs and policies.

While there are numerous direct observation systems, we describe only two here.

SOFIT: System for Observing Fitness Instruction Time

SOFIT is used primarily during instructional sessions (e.g., PE, dance, and sports) to simultaneously assess (a) *participant PA levels* (i.e., lying down, sitting, standing, walking/moderate, and vigorous); (b) *lesson/session context* (i.e., how lesson/session content is delivered, including time allocated for physical fitness, motor skill development, game play, knowledge, and session management); and (c) instructor *teacher/coach behavior* relative to the promotion of physical activities, skills, and fitness (McKenzie et al., 1991). Instructor gender, class/session location and gender composition, and number of participants are also typically recorded. The main focus of SOFIT is on individual participants, and observers are paced by a visual or audible signal using an interval recording format (e.g., 10-second observe/10-second record). Typical SOFIT outcome data include the number of minutes and proportion of session time participants spend in various postures (i.e., lying down, sitting, standing) and in walking/moderate and vigorous activity. Time in MVPA, lesson energy expenditure (kcal/kg), and energy expenditure rate (kcal/kg/min) can be estimated from the observed data. SOFIT also provides important information on (a) *lesson context* (i.e., minutes and % lesson time spent in management, instruction, fitness, skill drills, game play, and free play), and (b) *instructor behavior* (e.g., intervals instructors spend promoting PA, fitness, and skill engagement). SOFIT (and its adaptations) has been widely used in the U.S. (McKenzie & Smith, 2017) and internationally (Smith, McKenzie, & Hammons, 2018) for over 25 years.

SOPLAY: System for Observing Play and Leisure in Youth

SOPLAY provides objective data on the number of participants and their physical activity levels during play and leisure opportunities in predetermined targeted areas. It uses a group momentary time-sampling format (i.e., a series of observation "snapshots") to record the PA level (i.e., sedentary, walking/moderate, vigorous) and other characteristics of each individual (e.g., gender) and the target area using systematic scanning (McKenzie, 2016; McKenzie et al., 2000). Separate scans are made for males and females, and simultaneous entries for area contextual characteristics including their *accessibility* and *usability*, and whether or not *supervision*, *organized activities*, and *loose equipment* are available. These five specific characteristics are targeted for observation because they (a) impact the number of participants and their PA levels within specific spaces and (b) they are capable of being modified in order to assess specific policy, programing, and environmental interventions. An enhanced version of SOPLAY (i.e., SOPARC: System for Observing Physical Activity and Leisure Time in Communities) was designed to include the recording of the age (i.e., child, teen, adult, senior) and race/ethnicity (e.g., white, black, Latino, other) groupings of area users (McKenzie, Cohen, Sehgal, Williamson, & Golinelli, 2006). While SOPARC is employed most often to investigate parks and recreation (Cohen et al., 2016, 2020), it is useful in assessing school policies (Evenson, Jones, Holliday, Cohen, & McKenzie, 2016).

Recommendations

We believe that the primary focus for policy research related to child and youth physical activity should be on identifying how policies can support engaging children in sufficient health-enhancing physical activity. Thus, policy research is a complex and, nearly always, demands extensive collaborations among researchers and practitioners.

Involvement by practitioners is essential because they are the people that know the important questions that need answers and they are the ones primarily responsible for the creation of the policies, their implementation, their adoption, and their outcomes (including any consequences the policies do or do not produce). The generation of quality data also requires the cooperation of practitioners – they not only typically serve as key informants, and they also provide the access to written policies and to program facilities and participants.

We strongly recommend that physical activity policy research moves beyond being only descriptive and correlational. Action-oriented research is needed, and this requires a thorough examination of the both the implementation of policies (i.e., process measures) and their results (i.e., outcome measures). Subsequently, when possible, we recommend the use of direct measures in the actual setting (e.g., systematic observation of physical activity and environmental characteristics) over more distal and indirect methods (e.g., questionnaires).

Our intent in writing this chapter was to introduce policy and policy research, especially as they relate to the physical activity of young people in school and community environments. Further, we aimed to help readers understand the importance of policy as a strategy for increasing population-level physical activity and to provide insight into the complex nature of policies, their enactment, and their implementation. Lastly, and specifically for those interested in conducting physical activity policy research, we provided a brief overview of the nature of existing physical activity policy research and described tools we developed for use in our own research.

References

2018 Physical Activity Guidelines Advisory Committee. (2018). *2018 Physical activity guidelines advisory committee scientific report*. Washington, DC: U.S. Department of Health and Human Services.

Anderson, J. E. (2003). *Public policymaking: An introduction*. Boston, MA: Houghton.

Bauman, A. E., Nelson, D. E., Pratt, M., Matsudo, V., & Shoeppe, S. (2006). Dissemination of physical activity evidence, programs, policies, and surveillance in the international public health arena. *American Journal of Preventive Medicine, 31*(4), S57–S65.

Bauman, A. E., Sallis, J. F., & Owen, N. (2002). Environmental and policy measurement in physical activity research. In G. Welk (Ed.), *Physical activity assessments for health-related research* (pp. 241–251). Champaign, IL: Human Kinetics.

Boehmer, T. K., Luke, D. A., Haire-Joshu, D. L., Bates, H. S, & Brownson, R. C. (2008). Preventing childhood obesity through state policy: Predictors of bill enactment. *American Journal of Preventive Medicine, 34*(4), 333–340.

Brener, N. D., Demissie, Z., McManus, T., Shanklin, S. L., Queen, B., & Kann, L. (2017). *School health profiles 2016: Characteristics of health programs among secondary schools.* Atlanta, GA: Centers for Disease Control and Prevention.

Brownson, R. C., Baker, E. A., Housemann, R. A., Brennan, L. K., & Bacak, S. J. (2001). Environmental and policy determinants of physical activity in the United States. *American Journal of Public Health, 91*, 1995–2003.

Carlson, J. A., Sallis, J. F. Chriqui, J. F., Schneider, L., McDermid, L. C., & Argon, P. (2013). State policies about physical activity minutes in physical education or during school. *Journal of School Health, 83*(3), 150–156. doi:10.1111/josh.12010

Carlton, T. A., Kanters, M. A., Bocarro J. N., Floyd, M. F., Edwards, M. B., & Suau, L. J. (2017). Shared use agreements and leisure time physical activity in North Carolina public schools. *Preventive Medicine, 95*, S10–S16.

Centers for Disease Control and Prevention [CDC]. (2010). *The association between school based physical activity, including physical education, and academic performance.* Atlanta, GA: U.S. Department of Health and Human Services.

Centers for Disease Control and Prevention [CDC]. (2013). *Comprehensive school physical activity programs: A guide for schools.* Atlanta, GA: CDC.

Centers for Disease Control and Prevention [CDC]. (2017a). *POLARIS: Policy resources and materials.* Retrieved November 15, 2018 from https://www.cdc.gov/policy/polaris/policy-cdc-policy-process.html

Center for Disease Control and Prevention [CDC]. (2017b). *Results from the school health policies and practices study.* Atlanta, GA: Centers for Disease Control, Division of Adolescent School Health, 2016. Retrieved October 26, 2018 from https://www.cdc.gov/healthyyouth/data/shpps/pdf/shpps-results_2016.pdf

Cohen, D. A., Han, B., Nagel, C., Harnik, P., McKenzie, T. L., Evenson, K. R., . . . Katta, S. (2016). The first national study of neighborhood parks: Implications for physical activity. *American Journal of Preventive Medicine, 51*(4), 419–426. doi:10.1016/j.amepre.2016.03.021

Cohen, D. A., Han, B., Williamson, S., Nagel, C, McKenzie, T. L., Evenson, K. R., & Harnik, P. (2020). Playground features and physical activity in U.S. neighborhood parks. *Preventive Medicine, 131*, 105945.

Craddock, A. L., Barrett, J. L., Carnoske, C., Chriqui, J. F., Evenson, K. R., Gustat, J., . . . Zieff, S. G. (2013). Roles and strategies of state organizations related to school-based physical education and physical activity policies. *Journal of Public Health Management Practice, 19*(Suppl 3), S34–S40. doi:10.1097/PHH.0b013e3182840da2

Evenson, K. R., Jones, S, Holliday, K. Cohen, D, & McKenzie, T. L. (2016). Park characteristics, use, and physical activity: A review of studies using SOPARC (system for observing play and recreation in communities), *Preventive Medicine, 86*, 153–166.

Frank, L., Kerr, J., Chapman, J., & Sallis, J. (2007). Urban form relationships with walk trip frequency and distance among youth. *American Journal of Health Promotion, 21*(4S): 305–311.

Gordon-Larsen, P., Nelson, M. C., Page, P., & Popkin, B.M. (2006). Inequality in the built environment underlies key health disparities in physical activity and obesity. *Pediatrics, 117*(2), 417–424.

Hallal, P., & Ramirez, A. (2015). The Lancet physical activity observatory: Monitoring a 21st century pandemic. *Research in Exercise Epidemiology, 17*(1), 1–5.

Institute of Medicine. (2013). *Educating the student body: Taking physical activity and physical education to school.* Washington, DC: The National Academies Press.

Kanters, M. A., Bocarro, J. N., Filardo, M., Edwards, M., McKenzie, T. L., & Floyd, M. (2014). Shared use of school facilities with community organizations and afterschool physical activity program participation: A cost-benefit assessment. *Journal of School Health, 84*, 302–309.

Kim, J. (2012). Are physical education-related state policies and schools' physical education requirement related to children's physical activity and obesity? *Journal of School Health, 82*, 268–276.

Lillehoj, C. J., Daniel-Ulloa, J. D., & Nothwehr, F. (2016). Prevalence of physical activity policies and environmental strategies in communities and worksites: The Iowa community transformation grant. *Journal of Occupational and Environmental Medicine, 58*(1), e1–e5. doi:10.1097/JOM.0000000000000601

Lounsbery, M. A. F. (2017). School physical activity: Policy matters. *Kinesiology Review, 6*, 51–59.

Lounsbery, M. A. F., McKenzie, T. L., Morrow, J. R., Jr., Holt, K. A., & Budnar, R. G. (2013). School physical activity policy assessment. *Journal of Physical Activity and Health, 10*(4), 496–503.

Lounsbery, M. A. F., McKenzie, T. L., Morrow, J. R., Jr., Monnat, S., & Holt, K. (2013). District and school physical education policies: Implications for physical education and recess time. *Annals of Behavioral Medicine, 45*(Suppl 1), S131–S141.

Lyn, R. S., Sheldon, E. R., & Eriksen, M. P. (2017). Adopting state-level policy to support physical activity among school-aged children and adolescents: Georgia's SHAPE act. *Public Health Reports, 132*(Suppl 2), 9S–15S. doi:10.1177/0033354917719705

Machado-Rodrigues, A. M., Coelho-e-Silva, M. J., Mota, J., Santos, R. M., Cumming, S., & Malina, R. M. (2012). Physical activity and energy expenditure in adolescent male sport participants and non-participants aged 13–16 years. *Journal of Physical Activity and Health, 9*(5), 626–633.

Masse, L. C., Chriqui, J. F., Igoe, J. F., Atienza, A. A., Kruger, J., Kohl, H. W., III, . . . Yaroch, A. L. (2007). Development of a physical education–related state policy classification system (PERSPCS). *American Journal of Preventive Medicine, 33*(4S), S264–S276.

McKenzie, T. L. (2016). Context matters: Systematic observation of place-based physical activity. *Research Quarterly for Exercise and Sport, 87*(4), 334–341.

McKenzie, T. L., Cohen, D. A., Sehgal, A., Williamson, S., & Golinelli, D. (2006). System for Observing play and recreation in communities (SOPARC): Reliability and feasibility measures. *Journal of Physical Activity and Health, 3*(Suppl 1), S208–S222.

McKenzie, T. L., & Lounsbery, M. A. F. (2009). School physical education: The pill not taken. *American Journal of Lifestyle Medicine, 3*(3), 219–225.

McKenzie, T. L., & Smith, N. J. (2017). Studies of physical education in the United States using SOFIT: A review. *Research Quarterly for Exercise and Sport, 88*(4), 492–502.

McKenzie, T. L., Strikmiller, P. K., Stone, E. J., Woods, S. E., Ehlinger, S., Romero, K. A., & Budman, S. T. (1994). CATCH: Physical activity process evaluation in a multicenter trial. *Health Education Quarterly, 21*(Suppl 2), S73–S89.

McKenzie, T. L., & van der Mars, H. (2015). Top 10 research questions related to assessing physical activity and its contexts using systematic observation. *Research Quarterly for Exercise and Sport, 86*(1), 13–29.

McMillan, T. E. (2009). *Walking and biking to school, physical activity, and health outcomes. A research brief.* Princeton, NJ: Active Living Research.

Monnat, S. M., Lounsbery, M. A. F., & Smith, N. J. (2014). Correlates of state enactment of elementary school laws. *Preventive Medicine, 69*(S5–S11), 1–20. doi:10.1016/j.ypmed.2014.09.006

Municipal Research & Services Center of Washington. (1999). *Local government policy making process.* Seattle, WA: Author.

National Cancer Institute. (2014). *Classification of laws associated with school students.* Bethesda, MD: U.S. Department of Health and Human Services, National Institutes of Health. Retrieved October 26, 2018 from https://class.cancer.gov/

NFHS. (2018). *High school sports participation increases for 29th consecutive year.* Retrieved from https://www.nfhs.org/articles/high-school-sports-participation-increases-for-29th-consecutive-year/

Oh, A. Y., Hennessy, E., McSpadden, K. E., & Perna, F. M. (2015). Contextual influences on weight status among impoverished adolescents: Neighborhood amenities for physical activity and state laws for physical education time requirements. *Journal of Physical Activity and Health, 12*, 875–878. doi:10.1123/jpah.2013-0303

Olstad, D. L., Campbell, E. J., Raine, K. D., & Nykiforuk, C. I. J. (2015). A multiple case history and systematic review of adoption, diffusion, implementation, and impact of provincial daily physical activity policies in Canadian schools. *BMC Public Health, 15*, 385. doi:10.1186/s12889-015-1669-6

Perna, F. M., Oh, A., Chriqui, J. F., Masse, L. C., Atienza, A. A., Nebeling, L., . . . Dodd, K. W. (2012). The association of state law to physical education time allocation in US public schools. *American Journal of Public Health, 102*(8), 1594–1599.

Powers, H. S., Conway, T. L., McKenzie, T. L., Sallis, J. F., & Marshall, S. J. (2002). Participation in extracurricular physical activity programs in middle schools. *Research Quarterly for Exercise and Sport, 73*, 187–192.

Pühse, U., & Gerber, M. (2005). *International comparison of physical education. Concepts, problems, prospects.* New York, NY: Meyer & Meyer Sport.

Ramirez-Varela, A., Pratt, M., Powell, K., Lee, I. M., Bauman, A., Heath, G., . . . Hallal, P. (2017). Worldwide surveillance, policy, and research on physical activity and health: The global observatory for physical activity. *Journal of Physical Activity and Health, 14*, 701–709. doi:10.1123/jpah.2016-0626.

Sanchez-Vaznaugh, E. V., Goldman Rosas, L., Fernandez-Peña, J. R., Baek, J., Egerter, S., & Sanchez, B. N. (2017). Physical education policy compliance and Latino children's fitness: Does the association vary by school neighborhood socioeconomic advantage? *PLoS One, 12*(6), 1–11, e0178980. doi:10.1371/journal. pone.0178980

Schwartz, M. B., Lund, A. E., Grow, H. M., McDonnell, E., Probart, C., Samuelson, A., & Lytle, L. (2009). A comprehensive coding system to measure the quality of school wellness policies. *Journal of the American Dietetic Association, 109*, 1256–1262.

Saelens, B. E, & Handy, S. L. (2008). Built environment correlates of walking: A review. *Medicine & Science in Sports & Exercise, 40*(7 Suppl 1), S550–S566.

Sallis, J. F., Cervero, R. B., Ascher, W., Henderson, K. A., Kraft, M. K., & Kerr, J. (2006). An ecological approach to creating active living communities. *Annual Review of Public Health, 27*, 297–322. doi:10.1146/annurev.publhealth.27.021405.102100

Sallis, J. F., McKenzie, T. L., Beets, M. W., Beighle, A., H., Erwin, H., & Lee, S. (2012). Physical education's role in public health: Steps forward and backward over 20 years and HOPE for the future. *Research Quarterly for Exercise and Sport, 83*(2), 125–135.

Sallis, J. F., & Owen, M. (2015). Ecological models of health behavior. In K Glanz, B. Rimer, & K. Viswanath (Eds.), *Health behavior: Theory, research, and practice* (Fifth ed.). San Francisco, CA; Jossey-Bass.

SHAPE America – Society of Health and Physical Educators. (2016). *Shape of the nation: Status of physical education in the USA*. Reston, VA: SHAPE America. Retrieved October 26, 2018 from https://www.shapeamerica.org/uploads/pdfs/son/Shape-of-the-Nation-2016_web.pdf

Slater, S. J., Nicholson, L., Chriqui, J., Turner, L., & Chaloupka, F. (2012). The impact of state laws and district policies on physical education and recess practices in a nationally representative sample of US public elementary schools. *Archives of Pediatric Adolescent Medicine, 166*(4), 311–316. doi:10.1001/archpediatrics.2011.1133

Smith, N. J., McKenzie, T. L., & Hammons, A. J. (2018). International studies of physical education using SOFIT: A review. *Advances in Physical Education, 9*(1), 53–74.

Stokols, D. (1992). Establishing and maintaining healthy environments: Toward a social ecology of health promotion. *American Psychologist, 47*, 6–22.

Stylianou, M., & Walker, J. L. (2018). An assessment of Australian school physical activity and nutrition policies. *Australian and New Zealand Journal of Public Health, 42*(1), 16–21. doi:10.1111/1753-6405.12751

Taber, D. R., Chriqui, J. F., Perna, F. M., Powell, L. M., Slater, S. J., & Chaloupka, F. J. (2013). Association between state physical education (PE) requirements and PE participation, physical activity, and body mass index change. *Preventive Medicine, 57*, 629–633.

Thompson, H. R, Singh, B. K., Reed, A., Lounsbery, M. A. F., Winig, B.D., & Madsen, K. A. (2018). Impact of litigation on compliance with California physical education laws in elementary schools. *Journal of Physical Activity and Health*. Advance online publication. doi:10.1123/jpah.2017-0307

Tremblay, M. S., Barnes, J. D., Gonzalez, S. A., Katzmarzyk, P. T., Onywera, V. O., Reilly, J. J., . . . the Global Matrix 2.0 Research Team. (2016). Global Matrix 2.0: Report card grades on the physical activity of children and youth comparing 38 countries. *Journal of Physical Activity and Health, 13*(11 Suppl 2), s343–s366. doi:10.1123/jpah.2016-0594

Turner, L., Chriqui, J. F., & Chaloupka, F. J. (2013). Withholding recess from elementary school students: Policies matter. *Journal of School Health, 83*(8), 533–541.

United Nations Educational, Scientific and Cultural Organization [UNESCO]. (2014). *World-wide survey of school physical education*. Paris, France: UNESCO. Retrieved September 30, 2018 from http://unesdoc.unesco.org/images/0022/002293/229335e.pdf

United Nations Educational, Scientific and Cultural Organization [UNESCO]. (2015). *Quality physical education: Guidelines for policy-makers*. Paris, France: UNESCO. Retrieved September 24, 2018 from http://unesdoc.unesco.org/images/0023/002311/231101E.pdf

Weatherson, K., Bradford, B., Berg, S., & Sloboda, S. (2016). Dissemination of daily physical activity policy on school websites in Alberta and British Columbia. *Revue phenEPS/PHEnex Journal, 8*(2), 1–14. ISSN 1918-8927 [cited 26 September 2018]. Retrieved from http://ojs.acadiau.ca/index.php/phenex/article/view/1619/1361

Wickel, E. E., & Eisenmann, J. C. (2007). Contribution of youth sport to total daily physical activity among 6- to 12-yr-old boys. *Medicine & Science in Sports & Exercise, 39*(9), 1493–1500.

World Health Organization [WHO]. (2011). *Global recommendations on physical activity for health, 5–17 years old*. Geneva, Switzerland: World Health Organization.

World Health Organization [WHO]. (2018a). *Global action plan on physical activity 2018–2030: More active people for a healthier world*. Geneva, Switzerland: World Health Organization. Retrieved September 30, 2018 from http://apps.who.int/iris/bitstream/handle/10665/272722/9789241514187-eng.pdf

World Health Organization [WHO]. (2018b, February 18). *Physical activity: Key facts*. Retrieved November 17, 2018 from http://www.who.int/news-room/fact-sheets/detail/physical-activity

World Health Organization [WHO]. (2018c, February 16). *Obesity and overweight*. Retrieved November 17, 2018 from http://www.who.int/news-room/fact-sheets/detail/obesity-and-overweight

PART 4

Physical Activity Measurement

12

INTRODUCTION TO PHYSICAL ACTIVITY MEASUREMENT

Stuart J. Fairclough and Robert J. Noonan

Introduction

The ability to accurately measure youth physical activity is fundamental to any research study in the field. Five specific types of research related to physical activity and health are described in an adapted version of the Behavioral Epidemiology Framework (Sallis, Owen, & Fotheringham, 2000). These are basic research (e.g., mechanistic), health outcomes research (e.g., associations with health indicators), surveillance research (e.g., secular trends), theory and correlates research (e.g., factors that are associated with behaviors), and intervention research (e.g., evaluation of programs to improve behaviors or health) (Welk, Morrow, & Saint-Maurice, 2017). Physical activity measurement is located at the center of this framework because a prerequisite for each research type is the requirement for accurate estimates of the physical activity behaviors (Figure 12.1). Physical activity measurement methods need to be appropriately selected to address the research questions under consideration, to accommodate the resources available to the researcher, and to be suitable for the population of interest.

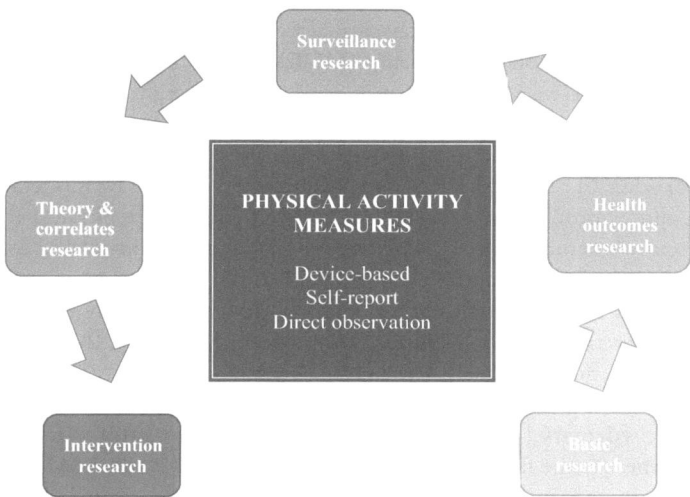

Figure 12.1 Behavioral epidemiology framework related to youth physical activity (Adapted from Welk et al., 2017)

Key Issues

Previous chapters have discussed the intermittent nature of youth physical activity which occurs across the full intensity spectrum. Over the course of a day, youth will spend varying amounts of time being sedentary[1] (e.g., sitting in class), and doing light (e.g., slow walking), moderate (e.g., brisk walking), and vigorous intensity physical activity (e.g., running, playing sports). The contribution of time spent in each physical activity intensity to total daily physical activity varies within and between individuals depending on the context, day of the week, environment, etc. Typically, there is an inverse relationship between physical activity intensity and time, whereby most time will be spent sedentary and the smallest proportion of time will be spent in moderate-to-vigorous intensity physical activity (MVPA). For example, it was recently reported that an international sample of over 1,700 youth aged 9–11 years, spent 36% of the day being sedentary, 21% in light intensity physical activity, and 4%–5% in MVPA (Dumuid et al., 2018). Youth engage in various forms of physical activities depending on a range of contextual factors. Physical activity is often unstructured and can encompass active travel (e.g., walking to school), free play (e.g., recess activities), as well as incidental activities, such as household chores. At other times, physical activity is structured and can be led by a teacher, instructor, or coach. Examples of these modes of physical activity include physical education classes, sports practices, swimming lessons, and gym workouts. While these forms of physical activity can be diverse, different physical activity measurement approaches are available to capture and quantify how much and what type of physical activity is undertaken (Hills, Mokhtar, & Byrne, 2014). These approaches typically aim to quantify some aspects of physical activity behavior, such as frequency, duration, intensity, and type, or estimate the physiological cost of physical activity (e.g., how much energy was expended).

Physical activity measurement approaches capture one or more dimension(s) of physical activity behavior (e.g., movement measured by an accelerometer; physiological response measured by a heart rate monitor) that can be analyzed and reported in raw form or translated to other units such as energy expenditure or minutes spent in MVPA. This calibration of raw activity data into intensity-related minutes or energy expenditure is based on the relationships between physical activity intensity and energy expenditure (i.e., the more intense the physical activity being performed, the more energy is expended per unit of time) (Welk et al., 2017). Algorithms based on these relationships can be built into physical activity measurement methods to convert raw movement data into more readily interpretable physical activity and/or energy expenditure metrics.

One such metric is metabolic equivalents (METs), which equate to oxygen consumption required at rest (assumed to be 3.5 mL/O_2/min per kg body weight). METs express energy expenditure or physical activity intensity as multiples of rest (i.e., 1 MET) and are therefore useful for categorizing and prescribing physical activities at different intensities (Schutz, Weinsier, & Hunter, 2001). For adults, light physical activity is defined as >1.5 METs, moderate physical activity as 3–6 METs, and vigorous physical activity as ≥6 METs. However, physical activity intensities are defined differently in youth due to variation in body composition-related resting energy expenditure, which is higher than in adults (Harrell et al., 2005). For example, 2 METs and 4 METs are commonly used as the thresholds for sedentary/light physical activity and light/moderate intensity activity, respectively (Saint-Maurice, Kim, Welk, & Gaesser, 2016; Welk et al., 2017). To reflect this principle more precisely, the National Collaborative on Childhood Obesity Research (NCCOR) in the US proposed age- and sex-specific adjusted MET thresholds for resting energy expenditure, sedentary behavior, and MVPA (Welk et al., 2017). For sedentary behavior, for 8–18-year olds, these range from 2.6 to 1.5 METs (boys) and 2.7 to 1.5 METs (girls). Similarly, MVPA MET values range from 5.3 to 3.0 (boys) and 5.4 to 3.0 (girls) (Welk et al., 2017). Though 2 METs and 4 METs have been used for some time, the NCCOR values arguably provide more precise MET estimates for researchers to apply to their measured physical activity data.

Unlike many stable health behaviors, youth physical activity varies naturally from day-to-day and between seasons (Aadland et al., 2017). The inherent goal with any physical activity measurement method is to capture the true random variation in the physical activity behavior, and minimize other sources of bias and error that obscure the true relationships in the data. Youth physical activity data measured in free-living settings will contain various components of systematic and random errors (e.g., coverage, sampling, non-response, and data processing errors) (Nusser et al., 2012). To obtain the best possible estimates of physical activity behaviors, the errors that impact the measurement process need to be quantified and accounted for. For example, it has been demonstrated that adjustment for physical activity survey nonresponse and measurement errors significantly influenced estimates of the percentage of adults achieving national physical activity guidelines in the US (Beyler & Beyler, 2017). Moreover, biased estimates of the true relationships between physical activity and health outcomes are likely when random measurement error is not accounted for (Nusser et al., 2012). Systematic error (e.g., recall inaccuracies compared to true activity) and random error (e.g., day-to-day (within-person) variation in reporting biases) are then critical influences on the precision of estimates from youth physical activity measurement methods. Thus, recognition of and adjustment for systematic and random measurement error sources are recommended to produce more accurate estimates of physical activity that researchers and research users, such as policy makers, commissioners, and practitioners, can use with confidence. These error sources can be modeled in the analysis of physical activity data using replicated measurements and appropriate statistical methods (Tooze, Troiano, Carroll, Moshfegh, & Freedman, 2013). For these reasons, true, error-free measurement of physical activity is extremely difficult to achieve, and so resultant physical activity data more likely reflect *estimates* of actual behavior.

Although sedentary behavior has been alluded to so far in the context of physical activity measurement, it is important to acknowledge that sedentary behaviors encompass a class of non-active behaviors that are distinct from physical activity. These have been presented by the Sedentary Behaviour Network (SBN), which defined the key terms of *physical inactivity, stationary behavior, sedentary behavior, standing, screen time, non-screen-based sedentary time, sitting, reclining, lying,* and *sedentary behavior pattern* (Tremblay et al., 2017). Youth routinely engage in a wide range of these behaviors, which underscores the importance of researchers using appropriate measurement methods. Fundamental to defining sedentary behavior are low energy expenditure ($\leq$1.5 METs in the SBN definition) and postural allocation (i.e., sitting, reclining, or lying postures) during waking hours (Tremblay et al., 2017). Therefore, obtaining estimates of sedentary time should theoretically encompass both of these features. Accurately capturing simultaneous estimates of energy expenditure and postural allocation provides specific challenges for youth sedentary behavior researchers.

Various validated methods are available to measure child physical activity that can present uncertainty when deciding which methods are most suitable. None of these methods are able to measure all domains and dimensions of physical activity (Dollman et al., 2009). When comparing physical activity measures it is important to consider their validity (i.e., accuracy) in relation to their feasibility (i.e., ease of use). This relationship is typically inverse with the more accurate methods (e.g., device-based and laboratory-based measures) tending to be less feasible due to their greater expense, technical complexity, time required, etc. Conversely, more feasible measures such as questionnaires which can be used with large numbers of participants, generally, are less accurate at estimating physical activity levels. The validity/feasibility continuum for physical activity measures (Figure 12.2) (Welk et al., 2017) is a useful basis for researchers when deciding on the most appropriate physical activity measurement tools (Dollman et al., 2009). The following chapters will provide a comprehensive overview of the various methods available to researchers. The next sections of this chapter will summarize key characteristics of self-report, device-based, and direct observation as the most common categories of measurement methods.

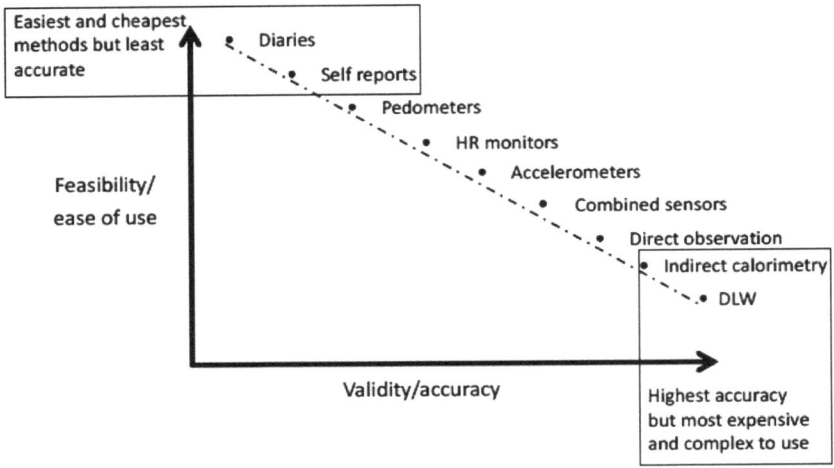

Figure 12.2 Feasibility-validity continuum of physical activity measurement methods (Adapted from Welk et al., 2017)

Measuring Physical Activity Using Self-Report

Self-report measures include questionnaires, diaries, and logs. Self-report measures are cost-effective and low burden, and provide a versatile, non-invasive, and time-effective way of collecting physical activity data from large numbers of youth (Loprinzi & Cardinal, 2011). Although self-report measures provide rich contextual information on activity mode (e.g., sport, transportation, or play) and domain (e.g., family-based or school-based) (Rachele, McPhail, Washington, & Cuddihy, 2012), they typically overestimate youth physical activity levels compared to objective measures (Adamo, Prince, Tricco, Connor-Gorber, & Tremblay, 2009; Hussey, Bell, & Gormley, 2007). Accurate recall is dependent on youth understanding and interpreting questions correctly (Janz, Lutuchy, Wenthe, & Levy, 2008). Shorter recalls provide more reliable estimates of physical activity than recalls of longer periods (Biddle, Gorely, Pearson, & Bull, 2011), and those which include questions on physical activity type rather than activity bout durations are also generally more reliable (Saint-Maurice, Welk, Beyler, Bartee, & Heelan, 2014). Computerized self-report measures have several advantages over paper-based formats (Saint-Maurice & Welk, 2014), including reduced financial and time cost, lower coding error, and provision for immediate data scoring and interpretation of results (Warren et al., 2010). Self-report measures are generally unable to accurately classify physical activity intensity (Rachele et al., 2012), but evidence does exist demonstrating the utility of calibrating self-report measures against accelerometers to convert self-report scores to time spent in physical activity intensities (Saint-Maurice & Welk, 2015). However, to date this approach has seldom been used.

Measuring Physical Activity Using Device-Based Methods

Pedometers are the simplest device-based measure of physical activity and provide estimates of the number of steps taken over a set time (Clemes & Biddle, 2013). Pedometers are relatively low cost, and their objectivity makes them feasible tools for measuring ambulatory physical activity in large-scale studies (Craig, Tudor-Locke, Cragg, & Cameron, 2010; Duncan, Scott-Duncan, &

Schofield, 2008; Laurson et al., 2008). However, pedometers provide no detail on physical activity intensity (Trost, 2007), and their output measure (i.e., steps taken) is not comparable between studies using different pedometer brands or across age groups due to differences in stride length (Corder, Ekelund, Steele, Wareham, & Brage, 2008). Pedometers cannot measure water-based activity, they are susceptible to data loss, device tampering, and reactivity unless sealed over the full data collection period (Scott, Morgan, Plotnikoff, Trost, & Lubans, 2013), and they have been shown to underestimate step frequency at slow walking speeds (Beets, Patton, & Edwards, 2005; Berlin, Storti, & Brach, 2006). Their accuracy is also compromised when placed at different body locations and used in younger populations and youth with gait impairments. Pedometers are insensitive to non-locomotive and upper body movements, which limits their use in studies investigating youth's free-living physical activity behavior (Rowlands & Eston, 2007; Warren et al., 2010).

Accelerometers are the most widely used device to measure youth physical activity (Cain, Sallis, Conway, Van Dyck, & Calhoon, 2013). Accelerometers provide estimates of physical activity frequency, intensity, and duration (Dollman et al., 2009). Accelerometers have time sampling capabilities which enables researchers to investigate active and inactive periods of the day (Fairclough, Beighle, Erwin, & Ridgers, 2012; Fairclough, Butcher, & Stratton, 2007) or week (Fairclough, Boddy, Mackintosh, Valencia-Peris, & Ramirez-Rico, 2015), as well as factors associated with physical activity during specific time periods and segments of the day including playtime (Ridgers, Timperio, Crawford, & Salmon, 2013), after school (Pearce, Page, Griffin, & Cooper, 2014), or weekends (McMinn, Griffin, Jones, & van Sluijs, 2013). Such capabilities are useful when assessing the effectiveness of physical activity interventions targeting specific periods of the day (Saint-Maurice, Welk, Russell, & Huberty, 2014). Accelerometers, though, are expensive, can be burdensome to wear, and provide limited contextual information on physical activity behavior (Dollman et al., 2009; Machado-Rodrigues et al., 2011). The Acti-Graph GT9X, GENEActiv, and Axivity accelerometers are water resistant but earlier models were not, which limited the ability to assess physical activity during water-based activities (i.e., swimming). Irrespective of wear site, incorrectly worn accelerometers provide biased physical activity level estimates. Hip-worn accelerometers underestimate cycling energy expenditure (Tarp, Andersen, & Østergaard, 2015) and misclassify non-ambulatory light-to-moderate intensity activities (e.g., playing catch) as sedentary time (Trost, Loprinzi, Moore, & Pfeiffer, 2011). Wrist-worn accelerometers have grown in popularity on the basis of improved wear compliance (Fairclough et al., 2016). The main drawback to accelerometers relates to data reduction as there is presently no uniform criteria for defining non-wear time, and reducing and scoring the data, which impacts on resultant physical activity estimates. The variation in scoring criteria and models used to measure physical activity across the research field also limits study comparability (Atkin et al., 2012; Cain et al., 2013), and confuses the application of accelerometer data for researchers and research users alike (e.g., when estimating compliance to physical activity guidelines) (Migueles et al., 2019).

The use of heart rate data to measure youth physical activity is centered on the linear relationship between heart rate and oxygen uptake (Hussey et al., 2007). The main strengths of heart rate monitors include their objectivity and ability to record data over time which provides a visual picture of the pattern and intensity of youth physical activity (Loprinzi & Cardinal, 2011). The relationship between heart rate and youth physical activity is weak at low intensities, and heart rate response typically lags behind changes in movement, which can cause measurement error (Armstrong & Welsman, 2006). Heart rate is also influenced by a range of other factors including age, body size, cardiorespiratory fitness, stress response, and hydration (Loprinzi & Cardinal, 2011). For these reasons, heart rate is often used in combination with other measures to estimate youth's daily physical activity (Collins, Al-Nakeeb, & Lyons, 2015; De Bock et al., 2010; Duncan, Badland, & Schofield, 2009; Eyre, Duncan, Birch, Cox, & Blackett, 2015).

Measuring Physical Activity Using Direct Observation

Direct observation allows for the study of youths' context-specific physical activity behaviors in settings such as playtime (Ridgers, Stratton, & McKenzie, 2010) and leisure-time (McKenzie, Cohen, Sehgal, Williamson, & Golinelli, 2006; McKenzie, Marshall, Sallis, & Conway, 2000). This rich contextual information can aid the interpretation of objective physical activity data (Warren et al., 2010). Direct observation has a high internal validity and has been widely used as a criterion measure for validating other physical activity measures such as pedometers and accelerometers (McKenzie & van der Mars, 2015). The main limitations to direct observation relate to the cost and time-intensive nature of the method both to train researchers and collect the data (Dale, Welk, & Matthews, 2002). Therefore, direct observation is only suitable for measuring physical activity behavior in small samples (McKenzie, 2002). Observer retraining is often required to reduce the potential of the observer's skills deteriorating over time to ensure reliable observer data monitoring (McKenzie, 2002). Observer presence can positively influence youth activity behavior, but this limitation can be minimized by conducting repeat observations (Trost, 2007).

Decisions for Researchers to Consider When Selecting Physical Activity Measurement Tools

Physical activity researchers have a wide range of measurement tools at their disposal, but this degree of choice can present challenges when selecting the most appropriate method. As discussed throughout the chapter and illustrated in Figure 12.3, there are several factors for researchers to consider when deciding the most appropriate measurement methods for a specific research project or question. Accuracy of the chosen method should be balanced against its ease of use in the context of the target population and the resources available to the researcher. Researcher expertise in the preparation, administration, and data processing is essential, irrespective of the measurement method. The decision-making process should be driven by the characteristics of the project design (e.g., population [e.g., preschoolers, adolescents], planned physical activity outcomes [e.g., steps taken, time spent in MVPA during school hours, context], study type [e.g., surveillance, intervention], level of burden the participants are prepared to accept, available resources [e.g., funding, staffing level, and expertise]), as well as an understanding of the strengths and weaknesses of each method. Combining methods may be appropriate in some studies, particularly where there are multiple planned physical activity outcomes (Troiano, Gabriel, Welk, Owen, & Sternfeld, 2012). However, combining methods brings additional participant burden, which can influence compliance to the monitoring protocol and impact on data reliability (Dollman et al., 2009).

This section aims to provide a comprehensive and contemporary overview of physical activity measurement methods that youth physical activity researchers can use to improve their understanding of the area and guide their decision-making when designing studies. The following chapters focus on the most commonly used youth physical activity measurement methods, which cover self-report, direct observation, pedometers, and accelerometers. Each chapter provides an overview of the issues and literature pertaining to each specific method, and concludes with a commentary of current and future challenges and developments. The final chapter in this section is devoted to the use of emerging technologies in youth physical activity measurement.

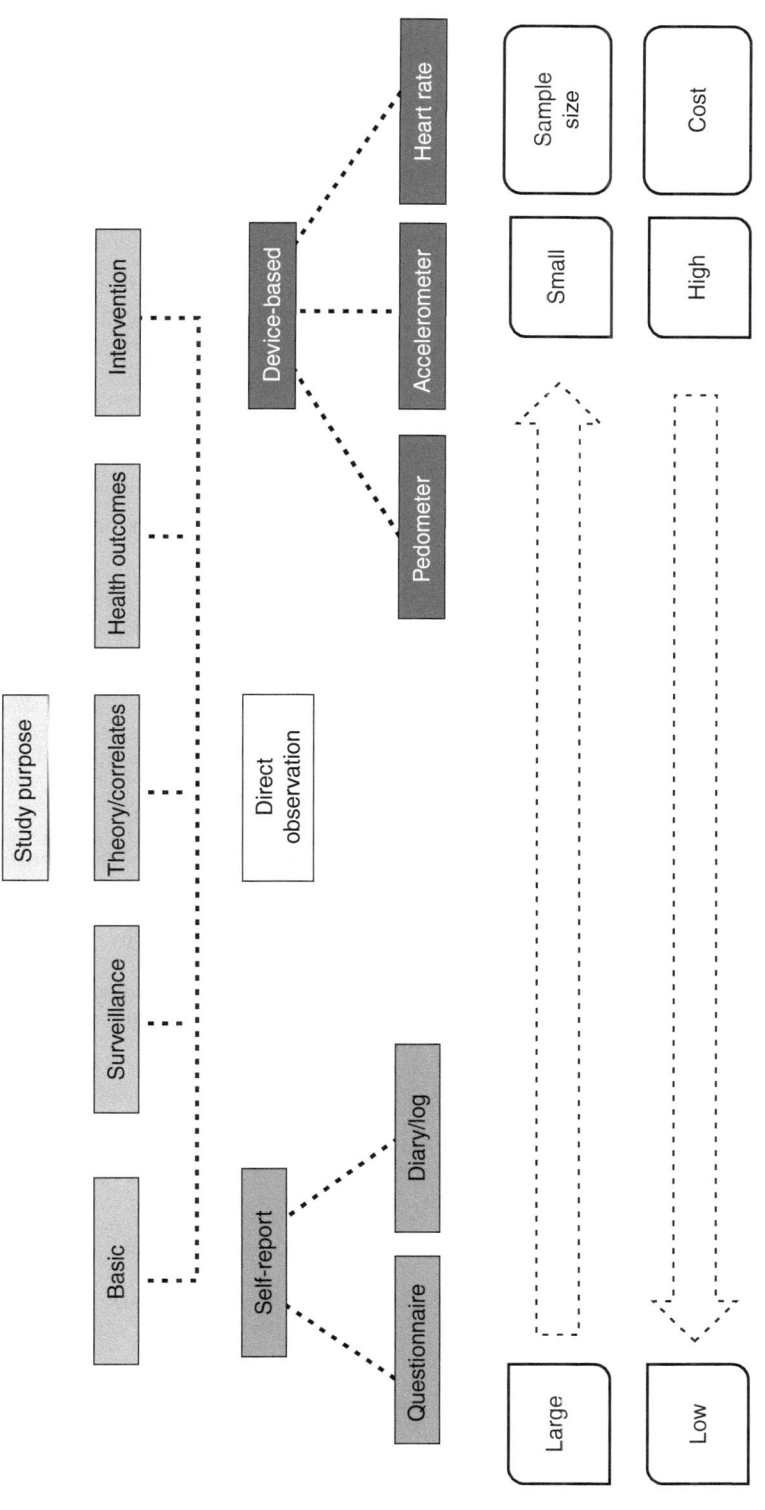

Figure 12.3 Flow chart of possible researcher decisions when selecting physical activity measurement approaches for use with youth (Adapted from Dollman et al., 2009)

Note

1 Although sedentary behavior describes a distinct group of behaviors separate from physical activity (Tremblay et al., 2017), in this chapter, the term sedentary behavior will refer the lower end of the physical activity intensity spectrum.

References

Aadland, E., Andersen, L. B., Skrede, T., Ekelund, U., Anderssen, S. A., & Resaland, G. K. (2017). Reproducibility of objectively measured physical activity and sedentary time over two seasons in children: Comparing a day-by-day and a week-by-week approach. *PLoS One, 12*(12), e0189304. doi:10.1371/journal.pone.0189304.

Adamo, K.B., Prince, S.A., Tricco, A.C., Connor-Gorber, S., & Tremblay, M.S. (2009). A comparison of indirect versus direct measures for assessing physical activity in the pediatric population: A systematic review. *International Journal of Pediatric Obesity, 4*, 2–27.

Armstrong, N., & Welsman, J. R. (2006). The physical activity patterns of European youth with reference to methods of assessment. *Sports Medicine, 36*(12), 1067–1086.

Atkin, A. J., Gorely, T., Clemes, S. A., Yates, T., Edwardson, C., Brage, S., . . . Biddle, S. J. H. (2012). Methods of measurement in epidemiology: Sedentary behaviour. *International Journal of Epidemiology, 41*, 1460–1471.

Beets, M., Patton, M., & Edwards, S. (2005). The accuracy of pedometer steps and time during walking in children, *Medicine & Science in Sports & Exercise, 37*, 513–520.

Berlin, J., Storti, K., & Brach, J. (2006). Using activity monitors to measure physical activity in free-living conditions. *Physical Therapy, 86*, 1137–1145.

Biddle, S. J. H., Gorely, T., Pearson, N., & Bull, F. C. (2011). An assessment of self-reported physical activity instruments in young people for population surveillance: Project ALPHA. *International Journal of Behavioral Nutrition and Physical Activity, 8*, 1.

Beyler, N., & Beyler, A. (2017). Adjusting for measurement error and nonresponse in physical activity surveys: A simulation study. *Journal of Official Statistics, 33*, 533–550).

Cain, K. L., Sallis, J. F., Conway, T. L., Van Dyck, D., & Calhoon, L. (2013). Using accelerometers in youth physical activity studies: A review of methods. *Journal of Physical Activity & Health, 10*, 437–450.

Clemes, S. A., & Biddle, S. J. H. (2013). The use of pedometers for monitoring physical activity in children and adolescents: Measurement considerations. *Journal of Physical Activity & Health, 10*, 249–262.

Collins, P., Al-Nakeeb, Y., & Lyons, M. (2015). Tracking the commute home from school utilizing gps and heart rate monitoring: Establishing the contribution to free-living physical activity. *Journal of Physical Activity & Health, 12*, 155–162.

Corder, K., Ekelund, U., Steele, R. M., Wareham, N. J., & Brage, S. (2008). Assessment of physical activity in youth. *Journal of Applied Physiology, 105*(3), 977–987.

Craig, C. L., Tudor-Locke, C., Cragg, S., & Cameron, C. (2010). Process and treatment of pedometer data collection for youth: The Canadian physical activity levels among youth study. *Medicine & Science in Sports & Exercise, 42*(3), 430–435.

Dale, D., Welk, G. J., & Matthews, C. E. (2002). Methods for assessing physical activity and challenges for research. In G. J. Welk (Ed.), *Physical activity assessments for health-related research*. Leeds, UK: Human Kinetics.

De Bock, F., Menze, J., Becker, S., Litaker, D., Fischer, J., & Seidel, I. (2010). Combining accelerometry and HR for assessing preschoolers' physical activity. *Medicine & Science in Sports & Exercise, 42*(12), 2237–2243.

Dollman, J., Okely, A. D., Hardy, L., Timperio, A., Salmon, J., & Hills, A. P. (2009). A hitchhiker's guide to assessing young people's physical activity: Deciding what method to use. *Journal of Science and Medicine in Sport, 12*, 518–525.

Dumuid, D., Stanford, T. E., Pedišić, Ž., Maher, C., Lewis, L. K., Martín-Fernández, J.-A., ... Olds, T. (2018). Adiposity and the isotemporal substitution of physical activity, sedentary time and sleep among school-aged children: A compositional data analysis approach. *BMC Public Health, 18*(1), 311. doi:10.1186/s12889-018-5207-1

Duncan, J. S., Badland, H. M., & Schofield, G. (2009). Combining GPS with heart rate monitoring to measure physical activity in children: A feasibility study. *Journal of Science and Medicine in Sport, 12*, 583–585.

Duncan, E., Scott-Duncan, J., & Schofield, G. (2008). Pedometer-determined physical activity and active transport in girls. *International Journal of Behavioral Nutrition and Physical Activity, 5*, 2.

Eyre, E. L. J., Duncan, M. J., Birch, S. L., Cox, V., & Blackett, M. (2015). Physical activity patterns of ethnic children from low socio-economic environments within the UK. *Journal of Sports Sciences, 33*(3), 232–242.

Fairclough, S. J., Beighle, A., Erwin, H., & Ridgers, N. D. (2012). School day segmented physical activity patterns of high and low active children. *BMC Public Health, 12*, 406.

Fairclough, S. J., Boddy, L. M., Mackintosh, K. A., Valencia-Peris, A., & Ramirez-Rico, E. (2015). Week-day and weekend sedentary time and physical activity in differentially active children. *Journal of Science and Medicine in Sport, 18*, 444–449.

Fairclough, S. J., Butcher, Z. H., & Stratton, G. (2007). Whole-day and segmented-day physical activity variability of northwest England school children. *Preventive Medicine, 44*, 421–425.

Fairclough, S. J., Noonan, R. J., Rowlands, A. V., van Hees, V., Knowles, Z., & Boddy, L. M. (2016). Wear compliance and activity in children wearing wrist- and hip-mounted accelerometers. *Medicine & Science in Sports & Exercise, 48*(2), 245–253.

Harrell, J. S., McMurray, R. G., Baggett, C. D., Pennell, M. L., Pearce, P. F., & Bangdiwala, S. I. (2005). Energy costs of physical activities in children and adolescents. *Medicine and Science in Sports and Exercise, 37*(2), 329–336.

Hills, A. P., Mokhtar, N., & Byrne, N. M. (2014). Assessment of physical activity and energy expenditure: an overview of objective measures. *Frontiers in Nutrition, 1*. doi:10.3389/fnut.2014.00005

Hussey, J., Bell, C., & Gormley, J. (2007). The measurement of physical activity in children. *Physical Therapy Reviews, 12*, 52–58.

Janz, K., Lutuchy, E., Wenthe, P., & Levy, S. (2008). Measuring activity in children and adolescents using self-report: PAQ-C and PAQ-A. *Medicine & Science in Sports & Exercise, 40*(4), 767–772.

Laurson, K., Eisenmann, J., Welk, G., Wickel, E., Gentile, D., & Walsh D. (2008). Evaluation of youth pedometer-determined physical activity guidelines using receiver operator characteristic curves. *Preventative Medicine, 46*, 419–424.

Loprinzi, P. D., & Cardinal, B. J. (2011). Measuring children's physical activity and sedentary behaviours. *Journal of Exercise Science & Fitness, 9*(1), 15–23.

Machado-Rodrigues, A. M., Coelho-E-Silva, M. J., Mota, J., Cyrino, E., Cumming, S. P., Riddoch, C., . . . Malina, R. M. (2011). Agreement in activity energy expenditure assessed by accelerometer and self-report in adolescents: Variation by sex, age, and weight status. *Journal of Sports Sciences, 29*(14), 1503–1514.

McKenzie, T. L. (2002). Use of direct observation to assess physical activity. In G. J. Welk (Ed.), *Physical activity assessments for health-related research*. Leeds, UK: Human Kinetics.

McKenzie, T. L., Cohen, D. A., Sehgal, A., Williamson, S., & Golinelli, D. (2006). System for observing play and recreation in communities (SOPARC): Reliability and feasibility measures. *Journal of Physical Activity & Health, 3*(Suppl 1), S208–S222.

McKenzie, T. L., Marshall, S. J., Sallis, J. F., & Conway, T. L. (2000). Leisure-time physical activity in school environments: An observation study using SOPLAY. *Preventive Medicine, 30*, 70–77.

McKenzie, T. L., & van der Mars, H. (2015). Top 10 research questions related to assessing physical activity and its contexts using systematic observation. *Research Quarterly for Exercise and Sport, 86*(1), 13–29.

McMinn, A. M., Griffin, S. J., Jones, A. P., & van Sluijs, E. M. F. (2013). Family and home influences on children's after-school and weekend physical activity. *The European Journal of Public Health, 23*(5), 805–810.

Migueles, J. H., Cadenas-Sanchez, C., Tudor-Locke, C., Löf, M., Esteban-Cornejo, I., Molina-Garcia, P., . . . Ortega, F. B. (2019). Comparability of published cut-points for the assessment of physical activity: Implications for data harmonization. *Scandinavian Journal of Medicine & Science in Sports, 29*, 566–574.

Nusser, S. M., Beyler, N. K., Welk, G. J., Carriquiry, A. L., Fuller, W. A., & King, B. M. (2012). Modeling errors in physical activity recall data. *Journal of Physical Activity & Health, 9*(Suppl 1), S56–S67.

Pearce, M., Page, A. S., Griffin, T. P., & Cooper, A. R. (2014). Who children spend time with after school: Associations with objectively recorded indoor and outdoor physical activity. *International Journal of Behavioral Nutrition and Physical Activity, 11*, 45.

Rachele, J. N., McPhail, S. M., Washington, T. L., & Cuddihy, T. F. (2012). Practical physical activity measurement in youth: A review of contemporary approaches. *World Journal of Pediatrics, 8*(3), 207–216.

Ridgers, N. D., Stratton, G., & McKenzie, T. L. (2010). Reliability and validity of the system for observing children's activity and relationships during play (SOCARP). *Journal of Physical Activity & Health, 7*(1), 17–25.

Ridgers, N. D., Timperio, A., Crawford, D., & Salmon, J. (2013). What factors are associated with adolescents' school break time physical activity and sedentary time? *PLoS One, 8*(2), e56838.

Rowlands. A., & Eston R. (2007). The measurement and interpretation of children's physical activity. *Journal of Sports Science and Medicine, 6*, 270–276.

Saint-Maurice, P. F., Kim, Y., Welk, G. J., & Gaesser, G. A. (2016). Kids are not little adults: What MET threshold captures sedentary behavior in children? *European Journal of Applied Physiology, 116*, 29–38.

Saint-Maurice, P. F., & Welk, G. J. (2014). Web-based assessments of physical activity in youth: Considerations for design and scale calibration. *Journal of Medical Internet Research, 16*(12), e269.

Saint-Maurice, P. F., & Welk, G. J. (2015). Validity and calibration of the youth activity profile. *PLoS One, 10*(12), e0143949.

Saint-Maurice, P. F., Welk, G. J., Beyler, N. K., Bartee, R. T., & Heelan, K. A. (2014). Calibration of self-report tools for physical activity research: The physical activity questionnaire (PAQ). *BMC Public Health, 14*, 461.

Saint-Maurice, P. F., Welk, G. J., Russell, D. W., & Huberty, J. (2014). Moderating influences of baseline activity levels in school physical activity programming for children: The ready for recess project. *BMC Public Health, 14*, 103.

Sallis, J. F., Owen, N., & Fotheringham, M. J. (2000). Behavioral epidemiology: A systematic framework to classify phases of research on health promotion and disease prevention. *Annals of Behavioral Medicine, 22*(4), 294–298.

Schutz, Y., Weinsier, R. L., & Hunter, G. R. (2001). Assessment of free-living physical activity in humans: An overview of currently available and proposed new measures. *Obesity Research, 9*(6), 368–379. doi:10.1038/oby.2001.48

Scott, J. J., Morgan, P. J., Plotnikoff, R. C., Trost, S. G., & Lubans, D. R. (2013). Adolescent pedometer protocols: Examining reactivity, tampering and participants' perceptions. *Journal of Sports Sciences, 32*(2), 183–190.

Tarp, J., Andersen, L. B., & Østergaard, L. (2015). Quantification of underestimation of physical activity during cycling to school when using accelerometry. *Journal of Physical Activity & Health, 12*(5), 701–707.

Tooze, J. A., Troiano, R. P., Carroll, R. J., Moshfegh, A. J., & Freedman, L. S. (2013). A measurement error model for physical activity level as measured by a questionnaire with application to the 1999–2006 NHANES questionnaire. *American Journal of Epidemiology, 177*(11), 1199–1208. doi:10.1093/aje/kws379

Tremblay, M. S., Aubert, S., Barnes, J. D., Saunders, T. J., Carson, V., Latimer-Cheung, A., . . . Chinapaw, M. (2017). Sedentary behavior research network (SBRN) – Terminology consensus project process and outcome. *International Journal of Behavioral Nutrition and Physical Activity, 14*(1), 75. doi:10.1186/s12966-017-0525-8

Troiano, R. P., Gabriel, K. K. P., Welk, G. J., Owen, N., & Sternfeld, B. (2012). Reported physical activity and sedentary behavior: Why do you ask? *Journal of Physical Activity & Health, 9*(Suppl 1), S68–S75.

Trost, S. G. (2007). State of the art reviews: Measurement of physical activity in children and adolescents. *American Journal of Lifestyle Medicine, 1*, 299–314.

Trost, S. G., Loprinzi, P. D., Moore, R., & Pfeiffer, K. A. (2011). Comparison of accelerometer cut-points for predicting activity intensity in youth. *Medicine and Science in Sports and Exercise, 43*(7), 1360–1368.

Warren, J. M., Ekelund, U., Besson, H., Mezzani, A., Geladas, N., & Vanhees, L. (2010). Assessment of physical activity – A review of methodologies with reference to epidemiological research: A report of the exercise physiology section of the European association of cardiovascular prevention and rehabilitation. *European Journal of Cardiovascular Prevention & Rehabilitation, 17*(2), 127–139.

Welk, G., Morrow, J. R., Jr., & Saint-Maurice, P. F. (2017). *Measures registry user guide: Individual physical activity*. Washington, DC: National Collaborative on Childhood Obesity Research.

13

REPORT-BASED MEASURES OF PHYSICAL ACTIVITY

Features, Considerations, and Resources

Pedro F. Saint-Maurice, Sonia Sousa, Gregory Welk,
Charles E. Matthews, and David Berrigan

Introduction

Report-based measures are one of the most widely used methods to assess physical activity (PA) due to their versatility, ease of administration, and low cost. Report-based methods imply the use of a measure (i.e. questionnaire, diary/log), a respondent, and sometimes, an interviewer. The actual assessment involves a form of some kind, paper or electronic, with a standard set of items that ask about PA according to one or more dimensions such as type of activity, frequency, duration, or intensity. These measures tend to include questions "organized in fixed order, and often with fixed answer options" (Groves et al., 2009). This chapter provides an introductory description of such measures along with their applications. It also describes emerging developments for report-based methods for use in youth PA research (age 10–17 years). Here we use "youth", "child", and "children" interchangeably when referring to this age group. Proxy measures of PA that are more commonly used among younger children (<10 years) and measures of sedentary behavior (SB) are not addressed in this chapter. Interested readers are referred to recent reviews of proxy measures (Hidding, Chinapaw, van Poppel, Mokkink, & Altenburg, 2018) and SB (Hidding, Altenburg, Mokkink, Terwee, & Chinapaw, 2017; Prince, LeBlanc, Colley, & Saunders, 2017).

Self-reports of PA in youth have proven to be invaluable in large-scale epidemiological studies aimed at exploring associations between PA and health outcomes. On the other hand, measurement error associated with self-reports tends to be large and there is considerable concern that the error confounds efforts to assess effects of interventions or to evaluate patterns of behavior for PA surveillance. The key message of this chapter is that report-based measures can add unique value if researchers/practitioners are familiar with their strengths and limitations and if such measures are carefully selected and aligned with the purpose of the study.

The chapter includes three main sections followed by summary remarks. We begin with an overview of the merits of self-reports, here referred to as "report-based" measures or "reports" throughout the chapter and include descriptions of the various types of report-based measures and their applications. This is followed by a discussion of three key considerations related to the use of these measures, including: (1) cognitive processes associated with the recall and reporting of PA, (2) understanding the sources of error that can affect estimates obtained from report-based measures, and (3) interpretation of the information obtained from reports (i.e. assigning intensity values to physical activities). The last section of the chapter describes recent developments in new technologies and a discussion of resources available to assist in instrument selection.

Overview of the Literature

Given the variety of measures available to assess PA, it is critical to understand why report-based measures are needed, their unique features (e.g. design), and how have they been used to assess activity levels in youth. Part two of this chapter provides an overview of the value of different types of report-based measures and illustrates their use with examples.

Using Report-Based Measures: Why and How?

This section reviews the strengths and limitations of report-based measures and contrasts these measures with device-based measures. Report-based measures have contributed (and will continue contributing) to advancing youth PA research. These assessments provide valuable characterizations of youth PA patterns, particularly if measures are selected to minimize known challenges and limitations to assessing PA in youth. Report-based measures can also vary substantially in their design and methods of administration and acceptable options/tools are available for many applications.

Advantages of Report-Based Measures

Report-based measures are inexpensive, easy to use, and have provided robust and replicable results concerning the health benefits of PA. This has made them the most popular measure when collecting information on PA. To date, most of what we know concerning PA is based on report-based measures such as questionnaires or self-reports. For example, information from reports was key when developing and tracking PA guidelines for Americans specifying that "Children and adolescents … should do 60 minutes (1 hour) or more of moderate-to-vigorous physical activity daily" (https://health.gov/paguidelines/second edition/pdf/Physical_Activity_Guidelines_2nd_edition.pdf).

PA has been historically defined as "… *any bodily movement produced by skeletal muscles that result in caloric expenditure*" (Caspersen, Powell, & Christenson, 1985) but more recently, a more comprehensive definition was proposed "… *behavior that involves human movement, resulting in physiological attributes including increased energy expenditure* …" (Bowles, 2012; Pettee Gabriel, Morrow Jr, & Woolsey, 2012). This definition acknowledges that PA is a behavior and reinforces the notion that PA is characterized by body "movement". The operationalization of PA definitions has implications for how it is assessed and indirectly acknowledges the value of report-based measures in contrast to device-based measures that only assess human movement. In the PA landscape, when estimating youth activity levels, key characteristics of PA behavior include a reference to activity frequency (i.e. number per week), duration (i.e. minutes per session), intensity (i.e. energy cost or effort), and type (e.g. aerobic or bone-strengthening-related activities). Report-based measures generally target two or more of these dimensions.

It is also important to consider that PA occurs in a given functional/physical/social context. These contexts help define where activities take place, with whom activities are carried out, and the purpose of specific activities (e.g. activities at school, with friends, and for fun). This contextual information is valuable to understand what factors promote or limit participation in PA. Report-based measures are the simplest, cheapest, and most flexible option available to gather such information.

Considerations for Assessing Physical Activity

A general consensus has emerged that there are three key measurement issues underlying efforts to assess PA behavior using reports: the period of recall (i.e. time frame), how the questions about activity are perceived by the child, and the challenges that the typically intermittent activity patterns of youth can create when using these measures to characterize PA levels. Each of these considerations is discussed in more detail below.

TIME FRAME

The measurement of PA requires that the time frame of the assessment is defined. Characterizations of PA can be as narrow in time as describing activity in (1) physical education or recess; (2) PA on the previous day; (3) PA on the previous week; or (4) broader in frames of reference including descriptions of "usual" or "typical" activity, in the past month or year. Each time frame has implications for recall and the longer the time frame, the greater the challenge for recall. In addition to defining what time frame is more relevant to a study, researchers need to consider the cognitive challenges associated with recalling longer or more distant time frames and consequently, the degree of error in the recalls obtained.

PERCEPTIONS OF ACTIVITY

When asking about participation in PA there is an implicit assumption that children/adolescents understand what is being asked and can define the behavior. Items asking about "moderate intensity" activities or activities that occurred in the "previous week" might be not well understood even though a child can generate a response to such questions. These terms need to be well defined along with the time frame implied (e.g. from Monday to Sunday). Ultimately, well defined terminology and time frames can improve children's perceptions about their past activity and elicit appropriate memories that can lead to more accurate reports of PA.

ACTIVITY PATTERNS

Assessing PA is challenging for all populations but it is particularly difficult among youth. Children have unique behavioral patterns of PA and are known to engage in more sporadic and intermittent activity than adults. For example, adults engage in more structured exercise activities (e.g. jogging) that are characterized by continuous and cyclic body movements. Children's PA is highly sporadic due to the random nature of play at young ages (e.g. playing tag). Activity bouts at young ages typically last for ≤6 seconds (Bailey et al., 1995) and are usually clustered within general activities such as free or unstructured play or games like soccer or tag. These activity patterns have important implications when trying to assess PA with report-based measures (Welk, Corbin, & Dale, 2000). Activity items designed to elicit general memories about participation in PA (e.g. activity done in the last week) are likely to omit youth participation in less structured and intermittent activity events since these will be harder to recall. Report-based measures for youth asking about PA behaviors should be carefully designed to elicit recalls of both structured and unstructured activities.

Types of Report-Based Measures

Report-based measures of PA can be defined according to the time frame being recalled and consequently, the detail of information that each can provide. Here we describe these measures as using short, medium, and long recall time frames:

Short-term recalls include measures that typically ask individuals to recall their activity in the last few hours or previous 1–2 days. Examples of measures using these time frames include Ecological Momentary Assessment (EMA) techniques, diaries/logs, or 24-hour recalls measures including time-use surveys. Short-term recalls facilitate recall and therefore are often used to obtain more comprehensive and dynamic descriptions of activity pattern, type, intensity, and domain (e.g. occupational, transportation, recreational, household). EMA assessments rely on technology (e.g. smartphones) to sample individual's PA at random throughout the day by asking about current behavior or PA done in the last hour or two. This approach increases the accuracy of reports by asking individual to provide real time descriptions of the PA when prompted to do so (Dunton, 2017). Short-term recall measures can provide more accurate and detailed information but can also involve greater respondent burden for instrument completion (usually 15–45 minutes). Such recalls have been used successfully in children as young as 9–10 years (Ridley, Olds, & Hill, 2006).

Reports using **medium recall time frames** include measures that ask about participation in PA in the last 7–30 days. These measures tend to be short by nature (e.g. 5–15 items) and usually take <15 minutes to complete. This type of report-based measure is commonly used in epidemiologic studies and for surveillance (e.g. national assessments of PA). One strength of these measures is that they provide a reasonable balance between participant burden and information that can be obtained from individual responses (Matthews, 2002).

Long-term recalls are usually characterized by use of few items (e.g. 1–4 items) that ask about participation in PA in the previous year or general descriptions of an individuals' "usual" or "typical" activity level. Some examples include global self-reports which descriptions are often limited to specific PA domains such as occupation or leisure-time. These types of report-based measures have also been popular among epidemiological studies (Matthews, 2002). Both medium- and long-term recalls have been used in Government health surveys such as National Health and Nutrition Examination Survey (NHANES) and Youth Risk Behavior Surveillance System (YRBSS) in the United States (https://www.cdc.gov/healthyyouth/data/yrbs/index.htm; https://www.cdc.gov/nchs/nhanes/index.htm).

Report-based measures can be administered using a variety of techniques (i.e. mode of administration) but historically these measures have been administered by mail for self-administered completion, by in-person or phone interviews. The mode of administration can influence response rate. For example, interviews can result in higher response rates while mailed surveys result in the lowest response rates (Grooves et al., 2009b). In early research, report-based measures were often conducted using in-person interviews (e.g. using a 7-day recall interview) (Matthews, 2002). However, given the feasibility of administering questionnaires to large samples, phone interviews and mailed questionnaires have become a more common approach. More recently, the mode of administration has expanded to include technology using the internet, where questions are administered using a computer or smartphone. This mode of administration has become very popular and has the potential to reach a large segment of the population at relatively low cost and provide innovative features for participant interaction with the questionnaire (Grooves et al., 2009b). One limitation of this mode of administration is that contributions, assistance, or completion by/from friends or family members could influence responses even when the investigator is not seeking a proxy report.

Research Applications of Report-Based Measures

Report-based measures are often well suited for large studies even though their use in small–scale studies is still common. Historically, these measures have been used in studies that examined the benefits of PA for health in youth (i.e. cohort studies) and even more prominently, have been used in national and international surveillance of PA participation. This section describes some examples of these applications in more detail.

Predicting Health Outcomes: Prospective Cohort Studies

Report-based measures have been widely used in prospective cohort studies and have contributed to the evidence on the benefits of PA for health (particularly in adults). A prospective cohort study consists of a set of individuals (cohort) that can be exposed or not to certain risk factor(s) being studied. The cohort is assessed at baseline on the risk factors of interest and followed prospectively for the occurrence of diseases onset and other health conditions. Cohort studies are ideally suited for assessing the temporal relation between a given risk factor and onset of disease, assuming health condition is assessed when participants enroll in the study. This temporal sequence is an advantage over cross-sectional studies. Cohort studies typically involve large samples and hence tend to consider feasibility more heavily so that individuals can be assessed on a variety of risk factors including PA. For this reason, PA has been typically assessed in cohorts using report-based measures.

An example of a prospective cohort study involving youth is the Amsterdam Growth and Health Longitudinal Study, an ancillary study examining the health benefits of PA among youth. The study was established in the late 1970s and enrolled 410 13–16-year-old adolescents to examine growth patterns in health-related lifestyle behaviors, including diet and PA, and associations with cardiovascular disease risk factors. This cohort study is still ongoing and participants (now in their ~40s) have been followed over time (Wijnstok, Hoekstra, van Mechelen, Kemper, & Twisk, 2013). The study includes follow-up assessments of PA using a questionnaire developed for this study and administered by interview. Information collected included participation in organized sports, active transportation, and activities at home/school/work (Kemper, Post, Twisk, & van Mechelen, 1999). Numerous individual investigations have been published based on this cohort. One example illustrating the benefits of long-term follow-up includes the finding that weight-bearing activities during adolescence (i.e. 13 years) were associated with higher amounts of bone mineral mass when participants were in their late ~20s (Welten et al., 1994). The 1993 Pelotas Birth Cohort is another example of a prospective cohort study that enrolled ~5,000 newborns, later assessed for leisure-time PA and active commuting when they were 11 years and followed until they were entering adulthood (i.e. 18 years). Leisure-time PA and active commuting were assessed using the long version of the International Physical Activity Questionnaire (IPAQ) and an additional questionnaire that included questions about commuting to/from school delivered using face-to-face interviews. The study found that boys in the highest tertile for active commuting (i.e. more active commuting) at age 11 had lower measures of central body fatness (i.e. waist circumference and trunk fat mass) at age 18 (Martinez-Gomez et al., 2014). Both the Amsterdam Growth and Health Study and the Pelotas Birth Cohort now use a combination of report- and device-based measures to assess PA.

Trends in Physical Activity: Surveillance Studies

Surveillance studies guide population level PA promotion efforts and generate etiological and socioecological hypotheses. These studies often target national samples to characterize trends in a set of behaviors and/or disease outcomes. Such results inform intervention priorities and can sometimes be used to evaluate impact of large-scale public health initiatives. For this reason, surveillance tends to be conducted by governmental entities and occur systematically over time (e.g. every 2 years) to capture changes in health parameters in the population. Cross-sectional survey designs are most common, although in the United States and other countries, longitudinal study designs have been used as in the US National Longitudinal Survey of Youth (https://www.bls.gov/nls/nlsy97.htm). Such studies can have the advantages of cohort studies along with the surveillance benefits of representative sampling frames. We provide a few examples of these studies in this section. Chapter 3 of this book provides a comprehensive review of previous/existent surveillance studies.

Table 13.1 Examples of surveys conducted in United States assessing youth physical activity levels

Survey	Mode of data collection	Target population	Frequency of data collection	Physical activity domains
NHIS	Personal interview	Adults and youth in United States (n = 100,000)	Annual	Leisure-time
NHANES	Interview/examination	Adults and youth (n = ~5,000–10,000)	Annual	Leisure, domestic, transportation
YRBSS	School-based survey	Adolescents (n = 15,000)	Every 2 years	Leisure, domestic, transportation
NHTS	Household survey	US households (n = 25,000)	Every 5–7 years	Transportation
SHPPS	Mail survey	School districts/state education organizations/school classrooms in United States	Periodic	Physical activity policies and domains

Reproduced from Lee and colleagues (Dishman, Heath, & Lee, 2013). Abbreviations: NHANES – National Health and Nutrition Examination Survey; NHIS – National Health Interview Survey; NHTS – National Household Transportation Survey; SHPPS – School Health Policies and Practices Study; YRBSS – Youth Risk Behavior Surveillance System.

Most of what we know from PA levels in the population is also generated from these studies. For example, we know from the YRBSS that, in the US, "… 15.4% of students had not been physically active for a total of at least 60 minutes on at least 1 day …", and that girls tend to be less active than boys (https://www.cdc.gov/healthyyouth/data/yrbs/pdf/2017/ss6708.pdf). These are examples of valuable information that surveillance studies can generate and that is very relevant for PA and public health researchers/professionals. The systematic nature of these studies and large sample sizes that are defined to represent national data require highly feasible measures. For this reason, report-based measures are frequently selected for applications of this nature and have been incorporated in surveys in the United States, as for example, the YRBSS and the NHANES (Table 13.1).

In the YRBSS the assessment of PA was primarily thought to inform national efforts in increasing the proportion of youth meeting the PA guidelines, participating in physical education daily, as well as reducing screen time (https://www.cdc.gov/mmwr/pdf/rr/rr6201.pdf). PA in the YRBSS is assessed using five questions included in the standard questionnaire. For example, one question captures participation in PA for 60 minutes or more in the previous 7 days:

> During the past 7 days, on how many days were you physically active for a total of at least 60 minutes per day? (Add up all the time you spent in any kind of physical activity that increased your heart rate and made you breathe hard some of the time.)

This item allows options from 0 to 7 days, but other items ask about number of days students go to physical education class on an average week, or about participation in sports teams in the previous 12 months (https://www.cdc.gov/healthyyouth/data/yrbs/pdf/2019/2019_YRBS-Standard-HS-Questionnaire.pdf). One common indicator is the percentage of students that did not participate in 60 minutes or more on at least 1 day. The Centers for Disease Control and Prevention (CDC) in the United States manages the YRBSS website where users can explore trends in PA among this population (https://www.cdc.gov/healthyyouth/data/yrbs/results.htm).

The NHANES, like most of the major health surveys in the United States, is administered by the National Center for Health Statistics (NCHS), which is also coordinated through the CDC (Flegal, Carroll, Kit, & Ogden, 2012). In the 2015–2016 NHANES wave, PA was assessed using a questionnaire (i.e. using the Global Physical Activity Questionnaire (GPAQ)). The question-naire was administered at home using interviews: specifically, a Computerized Assisted Personal Interview for children aged 2–11 years, or 16 years and older. Children/adolescents aged 12–15 years were interviewed directly during a visit to the mobile examination center (NHANES mobile for collecting information through physical examinations). The report-based measure used in NHANES asks for example about the number of days youth walk or bike for commuting, in a typical week, or time (minutes/day) spent in moderate or vigorous intensities on a typical day (see one example below; item for 12 years and older only).

> How much time (do you/does sample participant) spend doing moderate-intensity sports, fitness or recreational activities on a typical day?

Other items include activity participation in school sports, or if the child has physical education in their school, or recess and how often. Data and materials from NHANES are available freely for users at https://wwwn.cdc.gov/nchs/nhanes/Default.aspx.

A limitation with most national health surveys involves the reliance on reports and their associated challenges alluded to throughout this chapter. For example, the estimate of ~15% with inadequate activity generated from the YRBSS could be biased by the social desirability of appearing active or misconception of what being active represents. A recent workshop report on enhancing surveillance of PA in youth makes a strong case for incorporating routine device-based measurement of PA in national surveys along with continued use of report-based measures to capture specific activities and context (Dunton et al., 2019). Triangulation of multiple measurement modalities could increase confidence in the estimated prevalence statistics and trends in PA behavior.

In summary, attention to PA in health surveillance systems and cohort studies is important for diverse aspects of PA research in youth. Such studies may provide key instruments for measurement in intervention and evaluation research, can provide benchmarks for local health departments or school systems seeking support for PA-related health promotion, and of course can alert the public health community to pressing public health needs. The discussion in this chapter is focused on examples from the United States, but there are health interviews and health examination surveys in many countries worldwide.

Key Issues

When using report-based measures of PA researchers and practitioners need to be acquainted with a variety of issues and considerations including: (1) cognitive processes involved in the recall and reporting of PA, (2) sources of error in reports of PA, and (3) how to interpret activity scores obtained from reports. These three issues are described below and are key for an appropriate use of these measures and the information they can generate.

Cognitive Processes Involved in Recall and Reporting of Physical Activity

The processes and strategies that individuals rely on to generate their reports of activity events are highly subjective. Report-based measures must rely on respondents alone to report autobiographical descriptions of their PA participation. We think of the human brain as the "hardware" underlying the reports of PA. In this section we describe what we know about human memory and how cognitive processes associated with memory storage and retrieval may influence PA recall and reporting. The recruitment of memories in response to surveys is often called "recall".

Defining Memory and Recall

Memory is a complex construct with a diversity of subcomponents, capable of registering and storing information from multiple sensory modalities such as vision or hearing, and making it available for later retrieval (Baddeley, 2005). Memory is usually divided into short-term memory, long-term memory, and working memory (Atkinson & Shiffrin, 1968; Baddeley, 2002) (Figure 13.1). Episodic memory is a subcomponent of long-term memory and is the most relevant subcomponent of long-term memory for understanding the process of memory formation of PA events. Below we describe each of the three types of memories involved in the process of memory formation (see Figure 13.1, Table 13.2):

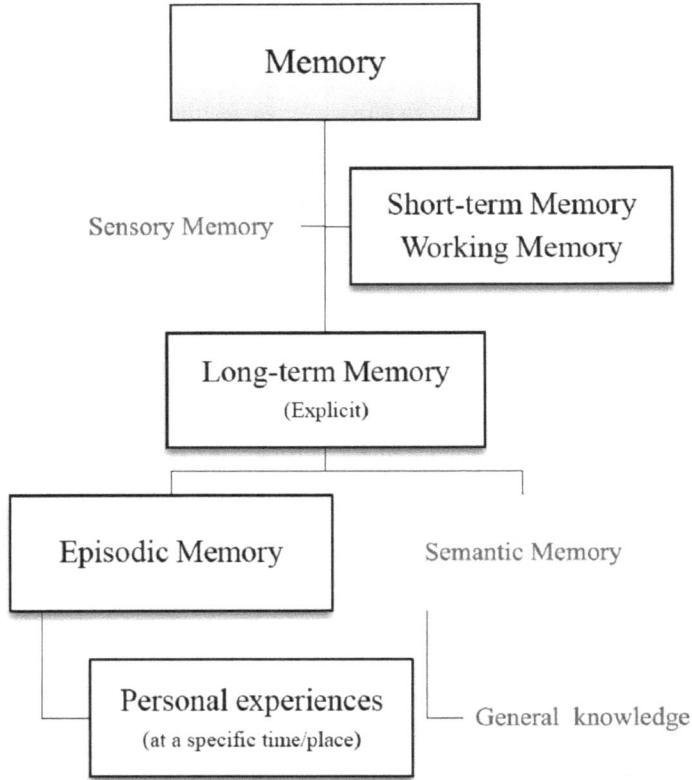

Figure 13.1 Representation of the memory construct. Adapted from Gazzaniga and colleagues (Gazzaniga et al., 2014)

Table 13.2 Characteristics of memory

Type of memory	Time frame	Capacity
Sensory	Milliseconds to seconds	High
Short-term/working	Seconds to minutes	Limited (7 ± 2 items)
Long-term (episodic)	Days to years	High

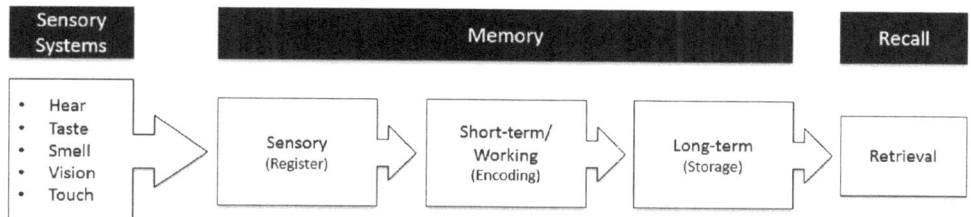

Figure 13.2 Mechanisms of memory formation

Short-term memory is described as a system with a limited storage capacity and is responsible for receiving initial information from the sensory systems (i.e. sensory memory) and holding this information for a short period of time (Baddeley, 2002).

Working memory is part of the short-term memory and represents a limited-capacity system that can maintain information over a short period of time and uses this information while engaging in a given task (also described as memory-in-action, e.g. driving to a place that we're not that familiar while remembering the route). This type of memory is also responsible for retrieving representations of past experiences from long-term storage (Baddeley, 1992; Miyake & Shah, 2009).

Episodic memory is responsible for storing a collection of past events, which occurred in a specific time and place (Baddeley, 1992; Baddeley, 2002). This type of memory is a subcomponent of long-term memory along with semantic memory (i.e. general knowledge) and is the most common memory type elicited in report-based measures that include retrospective assessments of individual's PA. Episodic memory relies on the hippocampus and other cognitive systems (e.g. working memory) and is sustained by a network of cerebral regions including the prefrontal cortex (Ghetti, DeMaster, Yonelinas, & Bunge, 2010; Keresztes, Ngo, Lindenberger, Werkle-Bergner, & Newcombe, 2018; Tang, Shafer, & Ofen, 2018).

Recall of autobiographical events is influenced by a variety of mechanisms, namely, memory encoding, storage, and retrieval/recall (Figure 13.2).

ENCODING

It is the stage in which new information from the sensory memory is transferred to the short-term memory, after a process of selective attention, generating memory traces or representations to be later stored in the long-term memory (Gazzaniga, Ivry, & Mangun, 2014; Miyake & Shah, 2009; Thompson, 2005).

STORAGE

It is the permanent archive of the initially encoded and consolidated information or memory traces (Gazzaniga et al., 2014).

RETRIEVAL AND RECALL

Retrieval represents the ability to access previously stored memory traces. Recall refers to the conscious process of accessing and retrieving information from long-term memory and using it to construct a representation of past experiences/knowledge (Gazzaniga et al., 2014; Ryan., Hoscheidt, & Nadel, 2008).

The recall of autobiographical events depends on both the maturation of brain structures and ability to recruit brain regions responsible for the recall processes (e.g. hippocampus). For example, both the hippocampus and the prefrontal cortex undergo changes in morphology and function with age, achieving full maturation only near early adulthood (Giedd et al., 1996; Gogtay et al., 2006; Lenroot & Giedd, 2006; Ostby et al., 2009). Children, adolescents, and adults also differentially recruit the hippocampus and other brain regions to accurately encode and retrieve episodic information (Ghetti et al., 2010; Guler & Thomas, 2013; Langnes et al., 2018; Sastre, Wendelken, Lee, Bunge, & Ghetti, 2016). These discrepancies are expected to lead to more inaccuracies in reports obtained from children when compared to adults and are attenuated after late adolescence. Adolescents are already capable of performing almost as well as adults, which may be associated with increasing stability of brain networks (Ghetti et al., 2010; Lee, Ekstrom, & Ghetti, 2014; Menon, Boyett-Anderson, & Reiss, 2005; Sastre et al., 2016; Shing & Lindenberger, 2011).

The Recall of Physical Activity in Children and Adolescents

The process of memory formation of past PA events involves the sensory register of the event such as the sights, sounds, and feelings associated with playing soccer; the encoding/consolidation of the event and contextual features (i.e. *what*; *when*; *where*; *with whom*); and the organization and retention of the information to be stored in the long-term memory. However, elements of this entire process can be challenged by constraints arising at each step that may contribute to later memory failure as well as influence responses provided in report-based instruments (Figure 13.3).

Figure 13.3 describes an example with a soccer activity. A memory is successfully stored in the long-term memory if key contextual descriptors of the activity event pass on through each of the memory types involved in the process of memory formation. Successful memory formation

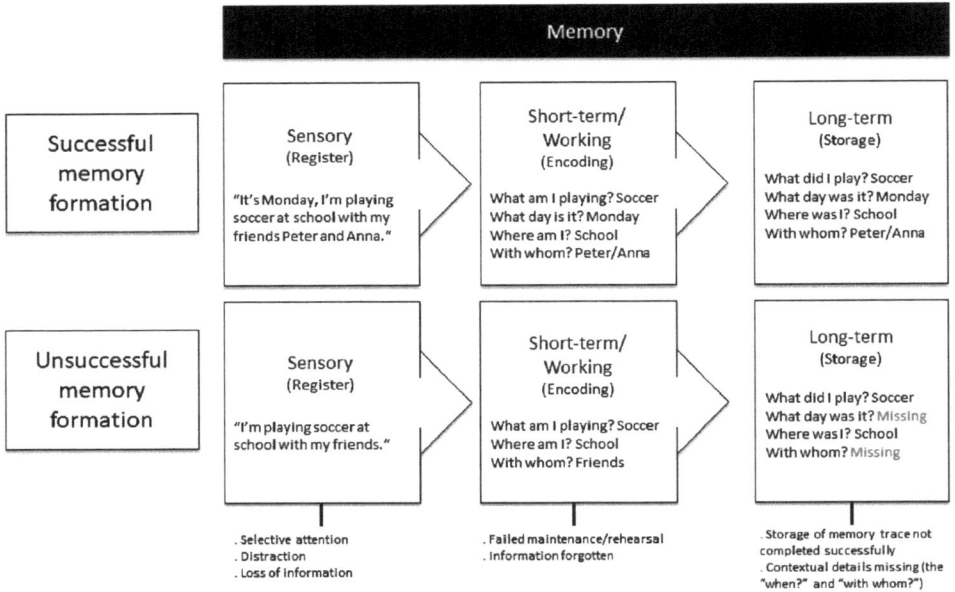

Figure 13.3 Conceptual illustration of successful vs. unsuccessful memory formation using a soccer activity

occurs when the child collects all relevant contextual information during early stages of memory formation (i.e. **sensory memory**) and then, the information is encoded and stored in long-term memory. In the situation that some contextual elements are not identified and encoded in long-term memory, this information may not be available for later recall. For example, incomplete encoding might occur if the child is distracted and did not situate the activity in time (i.e. which day of the week is it) and did not identify what other children were involved in the activity. This event would be encoded but without the "*when*" and "*with whom*" information. Processes associated with this omitted information in the sensory memory relate to selective attention, distraction, and loss of information.

Considering the limited capacity of the **short-term memory**, the information needs to go through what is known as maintenance/rehearsal – process of storing information through repetition. This process is important to stabilize or consolidate the memory traces so that they can be later transferred to long-term memory; otherwise the information might be forgotten. Using the earlier soccer example, if the child is not able to gather all the details of the event (i.e. *what*: playing soccer; *when:* yesterday at noon; *where:* at school; *with whom:* classmates) the specificities of this particular event might be forgotten and fail to be stored in the long-term memory.

At the final stage of memory formation, different components of the event are attached to form a single representation of the episode. Hence, if a bit of the contextual information (e.g. the *where*; *when*; *with whom* of the event) is lost during the process of memory consolidation, the successful retrieval of episodic memories might be disturbed. In our example, if the specifics of this particular event are not stored in **long-term memory**, generalization may occur. In this case the event may be assigned somewhat randomly to any day as one of myriad activities carried at some unspecified time. Hence, when questioned, the child will not be able to accurately recall the event of interest. This is a simplistic illustration of how information might be lost but there are many others. The key message is that memory formation and later retrieval require the collection of contextual descriptors and that this process seems to be more challenging for children, considering their tendency to collect a rather general knowledge of their experiences, and remembering fewer details of particular episodes (Bauer, 2015; Keresztes et al., 2018; Shing & Lindenberger, 2011).

Once memories are stored, the recall of an event relies on four main steps: question comprehension, event search and construction of the event skeleton (*what, when, where*), event elaboration and recall, and finally response. Consider the following question: **How much soccer did you play last week?** We selected this rather simplistic example in order to describe the recall process and more easily explain how this might be impacted by several factors. Most report-based instruments ask about general participation in activities of a certain intensity (i.e. moderate-to-vigorous intensity). The process described below also applies and will ultimately rely on the child's interpretation of what moderate intensity represents. Thus, the recall process will be more challenging when broader questions are used.

The **comprehension phase** requires that the child understands the time frame of the question (i.e. last week), identifies what soccer is, and that the question is asking about all soccer events that might have happened. At the **event search** phase, the child explores her/his long-term memories to find a specific memory that will correspond to the question asked: *what*: play soccer; *when*: last week; and *where*. In the specific question asked: "How much soccer did you play last week?" information about the *where* component of the event is not mentioned. Therefore, the child will have to search for all the activities he has done throughout the week and all the places she/he has been to find out if she/he played soccer and how much. This step will dictate what strategies are used for recall and whether the child is using episodic vs. generalized memories. The event **elaboration or retrieval phase** is when the child elaborates and reconstructs her/his memories by using some specific cues such as reference to the context (e.g. location) where activity might have happened.

Finally, a **response** is adjusted to address what is being asked. The elaboration or retrieval phase of this process is critical and might affect the accuracy of the response provided.

Report-based measures of PA tend to use either *when*, *what*, or/and *where* related cues to collect reported information on past PA events. Using our earlier example – **How much soccer did you play last week?** The *when* cue would be: "last week" while a *what* cue would be: "soccer". A *where* cue is not included but if this were added to the question: "How much soccer did you play last week when you were at school?". An immediate reaction might be that adding a *where* cue to the question seems to facilitate the recall and improve the accuracy of the response. Research within the field of cognitive psychology and neurodevelopment has shown that episodic memories are organized into relational networks linking new and past events that occurred in the same location – *where*. Also, episodic memory retrieval seems to be much more accurate when individuals are assisted with mental imagery and context-related cues where past events occurred (Bramao, Karlsson, & Johansson, 2017).

This section illustrates that youth performance when recalling past activity events changes as youth mature, and that this process is affected by the design of a given report instrument or single item. The inclusion of contextual references can facilitate recall and is key when assessing PA in this population with report-based measures. The general notion is that less detailed items such as those missing contextual cues will require greater cognitive effort in order to provide an answer, and result in less accurate responses (Tourangeau, Rips, & Rasinski, 2000). Unfortunately, such contextual cues are often left out of report-based measures of PA, which might explain the error that has been documented for these measures.

Sources of Error in Reports of Physical Activity

The error associated with reports has been attributed to individual's inability to accurately recall their past PA. However, the sources of error in these measures are not limited to the recall process alone and there are several properties beyond validity that need to be considered to minimize error in PA reports. This section introduces the reader to a qualitative framework for evaluating reports and includes descriptions of various sources of error that can contribute to inaccuracies in these measures.

Quality Assessment of Measures

Terwee and colleagues created a Quality Assessment of Physical Activity Questionnaire (QAPAQ) checklist intended to systematically evaluate the qualitative and measurement properties of PA questionnaires that need to be considered in order to minimize error (Terwee et al., 2010). According to this checklist, questionnaires should be examined based on nine major qualitative properties: construct, setting, recall period, purpose, target population, justification, format, interpretability, and ease of use (Table 13.3). Here we adopt this checklist to guide users when first identifying potential measures for their study. The checklist is not intended to provide a final answer to what measure should be selected and thus is particularly helpful at the first stages of measure selection and as users narrow their options to a few available measures. The selection of a given report-based measure is also not always straightforward and users might favor a combination of certain measurement properties while keeping in mind other study design considerations (e.g. age of participants, contact time allowed with participants to complete the questionnaire). Table 13.3 describes each of the nine qualitative properties to consider when first assessing the measurement properties of a given measure (Terwee et al., 2010). Other checklists have been proposed (Lohr, 2002; Mokkink et al., 2010; Terwee et al., 2007).

Table 13.3 Quality Assessment of Physical Activity Questionnaire (QAPAQ) Checklist

Qualitative properties	Example
Construct	What is the questionnaire intended to measure (e.g. energy expenditure, moderate-to-vigorous physical activity)?
Setting	What physical activity domain is being characterized (e.g. school)?
Recall	What is the defined time frame (e.g. previous 7 days)?
Purpose	What is the intended purpose of the questionnaire, rather to discriminate between populations, evaluate, or predict health-related events?
Target population	What are the characteristics of the sample with who the questionnaire was originally developed (e.g. age, social economic status, type of activities reported)?
Justification	Considering that there are a wide set of questionnaires available, it is also important to determine why a given questionnaire is more appropriate than existent alternatives (i.e. justification)
Format	Is the structure of the questionnaire adequate and intuitive? For example, with respect to the number of questions, number and type of response categories, and scoring algorithm
Interpretability	Can the questionnaire summary score be easily interpreted (e.g. are there norms available that allow for an interpretation of scores?)?
Ease of use	Includes the time required to complete the questionnaire, if there is a copy of the questionnaire available and, if instructions on how to use/fill the questionnaire are available

Total Survey Error

In addition to the properties described earlier more objective indicators have been used to quantify the error in these measures – including examinations of reliability and validity of a measure. These two are often the only properties reported when introducing new questionnaires and hence have been the focus among researchers when debating whether one measure is more appropriate than others. We will address reliability and validity in the context of Total Survey Error. Reliability and validity are two indicators of the total error associated with a given measure. This combined error is also known as **Total Survey Error** (term commonly used in survey statistics). Error can be generated at various stages from measure development/validation (i.e. validity) to data generation (i.e. measurement error), and data entry (i.e. processing error); hence, we find the Total Survey Error concept useful to better understand the various sources of error associated with report-based measures (Figure 13.4).

Validity of a given report-based measure of PA reflects the agreement between the "true" measure of PA and the report-based measure. This definition requires two key clarifications, how we define "true" and how we define "agreement". The concept of a "true measure of physical activity" is used conceptually here, as if we were to assess PA with the most accurate measure available that would be 100% accurate (i.e. free of error). This is of course unachievable, as every measure has error. Instead, use of the term "criterion measure" is more appropriate, as a measure that we establish as having considerably less error than the measure to be tested. The second key explanation is agreement. Agreement is defined by the amount of overlap that the report-based measure has with the criterion measure. Agreement is what ultimately provides a quantification for validity and is typically established using statistical parameters such as the Pearson-product correlation, test of mean differences, limits of agreement as proposed by Bland Altman, the standard error of estimate (SEE), and equivalence testing (Dixon et al., 2017; Zaki, Bulgiba, Ismail, & Ismail, 2012) (see Table 13.4).

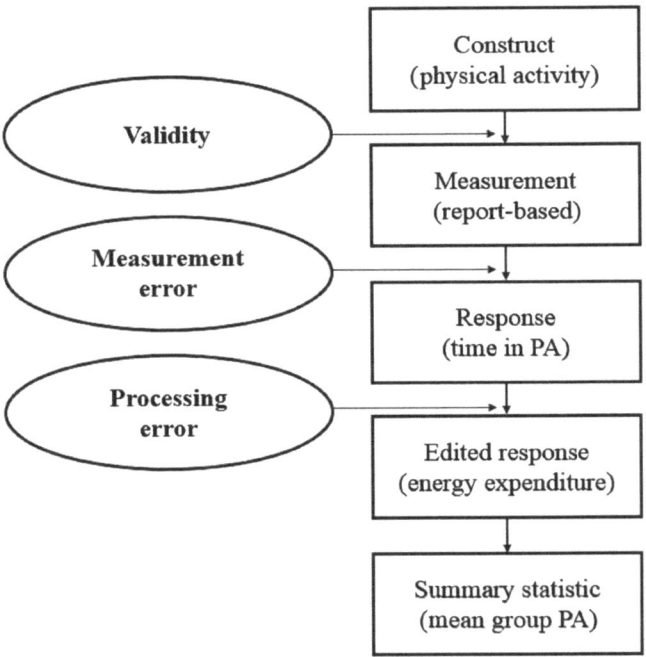

Figure 13.4 Total Survey Error scheme for physical activity measurement. Adapted from Groves and colleagues (Grooves et al., 2009a)

Table 13.4 Indices of Agreement Commonly Used in Validation Studies Involving Report-Based Measures

Pearson Product Moment	The report and the criterion measure are moderately and positively correlated (r = 0.50)
Test of Mean Differences	Report and criterion measure differ by a minimum amount, and the difference is not statistically significant
Bland Altman (Limits of Agreement)	The estimates of the report are within −450 and +560 kcal of that obtained from the criterion measure
Standard Error of Estimate	Estimates obtained from the report are ±10.0 units apart from those of the criterion measure
Equivalence Testing	Estimates obtained from the report are within 10% from those of the criterion measure

Adapted from National Collaborative on Childhood Obesity Research Measurement Guide – Individual Physical Activity (Welk, Morrow et al., 2017).

For example, validity for a report-based measure has been defined by comparing estimates of PA generated by a given questionnaire to those obtained from a device-based measure (i.e. criterion measure). Validity in these studies has been commonly demonstrated with Pearson correlations, a limited but necessary indicator that captures the ability of two instruments to rank individuals in similar order. We recommend the use of additional statistical indicators that can provide better representations of agreement, including agreement in absolute amounts of PA generated by the two instruments as those described in Table 13.4 (Dixon et al., 2017; Zaki et al., 2012).

Measurement error describes error that occurs during the measurement process. For example, socially undesirable behaviors tend to be underreported (this form of error is also known as bias). In youth, this might be less of a concern at very young ages but is more likely among older children. Error can also reflect the reproducibility of a measure – the ability of a measure/respondent to elicit similar estimates if the measure was administered on two different occasions. With report-based measures the assessment of reproducibility needs to be interpreted carefully as this can reflect both actual changes in behavior over time as well as inconsistent reports of PA.

Processing error can arise from the methods used to process or code the data (e.g. conversion of responses to numerical values). This can occur if a coder assigned a moderate-intensity Metabolic Equivalent of Task (MET) value (e.g. 4 METs) to one common sedentary activity (e.g. watching TV/screen time). It can also occur when converting reported physical activities to estimates of energy expenditure (EE). This source of error is usually minor but contributes to total error associated with report-based measures that require a data recording and conversion steps (see Figure 13.4). Checking distributions and flagging extreme observations are important in detecting this type of error.

Validity of Report-Based Measures

Validity has been the most extensive property examined for report-based measures, and more commonly for short-recall questionnaires. Historically, report-based measures have been tested for validity against device-based measures of PA (e.g. accelerometers) and only occasionally in comparison to direct observation or doubly labeled water. An example of a validation study is a test of the agreement between two measures for time spent in moderate-to-vigorous PA. However, fundamental differences between these two measures need to be introduced for the reader to appreciate the level of agreement found in validation studies of this nature.

Validation studies using device-based measures as criterion rely on the assumption that devices and reports can generate the same outcome (e.g. duration of PA). This is a reasonable assumption in some circumstances. However, such validation studies do not always adequately address differences between the two types of measures. For example, accelerometers measure total movement (across domains) while report-based measures are typically context or time specific (e.g. recess, after-school). These fundamental differences pose challenges when making direct comparisons between these two measures. Take the example of a report-based measure that asks about time spent commuting to and from school during the previous day. If a criterion measure was obtained from an accelerometer that a child wore for the full day, a direct comparison between the two measures would obviously conclude that the report-based measure generated substantially fewer minutes of activity (activity related to commuting alone) than those obtained from the accelerometer (total activity). This is a rather simplistic example, but the take home message is that report-based measures often measure domain-specific PA while accelerometers measure total PA. Hence, the two estimates might not be comparable unless the outcomes generated from the two measures are matched for domain or total PA.

Estimates of PA intensity based on calibrated activity counts may also be obtained from accelerometers. These crude measures are monitor specific and are based on the intensity of body movement at the waist, wrist, or other body site locations. Often, activity counts have been calibrated to measure specific types of activities, and these are not always reflective of free-living activity patterns, thus reducing their utility for validation of reported PA. For example, an accelerometer that has been calibrated to assess walking at different speeds will likely perform well when a child is walking, but its accuracy may be reduced when the child is doing other activities such as playing sports, playing tag, free play. Direct comparisons between reports of these activities and a device-based measure calibrated to assess walking would result in discrepant estimates and suggest that the report was inaccurate. However, it is also likely that the accelerometer did not identify or capture other activities that were possibly included in the report estimates. These examples illustrate that validation studies, while informative, need to be designed and interpreted carefully.

Many validation studies use device-based measures to validate reports of PA. Closer inspection of this literature suggests that few of these report-based measures have good utility with this population and few have acceptable indices of validity. Reviews and validation studies of report-based measures for youth suggest that the design features of report-based measures (e.g. time frame for recall, quality of items) can vary substantially and that attention to multiple design considerations previously described in this chapter can result in more accurate estimates obtained from report-based measures. For example, a review from Tessier, Vuillemin, and Briancon (2008) identified 30 questionnaires and concluded that the Physical Activity Questionnaire for Adolescents (PAQ-A), the Previous-day Physical Activity Recall (PDPAR), and the Modified Activity Questionnaire for Adolescents had the best indicators of validity with correlations greater than 0.60 (Tessier et al., 2008). A comprehensive review done by Chinapaw, Mokkink, van Poppel, van Mechelen, and Terwee (2010) included 56 self-report instruments and found correlations between self-reports and device-based measures to be low to moderate, but identified some questionnaires with acceptable validity coefficients. Validity indices were consistently higher among studies that included older children, for measures using shorter recall periods, and for measures that included items that are more likely to elicit episodic memories, and hence facilitate recall of previous PA events. The review of 89 self-report instruments by Biddle, Gorely, Pearson, and Bull (2011) identified the following three instruments as being the most suitable for surveillance research – the Physical Activity Questionnaire for Children/ Adolescents (PAQ-C/PAQ-A), Youth Risk Behavior Surveillance Survey (YRBS), and the Teen Health Survey (Biddle et al., 2011). The authors attributed the value of these measures in part to the inclusion of contextual questions (e.g. activity during recess) and concluded that that these cues can facilitate recall.

As suggested by the earlier reviews, one critical aspect of the accuracy of a given report-based measure is the process through which it elicits the use of appropriate memories essential for accurate recall of previous activity events. Important considerations include the use of contextual cues, reasonable time frames, and terms or concepts that can be easily understood. We have created a conceptual illustration of where the various report-based measures (previously grouped as using short, medium, and long recall time frames) would typically fall in relation to their quality (here defined as processes that elicit episodic memories and hence can facilitate recall) and feasibility (i.e. easy to use, cost of administration, time for completion) (see Figure 13.5).

The relation between feasibility and episodic memories for the examples provided can be enhanced by adapting some of the earlier measures and considering different modes of administration. For example, 7-day recalls can be enhanced if the measure is administered using interviews. However, this adaptation would also result in greater burden to the researcher (i.e. higher cost per administration) and participant (i.e. longer time to complete) and hence, would be less feasible. Our graphical representation of feasibility vs. episodic memories also assumes that recalls assessing longer time frames include more general inquiries about activity and therefore use fewer items and require less time to be completed. For example, a 1-year recall when compared to a 7-day recall is likely to include fewer items and ask for broader descriptions of activity (i.e. more feasible). However, items included in a 1-year recall are likely vague, ask about broader descriptions, and include fewer contextual cues. Such items are likely to elicit episodic memories to a lesser extent.

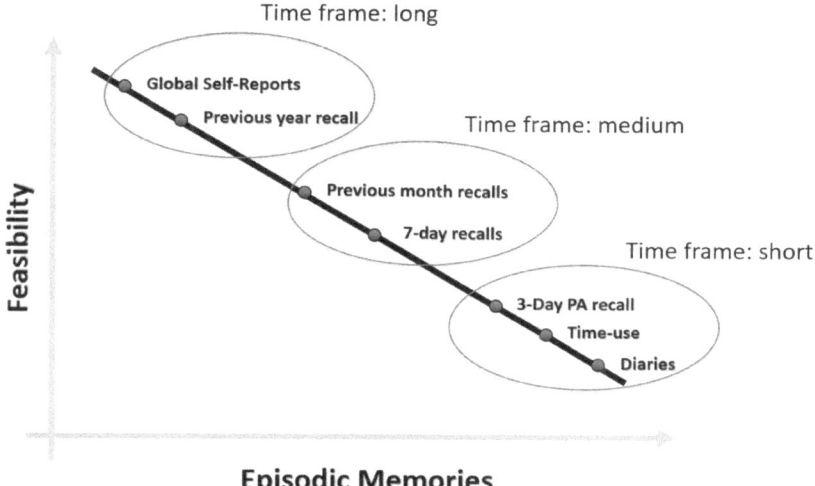

Figure 13.5 Conceptual illustration of the relation between feasibility and episodic memories that are likely to be elicited if the various types of report-based measures were used. Adapted from National Collaborative on Childhood Obesity Research Measurement Guide – Individual Physical Activity (Welk, Morrow et al., 2017)

Interpreting Reported Estimates of Physical Activity

Depending on the measure, reported PA can reflect either relative or absolute energy cost of the activities performed (Welk, Morrow, & Saint-Maurice, 2017). The energy cost of relative vs. absolute energy cost can lead to different representations of activity levels for the same individual. Nonetheless, most report-based measures are designed to describe the absolute intensity of youth activities. This section describes the concepts of relative vs. absolute intensity and the use of adult vs. youth generated absolute intensity thresholds and their implications for interpreting activity scores.

Absolute vs. Relative Intensity

Absolute vs. relative intensity refers to whether an intensity of an activity is defined in absolute terms using predefined intensity values (i.e. absolute intensity) or instead relative to the child's fitness level (i.e. relative intensity). PA intensity has been conveniently expressed as multiples of resting EE – MET (Howley, 2001). Historically, rest/sedentary is defined as an intensity of 1.0 to 1.4 METs, light intensity physical activities as from 1.5 to 2.9 METs, moderate-intensity physical activities range from 3.0 to 5.9 METs, and vigorous PA intensities are 6.0+ METs. These categories have been widely used to characterize the intensity of PA in various report-based forms. For example, a child can be asked to identify activities that he engaged during the day/week and these activities can be assigned energy cost values at posteriori. This is an example of a report-based measure that would include descriptions based on absolute intensity.

Questions about PA can also be framed to reflect a child's interpretation of the intensity associated with an activity event. For example, when asked to report the time spent in moderate-intensity physical activities while including definitions of intensities as being for example, activities eliciting an increase in heart rate or breathing rate, or activities that "make a sweat", the child response will reflect her/his perception of this level of intensity. Reports of activity to such items are likely to reflect a child's individual fitness level and hence, activity is reported in relative terms. For example, an activity reported by a fitter child as being light intensity may possibly be described as moderate intensity for a less fit child. This would be an example of report-based activities based on relative energy cost. The absolute vs. relative nuance is important for data generated from report-based measures and users should be aware of how the effort associated with an activity is quantified and described.

The Compendium of Youth Physical Activities

The Youth Physical Activity Compendium was developed to provide age-appropriate ways to process and interpret PA data in youth (Ainsworth et al., 2011; Butte et al., 2018). Researchers are often interested in estimating energy cost of activities alone, excluding resting metabolic rate and dietary thermogenesis. This measure, Activity Energy Expenditure (AEE), is of interest because it is more variable and susceptible to change via interventions or spontaneous changes in behavior. The associated energy cost of activities alone with the thermic effect of feeding, and resting EE add up to total energy cost (see Figure 13.6). The energy cost of activities has been standardized to absolute measures of EE using MET values so that they can be interpreted and their implications for health be better understood. The goal of estimating EE from report-based measures of activity led to the development of a compendium of physical activities, first for adults, later adapted for youth. The youth compendium was recently updated with many new measures of EE and with an effort to adjust for age specific reductions in resting EE.

MET values express energy cost of a given activity as multiples of energy cost over that required at rest. Historically, MET values were originally developed for adult applications and the required energy cost at rest for adults is assumed to be ~3.5 ml/kg/min. Hence, 1 MET = 3.5 ml/kg/min. This value at rest was derived for a 40-year old 70 kg (likely lean) individual back in 1940s (Byrne,

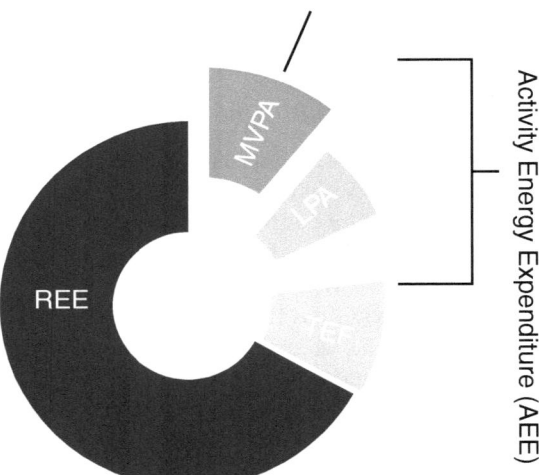

Figure 13.6 Conceptual description of energy expenditure components. Total energy expenditure includes resting energy expenditure (REE), thermic effect of feeding (TEF), and Activity Energy Expenditure (AEE). AEE includes energy expenditure associated with sedentary behaviors (SB), Light Physical Activity (LPA), and moderate-to-vigorous physical activity (MVPA). Many report-based measures of physical activity for youth limit their assessments to MVPA (e.g. free play, soccer)

Hills, Hunter, Weinsier, & Schutz, 2005; Gagge, Burton, & Bazett, 1941). However, resting EE is primarily determined by body composition including lean body fat mass, body size, and other factors such as age and sex (Byrne et al., 2005; Harrell et al., 2005; McMurray, Soares, Caspersen, & McCurdy, 2014; Molnar & Schutz, 1997). This variability is particularly problematic in younger children and adolescents who are undergoing biological maturation and hence consistent changes in body composition over time. The energy cost at rest for a 6-year old can be as high as ~6.5 ml/kg/min (i.e. almost twice as that of an adult). Values might be approximately 4.2 ml/kg/min for a 13-year old and decrease as adolescent reaches adult age of 18 (Ainsworth et al., 2018; Butte et al., 2018; Harrell et al., 2005; Pfeiffer et al., 2018; Ridley, Ainsworth, & Olds, 2008). This issue is illustrated in Figure 13.7 which shows the energy cost of various activities for youth. The figure also illustrates the systematic overestimation of METs that would arise if adult estimates of resting EE (3.5 ml/kg/min) were used. For example, MET values for sedentary activities (e.g. sitting in a chair reading) are all above 2.0 METs when adult estimates of METs are used. When energy cost of activities was standardized to resting EE values that were child age and sex specific, MET values were systematically attenuated and approximated those expected for sedentary (i.e. <1.5 METs), light (i.e. 1.5–2.9 METs), and moderate-intensity activities (≥3.0 METs) (Saint-Maurice, Kim, Welk, & Gaesser, 2016). These results show that using 3.5 ml/kg/min as the energy cost at rest for youth results in considerable overestimations of activity energy cost in youth (Figure 13.7). This is one example of discrepancies between adult and youth energy cost at rest that led to the revised and more comprehensive compendium of youth physical activities (Ainsworth et al., 2018; Butte et al., 2018).

The new youth compendium was developed by a team working with the National Collaborative on Childhood Obesity Research (NCCOR). The revised Youth Compendium of Physical Activities includes 196 activities using child-specific MET values with energy cost values presented separately for 6–9, 10–12, 13–15, and 16–18 years youth (Butte et al., 2018). The compendium is available at https://www.nccor.org/nccor-tools/youthcompendium/and provides EE values that can

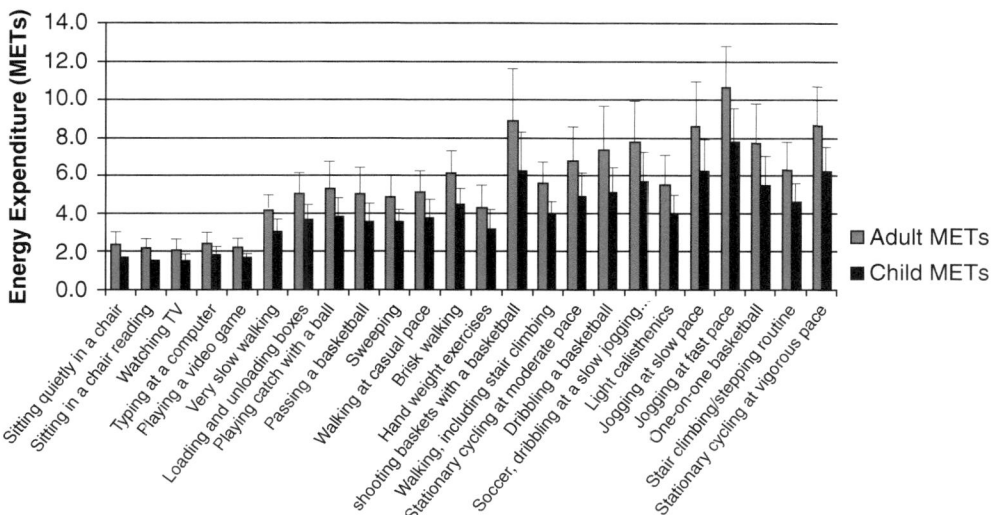

Figure 13.7 Activity Energy Expenditure for 102 7–13-year-old youth while performing various activities using adult (energy cost at rest assumed to be 3.5 ml/kg/min) and child MET values (energy cost at rest predicted using child's age and sex information – Schofield equation). Adapted from Lee, Saint-Maurice, Kim, Gaesser, and Welk (2016)

be assigned to a variety of activities that youth tend to engage. The compendium has great utility to improve comparability of studies using report-based measures by allowing transformation of activity classifications into time spent at various intensities or other units such as MET scores per day.

Recent Developments and Resources

In the final section of this chapter we highlight the need for exploring new technologies (e.g. internet-based platforms, smartphone apps) to increase both the accuracy and feasibility of PA recalls and to make use of available resources in order to standardize selection and evaluation of report-based measures. We first address the growing availability of internet and smartphone-based instruments and their potential for reducing costs and increasing the validity of PA data collection. Second, we discuss the development of diverse resources aimed at guiding the PA researcher and practitioners selecting the best possible measure, considering both study goals and available resources.

Web-Based Surveys

In the early 2000s, there were discussions about how the internet could replace traditional methods used in survey research (Couper, 2000). In 2000, approximately 50% of US adults were "connected" and now, nine out of ten adults have access to the internet (http://www.pewinternet.org/fact-sheet/internet-broadband/). Internet use has expanded across age groups and about 92% of adolescents aged 13–17 years have access to internet daily, while 24% are "constantly connected" (http://www.pewinternet.org/2015/04/09/teens-social-media-technology-2015/). Internet use has also become more popular among schools that use computers and the internet to promote interactive learning environments. With such availability, it has become clear that most children and adolescents in the United States and other developed countries have access to internet. Therefore, the potential of the internet to improve existing measures via interface design and ease of use and the possibility to reach out to hundreds or thousands of individuals with "one click" has sparked great interest among survey designers. Despite this promise, most report-based measures of PA are still limited to paper versions and were not designed and have not yet been adapted for internet applications.

There are a variety of uses of the internet for conducting surveys. In the realm of PA assessments, the internet can be used to send questionnaires to individuals, be completed offline, and sent back by email. Another application is to host a survey on the web and invite individuals to complete the survey online and submit once it is completed. The survey and responses are hosted in the server and the individual is online while completing the survey. Our descriptions of web surveys apply to the last example. One good example of a web survey designed for youth is the Youth Activity Profile (YAP; www.youthactivityprofile.org), a 15-item 7-day recall that includes questions about both PA and SBs. The YAP was also designed for school-based assessments and to provide educational value.

The YAP was designed for youth 4th–12th grades (10–17 years) and to generate estimates that would approximate those obtained from a device-based measure. The 15 items included in the YAP ask about general descriptions of time spent in PA and SB in various settings, including at school (i.e. transportation to school, recess, physical education, lunch, transportation from school), out-of-school (i.e. before school, after-school, and evening), and weekend (i.e. Saturday and Sunday). Scores from each item range from 1 to 5 and have been calibrated to minutes of moderate-to-vigorous PA per week and YAP estimates have demonstrated acceptable validity (Saint-Maurice & Welk, 2014, 2015; Saint-Maurice, Welk, Bartee, & Heelan, 2017; Saint-Maurice, Welk, Beyler, Bartee, & Heelan, 2014). The YAP was also designed to provide immediate feedback regarding a child's activity level. The survey uses a paging design where the screen changes as a child completes an item. The 15-item survey takes 5–7 minutes for completion and upon completion the screen displays summary PA scores for school, home, and for time spent in SBs (Figure 13.8).

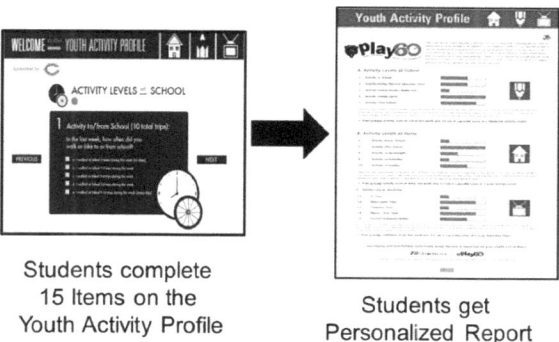

The web version of the YAP has facilitated the deployment of this tool at a large-scale. The tool has been integrated within FitnessGram – an internationally recognized web-based fitness platform developed in the United States – and integrated into a large participatory network of over 1,000 schools (NFL PLAY 60 FitnessGram Partnership Project https://fitnessgram.net/nflplay60/) (Welk, Bai, Saint-Maurice, Allums-Featherston, & Candelaria, 2016). The YAP was also used in the Family Life, Activity, Sun, Health, and Eating (FLASHE) study sponsored by the National Cancer Institute, United States, to assess PA/SB in ~1,500 youth aged 12–17 years (D'Angelo, Fowler, Nebeling, & Oh, 2017; Nebeling et al., 2017; Saint-Maurice, Kim, et al., 2017; Welk, Saint-Maurice et al., 2017). The YAP is also being used internationally in the United Kingdom and Czech Republic. In sum, the web has opened various venues for the short and validated PA instrument to be used for both national and international research and surveillance applications (http://www.youthactivitystudy.com).

Additional valuable applications of technology for PA assessments in children include the Multimedia Activity Recall for Children and Adolescents (MARCA). The MARCA is a time-use survey that can be completed offline using a computer and that allows a child to reproduce their previous day by indicating key time periods throughout their day (e.g. end of school, lunch) and select activities in blocks of five minutes that occurred throughout the 24-hour timeline. The anchoring of time periods provides a segmented approach that helps a child associate the context to a given activity and hence facilitate recall. Children as young as 9–10 years-old can select from over 500 activities, grouped into seven categories: inactivity, transport, play/sport, school work, self-care, chores, and "other" (Ridley et al., 2006). MARCA has been used quite a bit in New Zealand and Australia and provides very rich and detailed information about specific activities over the entire 24-hour day. These are unique examples of how report-based measures can benefit from web applications; however, more work is needed to extend these applications to other well-established reports of PA.

Measures Compilations and Training Materials

With the plethora of report-based measures available it becomes daunting to select the most appropriate measure for a given application. Here we emphasize the need to carefully consider the choice of exposure/outcome (e.g. intensity, volume, EE) as well as the degree of precision that is required. Presently, studies that should be assessing specific behaviors are pushed toward using device-based measures and studies that should be capturing total movement end up using inappropriate survey items when they could benefit from the use of 24-hour recalls or device-based measures. Together these inappropriate choices can lead to substantial wasted resources and perhaps misleading conclusions. As of 2019, there are several key resources available to aid in the selection of appropriate measures of PA in children and adolescents.

The US NCCOR has developed a searchable database of validation studies for measures of PA (https://tools.nccor.org/measures). This searchable database includes information on 479 papers concerning validation studies of instruments aimed at measuring various aspects of PA in children published between 1973 and 2018. The registry includes information on the type of measure, age range, context and measures of validity and reliability from the studies. NCCOR also supported the development of a monograph length guide to measuring PA in children (Welk, Morrow et al., 2017) and the aforementioned compendium of youth physical activities (Butte et al., 2018). These resources and related training materials including slide sets and short video presentations concerning key aspects of measurement posted on the NCCOR web site are intended to support selection of the best available measures for diverse research and evaluation projects concerning youth PA and obesity.

Additional compilations of measures and resources related to PA with less focus on children include the consensus measures for Phenotypes and Exposure (PhenX) tool kit (https://www.phenxtoolkit.org/index.php); the MRC PA downloads (http://www.mrc-epid.cam.ac.uk/physical-activity-downloads/); the Alberta Center for Active Living compilation of tools (https://www.centre4activeliving.ca/services/measurement-physical-activity/#tools); and the Active Living Research web site (https://activelivingresearch.org/). Presently there is a lack of consensus and precise guidance on matching specific measurement tools with specific populations and research questions. We recommend that researchers/practitioners take into consideration the project question and goals to guide their selection of the most appropriate measurement modality.

Summary

This chapter provides a comprehensive description of the various types of report-based methods and their applications to advance PA research. Report-based measures have had a long history in PA research and have informed about most of what we know about this topic. As use of device-based measurement increased, there was considerable focus on the perceived greater precision and accuracy of device-based measures of certain aspects of PA. More recently, a perspective is emerging that both report and device-based measures provide unique and valuable insights into human PA behaviors. This perspective leads naturally to a focus on selecting the most appropriate tool for measuring the PA outcome of interest in a given application. Section "Overview of the Literature" emphasizes the advantages of report-based measures, types of report-based measures, and their applications. While the applications might be obvious, this section provided specific examples of epidemiological studies that have relied on report-based measures to characterize activity levels in their sample and highlights the extensive use of report-based measures for surveillance of diverse aspects of PA in youth, where feasibility is critical.

Section "Key Issues" describes key topics related to report-based measures of PA, including the cognitive processes associated with recall, the sources of error that can impact estimates from reports, and how estimates obtained from reports can reflect absolute or relative intensity, depending on how the question is framed/scored. The neuro-cognitive processes underlying PA memory formations and the recall of these events are an understudied topic. It has been suggested that youth under 10 years are not able to recall past activity events, given the cognitive challenges of this task (Baranowski, Dworkin, & Cieslik, 1984; Sallis, 1991). This assumption has not been formerly tested but this section explored the cognitive challenges associated with recall among children and adolescents. This is a promising area for further work on improving measurement of PA in children.

Section "Key Issues" also described several measurement qualities central to report-based measures. Because of the plethora of available measures, systematic efforts to determine appropriate measures for specific research and surveillance topics are essential. Validity and reliability are often the decision factors when determining the value of a measure; however, users should consider other characteristics that might be equally relevant for the project that they have in mind. Examples include: (1) what is the setting of the PA of interest?; (2) over what time frame is the PA being assessed?; and (3) has the instrument been developed and validated for the population of interest? At the end of this section we introduce the newly updated Compendium of Physical Activities for Youth, a compilation of energy cost values for children and adolescents. The compendium is a valuable resource for studies using report-based measures to collect information on specific activities. It allows investigators to assign EE values to specific activities and compare the EE consequences of different combinations of activity patterns.

The final section of this chapter described recent research developments and resources addressing report-based measures. This section includes a description of the emerging interest and expansion of web-based surveys for PA assessments. Web-based surveys have been widely used in other fields (e.g. marketing research, political science) and are now becoming more popular for PA research. We provided a specific example, using the YAP, and described how this tool can generate automated feedback and adds value for school-based assessments of PA. Several key resources are also provided at the end of this section that we recommend the reader to explore. These are particularly helpful for assisting in selecting the most appropriate measure for a given project.

Report-based instruments are a vital aspect of the suite of available tools for assessing diverse aspects of youth PA. Improving such instruments to account for the development of cognitive capacity is an emerging research topic for PA measurement. Nevertheless, a variety of well documented and valid tools exist, along with resources to aid in understanding and selecting the appropriate measurement approach. Extra care in selecting the most appropriate measure for specific research and surveillance questions is highly worthwhile, and we hope this chapter will help the reader understand some of the main considerations involved in this selection process.

References

Ainsworth, B. E., Haskell, W. L., Herrmann, S. D., Meckes, N., Bassett, D. R., Jr., Tudor-Locke, C., . . . Leon, A. S. (2011). 2011 Compendium of physical activities: A second update of codes and MET values. *Medicine and Science in Sports and Exercise, 43*(8), 1575–1581. doi:10.1249/MSS.0b013e31821ece12

Ainsworth, B. E., Watson, K. B., Ridley, K., Pfeiffer, K. A., Herrmann, S. D., Crouter, S. E., . . . Fulton, J. E. (2018). Utility of the youth compendium of physical activities. *Research Quarterly for Exercise and Sport, 89*(3), 273–281. doi:10.1080/02701367.2018.1487754

Atkinson, R. C., & Shiffrin, R. M. (1968). Human memory: A proposed system and its control processes. *Psychology of Learning and Motivation, 2,* 89–195.

Baddeley, A. D. (1992). Working memory: The interface between memory and cognition. *Journal of Cognitive Neuroscience, 4*(3), 281–288. doi:10.1162/jocn.1992.4.3.281

Baddeley, A. D. (2002). The psychology of memory. In A. D. Baddeley, M. D. Kopelman, & B. A. Wilson (Eds.), *The handbook of memory disorders* (pp. 3–17). Chichester, UK: John Wiley & Sons.

Baddeley, A. D. (2005). What is memory? In A. D. Baddeley (Ed.), *Essentials of human memory* (pp. 1–18). London, UK: Taylor & Francis.

Bailey, R. C., Olson, J., Pepper, S. L., Porszasz, J., Barstow, T. J., & Cooper, D. M. (1995). The level and tempo of children's physical activities: An observational study. *Medicine and Science in Sports and Exercise, 27*(7), 1033–1041.

Baranowski, T., Dworkin, R., & Cieslik, C. (1984). Reliability and validity of self-report of aerobic activity: Family health project. *Research Quarterly for Exercise and Sport, 55*(4), 309–317.

Bauer, P. J. (2015). A complementary processes account of the development of childhood amnesia and a personal past. *Psychological Review, 122*(2), 204–231. doi:10.1037/a0038939

Biddle, S. J. H., Gorely, T., Pearson, N., & Bull, F. C. (2011). An assessment of self-reported physical activity instruments in young people for population surveillance: Project ALPHA. *International Journal of Behavioral Nutrition and Physical Activity, 8*, 1. doi:10.1186/1479-5868-8-1

Bowles, H. R. (2012). Measurement of active and sedentary behaviors: Closing the gaps in self-report methods. *Journal of Physical Activity and Health, 9*(Suppl 1), S1–S4.

Bramao, I., Karlsson, A., & Johansson, M. (2017). Mental reinstatement of encoding context improves episodic remembering. *Cortex, 94*, 15–26. doi:10.1016/j.cortex.2017.06.007

Butte, N. F., Watson, K. B., Ridley, K., Zakeri, I. F., McMurray, R. G., Pfeiffer, K. A., . . . Fulton, J. E. (2018). A youth compendium of physical activities: Activity codes and metabolic intensities. *Medicine and Science in Sports and Exercise, 50*(2), 246–256. doi:10.1249/MSS.0000000000001430

Byrne, N. M., Hills, A. P., Hunter, G. R., Weinsier, R. L., & Schutz, Y. (2005). Metabolic equivalent: One size does not fit all. *Journal of Applied Physiology, 99*(3), 1112–1119. doi:10.1152/japplphysiol.00023.2004

Caspersen, C. J., Powell, K. E., & Christenson, G. M. (1985). Physical activity, exercise, and physical fitness: Definitions and distinctions for health-related research. *Public Health Reports, 100*(2), 126–131.

Chinapaw, M. J., Mokkink, L. B., van Poppel, M. N., van Mechelen, W., & Terwee, C. B. (2010). Physical activity questionnaires for youth: A systematic review of measurement properties. *Sports Medicine, 40*(7), 539–563. doi:10.2165/11530770-000000000-00000

Couper, M. (2000). Web surveys: A review of issues and approaches. *Public Opinion Quarterly, 64*(4), 464–494.

D'Angelo, H., Fowler, S. L., Nebeling, L. C., & Oh, A. Y. (2017). Adolescent physical activity: Moderation of individual factors by neighborhood environment. *American Journal of Preventive Medicine, 52*(6), 888–894. doi:10.1016/j.amepre.2017.01.013

Dishman, R. K., Heath, G. W., & Lee, I. L. (2013). Measurement and surveillance of physical activity and fitness. In G. W. H. Rod, K. Dishman, & I-.M. Lee (Ed.), *Physical activity epidemiology* (2nd ed., pp. 37–74). Champaign, IL: Human Kinetics.

Dixon, P. M., Saint-Maurice, P. F., Kim, Y., Hibbing, P., Bai, Y., & Welk, G. J. (2017). A primer on the use of equivalence testing for evaluating measurement agreement. *Medicine and Science in Sports and Exercise.* doi:10.1249/MSS.0000000000001481

Dunton, G. F. (2017). Ecological Momentary Assessment in Physical Activity Research. *Exercise and Sport Sciences Reviews, 45*(1), 48–54. doi:10.1249/JES.0000000000000092

Dunton, G. F., Berrigan, D., Young, D. R., Pfeiffer, K. A., Lee, S. M., Slater, S. J., & Pate, R. R. (2019). Strategies to improve physical activity surveillance among youth in the United States. *The Journal of Pediatrics, 210*, 226–231.

Flegal, K. M., Carroll, M. D., Kit, B. K., & Ogden, C. L. (2012). Prevalence of obesity and trends in the distribution of body mass index among US adults, 1999–2010. *Journal of the American Medical Association, 307*(5), 491–497. doi:10.1001/jama.2012.39

Gagge, A. P., Burton, A. C., & Bazett, H. C. (1941). A practical system of units for the description of the heat exchange of man with his environment. *Science, 94*(2445), 428–430. doi:10.1126/science.94.2445.428

Gazzaniga, M. S., Ivry, R. B., & Mangun, G. R. (2014). Memory. In A. Javsicas & S. Snaveli (Eds.), *Cognitive neuroscience: The biology of the mind* (pp. 378–423). New York, NY: W. W. Norton & Company, Inc.

Ghetti, S., DeMaster, D. M., Yonelinas, A. P., & Bunge, S. A. (2010). Developmental differences in medial temporal lobe function during memory encoding. *Journal of Neuroscience, 30*(28), 9548–9556. doi:10.1523/JNEUROSCI.35000-09.2010

Giedd, J. N., Vaituzis, A. C., Hamburger, S. D., Lange, N., Rajapakse, J. C., Kaysen, D., . . . Rapoport, J. L. (1996). Quantitative MRI of the temporal lobe, amygdala, and hippocampus in normal human development: Ages 4–18 years. *Journal of Comparative Neurology, 366*(2), 223–230. doi:10.1002/(SICI)1096-9861(19960304)366:2<223::AID-CNE3>3.0.CO;2-7

Gogtay, N., Nugent, T. F., 3rd, Herman, D. H., Ordonez, A., Greenstein, D., Hayashi, K. M., . . . Thompson, P. M. (2006). Dynamic mapping of normal human hippocampal development. *Hippocampus, 16*(8), 664–672. doi:10.1002/hipo.20193

Grooves, R. M., Fowler, F. J., Couper, M. P., Lepkowski, J. M., Singer, E., & Tourangeau, R. (2009a). Inference and error in surveys. In R. M. Groves (Ed.), *Survey methodology* (pp. 39–67). Hoboken, NJ: John Wiley & Sons.

Grooves, R. M., Fowler, F. J., Couper, M. P., Lepkowski, J. M., Singer, E., & Tourangeau, R. (2009b). Methods of data collection. In R. M. Groves (Ed.), *Survey methodology* (pp. 149–181). Hoboken, NJ: John Wiley & Sons.

Groves, R. M., Fowler, F. J., Couper, M. P., Lepkowski, J. M., Singer, E., & Tourangeau, R. (2009). Questions and answers in surveys. In R. M. Groves (Ed.), *Survey methodology* (pp. 217–257). Hoboken, NJ: John Wiley & Sons.

Guler, O. E., & Thomas, K. M. (2013). Developmental differences in the neural correlates of relational encoding and recall in children: An event-related fMRI study. *Developmental Cognitive Neuroscience, 3,* 106–116. doi:10.1016/j.dcn.2012.07.001

Harrell, J. S., McMurray, R. G., Baggett, C. D., Pennell, M. L., Pearce, P. F., & Bangdiwala, S. I. (2005). Energy costs of physical activities in children and adolescents. *Medicine and Science in Sports and Exercise, 37*(2), 329–336.

Hidding, L. M., Altenburg, T. M., Mokkink, L. B., Terwee, C. B., & Chinapaw, M. J. (2017). Systematic review of childhood sedentary behavior questionnaires: What do we know and what is next? *Sports Medicine, 47*(4), 677–699. doi:10.1007/s40279-016-0610-1

Hidding, L. M., Chinapaw, M. J. M., van Poppel, M. N. M., Mokkink, L. B., & Altenburg, T. M. (2018). An updated systematic review of childhood physical activity questionnaires. *Sports Medicines, 48*(12), 2797–2842. doi:10.1007/s40279-018-0987-0

Howley, E. T. (2001). Type of activity: Resistance, aerobic and leisure versus occupational physical activity. *Medicine and Science in Sports and Exercise, 33*(6 Suppl), S364–S369; discussion S419–320.

Kemper, H. C., Post, G. B., Twisk, J. W., & van Mechelen, W. (1999). Lifestyle and obesity in adolescence and young adulthood: Results from the Amsterdam growth and health longitudinal study (AGAHLS). *International Journal of Obesity Related Metabolic Disorders, 23*(Suppl 3), S34–S40.

Keresztes, A., Ngo, C. T., Lindenberger, U., Werkle-Bergner, M., & Newcombe, N. S. (2018). Hippocampal maturation drives memory from generalization to specificity. *Trends in Cognitive Sciences, 22*(8), 676–686. doi:10.1016/j.tics.2018.05.004

Langnes, E., Vidal-Pineiro, D., Sneve, M. H., Amlien, I. K., Walhovd, K. B., & Fjell, A. M. (2018). Development and decline of the hippocampal long-axis specialization and differentiation during encoding and retrieval of episodic memories. *Cerebral Cortex.* doi:10.1093/cercor/bhy209

Lee, J. K., Ekstrom, A. D., & Ghetti, S. (2014). Volume of hippocampal subfields and episodic memory in childhood and adolescence. *Neuroimage, 94,* 162–171. doi:10.1016/j.neuroimage.2014.03.019

Lee, J. M., Saint-Maurice, P. F., Kim, Y., Gaesser, G. A., & Welk, G. J. (2016). Activity energy expenditure in youth: Sex, age, and body size patterns. *Journal of Physical Activity and Health, 13*(6 Suppl 1), S62–S70. doi:10.1123/jpah.2016-0014

Lenroot, R. K., & Giedd, J. N. (2006). Brain development in children and adolescents: Insights from anatomical magnetic resonance imaging. *Neuroscience Biobehavioral Reviews, 30*(6), 718–729. doi:10.1016/j.neubiorev.2006.06.001

Lohr, K. N. (2002). Assessing health status and quality-of-life instruments: Attributes and review criteria. *Quality of Life Research, 11*(3), 193–205.

Martinez-Gomez, D., Mielke, G. I., Menezes, A. M., Goncalves, H., Barros, F. C., & Hallal, P. C. (2014). Active commuting throughout adolescence and central fatness before adulthood: Prospective birth cohort study. *PLoS One, 9*(5), e96634. doi:10.1371/journal.pone.0096634

Matthews, C. E. (2002). Use of self-report instruments to assess physical activity. In G. J. Welk (Ed.), *Physical activity assessments for health-related research* (pp. 107–123). Champaign, IL: Human Kinetics.

McMurray, R. G., Soares, J., Caspersen, C. J., & McCurdy, T. (2014). Examining variations of resting metabolic rate of adults: A public health perspective. *Medicine and Science in Sports and Exercise, 46*(7), 1352–1358. doi:10.1249/MSS.0000000000000232

Menon, V., Boyett-Anderson, J. M., & Reiss, A. L. (2005). Maturation of medial temporal lobe response and connectivity during memory encoding. *Brain Research Cognitive Brain Research, 25*(1), 379–385. doi:10.1016/j.cogbrainres.2005.07.007

Miyake, A., & Shah, P. (2009). Models of working memory: An introduction. In A. Miyake & P. Shah (Eds.), *Models of working memory: Mechanisms of active maintenance and executive control* (pp. 1–27). New York, NY: Cambridge University Press.

Mokkink, L. B., Terwee, C. B., Knol, D. L., Stratford, P. W., Alonso, J., Patrick, D. L., . . . de Vet, H. C. (2010). The COSMIN checklist for evaluating the methodological quality of studies on measurement properties: A clarification of its content. *BMC Medical Research Methodology, 10,* 22. doi:10.1186/1471-2288-10-22

Molnar, D., & Schutz, Y. (1997). The effect of obesity, age, puberty and gender on resting metabolic rate in children and adolescents. *European Journal of Pediatrics, 156*(5), 376–381.

Nebeling, L. C., Hennessy, E., Oh, A. Y., Dwyer, L. A., Patrick, H., Blanck, H. M., . . . Yaroch, A. L. (2017). The FLASHE study: Survey development, dyadic perspectives, and participant characteristics. *American Journal of Preventive Medicine, 52*(6), 839–848. doi:10.1016/j.amepre.2017.01.028

Ostby, Y., Tamnes, C. K., Fjell, A. M., Westlye, L. T., Due-Tonnessen, P., & Walhovd, K. B. (2009). Heterogeneity in subcortical brain development: A structural magnetic resonance imaging study of brain maturation from 8 to 30 years. *Journal of Neuroscience, 29*(38), 11772–11782. doi:10.1523/JNEUROSCI.1242-09.2009

Pettee Gabriel, K. K., Morrow, J. R., Jr., & Woolsey, A. L. (2012). Framework for physical activity as a complex and multidimensional behavior. *Journal of Physical Activity and Health, 9*(Suppl 1), S11–S18.

Pfeiffer, K. A., Watson, K. B., McMurray, R. G., Bassett, D. R., Butte, N. F., Crouter, S. E., . . . CDC/NCI/NCCOR Research Group (2018). Energy cost expression for a youth compendium of physical activities: Rationale for using age groups. *Pediatric Exercise Science, 30*(1), 142–149. doi:10.1123/pes.2016-0249

Prince, S. A., LeBlanc, A. G., Colley, R. C., & Saunders, T. J. (2017). Measurement of sedentary behaviour in population health surveys: A review and recommendations. *PeerJ, 5*, e4130. doi:10.7717/peerj.4130

Ridley, K., Ainsworth, B. E., & Olds, T. S. (2008). Development of a compendium of energy expenditures for youth. *International Journal of Behavioral Nutrition and Physical Activity, 5*, 45. doi:10.1186/1479-5868-5-45

Ridley, K., Olds, T. S., & Hill, A. (2006). The multimedia activity recall for children and adolescents (MARCA): Development and evaluation. *International Journal of Behavioral Nutrition and Physical Activity, 3*, 10. doi:10.1186/1479-5868-3-10

Ryan, L., Hoscheidt, S., & Nadel, L. (2008). Perspectives on episodic and semantic memory retrieval. In E. Dere, A. Easton, L. Nadel, & J. P. Huston (Eds.), *Handbook of episodic memory* (pp. 5–19). Oxford, UK: Elsevier Press.

Saint-Maurice, P. F., Kim, Y., Hibbing, P., Oh, A. Y., Perna, F. M., & Welk, G. J. (2017). Calibration and validation of the youth activity profile: The FLASHE study. *American Journal of Preventive Medicine, 52*(6), 880–887. doi:10.1016/j.amepre.2016.12.010

Saint-Maurice, P. F., Kim, Y., Welk, G. J., & Gaesser, G. A. (2016). Kids are not little adults: What MET threshold captures sedentary behavior in children? *European Journal of Applied Physiology, 116*(1), 29–38. doi:10.1007/s00421-015-3238-1

Saint-Maurice, P. F., & Welk, G. J. (2014). Web-based assessments of physical activity in youth: Considerations for design and scale calibration. *Journal of Medical Internet Research, 16*(12), e269. doi:10.2196/jmir.3626

Saint-Maurice, P. F., & Welk, G. J. (2015). Validity and calibration of the youth activity profile. *PLoS One, 10*(12), e0143949. doi:10.1371/journal.pone.0143949

Saint-Maurice, P. F., Welk, G. J., Bartee, R. T., & Heelan, K. (2017). Calibration of context-specific survey items to assess youth physical activity behaviour. *Journal of Sports Sciences, 35*(9), 866–872. doi:10.1080/02640414.2016.1194526

Saint-Maurice, P. F., Welk, G. J., Beyler, N. K., Bartee, R. T., & Heelan, K. A. (2014). Calibration of self-report tools for physical activity research: The physical activity questionnaire (PAQ). *BMC Public Health, 14*, 461. doi:10.1186/1471-2458-14-461

Sallis, J. F. (1991). Self-report measures of children's physical activity. *Journal of School Health, 61*(5), 215–219.

Sastre, M., 3rd, Wendelken, C., Lee, J. K., Bunge, S. A., & Ghetti, S. (2016). Age- and performance-related differences in hippocampal contributions to episodic retrieval. *Developmental Cognitive Neuroscience, 19*, 42–50. doi:10.1016/j.dcn.2016.01.003

Shing, Y. L., & Lindenberger, U. (2011). The development of episodic memory: Lifespan lessons. *Child Development Perspectives, 5*(2), 148–155.

Tang, L., Shafer, A. T., & Ofen, N. (2018). Prefrontal cortex contributions to the development of memory formation. *Cerebral Cortex, 28*(9), 3295–3308. doi:10.1093/cercor/bhx200

Terwee, C. B., Bot, S. D., de Boer, M. R., van der Windt, D. A., Knol, D. L., Dekker, J., . . . de Vet, H. C. (2007). Quality criteria were proposed for measurement properties of health status questionnaires. *Journal of Clinical Epidemiology, 60*(1), 34–42. doi:10.1016/j.jclinepi.2006.03.012

Terwee, C. B., Mokkink, L. B., van Poppel, M. N., Chinapaw, M. J., van Mechelen, W., & de Vet, H. C. (2010). Qualitative attributes and measurement properties of physical activity questionnaires: A checklist. *Sports Medicine, 40*(7), 525–537. doi:10.2165/11531370-000000000-00000

Tessier, S., Vuillemin, A., & Briancon, S. (2008). Revue des questionnaires de mesure de l'activité physique validés chez les enfants et les adolescents. *Science & Sports, 23*(3–4), 118–125.

Thompson, R. F. (2005). In search of memory traces. *Annual Review of Psychology, 56*, 1–23. doi:10.1146/annurev.psych.56.091103.070239

Tourangeau, R., Rips, L. J., & Rasinski, K. (2000). The role of memory in survey responding. In L. J. Rips, R. Tourangeau, & K. Rasinki (Ed.), *The psychology of survey response* (pp. 62–99). New York, NY: Cambridge University Press.

Welk, G. J., Bai, Y., Saint-Maurice, P. F., Allums-Featherston, K., & Candelaria, N. (2016). Design and evaluation of the NFL PLAY 60 FITNESSGRAM partnership project. *Research Quarterly for Exercise and Sport, 87*(1), 1–13. doi:10.1080/02701367.2015.1127126

Welk, G. J., Corbin, C. B., & Dale, D. (2000). Measurement issues in the assessment of physical activity in children. *Research Quarterly for Exercise and Sport, 71*(2 Suppl), S59–S73.

Welk, G. J., Morrow, J., & Saint-Maurice, P. (2017). *Measures registry user guide: Individual physical activity.* In National Collaborative on Childhood Obesity Research (Ed.). Retrieved from https://www.nccor.org/wp-content/uploads/sites/2/2017/NCCOR_MR_User_Guide_Individual_PA-FINAL.pdf

Welk, G. J., Saint-Maurice, P. F., Kim, Y., Ellingson, L. D., Hibbing, P., Wolff-Hughes, D. L., & Perna, F. M. (2017). Understanding and interpreting error in physical activity data: Insights from the FLASHE study. *American Journal of Preventive Medicine, 52*(6), 836–838. doi:10.1016/j.amepre.2017.03.001

Welten, D. C., Kemper, H. C., Post, G. B., Van Mechelen, W., Twisk, J., Lips, P., & Teule, G. J. (1994). Weight-bearing activity during youth is a more important factor for peak bone mass than calcium intake. *Journal of Bone and Mineral Research, 9*(7), 1089–1096. doi:10.1002/jbmr.5650090717

Wijnstok, N. J., Hoekstra, T., van Mechelen, W., Kemper, H. C., & Twisk, J. W. (2013). Cohort profile: The Amsterdam growth and health longitudinal study. *International Journal of Epidemiology, 42*(2), 422–429. doi:10.1093/ije/dys028

Zaki, R., Bulgiba, A., Ismail, R., & Ismail, N. A. (2012). Statistical methods used to test for agreement of medical instruments measuring continuous variables in method comparison studies: A systematic review. *PLoS One, 7*(5), e37908. doi:10.1371/journal.pone.0037908

14

DIRECT OBSERVATION

Assessing Youth Physical Activity and Its Contexts

Hans van der Mars and Thomas L. McKenzie

You can observe a lot by just watching.

L.P. Berra

Introduction

Few children and adolescents meet the national/global physical activity (PA) recommendations (Active Healthy Kids Global Alliance, 2018; Katzmarzyk et al., 2018; USDHHS, 2018) and the need to track the type, amount, and intensity of PA is critical. As noted in an earlier chapter, engaging in health-enhancing PA may well be the most important and cost-effective investment in ensuring continued health and well-being. This applies across the lifespan. As interest in assessing PA has increased, so too has the assortment of data collection tools.

The words of the famous baseball player, Lawrence Peter "Yogi" Berra: "You can observe a lot by just watching" are at the heart of a data collection approach for PA assessment, called direct (or systematic) observation (DO). Compared with recent advances in tools such as accelerometers, pedometers, and wearables (discussed in detail elsewhere in this text), DO has a long history in a variety of disciplines, including anthropology, social psychology, clinical psychology, cross-cultural psychology, and Applied Behavior Analysis (e.g. Cooper, Heron, & Heward, 2007; van der Mars, 1989a) and it became the prevalent data collection method in studying teaching-learning processes in physical education in the 1970s (e.g. Locke, 1977).

The last 25 years have seen a rapid increase in the use of DO to measure PA, especially to assess interventions conducted in schools, parks, and community recreation settings (e.g. McKenzie, 1991, 2002; McKenzie, Sallis, & Nader, 1991; McKenzie, Cohen, Sehgal, Williamson, & Golinelli, 2006; McKenzie, Marshall, Sallis, & Conway, 2000; Ridgers, Stratton, & McKenzie, 2010). The DO systems used to assess PA have their roots in Applied Behavior Analysis (Cooper et al., 2007), which is heavily influenced by B. F. Skinner's (1953) studies of operant behavior. This is important, because, in addition to assessing PA behavior, we are interested in studying the environmental conditions that influence it. Environmental interventions include modifying the physical and social antecedents and consequences of PA.

In this chapter, we present an overview of the four basic DO data collection tactics, their key advantages and limitations, protocols used for observer training, and possible sources of observer error. We also provide an overview of five DO systems specifically designed for assessing PA and its contexts. In addition, we discuss issues related to observer reliability and data accuracy and emphasize capturing contextual data. Recent technological advances that can support using DO efficiently are then addressed, and we end the chapter by using the behavioral-ecological perspective (e.g. Hovell, Wahlgren, & Adams, 2009; Richard, Gauvin, & Rainie, 2011) to share several examples of using DO in PA research.

Overview of Direct Observation Tactics

Time spent in PA is a key metric in determining the impact of interventions and whether they are effective. A related metric is the time spent being sedentary. DO is an effective data collection approach for providing these data. It includes four main tactics: Event Recording (ER), Duration Recording (DR), Interval Recording (IR), and Momentary Time Sampling (MTS).

ER provides a frequency count of behavior and data are generally expressed as "rate per minute", "percent of all observed behavior", and/or as "ratios". ER should be the observation tactic of choice to use when assessing the number of people engaged in PA at various levels of intensity. Contextually, ER can also be used to assess environmental aspects such as the amount and type of equipment available, number of activity venues accessible and usable, and the different types of activities occurring.

DR provides data on the temporal dimension of behavior, and is the preferred method when assessing the length or continuity of a behavior (e.g. walking, cycling, swimming, jumping rope). Typically, the DR raw unit of measure is minutes and seconds and these are converted to "percent of (observed) time". For example, middle school students engaging in Moderate to Vigorous Physical Activity (MVPA) for 18 of a 50-minute physical education lesson would be in MVPA for 36% of the total lesson time. These 18 minutes could also be broken down by intensity levels (e.g. moderate, vigorous).

IR allows observers to assess the occurrence and nonoccurrence of PA during specified time intervals. While ER and DR provide precise measures of frequency and duration, IR data can provide only estimates of frequency and duration. IR intervals generally range from 3 to 10 seconds, with their length dependent on the complexity of the observation system (i.e. the number of observation categories). Converting raw IR data to "percent of intervals" allows for comparing results across observation sessions, including sessions of different lengths (e.g. PE lessons, coaching/sports practices).

When using IR, investigators have the option of using "whole-interval" and "partial-interval" recording. When recording PA using whole-interval recording, the observed person must be engaged in PA during the full length of the interval. When using partial-interval recording, the occurrence of PA would be recorded even it occurs only briefly (e.g. 2 seconds). IR provides only estimates of the actual occurrence of behavior and there is potential of whole-interval recording to underestimate the occurrence of PA and partial-interval recording to overestimate it.

Partial-interval recording provides two cueing options. In one, observers record target behaviors that are occurring exactly at a prerecorded "record" signal that is cued via verbal cues such as on a MP3 or MP4 audio file. A second procedure is the use of an alternating *observe-record* format which is commonly used with complex DO systems where observers must choose from a large number of behavior categories. An alternating "observe-record" cueing format paces observers to observe for a set time (e.g. 10 seconds) which is followed by a set time (e.g. 5 seconds) for them to record the data.

MTS involves recording the presence/absence of a target behavior at the end of each observed interval and it has the advantage of being able to assess the occurrence of behavior with either individuals or groups. When observing the behavior of groups of people, the method is often referred to as "Group Time Sampling" (GTS), and interval lengths can range from 1 minute to as much as 60 minutes. Staff in a fitness/recreation center, for example, could use GTS to track facility use throughout the day. At set time intervals (e.g. every 30 or 60 minutes), an observer could systematically walk through each PA area and record the number of people using it.

Observers can also simultaneously record additional relevant data (e.g. environmental conditions, activity type) with PA at the end of a GTS interval. When using MTS, the resulting raw data can be converted to the percent of intervals which allows for comparisons over time or among facilities. In addition, when groups of people are observed, the raw data can be converted to a percent/proportion of those engaging in a particular behavior (e.g. MVPA%).

Advantages of Using Direct Observation to Assess Physical Activity

Researchers assessing PA have numerous data collection tools from which to choose (e.g. accelerometers, pedometers, heart-rate monitoring, doubly labeled water). Choosing the appropriate tool(s) depends primarily on the research question being asked, available temporal and financial resources, and the scope of the project. For example, studies of large representative national samples have typically used self-report tools. Meanwhile, Cohen et al. (2016) used DO to assess a random representative sample of neighborhood parks and in addition to using MTS (via System for Observing Play and Recreation in Communities (SOPARC)), they included interviews of both park users and park managers.

McKenzie and van der Mars (2015) noted that, despite its long history of use in many different disciplines, researchers still avoid using DO as a method for assessing PA (e.g. Corder, Ekelund, Steele, Wareham, & Brage, 2008; Strath et al., 2013). Corder et al. (2008) speculated that not using DO might result from lack of familiarity with the method and the prevalence of a physiological orientation where overall Energy Expenditure (EE, an indirect measure) is the standard measure rather than PA itself. In contrast, PA researchers with a behavioral–ecological perspective typically are interested in the specifics of identifying the role of concurrent environmental antecedent and consequential stimuli that affect the PA (e.g. Cooper et al., 2007). Thus, in assessing the impact of (multi-level) intervention studies, DO is an attractive approach to data collection, especially when environmental and reinforcement variables are of interest. Moreover, DO has other key advantages, including: (a) strong internal validity, (b) ease in interpreting results, (c) limited need for sophisticated and expensive equipment, and (d) lack of burden placed on the people observed.

Strong Internal Validity

A major advantage of DO is that it is a direct method of data collection that produces objective information with strong internal (or face) validity. One can liken it to "WYSIWYG" (i.e. "What-You-See-Is-What-You-Get") which is not possible with methods such as heart-rate monitoring and doubly labeled water that do not assess PA itself. Meanwhile, pedometers and accelerometers do not function well in aquatic environments and they cannot be worn during high intensity activities involving physical contact (e.g. wrestling, American tackle football). Self-reported data (e.g. via questionnaires, interviews) also do not assess PA directly, but instead reflect people's *perceptions* of their own PA. In many cases, self-report data are far removed in both the time and location from when and where the actual PA behavior occurred. In contrast, DO assesses the environment and PA exactly when it occurs!

Data Are Easily Understood

As noted, DO data are generally expressed in easily understood measurement units (e.g. percentages of [observed] time). While this may appear mundane, consider practitioners (e.g. teachers, recreation leaders), administrators, and policy makers (e.g. school board members, state legislators) who receive and need to interpret the data. It would be inappropriate to confuse them by using F-values, R-square confidence interval values, Least Square Difference values, or p-values when a simple bar graph would suffice. In general, DO data, especially when presented graphically, require little explanation. Nonetheless, when needed, they can be manipulated using standard statistical procedures.

Technological Advances

With the advent of tablet and software Apps technology, observers can now more easily enter, store, and analyze data. We highlight these developments later in this chapter, but it is important to remember that adding technology increases the need for additional observer training (see below).

Minimal Burden

With few exceptions, DO can be used to assess PA in most settings (including aquatic environments). Importantly, as observers avoid being close and interfering with the ongoing environment, there is little, if any, burden on those being assessed. In contrast for example, HR monitors require time for researchers to place the instruments in the correct location, a problem in settings such as school physical education where lesson time is a precious commodity. In addition, placing instruments on some individuals (e.g. those with mental retardation or autism) might produce stress or emotional outbursts resulting in refusals to wear the devices. Meanwhile, observational data can be generated in public places (e.g. beaches, parks) without people being aware of it. Thus, any potential reactivity that might occur from wearing pedometers or accelerometers is eliminated. In addition, in case of tracking PA over time (multiple occasions), DO investigators need not worry about people losing their devices or forgetting to use them.

DO as a Criterion Measure for Validating Indirect PA Measures

The validity of data collection tools is important to the credibility of the results, and DO is often the "gold standard" (i.e. criterion measure) for validating less direct measures of PA (e.g. Finn & Specker, 2000; Sirard & Pate, 2001). Examples include assessing the accuracy of tools such as pedometers and accelerometers (e.g. McKenzie, Sallis, & Armstrong, 1994; Scruggs, 2013; Scruggs, Mungen, & Oh, 2010). Undoubtedly, technological advances will continue to produce new tools for assessing PA (e.g. more advanced wearables, nano-technology), but DO will still likely be an appropriate criterion measure for validating them.

Critical Advantage of DO: It's All in the Environment

PA is always "place-dependent" (or "place-based"). That is, PA does not just occur generally, but transpires in specific settings, each with its own natural (or built) physical and social characteristics (e.g. McKenzie, 2016; Sallis, 2009). A distinct advantage of DO is its ability to capture these contextual data. Home settings, for example, have environmental features that can either suppress PA (e.g. small indoor spaces) or facilitate it (e.g. large outdoor spaces with activity enhancing equipment). Similarly, schools, parks, and other settings may also suppress or promote PA, but generally PA is enhanced in outdoor areas (e.g. basketball and tennis courts, fields, fitness/running trails). Many factors affect the use of such settings, including their accessibility, the presence of lights, equipment, adult supervision, organized activities, and even amenities such as drinking fountains and toilet facilities (e.g. McKenzie, Cohen et al., 2006; McKenzie et al., 2000).

From a behavioral-ecological perspective, the environment is a strong determinant of people's PA (e.g. Sallis, Floyd, Rodriguez, & Saelens, 2012) and Bauer, Briss, Goodman, and Bowman (2014) pointed to an increased emphasis on determining the efficacy of environmental interventions

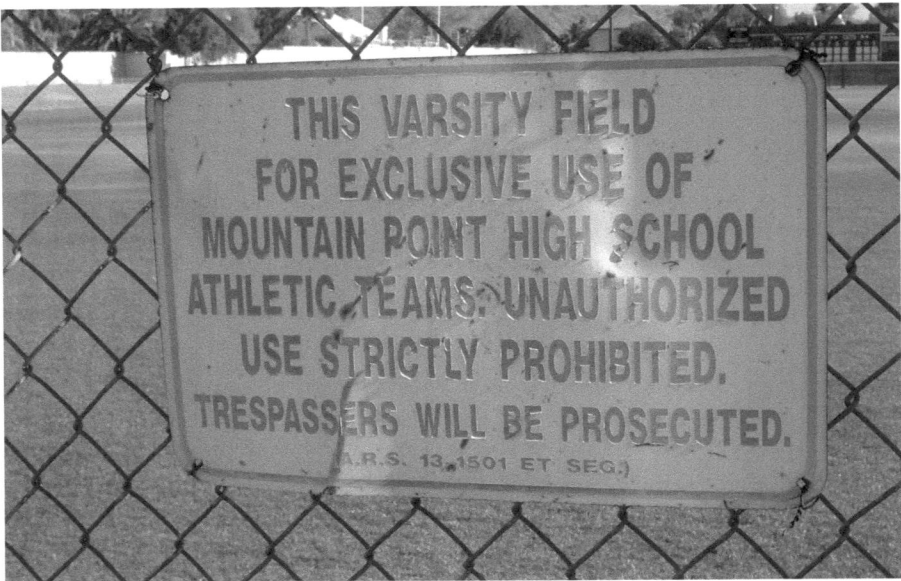

Figure 14.1   Posted sign limiting/suppressing PA

aimed at reducing the nation's health burden. One example is the improvement of access to PA settings on school campuses (Figure 14.1). This then makes the simultaneous data collection of PA behavior and environmental features through DO a powerful data collection approach (see also Sallis, Owen, & Fisher, 2008). In a later section, we provide a closer examination at why DO should be used in intervention research aimed at changing PA behavior.

Overview of Direct Observation Tools

This section provides an overview of five validated DO systems, main features of which are included in Table 14.1. The systems include: (a) *Behaviors of Eating and Activity for Children's Health: Evaluation System* (BEACHES; McKenzie, Sallis, Nader, Patterson et al., 1991), (b) the *System for Observing Fitness Instruction Time* (SOFIT; McKenzie, Sallis, & Nader, 1991), (c) the *System for Observing Play and Leisure Activity in Youth* (SOPLAY; McKenzie et al., 2000), (d) the SOPARC (McKenzie, Cohen et al., 2006), and (e) *System for Observing Children's Activity and Relationships during Play* (SOCARP; Ridgers et al., 2010). Full descriptions of these instruments and their coding protocols can be obtained for free through the Active Living Research Website (http://www.activelivingresearch.org).

PA Categories

All the systems in Table 14.1 have had their PA behavior categories validated and they are suitable for use across populations and age groups. Various criterion measures were used to establish PA category validity, including heart-rate monitoring and EE measured through oxygen consumption, pedometers, and accelerometers (e.g. Heath, Coleman, Lensegrav, & Fallon, 2006; McKenzie, Sallis, Nader, Patterson et al., 1991; McNamee & van der Mars, 2005; Pope, Coleman, Gonzalez, Barron, & Heath, 2002; Ridgers et al., 2010; Rowe, Schuldheisz, & van der Mars, 1997; Rowe, van der Mars, Schuldheisz, & Fox, 2004).

Table 14.1 Validated direct observation systems for assessing physical activity and its contexts

System features	BEACHES	SOFIT	SOPLAY	SOPARC	SOCARP
Observation tactic	• Momentary time sampling • Interval recording	• Momentary time sampling • Interval recording	Momentary time sampling	Momentary time sampling	• Momentary time sampling • Interval recording
Typical coding format	15 seconds obs./15 seconds rec.	10 seconds obs./10 seconds rec.	NA	NA	10 seconds obs./10 seconds rec.
Main target	Individual children	Individual students	All present in area	All present in area	Individual children
Main location	Home settings	Physical education lessons	School/recreation settings	Park/recreation settings	Playgrounds
Coding decision levels	• PA level • Social context • Physical context • Food ingestion • Media viewing	• PA level • Lesson Context (e.g. management, fitness, skill development, game play) • Instructor behavior	• PA level • Area context • Activity type	• PA level • Area context • Activity type	• PA level • Group size • Activity type • Interactions with peers
Demographic/ Context data	• Child location • Presence of others • PA prompts and consequences • Ingesting food • Viewing media	• Lesson content • Lesson location • Number of students • Student gender • Class gender composition • Teacher gender	• School • Temperature • Time of day (before school; lunch/recess, after school) • Area contexts (accessible, usable, organized, supervised, equipped)	• Park/recreation area • Temperature • Day & time of day • Gender • Age group • Race/ethnicity • Area contexts (accessible, usable, organized, supervised, equipped) • Area size	• Temperature • Area contexts (accessible, usable, organized, supervised, equipped) • Area size
First referenced	McKenzie, Sallis, Patterson et al. (1991)	McKenzie, Sallis, and Nader (1991)	McKenzie et al. (2000)	McKenzie, Cohen et al. (2006)	Ridgers et al. (2010)

Note: The five systems summarized above use the same five PA level codes; these have been validated using numerous measures. Their protocols can be downloaded free from Active Living Research (http://activelivingresearch.org/).

Adapted and reprinted with permission from McKenzie and van der Mars (2015).

As people with disabilities, from childhood through adulthood, are likely to be both more sedentary and more prone to chronic diseases than those without them (e.g. Rimmer & Marques, 2012; Rimmer, Schiller, & Chen, 2012; USDHHS, 2018), promoting PA in these populations is imperative. To that end, the PA categories in the various DO systems have also been validated for use with persons with disabilities (e.g. Faison-Hodge & Porretta, 2004; Kim & van der Mars, 2014; Sit, Capio, Cerin, & McKenzie, 2013) and they have also been validated for use in classroom settings (Honas et al., 2008).

Contextual Categories

The contextual categories within the systems are setting-specific (e.g. physical education classes, school campuses, school recess periods, parks) and users will need to select the DO instrument that best fits their interest and the setting where data are to be collected. The contextual categories within the instruments all have strong face validity, and sometimes they can be used with other DO systems.

Estimating Energy Expenditure

To help promote comparisons and generalizability (e.g. across settings or studies), DO researchers can calculate EE estimates (kcal/kg/min) for the sedentary, walking/moderate, and vigorous PA (VPA) categories by using the validated constants of 0.051, 0.096, and 0.144 kcal/kg/min, respectively (Bar-Or, 1983). These estimates can be used for both individuals and groups and can provide a supplementary means of discriminating between more and less active observation sessions (e.g. PA accrued in the home, physical education lessons, or team practice sessions).

When studying groups in school or park settings, SOPLAY or SOPARC is the DO system of choice. In this case, EE estimates are calculated by multiplying the total number of people counted in the sedentary, walking/moderate, and vigorous categories for each targeted activity area. The resulting estimates for walking/moderate and vigorous can also be summed to obtain an EE estimate of MVPA.

In the following paragraphs basic information is presented on the five DO systems identified in Table 14.2. More details on the use of these instruments can be found in their respective coding protocol, procedures, and training manuals.

BEACHES

The BEACHES (McKenzie, Sallis, Nader, Patterson et al., 1991) can be used to collect objective data on the PA and sedentary behaviors of children and selected environmental (social and physical) variables that may influence those behaviors in home settings. Given the complexity of BEACHES (i.e. the number of different categories), observers use an alternating 15-second observation and 15-second recording format that if used during a 90 minutes observation session would produce 180 observation samples. These are paced by prerecorded voice prompts (e.g. using an MP3 or MP4 file).

BEACHES includes the recording of a total of ten coding categories (dimensions) for each interval. These include: (a) home environment conditions including presence of adults (e.g. parents, peers), presence of food, and media (e.g. TV, computer, tablet, smartphone); (b) child location (e.g. inside or outside the home, on a playground); (c) child's PA level (i.e. lying down, sitting, standing, walking, or vigorous); (d) whether the child ingested food during the interval; (e) who prompted the child PA or eating behavior, (f) the type of prompt; (g) PA or eating behavior prompted;

(h) the child's response to the prompt; (i) presence of any subsequent reinforcing or punishing stimuli (i.e. consequences); and (j) the behavior receiving the consequence.

MTS is used to record the observed child's PA level and the remaining coding dimensions are scored using partial-interval recording. That is, these events are coded if they occur at any time during the 15-second "observe" interval. For example, events such as a child putting food in his/her mouth, a parent prompting the child to go play outside, and a peer prompting a child to play a computer game can all be captured.

SOFIT

The SOFIT (McKenzie, Sallis, & Nader, 1991) can be used to assess physical education classes and sports coaching settings. Observers simultaneously collect data on three main categories: (a) student/athlete PA level, (b) lesson/session context, and (c) instructor behavior (teacher/coach). PA engagement is a health-related goal of both physical education and sports and is the primary means toward becoming physically fit and physically skilled. The two other coding categories are critical, because MVPA is contingent on both what and how content is presented (i.e. lesson/session context) and the behavior of the instructor delivering it (i.e. teacher/coach behavior).

SOFIT enables researchers, teachers/coaches, and supervisors to determine the quantity and quality of physical education and team practice sessions, especially as it relates to program and session goals. This is reflected in the resulting outcome and process data. For example, outcome data can include the number of minutes and percent of lesson/team practice time spent in MVPA and/or VPA as well as estimated EE rate (kcal/kg/min).

SOFIT's context categories provide information on commonly studied process variables. For example, researchers and practitioners may both be interested relative to the scheduling of physical education lessons and how they are actually delivered (e.g. duration of scheduled and actual length of lessons, frequency of canceled lessons). In addition, the instrument provides information relative to the minutes and proportion session time spent in management vs. instruction, fitness, skill drills, game play, and other activities.

For instructor behavior, there are two versions of SOFIT. The first includes six instructor behavior categories (i.e. promotes fitness/PA [e.g. prompts, encourages, praises], demonstrates fitness [models], instructs generally, manages, observes, and other tasks). A simpler and more recent version focuses solely on participant PA engagement and includes only three instructor behavior categories (i.e. promotes in-class PA, fitness, or motor skills; promotes out-of-class PA, fitness, or motor skills; and does not promote in- or out-of-class PA, fitness, or motor skills). This latter version was developed specifically to assess instructor efforts in promoting out-of-session PA. Thus, it can be used to determine the percent of intervals that teachers/coaches spend promoting PA both during sessions (physical education/sports practices) and beyond.

SOPLAY

Beyond scheduled classes, students spend significant amounts of non-attached time on school campuses (i.e. before-school time, lunch periods, and after-school time) and the SOPLAY (McKenzie et al., 2000) was developed to collect data on the number of students (including their gender) and their PA levels in specified activity areas. As assessing PA in open spaces is complicated because of the rapidly changing number of students and their PA levels, prior to data collection campuses are mapped to identify available activity areas (some high schools have as many as 20 activity areas).

During data collection, observers visit each activity area in a set sequence and at designated times (e.g. before school, lunch time, and after school) to collect data on students' PA levels and environmental variables. At each area, observers use MTS to scan individuals and environmental conditions. During a scan, each person's PA level is coded as sedentary (lying down, sitting, or standing), walking/moderate, or vigorous using mechanical or electronic counters (e.g. with an App). Separate scans are typically made for females and males, but, depending on the research question, information can be generated as well for race/ethnicity and or age groupings. During each area visit, observers also make entries for specific environmental conditions including the time of day, temperature, area accessibility, area usability, and availability of adult supervision, organized activity (e.g. team practice session or game), and equipment. Following the observation period, the number of participants (by gender) and their activity levels can be determined within and across activity areas and by contextual condition (e.g. organized vs. unorganized activities). As noted earlier, summary score EE estimates (kcal/kg/min) can also be calculated for each activity area.

SOPARC

The SOPARC (McKenzie, Cohen et al., 2006) was designed to collect data in community park use, including the relevant concurrent characteristics of the parks and their users. As with SOPLAY, the park is mapped to identify the designated activity areas and observers use a set sequence of scans in each area. In each area, they collect data on the environmental conditions, including area accessibility and usability and the presence of supervision, organized activities, activity types, and activity equipment. They also count the number of park users and code their PA levels, gender, age, and race/ethnicity (if desired) via paper/pencil with a mechanical counter (see Figure 14.2; [http://denominatrocompany.com]), or the iSOPARC App (discussed later). Collected data are summarized similar to SOPLAY data.

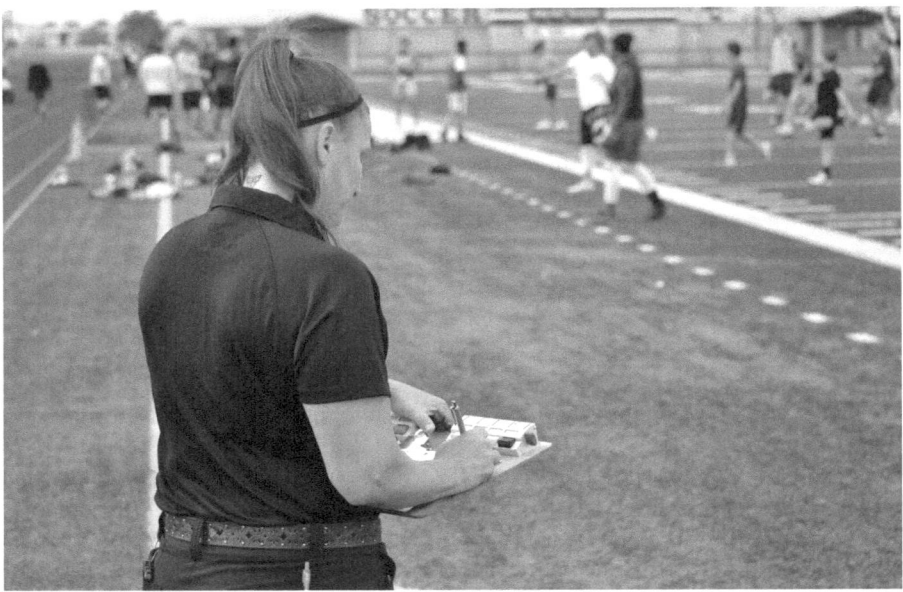

Figure 14.2 Data collector using SOPLAY counter board

SOCARP

The SOCARP (Ridgers et al., 2010) was designed to collect data on children's PA levels and interactions on playgrounds such as during recess. For each observation session, specific children can be targeted or they can be selected at random to mirror the population of those present. Demographic information such as the number of supervisors, availability of equipment, and temperature is captured. Observers also assess additional variables, including size of the social group, the main activity type, and pro-, and anti-social interactions with peers.

As with SOFIT, observers use an alternating 10-second observe, 10-second record interval coding format (e.g. using prerecorded prompts from a MP3 or MP4 file). The resulting data are converted to percent of intervals.

Key Issues When Using Direct Observation

DO users must consider several key issues. These include methodological considerations as well as observer training and maintenance, especially as it relates to reliability and independence. In addition, DO has several limitations that must be considered, including the investment of time, access to areas for observing and recording the target behavior(s), and observer error. These issues are discussed below.

Observer Reliability

In science, researchers must demonstrate collected data are credible (i.e. trustworthy). With DO, researchers need to present evidence of "observer reliability" (i.e. the consistency between observers to agree within and across observation sessions). Observer reliability is typically established in two different ways. The first is to assess the level of agreement of data recorded by two trained "independent" observers who record the same events at the same time. This is referred to as "inter-observer" reliability or inter-observer agreement (IOA).

A second approach requires researchers to obtain video records of events and then have the same observers code them on two separate occasions (typically at least 10–14 days apart). This is referred to as "intra-observer reliability". Video segments are recorded in the setting to be assessed and are later viewed and coded. One advantage of this procedure is that coding errors can be corrected if noticed, whereas specific errors made during "live" data collection are more challenging to fix. Another advantage is that observers can pause during coding, a tactic useful for preventing observer fatigue during lengthy sessions (e.g. longer than 45 minutes). Furthermore, observers can double-check the accuracy of their data entries by re-reviewing the coding manual. Finally, video records are durable and could possibly be used later for other research projects. One disadvantage of using video records is that the actual data coding might get put off until later causing delays in completing the research project. In experimental research such delays would not allow for tracking the impact of an intervention as it unfolds.

Calculating Observer Reliability

Observer reliability can be determined in numerous ways, including calculating: (a) Interval-by-Interval (I-I) percentages, (b) Intra-Class Correlation Coefficients (ICCs), and (c) Cohen's Kappa statistic. With the I-I method, each interval from two observers' data sets is compared. An agreement is counted when both observers entered the same code. A disagreement is identified when observers enter different codes, for example one codes a participant as "standing" and the other codes her as "vigorous". The number of agreements and disagreements is totaled and assessed using the equation shown in Figure 14.3.

$$\frac{\text{Agreements}}{\text{Agreements + Disagreements}} * 100 = \text{IOA Percentage}$$

Figure 14.3   Standard inter-observer agreement percentage formula

Calculating the ICC is another option for assessing observer reliability (i.e. consistency), and there are multiple ways to calculate ICCs. We recommend researchers use the "two-way mixed effects, absolute agreement, multiple raters/measurements" option, as suggested by Koo and Li (2016). ICC reliability values, at the 95% confidence interval, are typically interpreted as follows: 0.49 or less = *poor*, 0.5–0.74 = *moderate*, 0.75–0.89 = *good*, 0.90 or higher = *excellent*.

Cohen's Kappa (*k*) coefficient can also be used to assess agreement between two observers on categorical items. In general, Kappa coefficient values are lower than those produced with the I-I method, but is regarded the stronger measure because it accounts for possible chance agreements. Like Pearson correlation coefficients, *k*-values can range from +1 to −1. Negative values are uncommon, and a value of 0 reflects a level of agreement based on random chance. The following is a guide to determine whether the *k* value reflects an acceptable level of observer agreement: *k* values between 0.01 and 0.20 indicate *no agreement*, 0.21 and 0.39 *minimal agreement*, 0.40 and 0.59 *weak agreement*, 0.60 and 0.79 *moderate agreement*, 0.80 and 0.89 *strong agreement*, and 0.90 or higher reflects *almost perfect agreement* (McHugh, 2012).

The DO systems highlighted in this chapter are complex, and across the possible three indicators of observer reliability explained earlier, IOA percentages of 80% or higher are deemed acceptable. When using less complex systems (i.e. fewer behavior categories), observers should be expected to reach the 90% agreement threshold (Cooper et al., 2007; van der Mars, 1989b).

Observer Independence

During IOA checks, observer independence refers to the two observers being far enough apart so they cannot see each other's coding decisions. When using SOFIT, for example, observers are typically cued to alternate tasks via prerecorded 10-second "observe" and "record" prompts from earphones connected to a playback device (e.g. mp3/4 file on a smartphone or tablet). The observers can still be independent by connecting their earphones to the same source via a "Y" adaptor.

Observers using SOPLAY or SOPARC are not paced by prerecorded audio prompts; nonetheless they should start and stop their observational scans simultaneously. Once in position at the target area (e.g. dance studio, basketball court) and counters are reset to zero, the lead observer indicates the start of the scan using a signal such as "Ready...Go". The observers need to be sufficiently close so that each can view the entire target area from the same angle, but they should not be able to see the data codes each one enters.

Observer Training

Quality training is needed to produce accurate and reliable observers and this needs to occur before commencing data collection for a study. IOA checks, however, should occur periodically to ensure observer performance levels are maintained throughout the study. This is especially important when there are extended breaks such as during seasons or school vacations. In colder climates, for example, public parks may not be used during winter. Thus, after the seasonal layoff, observers should receive retraining booster sessions.

Table 14.2 includes the typical steps used for training observers using the DO systems presented in this chapter. Prior to the start of observer training, prospective observers should be provided

Table 14.2 Observer training protocol

Phase 1: Prior to data collection

Observer training includes the following stages:

1   *Orientation to DO and the specific tool to be used*:
    Observer trainees learn about the research project in general without specifics about research questions and study design (e.g. is it experimental, correlational). Included would also be topics such as observer etiquette, confidentiality, objectivity, and behaving ethically

2   *Memorizing behavior categories and accompanying coding symbols*:
    Trainees participate in directed video practice using all coding protocols (i.e. pacing, coding formats, and conventions)

3   *Video assessments using "gold standard" coding records*:
    Trainees code video segments previously scored by a certified observer and make comparisons to the "gold standard"

4   *Introduction to the use of digital data collection devices and software*:
    If, in lieu of the traditional paper and pencil methods along with counter boards, observers practice using study tablets and Apps (see later section on use of technology)

5   *"Live" field-based practice of using parts of and later the full observation system*:
    Trainers are available to direct observers, answer questions, provide feedback, and assess potential gaps in observers' performance

6   *Field-based observer reliability checks with a certified assessor*:
    Observers are assessed formally and starting actual data collection is contingent on them, successfully meeting established IOA levels

Phase 2: During data collection

7   *Observer reliability checks during data collection*:
    Periodic IOA checks should be conducted throughout all phases of a study. Retraining should occur after extended breaks (e.g. summers, school vacations)

---

with the observation system's Description and Coding Procedures Manual (see Table 14.3). Each manual includes an introduction to the system, behavior category definitions (including examples of each), related coding symbols, coding conventions (i.e. coding rules developed for specific situations that may arise during the observation session), sample coding forms, and suggested IOA calculations. The manuals also include a section on "frequently asked questions" (FAQs). Videos have been developed to support training for several of the systems and currently can be accessed free online (see Table 14.3). Faithful adherence to the training protocols not only ensures all observers receive the same training, but makes study results more generalizable such as being able to make valid comparisons to other studies using the same observation system (McKenzie & Smith, 2017; Smith, McKenzie, & Hammons, 2019).

Observer Reliability Procedures and Reporting

When reporting observer reliability results in papers, it is important to report the number of observers and the number of reliability checks that were taken throughout the data collection phase. A rule of thumb is to do reliability checks in at least 20% of all observation sessions (fewer if observers demonstrate consistent high reliability). Ideally, observation checks should be balanced across settings, selected at random, and during experimental studies be balanced across experimental phases/conditions. When employing intra-observer agreement checks, the amount of time in between observations should be reported as well.

Researchers should calculate and identify the agreement values for each behavior category being reported at the level for which the actual data are being reported (van der Mars, 1989b).

Table 14.3 Online resources for observer training

Observer coding protocols

BEACHES coding protocol:

https://activelivingresearch.org/beaches-behaviors-eating-and-activity-childrens-health-evaluation-system

SOFIT coding protocol:

https://activelivingresearch.org/sofit-system-observing-fitness-instruction-time

SOPLAY coding protocol:

https://activelivingresearch.org/soplay-system-observing-play-and-leisure-activity-youth

SOPARC coding Protocol:

   a https://activelivingresearch.org/soparc-system-observing-play-and-recreation-communities

   b http://www.rand.org/health/surveys_tools/soparc/user-guide.html

SOCARP coding protocol:

Contact lead author for a copy of the coding protocol

Selected online resources for observer training

SOFIT training video 1.1:

https://www.youtube.com/watch?v=HiYTB_ee3t0

SOFIT assessment video:

https://www.youtube.com/watch?v=ODMbP4n7ork

SOPLAY/SOPARC training video:

https://www.youtube.com/watch?v=Vci6eX_Nvng

Introduction to using digital versions of iSOPARC:

https://activelivingresearch.org/sites/activelivingresearch.sdsc.edu/files/2014_iSOPARC_Kanters.pdf

The Apple iTunes store has the following compilation of SOFIT and SOPLAY/SOPARC training materials available as Podcasts:

https://itunes.apple.com/us/itunes-u/soplay-soparc-3assessment/id529513043?i=115757894

Active Living Research Systematic Observation Webinar:

https://www.youtube.com/watch?v=k9RTbgH8bB8

For example, if a study using SOFIT includes data for all categories within the three coding levels (i.e. PA, lesson context, and teacher behavior), the researchers should report the observer agreement values for each of these categories. Whenever possible the means and ranges for values should be reported separately. Merely reporting an overall mean limits judgments being made about the accuracy and trustworthiness of reported data, and in the case of experimental studies brings the believability of the intervention effect into question. Reporting a range of observer reliability values is acceptable when reporting data on a large number of behavior and context categories if the range is narrow. When reliability values have wide variability among behavioral categories, the outliers (i.e. low frequency categories) should be identified and explained.

Methodological Considerations When Using Direct Observation

How many observation sessions do I need? How long should I observe? What should my interval length be? Researchers using DO need to consider these questions as they plan studies, as each could affect data accuracy, statistical power calculations, and the generalizability of results. They also need to consider various other factors. For example, what is/are the target population(s)?; what time(s) of day will observations take place?; what time of year (e.g. fall vs. spring vs. summer season); what will the weather conditions be? what setting(s) will be targeted (e.g. parks vs. schools, physical education lessons vs. total school campus)?

As noted earlier, PA behavior is place-based. Because there are no single best answers to these questions, researchers can make sound decisions about the frequency and length of observation sessions only after making numerous visits to the target environments prior to the start of data collection. Nonetheless, we offer the following evidence-based recommendations.

First, Bailey et al. (1995) found significant variability in the duration, frequency, and intensity of free-range PA in natural conditions among children (age 6–10). Data were collected in homes, school, cars, restaurants, sports events, and elsewhere. Slightly over 75% of all PA was of low intensity and only 3% was of high intensity, with 95% of the PA bouts being 15 seconds or less in duration. These findings were based on observations made for 4 hour blocks per day, across 9 days (distributed evenly between morning, afternoon, and early evening). Within each 4 hour block observers had a 3 minute break every 27 minutes. Given the wide variability in children's PA duration, frequency, and intensity, DO observers who study PA across different settings over the course of the day should follow a data collection schedule similar to the one of Bailey et al. (1995).

In a multi-site park study using SOPARC, Cohen et al. (2011) found that four observation sessions per day on 4 days a week provided representative data on the characteristics of park users, including their age, race/ethnicity, and PA levels. In addition, based on Levin, McKenzie, Hussey, Kelder, and Lytle's (2001) findings in physical education classes, researchers need to be mindful of how factors like lesson goals, content variation, facility size, and available type and amount of equipment within and across lessons impact students' PA. Finally, in home settings, Klesges et al. (1984) recommended a minimum of four observation sessions for estimating young children's PA patterns.

In terms of the number of observation samples needed within a single observation session, a general rule of thumb is that shorter interval lengths (e.g. 10 seconds) are better as they provide more samples and reduce the complexity of observers' decision making. However, researchers need to weigh decisions relative to the study goals, practicality, and the complexity of the observation system. For example, McNamee and van der Mars (2005) reported that when using MTS, interval lengths up to 90 seconds would provide acceptable data accuracy levels.

Another factor to consider in determining the appropriate interval length is the degree to which activity types change during an observation session. Activity types are substantially different in the amount PA they provide. For example, gymnastics generally has less motor engagement than soccer. And in physical education, the type of activity typically changes frequently. Moreover, there is built-in variability in the natural duration of activities. Certain ones are by nature discrete (i.e. short in duration), while others are continuous (e.g. running, rope-jumping, swimming, doing push-ups). A single physical education lesson typically includes both types. McKenzie and van der Mars (2015) made the following suggestion specific to this point:

> With more continuous activities (e.g., swimming, group exercise), data accuracy may be maintained even with MTS interval lengths that are well beyond the standard 20-s coding format. However, in activities that have many inherent breaks (e.g., tackle football), more samples (i.e., shorter intervals) per observation session are likely needed.
>
> *(p. 17)*

Specific to PA intensity-level categories reviewed earlier, SOFIT includes five levels, three of which reflect sedentary body positions (i.e. lying down, sitting, standing). The remaining two categories are walking/moderate and "vigorous" PA. Having these five categories offers a more fine-grained PA profile which may be of interest to both researchers and practitioners. Nonetheless, based on the EE values being similar for lying down, sitting, and standing, Rowe et al. (2004) determined that these three SOFIT sedentary PA categories could be merged into a single one ("sedentary"), and this is reflected in the three level PA coding systems of SOPLAY and SOPARC.

Limitations of Direct Observation

All data collection instruments for assessing PA have limitations, including DO. It is important that researchers using DO be mindful of the following limitations: time investment, access to certain settings, and issues surrounding observer error.

Time Investment

Time can be a barrier in multiple ways, including traveling to and from the observation sites to collect data and complete reliability measures. Observer training also takes time and this depends on the complexity of the system and the number of observers (e.g. McKenzie & van der Mars, 2015; Montoye, Kemper, Saris, & Washburn, 1996).

It includes several steps, with observers needing to demonstrate they can collect accurate data under increasingly more complex conditions (i.e. from coding video-based scenarios to live coding in diverse environments). In addition (like mechanical and digital devices such as treadmills and metabolic carts in exercise physiology studies), the accuracy of observers should be checked periodically throughout the project's data collection phase. Another aspect of time investment becomes pertinent in studies where PA needs to be observed for longer periods of time, such studies that focus on PA over the course of a full school day, or for full 24 hour periods. When data are obtained from video recordings, personnel time is almost doubled as it takes time to both video the sessions and code them.

Access to Settings

In some cases, observer access to certain settings is limited or not allowed. For example, they may not be allowed to observe athletes' PA when coaches conduct closed practices. Private clubs (e.g. tennis, golf) may also restrict access. When reporting research, researchers are encouraged to be explicit in noting cases of limited access in their Methods section and to return to this in the discussion of results. In studies where people's PA is to be observed over a full day, observations within some private homes may not be possible.

Observer Error

As noted earlier, data accuracy is a key criterion in determining the credibility or trustworthiness of all science. Because humans are the data collectors, they are susceptible to observer error and there are generally two types. First are errors of *"omission"*, where observers fail to see and record the occurrence of (a) behavior(s). This is more common when coding the (non)occurrence of a single behavior, but is unlikely to occur when observing PA.

In contrast to errors of omission are errors of "commission" and these occur when observers perceive they see an event and enter an incorrect behavior or contextual code. Such errors may occur in PA research using the tools presented in this chapter, because the observers must choose from multiple behavior categories. For example, depending on the tool used, there are 3–5 PA level categories (e.g. lying down, sitting, standing, walking, vigorous). Recording a youngster's PA as "sedentary" when the correct choice was "walking" or "vigorous" is an example of a commission error. Generally, commission errors occur because observers have misconceptions about category definitions. That is, they fail to correctly discriminate between categories, and additional training is then needed to eliminate the misunderstanding. Another type of commission occurs if/ when observers accidentally select/enter an incorrect coding symbol.

Observer errors can manifest themselves in various ways. First, *observation system complexity* increases observer error. That is, the higher the number of behavior and contextual categories included in the system, the greater the possibility that observers will commit errors in either observing and/or recording. Second, *environmental complexity* also increases the likelihood of observer error. For example, if there are many people in the setting, with many moving fast or in different directions, or if numerous activities are occurring simultaneously, data accuracy may be affected. During a football practice, for example, there may be as many as 80 people on the field and players may be doing different drills, including moving in varying directions. In addition, during a school lunchtime open gym session there may be well over 100 students moving about. In these cases, errors can be reduced by dividing the observation area into smaller target areas (sub-sections).

Third, despite proper training, *observer drift* may occur if observers inadvertently change coding rules or modify their interpretation of behavior categories (e.g. coding a person doing curl-ups as being moderately active and months later coding it as vigorous). This problem can be monitored through frequent observer reliability checks. Furthermore, periodic "booster" or "recalibration" sessions should be scheduled that include "gold standard checks" that require observers to demonstrate they still are adhering to the observation protocol.

Fourth, fatigue can cause observers to lose focus and concentration, and thus commit both observing and recording errors. We recommend, especially in environmentally complex situations, that data collectors limit their observation session to no more than three per day. In addition, when multiple observation sessions are included, observers should have sufficient time between sessions to relax. Fifth, *observer expectancy/-bias* can occur (even unintentionally) if, for example, observers are aware an intervention is aimed at changing the behavior of the target person(s).

Sixth, observers who are aware that a second, independent observer is present to conduct reliability checks may be susceptible to what is called *observer reactivity*. That is, they may pay more attention during that observation session. Conversely, if same observers know that "no one is watching", they may be less alert, thereby being less accurate. Depending on available resources, observer reactivity can be minimized by having two observers during as many observation sessions as possible. And seventh, there is a risk of *observer cheating*. There is no evidence that cheating is prevalent, but observers could cheat by fabricating data, and/or altering data (after the fact). While not technically a form of cheating, researchers may inadvertently calculate IOA percentages incorrectly (van der Mars, 1989b). Project leaders can minimize cheating by (a) having observers send completed data forms (hard copy or electronic) immediately upon completing the observation session, (b) doing unannounced random reliability checks, and (c) having a person other than the observers calculate IOA percentages. The emergence of electronic data collection devices which allow for automatic time- and location-stamping of files is now also a way of minimizing observer cheating.

Emerging Technological Issues and Advances in Using Direct Observation

Advances in video recording technology have made video recording and storage much easier. The once dominant reel-to-reel, VHS, and VHS-C cassette analog video recording devices have been replaced by digital technology (e.g. GoPro cameras, tablets) which are much less obtrusive and permit recording for extended periods of time. They also allow for more and larger files to be stored. Cloud-based storage (e.g. DropBox, iCloud) is also available, though users should consider data security issues. In addition, with sufficient funding, events can be recorded remotely (e.g. via pre-programmed cameras in recreation centers and parks), permitting researchers to increase the number of observation sites.

Relative to digital software, Castelliano, Perea, Alday, and Mendo (2008) reported an increase in the number of computer-based DO tools and provided five criteria for determining the quality and usability of digital software-based DO instruments: (a) user friendliness, which refers to users having the flexibility to *customize* the software to their needs instead of being locked into a "closed" system, (b) being able to *self-define* target behaviors and contextual variables, (c) having the option to *time-stamp* observed events to indicate the time, duration, and location of their occurrence, (d) being capable of *linking video-based observational data directly with the video record* which allows for quick retrieval of events for review, and (e) the availability of *basic analytical features* which allows descriptive data on the frequency and/or duration of events to be assessed. In recent years, the availability of compact, digital hardware like tablets (e.g. iPads) prompted a corresponding development of DO Apps such as iSOFIT (see Figure 14.3) and iSOPARC. These two free Apps are available through the iTunes App Store and work on iOS devices only.

The main advantages of using software technology are being able to enter, compile, summarize, and store data much faster. In addition, the raw data can be easily transferred to statistical software packages such as SPSS for in-depth analysis. Such advantages make these technologies more attractive to researchers who use DO in conducting multi-site research.

Technological advances now permit initial portions of observer training to be done using the internet, and this is especially attractive for multi-site, large-scale studies. This can also help reduce the initial costs associated with preparing observers. Nonetheless, researchers must remain vigilant when training people to employ digital software to collect the data (McKenzie & van der Mars, 2015). Not only must the observers be trained to observe and record accurately, they must also be trained on how to use the technology effectively. This adds new dimensions to training as observers must learn to select the correct coding keys on their screen, make corrections immediately when necessary, and save and transfer data files.

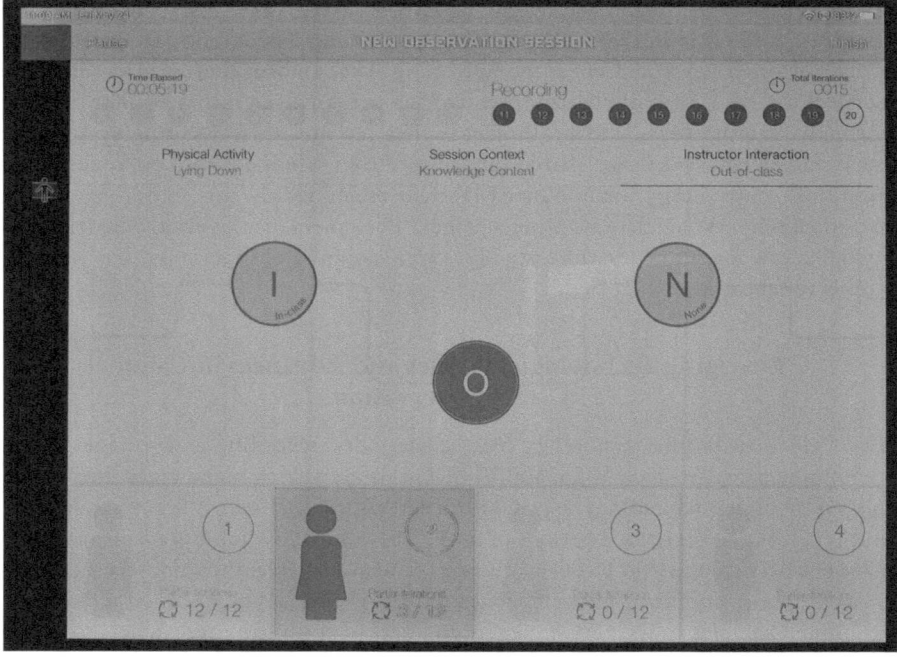

Figure 14.4   iSOFIT opening screen

Brief Overview of the Literature

The number of published research projects in which DO has been employed is far too expansive for all to be included in this chapter. However, the examples below offer answer to a key question: *Why use DO in PA Intervention/Surveillance Research?*

As noted earlier, studying the efficacy of environmental and policy interventions has become a major emphasis globally (e.g. Bauer et al., 2014). Given that context, DO provides a critical advantage over other data collection approaches by being able to assess the PA behavior of youth in diverse settings while simultaneously being able to capture data on the concurrent environmental contextual conditions that influence it. The behavioral-ecological perspective (Hovell et al., 2009) offers an appropriate framework for organizing examples of successful PA interventions where DO was used. Interventions aimed at changing the PA of individuals (or populations) can be targeted at multiple levels (i.e. individual, local, community, social/cultural).

The following examples include descriptive and intervention studies, in which the DO systems were used to assess youth PA behavior. (There is also growing evidence of similar successes with older age groups; however, that is beyond the scope of this chapter.)

Example 1: Home Environments

McKenzie, Sallis, Nader, Patterson et al. (1991) used BEACHES to collect baseline data on the physical and social environmental variables that were associated with young at-risk children's PA and sedentary behavior. Children spent almost 75% of their waking hours indoors and being sedentary. Only 11% of their waking hours were spent in VPA (e.g. running). When they were indoors, the children were typically sedentary, spending significant time viewing media (e.g. TV), and ingesting food. PA prompts were dependent on children's location, their gender, and the presence of an adult (e.g. parent, caretaker). Most PA-related prompts for boys who were indoors were to be sedentary (e.g. "stop jumping on the bed").

Example 2: School Physical Education Environment

Of all settings where DO has been used to assess PA interventions, physical education lessons have most extensive evidence base. Using SOFIT, Sallis, et al. (1997) demonstrated that ongoing professional development for physical education teachers and classroom teachers on the use of the SPARK curriculum produced significant increases in students' MVPA levels. Moreover, improvements in MVPA were sustained at least 2 years beyond the intervention phases (McKenzie, Sallis, Kolody, & Faucette, 1997). For a comprehensive review of SOFIT research in US physical education, see McKenzie and Smith (2017) and for international SOFIT studies see Smith et al. (2019).

More recently, Kahan and McKenzie (2015, 2017) used a combination of variables including those from DO (e.g. lesson frequency, length, student MVPA levels, and class size) to compare EE estimates of students in physical education with national PA recommendations and state policies. They reported that the EE during physical education in states with specific physical education time policy recommendations was significantly higher than in states without such a policy. In addition, even though more states had recently adopted policies for physical education minutes than had eliminated them, EE estimates in physical education had declined over a 4-year period (2017).

Example 3: School Campus Environment – School Day

SOPLAY was used to assess an intervention on 24 middle school campuses that targeted physical education lessons as well as the use of PA facilities throughout the school day (McKenzie et al.,

2000). While PA areas were almost always usable, they were accessible only about half the time and they were rarely equipped, provided structured activities, or had adult supervision. Use of the PA areas beyond physical education was greater during lunch periods but they were typically unused during before- and after-schools. More boys than girls used the areas during all measurement times and were more active when in school.

Example 4: School Campus Environment – After-School Time

After-school and youth sports programs are a dominant feature of secondary schools, and they have the potential to provide substantial PA opportunities. Nonetheless, these programs are often unregulated and most coaches are volunteers. There is preliminary evidence that PA levels in these programs are relatively low (e.g. Guagliano, Lonsdale, Kolt, Rosenkranz, & George, 2015; Leek et al., 2011; Sacheck et al., 2011).

Bocarro et al. (2012) used SOPLAY to compare the PA of youths in interscholastic programs with those participated in campus-based intramural sports programs. Boys, but not girls, in the intramural program schools were significantly more active than those in the interscholastic program schools. Self-contained programs on campuses (e.g. intramural sports programs) may be a more cost-effective means of increasing overall student participation and PA levels than interscholastic sports programs.

DO has also been used in other studies relative to policy implications for how sports programs targeting youth can best be structured and delivered. SOPARC, for example, has been used in numerous studies assessing school policies and practices, including shared-use agreements (Carlton et al., 2017), an after-school staff training program (e.g. Huberty, Beets, Beighle, & McKenzie, 2013), and the use of school playgrounds during out-of-school times (e.g. Colabianchi, Maslow, & Swayampakala, 2011).

Example 5: School Campus Environment-Recess

Recess during the school day provides PA opportunities for school-aged youths. Ridgers et al. (2010), for example, used SOCARP to assess how the social environment impacted students' PA levels during recess. They found that students, regardless of gender and weight status, engaged in MVPA well over 50% of recess time. Boys were more active than girls (particularly in VPA). Boys spent more time in sports-related activities (e.g. soccer), while girls were more likely to engage in playground games. Girls spent more time in small groups than boys and they engaged in more positive behavior. Boys exhibited more negative behavior involving physical contact. Statistically, boys and girls spent equal amounts of time in sedentary or locomotive activities. The findings have implications for how recess can be structured and how supervisors can be trained to monitor children's activities and their interactions. The latter is particularly pertinent relative to anti-social behavior such as bullying and fighting.

Example 6: Preschool-Aged Youth in Daycare Settings

The PA of preschool-aged children has received increased attention in recent years (Hnatiuk et al., 2018; Hnatiuk, Salmon, Hinkley, Okely, & Trost, 2014). Trost, Ward, and Senso (2010) noted that: (a) environmental variables such as staff education and training can have salient influences on preschoolers' MVPA, (b) larger, open play spaces positively influence MVPA, and (c) the quantity and quality of portable equipment (e.g. balls, jump ropes), but not fixed play equipment (e.g. climbing apparatus), influenced MVPA. The Observational System for Recording Physical

Activity in Children – Preschool Version (OSRAC-P; Brown et al., 2006) was used in several of the studies.

These six examples provide a glimpse of how DO has been used across different school levels, settings, and at different levels of the behavioral-ecological framework (Hovell et al., 2009). Research in which DO instruments are used provides evidence not only about PA but also about concurrent contextual variables. Importantly, these results can be used to inform practitioners (e.g. teachers, recreation leaders, child care providers, and sports coaches), as well as policy makers such as sports program administrators, school principals, school board members, and state legislators. We see DO as an invaluable tool for developing more and better evidence on PA levels and the effective delivery of programs that optimize them.

Emerging PA Research Directions When Using Direct Observation

McKenzie and van der Mars (2015) have provided a detailed overview of future PA research directions. These included suggestions to further our understanding of the methodological features of DO as well as the need to focus on the efficacy of interventions aimed at increasing PA behavior across persons and settings. Progress has been made in building a body evidence on PA in various contexts based on the use of DO. Nonetheless, as in all areas of science, there is need for further advancement and systematic replication (e.g. Makel & Plucker, 2014; Murad & Montori, 2013, Sidman, 1988). A brief summary is provided below.

Future Directions in Research on Direct Observation's Methodological Features

As noted earlier, there is a significant body of research that supports the validity of PA categories. Researchers have also shown how different interval lengths may result in under- or over-estimations of PA. However, since observer training is such a critical aspect of using DO, a legitimate question to ask is: how do observer training protocols and observer experience affect potential sources of error? There are advantages to using electronic versions of DO tools (Castelliano et al., 2008), but using them does not guarantee accurate and credible data. Ultimately, it is the observer who must make decisions about the occurrence, type, and intensity of PA behavior.

Little is known about specific aspects of observer training protocols. For example, what are the most efficient protocols for training observers in the use of electronic data collection tools. Should observers be required to employ the paper and pencil version of an observation system before being introduced to the electronic version? What is the best sequence for observer training modules? What is the optimal balance between video-based and live observation practice? How many and what type of video examples are necessary for observers to reach acceptable performance levels? And of special importance in longitudinal studies, after demonstrating observer proficiency, how frequent should IOA checks be conducted to guard against observer drift?

Relative to the use of electronic data collection tools, the most important question is: to what extent and how (if at all) does their use affect data accuracy? McKenzie and van der Mars (2015) summarized the role and potential of using technology in DO as follows:

> … technology advancements offer a number of attractive features for SO researchers. Decisions on the 'what' and 'how much' technology to use should depend on how data can be expediently collected with the best possible accuracy and with consideration given to the research question, costs, available resources, and the rigor of observer training.

(p. 20)

Future Directions in PA Research Using Direct Observation

There are several PA research areas where the use of DO would strengthen the quality of the evidence base. These include assessing: (a) PA levels on school campuses throughout the school day (e.g. before-, during-, and after-school times), (b) tracking PA at the surveillance (e.g. state, provincial, or national level, (c) the role of policies and laws on student PA in physical education at all school levels, (d) parks, recreation, and sports environments, and (e) home and child care settings.

Policy Research

Policy-focused research in physical education is one particular area where DO-based PA research is needed, especially because self-report measures have been the predominant data collection tool and these are often completed by people far removed from the school setting (e.g. school district-level or state-level personnel). Only a few studies have used DO to assess the link between PA levels and context-based policy and environmental variables (e.g. Lounsbery, Holt, Monnat, Funk, & McKenzie, 2014; Robinson, Wadsworth, Webster, & Bassett Jr, 2014). Obtaining more information through studies using DO would strengthen the evidence of the role and impact of school, district, and state-level policies and laws on the delivery of physical education. This is especially important as there is evidence that simply having national recommendations for minutes of physical education per week and state policies/laws (e.g. SHAPE America, 2015; Kahan & McKenzie, 2015, 2017; NPAPA, 2018) does not translate into adherence to them.

Surveillance Research

Doing surveillance on PA at the national, state and local levels is extremely important (National Academies of Sciences, Engineering, and Medicine, 2019). There have been a number of national surveillance studies on PA such as the YRBSS assessments that are conducted every other year since 1991 (see https://www.cdc.gov/healthyyouth/data/yrbs/data.htm). However, most of these are surveys using self-reports, and, to date, there have been no state-wide or national surveillance studies of PA levels using DO on school campus settings. One good example of a national level surveillance study using SOPARC is a study of 174 neighborhood parks in 25 major US cities, over two time points (2014 and 2106). The authors reported that males used neighborhood parks more often than females, older adults used neighborhood parks less than other age groups, approximately two-thirds of neighborhood park users were sedentary, and approximately one-third of neighborhood park users were physically active. DO studies of this magnitude are necessary in other areas as well (e.g. K-12 school physical education, youth sports, community sports).

PA on School Campuses throughout the School Day

There has been extensive study of students' PA levels in elementary and middle school physical education (e.g. McKenzie, 2001; McKenzie, Catellier et al., 2006; McKenzie et al., 2004; McKenzie & Smith, 2017). In recent years, with the emergence of whole-of-school initiatives to promote student PA, more DO research has targeted before-school times (e.g. Mahar, Vuchenich, Golden, DuBose, & Raedeke, 2011; Stylianou et al., 2016) and during-school periods (e.g. Mahar, 2011; Mahar et al., 2006; Ward, 2011). The emerging evidence base, however, remains relatively thin and systematic replication (e.g. across grade/school levels) is needed to assess the feasibility and sustainability of different programs.

PA in Parks/Recreation and Sports Environments

Parks, recreation centers, and sports programs are also key settings for population level PA. SOPARC has been used in numerous studies in park settings, including the impact of park improvements (e.g. Cohen et al., 2007, 2015, 2016; Cohen, Williamson, Sehgal, Marsh, & McKenzie, 2009). Recently, Cohen et al. (2016) completed the first-ever national surveillance study of a representative sample of 174 neighborhood parks in 25 major US cities.

In contrast to the preparation and licensing of physical education professionals, sports coaching is less regulated. And while coaches are encouraged to complete certification programs, few states require coaches to complete such programs. Consequently, little is known about the effectiveness of coaching education programs relative to the skill of coaches in designing practice sessions that provide optimal PA and skill and physical fitness development. As noted earlier in the chapter, there are few empirical studies in which athletes' practice behavior and PA have been assessed (e.g. McKenzie & Rushall, 1974; Kanters, McKenzie et al., 2014). In addition, there is some DO-based evidence that policies permitting the shared-use of school facilities by community members and schools focusing on intramural and club programs promote higher PA levels (Bocarro et al., 2012; Bocarro, Kanters, Edwards, Casper, & McKenzie, 2014; Kanters, Bocarro et al., 2014). Nonetheless, given the limited number of studies and schools, additional investigations are needed across different programs, sports, and regions.

PA Assessment in Home and Child Care Settings

Children's PA habits are shaped in the home and child care environments during the first few years of life. Unfortunately, these settings are understudied relative to children's PA levels and the physical and social conditions that impact their PA. For example, the readily available technology within the home may be a powerful environmental factor that suppresses children's PA. McKenzie et al. (2008) used DO to assess PA patterns of Mexican-American children (age 6) and related contextual factors in the home using BEACHES. They found that children were mostly indoors, and sedentary with little, if any, VPA. Extensions and replications of this study are needed in other home environments.

The *2018 United States Report Card on Physical Activity for Children and Youth* (NPAPA, 2018) did not provide a grade in the "family and peers" category on account of the lack of data. The National Physical Activity Plan's (NPAPA, 2016) Education Sector, however, does include strategies and objectives targeting child care and early childhood education settings. It includes a call for the development of standards that ensure appropriate amounts of PA in those settings, and DO would allow for direct assessment of PA and related environmental variables to determine whether such standards are met. Researchers would also be able to assess the efficacy of environmental interventions (e.g. changes in time allocations for PA or the type and amount of play equipment) in such settings.

Additional Recommendations for Researchers/Practitioners

As indicated in the previous section, DO has long history of success and is an essential tool for assessing the environmental physical and social contexts of PA. Careful consideration of its advantages and limitations will aid researchers in obtaining the best possible data. A concept called "Ground-truthing" is pertinent here. Ground-truthing has been a critical approach to collecting data in fields such as archeology and forestry. For example, as technology advanced in forestry, photographs taken from satellites orbiting the earth became common sources of data for forest conditions and characteristics. Such an approach is distal from the actual forest setting, forest researchers, and workers. Forestry researchers recognized that they still needed more proximal measures of conditions and most of this research is generated by observers directly in the environment. Similarly, in an effort to understand and improve the conditions in which PA occurs, ground-truthing is needed in which observers have "boots on the ground" in settings where the PA occurs. Only then can PA along with the environmental conditions be observed directly.

The utility of systematic DO as a method for practitioners (e.g. physical educators, sports coaches, recreation/fitness center workers) to obtain relevant information should not be overlooked. While it is unrealistic to expect practitioners to use the full protocols of the DO instruments identified in this chapter and elsewhere, they can use parts of them. For example, there is evidence that physical educators can reliably assess student PA levels in physical education while teaching when they use MTS with extended intervals (see Table 14.1) and dichotomous coding categories of "Yes MVPA" and "No MVPA" (e.g. McNamee & van der Mars, 2005; van der Mars, McNamee, & Timken, 2018). In addition, personnel in fitness-health clubs and recreation centers can easily use portions of the SOPLAY or SOPARC instruments to systematically track the use and conditions of their various activity areas.

Summary and Conclusion

In this chapter, we described the essential features of DO as used to collect PA data on youths in a variety of settings and provided a brief overview of five widely used DO systems. The notable advantage of DO is that it can be used to collect data on both the PA behavior of youths and the antecedent (and consequent) environmental factors that may influence it. We highlighted the importance of observer training and the strategies for calculating and report observer reliability and noted how advances in video and software technology allow for more efficient data entry, storage, and analysis. We closed the chapter with examples of studies that highlight how capturing data on both PA and environmental variables can provide important evidence.

This type of evidence collected using DO is essential for supporting teachers, coaches, recreation leaders, and other practitioners in the delivering of programs that provide optimal opportunities for youths to be physically active. In addition, the information can help inform the development of strong policies that support PA. As can be seen in recent national and global reports (Active Healthy Kids Global Alliance, 2018; Katzmarzyk et al., 2018), much work remains. DO systems are important tools that can help these efforts.

References

Active Healthy Kids Global Alliance. (2018). *Childhood physical inactivity reaches crisis levels around the globe.* Ottawa, Canada: Active Healthy Kids Global Alliance. Retrieved from https://www.activehealthykids.org/global-matrix/

Bailey, R. C., Olson, J., Pepper, S. L., Porszasz, J., Barstow, T. J., & Cooper, D. M. (1995). The level and tempo of children's physical activities: An observational study. *Medicine & Science in Sports & Exercise, 27,* 1033–1041.

Bar-Or, O. (1983). *Pediatric sports medicine for the practitioner.* New York, NY: Springer-Verlag.

Bauer, U. E., Briss, P. A., Goodman, R. A., & Bowman. B. A. (2014). Prevention of chronic disease in the 21st century: Elimination of the leading preventable causes of premature death and disability in the USA. *The Lancet, 384,* 45–52.

Bocarro, J. N., Kanters, M. A., Cerin, E., Floyd, M. F., Casper, J. M., Suau, L. J., & McKenzie, T. L. (2012). School sport policy and school-based physical activity environments and their association with observed physical activity in middle school children. *Health & Place, 18,* 31–38.

Bocarro, J. N., Kanters, M. A., Edwards, M. B., Casper, J. M., & McKenzie, T. L. (2014). Prioritizing school intramural and interscholastic programs based on observed physical activity. *American Journal of Health Promotion, 28*(3 Suppl), S65–S71.

Brown, W. H., Pfeiffer, K. A., McLver, K. L., Dowda, M., Almeida, M. J., & Pate, R. R. (2006). Assessing preschool children's physical activity: The observational system for recording physical activity in children–preschool version. *Research Quarterly for Exercise and Sport, 77*, 167–176.

Carlton, T. A., Kanters, M. A., Bocarro, J. N., Floyd, M. F., Edwards, M. B., & Suau, L. J. (2017). Shared use agreements and leisure time physical activity in North Carolina public schools. *Preventive Medicine, 95*, S10–S16.

Castelliano, J., Perea, A., Alday, L., & Mendo, A. H. (2008). The measuring and observation tool in sports. *Behavior Research Methods, 80*, 898–905.

Cohen, D. A., Han, B., Nagel, C., Harnik, P., McKenzie, T. L., Evenson, K. R., . . . Katta, S. (2016). The first national study of neighborhood parks: Implications for physical activity. *American Journal of Preventive Medicine, 51*, 419–426.

Cohen, D. A., McKenzie, T. L., Sehgal, A., Williamson, S., Golinelli, D., & Lurie, N. (2007). Contribution of public parks to physical activity. *American Journal of Public Health, 97*, 509–514.

Cohen, D. A., Williamson, S., Sehgal, A., Marsh, T., & McKenzie, T.L. (2009). Effects of park improvements on park use and physical activity: Policy and programming implications. *American Journal of Preventive Medicine, 37*, 475–480.

Colabianchi, N., Maslow, A. L., & Swayampakala, K. (2011). Features and amenities of school playgrounds: A direct observation of utilization and physical activity levels outside of school time. *International Journal of Behavioral Nutrition and Physical Activity, 8*, 32. doi:10.1186/1479-5868-8-32

Cooper, J. O., Heron, T., & Heward, W. L. (2007). *Applied behavior analysis* (2nd ed.). Columbus, OH: Merrill.

Corder, K., Ekelund, U., Steele, R. M., Wareham, N. J., & Brage, S. (2008). Assessment of physical activity in youth. *Journal of Applied Physiology, 105*, 977–987.

Faison-Hodge, J., & Porretta, D. L. (2004). Physical activity levels of students with mental retardation and students without disabilities. *Adapted Physical Activity Quarterly, 21*, 139–152.

Finn, K. J., & Specker, B. (2000). Comparison of Actiwatch activity monitor and children's activity rating scale in children. *Medicine and Science in Sports and Exercise, 32*, 1794–1797.

Guagliano, J. M., Lonsdale, C., Kolt, G. S., Rosenkranz, R. R., & George, E. S. (2015). Increasing girls' physical activity during a short-term organized youth sport basketball program: A randomized controlled trial. *Journal of Science and Medicine in Sport, 18*, 412–417.

Heath, E. M., Coleman, K. J., Lensegrav, T., & Fallon, J. A. (2006). Using momentary time sampling to estimate minutes of physical activity in physical education: Validation of scores for the system for observing fitness instruction time. *Research Quarterly for Exercise and Sport, 77*, 142–146.

Hnatiuk, J. A., Brown, H. E., Downing, K. L., Hinkley, T., Salmon, J., & Hesketh, K. D. (2018). Interventions to increase physical activity in children 0–5 years old: A systematic review, meta-analysis and realist synthesis. *Obesity Reviews*, 1–13. doi:10.1111/obr.12763

Hnatiuk, J. A., Salmon, J., Hinkley, T., Okely, A. D., & Trost, S. (2014). A review of preschool children's physical activity and sedentary time using objective measures. *American Journal of Preventive Medicine, 47*, 487–497.

Honas, J. J., Washburn, R. A., Smith, B. K., Greene, J. L., Cook-Wiens, G., & Donnelly, J. E. (2008). The system for observing fitness instruction time (SOFIT) as a measure of energy expenditure during classroom-based physical activity. *Pediatric Exercise Science, 20*, 439–445.

Hovell, M. F., Wahlgren, D. R., & Adams, M. A. (2009). The logical and empirical basis for the behavioral ecological model. In R. J. DiClemente, R. A. Crosby, & M. C. Kegler (Eds.), *Emerging theories in health promotion practice and research* (2nd ed., pp. 347–385). San Francisco, CA: Jossey-Bass.

Huberty, J. L., Beets, M. W., Beighle, A., & McKenzie, T. L. (2013). Association of staff behaviors and after-school program features to physical activity: Findings from Movin' afterschool. *Journal of Physical Activity and Health, 10*, 423–429.

Kahan, D., & McKenzie, T. L. (2015). The potential and reality of physical education in controlling overweight and obesity. *American Journal of Public Health, 105*, 653–659.

Kahan, D., & McKenzie, T. L. (2017). Energy expenditure estimates during school physical education: Potential vs. reality? *Preventive Medicine, 95*, 82–88.

Kanters, M. A., Bocarro, J. N., Filardo, M., Edwards, M. B., McKenzie, T. L., & Floyd, M. F. (2014). Shared use of school facilities with community organizations and afterschool physical activity program participation: A cost-benefit assessment. *Journal of School Health, 84*(5), 302–309.

Kanters, M. A., McKenzie, T. L., Edwards, M., Bocarro, J., Mahar, M., & Hodge, C. (2014). *Youth sport practice model gets more kids active with more time practicing skills* (Research brief). Retrieved from http://activelivingresearch.org/

Katzmarzyk, P. T., Denstel, K. D., Beals, K., Carlson, J., Crouter, S. E., McKenzie, T. L., . . . Wright. C. (2018). Results from the United States' 2014 report card on physical activity for children and youth. *Journal of Physical Activity and Health, 15*(Suppl 2), S422–S424.

Kim, S. Y., & van der Mars, H. (2014). Accuracy of various interval lengths for measuring physical activity levels of children with intellectual disabilities using SOFIT. *The ICHPER-SD Asia Journal of Research, 6*, 65–69.

Klesges, R. C., Coates, T. J., Moldenhauer-Klesges, L. M., Holzer, B., Gustavson, J., & Barnes, B. (1984). The FATS: An observational system for assessing physical activity in children and associated parent behavior. *Behavioral Assessment, 6*, 333–345.

Koo, T. K., & Li, M. Y. (2016). A guideline of selecting and reporting intraclass correlation coefficients for reliability research. *Journal of Chiropractic Medicine, 15*, 155–163.

Leek, D., Carlson, J. A., Cain, K. L., Henrichon, S., Rosenberg, D., Patrick, K., & Sallis, J. F. (2011). Physical activity during youth sports practices. *Archives of Pediatrics and Adolescent Medicine, 165*, 294–299.

Levin, S., McKenzie, T. L., Hussey, J. R., Kelder, S., & Lytle, L. (2001). Variability of physical activity in physical education lessons across elementary school grades. *Measurement in Physical Education and Exercise Science, 5*, 207–218.

Locke, L. F. (1977). Research on teaching physical education: New hope for a dismal science. *Quest, 28*, 2–16.

Mahar, M. T. (2011). Impact of short bouts of physical activity on attention-to-task in elementary school children. *Preventive Medicine, 52*, S60–S64. doi:10.1016/j.ypmed.2011.01.026

Mahar, M. T., Murphy, S. K., Rowe, D. A., Golden, J., Shields, A. T., & Raedeke, T. D. (2006). Effects of a classroom-based program on physical activity and on-task behavior. *Medicine & Science in Sports & Exercise, 38*, 2086–2094. doi:10.1249/01.mss.0000235359.16685.a3

Mahar, M. T., Vuchenich, M. L., Golden, J., DuBose, K. D., & Raedeke, T. D. (2011). Effects of a before-school physical activity program on physical activity and on-task behavior [Abstract]. *Medicine & Science in Sports & Exercise, 43*(Suppl 1–5), 24. doi:10.1249/01.MSS.0000402740.12322.07

Makel, M. C., & Plucker, J. A. (2014). Facts are more important than novelty: Replication in the education sciences. *Educational Researcher, 43*, 304–316. doi:10.3102/0013189X14545513

McHugh, M. L. (2012). Interrater reliability: The kappa statistic. *Biochemia Medica, 22*, 276–282.

McKenzie, T. L. (1991). Observational measures of children's physical activity. *Journal of School Health, 61*, 224–227.

McKenzie, T. L. (2001). Promoting physical activity in youth: Focus on middle school environments. *Quest, 53*, 326–334.

McKenzie, T. L. (2002). Use of direct observation to assess physical activity. In G. J. Welk (Ed.), *Physical activity assessments for health-related research* (pp. 179–195), Champaign, IL: Human Kinetics.

McKenzie, T. L. (2016). Context matters: Systematic observation of place-based physical activity. *Research Quarterly for Exercise and Sport, 87*, 334–341.

McKenzie, T. L., Baquero, B., Crespo, N., Arredondo, E., Campbell, N., & Elder, J. P. (2008). Environmental correlates of physical activity in Mexican-American children at home. *Journal of Physical Activity and Health, 5*, 579–591.

McKenzie, T. L., Catellier, D. J., Conway, T., Lytle, L. A., Grieser, M., Webber, L. A., . . . Elder, J. P. (2006). Girls' activity levels and lesson contexts in middle school PE: TAAG baseline. *Medicine & Science in Sports and Exercise, 38*, 1229–1235.

McKenzie, T. L., Cohen, D. A., Sehgal, A., Williamson, S., & Golinelli, D. (2006). System for observing play and leisure activity in communities (SOPARC): Reliability and feasibility measures. *Journal of Physical Activity and Health, 1*, S203–S217.

McKenzie, T. L., Marshall, S. J., Sallis, J. F., & Conway, T. L. (2000). Leisure-time physical activity in school environments: An observational study using SOPLAY. *Preventive Medicine, 30*, 70–77.

McKenzie, T. L., & Rushall, B. S. (1974). Effects of self-recording on attendance and performance in a competitive swimming environment. *Journal of Applied Behavior Analysis, 7*, 199–206.

McKenzie, T. L., Sallis, J. F., & Armstrong, C. A. (1994). Association between direct observation and accelerometer measures of children's physical activity during physical education and recess. *Medicine & Science in Sports & Exercise, 26*, S143.

McKenzie, T. L., Sallis, J. F., Kolody, B., & Faucette, F. N. (1997). Long-term effects of a physical education curriculum and staff development program: SPARK. *Research Quarterly for Exercise and Sport, 68*, 280–291.

McKenzie, T. L., Sallis, J. F., & Nader, P. R. (1991). SOFIT: System for observing fitness instruction time. *Journal of Teaching in Physical Education, 11*, 195–205.

McKenzie, T. L., Sallis, J. F., Nader, P. R., Patterson, T. L., Elder, J. P., Berry, C. C., . . . Nelson, J. A. (1991). BEACHES: An observational system for assessing children's eating and physical activity behaviors and associated events. *Journal of Applied Behavior Analysis, 24*, 141–151.

McKenzie, T. L., Sallis, J. F., Prochaska, J. J., Conway, T. L., Marshall, S. J., & Rosengard, P. (2004). Evaluation of a two-year middle-school physical education intervention: M-SPAN. *Medicine & Science in Sport and Exercise, 36*, 1382–1388.

McKenzie, T. L., & Smith, N. J. (2017). Studies of physical education in the United States using SOFIT: A review. *Research Quarterly for Exercise and Sport, 88*, 492–502. doi:10.1080/02701367.2017.1376028

McKenzie, T. L., & van der Mars, H. (2015). Top 10 research questions related to assessing physical activity and its contexts using systematic observation. *Research Quarterly for Exercise and Sport, 86*, 13–29. doi:10. 1080/02701367.2015.991264

McNamee, J., & van der Mars, H. (2005). Accuracy of momentary time sampling: A comparison of varying interval lengths using SOFIT. *Journal of Teaching in Physical Education, 24*, 282–292.

Montoye, H. J., Kemper, H., Saris, W., & Washburn, R. A. (1996). *Measuring physical activity and energy expenditure.* Champaign, IL: Human Kinetics.

Murad, H. H., & Montori, V. M. (2013). Synthesizing evidence: Shifting the focus from individual studies to the body of evidence. *Journal of the American Medical Association, 309*, 2217–2218. doi:10.1001/jama.2013.5616

National Academies of Sciences, Engineering, and Medicine. (2019). *Implementing strategies to enhance public health surveillance of physical activity in the United States.* Washington, DC: The National Academies Press. doi:10.17226/25444

National Physical Activity Plan Alliance (NPAPA). (2016). *National physical activity plan.* Retrieved from https://physicalactivityplan.org/docs/2016NPAP_Finalforwebsite.pdf

National Physical Activity Plan Alliance (NPAPA). (2018). *The 2018 United States report card on physical activity for children and youth.* Washington, DC: National Physical Activity Plan Alliance. Retrieved from https://www.physicalactivityplan.org/projects/reportcard.html

Pope, R. P., Coleman, K. J., Gonzalez, E. C., Barron, F., & Heath, E. M. (2002). Validity of a revised system of observing fitness instruction time (SOFIT). *Pediatric Exercise Science, 14*, 135–146.

Richard, L., Gauvin, L., & Rainie, K. (2011). Ecological models revisited: Their uses and evolution in health promotion over two decades. *Annual Review of Public Health, 32*, 307–326. doi:10.1146/annurev-publhealth-031210-101141

Ridgers, N. D., Stratton, G., & McKenzie, T. L. (2010). Reliability and validity of the system for observing children's activity and relationships during play (SOCARP). *Journal of Physical Activity and Health, 7*, 17–25.

Rimmer, J. H., & Marques, A. C. (2012). Physical activity for people with disabilities. *The Lancet, 380*, 193–195. doi:10.1016/S0140-6736(12)61028-9

Rimmer, J. H., Schiller, W., & Chen, M. D. (2012). Effects of disability-associated low energy expenditure deconditioning syndrome. *Exercise Sport Sciences Reviews, 40*, 22–29.

Robinson, L. E., Wadsworth, D. D., Webster, E. K., & Bassett, D. R., Jr. (2014). School reform: The role of physical education policy in physical activity of elementary school children in Alabama's black belt region. *American Journal of Health Promotion, 28*(3 suppl), S72–S76.

Rowe, P. J., Schuldheisz, J. M., & van der Mars, H. (1997). Measuring physical activity in physical education: Validation of the SOFIT direct observation instrument for use with first to eighth grade students. *Pediatric Exercise Science, 9*, 136–149.

Rowe, P., van der Mars, H., Schuldheisz, J. M., & Fox, S. (2004). Measuring physical activity in physical education: Validating SOFIT for use with high school students. *Journal of Teaching in Physical Education, 23*, 235–251.

Sacheck, J. M., Nelson, T. F., Ficker, L., Kafka, T., Kuder, J., & Economos, C. D. (2011). Physical activity during soccer and its contribution to physical activity recommendations in normal weight and overweight children. *Pediatric Exercise Science, 23*, 281–292.

Sallis, J. F. (2009). Measuring physical activity environments: A brief history. *American Journal of Preventive Medicine, 36*, S86–S92.

Sallis, J. F., Floyd, M. F., Rodriguez, D. A., & Saelens, B. E. (2012). Role of built environments in physical activity, obesity, and cardiovascular disease. *Circulation, 125*, 729–737. doi:10.1161/CIRCULATIONAHA.110.969022

Sallis, J. F., McKenzie, T. L., Alcaraz, J. E., Kolody, B., Faucette, N., & Hovell, M. F. (1997). The effects of a 2-year physical education program (SPARK) on physical activity and fitness in elementary school students. Sports, play and active recreation for kids. *American Journal of Public Health, 87*, 1328–1334.

Sallis, J. F., Owen, N., & Fisher, E. B. (2008). Ecological models of health behavior. In K. Glanz, B. K. Rimer, & K. Viswanath (Eds.), *Health behavior and health education: Theory, research, and practice* (4th ed., pp. 465–486). San Francisco, CA: Jossey-Bass.

Scruggs, P. W. (2013). Pedometer steps/min in physical education: Does the pedometer matter? *Journal of Science and Medicine in Sport, 16*, 36–39.

Scruggs, P. W., Mungen, J. D., & Oh, Y. (2010). Physical activity measurement device agreement: Pedometer steps/minute and physical activity time. *Measurement in Physical Education and Exercise Science, 14*, 151–163.

SHAPE America. (2015). *The essential components of physical education.* Reston, VA: SHAPE America.

Sidman, M. (1988). *Tactics of scientific research* (2nd ed.). Cambridge, MA: Cambridge Center for Behavioral Studies.

Sirard, J. R., & Pate, R. R. (2001). Physical activity assessment in children and adolescents. *Sports Medicine, 31*, 439–454.

Sit, C. H. P., Capio, C. M., Cerin, E., & McKenzie, T. L. (2013). Assessment of measures of physical activity of children with cerebral palsy at home and school: A pilot study. *Journal of Child and Adolescent Behavior, 1*, 112. doi:10.41172/jcalb.100112. Retrieved from http://esciencecentral.org/journals/assessment-of-measures-of-physical-activity-of-children-with-cerebral-palsy-at-home-and-school-a-pilot-study-2375-4494.1000112.pdf

Skinner, B. F. (1953). *Science and human behavior.* New York, NY: Free Press.

Smith, N. J., McKenzie, T. L., & Hammons, A. J. (2019). International studies of physical education using SOFIT: A review. *Advances in Physical Education, 9*, 53–74. doi:10.4236/ape.2019.91005

Strath, S. J., Kaminsky, L. A., Ainsworth, B. E., Ekelund, U., Freedson P. S., Gary, R. A., . . . Swartz, A. M. (2013). Guide to assessment of physical activity: Clinical and research applications: A scientific statement from the American Heart Association. *Circulation, 128*, 2259–2279.

Stylianou, M., Hodges-Kulinna, P., van der Mars, H., Mahar, M. T., Adams, M. A., & Amazeen, E. (2016). Before-school running/walking club: Effects on student on-task behavior. *Preventive Medicine Reports, 3*, 196–202. doi:10.1016/j.pmedr.2016.01.010

Trost, S. G., Ward, D. S., & Senso, M. (2010). Effects of child care policy and environment on physical activity. *Medicine and Science in Sports and Exercise, 42*, 520–525.

U.S. Department of Health and Human Services (USDHHS). (2018). *Physical activity guidelines for Americans* (2nd ed.). Washington, DC: U.S. Department of Health and Human Services.

van der Mars, H. (1989a). Systematic observation: An introduction. In P. W. Darst, D. Zakrajsek, & V. H. Mancini (Eds.), *Analyzing physical education and sport instruction* (2nd ed., pp. 3–18). Champaign, IL: Human Kinetics.

van der Mars, H. (1989b). Observer reliability: Issues and procedures. In P. W. Darst, D. Zakrajsek & V. H. Mancini (Eds.), *Analyzing physical education and sport instruction* (2nd ed., pp. 54–80). Champaign, IL: Kinetics.

van der Mars, H., McNamee, J., & Timken, G. (2018). Physical education meets teacher evaluation: Supporting secondary school physical educators in formal assessment of student outcomes. *The Physical Educator, 75*, 581–615. doi:10.18666/TPE-2018-V75-I4-8471

Ward, D. S. (2011). *School policies on physical education and physical activity – Research synthesis.* San Diego, CA: Active Living Research. Retrieved from https://www.activelivingresearch.org

15

PEDOMETERS FOR MEASURING PHYSICAL ACTIVITY IN CHILDREN AND ADOLESCENTS

Joseph J. Scott

Introduction

Pedometers are commonly used for measuring physical activity in child and adolescent populations because they are relatively robust, easy to use, require no initialization prior to use (or downloading after), and provide an easily interpretable measure in a standard metric (most commonly steps/day) (Beets, Bornstein, Beighle, Cardinal, & Morgan, 2010). Steps represent a fundamental unit of human activity (Bassett, Toth, LaMunion, & Crouter, 2017) and there is a consensus that measurement of cumulative steps over the course of a 24-hour period is an appropriate indicator of habitual physical activity (Craig, Tudor-Locke, Cragg, & Cameron, 2010; Trost, 2007; Tudor-Locke, McClain, Hart, Sisson, & Washington, 2009a). For these reasons, pedometers are commonly used for physical activity surveillance, screening, and intervention evaluation (Lubans et al., 2015; Trost, 2007).

Over the last 20 years, objective monitoring technology has rapidly advanced, leading to an abundance of activity monitors (such as accelerometers and heart rate monitors). However, as pedometers were designed to detect only vertical movements, they are logically the most sensitive to ambulatory activity (e.g. walking and running). Due to the low cost of pedometers per unit, they are often a more feasible option and hence remain commonly utilized by physical activity researchers (Ferguson, Rowlands, Olds, & Maher, 2015). The major limitation of most traditional pedometers is that they do not provide intensity or any contextual information of the activity completed (Chinapaw, Mokkink, van Poppel, van Mechelen, & Terwee, 2010; Lubans, Morgan, & Tudor-Locke, 2009).

Although pedometers have commonly been used to objectively measure youth, there are no standardized protocols for using pedometers in child and adolescent populations. Hence, this chapter explores the use of pedometers as a measurement tool in youth. It will review the history and existing literature of pedometer use. In addition, the chapter addresses current challenges when measuring youth, emerging issues, and recommendations for future research and practice.

Overview of the Literature

History of Pedometers as a Measure of Physical Activity

Step counting dates back to the 15th century when Leonardo da Vinci designed a device originally used to approximate distance traveled on foot by Roman military troops. The mechanical gear-driven device was worn on the thigh, and a pendulum arm would swing back and forth to detect motion of the leg and a step would be counted (Gibbs-Smith, 1978). Other well-known inventors such as Thomas Jefferson, Robert Hooke, and Abraham-Louis Perrelet have also been credited for further developments of pedometer-like step counting devices over the coming centuries. However, it wasn't until the early 1960s when Dr Yoshiro Hatano from the Japanese company "Yamax" designed a device known as the "10,000 step meter" that awareness and interest in pedometers flourished (Stunkard, 1960).

Over the next three decades, Yamax and other large companies developed a series of pedometers and in the early 1990s, physical activity researchers started to investigate the relationship between ambulatory movement (i.e. walking) and health outcomes (Bassett & Strath, 2002). This sparked greater interest in the devices from the perspective of health promotion and later in the subsequent use of pedometers in large-scale population surveillance studies to evaluate physical activity interventions and validate other physical activity measures such as questionnaires. This prompted investigation into pedometers' step counting precision and accuracy, and in 1995, led to the technological development of spring-lever pedometers with digital display screens (Bravata et al., 2007). These pedometers provide users with direct feedback of step counts and hence allow the participants to monitor their general physical activity level for health purposes.

Since 2010, there has also been the development of commercially available pedometers some of which (depending on the device) provide instant (or delayed) digital feedback of step counts via a small screen on the monitor, a computer program, or a smartphone application (Bassett et al., 2017). In recent years the market has been flooded with commercial-grade pedometers, and the sales of the monitors have grown exponentially. However, few studies have tested the validity of these measures. Preliminary validation studies have revealed that consumer-level pedometers can accurately assess step counts, but are less precise when it comes to measuring distance traveled and energy expenditure (Ferguson et al., 2015; Kooiman et al., 2015).

Steps as a Measure of Activity

Pedometer-determined step counts represent a fundamental unit of human activity (Bassett et al., 2017). The standard pedometer output in metric unit of steps/day is easily interpreted by researchers, and importantly, for health promotion and public health purposes, by the lay-person. This is an added advantage of pedometers over some of the more complex objective monitors, as participants have the ability to interpret their level of activity and self-monitor data over an extended period of time (e.g. days, weeks, or months). This sparked interest for pedometers to be used as a tool to enhance motivation and change in behavior in both youth and adults (Bravata et al., 2007; Lubans et al., 2009).

There is a lack of consensus regarding the minimum amount of daily step required for good health. The following questions have remained: how many steps are enough to prevent ill-health? The development of the Yamax's "10,000 step meter" device previously mentioned is responsible for the widely known recommendation of 10,000 steps/day. Although the recommendation was considered a reasonable amount of activity to reduce the risk of developing lifestyle-related diseases, it was not generalizable across population groups and researchers highlighted the need to develop pedometer-defined steps/day lifestyle indices for youth (Tudor-Locke, 2003).

Types of Pedometers

Traditional pedometers counted steps via an internal mechanism that was spring-levered. These pedometers did not measure acceleration, but worked by detecting vertical motion. When there is a change in vertical motion, a horizontal arm bounces up and down inside the unit causing the electrical circuit to open and close and a step to be recorded (Bassett et al., 2017). A major limitation of spring-levered pedometers is that they do not measure intensity or provide any contextual information of the activity completed, and consequently are not suitable for all studies, especially those investigating health outcomes and physical activity dose response relationships (Chinapaw et al., 2010; Lubans et al., 2009).

More recently, piezoelectric pedometers have been developed. These pedometers have an internal mechanism, which is a suspended beam and piezoelectric crystal that measures horizontal movement past the in-built threshold when subjected to movement. The movement (or step count) is then stored into the device's internal memory and displayed on a digital screen (McClain & Tudor-Locke, 2009). The step counts can then be recorded by the individual who is wearing the pedometer or by the researcher periodically during data collection or once the data collection period has been completed (if the device has the ability to automatically reset daily and store data over a series of days). In addition to steps, piezoelectric pedometers commonly have the ability to estimate distance covered, time spent in activity, and energy expenditure.

Pedometers as a Way to Quantify Activity in Youth

Pedometers have emerged as a popular and convenient tool for measuring physical activity in youth due to their feasibility, reliability, and validity (Clemes & Biddle, 2013; McNamara, Hudson, & Taylor, 2010). Validation studies have also shown that pedometer step counts are moderately associated with doubly labeled water, heart rate, and $VO_{2\,peak}$, and strongly associated with accelerometer output in youth (Beets et al., 2011; Eston, Rowlands, & Ingledew, 1998; Tudor-Locke, Williams, Reis, & Pluto, 2002). While pedometers can be worn on various parts of the body (upper arm, wrist, thigh, ankle), they are most commonly worn on the hip (Rowlands & Eston, 2007). Pedometers are relatively non-invasive, robust, easy to use, and hence are still commonly used to quantify activity in youth (Beets et al., 2010).

Step Count Recommendations and Physical Activity Guidelines for Youth

As mentioned earlier, there has been continued interest in identifying minimum daily step counts for health benefits across population subgroups, including youth. Over the past two decades, there has been inconsistency in step count recommendations for youth internationally for both boys and girls. Studies have provided daily step counts guidelines for youth ranging from 9,000 to 16,500 steps/day (Beets, Le Masurier, Beighle, & Rowe, 2008; Frank et al., 2017; Tudor-Locke & Bassett, 2004; Tudor-Locke et al., 2004). Due to the great variability, in 2010 the Public Health Agency of Canada commissioned a large-scale narrative literature review which collated normative data of objectively monitored step/defined activity to provide evidence-based guidelines for special populations including elderly, adults, children, and adolescents. The review highlighted that there were no definitive cut-points for minimum step counts for youth and concluded the more activity completed the better in relation to health outcomes. The researchers reported the expected values for children to be in the range from 12,000 to 16,000 steps/day for boys, and from 10,000 to 13,000 steps/day for girls. For adolescents, the authors reported expected values to be in the range from 10,000 to 11,700 steps/day and noted that there was a steady decline in steps/day for adolescents with 8,000–9,000 steps/day typically observed in 18 year olds (Tudor-Locke, Craig, Beets et al., 2011).

In recent years, there has been growing interest in intensity of physical activity and the relationship with health outcomes. This has led to international physical activity guidelines being based on intensity (most commonly, moderate-to-vigorous physical activity (MVPA)), rather than minimum step count cut-points. The World Health Organization's physical activity recommendations for young people state that youth aged 5–17 years should accumulate at least 60 minutes of MVPA daily, with most activity being aerobic. Vigorous-intensity activities should be incorporated, including those that strengthen muscle and bone, at least three times per week (World Health Organization, 2016).

Although the minimum recommendation of 60 minutes of MVPA daily for youth is reasonably consistent internationally, there remains variability in the type of activity recommended and amount of time spend in "vigorous" activity. It is important to note that the guidelines most commonly provide the time spent in activity rather than an easily interpretable step count recommendation. As the lay-person may not have the knowledge to distinguish intensity levels, these guidelines potentially remain unclear for the general population. To provide easily interpreted metric pedometer guidelines, researchers have attempted to translate 60 minutes of MVPA into steps/day and have identified 10,000–12,000 steps/day as a reasonable target for youth to meet the international physical activity guidelines (Colley, Janssen, & Tremblay, 2012; Tudor-Locke, Craig, Beets et al., 2011).

Use of Pedometers in Youth Physical Activity Research

Pedometers are relatively unobtrusive; hence they provide a practical and simple way to collect large amounts of physical activity data of young participants in free-living environments (Hamilton, Clemes, & Griffiths, 2008). Pedometers provide objective output which is comparable across studies, cohorts, and population groups. Moreover, the highly reproducible nature of the output has led to pedometers being commonly used for cross-sectional and longitudinal physical activity population studies (Stearns et al., 2016). Pedometers have also been commonly used to evaluate youth physical activity interventions by measuring change in behavior (Tudor-Locke et al., 2009a).

There is growing research to support that pedometers can be used to promote physical activity and improve health in children, adolescents, and adults (Bravata et al., 2007; Lubans et al., 2015). The basic principle is that participants are able to get instant feedback on their activity level throughout the day and through increased awareness are encouraged to self-monitor their activity pattern and make behavioral decisions to modify activity. This has led to increased interest in evaluating the association between the use of pedometers and participants' physical activity levels. A systematic review of 14 studies that used pedometers to promote physical activity in youth observed an increase in physical activity in 12 of the studies. In addition, the review identified three main pedometer-based interventions for promoting activity in youth: (i) self-monitoring and goal setting, (ii) open loop feedback, and (iii) integration into school programs. Based on their review of studies, the authors also noted that many of the interventions were not underpinned by a health behavior theory (e.g. social cognitive theory, self-determination theory), and second that there is no existing optimal guidelines for physical activity intervention for youth (Lubans et al., 2009).

Strengths and Limitations of Pedometers

Pedometers are robust and provide a valid, reliable, and cost-effective way to collect physical activity in free-living youth (Beets et al., 2010; Corder, Ekelund, Steele, Wareham, & Brage, 2008). Some pedometers, such as the Yamax Digi-Walker CW700 (Yamax Corporation, Kumamoto City, Japan), possess the ability to store data over a 7-day period and therefore do not require daily resets. This is an important advantage as participants are not required to self-report/log their step counts, which reduces reporting bias and risk of accidental resets (Bassett et al., 2017). Pedometers also provide a universally understood metric step count which is easily interpreted by youth (Hamilton et al., 2008). A further strength of pedometers is that they provide direct real-time feedback to the participants throughout the day on activity level and hence have the potential to motivate the participants to be more active (Mansi, Milosavljevic, Baxter, Tumilty, & Hendrick, 2014).

Despite the strengths of pedometers, there are some limitations that should be noted. It has been reported that: (i) wearing them can be considered invasive (Clemes & Biddle, 2013), (ii) they are insensitive to non-ambulatory movements and are normally not waterproof; hence they have to be removed for water activities (Miller, Brown, & Tudor-Locke, 2006), (iii) they are prone to data loss due to accidental resets, (iv) they are subject to potential reactivity participant tampering (i.e. shaking) (Scott, Hansen, Morgan, Plotnikoff, & Lubans, 2018; Scott, Morgan, Plotnikoff, Trost, & Lubans, 2014), (v) they do not provide intensity or any contextual information of the activity completed (Chinapaw et al., 2010; Lubans et al., 2009), and (vi) they normally require either the participant, teacher, or parent to log the daily step counts (Tudor-Locke et al., 2009a).

Key Issues

Despite their widespread use, there are no standardized protocols for the use of pedometers in adolescent populations (Clemes & Biddle, 2013; Lubans et al., 2015). There is need for the identification of optimal protocols to address the complex technical and behavioral challenges that exist when measuring youth with pedometers (Rowlands & Eston, 2007; Scott et al., 2014).

Low Adherence in Youth

Youth physical activity measurement has remained problematic due to low adherence levels in monitoring protocols (Kahan & Nicaise, 2011; McNamara et al., 2010; Troiano et al., 2008). Low adherence leads to large amounts of missing data during the monitoring period, making it difficult to obtain accurate estimates of habitual activity patterns (Sirard & Slater, 2009). To maximize sample sizes, researchers have attempted to identify the minimum number of days required to gain a valid estimate of habitual physical activity (Tudor-Locke, Craig, Beets et al., 2011). Studies with children (R= 0.87, CI= 0.84–0.89) and adolescents (R= 0.77, CI =0.72–0.82) have found that 7 days are needed to provide a reliable estimate of usual physical activity (Trost, Pate, Freedom, Sallis, & Taylor, 2000).

Further research has recommended the inclusion of at least one weekend day to allow for day-to-day variability (Rowlands, 2007), and that the minimum required amount of monitoring days and reliability estimates may differ depending on age and sex of participants (Fairclough, Butcher, & Stratton, 2007). To maximize sample size in youth, a protocol of 7 days of monitoring with a minimum of 4 valid days including 1 weekend day has been recommended (Lubans et al., 2015). While these recommendations have been made, there is general consensus that to identify a standardized recommendation for youth, further research with large data sets containing multiple days of pedometer monitoring and a range of different age groups is warranted (Craig et al., 2010).

Treatment of Missing Data

Procedures for managing missing pedometer data in youth have also remained problematic and research in this area is limited (McNamara et al., 2010). There is research to suggest that participants should be excluded from the analysis if the monitoring frame includes incomplete days and/or extended periods of non-wear time (Schmidt, Blizzard, Venn, Cochrane, & Dwyer, 2007). Conversely, other researchers have recommended replacing the missing day or incomplete day with the individual's mean daily step count and have shown this to be more accurate than applying the group mean (Kang, Zhu, Tudor-Locke, & Ainsworth, 2003). It has also been deemed appropriate to exclude extreme values and treat them as missing data. Rowe and colleagues proposed that to be considered a valid estimate of activity pattern, daily step counts must fall between 1,000 and 30,000/day; they suggested that values <1,000 and >30,000 are implausible and should be excluded (Rowe, Mahar, Raedeke, & Lore, 2004). Pedometer studies in youth show large variation in the way that missing values are addressed, treated, transformed, and analyzed (Tudor-Locke et al., 2009a).

Non-ambulatory activities such as cycling and swimming are not accurately recorded by pedometers, as there is little vertical movement at the hip (Miller et al., 2006). The relative contribution of non-ambulatory movement to daily activity remains largely underreported in the literature (McNamara et al., 2010). One solution is for participants to self-report their time spent in non-ambulatory activity. However, this can lead to further inaccuracies of activity estimates due to reporting bias and/or step conversion methods (Scott, Morgan, Plotnikoff, & Lubans, 2015). There remains no common approach to converting time spent in activity (commonly MVPA) to step counts with preliminary research requiring complex mathematical calculations (Miller et al., 2006). Further research is required to provide standardized protocols for the treatment of non-ambulatory data, conversion, and data imputation methods in youth.

Pedometer Placement

As pedometers were designed to detect vertical motion, they have commonly been worn at the hip. However, researchers have reported that pedometer tilt due to torso body fat may also diminish the accuracy of pedometers (Bassett et al., 2017; Mitre, Lanningham-Foster, Foster, & Levine, 2009). In an attempt to increase adherence in youth, researchers have trialed the effectiveness of different pedometer placement positions including the ankle, thigh, upper arm, chest, and back (Ehrler, Weber, & Lovis, 2016; Lubans et al., 2009). However, comparative studies on placement sites indicate that the accuracy is dependent on not only the angle (or tilt) of the pedometer but also the speed the participant is moving (Oliver, Schofield, Kolt, & Schluter, 2007; Park, Lee, Ku, & Tanaka, 2014). Wearing the pedometer on the wrist has also been trialed. Studies have shown there are less missing data when objective monitors are worn on the wrist when compared to the hip, with adolescent participants reporting a preference for the wrist as a placement site indicating it is less invasive to wear (Scott et al., 2017; Troiano et al., 2008).

Reactivity and Tampering

Reactivity is defined as a change in normal activity pattern when participants are aware that they are being monitored (Vincent & Pangrazi, 2002). Reactivity to pedometer monitoring is a potential threat to the validity of physical activity measurement in youth (Scott et al., 2014) Although many studies have explored participant reactivity to wearing pedometers, the findings have been mixed (Behrens, Dinger, Vesely, & Fields, 2007; Clemes, Matchett, & Wane, 2007; Matevey, Rogers, Dawson, & Tudor-Locke, 2006; Oliver et al., 2007; Ozdoba, Corbin, & Masurier, 2004; Vincent & Pangrazi, 2002; Wang & Quek, 2005). It has been suggested that if reactivity exists, it is expected that participants will exhibit an increase in activity at the start of the monitoring period and then return to a more stable pattern once they become accustomed to wearing the devices (Behrens et al., 2007). With some research showing support for reactivity in youth (Scott et al., 2014, 2018), a range of strategies have been used to limit reactivity in different populations. A common method used in youth has been sealing the pedometer using "zip ties" or "stickers" so that the participant cannot see their step count, thus eliminating the feedback effect (Matevey et al., 2006; Scott et al., 2014).

Researchers have investigated the impact of sealing pedometer on reactivity in children and concluded that, if the pedometers are sealed (thus ruling out feedback), reactivity does not occur (Clemes et al., 2007; Clemes & Parker, 2009; Oliver et al., 2007; Vincent & Pangrazi, 2002). In addition, the sealing of pedometers greatly reduces the risk of accidental reset which is a common problem in pedometer studies. Of note, a recent study with a sample of 123 adolescents found that participants that were asked to wear unsealed pedometers showed evidence of reactivity, whereas those who wore sealed pedometers did not (Scott et al., 2014). These findings suggest that the pedometer protocol utilized may influence participant behavior.

Device tampering is an additional threat to the accuracy of physical activity assessment using pedometers. Tampering involves the participant purposely attempting to inflate their step counts by manually shaking the device and/or putting the device on someone or something else (e.g. pets, cars, or machines) (Kahan & Nicaise, 2011; Scott et al., 2018). One pedometer study conducted with children found that participants tampered with their pedometers regardless of safe-guards such as seals (Inchley, Cuthbert, & Grimes, 2007). A further study examining adolescents adherence to a pedometer protocol found that 30 of the 43 participants self-reported that they tampered with their pedometers during the monitoring phase (Kahan & Nicaise, 2011). A recent qualitative study (n = 24) in youth using focus groups found that 87.5% of participants reported shaking their pedometers to increase their step counts (Scott et al., 2018). As reactivity and tampering are a potential threat to validity, researchers should implement strategies to minimize problematic behaviors in child and adolescent populations.

Participant Perceptions of the Pedometer Monitoring Process

Few studies have investigated why adherence to objective monitoring is so poor in adolescent populations (Kahan & Nicaise, 2011). Qualitative research using focus groups to explore young people's perceptions of objective monitoring has noted the following concerns: size of device and lack of comfort, unwanted attention and increased risk of being bullied, and feelings of embarrassment (Kirby et al., 2012; Scott et al., 2018). This differed from adults, who reported adult-specific issues such as occupational factors, for example discomfort when driving, work uniform/duties (Kirby et al., 2012; Perry et al., 2010). One study conducted with young people found that girls were more concerned about the look of the device than boys (Audrey, Bell, Hughes, & Campbell, 2012). A further study that investigated participants' perceptions of the pedometer monitoring process found that adolescents felt a perceived need to increase their step counts when being monitored; that they felt self-competition was a motivating factor; and that peer and social factors may also increase reactivity (Scott et al., 2018). Although there is limited existing qualitative research investigating young people's perceptions of pedometer monitoring, these findings provide valuable information for researchers attempting to measure physical activity in youth.

Emerging Issues

Pedometer Measurement Error

There is now a wide array of existing pedometers that vary in type, function, and accuracy making it difficult for researchers to select the most suitable instrument for their studies (McClain & Tudor-Locke, 2009). Studies that have investigated interchangeability of ten pedometer brands across five walking speeds found that there was good accuracy across brands; however, as speed increased to >3.2 km/hour (or 2 mph) the degree of error also increased (Beets, Patton, & Edwards, 2005; Schneider, Crouter, Lukajic, & Bassett, 2003). At even slower speeds of 1.6 km/hour (or 1 mph) most pedometers will only count 50%–75% of the steps taken (Bassett et al., 2017). To address this measurement error, some research-grade pedometers (such as the StepWatch) have customizable settings of cadence speed to improve sensitivity and accuracy of step counting; however these pedometers remain expensive and as a result underutilized. Although traditional spring-levered pedometers are more feasible, they are susceptible to double counting steps during movements. In an attempt to address this, some manufacturers (e.g. Yamax) have included a refractory period where a step will not be recorded if it too close to the previous step; however this is only sensitive to ambulatory movements (Bassett et al., 2017).

Although young people report a preference for wrist-worn devices (Scott et al., 2017; Troiano et al., 2008), hand movements throughout the day such as general house and desk/computer work, brushing teeth, and hand gestures can attribute to inaccurate step counting (Bassett et al., 2017). Behavioral measures such as wearing the device on the non-dominant hand have been recommended to limit inaccurate counts. However, to eliminate this error, enhanced movement detection via pattern recognition and inbuilt thresholds are required to improve the sensitivity for these false-positive step counts. With studies showing that on occasion pedometers can erroneously detect movement and under- or overestimate step counts (Crouter, Schneider, Karabalut, & Basset, 2003; Schneider et al., 2003), careful selection of pedometer is required so that parameters can be administered to limit measurement error.

Additional Pedometer Measures

Steps/day are the most commonly used pedometer output; however, newly developed piezo-electric pedometers have the ability to capture distance traveled, time spent in activity, calories burnt, and cadence (or stride rate). Previous research has shown inconsistencies with distance traveled, as the estimates are dependent on participants' stride length and frequency (Crouter et al., 2003; Schneider et al., 2003). As a result, some researchers have recommended that pedometer output should be expressed as steps/day without further estimation of distance or energy expenditure, as the level of inconsistencies may be unacceptably high for comparative purposes (Corder et al., 2008). Conversely, in the last decade there has been public health interest in these additional measures as they provide information on intensity of activities, rather than just total volume. As physical activity guidelines are based on intensity of daily activity (i.e. for youth 60 minutes of MVPA/day), there is growing interest in translating step counts/ minute into daily physical activity recommendations so that they are more easily interpreted by the general population.

The advancement of measures such as intensity and duration allows activity to be time-stamped throughout the day. A measure of step counts/min has commonly been termed "cadence". Cadence is an important measure as it can be used to test walking speed and rate of energy expenditure and is therefore valuable for health outcome and promotion research (Bassett et al., 2017). Researchers have tested the measure of cadence under controlled conditions (treadmill speed range 1.8–12.1 km/hour) and found that cadence is strongly associated with speed ($r = 0.97$) and intensity ($r = 0.94$) (Tudor-Locke, Craig, Brown et al., 2011). There is now consensus that a metabolic equivalent of task (MET) count of ≥ 3 is equal to moderate activity for adults (World Health Organization, 2014); however there has been considerable contentions in relation to minimum cut-points of moderate activity for youth with research suggesting it is closer to 4 METs (Ridley & Olds, 2008; Tudor-Locke et al., 2018; Welk, Morrow, & Saint-Maurice, 2017). For adults, a cadence of 100 steps/minute is considered a reasonable threshold for moderate ambulatory activity (i.e. equivalent to a MET of ≥ 3) (Tudor-Locke & Rowe, 2012). A recent study (n = 120, 6–20 year olds) that investigated cadence in a range of controlled settings with minimum thresholds of ≥ 4 METs for moderate, and ≥ 6 METs for vigorous activity, provided a recommended cadence for youth of 90–125 steps/minute for moderate activity, and 126–155 steps/minute for vigorous activity (Tudor-Locke et al., 2018). Therefore, to meet the minimum recommended international physical activity guidelines youth should be involved in activity that is at a cadence of at least 90 steps/minute for at least 60 minutes/day.

Consumer Level Pedometry and Connectivity

In recent years there has been a proliferation of consumer-grade pedometers that have been marketed to the general public as "activity" or "fitness" tracker. The market has been flooded with a variety of pedometers that are far cheaper than the research-grade pedometers. However, research on their accuracy remains relatively sparse. One of the largest producers of commercial-grade activity trackers is the company "FitBit". In 2010, FitBit sold approximately 60,000 devices globally. By 2014, sales were up to 10 million/year and in 2017 alone, FitBit sold over 15 million activity trackers worldwide (Statista, 2017). The continued technological developments and consumer demand have led to an abundance of monitoring devices that vary in design, type, appearance, and accuracy.

A recent study that compared popular consumer-grade pedometers such as the FitBit charge, Omron HJ-303, the walking FIT, and Sportline found an inverse relationship between cost and accuracy indicating that the more expensive the pedometers the less accurate they were (Husted & Llewellyn, 2017). A further study that compared additional consumer-grade pedometers including the wrist-worn Fitbit Charge HR, Garmin Vivosmart HR, Apple iWatch, Jawbone UP3, and the hip-worn Yamax Digi-Walker® found that the Digi-walker was the most accurate pedometer when collecting step counts over five different speeds. The findings also indicated the FitBit, Garmin, and Jawbone became increasingly inaccurate at higher speeds (Sears et al., 2017).

Many of the available consumer-level pedometers are accompanied by internet-based computer software or smartphone application connectivity. Some applications are free and can provide easily interpretable and accessible data on daily activity via handheld technology (smartphones or tablets) or computers. Commonly, wrist-worn pedometers have a digital screen which provides real-time direct feedback to the participant throughout the day but can cause reactivity and tampering (Scott et al., 2014). If the aim of the study is to motivate youth to be active, then the feedback provided by these devices will be of benefit (Lubans et al., 2009).

Considerations for Pedometer Use

Prior to selecting pedometers as the physical activity monitoring tool for youth, researchers should first answer the following questions.

What Is the Purpose of the Study?

Is it to obtain normal activity pattern, evaluate a physical activity intervention, observe population trends, or promote physical activity? For measurement purposes, participants should not see their steps, as this may result in reactivity and/or tampering leading to inaccurate estimates of normal activity pattern. If the goal is physical activity promotion, researchers may choose to promote self-monitoring via the feedback effect and in addition set step count goals and easily accessible feedback on daily trends.

Has the Pedometer Brand and Model Been Previously Validated?

Have previous validation studies shown that this device can accurately assess step counts (and other additional measures if applicable) in youth? If so, what are the recommended pedometer protocols for this pedometer? What is the battery life of the pedometer? Does the pedometer have the ability to store data over multiple days? Will it automatically reset each day or will this require participants to reset step counts?

What Is the Appearance of the Device?

What does the device look like? Youth have reported that the appearance of the pedometer is a factor that can influence their adherence. Is it large/bulky, comfortable/uncomfortable to wear? Is it discrete or could youth potentially find it embarrassing to wear?

What Is the Desired Objective Output?

Is the goal to obtain total volume of ambulatory activity, energy expenditure, time spent in activity, or cadence? This will direct what brand/model of pedometer is chosen. Researchers should also investigate if validation studies have been completed and support that the model of pedometer can accurately assess the step counts, intensities, and cadence.

How Many Days of Monitoring Will Be Required to Provide a Reliable Estimate of Activity Pattern?

What is the recommendation for the ages of participants involved in the study? Will partial wear-time on the first and last day be included or excluded? What constitutes a valid day of wear-time?

How Will Non-Wear Time and Non-Ambulatory Activity Be Managed?

How will activity when not wearing the pedometer be estimated or will non-wear days be excluded? Will participants self-report activity when involved in water activities and non-ambulatory movements? Will the participants be required to remove the pedometers for showering/swimming/sleeping? Will participants be reminded to put the pedometers back on if they are removed (e.g. daily reminder text message)? If the pedometer is removed, will the participant be required to self-report their step counts/activity data? Will a conversion method be required to estimate steps during non-wear times? Will data replacement strategies be used? Will extreme values (e.g. <1,000–30,000) be excluded?

How Will the Feedback Effect Be Managed?

Will the participants be able to obtain feedback during the monitoring phase? How will this be managed to limit reactivity and tampering? Will pedometers be unsealed or sealed? How will the pedometers be sealed (e.g. stickers, zip-ties).

By providing answers to the earlier questions, researchers can then determine first, if pedometers are the right objective monitoring tool for the purposes of their study, and second, what type/model is best suited to the needs of the study. Carefully selected pedometer protocols are required to accurately assess youth physical activity.

Recommendations for Researchers/Practitioners

Pedometers remain a feasible way to objectively measure young people's physical activity levels. However, there are no standardized pedometer protocols for measuring physical activity in young people using pedometers. Based on the existing literature and studies completed to date, the following protocols are recommended for youth (Table 15.1).

Table 15.1 Recommendations for pedometer protocols for youth

Factor	Recommendation
Pedometer	Choice of pedometer should align with study objectives. Pedometer should have the ability to record and store data over a series of days (e.g. Lifestyles NL-2000, Yamax CW-700) (Scott et al., 2014)
Placement site	To increase adherence and reduce risk of erroneous steps, pedometers should be worn on the non-dominant wrist (Bassett et al., 2017; Craig et al., 2010; Scott et al., 2017)
Number of valid days	Greater than 5 full days of pedometer monitoring is needed to capture habitual activity in children and adolescents (Clemes & Biddle, 2013; Lubans et al., 2015)
Activity feedback effect	Pedometers should be sealed with stickers or zip-ties to limit reactivity and tampering while attempting to obtain valid estimates of normal activity (Lubans et al., 2015; Scott et al., 2014)
Treatment of extreme values	Values of <1,000 and >30,000 should be excluded and treated as missing data (Rowe et al., 2004)
Wear duration	Participants are to wear pedometers for the duration of the day only removing them if required (e.g. water or contact sports). Any activity completed while the pedometer is not being worn is self-reported via a log/diary. If there are large amounts of missing data due to non-wear time data treatment, correction and imputation may be required. If the pedometer is removed for greater than an hour on any day, then this day should be removed and treated as missing data (Delisle Nystrom, Barnes, & Tremblay, 2018; Lubans et al., 2015; Tudor-Locke, McClain, Hart, Sisson, & Washington, 2009b)
Non-ambulatory movement	For population estimates of physical activity, research indicates that non-ambulatory movements account for a small portion of daily activity; hence it is not necessary to complete estimate step counts. However, if pedometers are used to evaluate physical activity interventions, then conversion of non-ambulatory movement to step count may be necessary. Non-ambulatory movement should be self-reported as "time spent in MVPA" and converted to step counts using validated conversion methods and added to daily step count (Miller et al., 2006)
Pedometer output	If investigating total volume of activity, a measure of steps/day is recommended. If investigating activity pattern, intensity, or cadence a measure of steps/minute is recommended
Cadence cut-point for moderate and vigorous activity	MET count of >4 for moderate activity and >6 for vigorous activity is recommended for youth. While using cadence as a measure, piezoelectric pedometers are recommended (Tudor-Locke et al., 2018)

The following suggestions are made for further research.

- There is a need for the identification of step-defined lifestyle index for youth to determine minimum required step counts to prevent ill-health. In addition, an appropriate and reliable conversion method is needed to accurately convert step counts and cadence (steps/minute) to daily MVPA to determine how youth are meeting the international physical activity guidelines.
- There is a need for greater refinement of step count accuracy for research-grade pedometers, especially for wrist placement which has been recommended recently as the preferred placement site for adolescents.
- The use of standardized pedometer protocols will help to address the current behavioral and technical measurement issues surrounding the use of pedometers in youth (e.g. reactivity,

tampering, poor adherence, treatment of missing data, and measurement error). As youth have reported that comfort and appearance of the pedometer influence adherence, careful selection of device and placement site on the body should be considered.

- Further qualitative research investigating participants exhibited behaviors while wearing pedometers and their perceptions of the monitoring process will provide insights into why young participants choose to tamper with their pedometers, change their activity pattern, or do not adhere to the pedometer protocol. This information will assist researchers to design and implement improved pedometer studies in the future. By investigating factors that may enhance the level of participant reactivity, researchers can better understand the best ways to motivate youth to be active via self-monitoring and the feedback effect.

- With the emergence of an abundance of consumer-grade pedometers, there is a need for continued validation and comparative studies to determine their value of these devices for researchers and physical activity studies. Further studies investigating the accuracy of additional measures such as distance traveled, intensity of activity, and cadence are warranted.

References

Audrey, S., Bell, S., Hughes, R., & Campbell, R. (2012). Adolescent perspectives on wearing accelerometers to measure physical activity in population-based trials. *The European Journal of Public Health.* doi:10.1093/eurpub/cks081

Bassett, D. R., & Strath, S. J. (2002). Use of pedometers to assess physical activity. In: G. J. Welk (Ed.), *Physical activity assessments for health-related research* (pp. 163–177). Champaign, IL: Human Kinetics.

Bassett, D. R., Toth, L. P., LaMunion, S. R., & Crouter, S. E. (2017). Step counting: A review of measurement considerations and health-related applications. *Sports Medicine, 47*(7), 1303–1315. doi:10.1007/s40279-016-0663-1

Beets, M. W., Bornstein, D., Beighle, A., Cardinal, B. J., & Morgan, C. F. (2010). Pedometer-measured physical activity patterns of youth: A 13-country review. *American Journal of Preventative Medicine, 38*(2), 208–216. doi:10.1016/j.amepre.2009.09.045

Beets, M. W., Le Masurier, G. C., Beighle A., & Rowe, D. A. (2008). Are current body mass index referenced pedometer step count recommendations applicable to U.S. youth? *Journal of Physical activity and Health, 5*(5), 665–674.

Beets, M. W., Morgan, C. F., Banda, J. A., Bornstein, D., Byun, W., Mitchell, J., . . . Erwin, H. (2011). Convergent validity of pedometer and accelerometer estimates of moderate-to-vigorous physical activity of youth. *Journal of Physical Activity & Health, 8*(Suppl 2), 298–305.

Beets, M. W., Patton, M., & Edwards, S. (2005). The accuracy of pedometer steps and time during in children. *Medicine and Science in Sports and Exercise, 37*(3), 513–520.

Behrens, T. K., Dinger, M. K., Vesely, S. K., & Fields, D. A. (2007). Accuracy of step recording in free-living adults. *Research Quarterly for Exercise and Sport, 78*(5), 542–547. doi:10.1080/02701367.2007.10599453

Bravata, D. M., Smith-Spangler, C., Sundaram, V., Gienger, A. L., Lin, N., Lewis, R., & Sirard, J. R. (2007). Using pedometers to increase physical activity and improve health: A systematic review. *The Journal of the American Medical Association, 298*(19), 2296–3204.

Chinapaw, M. J., Mokkink, L. B., van Poppel, M. N., van Mechelen, W., & Terwee, C. B. (2010). Physical activity questionnaires for youth: A systematic review of measurement properties. *Sports Medicine, 40*(7), 539–563. doi:10.2165/11530770-000000000-00000

Clemes, S. A., & Biddle, S. J. (2013). The use of pedometers for monitoring physical activity in children and adolescents: Measurement considerations. *Journal of Physical activity and Health, 10*(2), 249–262.

Clemes, S. A., Matchett, N., & Wane, S. (2007). Reactivity: An issue for short-term pedometer studies? *British Journal of Sports Medicine, 42*(1), 68–70.

Clemes, S. A., & Parker, R. A. (2009). Increasing our understanding of reactivity to pedometers in adults. *Medicine & Science in Sports & Exercise, 41*(3), 674–680.

Colley, R. C., Janssen, I., & Tremblay, M. S. (2012). Daily step target to measure adherence to physical activity guidelines in children. *Medicine & Science in Sports & Exercise, 44*(5), 977–982. doi:10.1249/MSS.0b013e31823f23b1

Corder, K., Ekelund, U., Steele, R. M., Wareham, N. J., & Brage, S. (2008). Assessment of physical activity in youth. *Journal of Applied Physiology, 105*(3), 977–987. doi:10.1152/japplphysiol.00094.2008

Craig, C., Tudor-Locke, C., Cragg, S., & Cameron, C. (2010). Process and treatment of pedometer data collection for youth: The Canadian physical activity levels among youth study. *Medicine and Science in Sports and Exercise, 42*(3), 430–435.

Crouter, S. E., Schneider, P. L., Karabalut, M., & Basset, D. R. (2003). Validity of 10 electronic pedometers for measuring steps, distance, and energy cost. *Medicine & Science in Sports & Exercise, 35*(8), 1455–1460.

Delisle Nystrom, C., Barnes, J. D., & Tremblay, M. S. (2018). An exploratory analysis of missing data from the Royal Bank of Canada (RBC) learn to play – Canadian assessment of physical literacy (CAPL) project. *BMC Public Health, 18*(Suppl 2), 1046. doi:10.1186/s12889-018-5901-z

Ehrler, F., Weber, C., & Lovis, C. (2016). Influence of pedometer position on pedometer accuracy at various walking speeds: A comparative study. *Journal of medical Internet research, 18*(10), e268. doi:10.2196/jmir.5916

Eston, R. G., Rowlands, A. V., & Ingledew, D. K. (1998). Validity of heart rate, pedometry, and accelerometry for predicting the energy cost of children's activities. *Journal of Applied Physiology, 84*(1), 362–371.

Fairclough, S. J., Butcher, Z. H., & Stratton, G. (2007). Whole-day and segmented-day physical activity variability of northwest England school children. *Preventive Medicine, 44*(5), 421–425. doi:10.1016/j.ypmed.2007.01.002

Ferguson, T., Rowlands, A. V., Olds, T., & Maher, C. (2015). The validity of consumer-level, activity monitors in healthy adults worn in free-living conditions: A cross-sectional study. *International Journal of Behavioral Nutrition and Physical Activity, 12*(1), 42. doi:10.1186/s12966-015-0201-9

Frank, L. D., Fox, E. H., Ulmer, J. M., Chapman, J. E., Kershaw, S. E., Sallis, J. F., . . . Schipperijn, J. (2017). International comparison of observation-specific spatial buffers: Maximizing the ability to estimate physical activity. *International Journal of Health Geographics, 16*(1), 4. doi:10.1186/s12942-017-0077-9

Gibbs-Smith, C. (1978). *The inventions of Leonardo da Vinci.* Oxford, UK: Phaidon Press.

Hamilton, S. L., Clemes, S. A., & Griffiths, P. L. (2008). UK adults exhibit higher step counts in summer compared to winter months. *Annals of Human Biology, 35*(2), 154–169. doi:10.1080/03014460801908058

Husted, H. M., & Llewellyn, T. L. (2017). The accuracy of pedometers in measuring walking steps on a treadmill in college students. *International Journal of Exercise Science, 10*(1), 146–153.

Inchley, J., Cuthbert, L., & Grimes, M. (2007). *An investigation of the use of pedometers to promote physical activity, and particularly walking, among school-aged children: Review of evidence and scoping study.* Edinburgh, Scotland: Child and Adolescent Health Research Unit.

Kahan, D., & Nicaise, N. (2011). Walk as directed! Adolescent adherence to pedometer intervention protocols. *Journal of Physical Activity & Health, 9*(7), 962–969.

Kang, M., Zhu, W., Tudor-Locke, C., & Ainsworth, B. E. (2003). An experimental determination of the best missing value recovery method in assessing physical activity using pedometers. *Research Quarterly for Exercise and Sport, 74*, 1–25.

Kirby, J., Tibbins, C., Callens, C., Lang, B., Thorogood, M., Tigbe, W., & Robertson, W. (2012). Young people's views on accelerometer use in physical activity research: Findings from a user involvement investigation. *ISRN Obesity, 2012*(Article ID 948504), 1–7. doi:10.5402/2012/948504

Kooiman, T. J. M., Dontje, M. L., Sprenger, S. R., Krijnen, W. P., van der Schans, C. P., & de Groot, M. (2015). Reliability and validity of ten consumer activity trackers. *BMC Sports Science, Medicine & Rehabilitation, 7*, 24. doi:10.1186/s13102-015-0018-5

Lubans, D. R., Morgan, P. J., & Tudor-Locke, C. (2009). A systematic review of studies using pedometers to promote physical activity among youth. *Preventative Medicine, 48*(4), 307–315. doi:10.1016/j.ypmed.2009.02.014

Lubans, D. R., Plotnikoff, R. C., Miller, A., Scott, J. J., Thompson, D., & Tudor-Locke, C. (2015). Using pedometers for measuring and increasing physical activity in children and adolescents: The next step. *American Journal of Lifestyle Medicine, 9*(6), 418–427. doi:10.1177/1559827614537774

Mansi, S., Milosavljevic, S., Baxter, G. D., Tumilty, S., & Hendrick, P. (2014). A systematic review of studies using pedometers as an intervention for musculoskeletal diseases. *BMC Musculoskeletal Disorders, 15*(1), 231. doi:10.1186/1471-2474-15-231

Matevey, C., Rogers, L. Q., Dawson, E., & Tudor-Locke, C. (2006). Lack of reactivity during pedometer self-monitoring in adults. *Measurement in Physical Education and Exercise Science, 10*(1), 1–11. doi:10.1207/s15327841mpee1001_1

McClain, J. J., & Tudor-Locke, C. (2009). Objective monitoring of physical activity in children: Considerations for instrument selection. *Journal of Science and Medicine in Sport, 12*(5), 526–533. doi:10.1016/j.jsams.2008.09.012

McNamara, E., Hudson, Z., & Taylor, S. J. (2010). Measuring activity levels of young people: The validity of pedometers. *British Medical Bulletin, 95*, 121–137. doi:10.1093/bmb/ldq016

Miller, R., Brown, W., & Tudor-Locke, C. (2006). But what about swimming and cycling? How to "count" non-ambulatory activity when using pedometers to assess physical activity. *Journal of Physical Activity and Health, 3,* 257–266.

Mitre, N., Lanningham-Foster, L., Foster, R., & Levine, J. A. (2009). Pedometer accuracy for children: Can we recommend them for our obese population? *Pediatrics, 123*(1), e127–e131. doi:10.1542/peds.2008-1908

Oliver, M., Schofield, G., Kolt, G., & Schluter, P. (2007). Pedometer accuracy in physical activity assessment of preschool children. *Journal of Science and Medicine in Sport, 10*(5), 303–310.

Ozdoba, R., Corbin, C. B., & Masurier, G. L. (2004). Does reactivity exist in children when measuring activity levels with unsealed pedometers? *Pediatric Exercise Science, 16,* 158–166.

Park, W., Lee, V. J., Ku, B., & Tanaka, H. (2014). Effect of walking speed and placement position interactions in determining the accuracy of various newer pedometers. *Journal of Exercise Science & Fitness, 12*(1), 31–37. doi:10.1016/j.Jesf.2014.01.003

Perry, M. A., Hendrick, P. A., Hale, L., Baxter, G. D., Milosavljevic, S., Dean, S. G., . . . Hurley, D. A. (2010). Utility of the RT3 triaxial accelerometer in free living: An investigation of adherence and data loss. *Applied Ergonomics, 41*(3), 469–476. doi:10.1016/j.apergo.2009.10.001

Ridley, K., & Olds, T. S. (2008). Assigning energy costs to activities in children: A review and synthesis. *Medicine & Science in Sports & Exercise, 40*(8), 1439–1446. doi:10.1249/MSS.0b013e31817279ef

Rowe, D. A., Mahar, M. T., Raedeke, T. D., & Lore, J. (2004). Measuring physical activity in children with pedometers: Reliability, reactivity, and replacement of missing data. *Pediatric Exercise Science, 16*(4), 343–354.

Rowlands, A. V. (2007). Accelerometer assessment of physical activity in children: An update. *Pediatric Exercise Science, 19,* 252–266.

Rowlands, A. V., & Eston, R. (2007). The measurement and interpretation of children's physical activity. *Journal of Sports Science and Medicine, 6,* 270–276.

Schmidt, M., Blizzard, L., Venn, A., Cochrane, J., & Dwyer, T. (2007). Practical considerations when using pedometers to assess physical activity in population studies. *Research Quarterly for Exercise and Sport, 78*(3), 162–170.

Schneider, P. L., Crouter, S. E., Lukajic, O., & Bassett, D. R., Jr. (2003). Accuracy and reliability of 10 pedometers for measuring steps over a 400-m walk. *Medicine & Science in Sports & Exercise, 35*(10), 1779–1784. doi:10.1249/01.mss.0000089342.96098.c4

Scott, J. J., Hansen, V., Morgan, P. J., Plotnikoff, R. C., & Lubans, D. R. (2018). Young people's perceptions of the objective physical activity monitoring process: A qualitative exploration. *Health Education Journal, 77*(1), 3–14. doi:10.1177/0017896917734576

Scott, J. J., Morgan, P. J., Plotnikoff, R. C., & Lubans, D. R. (2015). Reliability and validity of a single-item physical activity measure for adolescents. *Journal of Paediatrics and Child Health, 51*(8), 787–793. doi:10.1111/jpc.12836

Scott, J. J., Morgan, P. J., Plotnikoff, R. C., Trost, S. G., & Lubans, D. R. (2014). Adolescent pedometer protocols: Examining reactivity, tampering and participants' perceptions. *Journal of Sports Sciences, 32*(2), 183–190. doi:10.1080/02640414.2013.815361

Scott, J. J., Rowlands, A. V., Cliff, D. P., Morgan, P. J., Plotnikoff, R. C., & Lubans, D. R. (2017). Comparability and feasibility of wrist- and hip-worn accelerometers in free-living adolescents. *Journal of Science and Medicine in Sport.* doi:10.1016/j.jsams.2017.04.017

Sears, T., Avalos, E., Lawson, S., Mcalister, I., Eschbach, C., & Bunn, J. (2017). Wrist-worn physical activity trackers tend to underestimate steps during walking. *International Journal of Exercise Science, 10*(5), 764–773.

Sirard, J. R., & Slater, M. E. (2009). Compliance with wearing physical activity accelerometers in high school students. *Journal of Physical activity and Health, 6*(Supp 1), S148–S155.

Statista. (2017). Number of Fitbit devices sold worldwide. Retrieved from www.statista.com/statistics/472591/fitbitdevices-sold/

Stearns, J. A., Rhodes, R., Ball, G. D., Boule, N., Veugelers, P. J., Cutumisu, N., & Spence, J. C. (2016). A cross-sectional study of the relationship between parents' and children's physical activity. *BMC Public Health, 16*(1), 1129. doi:10.1186/s12889-016-3793-3

Stunkard, A. (1960). A method of studying physical activity in man. *The American Journal of Clinical Nutrition, 8*(5), 595–601. doi:10.1093/ajcn/8.5.595

Troiano, R. P., Berrigan, D., Dodd, K. W., Masse, L. C., Tilert, T., & McDowell, M. (2008). Physical activity in the United States measured by accelerometer. *Medicine & Science in Sports & Exercise, 40*(1), 181–188. doi:10.1249/mss.0b013e31815a51b3

Trost, S. G. (2007). State of the art reviews: The measurement of physical activity in children and adolescents. *American Journal of Lifestyle Medicine, 1,* 299–314.

Trost, S. G., Pate, R., Freedom, P., Sallis, J., & Taylor, W. (2000). Using objective physical activity measures with youth: How many days of monitoring are needed? *Medicine and Science in Sports and Exercise, 32*(2), 426–431.

Tudor-Locke, C., & Bassett, D. R., Jr. (2004). How many steps/day are enough? Preliminary pedometer indices for public health. *Sports Medicine, 34*(1), 1–8.

Tudor-Locke, C., Craig, C. L., Beets, M. W., Belton, S., Cardon, G. M., Duncan, S., & Blair, S. N. (2011). How many steps/day are enough? For children and adolescents *International Journal of Behavioral Nutrition and Physical Activity, 8*(78). doi:10.1186/1479-5868-8-78

Tudor-Locke, C., Craig, C. L., Brown, W. J., Clemes, S. A., De Cocker, K., Giles-Corti, B., . . . Blair, S. N. (2011). How many steps/day are enough? For adults. *The International Journal of Behavioral Nutrition and Physical Activity, 8*, 79. doi:10.1186/1479-5868-8-79

Tudor-Locke, C., McClain, J. J., Hart, T. L., Sisson, S. B., & Washington, T. L. (2009a). Pedometry methods for assessing free-living youth. *Research Quarterly for Exercise and Sport, 80*(2), 175–184.

Tudor-Locke, C., McClain, J. J., Hart, T. L., Sisson, D. B., & Washington, T. L. (2009b). Expected values for pedometer-determined physical activity in youth. *Research Quarterly for Exercise and Sport, 80*(2), 164–174.

Tudor-Locke, C., Pangrazi, R. P., Corbin, C. B., Rutherford, W. J., Vincent, S. D., Raustorp, A., . . . Cuddihy, T. F. (2004). BMI-referenced standards for recommended pedometer-determined steps/day in children. *Preventive Medicine, 38*(6), 857–864.

Tudor-Locke, C., & Rowe, D. A. (2012). Using cadence to study free-living ambulatory behaviour. *Sports Medicine, 42*(5), 381–398. doi:10.2165/11599170-000000000-00000

Tudor-Locke, C., Schuna, J. M., Han, H., Aguiar, E. J., Larrivee, S., Hsia, D. S., . . . Johnson, W. D. (2018). Cadence (steps/min) and intensity during ambulation in 6–20 year olds: The CADENCE-kids study. *International Journal of Behavioral Nutrition and Physical Activity, 15*(1), 20. doi:10.1186/s12966-018-0651-y

Tudor-Locke, C., Williams, J. E., Reis, J. P., & Pluto, D. (2002). Utility of pedometers for assessing physical activity. *Sports Medicine, 32*(12), 785–808.

Vincent, S., & Pangrazi, R. (2002). Does reactivity exist in children when measuring activity levels with pedometers? *Pediatric Exercise Science, 14*(1), 56–63.

Wang, J., & Quek, J. (2005). Measures of reliability and validity of school-based pedometer step counts in Singaporean children. *Asian Journal of Exercise & Sports Science, 2*(1), 17–24.

Welk, G. J., Morrow, J. R., Jr., & Saint-Maurice, P. F. (2017). *Measures registry user guide: Individual physical activity*. Washington, DC: National Collaborative on Childhood Obesity Research. Retrieved from http://www.nccor.org/downloads/NCCOR_MR_User_Guide_Individual_PA-v7.pdf

World Health Organization. (2014). *What is moderate-intensity and vigorous-intensity physical activity? Global Strategy on Diet, Physical Activity & Health*. Retrieved from www.who.int/dietphysicalactivity/physical_activity_intensity

World Health Organization. (2016). *Global strategy on diet, physical activity and health: Physical activity and young people*. World Health Organization. Retrieved from http://www.who.int/dietphysicalactivity/factsheet_young_people/en/

16

MEASURING PHYSICAL ACTIVITY WITH BODY-WORN ACCELEROMETERS

Alex V. Rowlands

Introduction

Physical behaviors across the 24 hour day can be categorized as sleep, sedentary behavior and physical activity. Movement, or lack of movement, due to these physical behaviors can be captured using accelerometry-based activity monitors (from herein: accelerometers) worn 24 hours a day. Accelerometers are small wearable motion sensors that measure the accelerations of the body part they are attached to and provide time-stamped data, facilitating assessment of temporal patterns of physical behaviors. Initially accelerometers were predominantly worn at the hip, but since 2010 wrist-worn monitors have increasingly been used. The aim of this chapter is to provide an overview of the use of accelerometers to measure physical behaviors, specifically, the history of their use to where we are now, and challenges for the future.

From Measurement of Waking Physical Activity to Measurement of 24 Hour Physical Behaviors

Historically, studies have focused on the importance of physical activity, particularly moderate-to-vigorous physical activity (MVPA), for children's health (Janssen & LeBlanc, 2010). Because of this, studies using accelerometers to measure physical activity usually only required them to be worn during waking hours (e.g. Troiano et al., 2008). More recently, studies have highlighted that low time spent in sedentary behaviors and sufficient sleep are also positively associated with children's health (Cappuccio et al., 2008; Tremblay et al., 2011). Further, as the duration of the day is finite, the time spent on any one of the three physical behaviors is co-dependent on the other behaviors (Chastin, Palarea-Albaladejo, Dontje, & Skelton, 2015), meaning changes in any one behavior will impact on at least one other. Consequently, there has been a shift to a focus on quantifying all physical behaviors across the entire 24 hour period rather than physical activity alone.

Concurrently, advancing technology has led to accelerometers that continuously sample and store data at very high resolution (up to 100 times per second [100 Hz]) becoming widely available. These accelerometers are waterproof and designed primarily for continuous wrist-wear enabling measurement of the full 24 hour profile of children's physical behaviors in large-scale studies (e.g. da Silva et al., 2014; Li, Kearney, Keane, Harrington, & Fitzgerald, 2017; Wake et al., 2014).

Overview of the Literature

A Brief History of the Use of Accelerometers for Measurement of Physical Activity

Probably the most widely used accelerometer in the physical activity research literature to date is the ActiGraph (ActiGraph LLC, Pensacola, FL, United States). The first model was the uniaxial (vertical axis, or up and down) 7164 in the early 1990s. This was followed in 1999 by the 71256 model, which had a greater memory capacity; in 2005, the memory was increased further in the GT1M model, and a second axis of measurement was incorporated (antero-posterior, or front-to-back), although this was not 'unlocked' until 2008. In 2009 the GT3X, the first triaxial ActiGraph model, was released, and in late 2010 the GT3X+, which had sufficient memory capacity to enable storage of multiple days of high-resolution raw acceleration data instead of pre-processed Acti-Graph proprietary counts. In 2014, the GT9X Link was released which also contains additional features (gyroscope, magnetometer and secondary accelerometer) that can be activated to give advanced information about movement, rotation and body position over short time periods (less than 1 day).

Other widely used models include: the triaxial Tritrac (Hemokinetics Professional Products, Reining, Madison, WI, United States), released in the early 1990s and succeeded in 2000 by the triaxial RT3 (Stayhealthy, Inc, Monrovia, CA, United States); the Actical (Phillips Respironics, Bend, OR, United States) an omnidirectional accelerometer (with the sensor positioned to be most sensitive to vertical accelerations) released around 2004; the GENEActiv triaxial raw acceleration monitor (Activinsights Ltd, Cambridgeshire, United Kingdom) in 2011; and most recently the Axivity AX3 triaxial raw acceleration monitor (Axivity, Newcastle, United Kingdom) in 2013.

The ActiGraph (7164, 71256, GT1M, GT3X), Tritrac, RT3 and Actical store data summarized over user-defined time intervals or epochs (e.g. 5 seconds, 15 seconds, 60 seconds) in the form of proprietary counts. The GT3X+, GT9X Link, GENEActiv and Axivity AX3 store non-proprietary raw acceleration signals. If required, the ActiGraph software (Actilife) can be used to obtain the ActiGraph proprietary counts from raw acceleration data collected using the ActiGraph GT3X+ or GT9X Link.

Count-Based Accelerometers

Accelerometers that store high-resolution raw accelerations for multiple days were not commercially available until after 2010. Until then, raw accelerations were processed on-board the accelerometer, and output was in proprietary counts. Accelerometer counts are an arbitrary dimensionless unit that are manufacturer-specific and therefore cannot be compared between different brands of accelerometer.

The signal from count-based accelerometers is integrated, processed and stored over a given time interval, or epoch. With raw acceleration accelerometers epoch size is selected post-data collection, but with count-based accelerometers it was necessary to select epoch size pre-data collection. This could be set as low as 1 second or as high as 60 seconds. Before the early 2000s, most studies set the epoch at 60 seconds, a pragmatic decision because the limitations of the memory size of accelerometers dictated that this was necessary to store 7 days of data.

Studies deploying count-based accelerometers were usually concerned with waking behaviors, primarily physical activity and, more recently, time spent in sedentary behaviors. Protocols generally requested the monitor was worn at the hip, during waking hours only, and removed for any water-based activities (Rowlands, 2007).

Determining Whether the Accelerometer Is Being Worn

When analyzing accelerometer output, it can be difficult to distinguish between times when the monitor has been removed and prolonged periods of inactivity. Failing to distinguish between non-wear and sedentary time can lead to inclusion bias and misclassification. For example misclassification of inactive time as monitor removal may lead to overestimation of activity and underestimation of inactivity, or alternatively may lead to participants failing to meet minimal wear requirements for the study and their exclusion leading to a biased sample; misclassification of monitor removal (e.g. to go swimming) as inactive time may lead to underestimation of physical activity and overestimation of inactivity.

With count-based accelerometers, monitor removal is usually assumed when there are prolonged strings of consecutive zero counts, indicating minimal movement for a sustained period. However, there is no real consensus on how long a string of zeros represents monitor removal. Some studies use periods as short as 10 minutes (Mattocks et al., 2007), but up to 180 minutes has been used (e.g. van Coervering, Harnack, Schmitz, Fulton, & Galuska, 2005). Strings of consecutive zeros lasting 60 minutes are perhaps the most widely used (e.g. Troiano et al., 2008) and have been recommended (Evenson & Terry, 2009).

Total Volume of Activity

The total volume of activity can be quantified by simply summing the total accelerometer counts accumulated over the day (TAC/d). This incorporates the full continuum of activity intensities by condensing the frequency, intensity and duration of activity bouts into a single metric (Bassett, Troiano, McClain, & Wolff, 2015). It is close to the parameter measured by the accelerometer (acceleration), therefore minimizing the error (Brage, Burton, Chastin, Penpraze, & Rowe, 2015). Further, although it is a proprietary metric, it is a physical activity output that can be compared across any study using the same brand of accelerometer (Bassett et al., 2015). Wolff-Hughes and colleagues (Wolff-Hughes, Bassett, & Fitzhugh, 2014; Wolff-Hughes, Fitzhugh, Bassett, & Churilla, 2015) generated age- and sex-specific population-referenced percentiles for ActiGraph TAC/d using NHANES 2003–2006 data (ActiGraph 7164), facilitating comparison of accelerometer outcomes to norms for US children and adults.

Cut-Points and Epoch Size

Count cut-points were developed to give biological meaning to accelerometer output by categorizing ranges of accelerometer counts as time spent at a given activity intensity (e.g. time spent in MVPA (Bassett, Rowlands, & Trost, 2012)). The amount of time spent in a given activity intensity (e.g. MVPA) is simply the time accumulated with accelerometer counts per epoch greater than the MVPA cut-point, making this an easy and efficient way for end users to convert accelerometer counts into more meaningful units. Best practices for calibrating and validating wearable activity monitors are presented by Bassett and colleagues (2012).

As previously noted, in the past the memory capacity of accelerometers restricted epoch size to 60 seconds when assessing activity for 7 days. A 60 seconds epoch is known to underestimate vigorous and high-intensity activity (Nilsson, Ekelund, Yngve, & Sjostrom, 2002) as more intense activities are typically undertaken in brief bursts. Brief bursts of high-intensity activity are smoothed out when assessed over 60 seconds epochs. This is particularly relevant in studies involving children because their physical activity patterns are characterized by short bursts of rapidly changing activity (Bailey et al., 1995). Following the early 2000s when memory capacity of accelerometers increased, studies were able to use shorter epochs to ensure capture of children's transitory activity patterns (e.g. Baquet, Stratton, van Praagh, & Berthoin, 2007; Blaes, Baquet, van Praagh, & Berthoin, 2011; Stone, Rowlands, Middlebrooke, Jawis, & Eston, 2009).

Cut-Point Conundrum

Count cut-points are specific to accelerometer brand due to the proprietary nature of counts. For each brand of accelerometer there are several sets of cut-points available for use; which of the available cut-points is selected can have a large effect on activity outcomes. For example, when analyzing ActiGraph data from a sample of 419 young children with five different sets of cut-points, Bornstein and colleagues (2011) reported that estimated MVPA varied from 22.5 to 269 minutes per day.

The variability in cut-points reflects the dependency of the cut-points on the calibration study used to generate them. Cut-points reflect the study sample and the activities included in the calibration (e.g. cut-points that are developed using only ambulatory activities will be higher than those developed using a range of lifestyle activities). This is because, for a given energy expenditure, accelerometer counts are lower for intermittent or lifestyle activities (e.g. household chores and sport) than for predominantly ambulatory continuous activities (Crouter, Clowers, & Bassett, 2006).

The International Children's Accelerometer Database

In 2008 the International Children's Accelerometry Database (ICAD) was initiated to address the lack of comparability of studies using the ActiGraph hip-worn accelerometer (http://www.mrc-epid.cam.ac.uk/research/studies/icad/). ICAD is a compilation of hip-worn ActiGraph accelerometer-derived estimates of children's physical activity from studies worldwide (Sherar et al., 2011). Large-scale surveys that have contributed data to ICAD include the US National Health and Nutrition Examination Survey (NHANES) 2003–2004 and 2005–2006 (Troiano et al., 2008), Avon Longitudinal Study of Parents and Children (ALSPAC) 2003–2005 (Riddoch et al., 2007) and the European Youth Heart Survey (EYHS) 2006 (Andersen et al., 2006).

Importantly, ICAD obtained the epoch level count data for each of the studies and the data were re-processed using consistent rules for classifying wear-time and intensity cut-points, making the outputs comparable. This harmonization of data from over 37,000 children across >20 studies worldwide has facilitated the investigation of diverse questions across international datasets. A list of publications can be found on the ICAD website (http://www.mrc-epid.cam.ac.uk/research/studies/icad/).

The Emergence of Raw Acceleration Monitors

The shift to commercial availability of raw acceleration monitors occurred in 2010/2011 and followed a general movement toward more transparent and open science. This led to a demand for accelerometer data that are collected and saved as raw signals, thus removing the proprietary nature of accelerometer output. The term 'raw' refers to the accelerometer data being expressed in m/s^2 or gravitational acceleration, instead of proprietary counts as in the previous generations of accelerometers (van Hees, 2018). Further, as raw data are stored, all data transformations are carried out post-data collection under the control of the researcher.

The availability of raw data presents physical activity researchers with a new and different challenge; without the 'black box' generation of proprietary counts, the researcher is now responsible for processing and analyzing huge amounts of data. One week of measuring at 100 Hz, as in most of these studies, generates over 180 million data points for each person. The researcher has responsibility for ensuring methods are transparent and replicable. To provide the expertise necessary to deal with these data, physical activity research benefits from an increasing number of researchers with backgrounds in mathematics, computer science, engineering and statistics as well as sports and exercise science.

The raw acceleration signal consists of a gravitational component (static acceleration), a movement component (dynamic acceleration) and noise (van Hees et al., 2013). To quantify accelerations due to physical activity it is necessary to attempt to remove the gravitational component of acceleration from the signal. However, when a person is inactive and there is no acceleration due to movement the orientation of the gravity vector can be used to determine the position and orientation of the monitor. This can be particularly useful for wrist-worn monitors as orientation of the monitor indicates the position of the wrist. This approach has been used to classify sleep (van Hees et al., 2015) and posture (Hurter et al., 2019; Rowlands et al., 2014).

There is an open-source package available, GGIR (Migueles, Rowlands, Huber, Sabia, & van Hees, 2019; Rowlands, Yates, Davies, Khunti, & Edwardson, 2016; van Hees et al., 2013, 2014, 2015), that enables researchers to process and analyze raw accelerometer signals in R (http://cran.r-project.org) using comprehensive, validated and transparent methods. Currently, GGIR can be used to process and analyze raw accelerometer signals from the GENEActiv, ActiGraph (GT3X+ and GT9X) and Axivity accelerometers. Signal processing includes quality control (automatic calibration, detection of sustained abnormally high values), detection of non-wear and calculation of a range of acceleration metrics that employ different methods of separating the movement and gravity components of acceleration (van Hees et al., 2013). The most widely used of these metrics is Euclidean Norm Minus One (ENMO) (e.g. da Silva et al., 2014; Doherty et al., 2017; Sabia et al., 2014; van Hees et al., 2011). A large range of outcome variables to describe the daily activity profile and sleep are also calculated.

A General Shift to Wrist-Wear

Unlike, the previous generation of accelerometers, raw acceleration monitors (e.g. GENEActiv, ActiGraph GT3X+ and GT9X, Axivity) are designed predominantly for wrist-wear and are suitable for wear during water-based activities including showering, bathing and swimming. This makes them suitable for 24 hour wear and studies have shown that compliance and acceptability are greater than for hip-worn monitors in children (Fairclough et al., 2016), adolescents (Scott et al., 2017) and adults (van Hees et al., 2011). Wear for the 24 hour period facilitates assessment of the 24 hour profile of physical behaviors (i.e. sedentary time and sleep as well as physical activity), and the greater compliance reduces the risks of measurement error and/or bias due to monitor removal (Price et al., 2018). Further, misclassification of non-wear is potentially reduced as raw acceleration output is more sensitive to small movements than the proprietary counts. For example, the non-wear detection method described by van Hees et al. (2011; and 'Procedure for non-wear detection' supplementary document, van Hees et al., 2013) estimates non-wear based on the standard deviation (SD) and value range of each axis, calculated for 60 minute windows with a 15-minute sliding window. The window is classified as non-wear if, for at least two out of the three axes, the SD is less than 3 mg or the value range is less than 50 mg. Given that the acceleration of the chest at rest from breathing has an amplitude of 10 mg and the vibrations resulting from the heart beating have a peak-to-peak amplitude of 80 mg (Phan, Bonnet, Guillemaud, Castelli, & PhamThi, 2008), the non-wear method described should detect even tiny wrist movements as wear (van Hees et al., 2011).

Although the shift to wrist-wear has brought advantages, it has also brought further challenges. In the past, accelerometers were most commonly worn close to the center of gravity of the body, usually the hip, to reflect whole body movement and thus energy expenditure (Westerterp, 1999). Accelerometer output differs by wear-site with, for example, higher magnitudes of acceleration generally found at the wrist (Hildebrand, van Hees, Hansen, & Ekelund, 2014; Rowlands et al., 2014); thus it is important that data analysis and interpretation is wear-site specific. It is not appropriate to simply apply methods that had been generated with hip-worn monitors to data from wrist-worn monitors. Further, when wearing monitors at the wrist, arm movements that do not reflect notable increases in energy expenditure will be recorded and may lead to lower accuracy leading to concerns that validity would be detrimentally affected. However, laboratory studies have shown similar correlations between energy expenditure and acceleration, irrespective of whether it was measured at the hip or wrist (Esliger et al., 2011; Phillips, Parfitt, & Rowlands, 2012; Hildebrand et al., 2014). Further, free-living studies have shown that a strong relationship exists between physical activity energy expenditure and wrist acceleration (White, Westgate, Wareham, Brage, & 2016).

It is also possible that the greater variety in wrist movements may also provide a richer, more detailed picture of a person's behaviors than is possible with waist-worn accelerometers (Rowlands et al., 2014). With the application of sophisticated analytical tools, wrist wear may offer considerable potential for classification of behavior types, particularly sedentary and light activities.

Deployment in Large-Scale Surveys

There is an increasing number of large-scale studies deploying raw acceleration accelerometers to assess children's physical activity including NHANES 2011–2014, the Pelotas Birth Cohort (da Silva et al., 2014), the Melbourne Child Health Checkpoint (Wake et al., 2014), the Millennium Cohort Study (Ipsos MORI, 2017), the Cork Children's Lifestyle Study (Li et al., 2017) and the International Study of Childhood Obesity, Lifestyle and the Environment (ISCOLE). All used a 24-hour wear protocol, with ISCOLE using the hip wear-site and the other studies using the wrist. The removal of proprietary accelerometer outcomes offers considerable potential for comparability between datasets and harmonizing data. Moving forward, where studies use the same wear-site, it would be beneficial to ensure data and results are comparable.

Key and Emerging Issues

Opportunities and Challenges with Accelerometry

Maximizing comparability of accelerometer outcome variables and the potential for data harmonization.

Inter-Device Comparability

The availability of raw acceleration data from research-grade accelerometers offers considerable potential for comparability between datasets and harmonizing data. This is an important step as harmonization enables researchers to combine and/or compare data acquired across diverse settings or populations for analysis, providing greater heterogeneity and increased statistical power relative to analysis of individual studies. For example, data harmonization has facilitated production of robust and generalizable estimates of risk for cardiovascular events, cardiovascular disease and mortality that have informed clinical and public health practice (e.g. Chen et al., 2013; Mons et al., 2015). Further, harmonization of physical activity data would enable comparison of risk prevalence (e.g. not meeting physical activity guidelines, across and within populations).

The availability of raw acceleration data from the monitors deployed in large studies and surveys potentially enables comparison of the data and findings. However, as stressed by Welk, McClain, and Ainsworth (2012), equivalence of raw acceleration output from different devices cannot be assumed and it is necessary to carry out rigorous equivalency testing to determine whether, and under which conditions, outputs from these monitors can be considered interchangeable.

Laboratory and free-living data collected from the GENEActiv, Axivity and ActiGraph contemporaneously indicates that while direct measures of acceleration can be considered equivalent between the GENEActiv and the Axivity (Rowlands, Mirkes et al., 2018), the magnitude of accelerations measured by the ActiGraph is approximately 10% lower (John, Sasaki, Staudenmeyer, Mavilia, & Freedson 2013; Rowlands et al., 2015, 2016; Rowlands, Mirkes et al., 2018). However, accumulating evidence from studies to date suggests that data from the frequency domain (i.e. underlying frequencies or repeating patterns, (John et al., 2013; Rowlands et al., 2015)) and the orientation of the monitor (Edwardson et al., 2016; Rowlands et al., 2014) are comparable between the GENEActiv and the ActiGraph.

While most studies using the wrist-site request participants wear the monitor on their non-dominant wrist, others have used the dominant wrist – most notably the adult UK Biobank study (Doherty et al., 2017). Preliminary evidence suggests that accelerations measured at the dominant wrist, in free-living participants, are approximately 10% higher than those measured concurrently at the non-dominant wrist (Rowlands, Plekhanova et al., 2019). It is early days and evidence will continue to accumulate regarding the extent to which accelerometer outputs from different devices can be considered equivalent. At present caution is advised when comparing the magnitude of accelerations measured: (a) by the ActiGraph to the Axivity or GENEActiv, and (b) at the dominant wrist to the non-dominant wrist.

Reporting Standardized Accelerometer Metrics

Another source of variability between studies is the physical behavior metrics generated from the raw accelerometer data. Given the richness of the data collected, there are vast possibilities for how it can be summarized or expressed. The most appropriate accelerometer metrics for a study will depend on the research question, so individual studies may use a variety of approaches and outcome measures and/or employ innovative metrics. To aid comparability between studies, it would be beneficial if researchers also made key standardized physical activity metrics available, much as other standard information such as age, height and mass is always given (Rowlands, 2018).

To fulfill this purpose, it has been proposed (Rowlands, 2018) that ideally the metrics should:

- Reflect directly measured acceleration. The further we move from the measured variable (e.g. by predicting energy expenditure or time spent in different activity intensities), the greater the scope for error (Brage et al., 2015).
- Consist of a single metric for 'How much?' or the volume of activity, and a single metric for 'How hard?' the intensity of activity.
- The volume metric should not be highly correlated with the intensity metric; this enables investigation into the relative importance of intensity and volume for health.
- The intensity metric should reflect the entire intensity profile. Widely used intensity metrics (e.g. time spent in MVPA and/or VPA) only cover a small fraction of the activity profile. Further, time accumulated above acceleration thresholds is highly correlated with activity volume, which complicates exploration of the relative contributions of volume and intensity of activity to health.
- The volume and intensity metrics should be possible to produce simply, using open-source freely available software that works with major brands of research-grade raw acceleration accelerometers.

As previously mentioned, a standardized metric of activity volume for counts assessed by the ActiGraph accelerometer is total accelerometer counts accumulated over the day (TAC/d) (Bassett et al., 2015; Wolff-Hughes et al., 2014, 2015). With 24 hour raw accelerometry data, the complete activity profile can be described using two standardized metrics: the average acceleration for volume of activity and the intensity gradient for the distribution of intensity across the 24 hour profile (Rowlands, 2018; Rowlands, Edwardson et al., 2018). Most of a child's day is spent in very low intensity activities, somewhat less time in light activities, less in moderate- and little in vigorous- and high-intensity activities, such that if you plot time accumulated against intensity you get a curvilinear plot (Figure 16.1). Taking the natural logs of time and intensity turns this into a straight-line graph. The intensity gradient describes the slope of this straight-line graph (Rowlands, Edwardson et al., 2018). The steeper the slope (the more negative), the worse the intensity profile, the shallower the slope (the less negative), the better the intensity profile. The intensity gradient reflects the whole profile of acceleration, rather than just a small fraction of it like MVPA.

Both average acceleration and the intensity gradient can be produced using the open-source freely available GGIR R-package (https://cran.r-project.org/web/packages/GGIR/index.html, van Hees et al., 2011, 2013). Note that as acceleration differs depending on the body site where it is measured, the values of metrics would be specific to wear-site (i.e. metrics generated from hip-worn accelerometers would not be comparable to metrics generated from wrist-worn monitors). Preliminary evidence suggests these two metrics can be considered equivalent for wrist-worn data from any of the three research-grade accelerometers usually deployed in large-scale surveys (Acti-Graph, GENEActiv, Axivity, (Rowlands, Mirkes et al., 2018; Rowlands, Plekhanova et al., 2019)) irrespective of wrist of wear, provided the average acceleration is decreased by 10% for monitors worn on the dominant wrist (Rowlands, Plekhanova et al., 2019).

Notably these two metrics are not highly correlated, unlike cut-point measures of intensity and activity volume, facilitating investigation of the relative importance of activity and volume for health. Cross-sectional analyses have shown that the intensity profile of activity is associated

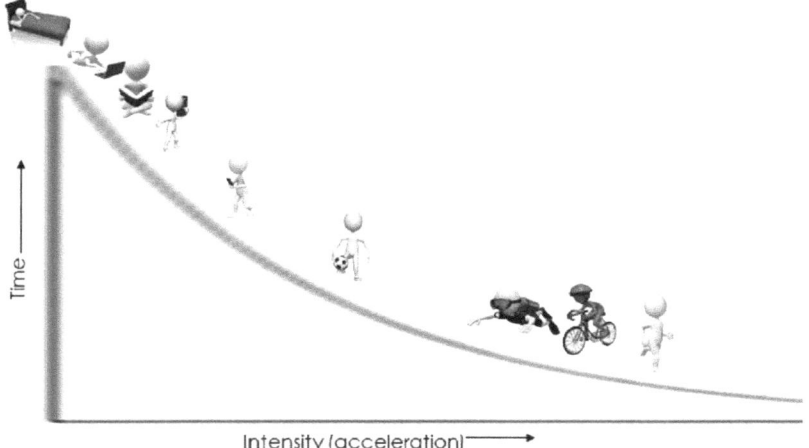

Figure 16.1 The curvilinear relationship between time accumulated (y-axis) and intensity of physical activity (x-axis): the majority of the day is usually spent in very low-intensity activities, somewhat less time in light activities, less in moderate and little in vigorous- and high-intensity activities. The intensity gradient describes the slope of the log-log plot of this curvilinear relationship (Rowlands, Edwardson et al., 2018). The steeper the slope (the more negative the intensity gradient) the worse the intensity profile, the shallower the slope (the less negative the intensity gradient) the better the intensity profile. Adapted from Rowlands (2018)

with adiposity independent of volume (Fairclough, Taylor, Rowlands, Boddy, & Noonan, 2019; Rowlands, Yates et al., 2019). The intensity profile of the leanest children was characterized by short periods of high-intensity activity (e.g. running/sprinting, accumulated across the day (Fairclough et al., 2019; Rowlands, Yates et al., 2019)). Similar analyses in adults have shown additive effects of volume and intensity of body fatness and interactive effects on bone health and physical function (Rowlands, Yates et al., 2019), highlighting the potential of using these two metrics to identify the differential effects of volume and intensity of physical activity for specific health outcomes and populations (Rowlands, Yates et al., 2019). The importance of vigorous physical activity for children's health is also demonstrated by Aadland, Kvalheim, Andessen, Resalan and Anderson's (2018) recent investigation of the association between the whole spectrum of physical activity intensities (multivariate physical activity signature) and metabolic health in 10 year olds.

Patterning of Physical Activity

The time-series nature of both count and raw accelerometer data provides the opportunity for detailed examination of the patterning of physical activity. This would be difficult to investigate with other methods. Researchers are increasingly applying sophisticated analyses that enable them to exploit these data to comprehensively phenotype children's physical activity levels. Goldsmith, Liu, Jacobson and Rundle (2016) examined the diurnal activity profile using Functional Data analysis (FDA), which takes into account the correlation of the accelerometer data points over time while maintaining the richness of the time-series accelerometer data. They reported time-specific associations between activity and a series of co-variates. For example girls are less active than boys in the daytime, but not in the evening; children born to US mothers were less active in the morning and more active in the afternoon than children of mothers born elsewhere, despite similar aggregate activity levels. This type of information could be important for tailoring activity interventions. Further, analyses that take into account the timing of physical behaviors could be particularly pertinent given that it is becoming increasingly clear that the timing of physical behaviors can be important for health. For example, it appears that preferred sleep timing, being a 'morning' or 'evening' person (chronotype), is linked to cardiometabolic health even after accounting for sleep duration (Merikanto et al., 2013).

This sequential nature of accelerometer data facilitates the investigation of whether variability in physical activity, as well as volume and intensity, is important for health. This was exploited by Millard, Tilling, Lawlor, Flach and Gaunt (2017) who used activity bigrams to capture how a child's activity changes from one moment to the next. Using minute-by-minute accelerometer count data from nearly 5,000 11-year-old children they showed that higher variation in physical activity from 1 minute to the next is associated with lower BMI, after accounting for time spent at intensity levels. If further research confirms a role of variability in physical activity on health, this could have an impact on physical activity recommendations that currently focus predominantly on volumes of MVPA.

Classification of Behavior Type

Due to the flexibility in data processing and rich array of features that can be extracted from raw acceleration data there is increased potential for classification of activity type from free-living data using pattern recognition and machine learning approaches (Troiano, McClain, Brychta, & Chen, 2014). This is possible as examination of the features of the raw acceleration signal, beyond the magnitude of acceleration alone, can give insight into the type of activity a person may be doing. For example a cyclic acceleration signal (showing repeating patterns) indicates a rhythmic activity (e.g. walking or running) and the orientation of the monitor can be determined from the gravitational component of the signal.

Machine learning is a branch of artificial intelligence and is an umbrella term covering techniques that fit algorithms based on patterns in data (e.g. patterns based on activity types) (Mooney & Pejaver, 2018), enabling automated predictions to be made on unseen data (e.g. predictions of what activity type someone is doing). The ability to exploit machine learning approaches to try and classify behavior type could be beneficial in a multitude of ways. For instance, knowledge of activity type could be useful for identifying how behaviors differ across population groups (e.g. age-groups, ethnicity, socio-economic status), designing and/or evaluating interventions by enabling evaluation and targeting of specific behaviors (Ellis, Kerr, Godbole, Staudenmeyer, & Lanckriet, 2016), or improving the estimation of energy expenditure by accounting for acceleration differing across activity types that have similar energy expenditure (e.g. cycling and intermittent lifestyle activities compared to walking/running).

Initially studies developing machine learning approaches for the classification of activity type trained algorithms only on laboratory data, with participants performing a choreographed routine of known structured activities (e.g. Zhang, Rowlands, Murray, & Hurst, 2012). But, despite high classification accuracy in a laboratory setting, accuracy tended to drop dramatically when the laboratory trained algorithms were applied to a free-living setting (Bastian et al., 2015; Sasaki et al., 2015; van Hees et al., 2013). Ideally the machine learning algorithms need to be trained on free-living data. The challenge when using free-living data is to find a criterion measure that is feasible to use with free-living participants and will not unduly impinge on their natural behaviors. Recently, researchers have obtained data from free-living participants wearing the SenseCam wearable camera and accelerometers concurrently for up to seven free-living days (Ellis et al., 2016; Kerr et al., 2016). Results show that classifiers trained on free-living data outperform those trained on laboratory data, but further research is needed as recognition accuracy of physical activity type from free-living data is still only modest (Pavey, Gilson, Gomersall, & Clark, 2017). Use of a dual-accelerometer system, with monitors affixed directly to the skin on both the thigh and the back, out-performed a single accelerometer for classification of non-ambulatory activities (Stewart et al., 2018), but is yet to be tested in a free-living setting. Given the high compliance achieved for the dual-accelerometer system in adults and children (Duncan et al., 2018; Schneller et al., 2017), it is important to ascertain the classification accuracy of the dual-accelerometer system during free-living.

Supervised machine learning, as used in the studies described earlier, use labeled data (i.e. where the activity the person is doing is known), where it is necessary to have a 'ground truth' measure of what the person is doing. More recently, unsupervised machine learning approaches (e.g. van Kuppevelt et al., 2019) have been used with free-living data. Instead of using labeled data these models are data-driven and allow for the identification of clusters or characteristic states present in the data. It may then be possible to explore the physical behaviors these states likely represent by examining the features of the accelerometer signal that characterize the clusters identified. Subsequently, it may be possible to explore how the clusters differ between groups, change over time and associate with health.

Public Health Friendly Translation of Accelerometer Outcomes

The World Health Organization's recent Global Activity Action Plan on Physical Activity 2018–2030 (WHO, 2018) highlights monitoring and surveillance, using robust and reliable data, as the cornerstone to the implementation and evaluation of national strategies. Accelerometers are increasingly used in national surveys globally. Yet, a lack of standardized, robust methods to create meaningful and easy to interpret outcome variables from accelerometer data is hampering important monitoring and evaluation activities within and across countries.

For the purposes of monitoring and surveillance, standardized, population-independent metrics that are derived directly from the measured acceleration are appropriate. For example, the average acceleration and the intensity gradient can be used to describe the volume and intensity distribution of the 24 hour profile. However, physical activity guidelines are expressed in terms of MVPA. For children, the recommendation is 60 minutes MVPA per day (Physical Activity Guidelines for Americans, 2018). Cut-points are generally used to assess meeting guidelines and the problems associated with this are well-documented: the cut-point conundrum (cut-points are population-specific limiting comparability across studies); participants score very differently if one has activity falling just above a cut-point and the other just below; participants may fail to obtain any activity above cut-points (particularly in the vigorous range), and simply score zero. An alternative approach is to identify the minimum acceleration value above which a child's most active 60 minutes ($M60_{ACC}$) is accumulated (Rowlands, Sherar et al., 2019). With this approach the metric is population-independent and derived from directly measured acceleration, thus not relying on assumptions as cut-points do. Meeting guidelines could be reported as the proportion of children whose $M60_{ACC}$ exceeded the acceleration magnitude associated with MVPA, or a brisk walk. This acceleration value could be obtained from calibration studies (e.g. Hildebrand et al., 2014).

Crucially, this approach shifts the population-specific translation and interpretation of accelerometer data to post processing/analysis. For example, if percentiles (e.g. 5th centile through to 95th centile) for $M60_{ACC}$ are reported, the results can be translated in light of any current or future calibration study. Using example data from the United Kingdom to illustrate this (Rowlands, Sherar et al., 2019), Figure 16.2a shows that, relative to Hildebrand et al.'s (2014) MVPA cut-point of 200 mg (equivalent to a brisk walk, lower black dashed horizontal line) just under 50% of 10-year-old girls (N = 83) accumulated 60 minutes of activity above this intensity (the 50th centile for $M60_{ACC}$ is just under 200 mg), this decreased to 25% for 11–12-year-old girls (N = 974, the 75th centile for $M60_{ACC}$ was 200 mg), and approximately 20% 13–14 year olds (N = 695, the 80th centile was around 200 mg). Applying the MVPA cut-point developed by Phillips et al. (2012) of 250 mg (upper dashed horizontal line), the percentages of girls meeting the guidelines were approximately 15%, 5% and <5% for 10, 11–12 and 13–14-year olds, respectively. For comparison, Figure 16.2b shows percentiles for the minimum acceleration for the most active 30 minutes ($M30_{ACC}$) for the same girls, highlighting the greater drop across age and spread across the percentiles when looking at the shorter time period. It is possible to evaluate the data relative to any published cut-points, or to use typical values for accelerations elicited by walking or running for a given age-group, to translate the findings with no need to access the original data.

As data accumulate it would be possible to generate standardized population-specific norms for each of these standardized metrics (i.e. for activity volume, intensity profile and for the most active 60 minutes (or other duration)). The metrics are easy to derive through open-source software and could facilitate global surveillance and dose-response studies (Rowlands, Sherar et al., 2019). To provide a public health friendly interpretation of the results the metrics can be translated in terms of indicative activities such as brisk walking.

It is important to note that currently guidelines are largely derived from self-report data (Troiano et al., 2014). It has been repeatedly demonstrated in studies that compare self-reported and accelerometer assessed physical activity that the measures have low to moderate correlations; this is because they are distinct physical activity assessment methods and their outcomes are not equivalent (Troiano et al., 2014). Despite this, studies using accelerometers to assess physical activity frequently compare their results to physical activity guidelines. Moving forward, as accelerometer and corresponding health data accumulate it will be possible to derive evidence-based physical activity guidelines directly from accelerometer data (Rowlands, Sherar et al., 2019).

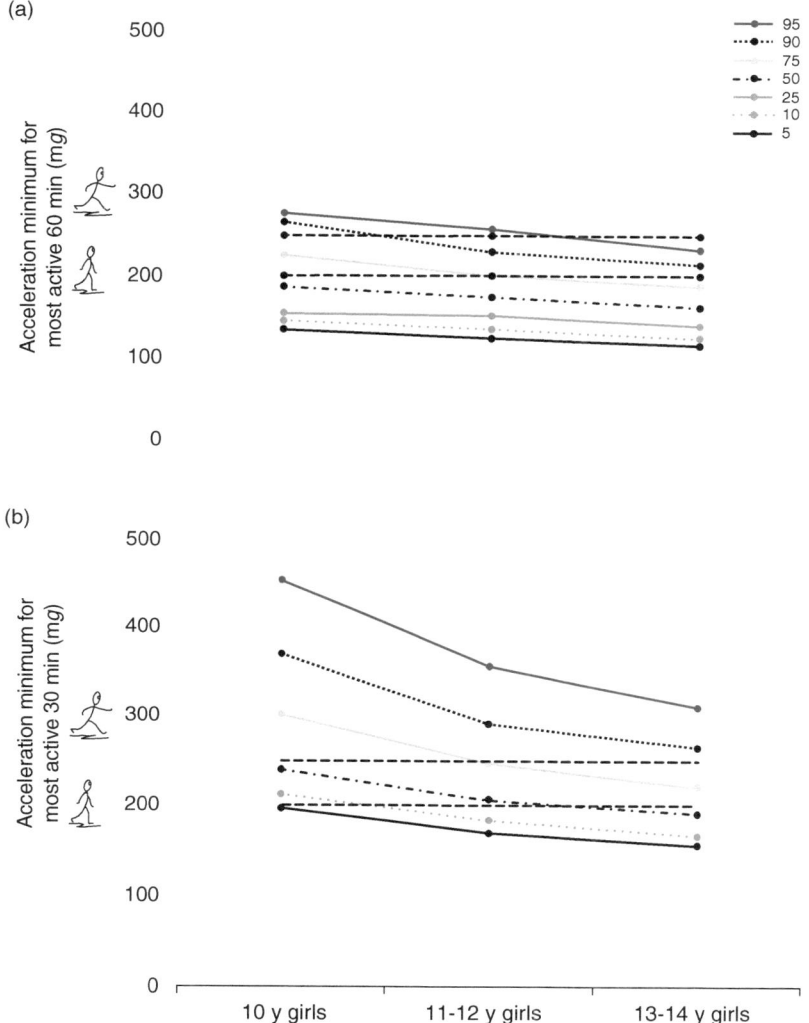

Figure 16.2 Percentiles for the magnitude of acceleration above which the children's most active (a) 60 and (b) 30 minutes are accumulated. Black dashed horizontal lines represent MVPA according to Hildebrand et al.'s (2014, lower) and Phillip et al.'s (2013, upper) cut-points

Summary

Over the last decade there has been very rapid progress in the use of accelerometers to assess physical activity and other physical behaviors. This chapter has given a brief history of the use of accelerometers to assess physical activity covering the shift from proprietary count-based acceler-ometers to raw accelerometers, and some of the key things to be aware of in relation to the pro-cessing and analysis of accelerometer data. Finally, the challenges and opportunities ahead were highlighted. These include taking advantage of the richness of the accelerometer data to provide comprehensive physical activity phenotyping and classify behaviors, but also to work toward ensuring that standardized, comparable metrics can be easily and routinely generated. Not only would this facilitate global monitoring and surveillance, but it would help build an evidence base to derive evidence-based physical activity guidelines directly from accelerometer data.

Recommendations for Researchers Using Body-Worn Accelerometers

- When reporting results from body-worn accelerometers ensure the protocol details are provided:
  - monitor used (make, model, firmware version), sampling frequency, wear-site, wear protocol/instructions (e.g. 24 hour, worn for water-based activities or not), orientation of monitor, handedness of participant (if the wrist wear-site is used).
  - software used to process data, data cleaning and processing decisions (e.g. calibration, epoch size; determination of non-wear; output metrics used (e.g. ENMO); cut-points applied (if cut-points are used), algorithms applied to the data).
- Where possible store the raw data file.
- The optimal physical behavior outcomes for a study will vary, but where possible report data-driven metrics (e.g. average acceleration (ENMO), intensity gradient, $M60_{ACC}$) alongside study specific physical behavior outcomes. This will aid in comparing between studies.
- For further information and to keep up-to-date, the International Society for the Measurement of Physical Behaviour (ISMPB) is highly recommended (http://www.ismpb.org). This Society brings together people who have an interest in measuring free-living physical behavior. It is a non-profit scientific society dedicated to ambulatory monitoring, wearable monitors, movement sensors, physical activity, sedentary behavior, movement behavior, body postures, sleep and constructs related to physical behaviors. It also hosts the International Conference on Ambulatory Monitoring and Physical Activity (ICAMPAM) every 2 years.

Acknowledgments

AVR is supported by the NIHR Leicester Biomedical Research Centre, and the Collaboration for Leadership in Applied Health Research and Care (CLAHRC) East Midlands. The views expressed are those of the authors and not necessarily those of the NHS, NIHR, or Department of Health.

References

Aadland, E., Kvalheim, O. M., Andessen, S. A., Resalan, G. K., & Anderson, L. B. (2018). The multivariate physical activity signature associated with metabolic health in children. *International Journal of Behavioural Nutrition, 15*, 77. doi:10.1186/s12966-018-0707-z

Andersen, L. B., Harro, M., Sardinha, L. B., Froberg, K., Ekelund, U., Brage, S., & Anderssen, S. A. (2006). Physical activity and clustered cardiovascular risk in children: A cross-sectional study (The European Youth Heart Study). *Lancet, 368*, 299–304.

Bailey, R. C., Olson, J., Pepper, S. L., Porszasz, J., Barston, T. J., & Cooper, D. M. (1995). The level and tempo of children's physical activities: An observational study. *Medicine and Science in Sports and Exercise, 27*, 1033–1041.

Baquet, G., Stratton, G., van Praagh, E., & Berthoin, S. (2007). Improving physical activity assessment in prepubertal children with high-frequency accelerometry monitoring: A methodological issue. *Preventive Medicine, 44*, 143–147.

Bassett, D. R., Rowlands, A. V., & Trost, S. G. (2012). Calibration and validation of wearable monitors. *Medicine and Science in Sports and Exercise, 44*, S32–S38.

Bassett, D. R., Troiano, R. P., McClain, J. J., & Wolff, D. L. (2015). Accelerometer-based physical activity: Total volume per day and standardised measures. *Medicine and Science in Sports and Exercise, 47*, 833–838. doi:10.1249/MSS.0000000000000468

Bastian, T., Maire, A., Dugas, J., Ataya, A., Villars, C., Gris, F., . . . Simon, C. (2015). Automatic identification of physical activity types and sedentary behaviors from triaxial accelerometer: Laboratory-based calibrations are not enough. *Journal of Applied Physiology, 118*(6), 716–722.

Blaes, A., Baquet, G., van Praagh, E., & Berthoin, S. (2011). Physical activity patterns in French youth – From childhood to adolescence – Monitored with high-frequency accelerometry. *American Journal of Human Biology, 23*, 353–358.

Bornstein, D. B., Beets, M. W., Byun, W., Welk, G., Bottai, M., Dowda, M., & Pate, R. (2011). Equating accelerometer estimates of moderate-to-vigorous physical activity: In search of the Rosetta Stone. *Journal of Science and Medicine in Sport, 14*, 404–410.

Brage, S., Burton, F., Chastin, S. F. M., Penpraze, V., & Rowe, D. A. (2015). Introduction to the objective measurement of physical activity and sedentary behaviour. doi:10.13140/RG.2.1.1829.3202. Retrieved from https://www.researchgate.net/publication/284186564_Introduction_to_the_Objective_Measurement_of_Physical_Activity

Cappuccio, F. P., Taggart, F. M., Kandala, N.-B., Currie, A., Peile, E., Stranges, S., & Miller, M. A. (2008). Meta-analysis of short sleep duration and obesity in children and adults. *Sleep, 31*(5), 619–626.

Chastin, S. F. M., Palarea-Albaladejo, J., Dontje, M. L., & Skelton, D. A. (2015). Combined effects of time spent in physical activity, sedentary behaviors and sleep on obesity and cardio-metabolic health markers: A novel compositional data analysis approach. *PLoS One, 10*(10), e0139984. doi:10.1371/journal.pone.0139984

Chen, Y., Copeland, W. K., Vedanthan, R., Grant, E., Lee, J. E., Gu, D., . . . Potter, J. D. (2013). Association between body mass index and cardiovascular disease mortality in East Asians and South Asians: Pooled analysis of prospective data from the Asia cohort consortium. *British Medical Journal, 347*, f5446.

Crouter, S. E., Clowers, K. G., & Bassett, D. R. (2006). A novel method for using accelerometer data to predict energy expenditure. *Journal of Applied Physiology, 100*, 1324–1331.

da Silva, I. C. M., van Hees, V. T., Ramires, V. V., Knuth, A. G., Bielemann, R. M., Ekelund, U., . . . Hallal, P. C. (2014). Physical activity levels in three Brazilian birth cohorts as assessed with raw triaxial wrist accelerometry. *International Journal of Epidemiology, 43*, 1959–1968.

Doherty, A., Jackson, D., Hammerla, N., Plotz, T., Olivier, P., Granat, M. H., . . . Wareham, N. J. (2017). Large scale population assessment of physical activity using wrist worn accelerometers: The UK biobank study. *PLoS One, 12*(2), e0169649. doi:10.1371/journal.pone.0169649

Duncan, S., Stewart, T., Mackay, L., Neville, J., Narayanan, A., Walker, C., . . . Morton, S. (2018). Wear-time compliance with a dual-accelerometer system for capturing 24-hour behavioural profiles in children and adults. *International Journal of Environmental Research and Public Health, 15*(7), 1296.

Edwardson, C. L., Rowlands, A. V., Bunnewell, S., Sanders, J., Esliger, D., Gorely, T., . . . Yates, T. (2016). Accuracy of posture allocation algorithms for thigh and waist-worn accelerometers. *Medicine and Science in Sports and Exercise, 48*, 1085–1090. doi:10.1249/MSS.0000000000000865

Ellis, K., Kerr, J., Godbole, G., Staudemeyer, J., & Lanckriet, G. (2016). Hip and wrist accelerometer algorithms for free-living behavior classification. *Medicine and Science in Sports and Exercise, 48*, 933–940.

Esliger, D. W., Rowlands, A. V., Hurst, T. L., Catt, M., Murray, P., & Eston, R. G. (2011). Validation of the GENEA accelerometer. *Medicine and Science in Sports and Exercise, 43*, 1085–1093.

Evenson, K., & Terry, J. W., Jr. (2009). Assessment of differing definitions of accelerometer non-wear time. *Research Quarterly for Exercise and Sport, 80*, 355–362.

Fairclough, S. J., Noonan, R., Rowlands, A. V., van Hees, V., Knowles, Z., & Boddy, L. M. (2016). Wear compliance and activity in children wearing wrist and hip mounted accelerometers. *Medicine and Science in Sports and Exercise, 48*, 243–253. doi:10.1249/MSS.0000000000000771

Fairclough, S. J., Taylor, S., Rowlands A. V., Boddy, L., & Noonan, R. (2019). Average acceleration and intensity gradient of primary school children and associations with indicators of health and wellbeing. *Journal of Sports Sciences, 37*, 2159–2167. doi:10.1080/02640414.2019.1624313

Goldsmith, J., Liu, X., Jacobson, J. S., & Rundle, A. (2016). New insights into activity patterns in children, found using functional data analyses. *Medicine and Science in Sports and Exercise, 48*(9), 1723–1729.

Hildebrand, M., van Hees, V. T., Hansen, B. H., & Ekelund, U. (2014). Age-group comparability of raw accelerometer output from wrist- and hip-worn monitors. *Medicine and Science in Sports and Exercise, 46*, 1816–1824.

Hurter, L., Rowlands, A. V., Fairclough, S. J., Knowles, Z. R., Porcellato, L. A., Cooper, A. M., & Boddy, L. M. (2019). Validating the sedentary sphere method in children: Does wrist or accelerometer brand matter. *Journal of Sport Sciences, 37*. doi:10.1080/02640414.2019.1605647.

Ipsos MORI. (2017). *CLS. Millennium cohort study sixth sweep (MCS6): Physical activity: Time use diary harmonised dataset.* London, UK: Centre for Longitudinal Studies, UCL Institute for Education.

Janssen, I., & LeBlanc, A. G. (2010). Systematic review of the health benefits of physical activity and fitness in school-aged children and youth. *International Journal of Behavioural Nutrition and Physical Activity, 7*, 7–40

John, D., Sasaki, J., Staudenmayer, J., Mavilia, M., & Freedson, P. S. (2013). Comparison of raw acceleration from the GENEA and ActiGraphTM GT3X+ activity monitors. *Sensors, 13*, 14754–14763.

Kerr, J., Patterson, R. E., Ellis, K., Godbole, S., Johnson, E., Lanckriet, G., & Staudenmeyer, J. (2016). Objective assessment of physical activity. *Medicine and Science in Sports and Exercise, 48*, 951–957.

Li, X., Kearney, P. M., Keane, E., Harrington, J. M., & Fitzgerald, A. P. (2017). Levels and sociodemographic correlates of accelerometer-based physical activity in Irish children: A cross-sectional study. *Journal of Epidemiology and Community Health*. doi:10.1136/jech-2016-207691

Mattocks, C., Leary, S., Ness, A., Deere, K., Saunders, J., Kirkby, J. . . . Riddoch, C. (2007). Intraindividual variation of objectively measured physical activity in children. *Medicine and Science in Sports and Exercise, 39*, 622–629.

Merikanto, I., Lahti, T., Puolijoki, H., Vanhala, M., Peltonen, M., Lattikainen, T., . . . Partonen, T. (2013). Associations of chronotype and sleep with cardiovascular diseases and type 2 diabetes. *Chronobiology International, 30*(4), 470–477.

Migueles, J. H., Rowlands, A. V., Huber, F., Sabia, S., & van Hees, V. (2019). GGIR: A research community-driven open-source R-package for generating physical activity and sleep outcomes from multi-day raw accelerometer data. *Journal for the Measurement of Physical Behaviours, 2*, 188–196. doi:10.1123/jmpb.2018-0063

Millard, A. C., Tilling, K. T., Lawlor, D. A., Flach, P. A., & Gaunt, T. R. (2017). Physical activity phenotyping with activity bigrams, and their association with BMI. *International Journal of Epidemiology, 46*, 1857–1860.

Mons, U., Müezzinler, A., Gellert, C., Schottker, B., Abnet, C. C., Bobak, M., . . . Brenner, H. (2015). Impact of smoking and smoking cessation on cardiovascular events and mortality among older adults: Meta-analysis of individual participant data from prospective cohort studies of the CHANCES consortium. *British Medical Journal, 350*, h1551. doi10.1136/bmj.h1551

Mooney, S. J., & Pejaver, V. (2018). Big data in public health: Terminology, machine learning, and privacy. *Annual Review of Public Health, 39*, 95–112.

Nilsson, A., Ekelund, U., Yngve, A., & Sjostrom, M. (2002). Assessing physical activity among children with accelerometers using different time sampling intervals and placements. *Pediatric Exercise Science, 14*, 87–96.

Pavey, T. G., Gilson, N. D., Gomersall, S. R., & Clark, B. (2017). Field evaluation of a random forest classifier for wrist-worn accelerometer data. *Journal of Science and Medicine in Sport, 20*, 75–80. doi:10.1016/j.jsams.2016.06.003

Phan, D. H., Bonnet, S., Guillemaud, R., Castelli, E., & PhamThi, N. Y. (2008). Estimation of respiratory waveform and heart rate using an accelerometer. *Conference Proceedings IEEE Engineering in Medicine and Biology Society, 2008*, 4916–4919.

Phillips, L. R. S., Parfitt, C. G., & Rowlands, A. V. (2012). Calibration of the GENEA accelerometer for assessment of physical activity intensity in children. *Journal of Science and Medicine in Sport, 16*, 124–128.

Physical Activity Guidelines for Americans. (2018) (2nd ed.). Washington, DC: US Department of Health and Human Services. Retrieved November 18, 2018 from https://health.gov/paguidelines/secondedition/pdf/Physical_Activity_Guidelines_2nd_edition.pdf

Price, L., Wyatt, K., Lloyd, J., Abraham, C., Creanor, S., Dean, S., & Hillsdon, M. (2018). Children's compliance with wrist worn accelerometry within a cluster randomised controlled trial: Findings from the healthy lifestyles programme (HeLP) *Pediatric Exercise Science, 30*, 281–287.

Riddoch, C., Mattocks, C., Deere, K., Saunders, J., Kirkby, J., Tilling, K., . . . Ness, A. R. (2007). Objective measurement of levels and patterns of physical activity. *Archives of Disease in Childhood, 92*, 963–969.

Rowlands, A. V. (2007). Accelerometer assessment of physical activity in children: An update. *Pediatric Exercise Science, 19*, 252–266.

Rowlands, A. V. (2018). Moving forward with accelerometer-assessed physical activity: Two strategies to ensure meaningful, interpretable & comparable measures. *Pediatric Exercise Science, 30*, 450–456. doi:10.1123/pes.2018-0201

Rowlands, A. V., Edwardson, C. L., Davies, M. J., Khunti, K., Harrington, D. M., & Yates, T. (2018). Beyond cut-points: Accelerometer metrics that capture the physical activity profile. *Medicine and Science in Sport and Exercise, 50*, 1323–1332. doi:10.1249/MSS.0000000000001561

Rowlands, A. V., Fraysse, F., Catt, M., Stiles, V. H., Stanley, R. M., Eston, R. G., & Olds, T. S. (2015). Comparison of measured acceleration output from accelerometry-based activity monitors. *Medicine and Science in Sports and Exercise, 47*, 201–210. doi:10.1249/MSS.0000000000000394

Rowlands, A. V., Mirkes, E., Yates, T., Clemes, S., Davies, M., Khunti, K., & Edwardson, C. L. (2018). Accelerometer assessed physical activity in epidemiology: Are monitors equivalent? *Medicine and Science in Sport and Exercise, 50*, 257–265. doi:10.1249/MSS.0000000000001435

Rowlands, A. V., Olds, T. S., Hillsdon, M., Pulsford, R., Hurst, T. L., Eston, R. G., . . . Langford, J. (2014). Assessing sedentary behaviour with the GENEActiv: Introducing the sedentary sphere. *Medicine and Science in Sports and Exercise, 46*, 1235–1247. doi:10.1249/MSS.0000000000000224

Rowlands, A. V., Plekhanova, T., Yates, T., Mirkes, E., Davies, M., Khunti, K., & Edwardson, C. E. (2019). Providing a basis for harmonisation of accelerometer-assessed physical activity outcomes across epidemiological datasets. *Journal for the Measurement of Physical Behaviour, 2*, 131–142. doi:10.1123/jmpb.2018-0073

Rowlands, A. V., Sherar, L., Fairclough, S., Yates, T., Edwardson, C. E., Harrington, D. M., . . . Stiles, V. H. (2019). A data-driven, meaningful, easy to interpret, population-independent accelerometer outcome variable for global surveillance. *bioRxiv*, 12 April 2019 doi:10.1101/604694.

Rowlands, A. V., Yates, T., Davies, M., Khunti, K., & Edwardson, C. L. (2016). Raw accelerometer data analysis with GGIR R-package: Does accelerometer brand matter? *Medicine and Science in Sports and Exercise, 48*, 1935–1941.

Rowlands, A. V., Yates, T., Edwardson, C. L., Fairclough, S., Davies, M. J., . . . Stiles, V. H. (2019). Activity intensity, volume & norms: Utility & interpretation of accelerometer metrics. *Medicine and Science in Sports and Exercise*, 51, 2410–2422. doi:10.1249/MSS.0000000000002047

Sabia, S., van Hees, V. T., Shipley, M. J., Trenell, M. I., Hagger-Johnson, G., Elbaz, A., . . . Singh-Manoux, A. (2014). Association between questionnaire- and accelerometer-assessed physical activity: The role of sociodemographic factors. *American Journal of Epidemiology, 179*(6), 781–790. doi:10.1093/aje/kwt330

Sasaki, J. E., Hickey, A., Staudenmayer, J., John, D., Kent, J. A., & Freedson, P. S. (2015). Performance of activity classification algorithms in free-living older adults. *Medicine and Science in Sports and Exercise, 48*, 941–950.

Schneller, M. B., Bentsen, P., Nielsen, G., Brond, J. C., Ried-Larsen, M., Mygind, E., & Schipperijn, J. (2017). Measuring children's physical activity: Compliance using skin-taped accelerometers. *Medicine and Science in Sport and Exercise, 49*(6), 1261–1269.

Scott, J. J., Rowlands, A. V., Cliff, D., Morgan, P. J., Plotnikoff, R. C., & Lubans, D. R. (2017). Comparability and feasibility of wrist- and hip-worn accelerometers in free-living adolescents. *Journal of Science and Medicine in Sport, 20*, 1101–1106. doi:10.1016/j.jsams.2017.04.017

Sherar, L., Griew, P., Esliger, D., Cooper, A. R., Ekelund, U., Judge, K., & Riddoch, C. (2011). International children's accelerometry database (ICAD): Design and methods. *BMC Public Health, 11*, 485. doi:10.1186/1471-2458-11-485

Stewart, T., Narayanan, A., Hedayatrad, L., Neville, J., Mackay, L., & Duncan, S. (2018). A dual-accelerometer system for classifying physical activity in children and adults. *Medicine and Science in Sport and Exercise, 50*, 2595–2602.

Stone, M. R., Rowlands, A. V., Middlebrooke, A. R., Jawis, N. M., & Eston, R. G. (2009). The pattern of physical activity in relation to health outcomes in children. *International Journal of Pediatric Obesity, 4*, 306–315.

Tremblay, M., LeBlanc, A., Kho, M., Saunders, T., Larouche, R., Colley, R., Goldfield, G., & Connor, G. S. (2011). Systematic review of sedentary behaviour and health indicators in school-aged children and youth. *International Journal of Behavioural Nutrition and Physical Activity, 8*(1), 98.

Troiano, R. P., Berrigan, D., Dodd, K. W., Mâsse, L. C., Tilert, T., & McDowell, M. (2008). Physical activity in the United States measured by accelerometer. *Medicine and Science in Sports and Exercise, 40*, 181–188.

Troiano, R. P., McClain, J. J., Brychta, R. J., & Chen, K. Y. (2014). Evolution of accelerometer methods for physical activity research. *British Journal of Sports Medicine, 48*(13), 1019–1023.

van Coervering, P. L., Harnack, K., Schmitz, J. E., Fulton, D. A., & Galuska, S. G. (2005). Feasibility of using accelerometers to measure physical activity in young adolescents. *Medicine and Science in Sports and Exercise, 37*, 867–871.

van Hees, V. (2018). Package 'GGIR'. Raw accelerometer data analysis. Retrieved November 26, 2018 from https://cran.r-project.org/web/packages/GGIR/GGIR.pdf

van Hees, V. T., Fang, Z., Langford, J., Assah, F., Mohammad, A., da Silva, I. C., . . . Brage, S. (2014). Auto-calibration of accelerometer data for free-living physical activity assessment using local gravity and temperature: An evaluation on four continents. *Journal of Applied Physiology, 117*(7), 738–744.

van Hees, V. T., Gorzelniak, L., Dean León, E. C., Eder, M., Pias, M., Taherian, S., . . . Brage, S. (2013). Separating movement and gravity components in an acceleration signal and implications for the assessment of human daily physical activity. *PLoS One, 8*(4), e61691. doi:10.1371/journal.pone.0061691

van Hees, V. T., Renstron, F., Wright, A., Gradmark, A., Catt, M., Chen, K. Y., . . . Franks, P. W. (2011). Estimation of daily energy expenditure in pregnant and non-pregnant women using a wrist-worn triaxial accelerometer. *PLoS One, 6*(7), e22922. doi:10.1371/journal.pone.0022922

van Hees, V. T., Sabia, S., Anderson, K. N., Denton, S. J., Oliver, J., Catt, M., . . . Singh-Manoux, A. (2015). A novel, open access method to assess sleep duration using a wrist-worn accelerometer. *PLoS One, 10*(11), e0142533. doi:10.1371/journal.pone.0142533 van Kuppevelt, D., Heywood, J., Hamer, M., Sabia, S., Fitzsimons, E., & van Hees, V. (2019). Segmenting accelerometer data from daily life with unsupervised machine learning. *PLoS One, 14*(1), e0208692. doi:10.1371/journal.pone.0208692

Wake, M., Clifford, S., York, E., Mensah, F., Gold, L. C., Burgner, D., . . . Zubrick, S. R. (2014). Introducing growing up in Australia's child health CheckPoint: A physical and biomarkers module for the longitudinal study of Australian children. *Family Matters, 94*, 15–23.

Welk, G. J., McClain, J., & Ainsworth, B. E. (2012). Protocols for evaluating equivalency of accelerometry-based activity monitors. *Medicine and Science in Sports and Exercise, 44*, S39–S49.

Westerterp, K. (1999). Physical activity assessment with accelerometers. *International Journal of Obesity, 23*, S45–S49.

White, T., Westgate, K., Wareham, N., & Brage, S. (2016). Estimation of physical activity energy expenditure during free-living from wrist accelerometry in UK adults. *PLoS One, 11*(12), e0167472. doi:10.1371/journal.pone.0167472

Wolff-Hughes, D. L., Bassett, D. R., & Fitzhugh, E. C. (2014). Population-referenced percentiles for waist-worn accelerometer-derived total activity counts in U.S. youth: 2003–2006 NHANES. *PLoS One, 9*(12), e115915. doi:10.1371/journal.pone.0115915

Wolff-Hughes, D. L., Fitzhugh, E. C., Bassett D. R., & Churilla, J. R. (2015). Waist-worn actigraphy: Population-referenced percentiles for total activity counts in U.S. adults. *Journal of Physical Activity and Health, 12*(4), 447–453.

World Health Organization. (2018). Global action plan on physical activity 2018–2030: More active people for a healthier world. Geneva: World Health Organization. Licence: CC BY-NC-SA 3.0 IGO. Retrieved November 25, 2018 from http://apps.who.int/iris/bitstream/handle/10665/272722/978924151 4187-eng.pdf

Zhang, S., Rowlands, A. V., Murray, P., & Hurst, T. L. (2012). Physical activity classification using the GENEA wrist-worn accelerometer. *Medicine and Science in Sports and Exercise, 44*, 742–748.

17

NEW PERSPECTIVES THROUGH EMERGING TECHNOLOGIES

Cain C. T. Clark, Maria Cristina Bisi, and Rita Stagni

Introduction

Since Galenus (129–201 AC, physician and philosopher in the Roman Empire) approached the study of physical exercise and training of gladiators, classifying muscles and their function in his *De Motu Musclorum*, the assessment of motor activity and physical function has been the object of innumerate applied research. Great minds such as Leonardo da Vinci (1452–1519), with his study of limb motion, and Galileo Galilei (1564–1642), in his *De Animalium Motibus*, opened the path to the systematic study of human motion, while Borelli, in his *De Motu Animalium* (1680; Figure 17.1), was the first to apply a traditionally biological topic to the rigorous analytic method developed by Galileo.

From a scientific perspective, the assessment of motor activity entails the definition and measurement of objective descriptors (e.g. number of repetitions, durations, distances, angles), intended to characterize function, and the essential introduction of objective measurement tools demonstrated its disruptive potential since the pioneering studies by Etienne-Jules Marey (1830–1904, physiologist and inventor) and Eadweard James Muybridge (1830–1904, photographer): their chrono-photogrammetric method exploited the innovation of the time in photographic technology to quantify, for the first time, segmental kinematics of living subjects during the execution of different motor tasks and is considered the starting point of modern quantitative motion analysis (Figure 17.2a and b).

Ever since, a number of different tools and approaches have been exploited to further develop and integrate the quantitative assessment of human motion, from the simple use of paper stripes and inked feet for the quantification of step and stride length, and chronographers for speed, to the more advanced technological solutions allowed by the spread use of personal computers in the early 1980s. The progressive advances in the field of electronics and computer sciences, together with the concurrent reduction of costs, led, in the following decades from the first two camera stereophotogrammetric systems, for the automatic quantification of segmental kinematics, to the most advanced modern systems integrating multiple cameras together with several other measurement devices such as load cells and platforms for the quantification of reaction forces, electromyography for muscle activity, pressure insoles, and many others.

Nowadays, integrated motion analysis systems have reached a high technological level and simplicity of use, becoming a *de facto* standard for the detailed and accurate quantification of human motion in laboratory conditions. They are extensively used for the characterization of motor alterations, the design and evaluation of clinical interventions, and the monitoring of the follow-up in specific pathological conditions (e.g. arthritis, stroke, cerebral palsy, Parkinson disease), as well

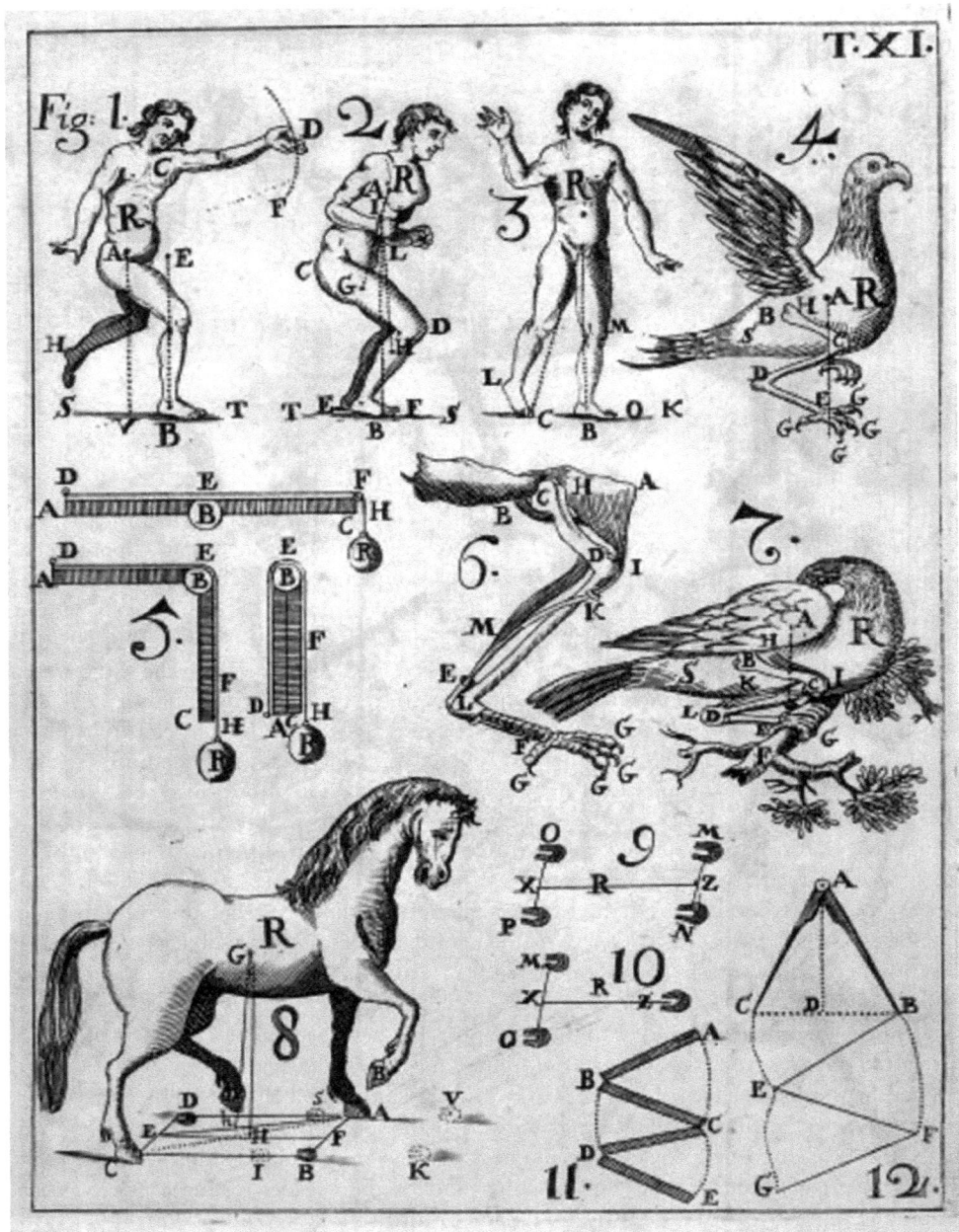

Figure 17.1   Giovanni Alfonso Borelli, *De Motu Animalium*

as for the evaluation of performance, the optimization of training, and the prevention of injuries in sport applications.

Despite the valuable quantitative information provided by these systems, their use remains limited to laboratory, or, at least, to controlled environment conditions, while the assessment of motor activity and performance is expected to describe what people do in real life.

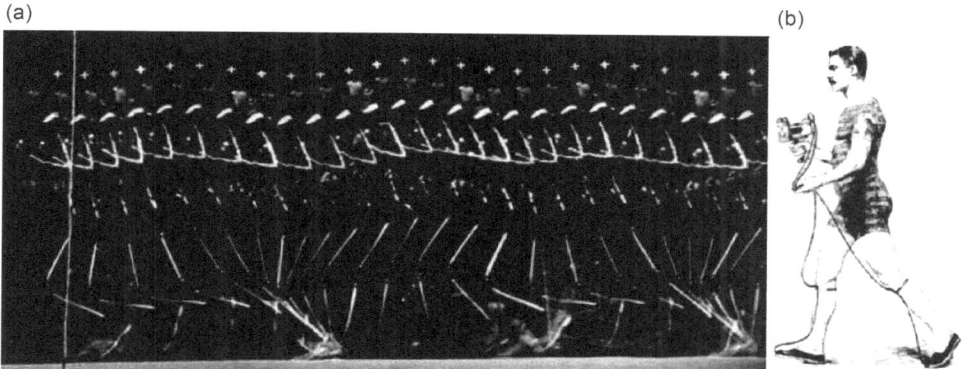

Figure 17.2 (a) Chrono-photogrammetry (E. J. Marey and E. J. Muybridge). (b) Device for the quantification of foot pressure (E. J. Marey)

The technological solution required to respond to this need must:

- be un–obstructive and self–contained, not to alter the natural performance of motor activities in real life conditions;
- allow long recordings with sufficient sampling frequency, to guarantee an appropriate description of motion and take into account physiological variability;
- be simple to use and low-cost, to support extensive assessment by non-technical operators in different contexts.

Despite the several attempts to produce measurement systems with these characteristics in the past decades (e.g. portable systems integrating electro-goniometers, foot switches, pressure insoles, and/or electromyography), none of them actually satisfied all the aforementioned requirements. Only in recent years, the disruptive development of mobile technologies provided the first effective response to the need for pervasive real-time motor assessment.

Wireless wearable sensors have become available on the market, ready to be exploited in a number of technological solutions aiming at the quantitative assessment of motor activity and performance. Among these, magneto-inertial measurement units have certainly gained a key role, providing miniaturized measurement units integrated in minimally invasive setups (i.e. a single wireless tri-axial sensor or a small network, mounted on bands or straps, with integrated power supply and data transmission), allowing the measurement and recording of real-time orientation, angular velocity, and acceleration of body segments in free environment. They have found application for different types of motion analysis assessment, from activity monitoring to traditional motion analysis, also opening the path to novel approaches to the objective assessment of motor control. In addition to this, an innovation coming from the gaming industry (Kinect, Microsoft) has served motion analysis researchers with the first low-cost video-based solution allowing the automatic reconstruction of segmental kinematics not requiring the placement of any markers on the analyzed subject.

All these novel emerging technologies have readily found application and have the breaking potential of priming a new era in the field of motor assessment. They certainly have the advantage of providing informative, quantitative data for the application of traditional approaches, reducing workload in terms of time, improving inter- and intra-rater reliability, enabling systematic analysis and objective evaluation of concurring factors, facilitating population classification, characterization, and longitudinal monitoring; but they are also opening the path to novel perspectives in the objective assessment of motion, as for the evidence-based characterization of specific aspects of motor control and development.

As exciting as the potential provided by these innovative technological tools can appear, its effective deployment to applied research requires a certain level of critical awareness; specific advantages and the possible limitations have to be considered to support the informed selection of the most suitable solution for each specific application. Different technological solutions have become available for certain types of assessment, and, on the other hand, the same devices can be exploited for different applications using different computational approaches.

Far from aiming to be conclusive, this chapter is intended to provide a synthetic overview of the broad and developing landscape of novel technological solutions for the measurement and assessment of youth physical activity (PA). Considering the continuous on-going advances in the field, the authors want to provide a schematic scope-oriented outline of the possible solutions, the basic references supporting further specific in-depth analysis, highlighting key advantages and limitations.

Overview of the Literature

Given the number of technological solutions proposed and available for the quantitative assessment of motor activity, they have been organized in a scope-oriented schematic outline in Tables 17.1 and 17.2, to summarize and organize the key concepts and terms, and introduce basic references. In particular, Table 17.1 outlines solutions proposed for quantitative activity monitoring, considering both product- and process-oriented approaches, while Table 17.2 refers to quantitative motion analysis, which is a detailed process-oriented description of specific motor tasks.

Activity Monitoring

Process-oriented assessment is considered an important tool in the development of youth PA programs, motor competence, and indeed physical development. Problematically, traditional assessments of child motor competence and PA have been conducted with either direct observation, or accelerometers, in the case of the latter. Technological development has progressed to a point where multi-disciplinary teams are utilizing engineering-based tools or analyses, applied to human movement, and while in its infancy, promising developments have prompted novel perspectives. In Barnes, Clark, Rees, Stratton, and Summers (2018), a magnetometer, which measures magnetism – either the magnetization of a magnetic material like a ferromagnet, or the direction, strength, or relative change of a magnetic field at a given location, affixed to the dominant wrist on children (10–12 years), was worn during a motor competence assessment. The raw signal output was treated with novel analytical techniques, namely Dynamic time warping (DTW), which enables two signals to be artificially matched (i.e. where children complete identical tasks but over a shorter or longer time-frame), facilitating direct comparison between signals, or, in this case, children, removing time-based discrepancies. Pairwise comparison across a cohort produces a similarity matrix of all child to child correlations. Visualization of the relative performance in three-dimensions, using multi-dimensional scaling of the similarity matrix, shows a 'performance sphere' (Barnes et al., 2018) in which children sit on concentric shells of increasing radius as performance deteriorates. The relative distance between children within the multi-dimensional scaling can then be used to create an automated sensor-based rank scoring. This technique was also shown to provide 'product' assessments; by reducing the dimensionality, removing process measures, product can be efficaciously plotted against time (Barnes et al., 2018). Further work highlighting our potential to assess process-oriented measures was demonstrated by Xiao and Menon (2014), who utilized a force sensitive resistor, and applied it to the upper extremities to

Table 17.1 Activity monitoring

Scope	Target	Target variable	Technology	Computational approach
Activity monitoring	Product	Space parameters	Magnetometer (Barnes et al., 2018)	Dynamic time warping; cross-correlation (Barnes et al., 2018)
	Process	Space parameters; time parameters	Magnetometer (Barnes et al., 2018); force sensitive resistor (Xiao & Menon, 2014)	Dynamic time warping (Barnes et al., 2018); contour mapping (Barnes et al., 2018); extreme learning machine classifier (Xiao & Menon, 2014)
	Daily living	Visual; time parameters; space parameters	Electrooculography (Bulling et al., 2011); gyroscope (Leutheuser et al., 2013); Radio frequency identification (Spinney et al., 2015)	Support vector machine (Bulling et al., 2011; Leutheuser et al., 2013); *k*-Nearest Neighbor classifier (Leutheuser et al., 2013); classification and regression tree (Leutheuser et al., 2013); linear correction (Spinney et al., 2015)
	PA intensities	Visual; tangible; frequency parameters	Magnetometer (Crossley et al., 2018); 3D printing (Khot et al., 2014); micro-electromechanical system (Clark et al., 2016, 2017)	Vector of dynamic body acceleration (Crossley et al., 2018); visual inspection (Crossley et al., 2018); arithmetic mean (Khot et al., 2014); spectral density (Clark et al., 2016, 2017); Fourier transformation (Clark et al., 2016, 2017)
	PA type/characterization	Time parameters; space parameters; visual	Heart rate + calorimeter (Duncan et al., 2011); video sensor (Loveday et al., 2016; Zhang et al., 2011); force sensitive resistor (Fulk & Sazonov, 2011); inclinometer (Crouter et al., 2018)	Feature extraction (Duncan et al., 2011); machine learning (Duncan et al., 2011); good features detector (Zhang et al., 2011); binary coding (Loveday et al., 2016); support vector machine (Fulk & Sazonov, 2011); feature extraction (Crouter et al., 2018)
	Global position	Space parameters	Wi-Fi real-time locating system (Loveday et al., 2016); global positioning system (Holliday et al., 2017); Wi-Fi + accelerometer (Kjaergaard et al., 2012)	Proximity (Loveday et al., 2016); location features detector (Holliday et al., 2017); hierarchical cluster analysis (Kjaergaard et al., 2012)

Definitions: *Magnetometer*: a device measuring the direction, strength, or relative change of a magnetic field at a given location; terrestrial magnetic field is usually assumed as reference. *Force sensitive resistor*: a material whose resistance changes when a force, pressure, or mechanical stress is applied. *Electrooculography*: a device for measuring the corneo–retinal standing potential that exists *between* the front and the back of the human eye. *Gyroscope*: a device used for measuring or maintaining orientation and angular velocity. *Radio frequency identification*: the use of electromagnetic fields to automatically identify and track tags attached to objects. *3D printing*: is where material is joined or solidified under computer control to create a 3D object. *Micro-electromechanical system*: microscopic devices merged at the nano-scale. *Calorimeter*: an object or device used for calorimetry, or the process of measuring the heat of chemical reactions or physical changes as well as heat capacity. *Inclinometer*: an instrument used for measuring angles of slope, elevation, or depression of an object with respect to gravity's direction. *Wi-Fi Real-time locating system*: uses a wireless network to automatically identify and track the location of objects or people in real time, usually within a building or other contained area. *Global positioning system*: a system that uses satellites to provide autonomous geo-spatial positioning. *Accelerometer*: a device which measures the acceleration of a body in its own instantaneous rest frame.

Table 17.2 Motion analysis

Scope	Task	Target	Target variables	Technology	Computational approach
Motion analysis	Gait	Gait events (foot contact and toe-off) and temporal parameters (stride, step, stance, swing time)	Acceleration; angular velocity; plantar pressure	*Wearable:* accelerometers (Caldas, Mundt, Potthast, Buarque de Lima Neto, & Markert, 2017; Pacini Panebianco, Bisi, Stagni, & Fantozzi, 2018; Taborri, Palermo, Rossi, & Cappa, 2016); gyroscopes (Caldas et al., 2017; Pacini Panebianco et al., 2018; Taborri et al., 2016); Foot switches (Taborri et al., 2016); foot pressure insoles (Taborri et al., 2016) *Non wearable:* markerless 2D video camera (Castelli, Paolini, Cereatti, & Della Croce, 2015; Verlekar, Soares, & Correia, 2018); Kinect (Latorre, Llorens, Colomer, & Alcañiz, 2018)	*Wearable:* peak identification (Pacini Panebianco et al., 2018); threshold identification(Pacini Panebianco et al., 2018; Taborri et al., 2016); artificial intelligence (Caldas et al., 2017); machine learning (Taborri et al., 2016) *Non wearable:* 2D markerless technique(Castelli et al., 2015); Kinect-based methods (Latorre et al., 2018)
		Kinematics	Joint angles	*Wearable:* IMUs (Caldas et al., 2017; Picerno, 2017; Teufl, Miezal, Taetz, Fröhlich, & Bleser, 2018) *Non wearable:* markerless 2D video cameras (Colyer, Evans, Cosker, & Salo, 2018); depth-sensing cameras (narrow-baseline binocular-stereo camera systems or active cameras) (Colyer et al., 2018)	*Wearable:* artificial intelligence (Caldas et al., 2017); sensor fusion (Teufl et al., 2018) *Non wearable:* machine learning; generative or discriminative algorithms (Colyer et al., 2018)
		Motor control performance	Variability structure of trunk/limb kinematics	*Wearable:* IMUs (Stergiou, 2016) *Non wearable:* markerless 2D video camera (Verlekar et al., 2018)	*Wearable:* nonlinear measures of human motion (Stergiou, 2016) *Non wearable:* markerless 2D video camera (Verlekar et al., 2018)
	Posture	Postural sway parameters	Trunk sway (acceleration and displacement)	Accelerometer (Mancini et al., 2012; Palmerini, Rocchi, Mellone, Valzania, & Chiari, 2011)	Frequency domain and time domain analysis (Mancini et al., 2012; Palmerini et al., 2011)
	Other tasks of daily living	Space–time parameters; joint kinematics; body segment kinematics	Joint angles; foot contacts; time events	IMUs (Bergmann, Mayagoitia, & Smith, 2009, 2010; Camomilla, Bergamini, Fantozzi, & Vannozzi, 2018; El-Gohary et al., 2013; Filippeschi et al., 2017; Fino, Frames, & Lockhart, 2015)	Computational approaches applied to the different gait target variables

Definitions – Foot switch: a pressure sensor used to detect on-off of ground contact of specific points under the foot. IMU: Inertial measurement unit, a device integrating a 3D accelerometer and a 3D gyroscope.

analyze force myographic signals of the forearm. The authors were able to accurately identify upper extremity movements during a controlled drinking task (92% accuracy). Xiao and Menon (2014) also utilized a form of machine learning to learn and classify the data, an extreme learning machine (ELM) classifier, where a training approach was taken, where the ELM classifier was 'taught' or 'trained' to model the force myography trace.

Daily Living

Developments have not only ensued for short-term, acute bouts of activity. Technological advancement and integration have facilitated novel perspectives into daily free-living activities. Bulling, Ward, and Gellersen (2011) reported an accuracy of 76% when identifying activities such as text copying, reading a printed paper, taking hand-written notes, watching a video, and browsing the web. The authors assert that recording the movements of human eyes, otherwise termed '*electrooculography*', can successfully be used to identify certain activities and may be feasible in wider applications such as accurately identifying non-traditional activities (e.g. rock climbing), which would inherently be missed by common sensing modalities. However, while promising, further investigations to corroborate the effectiveness of this technique are required in order to up-scale this technology. The application of cameras, in different forms, to characterize activity has demonstrated variable success when complemented with novel analyses. Leutheuser, Schuldhaus, and Eskofier (2013) utilized machine learning, in combination with feature extraction, on gyroscopic data and could correctly identify basic free-living PAs with up to 89.6% accuracy. The use of machine learning with gyroscopic signals appears to allow identification of specific movements with high accuracy. However, at present activity classification using this method appears to only be able to identify basic movements. Notwithstanding potential drawbacks, when integrated with more traditional sensor-based devices (e.g. accelerometers), the limitations of this approach are somewhat ameliorated (Leutheuser et al., 2013). Further evidence exists, not only in the form of wearables, but rather, 'nearables'; Spinney, Smith, Ucci, Fisher, and Konstantatou (2015) used Radio frequency identification (RFID) to successfully demonstrate patterns of PA, standing, and sitting by office workers. This study highlighted the relationship between location, light PA, and sitting, across multiple office environments, and although preliminary, the explanatory power of the technique is promising.

Physical Activity Intensities

Magnetometers have not only been applied in the assessment of process-based metrics, but preliminary studies in children have shown them to be useful in the assessment of turning, or altering direction (Crossley et al., 2018). Recently, it has been suggested that turning is power intensive, and given the sporadic and irregular movement patterns of children may be an important consideration for PA assessment. Crossley et al. (2018) first highlighted significantly higher energy expenditure when the angle and speed of turn were increased, and then demonstrated that magnetometry can be used to highlight where and when such turns take place. By incorporating accelerometry with novel technology (i.e. magnetometry), the additional energy expenditure as a result of turning can be taken into consideration. Additional wearable-based technology, in the form of micro-electromechanical system (MEMS) devices such as accelerometers or magnetometers that are microscopic fabrications, has shown promise in the assessment of PA intensities. MEMS devices were applied in either a controlled fitness test (Clark, Barnes, Holton, Summers, & Stratton, 2016) or in free-play (Clark et al., 2017), in children aged 3–11 years. The novel, microscopic technology was complemented with novel analytical procedures, where Fourier transformations facilitated the use of the frequency domain (as opposed to traditional time–space), in addition to hierarchical clustering of metrics. The resultant technology-analytics combination demonstrated that frequency-based metrics cluster with motor competence and PA levels (Clark et al., 2017) is indicative, and potentially predictive, of physical fitness (Clark et al., 2016). Novel wearable technology has been showcased to provide novel insights; however, 'tangible' technology has been shown to not only measure and enhance PA, but also improve knowledge and understanding of personal activity levels (Crossley, McNarry, Eslambolchilar, Knowles, & Mackintosh, 2019; Khot, Hjorth, & Floyd, 2014), where the Precaution Adoption Process Model (Weinstein, 1988), from the Stages of Change (Prochaska & DiClemente, 1992), suggests that an individual is unlikely to proceed to the contemplation stage unless they become aware that their behaviors are inadequate. Khot et al. (2014) advocate a novel approach for representing PA in the form of material, 3D printed, artifacts, where a 3D printing device was located in households and manufactured 3D 'print-outs' of corresponding heart rate data. This novel contribution of this work is the first to highlight a conceptual understanding of the relationship between material representations and PA, and is promising, given the suitability of being located across households, rather than research labs, potentially reducing participant burden. Further work, by Crossley et al. (2019), has also reported that, when supplied with 3D representations of PA, children and adolescents are able to identify whether they did or did not meet, or how close they were to meeting PA guidelines, and encouraged a healthier, more active lifestyle.

Physical Activity Characterization/Type

A further example of instruments used when attempting to characterize human movement with novel analytics is force sensitive resistors, which contains a material whose resistance changes when a force, pressure, or mechanical stress is applied. Fulk and Sazonov (2011), for example, mounted the device in the footwear of participants to measure plantar pressure and record the acceleration signal, thereby inferring postural activity in stroke victims. The raw signal from the device was analyzed using a support vector machine, which is a supervised machine learning technique that can use training examples to learn the dependencies in the data. The computer was taught how the signals from the sensors can predict postural activities, and the learned model was then applied to the recognition of previously unseen data (Fulk & Sazonov, 2011). Across all participants, accuracy in identifying postural activity of 99%–100% was found, indicating that with a modest sample size, and applying the combination of acceleration and pressure traces, postures may confidently be assessed. Conversely, when focusing more broadly on inferring activity type, and not specifically falls or basic movement, Duncan, Lester, and Migotsky (2011) achieved 97% accuracy in the assessment of walking and running in the laboratory and 84% accuracy in the field, using feature recognition. This particular method appears to be increasingly successful when energy expenditure assessment is combined, in order to infer activity type, rather than the accelerometer signal alone. However, once field testing was performed, the accuracy falls by 13 percentage points, indicating reliability issues outside of a controlled setting, and highlights the need for more robust machine learning techniques to be developed for free-living activity.

So far, novel technology has been showcased in the form of MEMS, 3D printing, force sensitive resistors, RFID, gyroscopes, and magnetometers. A further novel technology being pioneered in the assessment of PA in children is inclinometers that measure angles of slope, elevation, or depression of an object with respect to gravity's direction. Crouter, Hibbing, and LaMunion (2018) demonstrated, in a comprehensive evaluation of time spent in sedentary behaviors, utilizing inclinometers, accelerometers, and indirect calorimetry, that inclinometers can facilitate precise estimates of sedentary behavior during free-living activity in youth.

Global Position

Up to this point in the chapter, it is clear that refining and developing emerging technologies should remain a strong focus, so that adequate levels of accuracy and confidence may be established and further improved upon. Moreover, it is clear that the technologies and techniques by which PA can be measured will continue to proliferate. Cluster analysis has been utilized for the assessment of frequency-based metrics for microscopic technology (Clark et al., 2016, 2017). This analytical technique involves the use of algorithms to separate a population into clusters or groups based on various parameters such as activity behaviors. Kjaergaard, Wirz, and Roggen (2012) employed the same analytical protocol, yet focused on group activity, rather than individual activity, using 'flock detection' (i.e. multiple persons forming a cohesive whole) and Wi-Fi signals to identify and track pedestrian flocks with 87% accuracy. While the novel application of this technology is promising, problems emerged regarding flock proximity (i.e. the ability of the cluster analysis to successfully differentiate between flocks was encumbered when various groups become entwined or proximity was too high). This indicates that the mathematical modeling process applied to the novel technology requires further refinement.

The importance of location-based information, to better inform PA, has recently come to the fore, whether that be restricted to specific locations, such as an office, or wider. Holliday et al. (2017) sought to highlight necessary wear time for global positioning system devices. They demonstrated that in general, minutes of all PA intensities spent in a given location could be measured with over 80% reliability, including fitness facilities, schools, and footpaths (Holliday et al., 2017). However, in order to accurately monitor location-based activity in parks and roads, a wear time minimum of 5 days is required, and PA assessment in homes and commercial areas necessitates over 19 days of monitoring to yield accurate results (Holliday et al., 2017). Furthermore, this approach for the assessment of free-living PA in youth is likely feasible as current, global surveillance practices already utilize multi-day accelerometry, for example, the National Health and Nutrition Examination Survey (NHANES) in the United States (Freedson & John, 2013), Brazilian birth cohorts (da Silva et al., 2014), the Growing Up in Australia's Child Health Checkpoint (Wake et al., 2014), and Biobank investigations in the United Kingdom (http://www.ukbiobank.ac.uk/about-biobank-uk/). Moreover, numerous accelerometers include global positioning attachments, compatibility or in-built functionality, which represents the opportunity for a relatively straightforward adoption.

Finally, global position work in the form of Wi-Fi real-time locating systems, showcased in Loveday, Sherar, Sanders, Sanderson, and Esliger (2016), can be used to enable remote assessment of intervention adherence. The proximity-based assessment indicated that office workers may spend a proportion of working hours outside of their office. This, evidently, has implications for assessing the efficacy of office-based environmental interventions, and could be extended to children's time spent in classrooms, and adherence to location-based interventions. This novel technology may provide more robust means of assessing intervention efficacy, as opposed to comparatively time consumptive, participant burdensome, and inaccurate self-report measures. Although refinement and development are clearly necessary, the adoption of novel technologies will provide researchers with a more complete understanding of PA behaviors than has previously been available.

Video-Based

While actigraphy-based sensors have become the *de facto* tool for the objective assessment of PA, the use of other sensors (i.e. cameras, force sensitive resistors, electrooculography) to achieve the same or advancing outcomes has grown. It is evident that the aim of many emerging analytical technologies and techniques has been to aid in better detecting the quality and type of activity that a person is undertaking. Zhang, Li, and Jia (2011) incorporated motion cameras to automatically recognize patterns of movement, albeit in young adults, and demonstrated that basic motor movements could be recognized with 85% accuracy. Notwithstanding this promising accuracy, Zhang et al. (2011) asserted that this upper limit of accuracy could be an artifact of the device, as acquired images are often blurry and ineffective in capturing feature points, which may be an inherent limitation of cameras. Furthermore, contemporary work has also demonstrated that wearable cameras can be used to assess children's PA and behavior recall (Everson, Mackintosh, McNarry, Todd, & Stratton, 2019). However, particularly with respect to children and adolescents, wearable cameras carry some ethical and technical challenges; as Everson et al. (2019) highlighted, parents and children reported that wearable cameras are burdensome and invade privacy.

Further vision-based approaches for the assessment of PAs have been showcased by Loveday et al. (2016). While there is a plethora of reasons for the prevalence of sedentary behaviors, a possible contributing factor to our lack of intervention success is the current lack of behavioral context offered by accelerometers and posture sensors. Utilizing concurrent electrical energy monitoring and wearable cameras as measures of television viewing, Loveday et al. (2016) found that, on average, televisions were switched on for 202 minutes per day, yet only visible in just 90 minutes of wearable camera images with a further ~50 minutes where the participant is in their living room, but the television is not visible in the image. The authors highlighted that the high number of un-codable images from the wearable cameras (deployed on a lanyard or fixed to clothing) may therefore not be conducive to a reliable measure of television viewing. In order to counteract this limitation, the method of camera affixation, and therefore resultant field of view, must be acutely considered, but remains a promising novel technology in the assessment of PAs.

Within the same study, Loveday et al. (2016) utilized indoor monitoring with the same video monitors, to assess where individuals accumulated their sedentary time. Utilizing this novel technology and approach, quantifying time spent in specific rooms or communal areas becomes a realistic accomplishment. Given the potential, it would be advantageous to investigate the utility of this technology in settings that may offer more location possibilities with populations such as children and adolescents, who are likely to spend their time in varied locations.

Motion Analysis

Human motion analysis, with particular reference to the evaluation of gait, was traditionally process oriented, aiming at the quantitative assessment of joint kinematics and kinetics in time, to be compared with reference normality patterns for biomechanical analysis, diagnosis, and/or follow-up evaluation. Gait analysis is extensively used for the quantitative assessment of motor function in basic research as well as clinical and sport applications. The traditional implementation of motion analysis relies on laboratory instrumentation, stereophotogrammetry and force platforms being just the basic laboratory setup, but the availability of inertial measurement units (IMUs) rapidly gained a primary role for the ecological assessment out of the lab. Wearable, cheap, and self-contained, IMUs are now extensively exploited for the ambulatory evaluation of gait, as described through spatio-temporal parameters, joint kinematics, as well as newly proposed metrics for characterization of the underlying motor control (e.g. variability, stability, complexity, automaticity).

Spatio-Temporal Parameters (IMUs)

Gait timing is considered of primary importance for the characterization of gait alterations. The quantification of gait temporal parameters (GTP) (i.e. step and stance times) requires, first of all, to identify gait events (GE) (i.e. heel strike and toe off). GE can be estimated from measurements obtained using various portable sensing technologies such as foot switches, pressure insoles (in both cases identifying when the contact pressure under a specific area of the foot crosses a certain threshold), and IMUs. In particular, segment angular velocity and acceleration as quantified by IMUs led to the need for appropriate gait segmentation methods (Taborri, Palermo, Rossi, & Cappa, 2016) and to the development of a number of algorithms. These were proposed and applied in different conditions, exploiting different sensor positions, analyzing different variables, with different computational approaches. Recently, Pacini Panebianco et al. (2018) analyzed all these different implementation characteristics, highlighting how all these factors affect GE and GTP estimation. No proposed algorithm is generally preferred over the others, and specific characteristics have to be taken into account based on the experimental conditions (e.g. number/type/placement of sensors) and research questions (e.g. mean/variability of the selected gait variable).

Kinematics (IMUs)

Body-worn IMUs were also proposed for the estimation of segment orientation and joint angular kinematics (Picerno, 2017; Teufl et al., 2018). Using sensor fusion algorithms (e.g. variations of the Kalman filter or optimization-based methods (Teufl et al., 2018) or artificial intelligence methods (Caldas et al., 2017), it is possible to estimate the IMU's orientation in reference to a global coordinate system (Picerno, 2017; Teufl et al., 2018). Combining more IMUs attached to linked body segments, it is possible to estimate the joint kinematics of the specified segments. Commercially available solutions usually provide a 3D sensor's orientation or even protocols for estimating 3D joint kinematics during gait. In this case, the user must be aware of the issues related to ferromagnetic disturbances, to sensor-to-segment alignment, and to the proprietary sensor fusion algorithm's accuracy when estimating the 3D sensor's orientation.

The drawbacks concerning IMU systems when measuring human motion are mainly that IMU-based orientation estimation suffers from drift due to the integration of 'noisy' gyroscope measurements, and that the incorporation of magnetometer measurements is typically based on the assumption of a homogeneous magnetic field, which is often violated (Teufl et al., 2018). The main approaches (Picerno, 2017) proposed in literature for drift correction are (1) kinematical reset or sensor fusion, (2) by using a mixed approach of the two previous methodologies, and (3) by using neural network prediction. These approaches have been proven efficient in particular for the evaluation of low-frequency cycling gestures like walking. For the second limitation, there are efforts to develop methods for handling magnetic disturbances or completely omit magnetometer data but still no gold standard method has been identified because environmental settings are unpredictable and not very standardizable from this point of view.

Other Tasks

Similarly, wearable sensing supports the quantitative assessment of other non-gait human daily tasks (e.g. posture, stairs, turns), with the aim of assessing and defining the functional status of a person. Quantitative measures of (process) task performance, mainly proposed and used for clinical purposes (El-Gohary et al., 2013; Fino et al., 2015; Mancini et al., 2012; Palmerini et al., 2011), can be applied in several different contexts (e.g. for monitoring how personal postural oscillations vary during the day, after sports, and in relation to tiredness). For example, if static posture is accurately recognized during daily activities, a number of quantitative measures could characterize the quality of the postural oscillations, by means of one accelerometer positioned on the trunk. These measures allow quantification of postural displacement, acceleration, and, if of interest, tremor (e.g. in participants with Parkinson disease (Mancini et al., 2012; Palmerini et al., 2011)).

Continuous monitoring of turning, in terms of anatomical joint angles (El-Gohary et al., 2013), and type of turns (turning on the ipsilateral or on the contralateral turn, respectively) (Fino et al., 2015) during spontaneous daily activities were proposed to help clinicians and patients determining who is at risk of falls and could benefit from preventative intervention. A similar approach has been proposed for assessing the quality of stair ascent, allowing the identification of GE (initial contacts) (Bergmann et al., 2010) and lower limb joint angles (Bergmann et al., 2009). Last but not least, it is possible to focus on upper limb movement, in order to track and assess the quality of upper limb joint kinematics during the day (Filippeschi et al., 2017).

The earlier tasks are only some of the possible examples. By extracting classic biomechanical parameters (Camomilla et al., 2018), or developing specific algorithms for assessing limb coordination (Bisi, Pacini Panebianco, Polman, & Stagni, 2017) based on body segment acceleration/angular velocities, an automatic evaluation of subjective performance during PA and/or specific motor tasks is possible (e.g. for children's motor competence assessment (Bisi, Tamburini, Pacini Panebianco, & Stagni, 2018; Grimpampi, Masci, Pesce, & Vannozzi, 2016; Masci et al., 2013; Masci, Vannozzi, Getchell, & Cappozzo, 2012)).

Video-Based Motion Analysis

Recently, vision-based motion analysis methods within sports and rehabilitation applications have evolved substantially thanks to innovative (markerless) techniques developed primarily for entertainment purposes. This allowed biomechanical research to contribute a vast amount of meaningful information in sports and rehabilitation applications (Colyer et al., 2018). Literature shows that some of these systems are capable of measuring sagittal plane angles to within 2°–3° during walking gait (Colyer et al., 2018). However, accuracy requirements vary across different scenarios and the validity of markerless systems has yet to be fully established across different movements in varying environments.

The four major components of a markerless motion capture system are (1) the camera systems that are used, (2) the representation of the human body (the body model), (3) the image features used, and (4) the algorithms used to determine the parameters (shape, pose, location) of the body model (Colyer et al., 2018). Body pose on a given image is inferred by algorithms, which can be classified as 'generative' or 'discriminative': generative algorithms use model parameters to generate a hypothesis that is evaluated against image data and then iteratively refined to determine a best possible fit; discriminative algorithms start from image data to directly infer model parameters (Colyer et al., 2018).

Each of these components has limitations and, depending on the specific implementation choice, influences the final accuracy and validity of the reconstructed motion data. Accuracy evaluation, performed by comparing kinematic output variables obtained by markerless system and by marker-based optoelectronic ones, was mostly evaluated on slow movements (typically walking gait), highlighting that transverse plane rotations are currently difficult to extract accurately and reliably by markerless technologies. To verify the utility of these approaches in PA applications, much quicker movements need still to be thoroughly assessed.

Key and Emerging Issues

Activity Monitoring

Research into PA is expanding to incorporate a multitude of different technologies and analytical techniques, and within each approach exists a series of constraints that must be considered. This chapter has identified an array of technological developments, showcasing high accuracies across

PA measurement, with success in activity classification, success in identifying global position, success in quantifying intensity of movements, and even daily living, all while using various wearable, nearable, or tangible technology.

Notwithstanding, the application of such novel technology remains in its infancy; many of the studies were exploratory, under-powered, or require further development to establish reliable, accurate measures across larger samples, and this raises a number of key and emerging issues. Based on the findings highlighted in Table 17.1, four key issues were emergent, with reference to activity monitoring: (1) developing performance, reliability, and constraints, (2) scaling up of datasets/sample size, (3) utilization of interventionist study designs, and (4) integration of technologies.

First, an important consideration when classifying data is that large datasets obtained through novel sensing units will result in multiple features, which necessitates time-consuming data analysis, and may significantly impact the classification methods. In fact, large feature sets may need huge datasets for training computational methods that could be unavailable (the so-called 'curse of dimensionality') and, notwithstanding, would slow down the development of the classification system. This issue of developing the performance, reliability, and constraints from novel technology is exacerbated by the relatively small sample sizes currently recruited, given that a number of participants' data is often 'withheld' to 'train' appropriate analytical frameworks.

Given that usage of some technology for PA assessment is in its infancy, it is unsurprising that there exists an over-propensity of cross-sectional study designs, and a dearth of interventionist studies. This is likely an artifact of the stage of development and refinement. In order to progress the application and acceptance of novel technology for PA assessment, the performance and reliability of the technology and data output must be affirmed in response to interventions, to elucidate whether such novel outputs can be positively (or negatively) impacted, and likewise, to detect change and normative values over time, through the course of motor development, thereby highlighting the constraints that novel technology operates within.

A further emergent issue manifest in the activity monitoring literature is one of technology integration. Some studies utilized novel technology in isolation; yet a number of groups have advocated the combination of technology of different types, to better measure PA (Table 17.1). Novel technological approaches to PA measurement may be tentatively demarcated into wearable – specific to body-worn technology such as inclinometers or magnetometers, nearable – technology located 'near' participants, usually, to define position or proximity, and tangible – a physical output that the participant can feel and touch, where the physical form of the output is defined by preceding activities or intensities of movement. While integration of these technology types is pragmatic and attractive, the integration of multiple inputs and outputs brings difficulties, including time-alignment of sensor outputs, harmonization of different data, the pairing of data measured in different space (e.g. time versus frequency domain), and indeed, time taken to process multiple data sources. Notwithstanding the self-evident challenges, the integration of such technology is intertwined with the development of performance, reliability, and constraints, which must remain a strong focus.

Motion Analysis

As presented in the previous section, IMUs are a promising wearable solution for the characterization of different motor tasks out of the laboratory and during daily living activities. Among the analyzed tasks, gait is surely the most widely investigated in literature and, thus, is an example of the current and crucial issues with respect to motion analysis.

First, most of the developed algorithms for the estimation of (gait) space-temporal parameters were validated for healthy subjects in controlled environments. Thus, before effective widespread use of these methods, there are still some relevant questions to answer. For example, to what extent are the developed solutions ecologically valid (Pacini Panebianco et al., 2018)? How does their performance (in terms of sensitivity, specificity, accuracy, repeatability) change when used by people with an altered (gait) pattern (e.g. children, older adults) (Pacini Panebianco et al., 2018)? Recently, researchers started addressing these questions, suggesting that there is no 'perfect' algorithm fitting for all conditions, but probably that compromises are necessary depending on the specific goal. Clearly, further investigation is still needed in this area.

With respect to the estimation of segment orientation and joint angle kinematics, the main limitations concerning IMU systems are the drift affecting the numerical integration of the gyro-based segment's orientation and ferromagnetic disturbances. Sensor fusion methods and kinematical resets (Picerno, 2017) are the two main approaches used to efficiently handle the drift, especially during low-frequency cycling gestures like walking. On the other hand, compensation for ferromagnetic disturbances remains the biggest issue, because any alteration of the local magnetic field may introduce errors in the estimation. The unpredictability of ecological environment for a continuous activity monitoring remains an unsolved issue that cannot be handled using sensor fusion algorithms. The best solution thus far seems to be, when possible, to avoid using magnetometers at all, but by settling for a two-plane approach rather than 3D joint kinematics in order to have a significant signal-to-noise ratio (Picerno, 2017).

Besides kinematic analysis, in the last few years, IMUs have also been proposed for estimating ground reaction forces (GRFs) during movement, paving the way to kinetic analysis and sports performance testing outside of labs (Ancillao, Tedesco, Barton, & O'Flynn, 2018). This aspect is considered 'emerging' and not presented in the previous section given the major open issues that still need to be addressed. As outlined in the review by Ancillao and colleagues (Ancillao et al., 2018), the literature demonstrates the possibility of predicting GRFs from IMU data by using biomechanical models in conjunction with Newton's second law of motion, or machine learning approaches. These methods have been proposed for several motor tasks like walking, running, jumping, squatting. The most critical aspects in estimating GRF from kinematic data were synthesized as follows (Ancillao et al., 2018):

1   the number of sensors/body segments required for the biomechanical modeling
2   knowledge of the inertial properties of each body segment;
3   determining the antero-posterior and medio-lateral components of GRF;
4   determining the GRF acting on each foot in double support conditions and evaluating loading asymmetry;
5   even if a correlation between predicted and directly measured GRF exists, it is difficult to estimate.

Clearly, despite the above-mentioned open issues, the design of a small non-invasive wearable system or sensor network to estimate GRF represents a significant research challenge for PA assessment. Such a device would enable smart monitoring of training and of injuries or fatigue related to repeated loads on the lower limbs.

Besides the standard methods of movement analysis (kinematic and kinetic analysis of movement), a growing number of novel approaches have been proposed aiming at revealing intriguing properties of the motor control system and introduce new ways of thinking about variability, adaptability, health, and motor learning. These methods, often referred to as Nonlinear Analysis Methods for Human Movement Variability (Stergiou, 2016), have been proposed as descriptors of specific features characterizing the motor control underlying said realization of motor pattern. Examples of such nonlinear assessments include pattern regularity (recurrence quantification analysis, RQA (Sylos Labini, Meli, Ivanenko, & Tufarelli, 2012)), motor complexity (entropy-based measures (Bisi & Stagni, 2016; Costa, Peng, Goldberger, & Hausdorff, 2003)), gait stability (short Lyapunov exponents, (Rosenstein, Collins, & De Luca, 1993)), and rhythmicity or symmetry (harmonic ratio (Menz, Lord, & Fitzpatrick, 2003)). They have been often applied on trunk acceleration data, collected by a single IMU, for the investigation of postural control, gait, motor control, and motor development, in healthy adult populations (e.g. evaluating the influence of environmental conditions (Tamburini et al., 2017), in developing children (Bisi et al., 2018), and in elderly and pathologic patients (Stergiou, 2016), offering new insights about how conditions/development/age/pathology influence motor performance. Moreover, in combination with GTP, they were proposed as useful metrics for the monitoring of locomotor development in childhood (Bisi, Tabmurini, & Stagni, 2019).

However, despite the promising and intriguing results that these measures are revealing in several contexts, further research is needed to assess the influence of experimental implementation parameters on the estimated measures, in order to ensure their reliability and to understand their physiological correlates.

Wearable systems research to date has focused more on analysis and less on intervention as only a low number of works focused on wearable feedback. While wearable sensing enables gait assessment, wearable feedback can facilitate intervention. Wearable feedback has been proposed to facilitate gait changes in foot progression or joint loading, to improve postural stability for the elderly, and to assist in a variety of human learning tasks such as drumming, snowboarding, and jump landings (Shull, Jirattigalachote, Hunt, Cutkosky, & Delp, 2014).

Most studies of this type have been published in the last few years, and further research is needed to investigate on the effective advantages that this approach have in different context. However, it is plausible that the growth of wearable systems will extend into a diverse array of human movement applications (Shull et al., 2014).

When comparing wearable versus vision-based approaches, different advantages and/or limitations are present. Vision-based methods have the advantage that the setup is usually less complex (the subject needs to only move in front of the camera without any wearable sensors). On the other hand, IMU-based solutions allow an assessment without space restriction. Nowadays, IMU-based sensor system shows a better performance and a higher reliability than vision systems for the estimation of space-time parameters and joint angles (Kyrarini, Wang, & Gräser, 2015).

As introduced in the previous section, markerless techniques are evolving rapidly thanks to developments in computer vision methods, but it is not yet clear exactly what accuracy can be achieved and whether such systems can be effectively utilized in field-based and therefore, more externally valid settings. Accuracy requirements vary across different scenarios and the validity of markerless systems has yet to be fully established across different movements in varying environments. In particular, accuracy and validity of markerless approach have been investigated mainly on low speed movement (gait, stairs (Oh, Kuenze, Jacopetti, Signorile, & Eltoukhy, 2018), single leg stance (Asaeda, Kuwahara, Fujita, Yamasaki, & Adachi, 2018)) with results that are task specific and dependent on the variable of interest (e.g. joint angle, time parameters). For PA and sports applications, much quicker movements need still to be thoroughly assessed.

Recommendations for Research and Practice

Overall, the novel technology available in the field, acutely juxtaposed with the historical beginnings in the ancient Roman Empire, presents researchers with hitherto unseen options in the assessment of PA. Yet, this availability and ubiquity come with both positives and negatives. As evidenced in this chapter, novel technology, in the form of IMUs, magnetometers, gyroscopes, foot switches, RFID, Wi-Fi, inclinometers, oculography, 3D printing, and more, can be used to proffer new insights into how (well), why, where, and when we move, beyond that of current *de facto* standards. However, with novelty, often comes naivety, and there remains a number of outstanding issues to be resolved or improved upon, in order to advance assessment through novel technology. Following the presentation and discussion of key issues earlier, there emerged three broad recommendations for research, researchers, and practice.

First, given the innumerable technological and analytical options available, open source development, data, and analytics are essential to facilitate global benchmarking of novel technology and incumbent data. Second, there exists an over-predominance of cross-sectional-based empirical studies when novel technology is used. As such, a clear, realistic goal for research, researchers, and, eventually, practice is to conduct interventionist and longitudinal studies of data emerging from novel technology, in addition to advancing the application of such techniques from the lab, and into free-living environments. These study priorities will facilitate our understanding of the technology, and their eventual outputs. Third, the integration of technologies is both an attractive and powerful prospect, and, if successfully operationalized, would facilitate a greater, clearer picture of PA, theoretically enabling objective assessment of how (well), where, why, and when activity behaviors are performed (or not).

It is clear that the technology we use is a large piece of the 'physical activity' puzzle, however, concomitant to the technology is the analytical approach undertaken. As such, researchers must be acutely aware that any decision made in the analytical process will impact the outcome of any technological output, giving further credence to the assertion that open data, open source, transparent reporting and development, and inter-disciplinary collaboration between sports and exercise scientists, computer scientists, and engineers, among many others, are essential.

References

Ancillao, A., Tedesco, S., Barton, J., & O'Flynn, B. (2018). Indirect measurement of ground reaction forces and moments by means of wearable inertial sensors: A systematic review. *Sensors, 18*(8), 2564. doi:10.3390/s18082564

Asaeda, M., Kuwahara, W., Fujita, N., Yamasaki, T., & Adachi, N. (2018). Validity of motion analysis using the Kinect system to evaluate single leg stance in patients with hip disorders. *Gait & Posture, 62*, 458–462. doi:10.1016/j.gaitpost.2018.04.010

Barnes, C. M., Clark, C. C. T., Rees, P., Stratton, G., & Summers, H. D. (2018). Objective profiling of varied human motion based on normative assessment of magnetometer time series data. *Physiological Measurement.* doi:10.1088/1361-6579/aab9de

Bergmann, J. H. M., Mayagoitia, R. E., & Smith, I. C H. (2009). A portable system for collecting anatomical joint angles during stair ascent: A comparison with an optical tracking device. *Dynamic Medicine, 8*(1), 3. doi:10.1186/1476-5918-8-3

Bergmann, J. H. M., Mayagoitia, R. E., & Smith, I. C. H. (2010). A novel method for determining ground-referenced contacts during stair ascent: Comparing relative hip position to quiet standing hip height. *Gait & Posture, 31*(2), 164–168. doi:10.1016/j.gaitpost.2009.09.018

Bisi, M., Pacini Panebianco, G., Polman, R., & Stagni, R. (2017). Objective assessment of movement competence in children using wearable sensors: An instrumented version of the TGMD-2 locomotor subtest. *Gait & Posture, 56*, 42–48. doi:10.1016/j.gaitpost.2017.04.025

Bisi, M. C., & Stagni, R. (2016). Complexity of human gait pattern at different ages assessed using multiscale entropy: From development to decline. *Gait & Posture, 47*, 37–42. doi:10.1016/j.gaitpost.2016.04.001

Bisi, M., Tamburini, P., Pacini Panebianco, G., & Stagni, R. (2018). Nonlinear analysis of human movement dynamics offer new insights in the development of motor control during childhood. *Journal of Biomechanical Engineering.* doi:10.1115/1.4040939

Bisi, M., Tamburini, P., & Stagni, R. (2019, February). A 'fingerprint' of locomotor maturation: Motor development descriptors, reference development bands and data-set. *Gait Posture, 68*, 232–237. doi:10.1016/j.gaitpost.2018.11.036. Epub 2018 November 29.

Bulling, A., Ward, J. A., & Gellersen, H. (2011). Eye movement analysis for activity recognition using electrooculography. *IEEE Transactions on Pattern Analysis and Machine Intelligence, 33*(4), 741–753. doi:10.1109/TPAMI.2010.86

Caldas, R., Mundt, M., Potthast, W., Buarque de Lima Neto, F., & Markert, B. (2017). A systematic review of gait analysis methods based on inertial sensors and adaptive algorithms. *Gait & Posture, 57*, 204–210. doi:10.1016/j.gaitpost.2017.06.019

Camomilla, V., Bergamini, E., Fantozzi, S., & Vannozzi, G. (2018). Trends supporting the in-field use of wearable inertial sensors for sport performance evaluation: A systematic review. *Sensors, 18*(3), 873. doi:10.3390/s18030873

Castelli, A., Paolini, G., Cereatti, A., & Della Croce, U. (2015). A 2D markerless gait analysis methodology: Validation on healthy subjects. *Computational and Mathematical Methods in Medicine, 2015,* 1–11. doi:10.1155/2015/186780

Clark, C. C. T., Barnes, C. M., Holton, M., Summers, H. D., & Stratton, G. (2016). Profiling movement quality and gait characteristics according to body-mass index in children (9–11 y). *Human Movement Science, 49,* 291–300. doi:10.1016/j.humov.2016.08.003

Clark, C. C. T., Barnes, C. M., Swindell, N. J., Holton, M. D., Bingham, D. D., Collings, P. J., & Stratton, G. (2017). Profiling movement and gait quality characteristics in pre-school children. *Journal of Motor Behavior.* doi:10.1080/00222895.2017.1375454

Colyer, S. L., Evans, M., Cosker, D. P., & Salo, A. I. T. (2018). A review of the evolution of vision-based motion analysis and the integration of advanced computer vision methods towards developing a markerless system. *Sports Medicine – Open, 4*(1). doi:10.1186/s40798-018-0139-y

Costa, M., Peng, C.-K., L. Goldberger, A., & Hausdorff, J. M. (2003). Multiscale entropy analysis of human gait dynamics. *Physica A: Statistical Mechanics and Its Applications, 330*(1–2), 53–60. doi:10.1016/j.physa.2003.08.022

Crossley, S. G. M., Mackintosh, K. A., Wilson, R. P., Lester, L. J., Griffiths, I. W., & McNarry, M. A. (2018). Energy expenditure associated with walking speed and angle of turn in children. *European Journal of Applied Physiology.* doi:10.1007/s00421-018-3981-1

Crossley, S. G. M., McNarry, M., Eslambolchilar, P., Knowles, Z., & Mackintosh, K. (2019). The tangibility of personalized 3D-printed feedback may enhance youths' physical activity awareness, goal setting, and motivation: Intervention study. *Journal of Medical Internet Research, 21*(6), e12067. doi:10.2196/12067

Crouter, S. E., Hibbing, P. R, & LaMunion, S. R. (2018). Use of objective measures to estimate sedentary time in youth. *Journal for the Measurement of Physical Behaviour, 1,* 136–142.

da Silva, I. C., van Hees, V. T., Ramires, V. V., Knuth, A. G., Bielemann, R. M., Ekelund, U., . . . Hallal, P. C. (2014). Physical activity levels in three Brazilian birth cohorts as assessed with raw triaxial wrist accelerometry. *International Journal of Epidemiology, 43,* 1959–1968

Duncan, G. E., Lester, J., & Migotsky, S. (2011). Accuracy of a novel multi-sensor board for measuring physical activity and energy expenditure. *European Journal of Applied Physiology, 111*(9), 2025–2032. doi:10.1007/s00421-011-1834-2

El-Gohary, M., Pearson, S., McNames, J., Mancini, M., Horak, F., Mellone, S., & Chiari, L. (2013). Continuous monitoring of turning in patients with movement disability. *Sensors, 14*(1), 356–369. doi:10.3390/s140100356

Everson, B., Mackintosh, K. A., McNarry, M. A.; Todd, C., & Stratton, G. (2019). Can wearable cameras be used to validate school-aged children's lifestyle behaviours? *Children, 6,* 20.

Filippeschi, A., Schmitz, N., Miezal, M., Bleser, G., Ruffaldi, E., Stricker, D. (2017). Survey of motion tracking methods based on inertial sensors: A focus on upper limb human motion. *Sensors, 17*(6), 1257. doi:10.3390/s17061257

Fino, P., Frames, C., & Lockhart, T. (2015). Classifying step and spin turns using wireless gyroscopes and implications for fall risk assessments. *Sensors, 15*(5), 10676–10685. doi:10.3390/s150510676

Freedson, P. S., & John, D. (2013). Comment on "estimating activity and sedentary behavior from an accelerometer on the hip and wrist". *Medicine and Science in Sports and Exercise, 45,* 962–963.

Fulk, G. D., & Sazonov, E. (2011). Using sensors to measure activity in people with stroke. *Topics in Stroke Rehabilitation, 18*(6), 746–757. doi:10.1310/tsr1806-746

Grimpampi, E., Masci, I., Pesce, C., & Vannozzi, G. (2016). Quantitative assessment of developmental levels in overarm throwing using wearable inertial sensing technology. *Journal of Sports Sciences, 34*(18), 1759–1765. doi:10.1080/02640414.2015.1137341

Holliday, K. M., Howard, A. G., Emch, M., Rodríguez, D. A., Rosamond, W. D., & Evenson, K. R. (2017). Deriving a GPS monitoring time recommendation for physical activity studies of adults. *Medicine and Science in Sports and Exercise, 49*(5), 939–947. doi:10.1249/MSS.0000000000001190

Khot, R., Hjorth, L., & Floyd, M. (2014). Understanding physical activity through 3D printed material artifacts. *Conference on Human Factors in Computing Systems – Proceedings.* doi:10.1145/2556288.2557144

Kjaergaard, M. B., Wirz, M., & Roggen, D. (Eds.). (2012). *Detecting pedestrian flocks by fusion of multi-modal sensors in mobile phones.* Proceedings of 2012 ACM Conference on Ubiquitous Computing, New York, NY.

Kyrarini, M., Wang, X., & Gräser, A. (2015). Comparison of vision-based and sensor-based systems for joint angle gait analysis. In *2015 IEEE international symposium on Medical Measurements and Applications (MeMeA) proceedings* (pp. 375–379). doi:10.1109/MeMeA.2015.7145231

Latorre, J., Llorens, R., Colomer, C., & Alcañiz, M. (2018). Reliability and comparison of Kinect-based methods for estimating spatiotemporal gait parameters of healthy and post-stroke individuals. *Journal of Biomechanics, 72*, 268–273. doi:10.1016/j.jbiomech.2018.03.008

Leutheuser, H., Schuldhaus, D., & Eskofier, B. M. (2013). Hierarchical, multisensory based classification of daily life activities: Comparison with state-of-the-art algorithms using a benchmark dataset. *PLoS One, 8*(10), e75196. doi:10.1371/journal.pone.0075196

Loveday, A., Sherar, L. B., Sanders, J. P., Sanderson, P. W., & Esliger, D. W. (2016). Novel technology to help understand the context of physical activity and sedentary behavior. *Physiological Measurement, 37*(10), 1834–1851.

Mancini, M., Salarian, A., Carlson-Kuhta, P., Zampieri, C., King, L., Chiari, L., & Horak, F. B. (2012). ISway: A sensitive, valid and reliable measure of postural control. *Journal of NeuroEngineering and Rehabilitation, 9*(1), 59. doi:10.1186/1743-0003-9-59

Masci, I., Vannozzi, G., Bergamini, E., Pesce, C., Getchell, N., & Cappozzo, A. (2013). Assessing locomotor skills development in childhood using wearable inertial sensor devices: The running paradigm. *Gait & Posture, 37*(4), 570–574. doi:10.1016/j.gaitpost.2012.09.017

Masci, I., Vannozzi, G., Getchell, N., & Cappozzo, A. (2012). Assessing hopping developmental level in childhood using wearable inertial sensor devices. *Motor Control, 16*(3), 317–328.

Menz, H. B., Lord, S. R., & Fitzpatrick, R. C. (2003). Acceleration patterns of the head and pelvis when walking on level and irregular surfaces. *Gait & Posture, 18*(1), 35–46.

Oh, J., Kuenze, C., Jacopetti, M., Signorile, J. F., & Eltoukhy, M. (2018). Validity of the Microsoft Kinect™ in assessing spatiotemporal and lower extremity kinematics during stair ascent and descent in healthy young individuals. *Medical Engineering & Physics, 60*, 70–76. doi:10.1016/j.medengphy.2018.07.011

Pacini Panebianco, G., Bisi, M. C., Stagni, R., & Fantozzi, S. (2018). Analysis of the performance of 17 algorithms from a systematic review: Influence of sensor position, analysed variable and computational approach in gait timing estimation from IMU measurements. *Gait & Posture, 66*, 76–82. doi:10.1016/j.gaitpost.2018.08.025

Palmerini, L., Rocchi, L., Mellone, S., Valzania, F., & Chiari, L. (2011). Feature selection for accelerometer-based posture analysis in Parkinson's disease. *IEEE Transactions on Information Technology in Biomedicine, 15*(3), 481–490. doi:10.1109/TITB.2011.2107916

Picerno, P. (2017). 25 years of lower limb joint kinematics by using inertial and magnetic sensors: A review of methodological approaches. *Gait & Posture, 51*, 239–246. doi:10.1016/j.gaitpost.2016.11.008

Prochaska, J., & DiClemente, C. C. (1992). Stages of change in the modification of problem behaviors. *Progress in Behavior Modification, 28*, 183–218.

Rosenstein, M. T., Collins, J. J., & De Luca, C. J. (1993). A practical method for calculating largest Lyapunov exponents from small data sets. *Physica D: Nonlinear Phenomena, 65*(1), 117–134. doi:10.1016/0167-2789(93)90009-P

Shull, P. B., Jirattigalachote, W., Hunt, M. A., Cutkosky, M. R., & Delp, S. L. (2014). Quantified self and human movement: A review on the clinical impact of wearable sensing and feedback for gait analysis and intervention. *Gait & Posture, 40*(1), 11–19. doi:10.1016/j.gaitpost.2014.03.189

Spinney, R., Smith, L., Ucci, M., Fisher, A., & Konstantatou, M. (2015). Indoor tracking to understand physical activity and sedentary behaviour: Exploratory study in UK office buildings. *PLoS One, 10*(5), e0127688. doi:10.1371/journal.pone.0127688

Stergiou, N. (2016). *Nonlinear analysis for human movement variability.* Boca Raton, FL: Taylor & Francis Inc.

Sylos Labini, F., Meli, A., Ivanenko, Y. P., & Tufarelli, D. (2012). Recurrence quantification analysis of gait in normal and hypovestibular subjects. *Gait & Posture, 35*(1), 48–55. doi:10.1016/j.gaitpost.2011.08.004

Taborri, J., Palermo, E., Rossi, S., & Cappa, P. (2016). Gait partitioning methods: A systematic review. *Sensors, 16*(1), 66. doi:10.3390/s16010066

Tamburini, P., Storm, F., Buckley, C., Bisi, M. C., Stagni, R., & Mazzà, C. (2017). Moving from laboratory to real life conditions: Influence on the assessment of variability and stability of gait. *Gait & Posture, 59*, 248–252. doi:10.1016/j.gaitpost.2017.10.024

Teufl, W., Miezal, M., Taetz, B., Fröhlich, M., & Bleser, G. (2018). Validity, test-retest reliability and long-term stability of magnetometer free inertial sensor based 3D joint kinematics. *Sensors, 18*(7), 1980. doi:10.3390/s18071980

Verlekar, T., Soares, L., & Correia, P. (2018). Automatic classification of gait impairments using a markerless 2D video-based system. *Sensors, 18*(9), 2743. doi:10.3390/s18092743

Wake, M., Clifford, S., York, E., Mensah, F., Gold, L. H., Burgner, D., . . . Zubrick, S. (2014). Introducing growing up in Australia's child health checkpoint: A physical health and biomarkers module for the longitudinal study of Australian children. *Family Matters, 95*, 15–23.

Weinstein, N. (1988). The precaution adoption process. *Health Psychology, 7*(4), 355–386.

Xiao, Z. G., & Menon, C. (2014). Towards the development of a wearable feedback system for monitoring the activities of the upper-extremities. *Journal of NeuroEngineering and Rehabilitation, 11*(1), 2. doi:10.1186/1743-0003-11-2

Zhang, H., Li, L., & Jia, W. (2011). Physical activity recognition based on motion in images acquired by a wearable camera. *Neurocomputing, 74*(12–13), 2184–2192. doi:10.1016/j.neucom.2011.02.014

PART 5

Fitness and Motor Skill Assessment

18

FIELD-BASED FITNESS ASSESSMENT IN YOUTH

Lynne M. Boddy and Gareth Stratton

Introduction

Physical fitness is defined as 'a set of attributes that people have or achieve relating to their ability to perform physical activity' (Corbin, Pangrazi, & Franks, 2000, p. 4). There are 11 components of fitness split into two categories: (1) health-related fitness that is made of five components: body composition, cardiorespiratory fitness (CRF), muscular strength, local muscular endurance and flexibility, and (2) skill-related fitness made up of six components: coordination, balance, power, speed, agility and reaction time (Corbin et al., 2000). While the existence of 11 discrete components of fitness is the subject of constant debate, exercise scientists unequivocally recognize that a sufficient level of physical fitness is important for children's health, well-being and optimal growth and development. Moreover, physical fitness can be viewed as an 'enabling factor' that helps children achieve physical activity goals (Welk, 1999). Despite the well-established benefits of physical fitness in youth, there has been much debate about the value of physical fitness testing, especially in the school setting. Both CRF and muscular strength are related to health during childhood (Artero, Ruiz, et al., 2011; Jiminez-Pavon et al., 2012; Ruiz et al., 2007; Smith et al., 2014; Tomkinson, Lang, & Tremblay, 2017) and are independent of physical activity (Blaes, Baquet, Fabre, Van Praagh, & Berthoin, 2011). Low levels of physical fitness in children and young people are significantly associated with increased risk of cardiometabolic diseases (Dwyer et al., 2009; Knox et al., 2012), obesity (Ortega et al., 2011), quality of life (Morales et al., 2013), skeletal health (Moliner-Urdiales et al., 2010), and mental health (Ortega, Ruiz, Castillo, & Sjostrom, 2008) later in life. In addition, these fitness measures are also associated with the acquisition of skills essential to physical activity and sporting success (Armstrong & McManus, 2011; Ceschia et al., 2016). Importantly physical fitness also tracks moderately well from childhood through to adulthood (Cleland, Ball, Magnussen, Dwyer, & Venn, 2009; Kristensen et al., 2006). Therefore, tracking fitness levels among school children is important in the surveillance of health as well as for monitoring the growth and development of children. Health-related components of physical fitness are specifically associated with health outcomes (Ruiz et al., 2009) and can be measured using (i) gold standard laboratory methods that are limited in a school or community setting due to resource, technical, and time constraints or (ii) field-based measures that are time and cost-efficient for use in schools and population-level settings (Artero, Espana-Romero et al., 2011; Castro-Pinero et al., 2010; Ruiz et al., 2007). Numerous field-based assessment batteries have been developed to assess health-related fitness in children and young people over the past 70 years. Three of the most widely used over recent years are (i) FITNESSGRAM (Plowman & Meredith, 2013), (ii) Eurofit (Adam, Klissouras, Ravazzolo, Renson, & Tuxworth, 1988), and (iii) Assessing Levels of Physical

Activity (ALPHA) (Ruiz et al., 2011). All of these examples provide a battery of valid, reliable, and feasible field-based tests for the assessment of health-related fitness in children and young people (Castro-Pinero et al., 2010).

Overview of Key Literature and Key Issues

Cardiorespiratory Fitness

The most frequently evaluated health-related fitness component is CRF (Tomkinson et al., 2017). CRF, also called cardiovascular fitness, cardiorespiratory endurance, aerobic fitness or maximal aerobic power, is the overall capacity of the cardiovascular and respiratory systems to transport oxygen to the skeletal muscles and to utilize it to generate energy to support muscle activity during prolonged strenuous dynamic exercise (Armstrong, Tomkinson, & Ekelund, 2011; Tomkinson et al., 2017). In children and young people, low CRF is a predictor of cardiovascular disease risk factors such as abnormal blood lipids, high blood pressure, clustered cardiometabolic risk, and overall and central adiposity, as well as metabolic syndrome, arterial stiffness, cancer and poor mental health, later in life (Ortega et al., 2008; Ruiz et al., 2009). Furthermore, there is evidence of an interaction between CRF and adiposity, suggesting that high levels of CRF may reduce the effects of being overweight or obese in children and young people (Eisenmann, Wickel, Welk, & Blair, 2005; Parrett, Valentine, Arngrimsson, Castelli, & Evans, 2011). The modifiable component of CRF is a product of vigorous physical activity and provides insight into the levels of children's physical activity, as well as the capabilities of several bodily systems that are involved in the performance of physical activity and exercise (Ortega et al., 2008). In addition, CRF tracks from childhood through to adulthood moderately well (Malina, 2001), demonstrating that the measurement of CRF in children provides insight into current and future health.

Peak oxygen consumption ($VO_{2\,peak}$) obtained through a graded maximal exercise to voluntary exhaustion test is considered as the single best indicator of CRF in youth (Armstrong & Welsman, 2001). Indirect assessments of CRF such as shuttle run tests indirectly assess fitness, and are influenced by the assessment environment and motivation of the participants. The latter therefore represent a measure of aerobic performance rather than a direct assessment of CRF (Armstrong et al., 2011). Though this limitation is acknowledged, direct assessments of $VO_{2\,peak}$ using graded maximal exercise testing require specialist equipment, facilities, and are time consuming; therefore more feasible field-based methods are often used that allow CRF to be estimated in several participants at the same time. The most common worldwide field-based assessment and estimate of CRF in children and young people is the 20 m multistage shuttle run test (20 m MSRT) (Tomkinson et al., 2017). This test has been shown to be an excellent population-based surveillance and monitoring tool as it is time-, cost- and labor-efficient through its ability to test multiple individuals simultaneously with minimal equipment and across different testing locations (indoors, outdoors, smaller spaces). Further, the 20 m MSRT has been shown to display good validity and reliability (Artero, Espana-Romero, et al., 2011; Tomkinson & Olds, 2008), and $VO_{2\,peak}$ can be estimated from the score obtained in the 20 m MSRT with use of validated equations (Leger, Mercier, Gadoury, & Lambert, 1988). Levels of CRF measured using the 20 m MSRT in children and young people have declined in recent years (Boddy, Fairclough, Atkinson, & Stratton, 2012; Tomkinson et al., 2017). Boddy, Fairclough et al. (2012) reported a significant decline in CRF in children between 1998 and 2010, regardless of weight status and maturation. The study also reported that the observed mean declines in CRF of 1.34% for boys and 2.29% in girls were greater than those reported globally since the turn of the millennium (Tomkinson, Leger, Olds, & Cazorla, 2003; Tomkinson et al., 2017). As low CRF is significantly associated with health, declines are indicative of a diminishing population health (Ruiz et al., 2009), and therefore highlight the case for the monitoring of CRF in youth.

Muscular Strength

Muscular strength refers to the ability of a specific muscle or muscle group to generate maximum force against a resistance in a single contraction (Bouchard & Stephens, 1994). Muscular strength is an important aspect of fitness and health status and is a marker of vigorous intensity physical activities, including those that strengthen muscle and bone, which are included in recommended physical activity guidelines for children and young people globally (WHO, 2010). In children and young people, increased muscular strength has been associated with reductions in total and central adiposity and cardiovascular risk factors, and increases in bone health, self-esteem and perceived competence (Smith et al., 2014). In adults, emerging evidence suggests that handgrip strength is a strong predictor of all-cause mortality, morbidity and the expectancy of being able to live independently (Garcia-Hermoso et al., 2018). Consequently, more attention is now being given to assessing muscular strength in children, as a predictor of health outcomes and all-cause mortality (De Miguel-Etayo et al., 2014). As the generation of maximum force is determined by several factors (e.g. the number and size of muscles, the proportion of muscle fibers, the coordination of the muscle groups), there is no single test for measuring overall muscle strength (Ortega et al., 2008). However, the handgrip strength test is one of the most used tests for assessing muscular strength in experimental and epidemiological studies (De Miguel-Etayo et al., 2014; Moliner-Urdiales et al., 2010). Moreover, the handgrip strength test is correlated with many other measures of strength and is therefore a good indicator of total muscular strength (Wind, Takken, Helders, & Engelbert, 2010). Studies on handgrip strength as a measure of muscular strength have revealed its direct associations with chronic diseases, multi-morbidity and premature mortality (Volaklis, Halle, & Meisinger, 2015).

Akin to levels of CRF, levels of muscular strength in children and young people have declined globally (Cohen et al., 2011; De Miguel-Etayo et al., 2014; Moliner-Urdiales et al., 2010). Studies on Canadian children (Tremblay et al., 2010) and Spanish adolescents (Moliner-Urdiales et al., 2010) showed declines in grip strength. Further, a study in England, on 10-year old English children, also found a decline in grip strength between 1998 and 2008 (Cohen et al., 2011). Declines in grip strength suggest that activities that promote bone health and muscle strength in children and young people are insufficient. Concomitantly, as low muscular strength is significantly associated with key determinants of health (Volaklis et al., 2015), these reported declines are indicative of declines in children's health.

Body Size and Composition

Most physical fitness test batteries for children and young people incorporate a measure of body composition, specifically body mass index (BMI) (Artero, Espana-Romero, et al., 2011; Castro-Pinero et al., 2010). BMI, based on height and weight, is used in many studies to assess overweight and obesity, and is the most practical method for large-scale studies. BMI assessment in children is more complex than in adults as a child's BMI changes with age, and growth patterns differ between sexes. As such, BMI thresholds are often defined using z-scores that indicate how many units of the standard deviation the BMI is above or below the average BMI for that age group and sex. Children with high BMI z-score and classified as overweight or obese (Cole, 2000) are at risk of developing a number of obesity-related conditions (Reilly et al., 2003), including type 2 diabetes (Haines, Wan, Lynn, Barrett, & Shield, 2007), metabolic and cardiovascular complications (Cote, Harris, Panagiotopoulos, Sandor, & Devlin, 2013) and mental health disorders (Griffiths, Parsons, & Hill, 2010). It is well documented that childhood obesity continues into adolescence and adulthood (Park, Falconer, Viner, & Kinra, 2012). An increased BMI also directly affects the capacity of children to acquire skills associated with physical activities (Ceschia et al., 2016). High BMI and overweight and obesity are a result of an imbalance between energy intake and energy expenditure, resulting in an accumulation of energy stores, mainly as fat, in the body (Ceschia et al., 2016). Overweight and obesity are associated with a reduction in physical activity levels (Tremblay et al., 2011), and changes in food habits toward high-energy food consumption (Flatt, 2008), as well as an increase in overall energy intake (Livingstone, 2000) although these factors related to overweight and obesity differ by gender (Sheldrick, Tyler, Mackintosh, & Stratton, 2018). Encouragingly, there is compelling evidence that increased physical activity in children is associated with a reduced risk of being overweight or obese (Janz et al., 2009; Ortega et al., 2011).

Globally the prevalence of overweight and obesity has more than doubled between 1980 and 2014 (WHO, 2017). However, the prevalence of overweight and obesity varies depending on age, ethnicity and geographic region. A review of data from nine countries (Australia, China, England, France, Netherlands, New Zealand, Sweden, Switzerland and United States) suggested that the rise in the prevalence of overweight and obesity in children aged 2–19 years old has slowed appreciably, or even plateaued, and in some countries slightly decreased (Olds et al., 2011). Further to this, studies conducted in England (Boddy, Hackett, & Stratton, 2010; Stratton et al., 2007), using data from the Sports*Linx* project's data archives which involved assessments on approximately 5,000 9–10-year old children annually from 1998 to 2012, have described an initial increase in BMI and prevalence of overweight and obesity from 1998 to 2003/2004 (Stratton et al., 2007), then a slowing in the year-on-year increase between 2004 and 2006 (Boddy, Hackett, & Stratton, 2009), and confirmed the leveling off in BMI and prevalence between 2005 and 2008 (Boddy et al., 2010). Regardless of these findings, the presented levels of overweight and obesity are still high. Therefore, continued investment to promote and monitor health-related fitness, including BMI, in children and young people is needed.

In summary, various components of fitness are associated with the health and development of children and youth. The appropriate monitoring of children's and adolescents' fitness is important to allow population health to be examined, and appropriate policy and resourcing strategies to be put in place or maintained.

A Brief History of Fitness Assessments in the Field

A seminal article on the historiography of health and fitness in physical education (Williams, 1988) outlined the importance of health and fitness to the identity of the nation. During the first half of the 20th century the world was beset with war and conflict and the need for a fit and active military was paramount. This, in turn, affected the school curriculum of the day and mass drill was evident in physical education through to the end of World War II. As the Western world returned to normal, physical education curricula changed again and health and fitness, including measurement of motor fitness developed alongside existing measures of child and motor development. The start of fitness surveillance of children in the United States began in 1956 when President Eisenhower responded to low level of fitness in American compared to European children by calling a conference focused on the issue. This conference led to the creation of the President's Council on Physical Fitness and the development of the American Association of Health Physical Education, Recreation and Dance (AAHPERD). In 1966 the Presidential Physical Fitness Award was established, and subsequently the President's Challenge Youth Physical Fitness Awards Program. Much debate and discussion ensued for several years, with a range of different screening batteries and processes proposed by various different organizations. Despite this, in the United States state sponsored fitness assessment continued and the AAHPERD Youth Fitness Test was used in large-scale surveys of motor fitness in children and youth. In the 1980s, the National Children and Youth Fitness Studies (NCYFS; study 1 on 10–18-year olds; study 2 on 6–9-year olds) was used as a surveillance tool resulting in nationally representative measures of children's motor fitness. These measures ended in 1989 and FITNESSGRAM is now the most commonly used fitness assessment battery in the United States.

The increasing focus on fitness populated the UK physical education curriculum in the 1980s only to be overtaken by the increased focus on physical activity some years later (Stratton, 1995). In the United Kingdom there has been limited large-scale fitness screening programs in youth. The Northern Ireland National Fitness Survey was completed in 1990 (Riddoch, Murphy, Nicholls, van Wersche, & Cran, 1990) and since then only three studies have routinely collected fitness data on children in the United Kingdom. First, the SportsLinx project (Taylor, Hackett, Stratton, & Lamb, 2004) systematically assessed the fitness of over 65,000, 9–10-year old children in Liverpool between 1996 and 2013. The East of England Healthy Hearts study measured the fitness of over 6,000 10–16 year olds (Voss & Sandercock, 2010) and the Swanlinx project has recently measured the fitness of 5,000 children in South West Wales between 2013 and 2018 (Tyler et al., 2015). Much of the focus has shifted toward assessments of physical activity and sport participation in recent years, with surveys examining the prevalence of children and young people meeting physical activity guidelines rather than assessments of physical fitness on nationally representative levels. Despite this, recent evidence consistently highlights the associations between various components of fitness and health outcomes/variables; therefore highlighting the importance of fitness for health and, in turn, the monitoring of population fitness is important from a public health perspective.

Example Fitness Assessment Batteries

As previously mentioned, three of the most widely used field-based fitness assessment batteries over recent years are as follows:

i   FITNESSGRAM (Plowman & Meredith, 2013);
ii   Eurofit (Adam et al., 1988);
iii ALPHA (Ruiz et al., 2011).

Table 18.1 displays the components of fitness assessed by each of these batteries.

Table 18.1 Example fitness assessment batteries

	Fitness assessment battery		
Component	*FITNESSGRAM*	*Eurofit*	*ALPHA*
Body composition	Bioelectrical impedance Body mass index Skinfold measurement	Body mass index Skinfold measurement	Body mass index Waist circumference Skinfold measurement
Cardiorespiratory fitness/ aerobic capacity	One-mile run One-mile walk PACER	Bicycle ergometer Endurance shuttle run	20 m shuttle run test
Muscular strength and endurance	90° Push-ups Curl-ups Flexed arm hang Modified pull-ups Trunk lift	Bent arm hang Sit-ups Handgrip	Handgrip Standing long jump
Flexibility	Back saver sit and reach Shoulder stretch	Sit and reach	
Balance		Flamingo balance	
Power		Standing broad jump	
Speed and agility		Shuttle run 10 × 5 m Plate tapping	Shuttle Run 4 × 10 m

FITNESSGRAM

FITNESSGRAM was released in 1982 by the Cooper Institute. Originally FITNESSGRAM was developed as a 'report card' to provide fitness information to children and their parents (Plowman et al., 2006). FITNESSGRAM is an educational and reporting software system that is used to help teachers track health-related fitness and physical activity levels over time, and provide individual reports for children, parents and schools (Plowman et al., 2006). The battery currently consists of 10 motor tests divided into groups as well as measures of body composition (Table 18.1). Test scores are compared to criterion reference standards, known as Healthy Fitness Zones to ease interpretation and provide a valid and reliable comparison. There have been a number of amendments to the program since its inception, for example version 6 was the first to include a measure of physical activity (ACTIVITYGRAM), while version 8 included an ACTIVITY LOG that allows pedometer data to be inputted. Therefore, FITNESSGRAM represents a package of assessments that enable a range of health-related behaviors to be examined.

Eurofit

The first methodological guide of the Eurofit test battery for school-aged children was published in 1983 by the Council of Europe, Committee for the Development of Sport, with the full manual released in English and French in 1988 (Adam et al., 1988). Eurofit has been used extensively in Belgium, Estonia, Italy, Lithuania, Hungary, Netherlands, Poland, Northern Ireland, Spain and Turkey as well as in large studies in the United Kingdom. Eurofit consists of nine motor tests and measures of body composition (Table 18.1). One of the objectives of Eurofit was to motivate participants to take part in sports and exercise and maintain participation into adulthood. The developers encouraged the use of Eurofit in school physical education programs, irrespective of the relatively high demands this would place on time, personnel and resources. Eurofit data are typically compared to age- and sex-specific normative data, rather than criterion reference standards.

ALPHA Health-Related Fitness Test Battery

The ALPHA fitness testing battery (Ruiz et al., 2011) was developed in Spain in 2009 to provide a valid, reliable, safe and feasible set of field-based fitness tests for use with children and young people across Europe. Three versions of the battery are available which include fewer/more tests depending on the time available to complete the assessment sessions. The 'evidence based' version of the battery includes six assessments with an additional assessment of motor fitness (agility, 40×10 m shuttle run test) included in the 'extended version' of the battery (Table 18.1). Scores on the various assessments are compared to age- and sex-specific reference standards that classify fitness from 'very low' to 'very high' for each component assessed.

Other Approaches

To complement the more standard measures of fitness outlined in the Eurofit, FITNESSGRAM and ALPHA batteries there has been progress in the development of fitness assessment batteries that are more aligned to children's motor development experiences by developing test batteries that consist of compound items (e.g. Fjortoft et al., 2011). The items included in the example battery from Fjortoft et al. (2011) are described in Table 18.2. Compound items assess various combinations of the components of fitness, rather than dividing fitness into its component parts and assessing each one separately. This approach is thought to help maintain participant motivation as the assessments are more similar to children's usual behaviors. As a result, the compound items

Table 18.2 Example fitness assessment battery using compound items (Fjortoft et al., 2011)

Compound fitness component	Assessment
Power	Standing broad jump
Agility	Jumping a distance of 7 m on 2 feet as fast as possible
	Jumping a distance of 7 m on 1 foot as fast as possible
Object control	Throwing a tennis ball with one hand
Strength	Pushing a medicine ball (1 kg) with 2 hands as far as possible
Agility-coordination strength	Climbing up wall bars, crossing over 2 columns to the right, and climbing down the fourth column as fast as possible
Speed agility	10 × 5 m shuttle run
Speed	Running 20 m as fast as possible
Aerobic fitness	Reduced Cooper test. Run/walk around a marked rectangle measuring 9 × 18 m (the size of a volleyball field) for 6 minutes

are more intuitive and require fewer instructions so are less cognitively demanding than single component-based assessments. As the physical literacy concept continues to expand and develop (Edwards et al., 2018), it is likely that field-based assessment batteries will expand to examine skills and attributes that are more aligned to children's development and the mastery of complex movements. The assessment of movement skills is outlined in detail in Chapter 19.

Interpreting Fitness Data: Standards and Norms

Fitness tests are generally based on one of two types of standards: (1) criterion and (2) norm referenced. Norm-referenced fitness standards rank children's performance relative to peers of the same age and gender. The norms approach does not provide information to the practitioner, researcher or participant on whether the performance is sufficient for to maintain health (Plowman et al., 2006). Furthermore, norm standards are dependent on the population on which the norms were calculated. For example, consider whether it is 'good' for a child to achieve 'average' fitness if the average child is unfit. Sex- and age-specific normative values for nine Eurofit tests were recently published, based on data on approximately 2.8 million children and young people from 30 European countries. These norms allow the comparison of Eurofit data to representative European norms for the first time (Tomkinson et al., 2018). Though these are norm-referenced standards, links to health outcomes have been made. It is generally thought that the use of norm-referenced standards is not the optimum approach from a health or educational perspective, especially when participants may feel disheartened and demotivated by performing poorly in comparison to norm-referenced standards and/or their peers (Wiersma & Sherman, 2008).

Criterion-referenced standards measure fitness by comparing the student's level of fitness to a health standard (rather than a population standard), where a participant needs to attain a threshold level of performance before the student is considered healthy (Welk, De Saint-Maurice Maduro, Laurson, & Brown, 2011). Criterion-referenced evaluations have been included from version 5 of the FITNESSGRAM and the current version utilizes criterion-referenced standards on health-related components that were updated in 2011 (Welk et al., 2011). For other fitness assessment batteries or individual tests, studies have calculated thresholds that relate to health outcomes, for example weight status and/or cardiometabolic risk (Boddy, Thomas et al., 2012; Ruiz et al., 2016). Criterion-referenced standards are useful when aiming to understand the health status or risk of populations, and therefore are helpful when planning health promotion activities, intervention studies and providing individualized advice to participants. Criterion-referenced standards also provide meaningful information to participants, parents and teachers about the current fitness levels, so are thought to be more useful and educational in comparison to norm-referenced standards, as they avoid some of the issues associated with peer-comparison and the detrimental effects this can have on motivation.

Validity and Reliability of Fitness Tests

As with any form of assessment, the validity and reliability of fitness assessments are of key importance to allow practitioners to accurately assess the components of fitness. This is particularly important when examining the impact of interventions and policies designed to improve one or more components of fitness over time or when relating results to health outcomes. Though the reliability of fitness assessment batteries has been debated over several years, more compelling evidence linking components of fitness to health outcomes has accumulated, while a number of studies investigating reliability of batteries and individual components of fitness have been published. For example, one large-scale study investigated the reliability and validity of FITENSS-GRAM when assessments were administered by school teachers or an administrator rather than highly trained assessors (Morrow, Martin, & Jackson, 2010). The study reported very good to generally acceptable reliability levels for all FITNESSGRAM tests, with BMI demonstrating the greatest reliability, followed by assessments of CRF. The musculoskeletal assessments displayed the lowest levels of reliability, which may be due to differences and alternations in technique between and within participants, and the ability of the assessors to identify and correct poor technique when completing the assessments (Morrow et al., 2010). When considering validity, results were similar between teachers and highly trained assessors, suggesting acceptable validity for the teacher-administered FITNESSGRAM battery, though reliability for a number of items was better in teachers who had received FITNESSGRAM training, highlighting the beneficial effect of training practitioners to conduct assessments in the field (Morrow et al., 2010).

A comprehensive systematic review of field-based fitness tests used to assess cardiorespiratory, musculoskeletal and motor fitness (speed, agility, coordination and balance) in children and youth was published in 2011 (Artero, Espana-Romero, et al., 2011). The CRF assessments included in the review were the: 20 m MSRT, 1 mile run/walk, 5 minute run/walk and 6 minute run/walk. The review found strong evidence to suggest that the 20 m MSRT produced results with good test-retest reliability, whereas moderate evidence was available for the 1 mile walk/run test. Because of the small number of studies included in the review that used the 6 minute and 5 minute run/walk tests, preliminary evidence suggested good test-retest reliability for the 6-minute assessment, and that two familiarization trials were required for the 5 minute walk/run assessment. For musculoskeletal components, grip strength was commonly used and test-retest correlation coefficients were highly significant with small systematic bias between tests. Children in the lower quartile of performance demonstrated larger test-retest bias. For the other musculoskeletal components, fewer studies were included in the review. The limited evidence available suggested that the sit and reach test displayed larger mean test-retest difference in those who scored lower, but non-significant differences between test-retest scores were observed. Non-significant test-retest differences were also observed for the standing broad jump and trunk lift, with higher differences observed in the bent arm hang assessment evident for those who scored higher. There was also contrasting evidence about the reliability of the modified pull-up test (Artero, Espana-Romero, et al., 2011).

A small number of studies were also included in the review for the assessment of motor fitness. Despite this, the 4 × 10 m shuttle run test (agility), the slalom test and hurdle test (termed 'sport related functional tests') were reliable as were body size/composition measures such as BMI, skinfolds and circumferences and percent body fat estimated from skinfolds (Artero, Espana-Romero et al., 2011). Authors concluded that the 20 m MSRT is a reliable test to measure CRF, handgrip strength and standing broad jump are reliable tests to measure musculoskeletal fitness and 4 × 10 m or 10 × 5 m shuttle run tests are reliable measures of motor fitness. In summary the current evidence suggests that field-based fitness tests are robust measures of fitness and are reliable for use in children and youth.

Despite the wealth of evidence regarding the reliability and validity of field-based fitness assessments in older children (e.g. aged 9 years and above), there are few batteries that have been validated for use with children 3–6 years old because of the difficulty participants at this age have following instructions. The PREFIT assessment battery is one example that was developed for use in younger children aged 3–5 years (Ortega et al., 2015). As a result of reviewing fitness assessments conducted with preschool aged children, their reliability and validity and relationships with health outcomes, Ortega and colleagues recommended that the PREFIT fitness assessment battery was most fit for purpose. PREFIT includes the following tests: the 20 m MSRT (CRF), the handgrip strength and the standing long jump (musculoskeletal fitness) and the 4 × 10 m shuttle run and one-leg-stance test (motor fitness) (Ortega et al., 2015). In addition, assessments of weight, height and waist circumference are also included in PREFIT. Normative values for preschool children completing the PREFIT assessment battery have been published (Cadenas-Sanchez et al., 2018). Therefore, it may now be possible to reliably examine fitness in children aged 3–5 years using field-based approaches such as PREFIT and compare scores to age- and sex-specific reference values.

The validity and reliability for a range of individual fitness tests examining individual components of fitness have been explored, and batteries such as FITNESSGRAM have been extensively investigated for their reliability and validity. Therefore, in theory these tests provide an accurate assessment of children and youth's physical fitness. Despite this, the accuracy of fitness assessments is heavily influenced by the motivation of participants to perform to their best ability, the test environment and the correct administration of assessments by practitioners 'on the ground'; therefore there are a number of practical issues that warrant consideration.

Practical and Pedagogical Considerations

Fitness assessment in all its forms has been an integral part of the school physical education curriculum for over a century. In their paper 'physical fitness testing of children, a 30 year history of misguided efforts' Seefeldt and Vogel (1989) denounced the use of 'fitness-testing' of children and youth making claim that this approach provided no useful insight into children's physical activity behaviors or the relationships between physical fitness and health in children and young people (Seefeldt & Vogel, 1989). Whitehead, Pemberton, and Corbin (1990) discussed the use of fitness assessments in school and outlined a range of issues that could be associated with fitness assessments, which could have a positive or negative impact upon the participants involved depending on how the assessments were conducted and results/scores were interpreted (Whitehead et al., 1990). The debate continued throughout the 1990s and early 2000s as calls grew for a focus on physical activity rather than fitness. While the use of fitness assessments has a number of detractors, an appropriate pedagogical approach to its implementation is key to positive child development, learning, and to motivate participants to perform to their best ability during assessments. The appropriate uses of fitness assessments include personal fitness self-testing, data for parental reporting and personal tracking, while the inappropriate uses included using fitness scores for grading, evaluating teacher effectiveness or determining exclusions. Wiersma and Sherman (2008) outlined a number of possible approaches to improve the fitness assessment environment and experience for children and young people, which would, in turn, lead to a positive and enjoyable experience and optimize performance (Wiersma & Sherman, 2008). Understanding the motivation of participants is important to ensure that fitness assessments are performed with maximum effort. For example, practitioners may use motivational theory to help understand how to best motivate participants during fitness assessments. Goal-orientation theory, competence motivation and cognitive evaluation theory are all discussed in the context of fitness 'testing' (Wiseman & Sherman, 2008) providing useful insight into how practitioners could provide an appropriate fitness assessment environment for the benefit of the participants (Wiersma & Sherman, 2008). Motivation is important, but it is also important to consider the rationale for conducting fitness assessments as well as their educational nature. Moreover who interprets the data (child, parent, teacher, researcher) and the appropriateness of tests from a physical and cognitive development perspective when conducting fitness assessments in children and youth are important factors to consider when designing a fitness testing plan. Silverman, Keating, and Phillips (2008) suggested that a balanced approach to physical fitness testing within the PE curriculum is valuable and provided three useful recommendations for people considering fitness assessments in children and youth (Silverman et al., 2008):

i   Fitness assessment should be implemented as an integral part of fitness instruction.
ii Fitness results should be used to assess fitness instruction and student learning.
iii All children have the potential to meet basic health-related fitness standards.

Creating the appropriate pedagogical and motivational climate are therefore key issues to consider when conducting fitness assessments with children and youth. There are other more obvious practical issues to consider such as timing, space, equipment and staffing. The space available can limit both the number of components of fitness that can be assessed and the number of children and youth that can take part safely. When working with partner organizations such as schools or community clubs it is important to establish where the assessments will be conducted to understand what is possible given the space, time, equipment and workforce available. It is also important to consider issues such as the screening of participants to rule out any children at risk of injury, for example those with pre-existing injuries, or conditions such as asthma that may need additional support and/or to be excluded from some assessments. While it is important to create an inclusive and motivational climate, the safety of participants is of course paramount.

Summary and Emerging Issues

There are a range of field-based fitness assessment batteries available to assess physical fitness, though most assessments have been validated in older children and youth. If conducted correctly within an environment that is safe, positive and motivational, field-based fitness assessments can be conducted reliably providing important health screening information to public health practitioners and researchers, and importantly providing children and youth, their parents and teachers/coaches with useful information that can help provide feedback on health status and act as a motivational tool toward participation in physical activity to improve assessment scores in the future.

Recent evidence has clearly linked some of the components of fitness to health outcomes, especially body size/composition and CRF, with evidence emerging linking other components of health-related fitness to health outcomes or variables in children and youth; therefore the utility of fitness screening programs is clear from a public health perspective. While individual components of fitness are often assessed by fitness assessment batteries, the recent increase in interest in physical literacy may drive further evolution of fitness assessment batteries that are designed to reflect children and youth's physical development and typical movements. Furthermore, fitness assessment batteries such as FITNESSGRAM now go beyond simply assessing the components of fitness by integrating assessments of physical activity behaviors, thus providing a more comprehensive picture of children's health-related movement behaviors.

While fitness assessments remain a debated topic, their utility from an educational and health perspective is clear. Creating the optimum environment and support structures for participants is key to their effectiveness; therefore careful consideration of these issues is urged for people planning on undertaking fitness assessments with children and youth in the field.

Recommendations for Researchers and Practitioners

- There are strong associations between various components of fitness and the health of children and youth. Therefore, appropriately designed fitness assessment programs should be included in school physical education programs and community health initiatives.
- It is important to create the optimal environment for participants to succeed in the fitness tests and to ensure participants have a positive, meaningful experience. Using criterion-referenced norms and adopting child-centered and motivational pedagogical approaches are key.

References

Adam, C., Klissouras, V., Ravazzolo, M., Renson, R., & Tuxworth, W. (1988). *EUROFIT: European test of physical fitness.* Rome, Italy: Council of Europe, Committee for the Development of Sport.

Armstrong, N., & McManus, A. M. (2011). Physiology of elite young male athletes. In N. Armstrong & A. M. McManus (Eds.), *The elite young athlete* (pp. 23–46). Basel, Switzerland: Karger.

Armstrong, N., Tomkinson, G., & Ekelund, U. (2011). Aerobic fitness and its relationship to sport, exercise training and habitual physical activity during youth. *British Journal of Sports Medicine, 45*(11), 849–858. Retrieved from http://www.ncbi.nlm.nih.gov/pubmed/21836169, doi:10.1136/bjsports-2011-090200

Armstrong, N., & Welsman, J. R. (2001). Peak oxygen uptake in relation to growth and maturation in 11- to 17-year-old humans. *European Journal of Applied Physiology, 85*(6), 546–551. Retrieved from https://www.ncbi.nlm.nih.gov/pubmed/11718283, doi:10.1007/s004210100485

Artero, E. G., Espana-Romero, V., Castro-Pinero, J., Ortega, F. B., Suni, J., Castillo-Garzon, M. J., & Ruiz, J. R. (2011). Reliability of field-based fitness tests in youth. *International Journal of Sports Medicine, 32*(3), 159–169. Retrieved from https://www.ncbi.nlm.nih.gov/pubmed/21165805, doi:10.1055/s-0030-1268488

Artero, E. G., Ruiz, J. R., Ortega, F. B., Espana-Romero, V., Vicente-Rodriguez, G., Molnar, D., . . . on behalf of the HELENA Group. (2011). Muscular and cardiorespiratory fitness are independently associated with metabolic risk in adolescents: The HELENA study. *Pediatric Diabetes, 12*(8), 704–712. doi:10.1111/j.1399-5448.2011.00769.x

Blaes, A., Baquet, G., Fabre, C., Van Praagh, E., & Berthoin, S. (2011). Is there any relationship between physical activity level and patterns, and physical performance in children? *International Journal of Behavioral Nutrition and Physical Activity, 8.*

Boddy, L. M., Fairclough, S. J., Atkinson, G., & Stratton, G. (2012). Changes in cardiorespiratory fitness in 9- to 10.9-year-old children: SportsLinx 1998–2010. *Medicine and Science in Sports and Exercise, 44*(3), 481–486. Retrieved from http://www.ncbi.nlm.nih.gov/entrez/query.fcgi?cmd=Retrieve&db=PubMed&dopt=Citation&list_uids=21814150, doi:10.1249/MSS.0b013e3182300267

Boddy, L. M., Hackett, A. F., & Stratton, G. (2009). Changes in BMI and prevalence of obesity and overweight in children in Liverpool, 1998–2006. *Perspectives in Public Health, 129*(3), 127–131. doi:10.1177/1757913908094808

Boddy, L. M., Hackett, A. F., & Stratton, G. (2010). Changes in fitness, body mass index and obesity in 9–10 year olds. *Journal of Human Nutrition and Dietetics, 23*(3), 254–259.

Boddy, L. M., Thomas, N. E., Fairclough, S. J., Tolfrey, K., Brophy, S., Rees, A., . . . Stratton, G. (2012). ROC generated thresholds for field-assessed aerobic fitness related to body size and cardiometabolic risk in schoolchildren. *PLoS One, 7*(9), e45755. doi:10.1371/journal.pone.0045755

Bouchard, C. S. R. J., & Stephens, T. (1994). *Physical activity, fitness and health: The model and key concepts.* Champaign, IL: Human Kinetics.

Cadenas-Sanchez, C., Intemann, T., Labayen, I., Peinado, A. B., Vidal-Conti, J., Sanchis-Moysi, J., . . . PREFIT Project Group. (2018). Physical fitness reference standards for preschool children: The PREFIT project. *Journal of Science and Medicine in Sport.* Retrieved from https://www.ncbi.nlm.nih.gov/pubmed/30316738, doi:10.1016/j.jsams.2018.09.227

Castro-Pinero, J., Artero, E. G., Espana-Romero, V., Ortega, F. B., Sjostrom, M., Suni, J., & Ruiz, J. R. (2010). Criterion-related validity of field-based fitness tests in youth: A systematic review. *British Journal of Sports Medicine, 44*(13), 934–943. Retrieved from http://www.ncbi.nlm.nih.gov/entrez/query.fcgi?cmd=Retrieve&db=PubMed&dopt=Citation&list_uids=19364756, doi:10.1136/bjsm.2009.058321

Ceschia, A., Giacomini, S., Santarossa, S., Rugo, M., Salvadego, D., Da Ponte, A., . . . Lazzer, S. (2016). Deleterious effects of obesity on physical fitness in pre-pubertal children. *European Journal of Sport Science, 16*(2), 271–278.

Cleland, V. J., Ball, K., Magnussen, C., Dwyer, T., & Venn, A. (2009). Socioeconomic position and the tracking of physical activity and cardiorespiratory fitness from childhood to adulthood. *American Journal of Epidemiology, 170*(9), 1069–1077.

Cohen, D. D., Voss, C., Taylor, M. J., Delextrat, A., Ogunleye, A. A., & Sandercock, G. R. (2011). Ten-year secular changes in muscular fitness in English children. *Acta Paediatrica, 100*(10), e175–e177. Retrieved from https://www.ncbi.nlm.nih.gov/pubmed/21480987, doi:10.1111/j.1651-2227.2011.02318.x

Cole, T. J. (2000). Establishing a standard definition for child overweight and obesity worldwide: International survey. *BMJ, 320*(7244), 1240. doi:10.1136/bmj.320.7244.1240

Corbin, C. B., Pangrazi, R. P., & Franks, D. B. (2000). Definitions: Health, fitness, and physical activity. *President's Council on Physical Fitness and Sports Research Digest, 3*(9), 3–10.

Cote, A. T., Harris, K. C., Panagiotopoulos, C., Sandor, G. G., & Devlin, A. M. (2013). Childhood obesity and cardiovascular dysfunction. *Journal of the American College of Cardiology, 62*(15), 1309–1319. Retrieved from https://www.ncbi.nlm.nih.gov/pubmed/23954339, doi:10.1016/j.jacc.2013.07.042

De Miguel-Etayo, P., Gracia-Marco, L., Ortega, F. B., Intemann, T., Foraita, R., Lissner, L., . . . IDEFICS Consortium. (2014). Physical fitness reference standards in European children: The IDEFICS study. *International Journal of Obesity (London), 38*(Suppl 2), S57–S66. Retrieved from https://www.ncbi.nlm.nih.gov/pubmed/25376221, doi:10.1038/ijo.2014.136

Dwyer, T., Magnussen, C. G., Schmidt, M. D., Ukoumunne, O. C., Ponsonby, A. L., Raitakari, O. T., . . . Venn, A. (2009). Decline in physical fitness from childhood to adulthood associated with increased obesity and insulin resistance in adults. *Diabetes Care, 32*(4), 683–687.

Edwards, L. C., Bryant, A. S., Keegan, R. J., Morgan, K., Cooper, S. M., & Jones, A. M. (2018). 'Measuring' physical literacy and related constructs: A systematic review of empirical findings. *Sports Medicine, 48*(3), 659–682.

Eisenmann, J. C., Wickel, E. E., Welk, G. J., & Blair, S. N. (2005). Relationship between adolescent fitness and fatness and cardiovascular disease risk factors in adulthood: The aerobics center longitudinal study (ACLS). *American Heart Journal, 149*(1), 46–53. Retrieved from http://www.ncbi.nlm.nih.gov/pubmed/15660033, doi:10.1016/j.ahj.2004.07.016

Fjørtoft, I., Pedersen, A. V., Sigmundsson, H., & Vereijken, B. (2011). Measuring physical fitness in children who are 5 to 12 years old with a test battery that is functional and easy to administer. *Physical Therapy, 91*(7), 1087-1095.

Flatt, J. P. (2008). Macronutrient composition and food selection. *Obesity, 9*(2), 256S–262S.

Garcia-Hermoso, A., Cofre-Bolados, C., Andrade-Schnettler, R., Ceballos-Ceballos, R., Fernandez-Vergara, O., Vegas-Heredia, E. D., . . . Izquierdo, M. (2018). Normative reference values for handgrip strength in Chilean children at 8–12 years old using the empirical distribution and the lambda, mu, and sigma statistical methods. *Journal of Strength and Conditioning Research*. Retrieved from https://www.ncbi.nlm.nih.gov/pubmed/29863592, doi:10.1519/JSC.0000000000002631

Griffiths, L. J., Parsons, T. J., & Hill, A. J. (2010). Self-esteem and quality of life in obese children and adolescents: A systematic review. *International Journal of Pediatric Obesity, 5*(4), 282–304. Retrieved from https://www.ncbi.nlm.nih.gov/pubmed/20210677, doi:10.3109/17477160903473697

Haines, L., Wan, K. C., Lynn, R., Barrett, T. G., & Shield, J. P. (2007). Rising incidence of type 2 diabetes in children in the U.K. *Diabetes Care, 30*(5), 1097–1101. Retrieved from https://www.ncbi.nlm.nih.gov/pubmed/17259470, doi:10.2337/dc06-1813

Janz, K. F., Kwon, S., Letuchy, E. M., Eichenberger Gilmore, J. M., Burns, T. L., Torner, J. C., . . . Levy, S. M. (2009). Sustained effect of early physical activity on body fat mass in older children. *American Journal of Preventive Medicine, 37*(1), 35–40. Retrieved from http://www.ncbi.nlm.nih.gov/pubmed/19423269, doi:10.1016/j.amepre.2009.03.012

Jiminez-Pavon, D., Ortega, F. B., Valtuena, J., Castro-Piñero, J., Gomez-Martinez, S., Zaccaria, M., . . . Ruiz, J. R. (2012). Muscular strength and markers of insulin resistance in European adolescents: The HELENA study. *European Journal of Applied Physiology, 112*(7), 2455–2465.

Knox, G. J., Baker, J. S., Davies, B., Rees, A., Morgan, K., Cooper, S. M., . . . Thomas, N. E. (2012). Effects of a novel school-based cross-curricular physical activity intervention on cardiovascular disease risk factors in 11- to 14-year-olds: The activity knowledge circuit. *American Journal of Health Promotion, 27*(2), 75–83.

Kristensen, P. L., Wedderkopp, N., Moller, N. C., Andersen, L. B., Bai, C. N., & Froberg, K. (2006). Tracking and prevalence of cardiovascular disease risk factors across socio-economic classes: A longitudinal substudy of the European youth heart study. *BMC Public Health, 6*, 20. Retrieved from http://www.ncbi.nlm.nih.gov/entrez/query.fcgi?cmd=Retrieve&db=PubMed&dopt=Citation&list_uids=16441892

Leger, L. A., Mercier, D., Gadoury, C., & Lambert, J. (1988). The multistage 20 metre shuttle run test for aerobic fitness. *Journal of Sports Sciences, 6*(2), 93–101. Retrieved from http://www.ncbi.nlm.nih.gov/entrez/query.fcgi?cmd=Retrieve&db=PubMed&dopt=Citation&list_uids=3184250, doi:10.1080/02640418808729800

Livingstone, B. (2000). Epidemiology of childhood obesity in Europe. *European Journal of Pediatrics, 159*, S14–S34.

Malina, R. M. (2001). Physical activity and fitness: Pathways from childhood to adulthood. *American Journal of Human Biology, 13*(2), 162–172. Retrieved from http://www.ncbi.nlm.nih.gov/pubmed/11460860, doi:10.1002/1520-6300(200102/03)13:2<162::AID-AJHB1025>3.0.CO;2-T

Moliner-Urdiales, D., Ruiz, J. R., Ortega, F. B., Jimenez-Pavon, D., Vicente-Rodriguez, G., Rey-Lopez, J. P., . . . HELENA Study Group. (2010). Secular trends in health-related physical fitness in Spanish adolescents: The AVENA and HELENA studies. *Journal of Science and Medicine in Sport, 13*(6), 584–588.

Morales, P. F., Sanchez-Lopez, M., Moya-Martinez, P., Garcia-Prieto, J. C., Martinez-Andres, M., Garcia, N. L., & Martinez-Vizcaino, V. (2013). Health-related quality of life, obesity, and fitness in schoolchildren: The Cuenca study. *Quality of Life Research, 22*(7), 1515–1523.

Morrow, J. R., Jr., Martin, S. B., & Jackson, A. W. (2010). Reliability and validity of the FITNESSGRAM: Quality of teacher-collected health-related fitness surveillance data. *Research Quarterly for Exercise Sport, 81*(3 Suppl), S24–S30. Retrieved from https://www.ncbi.nlm.nih.gov/pubmed/21049835, doi:10.1080/02701367.2010.10599691

Olds, T., Maher, C., Shi, Z. M., Peneau, S., Lioret, S., Castetbon, K., . . . Summerbell, C. (2011). Evidence that the prevalence of childhood overweight is plateauing: Data from nine countries. *International Journal of Pediatric Obesity, 6*(5–6), 342–360.

Ortega, F. B., Cadenas-Sanchez, C., Sanchez-Delgado, G., Mora-Gonzalez, J., Martinez-Tellez, B., Artero, E. G., . . . Ruiz, J. R. (2015). Systematic review and proposal of a field-based physical fitness-test battery in preschool children: The PREFIT battery. *Sports Medicine, 45*(4), 533–555. Retrieved from https://www.ncbi.nlm.nih.gov/pubmed/25370201, doi:10.1007/s40279-014-0281-8

Ortega, F. B., Labayen, I., Ruiz, J. R., Kurvinen, E., Loit, H. M., Harro, J., . . . Sjostrom, M. (2011). Improvements in fitness reduce the risk of becoming overweight across puberty. *Medicine and Science in Sports and Exercise, 43*(10), 1891–1897. doi:10.1249/MSS.0b013e3182190d71

Ortega, F. B., Ruiz, J. R., Castillo, M. J., & Sjostrom, M. (2008). Physical fitness in childhood and adolescence: A powerful marker of health. *International Journal of Obesity (London), 32*(1), 1–11. Retrieved from http://www.ncbi.nlm.nih.gov/entrez/query.fcgi?cmd=Retrieve&db=PubMed&dopt=Citation&list_uids=18043605, doi:10.1038/sj.ijo.0803774

Park, M. H., Falconer, C., Viner, R. M., & Kinra, S. (2012). The impact of childhood obesity on morbidity and mortality in adulthood: A systematic review. *Obesity Reviews, 13*(11), 985–1000. Retrieved from https://www.ncbi.nlm.nih.gov/pubmed/22731928, doi:10.1111/j.1467-789X.2012.01015.x

Parrett, A. L., Valentine, R. J., Arngrimsson, S. A., Castelli, D. M., & Evans, E. M. (2011). Adiposity and aerobic fitness are associated with metabolic disease risk in children. *Applied Physiology Nutrition and Metabolism, 36*(1), 72–79.

Plowman, S. A., & Meredith, M. D. (2013). *FITNESSGRAM/ACTIVTYGRAM reference guide* (4th ed.). Dallas, TX: The Cooper Institute.

Plowman, S. A., Sterling, C. L., Corbin, C. B., Meredith, M. D., Welk, G. J., & Morrow, J. R., Jr. (2006). The history of FITNESSGRAM. *Journal of Physical Activity & Health, 3*(2), S5–S20.

Reilly, J. J., Methven, E., McDowell, Z. C., Hacking, B., Alexander, D., Stewart, L., & Kelnar, C. J. H. (2003). Health consequences of obesity. *Archives of Disease in Childhood, 88*(9), 748–752.

Riddoch, C. J., Murphy, N. A., Nicholls, A., van Wersche, A., & Cran, G. (1990). *The Northern Ireland Fitness Survey – 1989*. Belfast, Northern Ireland: Queen's University of Belfast.

Ruiz, J. R., Castro-Piñero, J., Artero, E., Ortega, F., Sjöström, M., Suni, J., & Castillo, M. (2009, January 21). Predictive validity of health-related fitness in youth: A systematic review. *British Journal of Sports Medicine*, Online first. doi:10.1136/bjsm.2008.056499

Ruiz, J. R., Castro-Pinero, J., Espana-Romero, V., Artero, E. G., Ortega, F. B., Cuenca, M. M., . . . Castillo, M. J. (2011). Field-based fitness assessment in young people: The ALPHA health-related fitness test battery for children and adolescents. *British Journal of Sports Medicine, 45*(6), 518–524. Retrieved from https://www.ncbi.nlm.nih.gov/pubmed/20961915, doi:10.1136/bjsm.2010.075341

Ruiz, J. R., Cavero-Redondo, I., Ortega, F. B., Welk, G. J., Andersen, L. B., & Martinez-Vizcaino, V. (2016). Cardiorespiratory fitness cut points to avoid cardiovascular disease risk in children and adolescents: What level of fitness should raise a red flag? A systematic review and meta-analysis. *British Journal of Sports Medicine, 50*(23), 1451–1458. Retrieved from https://www.ncbi.nlm.nih.gov/pubmed/27670254, doi:10.1136/bjsports-2015-095903

Ruiz, J. R, Ortega, F., Rizzo, N., Villa, I., Hurtig-Wennlof, A., Oja, L., & Sjöström, M. (2007). High cardiovascular fitness is associated with low metabolic risk score in children: The European youth heart study. *Pediatric Research, 61*(3), 350–355.

Seefeldt, V., & Vogel, P. (1989). Physical fitness testing of children: A 30-year history of misguided efforts? *Pediatric Exercise Science, 1,* 295–302.

Sheldrick, M. P. R., Tyler, R., Mackintosh, K. A., & Stratton, G. (2018). Relationship between sedentary time, physical activity and multiple lifestyle factors in children. *Journal of Functional Morphology and Kinesiology, 3*(1), 15.

Silverman, S., Keating, X. D., & Phillips, S. R. (2008). A lasting impression: A pedagogical perspective on youth fitness testing. *Measurement in Physical Education and Exercise Science, 12*(3), 146–166.

Smith, J. J., Eather, N., Morgan, P. J., Plotnikoff, R. C., Faigenbaum, A. D., & Lubans, D. R. (2014). The health benefits of muscular fitness for children and adolescents: A systematic review and meta-analysis. *Sports Medicine, 44*(9), 1209–1223.

Stratton, G. (1995). Dearing or derailing health related exercise in the national curriculum? Tracking physical education's changing role in the promotion of public health. *British Journal of Physical Education, 26*(1), 21–25.

Stratton, G., Canoy, D., Boddy, L. M., Taylor, S. R., Hackett, A. F., & Buchan, I. E. (2007). Cardiorespiratory fitness and body mass index of 9–11-year-old English children: A serial cross-sectional study from 1998 to 2004. *International Journal of Obesity, 31*(7), 1172–1178. Retrieved from http://www.ncbi.nlm.nih.gov/entrez/query.fcgi?cmd=Retrieve&db=PubMed&dopt=Citation&list_uids=17310222

Taylor, S., Hackett, A., Stratton, G., & Lamb, L. (2004). SportsLinx: Improving the health and fitness of Liverpool's youth. *Education and Health, 22*(1), 3–7.

Tomkinson, G. R., Carver, K. D., Atkinson, F., Daniell, N. D., Lewis, L. K., Fitzgerald, J. S., . . . Ortega, F. B. (2018). European normative values for physical fitness in children and adolescents aged 9–17 years: Results from 2 779 165 Eurofit performances representing 30 countries. *British Journal of Sports Medicine, 52*(22), 1445–14563. Retrieved from https://www.ncbi.nlm.nih.gov/pubmed/29191931, doi:10.1136/bjsports-2017-098253

Tomkinson, G. R., Lang, J. J., & Tremblay, M. S. (2017). Temporal trends in the cardiorespiratory fitness of children and adolescents representing 19 high-income and upper middle-income countries between 1981 and 2014. *British Journal of Sports Medicine.* Retrieved from https://www.ncbi.nlm.nih.gov/pubmed/29084727, doi:10.1136/bjsports-2017-097982

Tomkinson, G. R., Leger, L., Olds, T., & Cazorla, G. (2003). Secular trends in the performance of children and adolescents (1980–2000). *Sports Medicine, 33,* 285–300.

Tomkinson, G. R., & Olds, T. S. (2008). Field tests of fitness. In N. Armstrong & W. Van Mechelen (Eds.), *Paediatric exercise science and medicine* (2nd ed.). Oxford, UK: Oxford University Press.

Tremblay, M. S., LeBlanc, A. G., Kho, M. E., Saunders, T. J., Larouche, R., Colley, R. C., . . . Connor Gorber, S. (2011). Systematic review of sedentary behaviour and health indicators in school-aged children and youth. *International Journal of Behavioral Nutrition and Physical Activity, 8,* 98. Retrieved from http://www.ncbi.nlm.nih.gov/pubmed/21936895, doi:10.1186/1479-5868-8-98

Tremblay, M. S., Shields, M., Laviolette, M., Craig, C., Janssen, I., & Gorber, S. (2010). Fitness of Canadian children and youth: Results from the 2007–2009 Canadian health measures survey. *Health Reports, 21*(1), 7–20.

Tyler, R., Mackintosh, K. A., Brophy, S., Christian, D., Todd, C., Tuvey, S., . . . Stratton, G. (2015). *Swan-Linx: Fitness fun day report – Swansea schools.* Retrieved from https://www.swansea.ac.uk/media/Swan-Linx%20Swansea%20Schools'%20Fitness%20Fun%20Day%20feedback%20report%20(2015).pdf

Volaklis, K. A., Halle, M., & Meisinger, C. (2015). Muscular strength as a strong predictor of mortality: A narrative review *European Journal of Internal Medicine, 26*(5), 303–310.

Voss, C., & Sandercock, G. (2010). Aerobic fitness and mode of travel to school in English schoolchildren. *Medicine and Science in Sports and Exercise, 42*(2), 281–287. Retrieved from https://www.ncbi.nlm.nih.gov/pubmed/20083960, doi:10.1249/MSS.0b013e3181b11bdc

Welk, G. J. (1999). The youth physical activity promotion model: A conceptual bridge between theory and practice. *Quest, 51*, 5–23.

Welk, G. J., De Saint-Maurice Maduro, P. F., Laurson, K. R., & Brown, D. D. (2011). Field evaluation of the new FITNESSGRAM(R) criterion-referenced standards. *American Journal of Preventive Medicine, 41*(4 Suppl 2), S131–S142. Retrieved from https://www.ncbi.nlm.nih.gov/pubmed/21961613, doi:10.1016/j.amepre.2011.07.011

Whitehead, J. R., Pemberton, C. L., & Corbin, C. B. (1990). Perspectives on the physical fitness testing of children: The case for a realistic educational approach. *Pediatric Exercise Science, 2*, 111–123.

WHO. (2010). *Global recommendations on physical activity for health.* Retrieved from https://www.who.int/dietphysicalactivity/global-PA-recs-2010.pdf

WHO. (2017). *Facts and figures on childhood obesity.* Retrieved from https://www.who.int/end-childhood-obesity/facts/en

Wiersma, L. D., & Sherman, C. P. (2008). The responsible use of youth fitness testing to enhance student motivation, enjoyment and performance. *Measurement in Physical Education and Exercise Science, 12*(3), 167–183.

Williams, A. (1988). Historiography of health and fitness in physical education. *British Journal of Physical Education, 3*, 1–4.

Wind, A. E., Takken, T., Helders, P., & Engelbert, R. (2010). Is grip strength a predictor for total muscle strength in healthy children, adolescents, and young adults? *European Journal of Pediatrics, 169*(3), 281–287.

19

MOTOR COMPETENCE ASSESSMENT

Lisa M. Barnett, David F. Stodden, Ryan M. Hulteen,
and Ryan S. Sacko

Introduction

Background to Motor Competence Assessment

An Introduction to Terminology

Assessment of human movement has a long history with many different terms used to describe movement performance and its development across time. The aim of this section is to introduce terminology applied in motor competence assessment literature to provide researchers and practitioners with important contextual information on the purpose of assessment. Terms such as motor coordination, motor proficiency, motor fitness, motor performance, motor abilities, motor function, and fundamental/foundational motor skills/movements have been used seemingly interchangeably to assess a similar latent construct, voluntary and goal-oriented human movement. However, different operational definitions and rationale for terminology used to express "motor competence levels" in the literature across the years have created confusion in understanding what different assessment batteries are actually capturing from a movement perspective.

Clear differences in measurement outcomes are noted when assessing qualitative aspects of the movement process (e.g. movement coordination patterns relative to body position, kinematics, and relative timing of segmental movements) versus the result or product of a movement (e.g. projectile or body movement speeds/distance, successful trials, force, accuracy). However, the relationship between qualitative movement process assessment and the outcome of that movement has received surprisingly little attention until recently (see Section "The Broad Measurement Approaches of Product and Process"), presumably influenced by the surge in research examining associations among motor competence and aspects of health in children (Robinson et al., 2015). Notwithstanding clear differences between movement process- and product-oriented assessments, additional terminology issues remain.

An international group of motor development researchers addressed this terminology and measurement issue at the inaugural meeting of the International Motor Development Research Consortium (I-MDRC) in Le Boulard, France in 2015 and proposed that the term *motor competence* be used moving forward as it is a term that globally speaks to product- and process-oriented measurement of human movement; this definition was noted subsequently by Robinson et al. (2015). Thus, the use of this term serves to align research and reduce terminology inconsistencies in the field of motor development and the applications of this work to understand the impact of motor development on various health and other developmental outcomes. It is important to note that the term motor competence should not be used interchangeably with motor development. Motor development is the study of change in movement across the lifespan and the underlying mechanisms and interactions with the environment and other individuals that promote change (Clark & Whitall, 1989; Haywood & Getchell, 2014), whereas motor competence speaks only to the measurement aspect of movement.

Importance of Assessing Motor Competence

The development of locomotor, object control/projection, and balance/stability competence is critical to a child's overall growth and development (Gallahue, Ozmun, & Goodway, 2012) and is suggested to be a critical mechanism promoting participation in various types of physical activity across the lifespan. Developing balance and stability facilitates the development of locomotion via many different movement patterns (e.g. rolling, creeping, crawling, cruising), ultimately leading to various forms of bipedal locomotion (Clark, 2007). Bipedal locomotor skills facilitate body transport in a gravity-based environment (e.g. walk, run, skip, jump) and allow children to independently explore and navigate their environments. The parallel development of locomotor and continually evolving balance and stability are critical to the somewhat later development of object control/projection skills as these types of skills (e.g. kick, throw, strike, catch) are performed in an upright standing posture or in association with during bipedal locomotion skills (e.g. leap-kick, slide-throw, jump-strike, run-catch) (Clark, 2007). The development of a wide variety of skilled movement patterns serves as a foundation (i.e. building blocks) that can then be integrated into more complex movements (Clark & Metcalfe, 2002; Hulteen, Morgan, Barnett, Stodden, & Lubans, 2018; Robinson et al., 2015; Seefeldt, 1980). Without these building blocks, it is difficult to participate in many childhood activities that inherently require a minimal level of competence (Stodden et al., 2008). As success is a critical determinant of various aspects of self-concept and social-emotional development (Bandura, 1986; Deci & Ryan, 2008; Eccles, Wigfield, & Schiefele, 1998; Estevan & Barnett, 2018), the development of these building blocks should be a critical focus in parenting, early childhood development, physical education, youth sports (Barnett, Stodden et al., 2016). A multitude of models hypothesize the importance of developing motor competence to promote various aspects of physical health (e.g. physical activity, physical fitness, and body weight status) and self-concept (i.e. perceived competence, self-efficacy, self-worth, social-emotional development). There is also emerging evidence linking motor competence to cognitive (Alvarez-Bueno et al., 2017; Haapala, 2013; Haapala et al., 2014; Schmidt et al., 2017) and social-emotional health (van der Fels et al., 2015). Thus, the development of motor competence is emerging as potentially being critical to a foundation of holistic child health and well-being.

In 1980, Seefeldt proposed there was a minimal threshold of competence necessary (i.e. a proficiency barrier) in "fundamental" motor skills (i.e. locomotor, object control/projection, balance stability) to further develop more complex skills that could be applied in a variety of settings. Haubenstricker and Seefeldt (1986) also suggested this proficiency barrier may impact physical activity behaviors, specifically for vigorous physical activities. Years later, Clark and Metcalfe (2002) published a seminal paper titled the "Mountain of Motor Development" (2002), where the mountain is a metaphor for an individual's journey in their motor development across their lifespan. Some years later, Stodden et al. (2008) integrated linked aspects of motor and psychological development with Seefeldt's proficiency barrier and hypothesized that these factors would positively and reciprocally relate to longitudinal trajectories of physical activity, health-related fitness, and obesity. Seefeldt's proficiency barrier speaks to the significance of a widening gap in motor competence and health-related outcome variables (e.g. physical activity participation, physical fitness, obesity status) in the most (i.e. the "haves") and least (i.e. the "have-nots") competent individuals (De Meester et al., 2018; Stodden, True, Langendorfer, & Gao, 2013). Over time, higher levels of actual and perceived motor competence increase the likelihood that children will sustain participation in health-enhancing physical activity (Barnett, van Beurden, Morgan, Brooks, & Beard, 2009; Lima et al., 2017). Thus, synergistic development of motor competence and habitual physical activity promotes various aspects of physical fitness (musculoskeletal and cardiorespiratory fitness), healthy weight status, and continued development of motor competence across childhood and into adulthood. In contrast, children who do not acquire adequate levels of motor competence will be less likely to engage in physical activity, develop physical fitness, and increase their risk of becoming obese (Stodden et al., 2008).

History and Purpose of Motor Competence Assessment

The development, performance, and assessment of human movement have been a curiosity of scientists for centuries (Thurston, 1999) and can be traced back as far as 800BCE where Spartans performed evaluations of young men to determine their fitness for citizenship (Van Dalen & Bennett, 1971). Assessment of human movement allows researchers to elucidate potential biological (i.e. genetic reflexive movements, growth, maturation), social (e.g. physical education teachers, coaches, peers, culture), and environmental (e.g. opportunities for practice, built environment) mechanisms associated with the development of competence in a variety of skills that promote functional capability, health, and well-being across the lifespan (Clark & Metcalfe, 2002; Hulteen, Morgan et al., 2018; Seefeldt, 1980). Thus, the study of how change in movement occurs, and the underlying factors that influence change across time (i.e. motor development), is critical to our understanding of overall human development.

The origin of motor competence assessments can generally be traced back to two fields, neurophysiology and psychology, but to better understand the evolution of motor competence assessment, it is important to understand the history of the field of motor development. Clark and Whitall (1989) described the history of motor development in four consecutive periods: Precursor, Maturational, Normative/Descriptive, and Process-Oriented. The proceeding sections provide an understanding of how assessment strategies developed in tandem with the field.

The *Precursor* (1787–1928) period was noted for its impact more on developmental theory, rather than a focus on "motor" development. A link to motor development was noted in the emergence of baby biographies, which did not necessarily focus on the processes of motor development, but laid the foundation for a more specific and dedicated focus to changes in movement behaviors from infancy. During this same extended period, anthropometric measurement and physical performance testing were popularized (Fullerton & Cattell, 1892; Leuba & Chamberlain, 1909; Sargent, Seaver, & Savage, 1897; William & Harter, 1899). This work predated tests of global physical function (i.e. Playground Association of America Athletic Badge Test) for boys (Playground Association of America, 1913) and girls (1916; Bovard, Cozens, & Hagman, 1950) that included the measurement of motor performance in a variety of tasks including jumping, climbing, vaulting, balancing, throwing, and running. The primary influence for this testing was predicated on the increasing popularity of games and play promoted by the Playground Association of America and physical educators. The product-oriented emphasis of these and other tests continued through the "Normative/Descriptive period" (1946–1970) and was further influenced by the need for military readiness during World War I and II.

From 1928 to 1946 the *Maturational* period became popular via the influence of developmental psychology. Clark and Whitall (1989) note this period to be the most rapid period of growth in motor "development" literature where there was an emphasis on maturational and environmental influences on the rate and order of motor development (i.e. change across time), which also initiated the linkage between the process (Halverson, 1931; Wild, 1937) of development and its product (Gesell, 1928; McGraw, 1935; Pratt, 1936). During this same period, Nikolai Bernstein (Russian) and Erich von Holst (German) published seminal papers (not translated into English until the 1960s) that merged the fields of neurophysiology and motor behavior. Bernstein specifically addressed the importance of addressing the biomechanical, neurological, and contextual complexities of human movement and its development (Bernstein, 1967; Schmidt, Lee, Winstein, Wulf, & Zelaznik, 2018). This period of interest in the process of motor development lay dormant as the influence of product–oriented assessment again took center stage because of the need to address military readiness issues during World War II.

The *Normative/Descriptive* period (1946–1970) was dominated by the assessment of product-oriented motor performance in children (Espenschade, 1940), where there was an increasing emphasis on physical education. Product-oriented testing (Fitts, 1954; Fleishman, 1954) also dominated the assessment culture in adults. The influence of this period remains even today with the noted emphasis on product-oriented outcomes in many popular test batteries ((e.g. Körper-Koordinationstest für Kinder (KTK; Kiphard & Schilling, 2007), Movement Assessment Battery for Children (M-ABC; Henderson & Sugden, 1992), and the Bruininks-Oseretsky Test of Motor Proficiency (BOTMP; Bruininks & Bruininks, 2005)).

In the 1970s and 1980s, the *Process-Oriented* period (1970–present) was noted by a resurgence of motor development research that focused on understanding not only how motor skills changed across time, but on the mechanisms that promoted change. During this time, the emphasis on Stage Theory and Dynamic Systems Theory dominated motor development research and led to the examination of movement pattern changes (e.g. whole body developmental sequences, component developmental sequences, see Section "Component Versus Whole Body Approach") mainly in locomotor and object control/projection skills across childhood (Roberton & Halverson, 1977; Wickstrom, 1983). But there was a limited emphasis on lifespan change (VanSant, 1988; Williams, Haywood, & VanSant, 1990, 1998). This work resulted in more contemporary process–oriented assessments that are widely used today ((e.g. Test Gross Motor Development (TGMD; Ulrich, 2000, 2017), Get Skilled: Get Active (GSGA; New South Wales Department of Education and Training, 2000), Children's Activity and Movement in Preschool Study (CHAMPS) Motor Skills Protocol (Williams et al., 2009), Motorische Basiskompetenzen (MOBAK; Herrmann, Gerlach, & Seelig, 2015)).

Overview of the Literature

Considerations for the Assessment of Motor Competence

What Do We Know Already about Motor Competence,
Physical Activity, and Health?

The onset of the 21st century can be characterized by extensive efforts to understand the role of motor development as it relates to public health (Clark, 2017). Physical activity habits are dependent upon a network of intrinsic (e.g. motivation and aspects of self-concept) and extrinsic (e.g. environment and sociological) factors that can work together across the lifespan to form positive or negative health trajectories. Stodden and colleagues' (2008) conceptual model highlighted the need to consider the dynamic and synergistic role of motor competence on multiple factors important to public health (i.e. physical activity, fitness, obesity).

There are now multiple reviews on the relationship between motor competence and physical activity (Engel, Broderick, van Doorn, Parmenter, & Hardy, 2018; Figueroa & An, 2017; Holfelder & Schott, 2014; Logan, Webster, Getchell, Pfeiffer, & Robinson, 2015; Lubans, Morgan, Cliff, Barnett, & Okely, 2010), physical fitness/body weight status (Cattuzzo et al., 2016; Lubans et al., 2010), as well as a review of evidence specific to the original model hypotheses proposed by Stodden and colleagues (Robinson et al., 2015). There is also emerging evidence regarding motor competence and neural and behavioral cognitive outcomes (Alvarez-Bueno et al., 2017; Pesce, 2012; van der Fels et al., 2015). Overall, there is conclusive evidence of a positive association between motor competence and physical activity, physical fitness and body weight status. However, the strength of association between these constructs is highly variable. Amongst studies included in reviews by Holfelder and Schott (2014) and Logan and colleagues (2015), the strength of association between physical activity and motor competence ranged from weak ($r = 0.10$) to strong ($r = 0.92$), which is potentially due to variations in how both physical activity and motor competence were assessed.

Differences in the strength of association between motor competence and physical activity are hypothesized to increase across time (Stodden et al., 2008); however, the previously mentioned assessment issues make it difficult to confirm this hypothesis. The long-term impact of motor competence on physical activity participation during the adolescent and adult years is supported by a number of longitudinal studies conducted over the past decade (Aaltonen et al., 2015; Barnett, van Beurden, Morgan, Brooks et al., 2009; Elhakeem, Hardy, Bann, Kuh, & Cooper, 2018; Jaakkola, Yli-Piipari, Huotari, Watt, & Liukkonen, 2016; Lima et al., 2017; Jaakkola et al., 2019; Lopes, Rodrigues, Maia, & Malina, 2011; Pinto Pereira, Li, & Power, 2014; Smith, Fisher, & Hamer, 2015). Much of this evidence has physical activity and other health behaviors situated as the outcome variable but there is also evidence of a reciprocal relationship (Barnett, Lai et al., 2016; Barnett, Salmon, & Hesketh, 2016; Lima et al., 2017). It is important to note though that only three of the aforementioned longitudinal studies (Barnett, Salmon et al., 2016; Jaakkola et al., 2019; Lima et al., 2017) used objective measures of physical activity and that associations between motor competence and physical activity are affected by measurement choices for physical activity (e.g. pedometers, accelerometers – see Chapters 15 and 16) and motor competence (e.g. see Section "The Broad Measurement Approaches of Product and Process").

When We Assess Intensity and Duration of Physical Activity, What Are We Missing?

Measurement choices for the construct of physical activity can reflect a lack of understanding of the performance of discrete movements such as motor skills. The focus of physical activity assessment in the public health realm generally relates to the health-enhancing aspect of various intensities, as well as the duration of activity. The differences in intensity levels specifically relate to differences in energy expenditure and physiological processes that impact energy balance (i.e. homeostasis of caloric intake). While progress on the assessment of the physiological responses that occur during different intensities of acute and chronic bouts of physical activity continues to advance, gaps still remain. Specifically, the acute and chronic health-enhancing aspects of motor skills are not well understood (Sacko, McIver, Brian, & Stodden, 2018; Sacko et al., 2019). The Compendium of Physical Activities and The Compendium of Energy Expenditures for Youth (ages 6.0–17.9) have been used worldwide to provide researchers with intensity values for activities that have established energy expenditure normative values (Ainsworth et al., 2011; Butte et al., 2018; Ridley, Ainsworth, & Olds, 2008). Notably, much of this research has focused on adults. While a large variety of methods have been used to quantify energy expenditure (e.g. indirect calorimetry, accelerometers, surveys), and have been accepted as a valid means to assess activity intensity, a limitation of these methods is the lack of understanding on how the neuromuscular demand of an activity impacts energy expenditure, specifically in discrete movements that occur intermittently or in a repetitive fashion (Sacko et al., 2018, 2019).

Direct and systematic observation methods of physical activity assessment also have been validated for use in both free-living and school-based environments; yet the accuracy of direct and systematic observation tools to adequately assess physical activity during discrete movements has recently been brought into question. The intermittent nature of discrete movements with high neuromuscular demand is related to high levels of energy expenditure, but these levels may not be captured with current assessment tools (Sacko et al., 2018, 2019).

While accelerometers and pedometers provide a solution for a "relatively" inexpensive and objective estimation of activity intensity, the accuracy of current technology to assess intensity levels (i.e. energy expenditure) of various physical activities has been questioned (Sacko et al., 2019). The underestimation of activity intensity is due to the intermittent nature of object skill performance, as well as the lack of inclusion of activities in accelerometry/pedometry validation studies that require the high intensity locomotor movements (e.g. jumping, hopping, agility/acute change of direction) and object projection skills (e.g. throwing, kicking, striking). Thus, it is critical that physical activity researchers understand more about the physical demands of performing motor skills as this will give insight into the types of movements and activities that inherently require higher neuromuscular demand and also better inform physical activity assessment practices.

Introduction to Motor Competence Assessment

What Does a Competent Performer Look Like?

Competency in movement is assessed with regard to various aspects of movement with most definitions referring to some aspect of volitional human movement (i.e. process of movement) and with the purpose of achieving a goal (i.e. product or outcome). The demonstration of competence or skilled movement also speaks to the variability or consistency in repeated performances (e.g. shooting a free throw or archery), the efficiency of movement (i.e. minimizing energy expenditure) and, in many instances, the fluidity and rhythmicity of a movement (e.g. dance, ice skating).

Competent performers move effectively in a gravity-based environment that includes responding to environmental perturbations and changing task demands (i.e. open skills). The development of higher levels of various locomotor, object control, and balance/stability skills generally places an increased demand on the neuromuscular system to effectively coordinate, control, and transfer energy within the musculoskeletal system (Langendorfer, Roberton, & Stodden, 2011; Stodden, Gao, Langendorfer, & Goodway, 2014; Stodden et al., 2008). While increased performance and relatively simple manipulations of independent body segment movements (e.g. stepping with the contralateral foot instead of the ipsilateral foot in throwing) can be accomplished in a relatively short time skill acquisition), relatively permanent changes (i.e. learning/development) in coordination patterns and performance outcomes demand substantial practice. Specifically, altering specific aspects of coordination patterns (e.g. movement pattern sequencing, relative timing, and segmental inertial lag) that are a result of increased systemic energy being transferred through the system is extremely complex and is a process that results in permanent changes in the peripheral (i.e. intra- and intermuscular coordination mechanisms) and central nervous systems (e.g. neural networks) (Bernstein, 1967; Clark, 2007; Langendorfer et al., 2011). The relatively permanent learning/developmental changes that occur are augmented by appropriately constructed learning environments and practice schedules. All contemporary learning theories follow the notion that practice environments and schedules that integrate a progressive continuum of increased complexity and variability effectively promote learning. However, substantially altering established coordination patterns can temporarily result in increased movement variability and may temporarily impact performance negatively, rather than improving performance as the coordination dynamics of the system reorganize.

Adaptations to movement via context-specific demands (i.e. choice of movement pattern and force regulation) within changing environments also provide another aspect of movement competency that is rarely assessed but is important to address in future research. There is an assumption that a highly skilled individual can vary their movement performance with a variety of different coordination patterns and with effective force regulation (i.e. control), whereas a low skilled individual will not have this capability. In other words, a highly skilled individual can modify performance by demonstrating different (i.e. less or more advanced) coordination patterns and modified force that would be the most appropriate movement for meeting specific task demands (i.e. the goal of the movement). This "flexibility" or adaptability in movement performance capability demonstrates the highest form of movement skill that we, as a field, have not generally addressed from a measurement perspective. Thus, answering what a "competent mover" looks like is relative to task and how the task may change based on the specific goal of the task.

The Broad Measurement Approaches of Product and Process

Motor competence is generally evaluated from a product- or process-oriented perspective. A product-oriented assessment evaluates movement by measuring a component of a resulting outcome of a skill (Haywood & Getchell, 2014). Examples of product assessments include: object projection/reception outcomes (e.g. throwing or kicking ball speeds, accuracy or number of successful attempts), whole body movement outcomes (e.g. running speed, jump distance/height/, moving platforms, balancing), or fine motor outcomes (e.g. threading buttons, tapping test). Advantages of product scores include the convenience of direct assessment at the time of testing (e.g. using stopwatches, radar devices, tape measures, or direct counts). In addition, advanced technology (e.g. inertial sensors, force transducers, force plates, motion capture) provides a means to directly and reliably examine movement outcomes (see Section "Wearable Sensors/Emerging Technology"). Product-oriented assessments provide an advantage over process-oriented assessments as they generally provide continuous data that are highly sensitive for detecting change in movement performances in the short term (i.e. acute intervention) and across the lifespan. However, product measures do not provide information to individuals about how the movement pattern can improve. Also, product scores that assess the performance outcome are not necessarily strongly aligned with the movement process (i.e. coordination patterns) (Haubenstricker & Branta, 1997; Lane et al., 2018; Logan, Barnett, Goodway, & Stodden, 2017; Lorson, Stodden, Langendorfer, & Goodway, 2013; Nesbitt et al., 2017) and may or may not be linked to changes in movement patterns across the lifespan (Halverson, Roberton, & Langendorfer, 1982; Lorson et al., 2013; Roberton & Konczak, 2001; Stodden et al., 2008). For example, a product outcome may be reflective not only of changes in skill but also of changes in anthropometric measures associated with growth and maturation, e.g. skeletal growth has a small, yet significant influence on both process- and product-oriented assessments (Freitas et al., 2015, 2018; Haywood, Roberton, & Getchell, 2012). In addition, learning a more advanced movement pattern, specifically in most locomotor and object control/projection skills, may temporarily result in either increased or decreased performance and increased variability in the movement pattern based on the restructuring of the adaptations in coordination among various limb segments (Langendorfer et al., 2011).

Alternatively, process assessment allows us to understand how a movement is completed and therefore gives practitioners more specific information on how to improve movement specific aspects of a skill. A process-oriented assessment can evaluate highly specific or general aspects of movement coordination based on quantitative evaluations of biomechanical properties of movement (i.e. center of mass displacement, kinematic, relative temporal factors) or by qualitative analyses of segmental movements (e.g. component or whole body developmental sequences). Qualitative process assessments capture either dichotomous, i.e. is a movement present or not – TGMD

(Ulrich, 2000, 2017) or GSGA (New South Wales Department of Education and Training, 2000), or ordinal aspects of coordination patterns (i.e. ranked in order of development – developmental sequences). Quantitative and qualitative movement assessments typically are analyzed via some form of motion capture or video recorded data of a performer's movement.

Component Versus Whole Body Approach

Examining the process of movement has led to the development of many assessments that have been used in research and practice. Stage Theory posits that the development of movement patterns occurs with relative invariance in a specific sequence. These sequences have been examined from a whole body approach (Seefeldt & Haubenstricker, 1976) and via specific body components (Cohen, Goodway, & Lidor, 2012; Langendorfer & Roberton, 2002; Roberton, 1978; Roberton, Thompson, & Langendorfer, 2017; Ulrich, 2000). A whole body approach, first examined by Wild (1938), became popular in the United States during the 1970s as the field of motor development also increased in popularity across the United States. This whole body approach was generally replaced by the component approach as researchers determined that individual limb and trunk movement configurations could develop independently and not necessarily be linked to the development of other body movements. Both the whole body and component approaches note the appearance of more advanced movement levels across age, with the number of levels varying (generally between 3 and 5 levels) depending on the assessment. The process of identifying distinct developmental levels is first conducted using a pre-longitudinal screen and then fully validated with longitudinal data. There are a limited number of skills that have been validated with longitudinal data; however, this validation process spurred the development of additional process-oriented assessments ((TGMD (Ulrich, 2000), GSGA (New South Wales Department of Education and Training, 2000), CHAMPS (Williams et al., 2009)) that also examine somewhat similar aspects of body component movements. These types of assessments only have two levels per component (i.e. present or absent). Thus, the level of measurement discrimination across movement pattern developmental levels is decreased, but the relative ease of use allows for more skills to be analyzed in less time.

Relationship between Process and Product Approaches

The relationship between the process (i.e. coordination and control) and product (i.e. outcome) of movement is an important assessment topic to understand as evaluation of both aspects of movement provides a stronger assessment of motor competence. Overall, the strength of associations among product and process measures on the same movement tasks/skills (Lane et al., 2018; Logan et al., 2017; Nesbitt et al., 2017; Roberton & Konczak, 2001) is generally stronger than comparisons between assessments that measure different skills or different variations of the same skills (Logan et al., 2017; Logan, Robinson, & Getchell, 2011; Ré et al., 2018; Rudd et al., 2016). Attempts to explain low correlations between overall measurement scores from different assessment batteries are usually based on various operational definitions that have little, if any valid, evidence to support the claim and relate to the terminology issues described earlier (see Section "An Introduction to Terminology"). For example, tasks used in tests that purportedly assess "motor abilities" (e.g. M-ABC; Henderson & Sugden, 1992) are suggested to be heritable factors that are relatively stable, while underlying "motor coordination" is proposed to be a factor that can be improved across time and influence "motor performance" or "motor skill" levels. However, the proposed divergence in terminology and measurement constructs is problematic from both a theoretical and practical perspective when similar tasks are promoted across test batteries. For example, hopping is tested in the KTK (Kiphard & Schilling, 2007), TGMD (Ulrich, 2000, 2017) and via product scores (Nesbitt et al., 2017) in three different ways. Likewise, various forms of jumping and/or throwing are assessed in multiple test batteries. Interestingly, these same skills have been noted to assess "different" movement constructs (i.e. motor skill versus motor coordination versus motor ability). More research is needed in this area to understand their individual and collective contributions to motor competence levels and motor development across the lifespan (Utesch et al., 2016).

Key Issues

Considerations When Choosing an Instrument

Reducing Assessment Bias

How we administer skill assessments can influence a participant's actions. When assessing competence levels, we are attempting to elicit an individual's highest level of motor competence. Therefore, it is important to ensure that testing environments are optimized for that purpose and that evaluator bias is removed during the evaluation of an individual's skill performance.

When administering an assessment, it is important to adhere to the administration protocol and also to understand the intent of the testing. Eliciting a child's optimal performance level is paramount in any assessment environment. Promoting maximum effort and/or consistent focus is a necessity to demonstrate the most advanced levels in many types of skills, specifically in ballistic motor skills (e.g. jumping, throwing, hopping, striking), as the most advanced coordination levels are a function of the integration of complex biomechanical and neuromuscular mechanisms (Langendorfer et al., 2011). A background in human movement from an academic perspective (i.e. motor behavior, physical education, or exercise science) and real-world experience (e.g. physical education teacher, coach) is very helpful (although not essential) to assess motor competence. Even so, sufficient training is important, not only of the rules/directions of the testing protocols but also in understanding what the specific protocol is supposed to elicit. For example, catching is a skill that primarily requires hand/eye coordination, but not maximum physical effort, which is more critical for the demonstration of advanced performance levels of other skills such as running, kicking, jumping, hopping, and throwing.

Thus, understanding that providing a throw/toss that is similar in speed, trajectory, and with consistent preparatory toss characteristics is critical to the reliability and validity for assessing the task. In addition, understanding differences in the size, mass, density, and texture of a ball that is catching tossed, thrown, kicked, or struck in a task also can impact performance. The age of participants is an additional critical factor that needs to be considered, not only because age-related cognitive and growth characteristics are integrated with the aforementioned protocol specifics of the task and equipment, but also because of how research staff interact with participants. For example, while explicit instructional protocols and equipment are usually provided with assessment guidelines, the cognitive capabilities, emotions, and behaviors of a 4-year-old are not the same as a 14-year-old. As children are not simply "little adults", having the experience and understanding to effectively work with different age groups is important to consistently elicit the most advanced performance of individuals of all ages.

Skill assessments have protocols in place to either demonstrate a skill prior to a participant's performance or for only verbal instructions to be given. A demonstration is important for novice or early learners based on potential language/cognition barriers. Also, as young children may have little to no experience performing some skills, demonstration of a skill is important for children to "get the idea" of the task and to understand what they are supposed to perform. If a demonstration is required, live or pre-recorded modeling can be used. Live modeling has more potential for variability in the visual information provided, specifically if different modelers demonstrate the task with varying skill levels. Viewing the demonstration through electronic means (e.g. viewing on an iPad) provides more reliable modeling information and may be more preferable to children (Robinson & Palmer, 2017). However, understanding how children relate to a model may also impact the information children extract from it. Specifically, age, gender, race/ethnicity may influence children's perceptions and information extracted from modeling. Research is needed to better understand the potential influence of providing a model on assessment performance and how the modeling information is provided to children. As modeling is an important form of instruction (Wulf, Shea, & Lewthwaite, 2010), understanding its role in assessment is specifically important for young children and low skilled performers, both of whom may use the modeling information to perform the skill at a more advanced level than they would demonstrate without the model (Obrusnikova & Cavalier, 2018).

When assessing process-oriented skill levels (e.g. TGMD, GSGA, developmental sequences), verbal instructions relating to how specific aspects of the body should move (e.g. knowledge of performance) should not be allowed (e.g. swing your arms when you jump). In contrast, providing verbal protocol information that motivates individuals to provide their best effort for any assessment should be provided (e.g. positive reinforcement, knowledge of results) to elicit an individual's best performance. Being consistent with verbal information and explanations of tasks is important as the words we use can impact results. Understanding what verbal information to use in a protocol description is another future direction of research in assessment, as there is very little evidence to understand the impact that verbal protocol information has on performance.

Reliability and Validity

Valid and reliable motor skill assessments are essential to the field so there can be confidence in results obtained. Reliability refers to the degree a test produces consistent results. Validity refers to a test's appropriateness, meaningfulness, and usefulness in a population of interest (Burton & Miller, 1998). It is also important to remember that measurement properties of an assessment need to be established in the population of interest. While many motor competence assessments exist, higher forms of validity (e.g. criterion) and reliability (e.g. test-retest) values are not commonly reported (Cools, Martelaer, Samaey, & Andries, 2009; Hulteen et al., 2015; Robertson, Burnett, & Cochrane, 2014). Specific measurement properties of available motor skill assessments have been described elsewhere (Cools et al., 2009; Hulteen et al., 2015; Robertson et al., 2014). For example, see two recent reviews of the validity and reliability properties of motor skill assessments for children and adolescents (Griffiths, Toovey, Morgan, & Spittle, 2018; Scheuer, Herrmann, & Bund, 2019). Findings show that many different assessments for fundamental movement skills exist, though M-ABC, TGMD, and BOT have been the skill assessments most commonly used. This would seem to indicate that we have many "different" assessments that assess similar types of skills, but the measurement properties of these different skill batteries may not be well understood.

Scoring or coding of performance is a major factor with potential to influence the measurement of both product- and process-oriented skill assessments. In process-oriented assessments, researchers need to ensure that raters remain objective (e.g. ideally blinded to intervention and control group in intervention research) and that data collectors have sufficient training. While there is no definitive number of hours mandated for training, researchers should have confidence that raters are able to suitably demonstrate inter-rater agreement with expert raters (gold standard), and reliably with their own ratings (i.e. intra-rater agreement) (Barnett, van Beurden, Morgan, Lincoln et al., 2009). For example, Palmer and Brian (2016) showed that, even with training, expert and novice coders do not necessarily demonstrate sufficient levels of agreement on a skill assessment. Another study demonstrated that even with well-trained raters, it can be challenging to find adequate inter-rater agreement at the skill component level (Barnett, Minto, Lander, & Hardy, 2014). This reinforces the need for standardized training prior to data being analyzed.

Sensitivity and Discrimination

Sensitivity (i.e. the capability of a test to detect meaningful differences between performer and performances) and discrimination (i.e. the capability of a test to adequately differentiate skill levels) are other considerations for motor skill assessments. If a test lacks either of these elements, it can negatively impact the predictive utility of the test, which has implications for determining the impact of motor competence on various outcome measures. Notably, the skill assessment type (product or process) can impact sensitivity and discrimination in different ways. Thus, these properties will differ for product measures (e.g. continuous scores), ordinal data (e.g. developmental sequences with multiple levels for each component), or component level data (yes/no score for each component which are then added together to get a "higher" score).

Lack of discrimination within an assessment can result in a ceiling effect (i.e. too many participants scoring at the maximum) or floor effects (i.e. too many participants scoring at the lowest level) (i.e. measurement sensitivity issue). Though floor effects are important, in that they may also show that individuals cannot perform a skill (e.g. the skill is too complex for participants' current capability). Process-oriented assessments in particular can suffer from having floor and ceiling effects, especially if there are too few components or too few levels within components used to assess participants. Having only two levels of a specific skill component (e.g. present or absent) may be problematic from a measurement and developmental validity perspective (Logan et al., 2017). Alternatively, most product-oriented measures are scored on continuous scales, which provides adequate sensitivity of assessment and discrimination, but a similar product score does not necessarily indicate agreement between performers' movement coordination patterns to achieve the performance (Lane et al., 2018; Logan et al., 2017).

Feasibility

The feasibility of the instrument for a particular context is also a factor that is often overlooked but is important (Klingberg, Schranz, Barnett, Booth, & Ferrar, 2019). Teachers report that assessments need to be simple to use and quick to administer (van Rossum, Foweather, Richardson, Hayes, & Morley, 2019). As such, motor skill measures that require one on one administration for a lengthy period might not be appropriate for a physical education teacher on their own with a class of students (Lander, Hanna et al., 2017). In this case, a circuit-based motor skill assessment may be useful as it can be easily administered in the context of a physical education class (Hoeboer, Krijger-Hombergen, Savelsbergh, & De Vries, 2018; Lander, Morgan, Salmon, & Barnett, 2015; Longmuir et al., 2017). A recent systematic review identified that administration time, equipment, space, assessment type, number of items, training needed, and qualifications required were important feasibility aspects, specifically for preschool settings (Klingberg et al., 2019).

Potentially, the most ecological and valid assessment of performance would assess common motor skills as well as how they are applied (i.e. strategies and tactics) in a game play environment – although then there would be the complexity of being able to tease out the different "skills" that were necessary for success. To illustrate this idea further, a recent Australian study noted that game play was a stronger predictor of moderate-to-vigorous physical activity than ball skill competence (Miller, Eather, Duncan, & Lubans, 2019). Thus, the development of perceptual-cognitive skills to evaluate, understand, and interpret the information present in a complex game environment is a critical aspect of overall competence/skills that have important implications for continued development as well as their impact on important health outcomes (Miller et al., 2019).

These considerations will likely have different levels of importance in different contexts and for the individuals who are assessing. For example, a well-resourced researcher may not be concerned with expensive equipment needs or the time to conduct an assessment, whereas childcare staff with no training in motor assessment and a limited budget would consider such factors very important. This is where it becomes useful to use a decision guide approach to assessment that will allow researchers or practitioners to work through particular scenarios to identify the most appropriate assessment instrument.

Choosing an Instrument

With so many motor skill assessments available, it can be challenging to decide which one is the "best" one to use in a particular situation. Often the measurement properties of an instrument will be used as the first point of judgment (see Section "Reliability and Validity"). While measurement properties are integral to a decision, there are other practical factors which also need to be considered. The *best* instrument will depend on your particular aim and purpose and a host of other factors (e.g. practical application or research, the characteristics of the population, administrative and feasibility aspects). Decision guides have been developed for physical activity (Dollman et al., 2009), sedentary behavior (Hardy et al., 2013), and more recently, physical literacy (Barnett, van Beurden, Morgan, Lincoln et al., 2019) assessment that help users identify which assessment would be right for their circumstance. A similar approach (modeled from these approaches) was recently published for motor skill assessment for children and adolescents (Bardid, Vannozzi, Logan, Hardy, & Barnett, 2019) and provides a guide for researchers and practitioners in their selection of motor competence measures.

Bardid et al. (2019) present a range of scenarios that cover the different contexts in which motor skill measurement occurs (i.e. clinical, education, population screening and monitoring, and sports). For each scenario, the reader is guided through questions that should be asked and is then provided information regarding different methods of assessment that might be appropriate. The guide provides information on the limitations and practical considerations with regard to each method and also includes information on both objective (motion devices and direct observation) and subjective measures (self- and proxy-reports; see Figure 19.1).

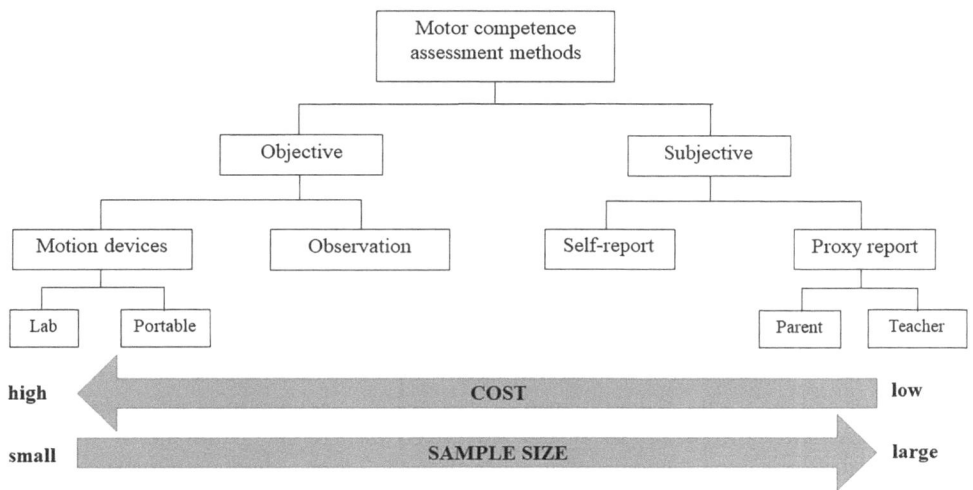

Figure 19.1 Flow chart for selecting methods to assess motor competence among young people. Taken with permission from "A hitchhiker's guide to assessing young people's motor competence: Deciding what method to use" (Bardid et al., 2019)

Emerging Issues

Developments in Motor Competence Assessment

Broadening Our Approach in Terms of Skills to Assess

When approaching motor development from a lifespan perspective, a traditional notion of children's fundamental motor skills (e.g. locomotor, object control/manipulation, balance/stability) provides only a small snapshot of skills that may be important for current and future physical activity participation into adulthood (Barnett, Stodden et al., 2016; Hulteen, Morgan et al., 2018). The limited representation of skills assessed within many assessments is in part due to the majority of research in motor development being focused from birth through adolescence. While any goal-directed human movement can be classified as assessing "motor competence", it is important to understand the most salient skills that can be linked to positive trajectories of other physical and psychological health outcomes across the lifespan (e.g. physical activity, health-related fitness, body weight status, self-concept) (Robinson et al., 2015). Therefore, the assessment of a wide variety of skills that are foundational to lifespan development is important. Alternative skills that are an important to an individual's physical activity behaviors include swimming skills (e.g. freestyle swim), cycling, and resistance training skills (e.g. squat, push-up, lunge), as well as functional (e.g. sit-to-stand, supine-to-stand, yoga) skills, all of which supplement daily levels of health-enhancing physical activity. Many of these skills can also be applied into more context-specific forms, thereby providing more choice and opportunity to participate in many types of physical activities (Hulteen, Morgan et al., 2018). For example, learning to swim is essential for water safety. However, once learned, these skills are applied within the context of other water-based activities (e.g. surfing, paddle boarding, kayaking). In essence, these ideas still resonate with previously established models of motor development (Gallahue et al., 2012; Seefeldt, 1980), where the initial development of many different types of skills is "foundational" to more complex movements and applicable to multiple contexts of movement.

Recent advancements such as the Lifelong Physical Activity Skills Battery (Hulteen, Barnett et al., 2018), Resistance Training Skills Battery (Barnett, Reynolds et al., 2015; Lubans, Smith, Harries, Barnett, & Faigenbaum, 2014) and Golf Swing and Putt Skill Assessment for Children (Barnett, Hardy, Brian, & Robertson, 2015) provide process-oriented measures for some of the skills that have not been routinely assessed from a research perspective. These skill batteries have recently been used in child and adolescent populations. Much like the traditional "fundamental" motor skills, recent evidence shows the majority of children and adolescents do not perform these skills at advanced levels (Duncan, Jones, O'Brien, Barnett, & Eyre, 2018; Furzer, Bebich-Philip, Wright, Reid, & Thornton, 2018; Hulteen, Barnett et al., 2018; Smith et al., 2018). As the development of movement skills does not "naturally occur" (Logan, Robinson, Wilson, & Lucas, 2012), our goal should be to ensure that individuals develop competency in a wide range of skills so that individuals can choose to be physically active in a variety of activities across the entire lifespan. Although it is important to note (and reflect on when using these assessments) that with skills such as a squat or lunge, a usual developmental progression across age may not be demonstrated as very young children can usually squat more effectively than adults. This is a case where a skill demonstrates developmental "regression" quite early in the lifespan due to allometric differences across childhood and growth patterns that dramatically redefine our anthropometric characteristics. In addition, sedentary behaviors and the lack of a physically demanding environment where full squatting is promoted via activities and exercise also can induce this movement pattern developmental regression.

Ecological Validity of Motor Competence Assessment

Adaptations to movement (i.e. choice of movement pattern and force regulation) based on context-specific demands within changing environments also provide another level of movement competency that is rarely assessed. Ecological validity is the degree to which performance on an assessment relates to real-world performance (Chaytor & Schmitter-Edgecombe, 2003). Franzen and Wilhelm (1996) outline two conceptual approaches to ecological validity: verisimilitude and veridicality. Applied to motor competence assessment, *verisimilitude* is how similar the motor skill demands of a test resemble the motor skill demands in everyday life, and *veridicality* is how accurately we can predict motor skill behavior in a real-world context. Therefore, research with a verisimilitude approach is concerned with the motor skill demands of a test and how this relates to real life as compared to research with a veridicality goal which uses statistical techniques to relate performance on a particular motor skill assessment to measures of real-world motor skill performance (e.g. success in a sports context).

Identifying the ecological validity of motor skill assessments is important as it means we are moving on from simply determining at what level a child is performing to considering the impact of their skill level and performance in other domains (e.g. physical health, cognitive and psychological health, interpersonal skills). If we consider different motor skill assessments in terms of a verisimilitude approach, they could exist on a continuum from low to high ecological validity. A test of jumping in a laboratory setting (e.g. requiring specialized equipment such as motion capture, Vertec or a force plate) has adequate ecological validity as performance reflects jumping in other contexts. A high effort jump performed in a playground setting and assessed using the TGMD would have better ecological validity as the child is in a real-life context. However, test scores based on the TGMD scoring criteria are not as sensitive or discriminative between participants as performances scored with the expensive laboratory equipment. A circuit-based assessment that links common motor skills together (Hoeboer et al., 2018; Klingberg et al., 2019; Lander, Morgan, Salmon, Logan, & Barnett, 2017) (including a jump) in a way that might reflect how a jump is used in a real-life game (e.g. a layup or rebound in basketball) could be ecologically valid, but will depend on the constraints of the task (e.g. does it require maximum effort?) and how the jump is scored based on specified criteria. Potentially, the most ecologically valid assessment would assess motor skills in a game play or other type of authentic environment with the added complexity of teasing out different levels of skills demanded for success and whether participants could correctly choose and execute the level of skill needed for success at various levels. For example, does a task require a high effort, advanced level movement pattern with a moderate degree of accuracy (e.g. long distance goal kick in football/soccer)? Or, is a more rudimentary movement pattern with low force and a high degree of accuracy required for successful completion of the goal (e.g. short underhand toss in baseball or softball)?

A recent review noted the challenge of conducting assessments that were both ecologically valid and well controlled (Buszard, Reid, Masters, & Farrow, 2016). They used the example of tennis, where a child's striking competence might be tested by requiring children to strike a ball coming from a ball machine – in this way, ball speed and direction are controlled. However, this approach doesn't reflect match conditions, which would require "rallying" with different types and speed of shots to reflect a verisimilitude approach. Yet this method brings in other issues such as the range of factors contributing to success in a match, and children needing a certain amount of skill to be able to participate (Buszard et al., 2016). In summary, striving for ecological validity is important, but the more ecologically valid a test is, the more likely there is a range of constraints that would include a range of exhibited skill levels, meaning we need to always consider what are we actually assessing and why are we assessing it in a particular way?

Wearable Sensors/Emerging Technology

As noted previously, one of the challenges with assessment, particularly process-oriented assessment, is the need to train researchers or staff to reach a certain degree of reliability. Accurately assessing skilled movement needs not only training and practice on a specific assessment, but some knowledge base in human movement, as there is a level of subjectivity involved in the various process-oriented motor skill assessments (see Section "The Broad Measurement Approaches of Product and Process").

Emerging technologies can potentially provide a more objective, sensitive, and reliable way to assess skill. Previous technology and cost limitations associated with examining kinematic, kinetic, and relative timing segmental movements (e.g. force plates and motion capture systems) were not feasible to assess these types of data on a large scale. However, emerging technology has the capability to incorporate instrumented versions of test batteries that integrate motion capture and observation methods to enhance the sensitivity and reliability of assessment of children's motor competence. For instance, recent papers from Italian researchers have reported the utility of wearable inertial sensor devices to assess running (Masci et al., 2013), hopping (Masci, Vannozzi, Getchell, & Cappozzo, 2012), standing long jump (Sgrò et al., 2017), and throwing (Grimpampi, Masci, Pesce, & Vannozzi, 2016) competence. In these studies, children performed the skill while wearing a number of inertial sensors located in different positions depending on the skill, e.g. wrist, trunk, and pelvis for the throw (Grimpampi et al., 2016). Biomechanical parameter data were used to develop algorithms that were compared to existing observational assessment data such as developmental sequences. In the study by Bisi, Panebianco, Polman, and Stagni (2017), children wore five such sensors mounted on the lower back, ankles, and wrists. Data from the sensors were compared to the standard assessment of the TGMD-2. Authors found the automated assessment was much quicker than standard subjective assessment and showed at least 87% agreement for each skill, and 77% agreement with the corresponding TGMD-2 performance criterion (Bisi et al., 2017). Another motion capture approach for objective assessment is use of the Kinect system (Ward, Thornton, Lay, & Rosenberg, 2017). Similar to studies using inertial sensors, one study categorized vertical jumping skill levels according to observational records. Then, these data were compared to kinematic and temporal parameters estimated using a biomechanical model derived from Kinect data (Sgrò, Nicolosi, Schembri, Pavone, & Lipoma, 2015). While these approaches using sensor wear are advancing motor skill measurement by making assessment more automotive and reliable, they can also be seen as a form of concurrent validity against other process-oriented observational instruments that are routinely used.

The previous examples are representative of a plethora of technological assessment possibilities with some assessments more applicable to research and/or clinical settings, e.g. raw accelerometry data, gyroscopes (Dobkin & Martinez, 2018), and some more applicable to field-based applications (e.g. two-dimensional motion capture and ball speed apps on phones, Kinect, or other gaming motion capture). These types of assessments are promising in terms of the potential to complete an assessment quickly and potentially, reliably; however, developmental validity should not be overlooked when integrating new assessment technology. There also are feasibility questions for widespread population monitoring. For sensors, considerations include: the number of sensors, where they are placed on the skin, whether children can place the sensors on themselves, and the cost of each sensor. For all of these assessments, the number of parameters considered important to determine a successful skill performance is an important consideration. Furthermore, some of the current analysis approaches (e.g. when using data from sensors) are complex, which could also limit widespread application (Sgrò et al., 2017). Bisi et al. (2017) allude to these issues by noting that future research will investigate the possibility of one single device with the data linked directly to an app on a smartphone. Finally, if technology is going to be used to make assessment more valid and reliable and that are valid from a developmental perspective, then it will be important to conduct concurrent validity studies using assessments that have adequate developmental validity.

Recommendations for Researchers and Practitioners

Twenty years ago, Burton and Miller (1998) provided a number of recommendations for the future in their well-known text on movement skill assessment. We will discuss some of these recommendations in terms of where we are today and our recommendations for the future.

The first recommendation was to focus on *program outcomes* when assessing motor competence. Considering program outcomes in terms of physical education and curricula standards has received more attention over the last 20 years. Yet in terms of motor assessment, we still have a long way to go in terms of international, national, or even state level representative motor skill data. Without such data it is difficult to monitor the impact of programs and policies or assess change over time. One exception is the Australian state level New South Wales Schools Physical Activity and Nutrition Survey (Hardy, Mihrshahi, Drayton, & Bauman, 2016; NSW Ministry of Health, 2011). In addition, the American National Health and Nutrition Education Survey recently added motor skill data to the Youth Fitness Survey (Kit, Akinbami, Isfahani, & Ulrich, 2017). Although a sample of 354 pre-schoolers is quite small to be considered a nationally representative sample, it is an important step to include motor assessment on a national survey. Many of the physical activity country-specific report cards report on motor skills (NCD Alliance, 2018), but the issue is whether the data used to form these reports can be considered as national or state representative data. Thus, our first recommendation is that we collect state, national, and international level representative motor skill data. Collecting these data will provide a valuable resource for understanding child development from a more holistic perspective as gross motor development is linked to other important aspects of development including cognition/academic achievement (Diamond, 2000; Haapala, 2013) and social-emotional development (Libertus & Hauf, 2017; Li, Kwan, & Cairney, 2019; Mancini, Rigoli, Roberts, & Piek, 2019).

Not only should there be a directed focus on collecting normative data, but it is also recommended that we collect longitudinal and experimental data on motor competence linked with other variables of interest to domains such as public health and education. This will be a critical step in understanding the potential impact that developing motor competence has on a variety of important outcomes. While physical activity levels can be transient, motor development results in permanent change to the central as well as the peripheral neuromotor system that also aligns with relatively permanent improvement in coordination patterns and performance. Aligned with growth and maturational processes, it is critical to understand both the short-term (motor skill acquisition) and long-term process of motor development (i.e. longitudinal trajectories) in order to understand both the role of relatively short (i.e. 6–12 week intervention references) and longer interventions (i.e. 1 year or more interventions; Cohen, Morgan, Plotnikoff, Barnett, & Lubans, 2015) and long-term impact that acquiring motor competence has on physical activity (Barnett, van Beurden, Morgan, Brooks et al., 2009; Lima et al., 2017; Lopes et al., 2011, 2019), health-related fitness, and body weight status (D'Hondt et al., 2013, 2014; Lima et al., 2017; Rodrigues, Stodden, & Lopes, 2016). More importantly, as negative motor competence trajectories (i.e. decreasing across time) parallel the general decreases in physical activity and increases in unhealthy body weight levels across childhood and into adolescence (D'Hondt et al., 2013, 2014; Lopes et al., 2011; Martins et al., 2010; Rodrigues et al., 2016) longitudinal investigations can provide valuable insight as to why general population data demonstrate these negative changes. For example, multiple longitudinal studies have demonstrated that higher levels of initial motor competence have a protective effect against decreasing physical activity levels and unhealthy weight gain (D'Hondt et al., 2013,

2014; Lima et al., 2017; Lopes et al., 2011; Rodrigues et al., 2016), while low levels of motor competence are associated with progressively worse trajectories of the same variables.

While traditional longitudinal designs demonstrate yearly follow-up intervals, shorter intervals of data collection (e.g. 3–6 months) are important to gain a better timescale of change in growth and motor development, specifically as this would allow better understanding of how other individual and environmental factors (e.g. growth, seasonality, school policies) relate to changes in children's motor development, body weight status, physical fitness, and physical activity patterns. It is also important that longitudinal studies utilize sophisticated modeling techniques so we can identify other factors that contribute to positive health trajectories. As an example, a recent longitudinal study provided insights into critical scaling factors (of the few measured in that study) regarding 6–9 year old children's stature and body mass changes that were associated with better motor competence. Authors identified that the greatest changes in motor competence over time were in children who were leaner and fitter, which led to authors recommending that physical educators also focus on fitness development (Dos Santos et al., 2018).

In addition, more studies are needed to help identify the minimal amount/level of motor competence that may be required to demonstrate adequate levels of other outcome variables (De Meester et al., 2018). De Meester et al. (2018) recently noted that children with high motor competence were 2.5 times more likely to meet the physical activity guidelines than children with low motor competence. It is also not clear if high levels of competence in one or two skills are more predictive of physical activity than moderate competency across a wider range of skills, or if some skills are more predictive than others (Jaakkola et al., 2019). Such advancements will further help to promote the importance of motor competence as a matter of public health.

Another recommendation from the Burton and Miller (1998) text was that product assessment may be better than process in terms of task achievement. They suggested that assessment methods may need to revert back to product assessment (common up until the 1960s, Section "History and Purpose of Motor Competence Assessment") because "movement function must ultimately be defined by product or outcome rather than process" (Burton and Miller, 1998, p. 324). However, 20 years later we would suggest it is critically important to understand the process of movement as it is central to understanding motor development and how to promote change via intervention. Furthermore, we do not view product or process assessment as either/or, but rather recommend the value of both assessment forms. In fact, recent suggestions are to recommend both product and process (Logan et al., 2017; Ré et al., 2018; Rudd et al., 2016) and to also consider other aspects such as the ecological validity of the assessment (i.e. authentic assessment) (see Section "Ecological Validity of Motor Competence Assessment").

Another recommendation by Burton and Miller was to use non-standardized tests, defined as informal assessment, e.g. manipulation of the task and/or environment (Burton & Miller, 1998). This was recommended because such modifications are said to allow a better understanding, in some circumstances, of a person's skill level (Burton & Miller, 1998). This recommendation has not generally been implemented as the field is seemingly more concerned with *valid, reliable, and replicable* assessments. There is one area, however, where informal assessment could be critically important, and that is when assessing children and youth with a disability. For instance, allowing the task to be manipulated or the instructions modified for children with disabilities (e.g. Autism Spectrum Disorder, visually impaired, and other movement disabilities) may provide a more contextually relevant picture of a child's motor skill level (Breslin & Liu, 2015). Aside from these circumstances, we recommend it is critical to continue to focus on valid, reliable, and replicable assessments.

The last recommendation from Burton and Miller (1998) was the application of technology. Technology is revolutionizing the way in which research is conducted and disseminated. For example, early researchers did not have hardware or software capable of quickly processing the vast quantities of data (via large samples) which is standard practice in research today. It is critical to continue to investigate the potential of emerging technologies to capture motor competence. At present, feasibility issues are specifically tied to a specific knowledge base in biomechanics and anatomy as well as being able to relate data to development. Thus, moving forward, having applications that can be used and interpreted for those with less knowledge in these areas (e.g. a primary school teacher) will be important. In the section on "Wearable Sensors/Emerging Technology" it was made clear that the assessment of motor competence is adapting with new technologies (and no doubt will continue to do so). Thus, we recommend that emerging technologies continue to be investigated with regard to their potential to appropriately capture motor competence levels and their implications for development.

Finally, while the use of process-oriented assessments coupled with product outcomes is an important step forward in assessment, and the integration of new technology will allow even greater advances in assessment, we caution and recommend researchers and practitioners to always consider whether the most critical and salient aspects of motor development are being captured. For example, two groups of researchers (Hands, McIntyre, & Parker, 2018; Utesch et al., 2016) have recently rekindled a long-standing debate relating to the development of skill being influenced by an underlying "general motor ability" or multiple different abilities; for a review see Hands et al. (2018). The notion of a general motor ability speaks to a "stable and relatively enduring trait" (Schmidt, 1991) that will influence the development of multiple skills, thus promulgating the concept of a "natural athlete" or "natural ability". However, the general motor ability idea was debunked via research noting the low correlations between "specific perceptuomotor abilities" (Fleishman, 1954). Unfortunately, the lack of adequate measurement techniques (e.g. biomechanical technologies), longitudinal data, and sophisticated statistical analysis techniques has limited the capacity of researchers to adequately address the argument (Hands et al., 2018). Thus, more sophisticated human movement measurement and statistical techniques such as Item Response Theory, structural equation modeling, and various forms of growth curve modeling will allow us to better understand and encapsulate what and how we assess changes in motor competence and what influences these changes across time. Finally, as this chapter demonstrates the need to improve motor competence assessment from validity, reliability, and feasibility perspectives to move the field of motor development forward, it leaves us with a question and direction for future research … Do current motor competence assessments adequately capture and explain changes in the development of skilled human movement?

References

Aaltonen, S., Latvala, A., Rose, R. J., Pulkkinen, L., Kujala, U. M., Kaprio, J., & Silventoinen, K. (2015). Motor development and physical activity: A longitudinal discordant twin-pair study. *Medicine and Science in Sports and Exercise, 47*(10), 2111–2118.

Ainsworth, B. E., Haskell, W. L., Herrmann, S. D., Meckes, N., Bassett, D. R., Jr., Tudor-Locke, C., . . . Leon, A. S. (2011). 2011 compendium of physical activities: A second update of codes and MET values. *Medicine and Science in Sports and Exercise, 43*(8), 1575–1581. doi:10.1249/MSS.0b013e31821ece12

Alvarez-Bueno, C., Pesce, C., Cavero-Redondo, I., Sanchez-Lopez, M., Martinez-Hortelano, J. A., & Martinez-Vizcaino, V. (2017). The effect of physical activity interventions on children's cognition and metacognition: A systematic review and meta-analysis. *Journal of the American Academy of Child and Adolescent Psychiatry, 56*(9), 729–738. doi:10.1016/j.jaac.2017.06.012

Bandura, A. (1986). *Social foundations of thought and action. A social cognitive theory.* Englewoods, NJ: Prentice-Hall.

Bardid, F., Vannozzi, G., Logan, S. W., Hardy, L. L., & Barnett, L. M. (2019). A hitchhiker's guide to assessing young people's motor competence: Deciding what method to use. *Journal of Science and Medicine in Sport, 22*(3), 311–318. doi:10.1016/j.jsams.2018.08.007

Barnett, L. M., Dudley, D. A., Telford, R. D., Lubans, D. R., Bryant, A. S., Roberts, W. M., . . . Keegan, R. J. (2019). Guidelines for the selection of physical literacy measures in physical education in Australia. *Journal of Teaching in Physical Education, 38*(2), 119–125. doi:10.1123/jtpe.2018-0219

Barnett, L. M., Hardy, L. L., Brian, A., & Robertson, S. J. (2015). The development and validation of a golf swing and putt skill assessment for children. *Journal of Sports Science and Medicine, 14*(1), 147–154.

Barnett, L. M., Lai, S. K., Veldman, S. L. C., Hardy, L. L., Cliff, D. P., Morgan, P. J., . . . Okely, A. D. (2016). Correlates of gross motor competence in children and adolescents: A systematic review and meta-analysis. *Sports Medicine, 46*(11), 1663–1688. doi:10.1007/s40279-016-0495-z

Barnett, L. M., Minto, C., Lander, N., & Hardy, L. L. (2014). Interrater reliability assessment using the test of gross motor development-2. *Journal of Science and Medicine in Sport, 17*(6), 667–670. doi:10.1016/j.jsams.2013.09.013

Barnett, L. M., Reynolds, J., Faigenbaum, A. D., Smith, J. J., Harries, S., & Lubans, D. R. (2015). Rater agreement of a test battery designed to assess adolescents' resistance training skill competency. *Journal of Science and Medicine in Sport, 18*(1), 72–76. doi:10.1016/j.jsams.2013.11.012

Barnett, L. M., Salmon, J., & Hesketh, K. D. (2016). More active pre-school children have better motor competence at school starting age: An observational cohort study. *BMC Public Health, 16*(1), 1068. doi:10.1186/s12889-016-3742-1

Barnett, L. M., Stodden, D. F., Cohen, K., E., Smith, J. J., Lubans, D., R., Lenoir, M., . . . Morgan, P. J. (2016). Fundamental movement skills: An important focus. *Journal of Teaching in Physical Education, 35*(3), 219–225. doi:10.1123/jtpe.2014-0209

Barnett, L. M., van Beurden, E., Morgan, P. J., Brooks, L. O., & Beard, J. R. (2009). Childhood motor skill proficiency as a predictor of adolescent physical activity. *Journal of Adolescent Health, 44*(3), 252–259. doi:10.1016/j.jadohealth.2008.07.004

Barnett, L. M., van Beurden, E., Morgan, P. J., Lincoln, D., Zask, A., & Beard, J. R. (2009). Interrater objectivity for field-based fundamental motor skill assessment. *Research Quarterly for Exercise and Sport, 80*(2), 363–368.

Bernstein, N. (1967). *The co-ordination and regulation of movements*. Oxford, UK: Pergamon Press Ltd.

Bisi, M. C., Panebianco, G. P., Polman, R., & Stagni, R. (2017). Objective assessment of movement competence in children using wearable sensors: An instrumented version of the TGMD-2 locomotor subtest. *Gait and Posture, 56*, 42–48.

Bovard, J. F., Cozens, F. W., & Hagman, E. P. (1950). *Tests & measurements in physical education*. Philadelphia, PA: WB Saunders Co.

Breslin, C. M., & Liu, T. (2015). Do you know what I'm saying? Strategies to assess motor skills for children with autism spectrum disorder. *Journal of Physical Education, Recreation & Dance, 86*(1), 10–15. doi:10.1080/07303084.2014.978419

Bruininks, R. H., & Bruininks, B. D. (2005). *Bruininks-Oseretsky test of motor proficiency* (2nd ed.). Minneapolis, MN: NCS Pearson.

Burton, A. W., & Miller, D. E. (1998). *Movement skill assessment*. Champaign, IL: Human Kinetics.

Buszard, T., Reid, M., Masters, R., & Farrow, D. (2016). Scaling the equipment and play area in children's sport to improve motor skill acquisition: A systematic review. *Sports Medicine, 46*(6), 829–843. doi:10.1007/s40279-015-0452-2

Butte, N. F., Watson, K. B., Ridley, K., Zakeri, I. F., McMurray, R. G., Pfeiffer, K. A., . . . Fulton, J. E. (2018). A youth compendium of physical activities: Activity codes and metabolic intensities. *Medicine and Science in Sports and Exercise, 50*(2), 246–256. doi:10.1249/mss.0000000000001430

Cattuzzo, M. T., Dos Santos Henrique, R., Re, A. H., de Oliveira, I. S., Melo, B. M., de Sousa Moura, M., . . . Stodden, D. F. (2016). Motor competence and health related physical fitness in youth: A systematic review. *Journal of Science and Medicine in Sport, 19*(2), 123–129. doi:10.1016/j.jsams.2014.12.004

Chaytor, N., & Schmitter-Edgecombe, M. (2003). The ecological validity of neuropsychological tests: A review of the literature on everyday cognitive skills. *Neuropsychology Review, 13*(4), 181–197. doi:10.1023/B:NERV.0000009483.91468.fb

Clark, J. E. (2007). On the problem of motor skill development: Motor skills do not develop miraculously from one day to the next. They must be taught and practiced. *Journal of Physical Education Recreation and Dance, 78*(5), 39–44.

Clark, J. E. (2017). Pentimento: A 21st century view on the canvas of motor development. *Kinesiology Review, 6*(3), 232–239. doi:10.1123/kr.2017-0020

Clark, J. E., & Metcalfe, J. S. (2002). The mountain of motor development: A metaphor. In J. E. Clark & J. H. Humphrey (Eds.), *Motor development: Research and reviews* (Vol. 2, pp. 163–190). Reston, VA: National Association for Sport and Physical Education.

Clark, J. E., & Whitall, J. (1989). What is motor development? The lessons of history. *Quest, 41*(3), 183–202. doi:10.1080/00336297.1989.10483969

Cohen, K. E., Morgan, P. J., Plotnikoff, R. C., Barnett, L. M., & Lubans, D. R. (2015). Improvements in fundamental movement skill competency mediate the effect of the SCORES intervention on physical activity and cardiorespiratory fitness in children. *Journal of Sports Sciences, 33*(18), 1908–1918. doi:10.108 0/02640414.2015.1017734

Cohen, R., Goodway, J. D., & Lidor, R. (2012). The effectiveness of aligned developmental feedback on the overhand throw in third-grade students. *Physical Education and Sport Pedagogy, 17*(5), 525–541. doi:10.10 80/17408989.2011.623230

Cools, W., Martelaer, K. D., Samaey, C., & Andries, C. (2009). Movement skill assessment of typically developing preschool children: A review of seven movement skill assessment tools. *Journal of Sports Science & Medicine, 8*(2), 154–168.

D'Hondt, E., Deforche, B., Gentier, I., De Bourdeaudhuij, I., Vaeyens, R., Philippaerts, R., & Lenoir, M. (2013). A longitudinal analysis of gross motor coordination in overweight and obese children versus normal-weight peers. *International Journal of Obesity (London), 37*(1), 61–67. doi:10.1038/ijo.2012.55

D'Hondt, E., Deforche, B., Gentier, I., Verstuyf, J., Vaeyens, R., Bourdeaudhuij, I., . . . Lenoir, M. (2014). A longitudinal study of gross motor coordination and weight status in children. *Obesity, 22*(6), 1505–1511.

De Meester, A., Stodden, D. F., Goodway, J. D., True, L., Brian, A., Ferkel, R., & Haerens, L. (2018). Identifying a motor proficiency barrier for meeting physical activity guidelines in children. *Journal of Science and Medicine in Sport, 21*(1), 58–62. doi:10.1016/j.jsams.2017.05.007

Deci, E. L., & Ryan, R. M. (2008). Self-determination theory: A macrotheory of human motivation, development, and health. *Canadian Psychology, 49*(3), 182–185.

Diamond, A. (2000). Close interrelation of motor development and cognitive development and of the cerebellum and prefrontal cortex. *Child Development, 71*(1), 44–56.

Dobkin, B. H., & Martinez, C. (2018). Wearable sensors to monitor, enable feedback, and measure outcomes of activity and practice. *Current Neurology and Neuroscience Reports, 18*(12), 87. doi:10.1007/ s11910-018-0896-5

Dollman, J., Okely, A. D., Hardy, L., Timperio, A., Salmon, J., & Hills, A. P. (2009). A hitchhiker's guide to assessing young people's physical activity: Deciding what method to use. *Journal of Science and Medicine in Sport, 12*(5), 518–525. doi:10.1016/j.jsams.2008.09.007

Dos Santos, M. A. M., Nevill, A. M., Buranarugsa, R., Pereira, S., Gomes, T., Reyes, A., . . . Maia, J. A. R. (2018). Modeling children's development in gross motor coordination reveals key modifiable determinants. An allometric approach. *Scandinavian Journal of Medicine and Science in Sports, 28*(5), 1594–1603. doi:10.1111/sms.13061

Duncan, M. J., Jones, V., O'Brien, W., Barnett, L. M., & Eyre, E. L. J. (2018). Self-perceived and actual motor competence in young British children. *Perceptual and Motor Skills, 125*(2), 251–264. doi:10.1177/0031512517752833

Eccles, J. S., Wigfield, A., & Schiefele, U. (1998). Motivation to succeed. In W. Damon & N. Eisenberg (Eds.), *Handbook of child psychology: Social, emotional, and personality development* (pp. 1017–1095). Hoboken, NJ: John Wiley & Sons Inc.

Elhakeem, A., Hardy, R., Bann, D., Kuh, D., & Cooper, R. (2018). Motor performance in early life and participation in leisure-time physical activity up to age 68 years. *Paediatric and perinatal epidemiology, 32*(4), 327–334.

Engel, A. C., Broderick, C. R., van Doorn, N., Parmenter, B. J., & Hardy, L. L. (2018). Exploring the relationship between fundamental motor skill interventions and physical activity levels in children: A systematic review and meta-analysis. *Sports Medicine, 48*(8), 1845–1857. doi:10.1007/s40279-018-0923-3

Espenschade, A. (1940). Motor performance in adolescence including the study of relationships with measures of physical growth and maturity. *Monographs of the Society for Research in Child Development, 5*(1), 1–126.

Estevan, I., & Barnett, L. M. (2018). Considerations related to the definition, measurement and analysis of perceived motor competence. *Sports Medicine, 48*(12), 2685–2694. doi:10.1007/s40279-018-0940-2

Figueroa, R., & An, R. (2017). Motor skill competence and physical activity in preschoolers: A review. *Maternal and Child Health Journal, 21*(1), 136–146. doi:10.1007/s10995-016-2102-1

Fitts, P. M. (1954). The information capacity of the human motor system in controlling the amplitude of movement. *Journal of Experimental Psychology, 47*(6), 381–391.

Fleishman, E. A. (1954). Dimensional analysis of psychomotor abilities. *Journal of Experimental Psychology, 48*(6), 437–454. doi:10.1037/h0058244

Franzen, M. D., & Wilhelm, K. L. (1996). Conceptual foundations of ecological validity in neuropsychological assessment. In R. J. Sbordone & C. J. Long (Eds.), *Ecological validity of neuropsychological testing* (pp. 91–112). Delray Beach, FL: Gr Press/St Lucie Press, Inc.

Freitas, D. L., Lausen, B., Maia, J. A., Gouveia, E. R., Antunes, A. M., Thomis, M., . . . Malina, R. M. (2018). Skeletal maturation, fundamental motor skills, and motor performance in preschool children. *Scandinavian Journal of Medicine and Science in Sports, 28*(11), 2358–2368. doi:10.1111/sms.13233

Freitas, D. L., Lausen, B., Maia, J. A., Lefevre, J., Gouveia, É. R., Thomis, M., . . . Malina, R. M. (2015). Skeletal maturation, fundamental motor skills and motor coordination in children 7–10 years. *Journal of Sports Sciences, 33*(9), 924–934. doi:10.1080/02640414.2014.977935

Fullerton, G. S., & Cattell, J. M. (1892). *On the perception of small differences, with special reference to the extent, force, and time of movement.* Baltimore, MD: University of Pennsylvania Press.

Furzer, B. J., Bebich-Philip, M. D., Wright, K. E., Reid, S. L., & Thornton, A. L. (2018). Reliability and validity of the adapted resistance training skills battery for children. *Journal of Science and Medicine in Sport, 21*(8), 822–827.

Gallahue, D. L., Ozmun, J. C., & Goodway, J. D. (2012). *Understanding motor development : Infants, children, adolescents, adults* (7th ed.). New York, NY: McGraw-Hill.

Gesell, A. (1928). Infancy and human growth. New York, NY: Macmillan.

Griffiths, A., Toovey, R., Morgan, P. E., & Spittle, A. J. (2018). Psychometric properties of gross motor assessment tools for children: A systematic review. *BMJ Open, 8*(10), e021734. doi:10.1136/bmjopen-2018-021734

Grimpampi, E., Masci, I., Pesce, C., & Vannozzi, G. (2016). Quantitative assessment of developmental levels in overarm throwing using wearable inertial sensing technology. *Journal of Sports Sciences, 34*(18), 1759–1765. doi:10.1080/02640414.2015.1137341

Haapala, E. A. (2013). Cardiorespiratory fitness and motor skills in relation to cognition and academic performance in children – A review. *Journal of Human Kinetics, 36*(1), 185–189. doi:10.2478/hukin-2013-0006

Haapala, E. A., Poikkeus, A. M., Tompuri, T., Kukkonen-Harjula, K., Leppanen, P. H., Lindi, V., & Lakka, T. A. (2014). Associations of motor and cardiovascular performance with academic skills in children. *Medicine and Science in Sports and Exercise, 46*(5), 1016–1024. doi:10.1249/mss.0000000000000186

Halverson, H. M. (1931). An experimental study of prehension in infants by means of systematic cinema records. *Genetic Psychology Monographs, 10*, 107–286.

Halverson, L. E., Roberton, M. A., & Langendorfer, S. (1982). Development of the overarm throw: Movement and ball velocity changes by seventh grade. *Research Quarterly for Exercise and Sport, 53*(3), 198–205.

Hands, B., McIntyre, F., & Parker, H. (2018). The general motor ability hypothesis: An old idea revisited. *Perceptual and Motor Skills, 125*(2), 213–233. doi:10.1177/0031512517751750

Hardy, L. L., Hills, A. P., Timperio, A., Cliff, D., Lubans, D., Morgan, P. J., . . . Brown, H. (2013). A hitchhiker's guide to assessing sedentary behaviour among young people: Deciding what method to use. *Journal of Science and Medicine in Sport, 16*(1), 28–35. doi:10.1016/j.jsams.2012.05.010

Hardy, L. L., Mihrshahi, S., Drayton, B. A., & Bauman, A. (2016). *NSW schools physical activity and nutrition survey (SPANS) 2015: Full report.* Sydney, Australia: NSW Department of Health.

Haubenstricker, J. L., & Branta, C. F. (1997). The relationship between distance jumped and developmental level on the standing long jump in young children. *Motor Development: Research & Reviews, 1*, 64–85.

Haubenstricker, J. L., & Seefeldt, V. (1986). Acquisition of motor skills during childhood. In S. Seefeldt (Ed.), *Physical activity and well-being* (pp. 41–92). Reston,VA: American Alliance for Health, Physical Education, Recreation, and Dance.

Haywood, K., & Getchell, N. (2014). *Life span motor development* (Sixth ed.). Champaign, IL: Human Kinetics.

Haywood, K., Roberton, M. A., & Getchell, N. (2012). *Advanced analysis of motor development.* Champaign, IL: Human Kinetics.

Henderson, S. E., & Sugden, D. A. (1992). *Movement assessment battery for children* (1st ed.). London, UK: The Psychological Corporation.

Herrmann, C., Gerlach, E., & Seelig, H. (2015). Development and validation of a test instrument for the assessment of basic motor competencies in primary school. *Measurement in Physical Education and Exercise Science, 19*(2), 80–90.

Hoeboer, J., Krijger-Hombergen, M., Savelsbergh, G., & De Vries, S. (2018). Reliability and concurrent validity of a motor skill competence test among 4-to 12-year old children. *Journal of Sports Sciences, 36*(14), 1607–1613. doi:10.1080/02640414.2017.1406296

Holfelder, B., & Schott, N. (2014). Relationship of fundamental movement skills and physical activity in children and adolescents: A systematic review. *Psychology of Sport and Exercise, 15*(4), 382–391. doi:10.1016/j.psychsport.2014.03.005

Hulteen, R. M., Barnett, L. M., Morgan, P. J., Robinson, L. E., Barton, C. J., Wrotniak, B. H., & Lubans, D. R. (2018). Development, content validity and test-retest reliability of the lifelong physical activity skills battery in adolescents. *Journal of Sports Sciences, 36*(20), 2358–2367. doi:10.1080/02640414.2018.1458392

Hulteen, R. M., Lander, N. J., Morgan, P. J., Barnett, L. M., Robertson, S. J., & Lubans, D. R. (2015). Validity and reliability of field-based measures for assessing movement skill competency in lifelong physical activities: A systematic review. *Sports Medicine, 45*(10), 1443–1454. doi:10.1007/s40279-015-0357-0

Hulteen, R. M., Morgan, P. J., Barnett, L. M., Stodden, D. F., & Lubans, D. R. (2018). Development of foundational movement skills: A conceptual model for physical activity across the lifespan. *Sports Medicine, 48*(7), 1533–1540. doi:10.1007/s40279-018-0892-6

Jaakkola, T., Hakonen, H., Kankaanpää, A., Joensuu, L., Kulmala, J., Kallio, J., . . . Tammelin, T. H. (2019). Longitudinal associations of fundamental movement skills with objectively measured physical activity and sedentariness during school transition from primary to lower secondary school. *Journal of Science and Medicine in Sport, 22*(1), 85–90. doi:10.1016/j.jsams.2018.07.012

Jaakkola, T., Yli-Piipari, S., Huotari, P., Watt, A., & Liukkonen, J. (2016). Fundamental movement skills and physical fitness as predictors of physical activity: A 6-year follow-up study. *Scandinavian Journal of Medicine & Science in Sports, 26*(1), 74–81.

Kiphard, E. J., & Schilling, F. (2007). *Körperkoordinationstest für Kinder: KTK*. Weinhem, Germany: Beltz-Test.

Kit, B. K., Akinbami, L. J., Isfahani, N. S., & Ulrich, D. A. (2017). Gross motor development in children aged 3–5 years, United States 2012. *Maternal and Child Health Journal, 21*(7), 1573–1580. doi:10.1007/s10995-017-2289-9

Klingberg, B., Schranz, N., Barnett, L. M., Booth, V., & Ferrar, K. (2019). The feasibility of fundamental movement skill assessments for pre-school aged children. *Journal of Sports Sciences, 37*(4), 378–386. doi:10.1080/02640414.2018.1504603

Lander, N. J., Hanna, L., Brown, H., Telford, A., Morgan, P. J., Salmon, J., & Barnett, L. M. (2017). Physical education teachers' perspectives and experiences when teaching FMS to early adolescent girls. *Journal of Teaching in Physical Education, 36*(1), 113–118. doi:10.1123/jtpe.2015-0201

Lander, N. J., Morgan, P. J., Salmon, J., & Barnett, L. M. (2015). Teachers' perceptions of a fundamental movement skill assessment battery in a school setting. *Measurement in Physical Education and Exercise Science, 20*(1), 50–62.

Lander, N. J., Morgan, P. J., Salmon, J., Logan, S. W., & Barnett, L. M. (2017). The reliability and validity of an authentic motor skill assessment tool for early adolescent girls in an Australian school setting. *Journal of Science and Medicine in Sport, 20*(6), 590–594. doi:10.1016/j.jsams.2016.11.007

Lane, A. P., Molina, S. L., Tolleson, D. A., Langendorfer, S. J., Goodway, J. D., & Stodden, D. F. (2018). Developmental sequences for the standing long jump landing: A pre-longitudinal screening. *Journal of Motor Learning and Development, 6*(1), 114–129. doi:10.1123/jmld.2016-0058

Langendorfer, S. J., & Roberton, M. A. (2002). Individual pathways in the development of forceful throwing. *Research Quarterly for Exercise and Sport, 73*(3), 245–256. doi:10.1080/02701367.2002.10609018

Langendorfer, S. J., Roberton, M. A., & Stodden, D. F. (2011). Chapter 9: Biomechanical aspects of the development of object projection skills. In D. S. C. Korff (Ed.), *Paediatric biomechanics and motor control: Theory and application*. Oxford, UK: Routledge.

Leuba, J. H., & Chamberlain, E. (1909). The influence of the duration and of the rate of arm movements upon the judgement of their length. *The American Journal of Psychology, 20*(3). 374–385. doi:10.2307/1413368

Li, Y. C., Kwan, M. Y. W., & Cairney, J. (2019). Motor coordination problems and psychological distress in young adults: A test of the environmental stress hypothesis. *Research in Developmental Disabilities, 84*, 112–121. doi:10.1016/j.ridd.2018.04.023

Libertus, K., & Hauf, P. (2017). Editorial: Motor skills and their foundational role for perceptual, social, and cognitive development. *Frontiers in Psychology, 8*(301), 1–4. doi:10.3389/fpsyg.2017.00301

Lima, R. A., Pfeiffer, K., Larsen, L. R., Bugge, A., Moller, N. C., Anderson, L. B., & Stodden, D. F. (2017). Physical activity and motor competence present a positive reciprocal longitudinal relationship across childhood and early adolescence. *Journal of Physical Activity and Health, 14*(6), 440–447. doi:10.1123/jpah.2016-0473

Logan, S. W., Barnett, L. M., Goodway, J. D., & Stodden, D. F. (2017). Comparison of performance on process- and product-oriented assessments of fundamental motor skills across childhood. *Journal of Sports Sciences, 35*(7), 634–641. doi:10.1080/02640414.2016.1183803

Logan, S. W., Robinson, L. E., & Getchell, N. (2011). The comparison of performances of preschool children on two motor assessments. *Perceptual and Motor Skills, 113*(3), 715–723. doi:10.2466/03.06.25.pms.113.6.715-723

Logan, S. W., Robinson, L. E., Wilson, A. E., & Lucas, W. A. (2012). Getting the fundamentals of movement: A meta-analysis of the effectiveness of motor skill interventions in children. *Child: Care, Health and Development, 38*(3), 305–315. doi:10.1111/j.1365-2214.2011.01307.x

Logan, S. W., Webster, E. K., Getchell, N., Pfeiffer, K. A., & Robinson, L. E. (2015). Relationship between fundamental motor skill competence and physical activity during childhood and adolescence: A systematic review. *Kinesiology Review, 4*(4), 416–426. doi:10.1123/kr.2013-0012

Longmuir, P. E., Boyer, C., Lloyd, M., Borghese, M. M., Knight, E., Saunders, T. J., . . . Tremblay, M. S. (2017). Canadian Agility and Movement Skill Assessment (CAMSA): Validity, objectivity, and reliability evidence for children 8–12 years of age. *J Sport Health Sci, 6*(2), 231–240. doi:10.1016/j.jshs.2015.11.004.

Lopes, L., Silva Mota, J. A. P., Moreira, C., Abreu, S., Agostinis Sobrinho, C., Oliveira-Santos, J., . . . Santos, R. (2019). Longitudinal associations between motor competence and different physical activity intensities: LabMed physical activity study. *Journal of Sports Sciences, 37*(3), 285–290. doi:10.1080/02640 414.2018.1497424

Lopes, V. P., Rodrigues, L. P., Maia, J. A. R., & Malina, R. M. (2011). Motor coordination as predictor of physical activity in childhood. *Scandinavian Journal of Medicine & Science in Sports, 21*(5), 663–669. doi:10.1111/j.1600-0838.2009.01027.x

Lorson, K. M., Stodden, D. F., Langendorfer, S. J., & Goodway, J. D. (2013). Age and gender differences in adolescent and adult overarm throwing. *Research Quarterly for Exercise and Sport, 84*(2), 239–244. doi:10.1 080/02701367.2013.784841

Lubans, D. R., Morgan, P. J., Cliff, D. P., Barnett, L. M., & Okely, A. D. (2010). Fundamental movement skills in children and adolescents: Review of associated health benefits. *Sports Medicine, 40*(12), 1019–1035. doi:10.2165/11536850-000000000-00000

Lubans, D. R., Smith, J. J., Harries, S., Barnett, L. M., & Faigenbaum, A. D. (2014). Development, test-retest reliability and construct validity of the resistance training skills battery. *The Journal of Strength & Conditioning Research, 28*(5), 1373–1380.

Mancini, V., Rigoli, D., Roberts, L., & Piek, J. (2019). Motor skills and internalizing problems throughout development: An integrative research review and update of the environmental stress hypothesis research. *Research in Developmental Disabilities, 84*, 96–111. doi:10.1016/j.ridd.2018.07.003

Martins, D., Maia, J., Seabra, A., Garganta, R., Lopes, V., Katzmarzyk, P., & Beunen, G. (2010). Correlates of changes in BMI of children from the Azores islands. *International Journal of Obesity (London), 34*(10), 1487–1493. doi:10.1038/ijo.2010.56

Masci, I., Vannozzi, G., Bergamini, E., Pesce, C., Getchell, N., & Cappozzo, A. (2013). Assessing locomotor skills development in childhood using wearable inertial sensor devices: The running paradigm. *Gait and Posture, 37*(4), 570–574. doi:10.1016/j.gaitpost.2012.09.017

Masci, I., Vannozzi, G., Getchell, N., & Cappozzo, A. (2012). Assessing hopping developmental level in childhood using wearable inertial sensor devices. *Motor Control, 16*(3), 317–328.

McGraw, M. B. (1935). Growth: A study of Johnny and Jimmy (Preface by F. Tilney; introduction by J. Dewey.). Oxford, UK: Appleton-Century.

Miller, A., Eather, N., Duncan, M., & Lubans, D. R. (2019). Associations of object control motor skill proficiency, game play competence, physical activity and cardiorespiratory fitness among primary school children. *Journal of Sports Sciences, 37*, 173–179. doi:10.1080/02640414.2018.1488384

NCD Alliance. (2018). Report cards on physical activity for children and youth confirm global inactivity crisis Retrieved from https://ncdalliance.org/news-events/news/report-cards-on-physical-activity-for-children-and-youth-confirm-global-inactivity-crisis

Nesbitt, D., Molina, S. L., Cattuzzo, M. T., Robinson, L. E., Phillips, D., & Stodden, D. F. (2017). Assessment of a supine-to-stand (STS) task in early childhood: A measure of functional motor competence. *Journal of Motor Learning and Development, 5*(2), 252–266. doi:10.1123/jmld.2016-0049

New South Wales Department of Education and Training. (2000). *Get skilled: Get active.* Sydney, Australia: DET Product No.: 10614/DVD.

NSW Ministry of Health. (2011). *NSW schools physical activity and nutrition survey (SPANS) 2010 full report.* Sydney, Australia. Retrieved from: http://www.health.nsw.gov.au/pubs/2011/pdf/spans_2010_summary.pdf

Obrusnikova, I., & Cavalier, A. (2018). An evaluation of videomodeling on fundamental motor skill performance of preschool children. *Early Childhood Education Journal, 46*(3), 287–299. doi:10.1007/s10643-017-0861-y

Palmer, K. K., & Brian, A. (2016). Test of gross motor development-2 scores differ between expert and novice coders. *Journal of Motor Learning and Development, 4*(2), 142–151.

Pesce, C. (2012). Shifting the focus from quantitative to qualitative exercise characteristics in exercise and cognition research. *Journal of Sports and Exercise Psychology, 34*(6), 766–786.

Pinto Pereira, S. M., Li, L., & Power, C. (2014). Early-life predictors of leisure-time physical inactivity in midadulthood: Findings from a prospective British birth cohort. *American Journal of Epidemiology, 180*(11), 1098–1108.

Playground Association of America. (1913). The athletic badge test for boys. *The Playground, 7*(33–37), 57–60.

Playground Association of America. (1916). The athletic badge test for girls. *The Playground, 10*, 165–171.

Ré, A. H., Logan, S. W., Cattuzzo, M. T., Henrique, R. S., Tudela, M. C., & Stodden, D. F. (2018). Comparison of motor competence levels on two assessments across childhood. *Journal of Sports Sciences, 36*(1), 1–6.

Ridley, K., Ainsworth, B. E., & Olds, T. S. (2008). Development of a compendium of energy expenditures for youth. *International Journal of Behavioral Nutrition and Physical Activity, 5*(1), 45. doi:10.1186/1479-5868-5-45

Roberton, M. A. (1978). Longitudinal evidence for developmental stages in the forceful overarm throw. *Journal of Human Movement Studies, 4*(2), 167–175.

Roberton, M. A., & Halverson, L. E. (1977). The developing child: His changing movement. In B. Logsdon (Ed.), *Physical education for children: A focus on the teaching process* (pp. 24–60). Philadelphia, PA: Lea and Febiger.

Roberton, M. A., & Konczak, J. (2001). Predicting children's overarm throw ball velocities from their developmental levels in throwing. *Research Quarterly for Exercise and Sport, 72*(2), 91–103.

Roberton, M. A., Thompson, G., & Langendorfer, S. J. (2017). Initial steps in creating a developmentally valid tool for observing/assessing rope jumping. *Physical Education and Sport Pedagogy, 22*(2), 187–196. doi:10.1080/17408989.2016.1165193

Robertson, S. J., Burnett, A. F., & Cochrane, J. (2014). Tests examining skill outcomes in sport: A systematic review of measurement properties and feasibility. *Sports Medicine, 44*(4), 501–518.

Robinson, L. E., & Palmer, K. (2017). Development of a digital-based instrument to assess perceived motor competence in children: Face validity, test-retest reliability, and internal consistency. *Sports, 5*(3), 48.

Robinson, L. E., Stodden, D. F., Barnett, L. M., Lopes, V. P., Logan, S. W., Rodrigues, L. P., & D'Hondt, E. (2015). Motor competence and its effect on positive developmental trajectories of health. *Sports Medicine, 45*(9), 1273–1284. doi:10.1007/s40279-015-0351-6

Rodrigues, L. P., Stodden, D. F., & Lopes, V. P. (2016). Developmental pathways of change in fitness and motor competence are related to overweight and obesity status at the end of primary school. *Journal of Science and Medicine in Sport, 19*(1), 87–92. doi:10.1016/j.jsams.2015.01.002

Rudd, J., Butson, M. L., Barnett, L. M., Farrow, D., Berry, J., Borkoles, E., & Polman, R. (2016). A holistic measurement model of movement competency in children. *Journal of Sports Sciences, 34*(5), 477–485. doi:10.1080/02640414.2015.1061202

Sacko, R. S., Brazendale, K., Brian, A., McIver, K., Nesbitt, D., Pfeifer, C., & Stodden, D. F. (2019). Comparison of indirect calorimetry- and accelerometry-based energy expenditure during object project skill performance. *Measurement in Physical Education and Exercise Science, 23*(2), 148–158. doi:10.1080/1091367X.2018.1554578

Sacko, R. S., McIver, K., Brian, A., & Stodden, D. F. (2018). New insight for activity intensity relativity, metabolic expenditure during object projection skill performance. *Journal of Sports Sciences, 36*(21), 2412–2418. doi:10.1080/02640414.2018.1459152

Sargent, D. A., Seaver, J. W., & Savage, W. L. (1897). Intercollegiate strength-tests. *American Physical Education Review, 2*, 216–220.

Scheuer, C., Herrmann, C., & Bund, A. (2019). Motor tests for primary school aged children: A systematic review. *Journal of Sports Sciences, 37*(10), 1097–1112. doi:10.1080/02640414.2018.1544535

Schmidt, M., Egger, F., Benzing, V., Jäger, K., Conzelmann, A., Roebers, C. M., & Pesce, C. (2017). Disentangling the relationship between children's motor ability, executive function and academic achievement. *PLoS One, 12*(8), e0182845.

Schmidt, R. A. (1991). *Motor learning and performance: From principles to practice*. Champaign, IL: Human Kinetics Publishers.

Schmidt, R. A., Lee, T. D., Winstein, C., Wulf, G., & Zelaznik, H. N. (2018). *Motor control and learning: A behavioral emphasis* (4th ed.). Champaign, IL: Human Kinetics.

Seefeldt, V. (1980). Developmental motor patterns: Implications for elementary school physical education. In W. H. C. Nadeau, K. Newell, & G. Roberts (Ed.), *Psychology of motor behavior and sport* (pp. 314–323). Champaign, IL: Human Kinetics.

Seefeldt, V., & Haubenstricker, J. L. (1976). *Developmental sequences of fundamental motor skills*. Michigan State University. Unpublished research. East Lansing, MI.

Sgrò, F., Mango, P., Pignato, S., Schembri, R., Licari, D., & Lipoma, M. (2017). Assessing standing long jump developmental levels using an inertial measurement unit. *Perceptual and Motor Skills, 124*(1), 21–38. doi:10.1177/0031512516682649

Sgrò, F., Nicolosi, S., Schembri, R., Pavone, M., & Lipoma, M. (2015). Assessing vertical jump developmental levels in childhood using a low-cost motion capture approach. *Perceptual and Motor Skills, 120*(2), 642–658. doi:10.2466/10.PMS.120v12x7

Smith, J. J., DeMarco, M., Kennedy, S. G., Kelson, M., Barnett, L. M., Faigenbaum, A. D., & Lubans, D. R. (2018). Prevalence and correlates of resistance training skill competence in adolescents. *Journal of Sports Sciences, 36*(11), 1241–1249. doi:10.1080/02640414.2017.1370822

Smith, L., Fisher, A., & Hamer, M. (2015). Prospective association between objective measures of childhood motor coordination and sedentary behaviour in adolescence and adulthood. *International Journal of Behavioral Nutrition and Physical Activity, 12*(1), 75.

Stodden, D. F., Gao, Z., Langendorfer, S. J., & Goodway, J. D. (2014). Dynamic relationships between motor skill competence and health-related fitness in youth. *Pediatric Exercise Science, 26*(3), 231–241. doi:10.1123/pes.2013-0027

Stodden, D. F., Goodway, J. D., Langendorfer, S. J., Roberton, M. A., Rudisall, M. E., Garcia, C., & Garcia, L. E. (2008). A developmental perspective on the role of motor skill competence in physical activity: An emergent relationship. *Quest, 60*(2), 290–306.

Stodden, D. F., True, L., K., Langendorfer, S. J., & Gao, Z. (2013). Associations among selected motor skills and health-related fitness: Indirect evidence for Seefeldt's proficiency barrier in young adults? *Research Quarterly for Exercise and Sport, 84*(3), 397–403. doi:10.1080/02701367.2013.814910

Thurston, A. J. (1999). Giovanni Borelli and the study of human movement: An historical review. *Australian and New Zealand Journal of Surgery, 69*(4), 276–288. doi:10.1046/j.1440-1622.1999.01558.x

Ulrich, D. A. (2000). *Test of gross motor development* (2nd ed.). Austin, TX: Pro-Ed.

Ulrich, D. A. (2017). Introduction to the special section: Evaluation of the psychometric properties of the TGMD-3. *Journal of Motor Learning and Development, 5*(1), 1–4. doi:10.1123/jmld.2017-0020

Utesch, T., Bardid, F., Huyben, F., Strauss, B., Tietjens, M., De Martelaer, K., . . . Lenoir, M. (2016). Using rasch modeling to investigate the construct of motor competence in early childhood. *Psychology of Sport and Exercise, 24*, 179–187. doi:10.1016/j.psychsport.2016.03.001

Van Dalen, D. B., & Bennett., B. L. (1971). *A world history of physical education : Cultural, philosophical, comparative* (Second ed.). Englewood Cliffs, NJ: Prentice-Hall.

van der Fels, I. M., Te Wierike, S. C., Hartman, E., Elferink-Gemser, M. T., Smith, J., & Visscher, C. (2015). The relationship between motor skills and cognitive skills in 4–16 year old typically developing children: A systematic review. *Journal of Science and Medicine in Sport, 18*(6), 697–703. doi:10.1016/j.jsams.2014.09.007

van Rossum, T., Foweather, L., Richardson, D., Hayes, S. J., & Morley, D. (2019). Primary teachers' recommendations for the development of a teacher–oriented movement assessment tool for 4–7 years children. *Measurement in Physical Education & Exercise Science, 23*(2), 124–134. doi:10.1080/1091367X.2018.1552587

VanSant, A. F. (1988). Age differences in movement patterns used by children to rise from a supine position to erect stance. *Physical Therapy, 68*(9), 1330–1338. doi:10.1093/ptj/68.9.1330

Ward, B. J., Thornton, A., Lay, B., & Rosenberg, M. (2017). Protocols for the investigation of information processing in human assessment of fundamental movement skills. *Journal of Motor Behavior, 49*(6), 593–602. doi:10.1080/00222895.2016.1247033

Wickstrom, R. (1983). *Fundamental motor patterns* (3rd ed.). Philadelphia, PA: Lea & Febiger.

Wild, M. R. (1937). *The behavior pattern of throwing and some observations concerning its course of development in children* (Unpublished doctoral dissertation). University of Wisconsin, Madison.

Wild, M. R. (1938). The behavior pattern of throwing and some observations concerning its course of development in children. *Research Quarterly. American Association for Health and Physical Education, 9*(3), 20–24.

William, L. B., & Harter, N. (1899). Studies on the telegraphic language: The acquisition of a hierarchy of habits. *Psychological Review, 6*(4), 345–375. doi:10.1037/h0073117

Williams, H. G., Pfeiffer, K. A., Dowda, M., Jeter, C., Jones, S., & Pate, R. R. (2009). A field-based testing protocol for assessing gross motor skills in preschool children: The children's activity and movement in preschool study motor skills protocol. *Measurement in Physical Education and Exercise Science, 13*(3), 151–165.

Williams, K., Haywood, K., & VanSant, A. (1990). Movement characteristics of older adult throwers. In J. E. Clark & J. H. Humphrey (Eds.), *Advances in motor development research* (pp. 29–44). New York, NY: AMS Press.

Williams, K., Haywood, K., & VanSant, A. (1998). Changes in throwing by older adults: A longitudinal investigation. *Research Quarterly for Exercise and Sport, 69*(1), 1–10. doi:10.1080/02701367.1998.10607661

Wulf, G., Shea, C., & Lewthwaite, R. (2010). Motor skill learning and performance: A review of influential factors. *Medical Education, 44*(1), 75–84. doi:10.1111/j.1365-2923.2009.03421.x

PART 6

Introduction to Interventions

20

YOUTH PHYSICAL ACTIVITY INTERVENTION DESIGN

Kirsten Corder, Sonja Klingberg, and Esther van Sluijs

Introduction

Importance of Intervention Design

Intervention design and subsequent implementation represent an important interchange between observational evidence and trial efficacy. This area between these two rigorously prepared evidence bases is often poorly reported, and is rarely given the gravitas that it deserves in the scientific literature. Intervention design often appears to be a covert process conducted behind closed doors. Increasingly there are criticisms of the apparently clandestine nature of intervention design with calls for transparency and the publication of adequate information to enable replication and development of programs by other researchers and practitioners. It is important for researchers to be able to build on, iterate and improve previous programs in order to advance the evidence base rather than risking repeating previous work. Intervention design is an incredibly important and exceptionally challenging process, often with no right answer or exact strategy to follow. The apparent 'black-box' nature of many interventions is likely to be at least partly due to the difficulty and multifaceted nature of the intervention design process, including the infinite number of processes and possible outcomes that are difficult to describe succinctly. Increasingly, calls for transparency are enabling more adequate descriptions of intervention design processes to be present in the peer-reviewed scientific literature and there are increasing numbers of strategies, models, frameworks and theories to aid with the intellectually challenging task of intervention design. This chapter summarizes some key considerations when approaching intervention design and suggests various strategies which may help researchers to bridge the gap between observational evidence and assessment of intervention efficacy.

Why We Need Physical Activity Promotion and Where Do We Start?

Despite much previous work aiming to increase physical activity among young people, many youth are insufficiently active (Bell et al., 2018). As childhood inactivity appears to track into adulthood (Lewandowski et al., 2015; Telema et al., 2005) increasing the risk of diabetes, cancer and mortality (Engle et al., 2014; Khaw et al., 2008), physical activity promotion is a public health priority (All-Party Commission on Physical Activity, 2014; Davis, Chen, Leon, Darst, &

Campbell, 2015). An individual's physical activity behavior is influenced by factors operating at different levels of influence, including individual, interpersonal and institutional levels as highlighted in the social ecological model (Golden & Earp, 2012). Reviews of physical activity determinants also suggest that a multitude of factors from different domains are associated with young people's physical activity levels and may therefore be important intervention targets (Craggs, Corder, van Sluijs, & Griffin, 2011). Beyond individual-level variables, these include those related to the school, neighborhood and family, as well as the increasing relevance of the online environment. As one of the main settings where children spend their time, the educational system has been identified as playing an important role in shaping children's health behaviors. Evidence suggests that on average English primary schoolchildren accumulate 39% of their daily activity (Brooke, Atkin, Corder, Ekelund, & van Sluijs, 2016) at school, so while schools are an important context, it is not the only one that warrants research attention. Children's activity is also influenced by the encouragement children receive from their parents, and modeled upon their parents' own behavior, which is, in turn, affected by, for example, the time parents are available for such pursuits, and access to recreational facilities (Davison & Birch, 2001). Every part of a young person's life is a potential avenue for intervention; physical activity appears to be continuing to decline at faster rates in more recent generations of youth (Knuth & Hallal, 2009) so continued pursuit of effective strategies in school, family, environmental and policy domains is still high up the research agenda.

Youth Physical Activity Promotion: Efficacy Summary

Recent reviews conclusively confirm the ineffectiveness of physical activity promotion strategies in young people (Beets et al., 2016; Borde, Smith, Sutherland, Nathan, & Lubans, 2017; Love, Adams, & van Sluijs, 2019; Metcalf et al., 2012). In a meta-analysis examining the effectiveness of physical activity promotion interventions in youth, 30 studies with objective outcomes were included (Metcalf et al., 2012) and only showed an effect size of 4 minutes/day (Metcalf et al., 2012). A further systematic review focusing on the impact of school-based interventions on objectively measured physical activity concluded small and non-significant pooled effects for total activity and moderate-to-vigorous physical activity (MVPA) (Borde et al., 2017). Focusing on those over 10 years old, and including 12 studies in meta-analyses, the authors concluded stronger effects with a smaller sample and higher accelerometer compliance (Borde et al., 2017). A recent systematic review re-analyzed data from 17 school-based cluster-randomized controlled trials and calculated a mean change score in accelerometer-assessed MVPA from baseline to follow-up by gender, and by socio-economic position (Love et al., 2019). This re-analysis definitively concluded that the summary effect of the 17 school-based trials providing data for re-analysis was ineffective, also highlighting that there was no evidence of differential effectiveness for boys and girls or for those of different socio-economic position (Love et al., 2019). Therefore, although schools do appear to have potential to offer a universal context to access and influence all children, school-based efforts to increase MVPA across the full day currently appear unable to do this (Love et al., 2019).

Research aiming to explain the apparent lack of effectiveness of school-based interventions has examined the mechanisms hypothesized to lead to change in youth physical activity (Beets et al., 2016). It has been suggested that for a school-based intervention to work, it needs to include a mechanism from at least one of three categories outlined in the Theory of Expanded, Extended and Enhanced Opportunities (TEO) (Beets et al., 2016). First, 'expansion' suggests providing new occasions to be active by replacing sedentary time for physical activity, an example of this would be substituting seated school work with active learning tasks in classrooms. The second suggested mechanism is 'extension' and suggests lengthening time currently allocated to activity, such as by adding extra weekly physical education lessons or extending break times. Finally, 'enhancement' refers to altering an existing physical activity offering to increase the amount of activity within a particular time allocation such as reducing waiting times during existing physical education classes (Beets et al., 2016).

Although the majority of previous youth physical activity promotion has been school-based, the limited effectiveness of many school-based approaches has prompted increasing calls for strategies targeted at other contexts (Kipping et al., 2014; van Sluijs, Kriemler, & McMinn, 2011). Observational evidence also suggests that non-school strategies may be particularly important as activity is often seen to particularly decline outside of school time and at weekends (Bobrowski et al., 2013; Brooke, Corder, Atkin, & van Sluijs, 2014; Dumith, Gigante, Domingues, & Kohl, 2011). Reviews specific to particular non-school contexts including family-based settings (Brown et al., 2016) and digital interventions (Rose et al., 2017) indicate the promise of these areas for future work. Goal-setting, reinforcement techniques and spending time active as a family have been identified as important for future use in family-based approaches, with education-only programs deemed potentially ineffective (Brown et al., 2016). The wide range of diverse community approaches is difficult to synthesize but there are calls for these approaches to be individually tailored to the particular target community and the cultural context of the community in question. For example, a faith-based family intervention is likely to need to be different to a youth center program aimed at older adolescents not in further education or training. Community-based approaches should also take account of multiple levels of influence such as parents, family, community leaders and policy (Glanz & Yaroch, 2004; Klassen, MacKay, Moher, Walker, & Jones, 2000; Mittelmark, Hunt, Heath, & Schmid, 1993; Stevens, De Bourdeaudhuij, & Van Oost, 2001). A recent bibliometric study has highlighted the rapid growth of the eHealth and mHealth fields, including increased use of social media for promoting physical activity (Muller et al., 2018). There are a limited number of well-designed trials surrounding apps, texts message and social media to promote physical activity among young people despite increasing use of these for behavior change (Rose et al., 2017).

The Need for More Rigor and Transparency

One potential reason for the lack of effectiveness of physical activity promotion interventions is likely to be poor design and implementation. Moreover, the lack of knowledge about this ineffectiveness is likely to be because of poor reporting and lack of transparency in much of the literature. If publications do not contain enough information for other researchers to understand and potentially replicate work then scientific knowledge will be lost and further efforts may repeat ineffective, infeasible or non-acceptable strategies (Romo-Nava et al., 2013). Building adequate scientific knowledge relies on transparency and replication. Therefore, it is good practice to provide sufficient description for others to repeat interventions (Schulz, Altman, Moher, & CONSORT Group, 2010). However, it has been reported that description of interventions is generally poor with adequate reporting only present in papers, appendices or websites for 39% of 137 trials of non-drug interventions reviewed (Hoffmann et al., 2014). Transparency is improving with guidance now available for intervention protocols (Chan, Tetzlaff, Altman, Dickersin, & Moher, 2013; Chan, Tetzlaff, Altman, Laupacis et al., 2013; Chan, Tetzlaff, Gotzsche et al., 2013) and for describing interventions in sufficient detail to allow replication (Hoffmann et al., 2014). Frameworks focusing on intervention development and implementation provide guidance promoting best practice throughout the design process (e.g. Intervention Mapping, Template for Intervention Description and Replication (TIDieR), PRACTical planning for Implementation and Scale-up (PRACTIS)) (Craig et al., 2008; Hoffmann et al., 2014; Koorts et al., 2018).

Overview of the Literature

Context-Specific Issues in Intervention Design

As illustrated by the social ecological model, it is important to consider the wider socio-ecological context of behaviors and interventions. Furthermore, in designing evidence-based physical activity interventions, the context also delineates what evidence is available to be applied in the design process. The maturity of the evidence base depends both on the exact behavior and intervention type of interest, but also on the geographic location and specific population. For example, there is a wealth of literature on behavioral correlates and school-based physical activity interventions from high income countries like the United States or the United Kingdom but far less on the same topic from low and middle income countries (Barbosa Filho et al., 2016; Hoffmann et al., 2014; van Sluijs, McMinn, & Griffin, 2007).

The behavioral epidemiology framework aims to highlight the contributions of behavioral science in addressing mortality and morbidity (Sallis, Owen, & Fotheringham, 2000). It involves a mapping of the kind of evidence that is needed at five different phases of health promotion. Designing and evaluating interventions are the fourth phase in the process from establishing the links between specific behaviors and health through to translating research into practice. Therefore, when designing interventions one needs to not only consider what evidence there is from previous interventions but whether there is enough context-specific evidence about the behavior the intervention is targeting, including how well it can be measured, and the links between the behavior and health. There is generally a large body of evidence of the links between physical activity and health, the measurement of physical activity, and factors that influence physical activity. However, much of this supporting evidence that feeds into intervention design is specific to the context in which the intervention is expected to work, or a particular age group, and thus some research may be needed in the earlier phases of the behavioral epidemiology framework as well. An assessment of the state of the evidence is important to do very early in the process of intervention design.

School-Based Programs

Physical activity promotion through schools may be achieved through the curriculum, but also through the social, policy and physical environments that schools provide (Morton, Atkin, Corder, Suhrcke, & van Sluijs, 2016). At a public health level, the ubiquity of school for youth makes it likely that the school is a part of the solution to prevent physical activity declines during childhood. However, as children spend most of their time out of school, other contexts also require consideration. The key focus of the wider educational system, of which schools are a part, is to improve academic outcomes for all children. Current physical activity promotion efforts frequently fail to recognize this, which impacts on their effectiveness. Effective preventative efforts should aim to align with the priorities of the educational system as a whole, and not distract it from its multiple core deliverables (such as education and safeguarding). Physical activity may come low down the list of priorities for many school-related stakeholders and we should be aware of that in all stages of our work with schools (Morton et al., 2017). Schools and teachers have many conflicting priorities and it is important that we design our interventions as simple to understand and as easy to implement as possible, with an aim to minimize any burden for teachers. During the intervention design process, it is also sensible to be aware of the need for flexibility as interventions must fit into an already crowded school schedule; we should allow schools the flexibility they need to deliver our programs. Recent high profile studies suggest the lack of effectiveness of school-based physical activity promotion strategies (Adab et al., 2018) and the limited scope for further research. It is likely that the school is still an important avenue for population-based health promotion but an outside-the-box approach to create novel multilevel strategies appears necessary with more attention given to the understanding of the wider school culture (Morton et al., 2016).

School-specific models and frameworks for school-based intervention design highlight the importance of working across multiple levels of the wider school and community system (Lewallen, Hunt, Potts-Datema, Zaza, & Giles, 2015; Moore et al., 2018; Rooney, Videto, & Birch, 2015). Following the principles included in these frameworks, coupled with more attention to implementation science, may illuminate some useful pathways for school-based intervention design.

The Comprehensive School Physical Activity Program (CSPAP) framework is a tool for planning and organizing physical education and physical activity activities in a school context. The CSPAP approach is multicomponent and aims to encourage schools to use all opportunities (in and out of school time) for student activity with an aim of all students meeting physical activity recommendations of 60 minutes/day of MVPA. This framework encourages development of knowledge, skills and confidence across all contexts (e.g. school time, before and after school) and stakeholders (e.g. school staff, family and community). Although based on physical education as an academic subject, this framework aims to broaden this out to other aspects of children's lives through five components: physical education classes, other school-based activity (e.g. recess, breaks), before and after school provision (including active travel and clubs), staff involvement (e.g. employee wellness) and family and community engagement (e.g. family activity outings). This framework predominantly includes resources aimed at public health practitioners and school officials and there has been criticism of a lack of implementation monitoring; implementation frameworks have been proposed to address this (Moore et al., 2018). This is a resource developed in the United States as a government initiative (Center for Disease Control and Prevention (CDC)) with further details available on their website (https://www.cdc.gov/healthyschools/professional_development/e-learning/cspap.html). This initiative has substantial impetus at a government level, and the available resources, together with the recently published Quality Implementation Framework (Moore et al., 2018), provide a set of useful guidelines.

The Whole School, Whole Community, Whole Child (WSCC) model aims to align health and educational approaches to target various salient health behaviors among school students, and also has a physical activity component. This model focuses on five tenets, valued by a wide group of stakeholders throughout the school system: keeping pupils healthy, safe, engaged, supported and challenged. Although this model was developed for the US context, the principles and steps have wider relevance by aiming for a collaborative and unified approach by incorporating learning from multiple fields across health and education to improve health and well-being across schools. This model highlights the importance of support, planning, communication and collaboration throughout multiple levels of the school and wider community systems (Rooney et al., 2015). Importance is also given to learning from previous successes and challenges. By incorporating a detailed planning process, this aligns with best practice of identifying strengths and weaknesses across key areas, and of gathering relevant data before implementing strategies. Post-planning prioritization phases, including identification of resource availability and the generation of a stakeholder-led timeline, in addition to clear multilevel communication throughout, make this model useful for those aiming to intervene in the school context (Lewallen et al., 2015; Rooney et al., 2015).

Non-School Design Issues

Family

There have been calls for increased emphasis on family-based interventions (van Sluijs et al., 2011). This is partly due to the lack of intervention efficacy of school-based approaches and also observational evidence including larger declines of activity during youth in out of school time

(Corder et al., 2013). The family-based intervention literature indicates an over-representation of pilot studies targeting this setting (O'Connor, Jago, & Baranowski, 2009), which may be partly due to the challenges of recruiting and retaining families in research. Correlates research consistently identifies that parental support is associated with physical activity among children (van der Horst, Chin, Paw, Twisk, & van Mechelen, 2007) and that the addition of a family component to a school-based intervention appears to be efficacious (van Sluijs et al., 2007). However, the diversity of previous family-based research which includes a very wide range of target populations, behavior change techniques (BCTs) and strategies can make it challenging to glean insights to tangibly inform intervention design (Brown et al., 2014).

A systematic review of family-based physical activity promotion approaches included 47 studies with participants 5–12 years old. Of the included studies, 66% demonstrated an effect, although only a small effect was demonstrated overall (Brown et al., 2016). This review also included a realist synthesis which aimed to understand how these previous interventions operated while considering the interaction between context, mechanism and outcome to enable insight into 'what works for whom, under what circumstances, how and why?' (Brown et al., 2016). Strategies that were identified as showing particular promise for incorporating in family-based physical activity promotion interventions included goal-setting, reinforcement techniques and those focusing on spending time active as a family (Brown et al., 2016). Education-based programs without additional strategies were concluded as potentially ineffective (Brown et al., 2016).

Family-based interventions include into several different subtypes, including whole family approaches (van Sluijs et al., 2016) and those targeting particular family members such as dads and daughters (Morgan et al., 2018) and mums and daughters (Corr, Morgan, McMullen, Barnes, & Murtagh, 2018). Despite great variation in context, strategies and targeted mechanisms, the realist synthesis suggested pointers for designing family programs in general (Brown et al., 2016). This review further concluded that families are difficult to recruit, engage and retain in research (O'Connor et al., 2009) with little information regarding recruitment uptake published (Brown, Schiff, & van Sluijs, 2015). As with many other types of research, it is likely that the families who do take part in these programs are not particularly representative of those who are in most need of health promotion. Therefore, challenges of recruiting, retaining and engaging families to health promotion research may need further exploring to progress the family-based intervention design literature.

Community

It has been suggested that interventions should target multiple ecological levels (community, family, school and individual) to have greater success (Gentile et al., 2009) and this means that at least part of many multicomponent interventions falls into the community arena. Community-based projects have seen mixed success when working with the built environment such as when promoting active travel (Coombes & Jones, 2016), when working in specific community settings such as universities (Morgan et al., 2018) or community centers (Elder et al., 2014) or when taking a natural experiment approach (Benjamin Neelon et al., 2015). The community environment may influence child activity through many multilevel factors, including via community recreational facilities, green space, playgrounds as well as how these factors interact with those from other domains such as parental support for taking children to places for activity or allowing children outside to play. Community settings may be incorporated in intervention design in a myriad of diverse ways including organization or promotion of community facilities and programs, by way of policy and directly by altering the built environment. Reviews of health behavior change among children in other areas of research have highlighted the need for individually tailored community-specific interventions (Klassen et al., 2000), also involving parents and family (Stevens et al., 2001) and the importance of support of community leaders through community endorsement and in the recruitment/involvement of other local leaders (Glanz & Yaroch, 2004; Mittelmark et al., 1993). The wide variation of approaches makes this an exciting and increasingly researched diverse setting for health promotion; however, community approaches can still be hampered by poor implementation and study design (Salmon, Booth, Phongsavan, Murphy, & Timperio, 2007). In addition, the wide variety of community-based settings and a suite of context-specific-related issues make intervention design a challenge. These issues are amplified by the existence of a relatively narrow evidence base for any particular specific context and therefore less observational evidence from which to draw upon in the design process. Extensive context-specific experience and knowledge will be necessary if aiming to design an intervention in a particular setting, especially if the context is particularly niche with a limited evidence base.

Digital

Physical activity promotion interventions are increasingly incorporating digital methods, especially among adolescents (Rose et al., 2017). US data from 2015 suggest that 92% of adolescents access the internet daily with 24% stating almost constant use (Lenhart, 2015) so the development of this evidence base is likely to be increasingly salient. Text messaging interventions are known to be acceptable to adolescents but the content, frequency and timing of text message use vary (Keating & McCurry, 2015). As text messages often form part of multicomponent interventions, it is often difficult to establish the efficacy of any particular component unless the trial is designed to do so (Keating & McCurry, 2015). Further research is necessary to better understand the potential of text message use for health promotion (Keating & McCurry, 2015). A review of randomized controlled trials (RCTs) aiming to increase physical activity including a range of technology-based intervention components identified 12 studies in youth, with seven identifying some positive effects on activity (Lappan, Yeh, & Leung, 2015). Although the variability in the included studies made comparisons difficult, these results do provide indications of small effects from digital interventions among adolescents and that digital platforms have been shown to support change in physical activity (Lappan et al., 2015). Approaches incorporated into interventions targeted at adolescents included stand-alone websites, mobile apps and text messages, and combinations of these; no particular approach stood out as being particularly promising (Lappan et al., 2015). Among 5–14-year-old children, only three physical activity promotion trials were identified and all included a supplemental text message as part of a wider intervention; none were concluded to increase activity (Fassnacht, Ali, Silva, Goncalves, & Machado, 2015; Shapiro et al., 2008; Silva et al., 2015). More work is needed on how technology can be incorporated into interventions designed to target both young children and adolescents.

Theory Overview

> The key challenge for practitioners is not simply to base their work on theory (they always work from implicit assumptions and rationales, whether or not they do so consciously), but to make explicit the informal and formal theories they are actually using.
>
> *(Davidoff, Dixon-Woods, Leviton, & Michie, 2015, p. 229)*

Using theory can seem challenging but theories are meant to support and inform research and intervention design, and as such should be approached as a useful resource, and something we are probably using already without realizing, rather than something that hinders our work (Davidoff et al., 2015). Particularly when it comes to behavioral interventions, it is extremely valuable (and arguably essential to success) to utilize the wealth of theories that both help us make sense of human behavior and provide us with tools for achieving behavior change.

Choice and Combination of Theories

Having a basic understanding of mainstream theories (see section below) is useful for getting started but there is generally no one correct theory, and often a combination of different theories may be best for capturing the specific problem or solution in focus. If one theory seems to explain everything it is important to reflect on whether the complexity of the situation is being accurately represented, or if it is being fitted to the theory for convenience. Finding a good theoretical fit has no inherent value if it means overlooking aspects of reality that do not match the theory of choice.

It is often best to approach theories with some flexibility, and a preparedness to adapt, combine and generate new theory depending on the context. What is perhaps most essential is to consider the purpose and origin of theories we want to utilize, as there is generally a difference between theories that help to *understand* behavior, and theories that aim to *change* behavior. The mechanisms of why we behave in certain ways do not necessarily lend themselves to changing behaviors, although some theoretical frameworks address both aspects (Bandura, 1986, 1991). There are also different theories for different levels of the social ecological model, and it is thus important to be clear about what levels the intervention is expected to target. By approaching theories as a resource rather than a constraint, they can be utilized at different phases of intervention design and behavioral epidemiology from understanding the problem to developing solutions (Bartholomew, Parcel, Kok, & Gottlieb, 2006; Sallis et al., 2000). In the section below, using examples, we will discuss how theories and frameworks can be adapted and used in combination. We will also illustrate the importance of combining theory-based rigor with awareness of setting-specific issues.

Key Issues

Incorporating Prior Knowledge from Multiple Sources

Replication, Adaptation or a Clean Slate?

There are many key decisions that need to be made early on in the intervention design process and realistically the flexibility available will depend whether adapting an existing program, and the level of participant and stakeholder involvement. It can be tempting to jump straight in with intervention design but it is important to first assess whether there is enough evidence to allow you to understand the problem and potential solution, and if not then it is important to take a few steps back. A thorough and systematic analysis of the literature (preferably via a systematic review) and critical use of existing analyses, ideally with creative use of available data, are important precursors to intervention design (Corder, Schiff, Kesten, & van Sluijs, 2015). Existing observational and qualitative evidence should be combined thoughtfully and purposefully. It is likely that intervention design from scratch may be unnecessary as there may be a suitable program in a similar population and much of the learning and initial acceptability, feasibility and efficacy testing may already have been done. We recommend considering adapting existing interventions, as it may be that the form of an intervention may need adapting but that the function can stay the same. For example, by maintaining key functions of a component (such as increasing self-efficacy) but thoughtfully changing the form (for example, from class-sessions to after-school sessions) might allow flexibility and more comprehensive use of existing literature (Hawe, Shiell, & Riley, 2004).

Some key decisions and suggestions for deciding on different aspects of early stage intervention design have been outlined in Table 20.1 and include identification of target group, context, timing, behavioral target, main outcome, theoretical basis, framework and behavior change strategies.

Table 20.1 Initial intervention design: evidence and expert informed key questions

Key decision	Key questions
Adapting a program or designing from scratch	Is there a need to design a new program or could an existing one be adapted?
Target behavior	What is the target behavior, for example, overall PA, LPA, MVPA or VPA?
	Consider physical activity as a behavior and as a proximal outcome (e.g. as active travel and MVPA)
	Consider your target behavior and how this will form an outcome measure?
	What evidence is there to justify this target? Are there particular links to health/ other outcomes?
Target group	Who is the target group? Consider whole population approaches versus specific groups?
	Is this decision based on evidence? For example, does a particular age group or social group experience a particularly detrimental change in behavior?
Setting of delivery	Where will the intervention be delivered?
	Who will be delivering it?
	Is training possible in that setting?
	Incorporate expert and stakeholder experience of the setting early in the design process
Setting of proposed behavior change	Where will the proposed behavior change occur? Is the delivery site the same as the site of the proposed activity increase?
	Will the activity be delivered in a session or will the intervention target activity in other settings (or in addition to the delivery setting)
Theoretical basis	Has the work got a theoretical basis which is appropriate for your target group?
Theoretical framework	Is a framework, or elements of multiple frameworks, being incorporated into the design?
Behavior change strategies	How will the proposed intervention align with behavior change strategies?
	Try to align intervention components with the behavior change taxonomy
Fit with TEO steps	Is your intervention likely to fit with at least one of the three TEO steps
Involvement of target group	How will the opinions and experiences of the target group be incorporated?
	What level of approach is appropriate for your population and setting?
Process evaluation	Clearly outlining outcomes, behavior change strategies and key tenets of the intervention will aid process evaluation
	Design intervention components to map onto key outcomes/mechanisms
Appeal	You are probably older than your target group; consider the appeal to your target group at all stages and don't forget common sense and fun
Think bigger	Consider how the intervention may last long term: think wider scale from the beginning including implementation, scale-up, economic evaluation

Note: PA=physical activity; LPA=light intensity physical activity; MVPA=moderate-to-vigorous physical activity; VPA=vigorous physical activity; TEO=Theory of expanded, extended, and enhanced opportunities for youth physical activity promotion (Beets et al., 2016)

All of these decisions should ideally be informed by the literature, incorporated with expert experience and opinion, while keeping a clear understanding of proposed target group and context. These initial decisions should be viewed as preliminary to be taken further and developed using a form of participant focused approach. Participant-led approaches can involve focus groups and interviews with potential participants and stakeholders but there are increasingly creative and innovative ways in which to incorporate which will be discussed in more detail later.

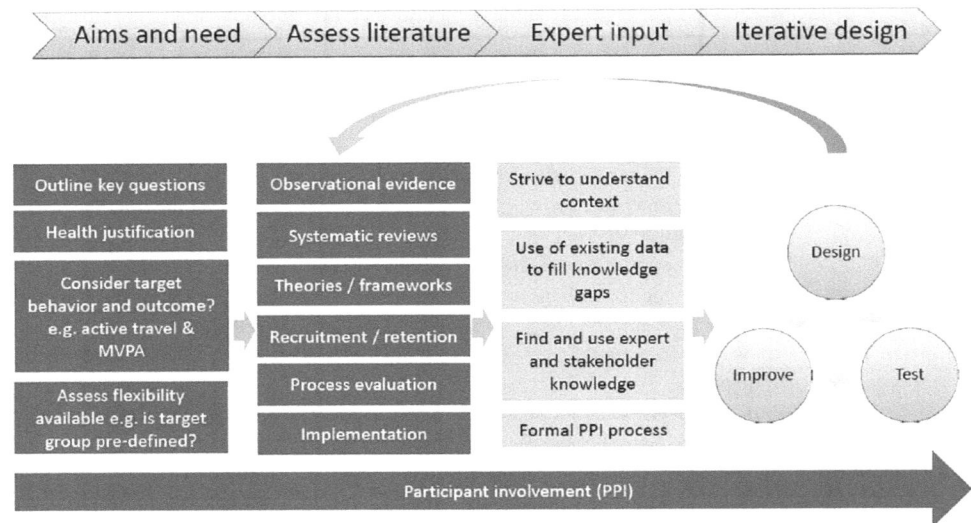

Figure 20.1   A proposed best-practice process of combining multiple sources of existing evidence, participant opinion, local knowledge and the wider context in the design process

Implementation or replication of previously successful interventions is challenging in the context
of the rapidly changing social and digital environments young people live in, and intervention
strategies or approaches may rapidly appear 'old-fashioned' to a new generation. However, although we may need to adapt the form (e.g. delivery method), it is plausible that the function may
stay the same (Hawe et al., 2004). This may increasingly be the case among young people as the
continual development of online-centric communication strategies diverges from that which the
scientific community has first-hand experience of; this makes the incorporation of target participant perspectives into the design process increasingly salient.

A proposed best-practice process of combining multiple sources of existing literature, qualitative work, local knowledge and the wider context and personal experience in the design process
is illustrated in Figure 20.1.

Design Thinking

The word 'design' is often used interchangeably with planning or development in the context of
public health interventions but few researchers or practitioners engaged in intervention design
tend to describe themselves as designers. Intervention design in the planning or development sense
can be characterized as deductive, scientific and guided by the search for effectiveness, whereas
creativity and new human experiences are not necessarily seen as central to the process. However,
there are many lessons to be learnt from the work of people who do describe themselves as designers, and other fields have already realized this (Dorst, 2011; Johansson-Sköldberg, Woodilla, &
Çetinkaya, 2013; Liedtka, 2018; Roberts, Fisher, Trowbridge, & Bent, 2016). Approaches like
design thinking have become popular in the world of business, and while the rationale for large
corporations to learn from design disciplines is likely driven by different objectives than public
health, it is worth noting that behavior change is as relevant to large technology companies or
the food industry as it is to those of us who are interested in promoting physical activity among
young people. A central appeal of design thinking is that the approach allows groups of people to
identify and generate solutions to a specific problem, in the same way that many health promotion

frameworks do, but with a specific emphasis on fostering creativity and innovation, and not limiting the process to what already exists or what has already been done. It is possible to allow space for new solutions even when tailoring or adapting existing interventions, and we particularly encourage researchers and practitioners to do this through inviting the envisaged intervention participants to contribute to the design process.

Incorporating Stakeholder and Target Group Opinions

For both ethical and practical reasons, it is essential to consider the specific needs, preferences and perspectives of the target group when designing youth physical activity interventions. This goes beyond finding out what a certain age group is likely to find interesting or 'cool'. Engaging participants who reflect the target group at the design stage is a vital part of intervention development and relevant to intervention content, participation and refinement (Craig et al., 2008; O'Cathain, Thomas, Drabble, Rudolph, & Hewison, 2013). Generally, the best way to incorporate stakeholder and target group opinion is to ask them about their views and involve them in the design process.

The need for formative work with the target group is highlighted by a systematic review which concluded that only a minority of qualitative work within RCTs is undertaken at the pre-trial stage but that this is important for optimizing interventions and trials (O'Cathain et al., 2013). Often referred to as Patient and Public involvement (PPI), this process refers to research conducted 'with' or 'by' participants rather than 'to', 'about' or for them (www.invo.org.uk). Participants actively contribute to the research process through discussion, ideally regarding all aspects from initial design, acceptability and relevance through to dissemination. In reality, the level of participant involvement varies from informal discussions to participants occasionally leading or doing the research themselves. Country-specific guidance on PPI best practice is increasingly available for researchers starting a study (Hoddinott et al., 2018). Steps for involving participants in research have been outlined and include ensuring that the research questions and outcomes really matter to the target group and making sure that the proposed research will be acceptable to participants so that they will be willing to participate (Hoddinott et al., 2018). Some examples are also included in the previously cited paper about how this process can work in practice (Hoddinott et al., 2018). Increasingly funding bodies are emphasizing the importance of PPI throughout the research process, and as a result the literature offering recommendations and advice for incorporating participant views in intervention design is increasing.

The Level of Participant Involvement

There are various levels and methods of participatory intervention design. Inviting a diverse group of stakeholders to consult and advise the design process early on is often recommended in intervention development frameworks (e.g. Intervention Mapping, PRACTIS) (Bartholomew et al., 2006; Craig et al., 2008; Koorts et al., 2018) but there are also different research methods that facilitate the incorporation of participant views. Qualitative research can capture lived experiences and an in-depth understanding of the individuals' or groups' perspectives (Green & Thorogood, 2018; Sparkes & Smith, 2014; Taylor & Francis, 2013). Data collection methods such as focus group discussions or different qualitative interviews are useful for this purpose and should be selected based on the specific aims of the qualitative inquiry, and with appropriate consideration of the theoretical and philosophical underpinnings of different methods.

Whatever the chosen approach and methods are, the most important components of successfully incorporating the views of the target group are to speak to the participants and actually listen, letting them inform your decisions, and not allowing preconceived plans or expectations to outweigh what you learn from speaking to the target group. It is worth dedicating time early on to planning exactly how insights from those the intervention is intended to benefit will be utilized, and considering how potential challenges, such as contradictory views from different individuals or groups, will be handled. More creative data collection methods such as asking young people to draw, take photos or in other ways represent ideal intervention components can foster innovation but without a plan for how to analyze and make use of qualitative data in different formats, the contributions of research participants may be wasted, which is not only a pity but also ethically problematic.

While some qualitative research methods may come across as simple or quick because sample sizes tend to be smaller than in quantitative studies, it may be very challenging and time-consuming to make sense of findings. The depth of understanding that qualitative research has the potential to deliver may result in researchers having to re-think key aspects of a proposed intervention such as who to target. The characteristics that define a target group from a research or practitioner point of view do not guarantee that the group is homogenous in views, interests or ability to contribute to research activities (Hamed, Klingberg, Mahmud, & Bradby, 2018). Critical reflection on how the researchers' expectations or experiences play into the dynamics and practice of qualitative research is also an essential part of the process, particularly when it comes to cross-cultural research or settings that are in some other way unfamiliar to the researcher (Green & Thorogood, 2018; Liamputtong, 2010).

As discussed earlier, in the medical and public health fields, PPI (Hoddinott et al., 2018) has become a key channel for driving participation in research and health promotion but other fields and disciplines have also developed various approaches to designing with the target group in mind that may be useful to draw from in designing youth physical activity interventions. For example, human- or user-centered design, and co-design describe approaches to user involvement in a product or service design process (Bazzano, Martin, Hicks, Faughnan, & Murphy, 2017; Gustavsson & Andersson, 2019; Matheson, Pacione, Shultz, & Klugl, 2015), whereas community-based participatory research (CBPR) refers to involving the intended beneficiaries of a program or project in the planning stages (Wallerstein & Duran, 2010). It may not be feasible to directly adopt methods from different fields but it is useful to consider benefits and shortcomings of various approaches to involving the target group.

Opportunities and Challenges of Different Approaches

Community-Based Participatory Research

OPPORTUNITIES

CBPR is an equity-oriented approach to doing research in partnership with a community, enabling researchers to benefit from an in-depth understanding of community needs. This can ensure interventions are acceptable, include relevant components and achieve buy-in or a sense of ownership from community members.

CHALLENGES

Any group or community will involve certain power dynamics, and potentially conflicting interests or different ideas about what membership in the group or community entails. Community cohesion or homogeneity cannot be assumed, and researchers should remember that a community in itself is a construct, and not necessarily an identity shared by those perceived by outsiders as belonging to a certain community (Hamed et al., 2018). For interested readers, there are further resources which include more detailed information about this approach (Wallerstein & Duran, 2010; Wallerstein, Duran, Oetzel, & Minkler, 2017).

Delphi Studies

OPPORTUNITIES

The Delphi method involves consulting experts in a specific field through, for example, online surveys, and condensing responses for further rounds of expert consultation in order to arrive at some degree of consensus. This relatively cheap and potentially quick method, which can be applied internationally, is useful for scoping priorities on topics in which expert consensus can advance the research or health promotion agenda.

CHALLENGES

Harmonizing diverse and complex views is difficult, perhaps even impossible in some cases. Delphi methods are not generally intended to be used for lay consultations, and such applications may create a false sense of agreed priorities among people who may not have enough expertise to provide recommendations or make an informed commitment to specific alternatives. These resources include further information and examples about this approach (Morton et al., 2017; Turner, Ollerhead, & Cook, 2017).

Focus Groups

OPPORTUNITIES

Focus groups or focus group discussions are moderated interactions between individuals who have been selected to participate based on certain shared characteristics (e.g. age, gender, experience), or who are already part of an existing group ('natural group'), in order to gain insights into group dynamics, shared norms and typical views or responses. When dividing participants into groups by, for example, profession, it is possible to make comparisons between different groups' views.

CHALLENGES

For inexperienced qualitative researchers, it may appear tempting to conduct focus group discussions instead of individual interviews in order to get a larger sample size but this is not an appropriate substitution as different methods cater to different needs and aims. Focus group discussions are not necessarily ideal for sensitive topics, and there is always the risk of dominant individuals taking up too much space in the group discussion or steering other people's responses. These additional references provide further details of this approach (Green & Thorogood, 2018; Liamputtong, 2010) and talk about potential conflicts and issues with group dynamics (Smithson, 2000).

Visual Data or Novel Methods

OPPORTUNITIES

The design process of interventions targeting children or young people may benefit from using videos, photos, drawings or mapping exercises to capture children's ideas or perspectives. This can be particularly useful if targeting young children for whom discussion- or interview-based methods may not be appropriate.

CHALLENGES

Involving young children in research requires specific ethical considerations, and there may not be enough time or resources for the bureaucratic demands involved. Another challenge is analyzing and making use of the data in practical and accurate ways, as using novel forms of data may necessitate expertise that the research team does not possess. This challenge can be overcome by collaborating across disciplines and fields, which is a useful option to consider even without specific data challenges. Resources providing further detail and examples regarding these techniques are available (Bland, 2018; Hall, 2015; Holm, 2014; Mayaba & Wood, 2015; Winton, 2016).

Ethnography

OPPORTUNITIES

Ethnography aims to elicit a deep understanding of how a certain group operates or what it is like to be a particular person. This may be the most effective way for someone outside of a situation, or particular target group, to develop a deep understanding of the spoken and unspoken nature of a culture (Grossoehme, 2014).

CHALLENGES

This is a particularly specialist approach requiring sensitive anthropological training and expertise. However, the learning from this type of approach, while specific to the individuals or group observed, is able to provide an incomparable depth of understanding. Further details of this approach are discussed in more detail elsewhere (Coffey, 2018; Taylor & Francis, 2013).

Intervention Design and Development Frameworks

Various frameworks for the development of health promotion interventions have been suggested including Intervention Mapping, the behavioral epidemiology framework, and the Medical Research Council (MRC) framework for developing and evaluating complex interventions (Bartholomew et al., 2006; Craig et al., 2008; Sallis et al., 2000). Existing frameworks generally suggest basing strategies on behavior change theory, existing evidence and conducting formative research with the target group. It may not be possible to follow one specific framework from start to finish but consulting intervention development frameworks is valuable for avoiding running into common problems, and identifying what information will be needed for the design process to be as successful and transparent as possible. Every setting is different and blindly following a framework for the sake of using one is unlikely to be the best solution. Indeed, frameworks like Intervention Mapping highlight context-specific, non-linear and iterative processes rather than being purely prescriptive (Bartholomew et al., 2006). Table 20.2 provides an overview of three relevant frameworks to consider when designing physical activity interventions.

Theories to Explain Behavior

We have provided a brief overview rather than try to provide a comprehensive account; the summaries below contain references to obtain more detail on these theories. This selection includes those commonly applied in physical activity promotion in youth but is not exhaustive.

Table 20.2 Characteristics, benefits and challenges of intervention development frameworks

Framework	MRC Complex Interventions (Craig et al., 2008)	Intervention Mapping (Bartholomew et al., 2006)	PRACTIS (Koorts et al., 2018)
Origin or underpinning	UK Medical Research Council guidance. Builds on drug development and pharmaceutical trial processes	Social ecological model, systems thinking	Based on implementation science, and specifically focused on PA
Main components	Intervention development: – Identifying existing evidence – Identifying and developing theory – Modeling process and outcomes Feasibility and piloting Evaluation Implementation	Step 1. Logic model of the problem Step 2. Logic model of change Step 3. Program design Step 4. Program production Step 5. Program implementation plan Step 6. Evaluation plan	Step 1. Characterize the parameters of the implementation setting Step 2. Identify and engage key stakeholders across multiple levels within the delivery system(s) Step 3. Identify contextual barriers and facilitators to implementation Step 4. Address potential barriers to effective implementation
Specific benefits	Widely used, flexible, and acknowledges the complex nature of real world interventions	Involves a thorough consideration of potential risks and key factors likely to determine success of an intervention. The framework builds on a log frame approach that traces key considerations backwards from the ultimate aim of an intervention	Prioritizes translation of research into practice, and thus gears intervention design process toward anticipating and mitigating potential implementation challenges
Potential challenges	While this framework provides useful guidance for considerations at different stages of intervention design and development, it does not cover practical instructions for specific processes or decision-making. This acknowledges that the design process cannot be prescribed in detail as contexts and interventions vary greatly	Making full use of this framework is labor-intensive and involves the development of numerous log frames and mappings. This may promote a box-ticking approach to the design process, and so care should be taken to really reflect on each decision with the context in mind, as opposed to just what seems logical when mapped out using tables	This framework provides a comprehensive set of instructions, considerations and checklists for real world problem-solving but the use of theory is not elaborated on much in the framework, although theories may support the process of anticipating implementation challenges

Note: PA=physical activity

HEALTH BELIEF MODEL

This theory conceptualizes people's health behaviors and health-related decision-making as being guided by four key psychological constructs related to beliefs about a health condition and related behaviors: perceived susceptibility, perceived severity, perceived benefits and perceived barriers

(Janz & Becker, 1984). As a simple model that helps to make sense of behavior, it can also be a useful starting point for thinking about behavior change, as changing one or more of the four constructs may form part of a behavior change intervention.

THEORY OF PLANNED BEHAVIOR

The theory of planned behavior is also a simple way to conceptualize people's health-related behavior with the help of psychological constructs (Ajzen, 1991). The most central one is intention, as the theory highlights the importance of intention as determining actions or behavior. According to the theory, three other constructs, namely attitude, subjective norms and behavioral control, influence people's health-related intentions. Attitude consists of perceptions or beliefs regarding the health behavior, while subjective norms refer to beliefs about what other people whose opinions are valued or considered relevant think about the behavior. Behavioral control captures perception about their own ability to perform a specific behavior.

Theories of Behavior Change

SOCIAL COGNITIVE THEORY

This is a widely used theory that can be applied to both understanding and changing behavior (Bandura, 1986, 1991). The main constructs it builds on are outcome expectations, outcome expectancies, self-efficacy, behavioral capability, perceived behavior of others and the environment. Outcome expectations differ from outcome expectancies in that the first is expected consequences of a behavior, while the second is concerned with how important those consequences are to an individual. Self-efficacy refers to how much confidence an individual has in their own ability to perform a certain behavior. Behavioral capability, in turn, refers to the individual's actual ability.

TRANSTHEORETICAL MODEL OF BEHAVIOR CHANGE

This is a theoretical model specifically concerned with changing behavior. It consists of multiple phases considered to be part of behavior change, and divides them into two categories: stages of change, and processes of change (Prochaska & Velicer, 1997). This means that behavior change is seen as following specific stages (e.g. preparation), and in order to progress through the stages specific processes (e.g. consciousness raising) need to take place.

SELF-DETERMINATION THEORY (SDT)

This is a theory of motivation concerned with supporting inherent tendencies to behave healthily (Ryan & Deci, 2000). SDT suggests that contextual social factors such as teacher behavior toward students can affect individuals' (students) motivation by targeting three psychological needs (Lonsdale et al., 2016). These three needs are autonomy (acting in a self-directed way), competence (interacting effectively with the environment) and relatedness (connectedness with others). This theory focuses on two types of motivation, first controlled motivation which stems from external or internal pressure (e.g. parental pressure or guilt, respectively). Second, autonomous motivation occurs because of enjoyment, interest or perceiving value and is positively associated with activity (Lonsdale et al., 2016). Strategies which may target autonomous motivation include promoting activity choice and establishing the relevance of being active to an individual.

DIFFUSION OF INNOVATIONS THEORY (NETWORK INTERVENTIONS)

All people are part of a social network, including friends, family and contemporary school students. Many interventions do not account for the underlying social interactions, or social networks which are inherently present in the design process (Hunter et al., 2015). Although seldom used with regard to physical activity, making use of social network knowledge in intervention design could improve effectiveness by generating social influence and accelerating behavior change (Buller et al., 1999; Campbell et al., 2008). Although there are indications of promise of using network theory in physical activity interventions in young people (Sebire et al., 2018) effectiveness of this approach has yet to be proved in full scale physical activity research (van Woudenberg et al., 2018). Network interventions are based on diffusion of innovations theory which explains how new ideas and practices spread within and between communities (Valente, 2012).

Organizational change theories   When trying to achieve behavior change within a wider social ecological context (Valente, 2012), and for example in a school setting, it may be useful to consider theories that address the institutional level as opposed to individuals alone. These theories capture determinants of behavior such as structures or cultures within the organization, and utilize similar constructs as individual theories, such as outcome expectations, skills and attitudes but with a focus on changing these through organizational change (Cummings & Worley, 2014).

For more detailed summaries of these and other theories of relevance to designing physical activity interventions for young people we recommend the resource book for the Intervention Mapping framework: 'Planning Health Promotion Programs: An Intervention Mapping Approach (4th edition)' (Bartholomew et al., 2006). The authors also provide helpful considerations for using theories at different stages of the design process.

Case Study

A school-based health promotion intervention targeting physical activity and dietary behavior in 12-year-old learners in Eastern Cape, South Africa, successfully combined context-specific formative research in the form of 'targeted ethnography', and theory-based rigor to develop the behavioral intervention (Jemmott et al., 2011). Even in the absence of existing high-quality evidence of successful physical activity interventions in South Africa or other African countries (Klingberg, Draper, Micklesfield, Benjamin-Neelon, & van Sluijs, 2019), the use of social cognitive theory, the theory of planned behavior and insights from and about the specific target group allowed the research team to develop an intervention which successfully increased self-reported physical activity, and improved self-reported dietary behaviors. Utilizing these theories also enabled the research team to conceptualize and measure the behavioral mediators through which the behavior change was expected to occur. Thus, even if the intervention had been less successful, the theoretical basis could have served as a map through which the shortcomings of the intervention could have been traced. Using appropriate theories is thus useful both for designing and evaluating physical activity interventions.

Behavioral Change Strategies

To aid transparency and replication to advance behavior change science, a taxonomy of BCTs is often used to consistently classify the specific BCTs, or 'active ingredients', used within an intervention and proposed as the mechanisms of change (Abraham & Michie, 2008; Abraham et al., 2015; Michie et al., 2015). In a design context, the use of this taxonomy has the potential to facilitate a structured and thorough process through all aspects of the intervention lifecycle.

An intervention designer can decide what determinants should be targeted, how these can be operationalized and identify which techniques of the BCT taxonomy these map on to. This will also allow the designer to see how their approach aligns with previous and contemporary programs and perhaps more easily draw upon existing evidence and available advice related to those particular components. The use of the BCT taxonomy also has the potential to facilitate process evaluation by identifying particular components that should be monitored during implementation. The use of the taxonomy in intervention reporting further aids consistency and comparability of published work to improve transparency and therefore increase the potential for the intervention to be replicated or adapted. There are suggestions that use of this taxonomy has resulted in improved clarity and replicability (Wood et al., 2016) but written descriptions of intervention components may still not be adequately reported to allow replication (Johnston et al., 2018). It is hoped that a refined taxonomy including 40-items specific to physical activity will better allow specification and replication of intervention components to strengthen behavior change science (Michie et al., 2011).

Emerging Issues

Flexibility Versus Replication: Should an Intervention be Expected to Work in Multiple Settings?

Many researchers strive for replicability, both for other researchers to be able to repeat and improve work, but also so that interventions can be scalable. We often aim for the same interventions to be rolled out widely, for example across many schools. This is where we find ourselves at an impasse striving for maximum replicability to advance the scientific field but perhaps having unrealistic expectations of sufficient similarities across settings to allow it. Taking the example of schools, while on the surface a school is relatively similar to other schools in many ways, there is likely to be an underlying culture which will be different for every individual school. For example, the opinions of the leadership, teachers and students about any particular issues, including physical activity, will be a combination of an infinite number of different factors, influences, opinions, at all levels of the system and community, and even the particular historical and local context of the individual school. This highlights the importance of gaining a deep understanding of the particular issues specific to any particular context during intervention design and the importance of incorporating participant and stakeholder opinion into intervention design. Although it can be tempting to rush into intervention design and implementation, planning implementation and scalability during the initial design process is incredibly important. Decisions about whether a particular intervention needs to be scalable, and if so, what issues are likely to be raised when this intervention is implemented more widely should be considered early on in the design phase.

This challenge of designing an intervention which is replicable versus the flexibility needed in many settings is demonstrated by the feasibility and pilot studies that appear to be successful on a small scale but which are then not effective when scaled up to full trials (Adab et al., 2018; Jago et al., 2015; Kipping et al., 2014). This is despite the fact that these interventions have already been iteratively tested and often refined or improved before use in an increased number of settings. There are likely to be multiple reasons for this phenomenon, including greater distance from the research team to the target population, especially in the United Kingdom where intervention delivery is not an eligible research grant cost, often requiring non-research organizations to fund and organize intervention delivery. The efficacy and effectiveness of some school-based interventions on a large scale have been demonstrated (Sutherland et al., 2016) but strong evidence is needed to shed light on how these interventions can be understood and scaled up, or disseminated, implemented and adopted more widely.

Further, even fewer efficacious interventions are successfully translated and sustained in policy and practice (Koorts et al., 2018). Implementation research is rapidly growing momentum; the PRACTIS guide focuses on physical activity interventions in multiple settings and highlights the importance of addressing differences between the research and practice contexts throughout the development process and considering potential barriers and facilitators to implementation early on (Koorts et al., 2018). The school-specific CSPAP and WSCC also provide guidance for working on a systems level and considering implementation at an early stage.

Due to the limited success of school-based physical activity promotion to date (Love et al., 2019), there definitely needs to be a step-change in how we approach school-based physical activity promotion. All schools are unique systems and although researchers often consider lack of success of a full trial to be 'the end of the line', it is perhaps not realistic to expect an intervention to be replicable in a similar form across multiple unique systems. While appropriate for trials of pharmacological interventions, perhaps it is inappropriate to consider a cluster RCT as the gold-standard test for a school-based intervention as currently the field is gaining incremental advances with this approach. There is a lot we can learn from success of a pilot or feasibility study and it may not always be appropriate for complex interventions to be implemented across many settings without substantial tailoring which may cause issues when using RCTs for evaluation (Hawe et al., 2004). This may particularly be the case for complex interventions which have had a lot of context-specific participant involvement during the design process and are highly tailored to a particular institution. It may be possible to make a complex intervention scalable by thoughtfully defining key intervention components and aligning underlying functions but allowing flexibility in form, but this needs to be considered early in the design process (Hawe et al., 2004). Even a relatively simple intervention is likely to be altered in some way when it is implemented in different schools. These may be acceptable, and in many cases essential, changes, but often the details of these changes are poorly recorded and reported in the literature. More detailed process evaluation and use of implementation science will hopefully begin to elucidate how intervention design can best navigate these issues in striving for a balance between replicability and tailoring.

Social Media: Do We Know Enough to Effectively Embrace This in Our Intervention Design?

As of January 2018, 42% of people worldwide were active social media users; this had risen 13% worldwide over the previous year (Smart Insights, 2018). The largest increase in social media use is occurring in Saudi Arabia (32% annual increase), with India and Indonesia along with the United Kingdom, South Korea, and the UAE experiencing the slowest annual growth (Hootsuite, 2017). In the United Kingdom, social media use may already have nearly reached saturation among older adolescents with 96% of 16–24 year-olds reporting being active users of social networking sites in 2017 (Office of National Statistics, 2017).

This high prevalence of use means that social media-based health promotion has the potential for incredibly large reach at relatively low cost (Gough et al., 2017). Despite a relatively limited evidence base, social media is increasingly used as part of behavioral interventions (Rose et al., 2017). Compared to interventions targeting other health behaviors, social media appears to be relatively little used in physical activity promotion among youth although there are some examples (Pumper et al., 2015) with somewhat limited acceptability (Saez et al., 2018; van Woudenberg et al., 2018). The one social media (Facebook intervention) identified in a recent review of digital interventions among adolescents showed no increase in objectively measured physical activity (Wojcicki, Grigsby-Toussaint, Hillman, Huhman, & McAuley, 2014).

It is hypothesized that social media use can influence behavior and health, via some of the principles that apply to social networks and diffusion of innovation theory. There are four proposed categories by which network data can be used in intervention design (Valente, 2012). The initial strategy is to identify individuals or 'nodes' within a network with certain characteristics, for example opinion leaders. 'Segmentation' suggests that an intervention can be directed toward a particular group of people with certain characteristics (e.g. cliques). The principle of 'induction' refers to the formation of new links between people within a network (e.g. stimulating peer to peer links to cascade information) whereas 'alteration' aims to change the structure of the network (e.g. by introducing a new 'healthy' mentor) (Valente, 2012). One way in which this theory could be applied to social media to influence behavior is by identifying online influencers and using them to cascade information to followers (Valente, 2012). Although the idea of an influential blogger or vlogger passing on important health information to a hard-to-reach at-risk group at low cost seems like a win-win potential strategy in intervention design, in reality the complex nature of the social media environment needs a deep understanding before embarking on this type of project. To add complication to the idea of information provision online, there is increased skepticism of academic-related health information, with falsehoods spreading more easily than truth online (Vosoughi, Roy, & Aral, 2018).

Further, those aiming to incorporate social media into intervention design should be aware of the complicated relationship between social media use and health and well-being, with indications of potential negative effects of social media use on body image but potentially positive impacts on self-esteem and social support (Easton, Morton, Tappy, Francis, & Dennison, 2018). Among adolescents and young adults, it is becoming popular to post 'fitspirational' content supposedly showing 'healthy behaviors' including physical activity and diet (Easton et al., 2018). Studies examining content analysis of supposedly health online trends have suggested that they can perpetuate unhealthy body image ideals but may increase social support and motivation (Deighton-Smith & Bell, 2017). Those designing interventions should be aware that there may be a very thin line between our health promotion messages and potentially harmful interpretations of that content (such as promoting body dissatisfaction). Whether it has positive or negative consequences, there is an increasing amount of social media–driven behavior change occurring outside of the research-arena, which researchers could learn from in an attempt to keep our behavior change efforts contemporary and broadly appealing to our target audience.

Despite the huge potential for physical activity research, there are several overarching issues with the incorporation of social media into intervention design. This stems from social media data being present on a platform owned by a commercial organization and being composed of interactions between multiple individuals who may not have provided consent for any particular study. Currently, there is no consensus about how to deal with these types of ethical issues as this legislation is lagging behind the advancements of these new technologies (Hunter et al., 2018). Terms and conditions of social media platform use tend to be very long and people may agree to the conditions without really knowing what they are agreeing to; even though users may technically own their content, the owners of the platform are legally able to alter and use the data however they want (Hunter et al., 2018). Anonymity of data is crucial in research but even if names are removed from social media data, the linked data may include other identifiable information. Further ethical issues stem from social media posts consisting of a wide range of information types (including photos and videos) which may include non-consented individuals. It is relatively easy to create a fake social media profile and for automated bots to post content; therefore, there may be no guarantee of the validity of any informed consent. As social media transcends international boundaries, the exact laws which govern the use are unclear and each county will be subject to specific online cultures and commercial interests.

Physical activity promotion research among youth is playing catch-up with the social media trend, although there is now guidance on behavior change theory specific to digital interventions (Michie, Yardley, West, Patrick, & Greaves, 2017). The pervasiveness of social media warrants future research in terms of how it can potentially be used for health promotion but also to elucidate any intended or unintended consequences of social media use in all elements of behavior change work. Further research is urgently needed to understand the complex associations of social media and young people's behavior and subsequently how we can best harness the ubiquitous nature of social media for behavior change.

Recommendations for Researchers and Practitioners

Although intervention design is challenging, and often feels like a daunting task, there are an increasing number of resources available to guide researchers throughout the process. While the number of these resources can also feel overwhelming, we provide a checklist to aid with the initial process as establishing a starting point and the opportunities for flexibility can help to illuminate a clearer path. We highlight the importance of utilizing existing literature and available data to fill knowledge gaps before embarking on intervention design. It is important to incorporate participant views from the start and to include formal participant involvement, ideally using a range of methods. In addition to incorporating participant views, the whole design process should be conducted as openly as possible, asking for advice from experts, stakeholders and practitioners throughout. Recommending an awareness of a whole-system socio-ecological approach, we summarize and suggest resources for finding the place of theories and frameworks in your particular design process. Retaining scientific rigor throughout is equally as important as thinking 'outside the box' wherever possible, including by incorporating relevant techniques from other research areas and using novel suggestions from your target group. It is easy to forget that an intervention should live on after initial testing so when embarking on a design process, remember to consider implementation and scalability from the start. Although intervention design can be daunting, it is also an exciting opportunity to use our scientific knowledge to improve health. It is appropriate that intervention design should be challenging as so many decisions are required which rarely have an obvious answer but being thoughtful about the process is the best place to start.

References

Abraham, C., & Michie, S. (2008). A taxonomy of behavior change techniques used in interventions. *Health Psychology, 27*(3), 379–387. doi:10.1037/0278-6133.27.3.379

Abraham, C., Wood, C. E., Johnston, M., Francis, J., Hardeman, W., Richardson, M., & Michie, S. (2015). Reliability of identification of behavior change techniques in intervention descriptions. *Annals of Behavioral Medicine, 49*(6), 885–900. doi:10.1007/s12160-015-9727-y

Adab, P., Pallan, M. J., Lancashire, E. R., Hemming, K., Frew, E., Barrett, T., . . . Cheng, K. K. (2018). Effectiveness of a childhood obesity prevention program delivered through schools, targeting 6 and 7 year olds: Cluster randomized controlled trial (WAVES study). *BMJ, 360,* k211. doi:10.1136/bmj.k211

Ajzen, I. (1991). The theory of planned behavior. *Organizational Behavior and Human Decision Processes, 50,* 179–211.

All-Party Commission on Physical Activity. (2014). Tackling physical inactivity – A coordinated approach. Retrieved from https://parliamentarycommissiononphysicalactivity.files.wordpress.com/2014/04/apco-pa-final.pdf

Bandura, A. (1986). *Social foundations of thought and action: A social cognitive theory.* Englewood Cliffs, NJ: Prentice Hall.

Bandura, A. (1991). Social cognitive theory of self-regulation. *Organizational Behavior and Human Decision Processes, 50,* 248–287.

Barbosa Filho, V. C., Minatto, G., Mota, J., Silva, K. S., de Campos, W., & Lopes Ada, S. (2016). Promoting physical activity for children and adolescents in low- and middle-income countries: An umbrella systematic review: A review on promoting physical activity in LMIC. *Preventive Medicine, 88,* 115–126. doi:10.1016/j.ypmed.2016.03.025

Bartholomew, L., Parcel, G., Kok, G., & Gottlieb, N. (2006). *Planning health promotion programs. An intervention mapping approach* (2nd ed.). San Francisco, CA: Jossey-Bass. A Wiley Imprint.

Bazzano, A. N., Martin, J., Hicks, E., Faughnan, M., & Murphy, L. (2017). Human-centred design in global health: A scoping review of applications and contexts. *PLoS One, 12*(11), e0186744. doi:10.1371/journal.pone.0186744

Beets, M. W., Okely, A., Weaver, R. G., Webster, C., Lubans, D., Brusseau, T., . . . Cliff, D. P. (2016). The theory of expanded, extended, and enhanced opportunities for youth physical activity promotion. *International Journal of Behavioral Nutrition and Physical Activity, 13*(1), 120. doi:10.1186/s12966-016-0442-2

Bell, J. A., Hamer, M., Richmond, R. C., Timpson, N. J., Carslake, D., & Davey Smith, G. (2018). Associations of device-measured physical activity across adolescence with metabolic traits: Prospective cohort study. *PLoS Medicine, 15*(9), e1002649. doi:10.1371/journal.pmed.1002649

Benjamin Neelon, S. E., Namenek Brouwer, R. J., Ostbye, T., Evenson, K. R., Neelon, B., Martinie, A., & Bennett, G. (2015). A community-based intervention increases physical activity and reduces obesity in school-age children in North Carolina. *Childhood Obesity, 11*(3), 297–303. doi:10.1089/chi.2014.0130

Bland, D. (2018). Using drawing in research with children: Lessons from practice. *International Journal of Research & Method in Education, 43*(3), 342–352.

Bobrowski, A., Spitzner, M., Bethge, S., Mueller-Graf, F., Vollmar, B., & Zechner, D. (2013). Risk factors for pancreatic ductal adenocarcinoma specifically stimulate pancreatic duct glands in mice. *American Journal of Pathology, 182*(3), 965–974. doi:10.1016/j.ajpath.2012.11.016

Borde, R., Smith, J. J., Sutherland, R., Nathan, N., & Lubans, D. R. (2017). Methodological considerations and impact of school-based interventions on objectively measured physical activity in adolescents: A systematic review and meta-analysis. *Obesity Reviews, 18*(4), 476–490. doi:10.1111/obr.12517

Brooke, H. L., Atkin, A. J., Corder, K., Ekelund, U., & van Sluijs, E. M. (2016). Changes in time-segment specific physical activity between ages 10 and 14 years: A longitudinal observational study. *Journal of Science and Medicine in Sport, 19*(1), 29–34. doi:10.1016/j.jsams.2014.10.003

Brooke, H. L., Corder, K., Atkin, A. J., & van Sluijs, E. M. (2014). A systematic literature review with meta-analyses of within- and between-day differences in objectively measured physical activity in school-aged children. *Sports Medicine, 44*(10), 1427–1438. doi:10.1007/s40279-014-0215-5

Brown, H. E., Atkin, A. J., Panter, J., Corder, K., Wong, G., Chinapaw, M. J., & van Sluijs, E. (2014). Family-based interventions to increase physical activity in children: A meta-analysis and realist synthesis protocol. *BMJ Open, 4*(8), e005439. doi:10.1136/bmjopen-2014-005439

Brown, H. E., Atkin, A. J., Panter, J., Wong, G., Chinapaw, M. J., & van Sluijs, E. M. (2016). Family-based interventions to increase physical activity in children: A systematic review, meta-analysis and realist synthesis. *Obesity Reviews, 17*(4), 345–360. doi:10.1111/obr.12362

Brown, H. E., Schiff, A., & van Sluijs, E. M. (2015). Engaging families in physical activity research: A family-based focus group study. *BMC Public Health, 15*, 1178. doi:10.1186/s12889-015-2497-4

Buller, D. B., Morrill, C., Taren, D., Aickin, M., Sennott-Miller, L., Buller, M. K., . . . Wentzel, T. M. (1999). Randomized trial testing the effect of peer education at increasing fruit and vegetable intake. *Journal of the National Cancer Institute, 91*(17), 1491–1500.

Campbell, R., Starkey, F., Holliday, J., Audrey, S., Bloor, M., Parry-Langdon, N., . . . Moore, L. (2008). An informal school-based peer-led intervention for smoking prevention in adolescence (ASSIST): A cluster randomized trial. *Lancet, 371*(9624), 1595–1602. doi:10.1016/S0140-6736(08)60692-3

Chan, A. W., Tetzlaff, J. M., Altman, D. G., Dickersin, K., & Moher, D. (2013). SPIRIT 2013: New guidance for content of clinical trial protocols. *Lancet, 381*(9861), 91–92. doi:10.1016/S0140-6736(12)62160-6

Chan, A. W., Tetzlaff, J. M., Altman, D. G., Laupacis, A., Gotzsche, P. C., Krleza-Jeric, K., . . . Moher, D. (2013). SPIRIT 2013 statement: Defining standard protocol items for clinical trials. *Annals of Internal Medicine, 158*(3), 200–207. doi:10.7326/0003-4819-158-3-201302050-00583

Chan, A. W., Tetzlaff, J. M., Gotzsche, P. C., Altman, D. G., Mann, H., Berlin, J. A., . . . Moher, D. (2013). SPIRIT 2013 explanation and elaboration: Guidance for protocols of clinical trials. *BMJ, 346*, e7586. doi:10.1136/bmj.e7586

Coffey, A. (2018). *Doing ethnography.* London, UK: Sage.

Coombes, E., & Jones, A. (2016). Gamification of active travel to school: A pilot evaluation of the beat the street physical activity intervention. *Health Place, 39*, 62–69. doi:10.1016/j.healthplace.2016.03.001

Corder, K., Craggs, C., Jones, A. P., Ekelund, U., Griffin, S. J., & van Sluijs, E. M. (2013). Predictors of change differ for moderate and vigorous intensity physical activity and for weekdays and weekends: A longitudinal analysis. *The International Journal of Behavioral Nutrition and Physical Activity, 10*, 69. doi:10.1186/1479-5868-10-69

Corder, K., Schiff, A., Kesten, J. M., & van Sluijs, E. M. (2015). Development of a universal approach to increase physical activity among adolescents: The GoActive intervention. *BMJ Open, 5*(8), e008610. doi:10.1136/bmjopen-2015-008610

Corr, M., Morgan, P. J., McMullen, J., Barnes, A., & Murtagh, E. (2018). Maternal influences on adolescent daughters to increase physical activity (supporting our lifelong engagement: Mothers and teens exercising [SOLEMATES]): A feasibility study. *Lancet, Meeting Abstracts, 392*, S5.

Craggs, C., Corder, K., van Sluijs, E. M., & Griffin, S. J. (2011). Determinants of change in physical activity in children and adolescents: A systematic review. *American Journal of Preventive Medicine, 40*(6), 645–658.

Craig, P., Dieppe, P., Macintyre, S., Michie, S., Nazareth, I., & Petticrew, M. (2008). Developing and evaluating complex interventions: The new medical research council guidance. *BMJ, 337*, a1655. doi:10.1136/bmj.a1655

Cummings, T., & Worley, C. (2014). *Organization development and change* (10th ed.). Stamford, CT: CENGAGE Learning.

Davidoff, F., Dixon-Woods, M., Leviton, L., & Michie, S. (2015). Demystifying theory and its use in improvement. *BMJ Quality and Safety, 24*(3), 228–238. doi:10.1136/bmjqs-2014-003627

Davis, E., Chen, J., Leon, K., Darst, S. A., & Campbell, E. A. (2015). Mycobacterial RNA polymerase forms unstable open promoter complexes that are stabilized by CarD. *Nucleic Acids Research, 43*(1), 433–445. doi:10.1093/nar/gku1231

Davison, K. K., & Birch, L. L. (2001). Childhood overweight: A contextual model and recommendations for future research. *Obesity Reviews, 2*(3), 159–171.

Deighton-Smith, N., & Bell, B. (2017). Objectifying fitness: A content and thematic analysis of #fitspiration images on social media. *Psychology of Popular Media Culture, 7*(4), 467–483.

Dorst, K. (2011). The core of 'design thinking' and its application. *Design Studies, 32*(6), 521–532.

Dumith, S. C., Gigante, D. P., Domingues, M. R., & Kohl, H. W., 3rd. (2011). Physical activity change during adolescence: A systematic review and a pooled analysis. *International Journal of Epidemiology, 40*(3), 685–698. doi:10.1093/ije/dyq272

Easton, S., Morton, K., Tappy, Z., Francis, D., & Dennison, L. (2018). Young people's experiences of viewing the fitspiration social media trend: Qualitative study. *Journal of Medical Internet Research, 20*(6), e219. doi:10.2196/jmir.9156

Elder, J. P., Crespo, N. C., Corder, K., Ayala, G. X., Slymen, D. J., Lopez, N. V., . . . McKenzie, T. L. (2014). Childhood obesity prevention and control in city recreation centers and family homes: The MOVE/me Muevo project. *Pediatric Obesity, 9*(3), 218–231. doi:10.1111/j.2047-6310.2013.00164.x

Engle, T. B., Jobman, E. E., Moural, T. W., McKnite, A. M., Bundy, J. W., Barnes, S. Y., . . . Ciobanu, D. C. (2014). Variation in time and magnitude of immune response and viremia in experimental challenges with Porcine circovirus 2b. *BMC Veterinary Research, 10*, 286. doi:10.1186/s12917-014-0286-4

Fassnacht, D. B., Ali, K., Silva, C., Goncalves, S., & Machado, P. P. (2015). Use of text messaging services to promote health behaviors in children. *Journal of Nutrition Education and Behavior, 47*(1), 75–80. doi:10.1016/j.jneb.2014.08.006

Gentile, D. A., Welk, G., Eisenmann, J. C., Reimer, R. A., Walsh, D. A., Russell, D. W., . . . Fritz, K. (2009). Evaluation of a multiple ecological level child obesity prevention program: Switch what you do, view, and chew. *BMC Medicine, 7*, 49.

Glanz, K., & Yaroch, A. L. (2004). Strategies for increasing fruit and vegetable intake in grocery stores and communities: Policy, pricing, and environmental change. *Preventive Medicine, 39*(Suppl 2), S75–S80.

Golden, S. D., & Earp, J. A. (2012). Social ecological approaches to individuals and their contexts: Twenty years of health education & behavior health promotion interventions. *Health Education and Behavior, 39*(3), 364–372. doi:10.1177/1090198111418634

Gough, A., Hunter, R. F., Ajao, O., Jurek, A., McKeown, G., Hong, J., . . . Kee, F. (2017). Tweet for behavior change: Using social media for the dissemination of public health messages. *JMIR Public Health and Surveillance, 3*(1), e14. doi:10.2196/publichealth.6313

Green, J., & Thorogood, M. (2018). *Qualitative methods for health research*. London, UK: Sage Publications Ltd.

Grossoehme, D. H. (2014). Overview of qualitative research. *Journal of Health Care Chaplain, 20*(3), 109–122. doi:10.1080/08854726.2014.925660

Gustavsson, S., & Andersson, T. (2019). Patient involvement 2.0: Experience-based co-design supported by action research. *Action Research, 17*(4), 469–491.

Hall, E. (2015). The ethics of 'using' children's drawings in research. In E. Stirling & D. Yamada-Rice (Eds.), Visual methods with children and young people (pp. 140–163). London, UK: Palgrave Macmillan.

Hamed, S., Klingberg, S., Mahmud, A. J., & Bradby, H. (2018). Researching health in diverse neighbourhoods: Critical reflection on the use of a community research model in Uppsala, Sweden. *BMC Research Notes, 11*(1), 612. doi:10.1186/s13104-018-3717-7

Hawe, P., Shiell, A., & Riley, T. (2004). Complex interventions: How "out of control" can a randomized controlled trial be? *BMJ, 328*(7455), 1561–1563. doi:10.1136/bmj.328.7455.1561

Hoddinott, P., Pollock, A., O'Cathain, A., Boyer, I., Taylor, J., MacDonald, C., . . . Donovan, J. L. (2018). How to incorporate patient and public perspectives into the design and conduct of research. *F1000Res, 7,* 752. doi:10.12688/f1000research.15162.1

Hoffmann, T. C., Glasziou, P. P., Boutron, I., Milne, R., Perera, R., Moher, D., . . . Michie, S. (2014). Better reporting of interventions: Template for intervention description and replication (TIDieR) checklist and guide. *BMJ, 348,* g1687. doi:10.1136/bmj.g1687

Holm, G. (2014). Photography as a research method. In P. Leavy (Ed.), *The Oxford handbook of qualitative research* (pp. 380–402). Oxford, UK: Oxford University Press.

Hootsuite. (2017). Retrieved November 28, 2018 from https://hootsuite.com/en-gb/newsroom/press-releases/digital-in-2017-report

Hunter, R. F., Gough, A., O'Kane, N., McKeown, G., Fitzpatrick, A., Walker, T., . . . Kee, F. (2018). Ethical issues in social media research for public health. *American Journal of Public Health, 108*(3), 343–348. doi:10.2105/AJPH.2017.304249

Hunter, R. F., McAneney, H., Davis, M., Tully, M. A., Valente, T. W., & Kee, F. (2015). "Hidden" social networks in behavior change interventions. *American Journal of Public Health, 105*(3), 513–516. doi:10.2105/AJPH.2014.302399

Jago, R., Edwards, M. J., Sebire, S. J., Tomkinson, K., Bird, E. L., Banfield, K., . . . Blair, P. S. (2015). Effect and cost of an after-school dance program on the physical activity of 11–12 year old girls: The Bristol Girls Dance project, a school-based cluster randomized controlled trial. *International Journal of Behavioral Nutrition and Physical Activity, 12,* 128. doi:10.1186/s12966-015-0289-y

Janz, N. K., & Becker, M. H. (1984). The health belief model: A decade later. *Health Education Quarterly, 11*(1), 1–47. doi:10.1177/109019818401100101

Jemmott, J. B., 3rd, Jemmott, L. S., O'Leary, A., Ngwane, Z., Icard, L., Bellamy, S., . . . Makiwane, M. B. (2011). Cognitive-behavioral health-promotion intervention increases fruit and vegetable consumption and physical activity among South African adolescents: A cluster-randomized controlled trial. *Psychology and Health, 26*(2), 167–185. doi:10.1080/08870446.2011.531573

Johansson-Sköldberg, U., Woodilla, J., & Çetinkaya, M. (2013). Design thinking: Past, present and possible futures. *Creativity and Innovation Management, 22*(2), 121–146.

Johnston, M., Johnston, D., Wood, C. E., Hardeman, W., Francis, J., & Michie, S. (2018). Communication of behavior change interventions: Can they be recognized from written descriptions? *Psychology and Health, 33*(6), 713–723. doi:10.1080/08870446.2017.1385784

Keating, S. R., & McCurry, M. K. (2015). Systematic review of text messaging as an intervention for adolescent obesity. *Journal of American Association of Nurse Practitioners, 27*(12), 714–720. doi:10.1002/2327-6924.12264

Khaw, K.-T., Wareham, N., Bingham, S., Welch, A., Luben, R., & Day, N. (2008). Combined impact of health behaviors and mortality in men and women: The EPIC-Norfolk prospective population study. *PLoS Medicine, 5*(1), e12.

Kipping, R. R., Howe, L. D., Jago, R., Campbell, R., Wells, S., Chittleborough, C. R., . . . Lawlor, D. A. (2014). Effect of intervention aimed at increasing physical activity, reducing sedentary behavior, and increasing fruit and vegetable consumption in children: Active for life year 5 (AFLY5) school based cluster randomized controlled trial. *BMJ, 348,* g3256. doi:10.1136/bmj.g3256

Klassen, T. P., MacKay, J. M., Moher, D., Walker, A., & Jones, A. L. (2000). Community-based injury prevention interventions. *Future of Children, 10*(1), 83–110.

Klingberg, S., Draper, C., Micklesfield, L., Benjamin-Neelon, S., & van Sluijs, E. (2019). Childhood obesity prevention in Africa: A systematic review of intervention effectiveness and implementation. *International Journal of Environmental Research and Public Health, 16*(7), 1212. doi:10.3390/ijerph16071212

Knuth, A. G., & Hallal, P. C. (2009). Temporal trends in physical activity: A systematic review. *Journal of Physical Activity and Health, 6*(5), 548–559.

Koorts, H., Eakin, E., Estabrooks, P., Timperio, A., Salmon, J., & Bauman, A. (2018). Implementation and scale up of population physical activity interventions for clinical and community settings: The PRACTIS guide. *International Journal of Behavioral Nutrition and Physical Activity, 15*(1), 51. doi:10.1186/s12966-018-0678-0

Lappan, L., Yeh, M.-C., & Leung, M. (2015). Technology as a platform for improving healthy behaviors and weight status in children and adolescents: A review. *Obesity Open Access, 1*(3). doi:10.16966/2380-5528.109

Lenhart, A. (2015). *Teens, social media & technology overview 2015.* Washington, DC: Pew Internet & American Life Project.

Lewallen, T. C., Hunt, H., Potts-Datema, W., Zaza, S., & Giles, W. (2015). The whole school, whole community, whole child model: A new approach for improving educational attainment and healthy development for students. *Journal of School Health, 85*(11), 729–739. doi:10.1111/josh.12310

Lewandowski, A. J., Davis, E. F., Yu, G., Digby, J. E., Boardman, H., Whitworth, P., . . . Leeson, P. (2015). Elevated blood pressure in preterm-born offspring associates with a distinct antiangiogenic state and microvascular abnormalities in adult life. *Hypertension, 65*(3), 607–614. doi:10.1161/HYPERTENSIONAHA.114.04662

Liamputtong, P. (2010). *Performing qualitative cross-cultural research.* Cambridge, UK: Routledge.

Liedtka, J. (2018). Why design thinking works. *Harvard Business Review, 96,* 72–79.

Lonsdale, C., Lester, A., Owen, K. B., White, R. L., Moyes, I., Peralta, L., . . . Lubans, D. R. (2016). An internet-supported physical activity intervention delivered in secondary schools located in low socioeconomic status communities: Study protocol for the activity and motivation in physical education (AMPED) cluster randomized controlled trial. *BMC Public Health, 16,* 17. doi:10.1186/s12889-015-2583-7

Love, R., Adams, J., & van Sluijs, E. M. F. (2019). Are school-based physical activity interventions effective and equitable? A meta-analysis of cluster randomized controlled trials with accelerometer-assessed activity. *Obesity Reviews.* doi:10.1111/obr.12823

Matheson, G. O., Pacione, C., Shultz, R. K., & Klugl, M. (2015). Leveraging human-centered design in chronic disease prevention. *American Journal of Preventive Medicine, 48*(4), 472–479. doi:10.1016/j.amepre.2014.10.014

Mayaba, N., & Wood, L. (2015). Using drawings and collages as data generation methods with children: Definitely not child's play. *International Journal of Qualitative Methods, 14,* 1–10.

Michie, S., Ashford, S., Sniehotta, F. F., Dombrowski, S. U., Bishop, A., & French, D. P. (2011). A refined taxonomy of behavior change techniques to help people change their physical activity and healthy eating behaviors: The CALO-RE taxonomy. *Psychology and Health, 26*(11), 1479–1498. doi:10.1080/08870446.2010.540664

Michie, S., Wood, C. E., Johnston, M., Abraham, C., Francis, J. J., & Hardeman, W. (2015). Behavior change techniques: The development and evaluation of a taxonomic method for reporting and describing behavior change interventions (a suite of five studies involving consensus methods, randomized controlled trials and analysis of qualitative data). *Health Technology Assessment, 19*(99), 1–188. doi:10.3310/hta19990

Michie, S., Yardley, L., West, R., Patrick, K., & Greaves, F. (2017). Developing and evaluating digital interventions to promote behavior change in health and health care: Recommendations resulting from an international workshop. *Journal of Medical Internet Research, 19*(6), e232. doi:10.2196/jmir.7126

Mittelmark, M. B., Hunt, M. K., Heath, G. W., & Schmid, T. L. (1993). Realistic outcomes: Lessons from community-based research and demonstration programs for the prevention of cardiovascular diseases. *Journal of Public Health Policy, 14*(4), 437–462.

Moore, J., Carson, R., Webster, C., Singletary, C., Castelli, D., Pate, R., . . . Beighle, A. (2018). The application of an implementation science framework to comprehensive school physical activity programs: Be a champion! *Front Public Health.* doi:10.3389/fpubh.2017.00354

Morgan, P. J., Young, M. D., Barnes, A. T., Eather, N., Pollock, E. R., & Lubans, D. R. (2018). Engaging fathers to increase physical activity in girls: The "dads and daughters exercising and empowered" (DADEE) randomized controlled trial. *Annals of Behavioral Medicine.* doi:10.1093/abm/kay015

Morton, K. L., Atkin, A. J., Corder, K., Suhrcke, M., Turner, D., & van Sluijs, E. M. (2017). Engaging stakeholders and target groups in prioritizing a public health intervention: The creating active school environments (CASE) online Delphi study. *BMJ Open, 7*(1), e013340. doi:10.1136/bmjopen-2016-013340

Morton, K. L., Atkin, A. J., Corder, K., Suhrcke, M., & van Sluijs, E. M. (2016). The school environment and adolescent physical activity and sedentary behavior: A mixed-studies systematic review. *Obesity Reviews, 17*(2), 142–158. doi:10.1111/obr.12352

Muller, A. M., Maher, C. A., Vandelanotte, C., Hingle, M., Middelweerd, A., Lopez, M. L., . . . Wark, P. A. (2018). Physical activity, sedentary behavior, and diet-related eHealth and mHealth research: Bibliometric analysis. *Journal of Medical Internet Research, 20*(4), e122. doi:10.2196/jmir.8954

Metcalf, B., Henley, W, Wilkin, T. Effectiveness of intervention on physical activity of children: systematic review and meta-analysis of controlled trials with objectively measured outcomes (EarlyBird 54). BMJ 2012 Sep 27;345:e5888. doi: 10.1136/bmj.e5888.

O'Cathain, A., Thomas, K. J., Drabble, S. J., Rudolph, A., & Hewison, J. (2013). What can qualitative research do for randomized controlled trials? A systematic mapping review. *BMJ Open, 3*(6). doi:10.1136/bmjopen-2013-002889

O'Connor, T. M., Jago, R., & Baranowski, T. (2009). Engaging parents to increase youth physical activity: A systematic review. *American Journal of Preventive Medicine, 37*(2), 141–149.

Office of National Statistics. (2017). Internet access – Households and individuals. Retrieved November 28, 2018 from https://www.ons.gov.uk/peoplepopulationandcommunity/householdcharacteristics/homeinternetandsocialmediausage/bulletins/internetaccesshouseholdsandindividuals/2017

Prochaska, J., & Velicer, W. (1997). The transtheoretical model of health behavior change. *American Journal of Health Promotion, 12*(1), 38–48.

Pumper, M. A., Mendoza, J. A., Arseniev-Koehler, A., Holm, M., Waite, A., & Moreno, M. A. (2015). Using a Facebook group as an adjunct to a pilot mHealth physical activity intervention: A mixed methods approach. *Studies in Health Technology and Informatics, 219*, 97–101.

Roberts, J. P., Fisher, T. R., Trowbridge, M. J., & Bent, C. (2016). A design thinking framework for healthcare management and innovation. *Healthcare (Amsterdam), 4*(1), 11–14. doi:10.1016/j.hjdsi.2015.12.002

Romo-Nava, F., Hoogenboom, W. S., Pelavin, P. E., Alvarado, J. L., Bobrow, L. H., Macmaster, F. P., . . . Shenton, M. E. (2013). Pituitary volume in schizophrenia spectrum disorders. *Schizophrenia Research, 146*(1–3), 301–307. doi:10.1016/j.schres.2013.02.024

Rooney, L. E., Videto, D. M., & Birch, D. A. (2015). Using the whole school, whole community, whole child model: Implications for practice. *Journal of School Health, 85*(11), 817–823. doi:10.1111/josh.12304

Rose, T., Barker, M., Maria Jacob, C., Morrison, L., Lawrence, W., Strommer, S., . . . Baird, J. (2017). A systematic review of digital interventions for improving the diet and physical activity behaviors of adolescents. *Journal of Adolescent Health, 61*(6), 669–677. doi:10.1016/j.jadohealth.2017.05.024

Ryan, D., & Deci, E. (2000). Self-determination theory and the facilitation of intrinsic motivation, social development, and well-being. *American Psychologist, 55*, 68–78.

Saez, L., Langlois, J., Legrand, K., Quinet, M. H., Lecomte, E., Omorou, A. Y., . . . PRALIMAP-INES Trial Group. (2018). Reach and acceptability of a mobile reminder strategy and Facebook group intervention for weight management in less advantaged adolescents: Insights from the PRALIMAP-INES trial. *JMIR Mhealth Uhealth, 6*(5), e110. doi:10.2196/mhealth.7657

Sallis, J. F., Owen, N., & Fotheringham, M. J. (2000). Behavioral epidemiology: A systematic framework to classify phases of research on health promotion and disease prevention. *Annals of Behavioral Medicine, 22*(4), 294–298.

Salmon, J., Booth, M. L., Phongsavan, P., Murphy, N., & Timperio, A. (2007). Promoting physical activity participation among children and adolescents. *Epidemiologic Reviews, 29*, 144–159.

Schulz, K. F., Altman, D. G., Moher, D., & CONSORT Group. (2010). CONSORT 2010 statement: Updated guidelines for reporting parallel group randomized trials. *Obstetrics and Gynecology, 115*(5), 1063–1070. doi:10.1097/AOG.0b013e3181d9d421

Sebire, S. J., Jago, R., Banfield, K., Edwards, M. J., Campbell, R., Kipping, R., . . . Hollingworth, W. (2018). Results of a feasibility cluster randomized controlled trial of a peer-led school-based intervention to increase the physical activity of adolescent girls (PLAN-A). *International Journal of Behavioral Nutrition and Physical Activity, 15*(1), 50. doi:10.1186/s12966-018-0682-4

Shapiro, J. R., Bauer, S., Hamer, R. M., Kordy, H., Ward, D., & Bulik, C. M. (2008). Use of text messaging for monitoring sugar-sweetened beverages, physical activity, and screen time in children: A pilot study. *Journal of Nutrition Education and Behavior, 40*(6), 385–391. doi:10.1016/j.jneb.2007.09.014

Silva, C., Fassnacht, D. B., Ali, K., Goncalves, S., Conceicao, E., Vaz, A., . . . Machado, P. P. (2015). Promoting health behavior in Portuguese children via short message service: The efficacy of a text-messaging program. *Journal of Health Psychology, 20*(6), 806–815. doi:10.1177/1359105315577301

Smart Insights. (2018). Global social media research summary 2018. Retrieved November 28, 2018 from https://www.smartinsights.com/social-media-marketing/social-media-strategy/new-global-social-media-research/

Smithson, J. (2000). Using and analysing focus groups: Limitations and possibilities. *International Journal of Social Research Methodology, 3*, 103–119.

Sparkes, A., & Smith, B. (2014). *Qualitative research methods in sport, exercise and health from process to product.* Oxford, UK: Routledge.

Stevens, V., De Bourdeaudhuij, I., & Van Oost, P. (2001). Anti-bullying interventions at school: Aspects of program adaptation and critical issues for further program development. *Health Promotion International, 16*(2), 155–167.

Sutherland, R. L., Campbell, E. M., Lubans, D. R., Morgan, P. J., Nathan, N. K., Wolfenden, L., . . . Wiggers, J. H. (2016). The physical activity 4 everyone cluster randomized trial: 2-Year outcomes of a school physical activity intervention among adolescents. *American Journal of Preventive Medicine, 51*(2), 195–205. doi:10.1016/j.amepre.2016.02.020

Taylor, B., & Francis, K. (2013). *Qualitative research in the health sciences: Methodologies, methods and processes.* Oxford, UK: Routledge.

Telema, R., Yang, X., Viikari, J., Valimaki, I., Wanne, O., & Raitakari, O. (2005). Physical activity from childhood to adulthood a 21-year tracking study. *American Journal of Preventive Medicine, 28*(3), 267–273.

Turner, S., Ollerhead, E., & Cook, A. (2017). Identifying research priorities for public health research to address health inequalities: Use of Delphi-like survey methods. *Health Research Policy and Systems, 15*(1), 87. doi:10.1186/s12961-017-0252-2

Valente, T. W. (2012). Network interventions. *Science, 337*(6090), 49–53. doi:10.1126/science.1217330

van der Horst, K., Chin, A., Paw, M. J., Twisk, J. W. R., & van Mechelen, W. (2007). A brief review on correlates of physical activity and sedentariness in youth. *Medicine and Science in Sports and Exercise, 39*(8), 1241–1250.

van Sluijs, E. M. F., Kriemler, S., & McMinn, A. M. (2011). The effect of community and family interventions on young people's physical activity levels: A review of reviews and updated systematic review. *British Journal of Sports Medicine, 45*(11), 914–922. doi:10.1136/bjsports-2011-090187

van Sluijs, E. M. F., McMinn, A. M., & Griffin, S. (2007). Effectiveness of interventions to promote physical activity in children and adolescents: Systematic review of controlled trials. *British Medical Journal, 6*(335), 703.

van Sluijs, E. M. F., Wilson, E. C., Brown, H., Morton, K., Jones, A., & Hughes, C. (2016). *The impact of a family-based physical activity promotion program on child physical activity: Feasibility and pilot of the families reporting every step to health (FRESH) intervention* University of Cambridge: NIHR-PHR 15/01. Retrieved from https://www.journalslibrary.nihr.ac.uk/programmes/phr/150119/#/

van Woudenberg, T. J., Bevelander, K. E., Burk, W. J., Smit, C. R., Buijs, L., & Buijzen, M. (2018). A randomized controlled trial testing a social network intervention to promote physical activity among adolescents. *BMC Public Health, 18*(1), 542. doi:10.1186/s12889-018-5451-4

Vosoughi, S., Roy, D., & Aral, S. (2018). The spread of true and false news online. *Science, 359*(6380), 1146–1151. doi:10.1126/science.aap9559

Wallerstein, N., & Duran, B. (2010). Community-based participatory research contributions to intervention research: The intersection of science and practice to improve health equity. *American Journal of Public Health, 100*(Suppl 1), S40–S46. doi:10.2105/AJPH.2009.184036

Wallerstein, N., Duran, B., Oetzel, E., & Minkler, M. (Eds.). (2017). *Community-based participatory research for health: Advancing social and health equity* (3rd ed.). San Francisco, CA: Jossey-Bass (Wiley).

Winton, A. (2016). Using photography as a creative, collaborative research tool. *The Qualitative Report, 21*(2), 428–449.

Wojcicki, T. R., Grigsby-Toussaint, D., Hillman, C. H., Huhman, M., & McAuley, E. (2014). Promoting physical activity in low-active adolescents via Facebook: A pilot randomized controlled trial to test feasibility. *JMIR Research Protocols, 3*(4), e56. doi:10.2196/resprot.3013

Wood, C. E., Hardeman, W., Johnston, M., Francis, J., Abraham, C., & Michie, S. (2016). Reporting behavior change interventions: Do the behavior change technique taxonomy v1, and training in its use, improve the quality of intervention descriptions? *Implementation Science, 11*(1), 84. doi:10.1186/s13012-016-0448-9

21

IMPLEMENTATION AND SCALE-UP OF SCHOOL-BASED PHYSICAL ACTIVITY INTERVENTIONS

Sarah G. Kennedy*, Heather A. McKay*, Patti Jean Naylor, and David R. Lubans

An effective school health program can be one of the most cost-effective investments a nation can make to simultaneously improve education and health.

(World Health Organization, 2018a)

We are at a time in human history like no other. Longevity is an unprecedented societal achievement and we have unlocked strategies that can effectively reduce the risk of common chronic diseases and improve health and well-being at every age. For the first time, the World Health Organization, many countries and their regions have invested time and resources in developing evidence informed global physical activity strategies and action plans (Australian Sports Commission, 2018; National Physical Activity Plan Alliance, 2016; Spence, Faulkner, Bradstreet, Duggan, & Tremblay, 2015; World Health Organization, 2018b). Among them 'whole of school' physical activity programs have been cited as one of seven best investments to improve child health at a population level (Global Advocacy for Physical Activity & Advocacy Council of the International Society for Physical Activity and Health, 2011).

However, despite approximately four decades of investing in 'what works' and the emergence of many effective school-based physical activity interventions, few are ever implemented at scale (Glasgow, Klesges, Dzewaltowski, Bull, & Estabrooks, 2004; Reis et al., 2016). Further, we are unaware of any school physical activity programs that are part of institutionalized school-health promotion practice on a national scale.

Enhancing the uptake, reach and sustainability of evidence-based school physical activity interventions is a societal imperative – as healthy behaviors established in childhood are sustained throughout the life course (Craigie, Lake, Kelly, Adamson, & Mathers, 2011). This demands we invest in unearthing strategies that bridge a 'know-do-scale-up' gap between evidence that something works (effectiveness) and broad scale-up of effective interventions (Durlak & DuPre, 2008; Milat, King et al., 2014).

There are many terms used to describe the transfer of research knowledge to the community setting. These include knowledge translation, knowledge exchange, knowledge mobilization, implementation, implementation science and research utilization (Straus, Tetroe, & Graham, 2009). Common to these definitions is the understanding that knowledge transfer requires a

---

*Sarah G. Kennedy and Heather A. McKay co-first authored this chapter.

socio-ecologic approach to health behavior change with multiple levels of influence that intersect to affect behavior and/or organizational change (Sallis, Owen, & Fisher, 2015).

Although scale-up science is emerging, we know relatively little about the broad range of contextual factors that promote or sustain health outcomes at scale in various settings and systems, including schools (Durlak & DuPre, 2008). These systems comprise 'real world' settings, with shifting political and policy environments, and other pressing priorities and competing interests (Milat, King, Bauman, & Redman, 2012; Norton & Mittman, 2010). Thus, scaling up becomes a thoughtful balance between planning for desired outcomes while adapting to contextual and environmental constraints (World Health Organization, 2010b).

Therefore, in this chapter we seek first to introduce the implementation continuum, different pathways to scale-up and types of scale-up. Second, we tackle key issues related to implementation and scale-up, as they apply to physical activity innovations in the school setting. Within this section, we provide working definitions for common terminology (e.g. implementation science, scalability and scale-up). In addition, we present relevant implementation and scale-up conceptual models and frameworks, and process frameworks that apply to scale-up of physical activity interventions/innovations in the school setting. Outcomes and determinants relevant for evaluating implementation in the school setting are also introduced within this part of the chapter. Third, we offer recommendations for researchers/practitioners, providing the reader with examples of school-based interventions that have progressed through to scale-up. Sustainability and institutionalization are also briefly discussed, as the ultimate end goal of implementation and scale-up research. By chapters end, we hope that readers, whose research encompasses physical activity promotion in the broader *school community* setting, will take away, think about and adopt learnings to guide them toward bridging the know-do-scale-up gap.

Overview of the Literature

The Implementation and Evaluation Continuum

Evaluation stages traditionally range from *formative evaluation* – during development of an intervention, to *outcome and process evaluation* – to establish efficacy, to *process and impact evaluation* – to evaluate effectiveness, to an almost exclusive focus on *implementation processes and reach* at the dissemination or scale-up stage (Bauman & Nutbeam, 2013). The ultimate goal beyond dissemination or scale-up is institutionalization, when programs or behaviors become routinely embedded in a system (think seat belts) (Rohrbach, Graham, & Hansen, 1993). Evaluation at this latter stage is most closely linked to monitoring implementation of a program or practice delivered at broad scale to a targeted population, often across settings and organizations (Bauman & Nutbeam, 2013).

Different Pathways to Scale-Up

While stages can be neatly described in logical succession, few research programs follow the progression in an orderly fashion along the evaluation continuum. In reality, research studies most commonly begin and end as formative evaluations or efficacy trials. Typical scale-up pathways were recently compared across four stages of scaling up – (i) development, (ii) efficacy testing, (iii) real-world trial and (iv) dissemination in a recent review (Indig, Lee, Grunseit, Milat, & Bauman, 2018). The pathways were referred to as (i) comprehensive, (ii) efficacy omitter, (iii) trial omitter and (iv) at-scale dissemination (names do not exactly roll off the tongue). The most common pathway to scale-up was 'comprehensive' (55% of studies), where all four stages were followed (Indig et al., 2018). Action! Schools BC (McKay et al., 2014) is an example of a school-based study that evaluated impact and implementation from efficacy to scale-up. Conversely, Project Energize (Rush et al., 2012) is a school-based intervention that was launched immediately as a large,

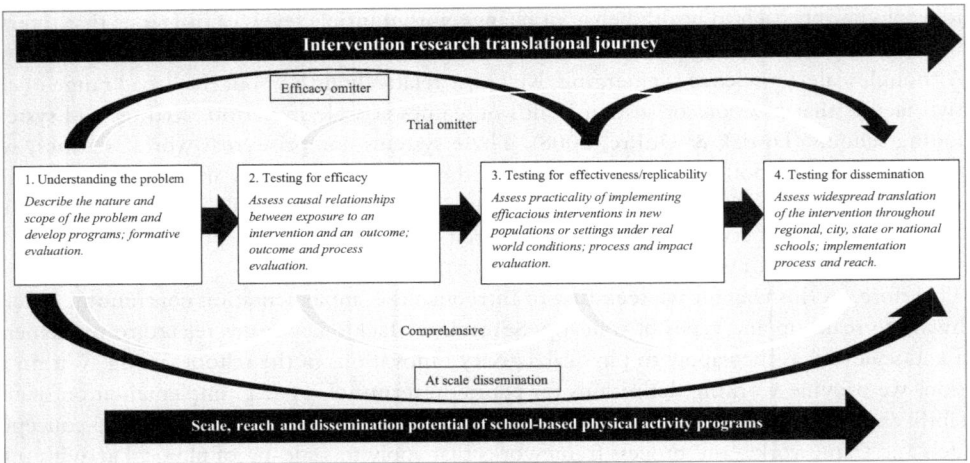

Figure 21.1   School-based physical activity intervention research progression model, including potential pathways, as described by Indig et al. (2018). Adapted from Kennedy et al. (2018). Originally adapted from Milat, Bauman, Redman, and Curac (2011) and Bauman and Nutbeam (2013)

real-world (effectiveness) trial. Only 5% of trials followed the 'efficacy omitter' pathway (Indig et al., 2018). In the 'trial omitter' pathway (25% of studies), dissemination of an intervention immediately followed an efficacy study (no effectiveness trial) (Indig et al., 2018). Finally, at-scale dissemination trials such as 'Exercise Your Options' (Dunton, Lagloire, & Robertson, 2009) and 'The Daily Mile' (Chesham et al., 2018) progressed directly from development to widespread roll-out; 15% of studies followed this pathway (Indig et al., 2018). Figure 21.1 presents an insight into the evaluation stages and how Indig et al.'s (2018) pathways align with these stages.

What Do We Mean by Implementation and Scale-Up?

At the outset, we acknowledge that implementation science has been a core part of research in many sectors including health services, health promotion, mental health and addictions, education and child development (among others) for over three decades. This surfaces time and again in how terms are defined and language is used differently across disciplines, sectors and settings (we provide a few examples of this below). This can wreak havoc among scientists newly entering the field. Thus, our goal is not to reinvent the wheel or take ownership where countless other distinguished scholars have tread before us. Rather, we endeavor to borrow, adapt, apply and where we can, clarify learnings from implementation and scale-up science for use in the school-based physical activity sector. We thank all those who have come before us in this field for lighting the way.

Types of Scale-Up

Vertical Scale-Up

Vertical scale-up introduces an intervention concurrently across the whole system toward institutionalization through policy and system level change. Vertical scale-up is often coordinated in collaboration with state/provincial-level government such as departments/ministries of education and health. Participation may be mandated within policy (such as the daily physical activity policies in several provinces in Canada) (Olstad, Campbell, Raine, & Nykiforuk, 2015). Based on the substantial cost, scale-up is most often supported by government resources. Rapid vertical scale-up, as sometimes occurs, may limit thoughtful planning and engagement, evaluation and adaptation to diverse contexts (e.g. inner city, rural) or populations (e.g. different cultures and abilities) (World Health Organization, 2010b).

Horizontal Scale-Up

Horizontal scale-up, also called expansion or replication, is a phased approach to implementation across different settings. This creates an opportunity to adapt the intervention to population and setting as scale-up progresses. Horizontal scale-up creates space for feedback so that implementation strategies can be adapted to enhance effectiveness (Milat, Newson, & King, 2014) or to accommodate limited resources. Adequate resources are an essential component of this and all other approaches (World Health Organization, 2010b).

Key Issues

The Murky World of Terminology

There is a need to elaborate on common terms and definitions from implementation and scale-up science, to provide a language with which to interact, compare and discuss. The waters are currently murky as the same terms are defined differently across sectors or groups, and the same definition is sometimes used to define different terms. In Table 21.1, we illustrate differences in how some terms are defined across sectors, while highlighting [a] definitions we recommend for those conducting school-based physical activity implementation or scale-up studies.

Table 21.1 Implementation and scale-up science terms and definitions from across sectors

Term	Definition
Implementation science	**Health care/service sector**
	1 The scientific study of methods to promote the systematic uptake of research findings and other evidence-based practices into routine practice, and, hence, to improve the quality and effectiveness of health services (Eccles & Mittman, 2006)
	2 The scientific study of methods to promote the integration of research findings and evidence-based interventions into healthcare practice and policy. It seeks to understand the behavior of healthcare professionals and support staff, healthcare organizations, healthcare consumers and family members, and policy makers in context as key variables in the adoption, implementation and sustainability of evidence-based interventions and guidelines (United States National Institutes of Health, 2016)
	Population and public health sector
	3 The study of methods and strategies to promote the uptake of interventions that have proven effective into routine practice, with the aim of improving population health (Global Alliance for Chronic Diseases, 2018).
	4 [a]The study of factors that influence the full and effective use of innovations in practice. The goal is not to answer factual questions about what is, but rather to determine what is required. This definition of implementation science emphasizes the study of factors that are action oriented and mission driven. In implementation science, implementation factors are identified or developed and demonstrated in practice, to 'influence the full and effective use of innovations'. (National Implementation Research Network, 2015)

(Continued)

Term	Definition
Implementation	**Dictionary definition** The process of putting a decision or plan into effect; execution. **Health care/service sector** 1 The integration of a new practice within a specific setting or context. Implementation involves the use of strategies to adopt and integrate evidence-based interventions and change practice patterns within specific settings (Glasgow et al., 2012) **Population and public health sector** 2 All the steps needed to put health promotion strategies and interventions into place and make them available (Centers for Disease Control and Prevention, 2015) 3 [a]At the setting level, implementation (within efficacy, effectiveness or scale-up studies) includes intervention agents' fidelity to the various elements of an intervention protocol. This includes consistency of delivery as intended and the time and cost of the intervention (Baranowski & Stables, 2000; Farris, Will, Khavjou, & Finkelstein, 2007; Glasgow, Vogt, & Boles, 1999; Linnan & Steckler, 2002)
Scale-up	**Population and public health sector** 1 The process by which efficacious health interventions are expanded under real-world conditions into broader policy or practice (Milat, King et al., 2014; Milat et al., 2013) 2 [a]Deliberate efforts to increase the impact of health innovations tested in pilot or experimental projects to benefit more people and foster policy and program development on a lasting basis (World Health Organization, 2010a)
Scaling-out	The implementation of interventions in new populations, new systems or both (Aarons, Sklar, Mustanski, Benbow, & Brown, 2017).
Scalability	The *ability* of a health intervention shown to be efficacious on a small scale and/or under controlled conditions to be expanded to real-world conditions to reach a greater proportion of the eligible population, while retaining effectiveness (Milat et al., 2012)
Scale-up science	A term we introduce to refer to the study of factors that influence the full and effective scale-up of innovations into practice under real-world conditions
Dissemination	1 Purposive distribution of information and intervention materials to a specific public health or clinical practice audience. The intent is to spread information and the associated evidence-based interventions (National Institutes of Health, 2011) 2 The communication or spread of new or existing knowledge through a planned or systematic process (Basch, Eveland, & Portnoy, 1986) 3 [a]A planned process that involves consideration of target audiences and the settings in which research findings are to be received and, where appropriate, communicating and interacting with wider policy and health service audiences in ways that will facilitate research uptake in decision-making processes and practice (Wilson et al., 2010)

a Definition we recommend when more than one is provided.

Importantly, we urge researchers to clarify for themselves at what stage they will assess implementation of an intervention along the continuum from formative evaluation to efficacy to scale-up. It is important to make this distinction because definitions, processes and the focus of the evaluation will vary between these study designs.

Theoretical Frameworks That Have Relevance for the School-Based Setting

Theories and frameworks provide necessary scaffolding on which to build and organize factors that influence whether implementation at scale succeeds or fails (Nilsen, 2015). These factors, once measured, link back to strategies that can be designed or adapted to improve outcomes. Indeed, adopting frameworks and guidelines was cited as one of five key enablers to implementation of school-based physical activity interventions (Hung, Chiang, Dawson, & Lee, 2014). Moreover, there is compelling evidence that the level of implementation success influences program outcomes (Durlak & DuPre, 2008; Naylor et al., 2015). Enhanced likelihood of implementation success and subsequent improvements in outcomes highlights the need for frameworks to design and deliver school-based physical activity interventions.

Over the last decade many implementation theories, models and frameworks have emerged from health services and business innovation sectors, fewer from within health promotion and education. Some are derived from classic models developed in sociology, psychology and organizational theory (Bandura, 1986; Deci & Ryan, 2002; Nilsen, 2015; Rogers, 2003). There are now more than 60 published theories, models and frameworks related to implementation and scale-up (Tabak, Khoong, Chambers, & Brownson, 2012). In the 7 years since the Tabak et al. (2012) review, even more have been published. With respect we contend that we might have enough now. Perhaps it is time for the focus to shift to application and adaption of frameworks from different contexts and their alignment with indicators and measures.

It is no wonder those of us who work in the field – or would like to – get lost among classic conceptual or theoretical frameworks (Rogers, 2003). Approaches span implementation to dissemination (Wandersman et al., 2008) with some elements of sustainability thrown in (Greenhalgh, Robert, Macfarlane, Bate, & Kyriakidou, 2004). There are also more clearly defined implementation determinants, frameworks and models (Damschroder et al., 2009; Durlak & DuPre, 2008) and process or 'how to' frameworks (Milat, Newson et al., 2014), a murky pool indeed.

Three years following the Tabak et al. (2012) paper, Nilsen (2015) rose to the challenge and sought to more clearly categorize 'frameworks'. Nilsen (2015) identified and defined five categories of theories, models and frameworks used in implementation science. They included, (i) process models, (ii) determinant frameworks, (iii) classic theories, (iv) implementation component-based frameworks and (v) evaluation frameworks. We utilize these five categories and definitions in Table 21.2 to guide us. We also provide examples of frameworks relevant to the school setting within each classification.

Classifying Implementation and Scale-Up Frameworks

As a means to provide some clarity and to zero in on frameworks of value to implementation and scale-up scientists in the physical activity sector (but not exclusive to schools), we conducted a five-round Delphi process. Participants were implementation science 'experts' in physical activity and behavioral nutrition from around the world. We qualify the term 'expert', as participants had from one to more than 20 years of experience in implementation science. Their task was to identify frameworks, determinants and outcomes they deemed most relevant (or had used personally) in physical activity and healthy eating interventions. Although defined differently in the literature, we use the term frameworks to represent both models and frameworks (Tabak et al., 2012).

We applied Nilsen's (2015) system to classify frameworks cited in the Delphi process (McKay et al., 2019). We also noted additional frameworks that the most senior Delphi participants (>10 years of experience) believed relevant for physical activity and healthy eating researchers (Table 21.2). Notably, scale-up frameworks are missing from Nilsen's (2015) classification system, although some scale-up frameworks fall within his process frameworks classification. Therefore, we added a specific scale-up frameworks category to the classification system. As a side note, to our knowledge only the Conceptual Framework for Maximizing Implementation Quality (Domitrovich et al., 2008) was specifically designed for the school setting. However, the other frameworks we present in Table 21.2 can all be readily adapted to the school setting.

Table 21.2 Implementation and scale-up theories and frameworks that have relevance for physical activity and healthy eating researchers (italics). For clarity, we adopt a modified classification system as per Nilsen (2015)

Type of theory/ framework	Descriptions and examples
Classic theories and comprehensive frameworks	Originate from fields external to implementation science (e.g. psychology, sociology and organizational theory); explain some aspects of implementation • Diffusion of innovations (Rogers, 2003)
Determinants frameworks	Explain influences on implementation outcomes; predict outcomes or interpret outcomes retrospectively • Framework for Effective Implementation (Durlak & DuPre, 2008) • Consolidated Framework for Implementation Research (Damschroder et al., 2009) • Conceptual Framework for Maximizing Implementation Quality (Domitrovich et al., 2008)
Process models that guide implementation and/or scale-up	Describe and often guide the step by step process of translating research into practice. An action model is a type of process model that guides planning and execution of implementation strategies • Scaling up health service delivery: from pilot innovations to policies and programs (Simmons, Fajans, & Ghiron, 2007) • Quality Implementation Framework (Meyers, Durlak, & Wandersman, 2012) • Increasing the scale of population health interventions (Milat, Newson et al., 2014) • The Practical planning for Implementation and Scale-up (PRACTIS guide) (Koorts et al., 2018)
Scale-up frameworks that address multiple interventions and varied end-users	Describes key elements and relationships essential to move effective interventions into practice on a broad scale • Scaling up health service innovations: a framework for action (Simmons & Shiffman, 2007) • Interactive Systems Framework for Dissemination and Implementation (Wandersman et al., 2008) • Scaling Up Global Health Interventions (Yamey, 2011) • Knowledge-to-Action Cycle (Graham et al., 2006)

Implementation and Scale-Up Frameworks for the School Setting

First, we pay homage to classic theories, including Rogers' (2003) Diffusion of Innovations; however we direct our attention more fully to describing frameworks that can be applied to the scale-up of school-based physical activity interventions.

Classic Theories

DIFFUSION OF INNOVATIONS (ROGERS, 2003)

Rogers' (2003) landmark theory influenced many other conceptual, implementation and scale-up frameworks. Among these the conceptual model for the spread and sustainability of innovations in service delivery and organization is notable (Greenhalgh et al., 2004). Rogers' (2003) theory proposes that diffusion occurs as information related to an innovation is communicated throughout a social system, resulting in social change – altering the structure and functionality of that system. The four main elements of Rogers' classic theory are innovation (i.e. the program/practice), communication channels (i.e. process of sharing information between those involved), time (i.e. the innovation-decision process) and social system (i.e. the adopters). Rogers (2003) describes varying characteristics of adopters, dependent on the time it takes to progress through the innovation–decision process. Early adopters are generally more educated, have a more positive attitude toward change, and are more socially mobile than those who adopt later (laggards), or not at all.

Implementation Frameworks

FRAMEWORK FOR EFFECTIVE IMPLEMENTATION (DURLAK & DUPRE, 2008)

This framework places factors that influence implementation of the 'innovation' (delivery, support and research systems) at the core of successful implementation – as described in Wandersman et al.'s (2008) Interactive Systems Framework (ISF). The innovation is embedded within a socio-ecologic framework where larger organizational and socio–political–economic contexts (called provider characteristics and community factors) interact with evidence to influence implementation and scale-up (Durlak & DuPre, 2008). Among all the frameworks we reviewed and from our collective experience, we settled upon the Framework for Effective Implementation as one accessible model that is highly adaptable to the school setting.

CONSOLIDATED FRAMEWORK FOR IMPLEMENTATION RESEARCH (DAMSCHRODER ET AL., 2009)

Another broadly adopted framework is the Consolidated Framework for Implementation Research (CFIR) (Damschroder et al., 2009). CFIR reflects many elements of the classic theories discussed earlier, and consolidates previous frameworks into five broad domains related to implementation: (1) intervention characteristics, (2) the inner setting, (3) the outer setting, (4) individuals and (5) process of implementation. These five domains are comprised of different constructs that range from (for example) adaptability, trialability and complexity of the intervention, to structural characteristics, culture and climate in the inner setting to external policies and incentives in the outer settings to an individuals' self-efficacy and belief system to, finally, planning, executing and evaluating the implementation process itself. These indicators can then be aligned with measures and tools for evaluation (Leeman et al., 2018). CFIR was designed to be adapted to different contexts, and as a means to categorize factors that facilitate or create barriers to implementation. We apply the CFIR framework to the school setting, using terms more familiar to school-based physical activity researchers in Figure 21.2.

CONCEPTUAL FRAMEWORK FOR MAXIMIZING IMPLEMENTATION QUALITY (DOMITROVICH ET AL., 2008)

The Conceptual Framework for Maximizing Implementation Quality described by Domitrovich et al. (2008) considers macro-, school- and individual-level factors that influence implementation. Domitrovich and colleagues (2008) acknowledge that factors influencing implementation differ according to stage of implementation. As per other frameworks, this one also places the quality of the innovation and its delivery at the core of successful implementation, while acknowledging individual to macro-level influences in the outer contexts.

Scale-Up Frameworks

INTERACTIVE SYSTEMS FRAMEWORK FOR DISSEMINATION AND IMPLEMENTATION (WANDERSMAN ET AL., 2008)

The Interactive Systems Framework for Dissemination and Implementation resides within the inner core (innovation characteristics) of Durlak and Dupre's (2008) Framework for Effective Implementation.

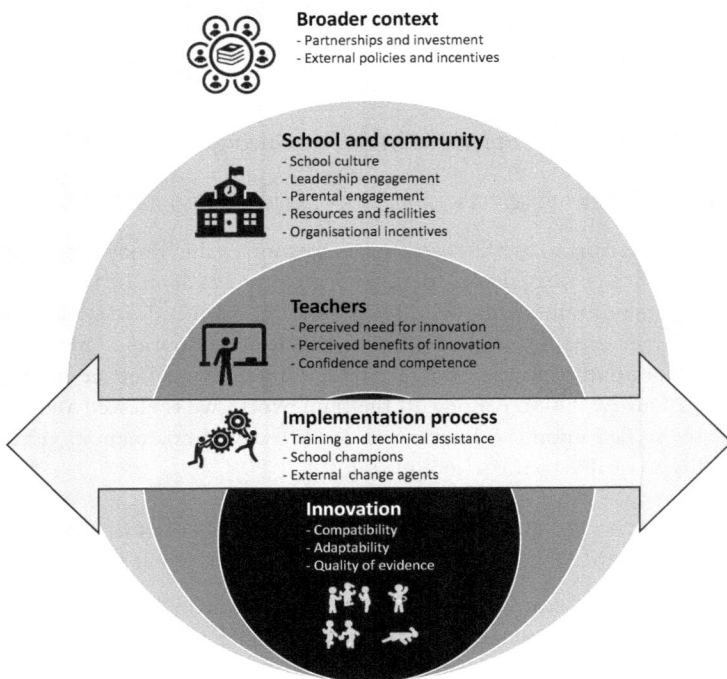

Figure 21.2   An implementation framework adapted from Damschroder et al. (2009) for the school setting

The ISF centers on three different prevention systems (i.e. delivery, support and synthesis & translation) required for effective dissemination and implementation (Wandersman et al., 2008).

Briefly, in school-based physical activity interventions, although we ultimately aim to improve the health of students, the focus of implementation at scale is training and technical support within schools (teachers and administrators) that comprise the prevention delivery system. The prevention support system can be an academic group, a government agency (e.g. Department/ Ministry of Education or Health) or a non-governmental organization (NGO) that has knowledge and experience implementing and sustaining programs in the school setting. The knowledge synthesis and translation system often comprises university or third party research groups. Ideally at scale-up, these systems are integrated through effective training, communication and constant feedback loops within the larger context of funding, policy, evidence and organizational climate – effective integration is essential for implementation to positively affect student health at the population level.

ELEMENTS OF SCALING UP (SIMMONS & SHIFFMAN, 2007)

As part of a broader set of WHO ExpandNet scale-up resources, Simmons and Shiffman (2007) developed a framework that described critical elements of scale-up. These elements include the innovation (the intervention being delivered at scale), the user organization/team (those adopting the innovation), the scale-up strategy (communication and promotion) and the environment (the larger socio-political, economic and cultural environments in which scale-up takes place). Embedded in their work are detailed action strategies; for instance, they highlight the importance of having a resource team that

Table 21.3 Factors that contribute to successful scale-up adapted from Simmons and Shiffman (2007) and Yamey (2011)

Category	Factors
Attributes of the innovation	1 Simplicity
	2 Scientifically robust technical policies
Attributes of the implementers	1 Strong leadership and governance
	2 Engaged local implementers and other stakeholders
	3 Both state and non-state actors as implementers
Chosen delivery system	1 Application of diffusion and social network theories
	2 Phased approaches to scale-up
	3 Tailoring scale-up to the local situation, and decentralizing delivery
	4 Integrated approach to scale-up
Attributes of the 'Adopting' community	An engaged, 'activated' community
Socio-political context	1 Political will and national policies
	2 Country ownership
Research context	Incorporation of research into implementation ('learning and doing')

provides motivating leadership and has credibility within the delivery system among others. Many of these factors are outlined in Greenhalgh et al.'s (2004) comprehensive model (a must read).

SCALING UP GLOBAL HEALTH INTERVENTIONS (YAMEY, 2011)

Although designed for scale-up of global health innovations in low and middle income countries, (such as HIV interventions in Africa), Yamey's (2011) simple and accessible framework is readily understandable and can be applied across settings and populations. This framework provides a sort of recipe book for successful scale-up where all ingredients are needed for a successful outcome. Six categories of factors contribute to successful scale-up including: (i) attributes of the innovation, (ii) attributes of the implementers, (iii) the delivery system, (iv) attributes of the adopting community, within (v) socio-political and (vi) research contexts (Yamey, 2011). Given their similarities, we provide a list of factors within each category that contribute to successful scale-up as outlined by the Simmons and Shiffman's (2007) and Yamey's (2011) frameworks (Table 21.3).

How to Choose a Framework and Indicators Relevant to Your Setting and Population

It is not surprising that many frameworks across sectors have similar categories, elements or factors, as Rogers' (2003) Diffusion of Innovations Theory serves as the predecessor to most of them (Wilson, Petticrew, Calnan, & Nazareth, 2010). A few frameworks are remarkably similar and differ only in the sector or population for which they were developed (e.g. health services versus community settings). Therefore, as a researcher, choose a framework based on which one resonates most within the setting and the population you are studying. Also consider the level of evaluation that matters most to your research. Your focus could potentially span students, teachers, parents, school administrators, NGOs or government agencies, or even larger systems.

Key questions for researchers to consider when selecting a framework include: which framework aligns with your research questions? What outcomes and determinants align with your selected framework and are indicators that your research team, school community or government stakeholders identify as key? At what level do you wish to evaluate? That is, do you wish to

Table 21.4 A minimum data set of outcomes, as defined by McKay et al. (2019, p. 7)

Implementation outcomes	Delivery of interventions	Delivery of implementation strategies
	Definitions	*Definitions*
Adoption	The proportion and representativeness of providers or delivery teams that deliver an intervention	The proportion and representativeness of providers or delivery teams that utilize implementation strategies
Dose delivered	The amount or number of intended units of each intervention component delivered to participants by delivery teams	The amount or number of intended units of each implementation strategy delivered to delivery teams by support teams
Reach	The proportion of the intended priority audience (i.e. participants) that participates in the intervention	The proportion of the intended priority populations (organizations or participants) that participate in the intervention
Fidelity	The extent to which an intervention is implemented by the delivery team as prescribed in the original protocol	The extent to which implementation strategies are implemented by the support team as prescribed in the implementation plan
Sustainability	The extent to which an intervention continues to be delivered and/or individual behavior change is maintained; the intervention and individual behavior change may evolve or adapt while continuing to produce benefits for individuals/systems, after a defined period of time	The extent to which implementation strategies continue to be delivered and/or behavior changes at the system levels are maintained; the implementation strategies and behavior changes at the system level may evolve or adapt while continuing to produce benefits for systems, after a defined period of time

consider the influence of teachers, school, government policy (or other factors) on implementation success and impact at the student level? The answers to these questions become an integral part of preplanning – which is in itself a fine balance between the context and needs of stakeholders and what the evidence suggests will work and should be measured.

Finally, few frameworks exist to specifically guide *scale-up* in the school setting. Therefore, we invite readers to consider all the models we have presented. Although specific scale-up frameworks include key (often similar) components to other implementation frameworks, they adopt slightly different sector-based approaches. So again, select the one that more closely applies to your research questions, population and setting.

As for choosing the right indicators, Tables 21.4 and 21.5 are a good place to start. We draw your attention later to the importance of partnerships as you design, implement and evaluate your school-based intervention at scale. Consider that your most important question as a researcher (did it work to improve the health/performance of students?) may be quite different than what is most important to policy makers (what is the reach? can it be scaled up at low cost?).

Implementation Determinants and Outcomes

If you thought the maze of frameworks was baffling to navigate welcome to the kingdom of outcomes and determinants, where depending on your research question and your study design (implementation of the innovation in an efficacy, effectiveness or scale-up study) indicators might be a determinant, an outcome or both. For example, perceived appropriateness, feasibility and implementation cost are likely determinants of perceived acceptability (an outcome)

Table 21.5 A minimum data set of determinants, as defined by McKay et al. (2019, p. 7)

Implementation determinants	Delivery of interventions	Delivery of implementation strategies
Acceptability	Perceptions among delivery teams that a given intervention/implementation strategies are agreeable, palatable or satisfactory	Perceptions among support team that the implementation strategies are agreeable, palatable or satisfactory
Adaptability	The extent to which an intervention can be adapted, tailored, refined or reinvented to meet local needs	The extent to which implementation strategies can be adapted, tailored, refined or reinvented to meet the needs of scale-up organizations
Feasibility	Perceptions among delivery teams that an intervention can be successfully used or carried out within a given organization or setting	Perceptions among support teams that implementation strategies can be successfully used or carried out at scale within different scale-up organizations or settings
Compatibility	The extent to which an intervention fits with the mission, priorities and values of implementation organizations	The extent to which implementation strategies fit with the mission, priorities and values of scale-up organizations
Cost	The amount of money spent on the design, adaptation and implementation of an intervention	The amount of money spent on the design, adaptation and delivery of implementation strategies
Culture	Organizations' norms, values and basic assumptions of the health issues of interest	Scale-up organizations' norms, values and basic assumptions of the implementation strategies
Dose (Satisfaction)	Delivery teams' satisfaction with an intervention and interactions with support teams	Support teams' satisfaction with the implementation strategies and interactions with research teams
Complexity	Perceptions among delivery teams that a given intervention is relatively difficult to understand and use; number of different components	Perceptions among support teams that the implementation strategies are relatively difficult to understand and use; number of different components
Self-efficacy	Delivery teams' belief in their own capability to execute courses of action to achieve implementation goal	Support teams' belief in their own capability to execute courses of action to achieve implementation goal
Context	Aspects of the larger social, political and economic environment that may influence intervention implementation	Aspects of the larger social, political and economic environment that may influence delivery of the implementation strategies

(Proctor et al., 2011). Acceptability, in turn, may serve as determinant for adoption, penetration and sustainability (Proctor et al., 2011). Importantly, implementation indicators (like acceptability and adoption) may also serve as determinants of **health outcomes** in scale-up studies.

Further, depending on the sector or context within which indicators are applied, two different outcomes may have been given the same definition or the same outcome may have two (or more) definitions. There is also little clarity as to when indicators refer to scale-up (and if their definitions change as a result). Currently most refer to implementation of an intervention at small scale. Not surprising given these inconsistencies these indicators, terms and their application are often difficult to navigate. Therefore, for this part we rely upon results from our Delphi process to guide us all toward the light (McKay et al., 2019).

To set the stage and for the purposes of this chapter, we define implementation **outcomes** as 'the effect of deliberate and purposive actions to implement new treatments, practices, and services' (Proctor et al., 2011). However, Proctor and colleagues (2011) consider that proximal indicators related to implementation strategies and the implementation process, as well as intermediate measures of effective implementation are all outcomes. We recommend a more traditional public health approach that identifies indicators such as acceptability and feasibility as **determinants**. Determinants are factors that help explain implementation effectiveness and precede implementation outcomes in the causal chain.

There is an important and necessary shift when the plan becomes to deliver effective interventions at a broader scale. The focus becomes less on the intervention (researchers may have already demonstrated intervention effectiveness), and more so on implementation strategies at scale-up. Scale-up encompasses a wider range of contextual factors that need to be considered across diverse settings and more diverse populations for implementation at larger scale to succeed. That said, some 'non-essential elements' of the intervention itself (not just implementation strategies) may need to be adapted for scale-up (Blase & Fixsen, 2013), and some outcomes may be selectively monitored.

Lessons Learned from a Delphi Process

You are not alone in navigating the maze of theories, frameworks, determinants and outcomes. Our Delphi study sought to coalesce how those in physical activity and healthy eating research were evaluating implementation and scale-up. McKay and colleagues aimed to generate a *minimum data set* of indicators that researchers recommend be evaluated in physical activity implementation and scale-up studies (McKay et al., 2019). From the Delphi process, five outcomes and ten determinants (indicators) comprised the minimum data (McKay et al., 2019). This list provides researchers a recommended place to start when choosing indicators to assess when conducting physical activity implementation and scale-up studies.

Interestingly, study results unveiled an apparent paradox. That is, many components that comprised the top ranked implementation and scale-up frameworks were not represented in the top ranked indicators (McKay et al., 2019). Ideally, accessible and relevant frameworks would align with important indicators. In turn, key indicators would align with flexible, standardized (where possible) measurement approaches or tools. Currently, researchers might 'customize' frameworks or measures to assess an assortment of indicators. Although some adaptation to context is inevitable, a broad array of approaches prohibits comparison across studies. It seems crucial that implementation scientists in health promotion put their minds to tackling this 'alignment' paradox in the near future.

Importantly, the Delphi study clearly delineated between how an indicator is defined during implementation of efficacy or effectiveness trials (where the target population or intervention participant is the focus) and how the indicator is defined during implementation at scale (where implementation success at broad scale is the focus) (Tables 21.4 and 21.5) (McKay et al., 2019).

Implementation Outcomes and Determinants in the School Setting

One key take away message is that although scale-up studies share core indicators with efficacy and effectiveness studies, they are different. At scale-up, the focus shifts toward factors that influence the process of implementation (from internal to external validity); these are conceptually and empirically different to impact outcomes (such as physical activity) at the individual level (Proctor et al., 2011). That said, many researchers will likely choose to measure implementation **and** impact outcomes across the continuum of intervention study designs from feasibility studies to scale-up studies.

The minimum data set of outcomes (Table 21.4) and determinants (Table 21.5) generated for implementation and scale-up studies readily apply to the school setting. Many indicators align with Proctor et al. (2011), although these authors did not distinguish between determinants and outcomes among eight implementation indicators. The minimum data set also closely aligns with findings from other studies. Nathan et al. (2017) identified ten scale-up indicators specific to the school setting, and Milat, Newson et al. (2014) described six components that are critical to evaluate and monitor for implementation at scale.

Adaptation Versus Fidelity: A Dynamic Tension

During scale-up, adaptation is both inevitable and appropriate. Program/intervention adaptation guidelines seek to balance program fidelity with (most often) process-based adaptations to align with the local context, while maintaining program outcomes (Proctor et al., 2009). Approaches often recognize a complex balance between preserving core content and delivery components while enhancing 'fit' within a local environment (Castro, Barrera, & Martinez, 2004). This 'dynamic tension' (Castro et al., 2004) becomes more apparent as we move along the continuum from efficacy to scale-up studies, as researchers work to consider the core ingredients of an intervention to effectively integrate programs into real-world settings (Proctor et al., 2011). The 'fidelity-adaptation dilemma' (Brownson, Colditz, & Proctor, 2018) is a fascinating part of scale-up science and we discuss it further later in the chapter.

Recommendations for Researchers/Practitioners

Implementation and Scale-Up of School-Based Interventions

Here we provide some real-world examples of school-based physical activity and health promotion studies that traversed efficacy to effectiveness to scale-up.

CATCH

Child and Adolescent Trial for Cardiovascular Health (CATCH) is the most widely published, school-based health promotion intervention. CATCH started in 1991 and is still going in some schools! CATCH served as an inspiration (at the very least a template) for many researchers who have since entered the realm of school-based physical activity research and adopted a whole of school/comprehensive approach. Guided by Diffusion of Innovations Theory (Rogers, 2003), this multisite intervention study was conducted in the United States and targeted children in Grades 3–5. The focus was on cardiovascular disease prevention, healthy eating, physical activity and cigarette smoking. CATCH employed changes to the classroom and physical education (PE) curricula (the target for increased physical activity), altered school environments and offered family programs for each grade level. CATCH was originally evaluated using a randomized controlled trial (RCT) design (Luepker et al., 1996), and subsequently was adapted for scale-up into new communities (Heath & Coleman, 2003; Hoelscher et al., 2010). After 20 years CATCH was institutionalized in some jurisdictions such as Texas (Heath & Coleman, 2003; Hoelscher et al., 2001).

SPARK

Sports, Play, and Active Recreation for Kids (SPARK) was another brain trust of McKenzie and Sallis (of CATCH pre-eminence) (Sallis et al., 1993, 1997). In 2014 SPARK was touted as the most widely published study ever in K-8 PE. The SPARK PE curriculum was designed as a practical resource for classroom PE teachers, and included staff development and support (McKenzie, Sallis, & Rosengard, 2009). Dissemination of SPARK occurred through providing schools with hands-on staff development workshops, and follow-up support from SPARK staff (Dowda, Sallis, McKenzie, Rosengard, & Kohl III, 2005; McKenzie et al., 2009). Dissemination of SPARK from 1994 to 2009 engaged an estimated one million students (McKenzie et al., 2009). Of those schools that adopted SPARK, approximately 80% sustained implementation up to 4 years later (Dowda et al., 2005).

Action Schools! BC

Action Schools! British Columbia (AS! BC) is a whole of school physical activity and healthy eating model that embraced a socio-ecological framework. For dissemination, AS! BC adopted many essential elements from the Diffusion of Innovations Theory (Rogers, 2003) and communities of practice sustained implementation model (Wenger, 1999). AS! BC reflected an interdisciplinary research, cross-sectoral school, community and British Columbia government collaboration (Ministry of Health funded; Ministry of Education supported). The goals of AS! BC were to: (a) provide a school environment where students had more opportunities to be more active and make healthy choices more often, and (b) facilitate a supportive community and provincial-level environment. Partners cycled through interactive phases of knowledge and product development, transmission (efficacy study) and dissemination (effectiveness and dissemination studies) embedded within a continuous process of stakeholder input and adaptation of the model. Teacher training, ongoing support and resources were provided to schools (McKay et al., 2014). AS! BC improved children's physical activity, bone and cardiovascular health (McKay et al., 2014). Importantly, AS! BC received high ratings from teachers and principals. After 10 years of scale-up, 100% of 1,600 BC schools were registered AS! BC schools, 89% of teachers had received AS! BC training and approximately 400,000 children were engaged in AS! BC through their schools.

iPLAY

Success of the Supporting Children's Outcomes using Rewards, Exercise and Skills (SCORES) program (Cohen, Morgan, Plotnikoff, Callister, & Lubans, 2015; Lubans et al., 2012) spawned a comprehensive school physical activity program known as iPLAY (Internet-based Professional Learning to help teachers to support Activity in Youth) (Lonsdale et al., 2016). Researchers secured funding from the New South Wales Department of Education and the National Health and Medical Research Council to scale up a modified version of the original SCORES intervention. The intervention includes three curricular (i.e. quality PE and school sport, classroom movement breaks and physically active homework) and three non-curricular (i.e. active playgrounds, community physical activity links and parent/caregiver engagement) physical activity promotion strategies. Teachers are provided with online professional learning and resources to support their implementation. Experienced PE teachers (known as Mentors) deliver professional learning workshops and provide individualized mentoring to primary teachers (i.e. Kindergarten – Year 6) and teachers responsible for supporting implementation of non-curricular strategies (known as Leaders). Two complementary (implementation and impact) evaluations of iPLAY are currently underway (i.e. cluster RCT involving 22 schools and scale-up study with 135 schools).

Schools Are Complex Settings, 'Constantly Shifting Broader Contexts'

Understanding factors that influence adoption and implementation within the school-setting is challenging (Newland, Dixon, & Green, 2013). Not least of all because schools and education systems 'sit within constantly shifting broader contexts' (Butler et al., 2010). Factors that influence educational practitioners and policy makers in the larger school community context need to be considered (Figgis, Zubrick, Butorac, & Alderson, 2000; Fullan, 2006; McMeniman, Cumming, Wilson, Stevenson, & Sim, 2000). For example, integrating new knowledge and skills into practice, within dynamic, nonlinear change processes is no easy task (Figgis et al., 2000; Fullan, 2006; McMeniman et al., 2000). The challenge is magnified at scale, as dissemination encompasses a complex web of policies, practices and relationships among researchers, practitioners, organizations, within dynamic systems and society generally (Butler et al., 2010).

Policy, Political Climate and Timing

Policy matters. Indeed, interventions have the best chance of being scaled up if they are aligned with policy priorities (World Health Organization, 2010b). However, it is unlikely that school-based policy changes without supportive environments (e.g. support of school principals) will be implemented (Sallis, 2018). Yamey (2011) highlights the benefits of tailoring an intervention to the local context and integrating activities into existing 'systems'. To illustrate, mandated PE or daily physical activity policies require the capacity of teachers to deliver and their will to do so (organizational environment and social climate). This is often achieved through training and ongoing technical support, a positive environment for delivery (supportive environments) and appropriate equipment (adequate physical environment) (Sallis, 2018).

Partnerships

Authentic partnerships are key. They will exist at multiple levels and be developed over time among groups committed to achieving a common goal. Relationships across sectors that align with levels of influence are imperative for successful implementation and scale-up of school-based physical activity interventions. Most proximally, these include those in the prevention delivery and support systems such as wellness champions, teachers, future intervention facilitators and executive staff (Leeman et al., 2018). More distally in what we refer to as the broader context, partnerships may encompass academics, policy makers, government officials, health promotion professionals, educational professionals, parents and students (Butler et al., 2010). Key partnership activities may take the form of policy briefings, engaging opinion leaders, input into policy and budgetary processes and establishing advisory boards made up of key influencers.

A crucial part of implementation or scale-up of any initiative is preplanning. In the health services sector, programs with 6 months of preplanning demonstrated the greatest implementation success (Saldana, Chamberlain, Wang, & Brown, 2012). A large part of preplanning is having enough lead time to engage partners in a meaningful way, as a single organization seldom has the knowledge, tools and resources needed to support scale-up of an intervention (Kohl & Cooley, 2003; Milat et al., 2012; Norton & Mittman, 2010). During preplanning, priorities of partners can be discussed as different outcomes have relevance for different stakeholders. For policy makers, cost may be of utmost importance, while program directors and delivery agents may look to feasibility, flexibility and appropriateness. Researchers, on the other hand, often have their eye on fidelity. Processes (Keller-Margulis, 2012; Proctor et al., 2009) and strategies that guide development of meaningful partnerships have been discussed at length elsewhere (Milat, Newson et al., 2014), so we delve no deeper into them here.

Co-Creation and 'Design for Dissemination'

Linked closely with partnerships is co-creation of an intervention with local stakeholders. Stakeholder groups are quite often dissemination agents over the longer term as they provide resources, knowledge or skills. Co-creation happens early on in the design stage, as a means to understand the context where the intervention will be implemented. There is no road map that clearly outlines co-creation approaches beyond investing substantial time to customize co-creation methods for stakeholder groups and settings. At the end of the day, co-creation is about working closely with partners to better understand their needs, motivation and level of commitment (Beran et al., 2018; Syed, 2018). Within the school setting, context influences the quality and viability of school-based interventions and their dissemination. Although co-creation approaches are often overlooked, they should not be. Especially when health promotion professionals enter the educational context, such is the case with school-based physical activity interventions (Butler et al., 2010).

Adaptation

Inevitably at scale-up, interventions and implementation strategies will need to be adapted to suit local contexts (Kohl & Cooley, 2003; Milat et al., 2012). In many cases, this entails simplifying an already flexible intervention to different cultures, social or physical environments while creating efficiencies and reducing costs. Thus surfaces the 'tug of war' between fidelity versus adaptation of evidence-based programs (Bopp, Saunders, & Lattimore, 2013; Cook, Dinnen, Thompson, Simiola, & Schnurr, 2014). We define fidelity and adaptation in Tables 21.4 and 21.5, respectively.

The first challenge is to identify and retain elements of the intervention that are considered to be 'essential' to maintain effectiveness (Milat, Newson et al., 2014). Given that many school-based studies evaluate a program's overall effect or include multiple components we seldom know the effect of individual components. Decisions as to what components are essential may therefore be based on an inadequate literature or best guess by experts. Further, there are many dimensions of fidelity that include the broad domains of content, quality, quantity and process (Sanetti & Kratochwill, 2009) – all dimensions are seldom measured. Indeed, dose and quality are most often measured to assess intervention fidelity (Ransford, Greenberg, Domitrovich, Small, & Jacobson, 2009). Finally, we do not know how good is 'good enough'. Durlak and DuPre (2008) suggest that programs implemented with 60% integrity may be effective.

The second challenge is to identify essential implementation strategies and processes that can be, or need to be, adapted for wide scale implementation within complex systems such as schools (Fullan, 2006; Hawe, Shiell, & Riley, 2004; Pawson, Tilley, & Tilley, 1997). Adaptation is closely linked to and a central part of planning for dissemination (Lomas, 1997; NHS Centre for Reviews and Dissemination, 1999). Thus, processes such as co-creation also apply here. School-based partners know their local context best, and can guide adaptation strategies (Leeman et al., 2018). Further, educational practitioners and policy makers' critical judgment is essential to effectively integrate key elements into programs, and disseminate programs across diverse settings.

The adaptation versus fidelity health promotion literature is sparse, but emerging. It entails a constant cycle of adaptation, implementation and evaluation as per the Knowledge-to-Action Cycle (Graham et al., 2006). A number of adaptation frameworks exist (Carroll et al., 2007; Pérez, Van der Stuyft, del Carmen Zabala, Castro, & Lefèvre, 2015; Stirman, Miller, Toder, & Calloway, 2013) that can be (dare we say) adapted to the school setting.

Research Design/Methods, Approaches and Outcomes

Implementation and scale-up science in health promotion is fast emerging into a well-conceived and accepted discipline. Notwithstanding that most implementation science studies still reside within the healthcare field (Landsverk et al., 2012). However, consensus has yet to be reached as to what approaches are most appropriate to assess implementation processes and strategies. It is well beyond the scope of our chapter to engage meaningfully in this discussion or to provide definitive answers. Instead we refer you to some excellent resources (Bauman & Nutbeam, 2013; Brownson et al., 2018; Society for Implementation Research Collaboration, 2018).

Very simply, 'hybrid' studies (Curran, Bauer, Mittman, Pyne, & Stetler, 2012) that evaluate both impact (effectiveness) of the intervention and implementation processes provide us the opportunity to better interpret outcomes and/or replicate school-based physical activity scale-up studies in the future. Hybrid studies by nature imply a mixed methods approach that morphs from an emphasis on quantitative outcomes in RCTs to using more qualitative approaches at scale-up. The current reality does not preclude that in some cases (but not often enough) implementation processes are evaluated in RCTs and impact is evaluated at scale-up. Indeed, we urge researchers to step up – as fewer than 5% of 1,200 studies reviewed assessed implementation (Durlak, 1997; Durlak & Wells, 1997). We refer you back to the evaluation continuum, which acknowledges types of studies and related methodologies often implemented in a nonlinear fashion.

In summary, for scale-up studies, we turn away from an exclusive focus on internal validity toward external validity (from fidelity to adaptation), from efficacy to feasibility, from exclusively impact toward cost and from adoption to sustainability (Glasgow & Emmons, 2007). Scale-up science is rife with strategic challenges, networking potential and all manner of new research possibilities for students, emerging and established researchers alike – what's not to love.

Sustainability and Institutionalization

There is a need to understand how best to implement, scale-up and **sustain** school-based physical activity interventions – while the ultimate goal remains the health of children at the population level. We briefly describe the Holy Grail – long-term sustainability and institutionalization of effective school-based physical activity interventions.

Sustainability is when an innovation becomes routine until it reaches obsolescence (Greenhalgh et al., 2004). Importantly, should scaled-up programs show evidence of sustained impact, schools are more likely to believe they are worth investing in and as a result more likely to adopt them (Dowda et al., 2005). However, the longer an organization sustains an innovation, the less likely it is to adopt a new one (Greenhalgh et al., 2004). All in, there is a dearth of research into the sustainability of school-based physical activity programs (Dowda et al., 2005).

Institutionalization is the 'long-term viability and integration of a new program within an organization' (Rohrbach et al., 1993) and ensures long-term use. Institutionalization is a lot like Santa Claus – we want to believe that the possibility exists but definitive evidence of its existence is very elusive. Institutionalization takes a long view and requires prolonged planning and resource provision, often supported by organizational or government policies (Hoelscher et al., 2004). As an intervention progresses to scale-up and should it become part of regular practice (institutionalized), there is a continued need for ongoing evaluation (Oldenburg, Sallis, French, & Owen, 1999). As in the scale-up space, institutionalization research allows delivery and support systems to adapt implementation processes and strategies to sustain implementation effectiveness and maintain engagement with stakeholders who are providing support for the intervention (Milat, Newson et al., 2014).

References

Aarons, G. A., Sklar, M., Mustanski, B., Benbow, N., & Brown, C. H. (2017). "Scaling-out" evidence-based interventions to new populations or new health care delivery systems. *Implementation Science, 12*(1), 111.

Australian Sports Commission. (2018). *Find your 30*. Canberra: Australian Government Retrieved from https://www.sportaus.gov.au/findyour30

Bandura, A. (1986). *Social foundation of thought and actions: A cognitive social theory*. Englewood Cliffs, NJ: Prentice Hall.

Baranowski, T., & Stables, G. (2000). Process evaluations of the 5-a-day projects. *Health Education & Behavior, 27*(2), 157–166.

Basch, C. E., Eveland, J., & Portnoy, B. (1986). Diffusion systems for education and learning about health. *Family & Community Health: The Journal of Health Promotion & Maintenance, 9*, 1–26.

Bauman, A., & Nutbeam, D. (2013). *Evaluation in a nutshell: A practical guide to the evaluation of health promotion programs.* Sydney, Australia: McGraw Hill.

Beran, D., Lazo-Porras, M., Cardenas, M. K., Chappuis, F., Damasceno, A., Jha, N., . . . Pastrana, N. A. (2018). Moving from formative research to co-creation of interventions: Insights from a community health system project in Mozambique, Nepal and Peru. *BMJ Global Health, 3*(6), e001183.

Blase, K., & Fixsen, D. (2013). *Core intervention components: Identifying and operationalizing what makes programs work.* ASPE Research Brief. Washington, DC: US Department of Health and Human Services.

Bopp, M., Saunders, R. P., & Lattimore, D. (2013). The tug-of-war: Fidelity versus adaptation throughout the health promotion program life cycle. *The Journal of Primary Prevention, 34*(3), 193–207.

Brownson, R. C., Colditz, G. A., & Proctor, E. K. (2018). *Dissemination and implementation research in health: Translating science to practice.* Oxford, UK: Oxford University Press.

Butler, H., Bowes, G., Drew, S., Glover, S., Godfrey, C., Patton, G., . . . Bond, L. (2010). Harnessing complexity: Taking advantage of context and relationships in dissemination of school-based interventions. *Health Promotion Practice, 11*(2), 259–267.

Carroll, C., Patterson, M., Wood, S., Booth, A., Rick, J., & Balain, S. (2007). A conceptual framework for implementation fidelity. *Implementation Science, 2*(1), 40.

Castro, F. G., Barrera, M., & Martinez, C. R. (2004). The cultural adaptation of prevention interventions: Resolving tensions between fidelity and fit. *Prevention Science, 5*(1), 41–45.

Centers for Disease Control and Prevention. (2015). *Workplace health promotion.* Atlanta, GA: Centers for Disease Control and Prevention. Retrieved from https://www.cdc.gov/workplacehealthpromotion/model/implementation/index.html

Chesham, R. A., Booth, J. N., Sweeney, E. L., Ryde, G. C., Gorely, T., Brooks, N. E., & Moran, C. N. (2018). The daily mile makes primary school children more active, less sedentary and improves their fitness and body composition: A quasi-experimental pilot study. *BMC Medicine, 16*(64), 1–13.

Cohen, K. E., Morgan, P. J., Plotnikoff, R. C., Callister, R., & Lubans, D. R. (2015). Physical activity and skills intervention: SCORES cluster randomized controlled trial. *Medicine and Science in Sports and Exercise, 47*(4), 765–774.

Cook, J. M., Dinnen, S., Thompson, R., Simiola, V., & Schnurr, P. P. (2014). Changes in implementation of two evidence-based psychotherapies for PTSD in VA residential treatment programs: A national investigation. *Journal of Traumatic Stress, 27*(2), 137–143.

Craigie, A. M., Lake, A. A., Kelly, S. A., Adamson, A. J., & Mathers, J. C. (2011). Tracking of obesity-related behaviours from childhood to adulthood: A systematic review. *Maturitas, 70*(3), 266–284.

Curran, G. M., Bauer, M., Mittman, B., Pyne, J. M., & Stetler, C. (2012). Effectiveness-implementation hybrid designs: Combining elements of clinical effectiveness and implementation research to enhance public health impact. *Medical Care, 50*(3), 217–226.

Damschroder, L. J., Aron, D. C., Keith, R. E., Kirsh, S. R., Alexander, J. A., & Lowery, J. C. (2009). Fostering implementation of health services research findings into practice: A consolidated framework for advancing implementation science. *Implementation Science, 4*(1), 50.

Deci, E. L., & Ryan, R. M. (2002). *Handbook of self-determination research.* Rochester, NY: University Rochester Press.

Domitrovich, C. E., Bradshaw, C. P., Poduska, J. M., Hoagwood, K., Buckley, J. A., Olin, S., . . . Ialongo, N. S. (2008). Maximizing the implementation quality of evidence-based preventive interventions in schools: A conceptual framework. *Advances in School Mental Health Promotion, 1*(3), 6–28.

Dowda, M., Sallis, J. F., McKenzie, T. L., Rosengard, P., & Kohl III, H. W. (2005). Evaluating the sustainability of SPARK physical education: A case study of translating research into practice. *Research Quarterly for Exercise and Sport, 76*(1), 11–19.

Dunton, G. F., Lagloire, R., & Robertson, T. (2009). Using the RE-AIM framework to evaluate the statewide dissemination of a school-based physical activity and nutrition curriculum: "Exercise your options". *American Journal of Health Promotion, 23*(4), 229–232.

Durlak, J. A. (1997). *Successful prevention programs for children and adolescents.* Boston, MA: Springer Science & Business Media.

Durlak, J. A., & DuPre, E. P. (2008). Implementation matters: A review of research on the influence of implementation on program outcomes and the factors affecting implementation. *American Journal of Community Psychology, 41*(3–4), 327–350.

Durlak, J. A., & Wells, A. M. (1997). Primary prevention mental health programs for children and adolescents: A meta-analytic review. *American Journal of Community Psychology, 25*(2), 115–152.

Eccles, M. P., & Mittman, B. S. (2006). Welcome to implementation science. *Implementation Science, 1*(1), 1–3.

Farris, R. P., Will, J. C., Khavjou, O., & Finkelstein, E. A. (2007). Beyond effectiveness: Evaluating the public health impact of the WISEWOMAN program. *American Journal of Public Health, 97*(4), 641–647.

Figgis, J., Zubrick, A., Butorac, A., & Alderson, A. (2000). Backtracking practice and policies to research. In *The impact of educational research* (pp. 279–374). Canberra, Australia: Australian Government, Department of Education, Training and Youth Affairs.

Fullan, M. (2006, May 24). *Beyond turnaround leadership.* Birmingham, UK: Priestly Lecture, University of Birmingham.

Glasgow, R. E., & Emmons, K. M. (2007). How can we increase translation of research into practice? Types of evidence needed. *Annual Review of Public Health, 28*, 413–433.

Glasgow, R. E., Klesges, L. M., Dzewaltowski, D. A., Bull, S. S., & Estabrooks, P. (2004). The future of health behavior change research: What is needed to improve translation of research into health promotion practice? *Annals of Behavioral Medicine, 27*(1), 3–12.

Glasgow, R. E., Vinson, C., Chambers, D., Khoury, M. J., Kaplan, R. M., & Hunter, C. (2012). National Institutes of Health approaches to dissemination and implementation science: Current and future directions. *American Journal of Public Health, 102*(7), 1274–1281.

Glasgow, R. E., Vogt, T. M., & Boles, S. M. (1999). Evaluating the public health impact of health promotion interventions: The RE-AIM framework. *American Journal of Public Health, 89*(9), 1322–1327.

Global Advocacy for Physical Activity, & Advocacy Council of the International Society for Physical Activity and Health. (2011). *NCD prevention: Investments that work for physical activity.* Retrieved from www.globalpa.org.uk/investmentsthatwork

Global Alliance for Chronic Diseases. (2018). *Implementation science.* Retrieved from https://www.gacd.org/research/implementation-science

Graham, I. D., Logan, J., Harrison, M. B., Straus, S. E., Tetroe, J., Caswell, W., & Robinson, N. (2006). Lost in knowledge translation: Time for a map? *Journal of Continuing Education in the Health Professions, 26*(1), 13–24.

Greenhalgh, T., Robert, G., Macfarlane, F., Bate, P., & Kyriakidou, O. (2004). Diffusion of innovations in service organizations: Systematic review and recommendations. *The Milbank Quarterly, 82*(4), 581–629.

Hawe, P., Shiell, A., & Riley, T. (2004). Complex interventions: How "out of control" can a randomised controlled trial be? *BMJ: British Medical Journal, 328*(7455), 1561–1563.

Heath, E. M., & Coleman, K. J. (2003). Adoption and institutionalization of the child and adolescent trial for cardiovascular health (CATCH) in El Paso, Texas. *Health Promotion Practice, 4*(2), 157–164.

Hoelscher, D. M., Feldman, H. A., Johnson, C. C., Lytle, L. A., Osganian, S. K., Parcel, G. S., . . . Nader, P. R. (2004). School-based health education programs can be maintained over time: Results from the CATCH institutionalization study. *Preventive Medicine, 38*(5), 594–606.

Hoelscher, D. M., Kelder, S. H., Murray, N., Cribb, P. W., Conroy, J., & Parcel, G. S. (2001). Dissemination and adoption of the child and adolescent trial for cardiovascular health (CATCH): A case study in Texas. *Journal of Public Health Management and Practice: JPHMP, 7*(2), 90–100.

Hoelscher, D. M., Springer, A. E., Ranjit, N., Perry, C. L., Evans, A. E., Stigler, M., & Kelder, S. H. (2010). Reductions in child obesity among disadvantaged school children with community involvement: The Travis County CATCH trial. *Obesity, 18*(S1), S36–S44.

Hung, T. T. M., Chiang, V. C. L., Dawson, A., & Lee, R. L. T. (2014). Understanding of factors that enable health promoters in implementing health-promoting schools: A systematic review and narrative synthesis of qualitative evidence. *PLoS One, 9*(9), e108284.

Indig, D., Lee, K., Grunseit, A., Milat, A., & Bauman, A. (2018). Pathways for scaling up public health interventions. *BMC Public Health, 18*(1), 68. doi:10.1186/s12889-017-4572-5

Keller-Margulis, M. A. (2012). Fidelity of implementation framework: A critical need for response to intervention models. *Psychology in the Schools, 49*(4), 342–352.

Kennedy, S. G., Smith, J. J., Hansen, V., Lindhout, M. I., Morgan, P. J., & Lubans, D. R. (2018). Implementing resistance training in secondary schools: An exploration of teachers' perceptions. *Translational Journal of the American College of Sports Medicine, 3*(12), 85–96.

Kohl, R., & Cooley, L. (2003). *Scaling up – A conceptual and operational framework.* Washington, DC: Management Systems International.

Koorts, H., Eakin, E., Estabrooks, P., Timperio, A., Salmon, J., & Bauman, A. (2018). Implementation and scale up of population physical activity interventions for clinical and community settings: The PRACTIS guide. *International Journal of Behavioral Nutrition and Physical Activity, 15*(1), 51.

Landsverk, J., Brown, C. H., Chamberlain, P., Palinkas, L., Ogihara, M., Czaja, S., . . . Horwitz, S. (2012). Design and analysis in dissemination and implementation research. In R. C. Brownson, G. A. Colditz, & E. K. Proctor (Eds.), *Dissemination and implementation research in health: Translating science to practice* (pp. 225–260). New York, NY: Oxford University Press.

Leeman, J., Wiecha, J. L., Vu, M., Blitstein, J. L., Allgood, S., Lee, S., & Merlo, C. (2018). School health implementation tools: A mixed methods evaluation of factors influencing their use. *Implementation Science, 13*(1), 48.

Linnan, L., & Steckler, A. (2002). *Process evaluation for public health interventions and research.* San Francisco, CA: Jossey-Bass.

Lomas, J. (1997). *Improving research dissemination and uptake in the health sector: Beyond the sound of one hand clapping.* Hamilton, ON: Centre for Health Economics and Policy Analysis.

Lonsdale, C., Sanders, T., Cohen, K. E., Parker, P., Noetel, M., Hartwig, T., . . . Salmon, J. (2016). Scaling-up an efficacious school-based physical activity intervention: Study protocol for the 'Internet-based professional learning to help teachers support activity in youth' (iPLAY) cluster randomized controlled trial and scale-up implementation evaluation. *BMC Public Health, 16*(1), 873.

Lubans, D. R., Morgan, P. J., Weaver, K., Callister, R., Dewar, D. L., Costigan, S. A., . . . Plotnikoff, R. C. (2012). Rationale and study protocol for the supporting children's outcomes using rewards, exercise and skills (SCORES) group randomized controlled trial: A physical activity and fundamental movement skills intervention for primary schools in low-income communities. *BMC Public Health, 12*(1), 427.

Luepker, R. V., Perry, C. L., McKinlay, S. M., Nader, P. R., Parcel, G. S., Stone, E. J., . . . Johnson, C. C. (1996). Outcomes of a field trial to improve children's dietary patterns and physical activity: The child and adolescent trial for cardiovascular health (CATCH). *JAMA, 275*(10), 768–776.

McKay, H. A., Macdonald, H. M., Nettlefold, L., Masse, L. C., Day, M., & Naylor, P.-J. (2014). Action schools! BC implementation: From efficacy to effectiveness to scale-up. *British Journal of Sports Medicine.* doi:10.1136/bjsports-2013-093361

McKay, H. A., Naylor, P.-J., Lau, E., Gray, S. M., Wolfenden, L., Milat, A., . . . Sims-Gould, J. (2019). Implementation and scale-up of physical activity and behavioural nutrition interventions: An evaluation roadmap. *International Journal of Behavioral Nutrition and Physical Activity, 16*(102), doi:10.1186/s12966-019-0868-4

McKenzie, T. L., Sallis, J. F., & Rosengard, P. (2009). Beyond the stucco tower: Design, development, and dissemination of the SPARK physical education programs. *Quest, 61*(1), 114–127.

McMeniman, M., Cumming, J., Wilson, J., Stevenson, J., & Sim, C. (2000). Teacher knowledge in action. *The Impact of Educational Research, 2*, 377–547.

Meyers, D. C., Durlak, J. A., & Wandersman, A. (2012). The quality implementation framework: A synthesis of critical steps in the implementation process. *American Journal of Community Psychology, 50*(3–4), 462–480.

Milat, A. J., Bauman, A. E., Redman, S., & Curac, N. (2011). Public health research outputs from efficacy to dissemination: A bibliometric analysis. *BMC Public Health, 11*(1), 934.

Milat, A. J., King, L., Bauman, A. E., & Redman, S. (2012). The concept of scalability: Increasing the scale and potential adoption of health promotion interventions into policy and practice. *Health Promotion International, 28*(3), 285–298.

Milat, A. J., King, L., Newson, R., Wolfenden, L., Rissel, C., Bauman, A., & Redman, S. (2014). Increasing the scale and adoption of population health interventions: Experiences and perspectives of policy makers, practitioners, and researchers. *Health Research Policy and Systems, 12*(1), 18.

Milat, A. J., Laws, R., King, L., Newson, R., Rychetnik, L., Rissel, C., . . . Bennie, J. (2013). Policy and practice impacts of applied research: A case study analysis of the New South Wales health promotion demonstration research grants scheme 2000–2006. *Health Research Policy and Systems, 11*(1), 5.

Milat, A., Newson, R., & King, L. (2014). *Increasing the scale of population health interventions: A guide.* North Sydney, Australia: NSW Ministry of Health.

Nathan, N., Elton, B., Babic, M., McCarthy, N., Sutherland, R., Presseau, J., . . . Yoong, S. L. (2017). Barriers and facilitators to the implementation of physical activity policies in schools: A systematic review. *Preventive Medicine, 107*, 45–53.

National Implementation Research Network. (2015). *Implementation science defined.* Retrieved from https://nirn.fpg.unc.edu/module-1/summary

National Institutes of Health. (2011). *Dissemination and implementation science.* Bethesda, MD: U.S. National Library of Medicine. Retrieved from https://hsric.nlm.nih.gov/hsric_public/display_links/790

National Physical Activity Plan Alliance. (2016). *National physical activity plan.* Retrieved from physicalactivityplan.org/docs/2016NPAP_Finalforwebsite.pdf

Naylor, P.-J., Nettlefold, L., Race, D., Hoy, C., Ashe, M. C., Higgins, J. W., & McKay, H. A. (2015). Implementation of school based physical activity interventions: A systematic review. *Preventive Medicine, 72*, 95–115.

Newland, B., Dixon, M. A., & Green, B. C. (2013). Engaging children through sport: Examining the disconnect between program vision and implementation. *Journal of Physical Activity and Health, 10*(6), 805–812.

NHS Centre for Reviews and Dissemination. (1999). *Effective health care: Getting evidence into practice* (Vol. 5). York, UK: University of York.

Nilsen, P. (2015). Making sense of implementation theories, models and frameworks. *Implementation Science, 10*(1), 53.

Norton, W., & Mittman, B. (2010). *Scaling-up health promotion/disease prevention programs in community settings: Barriers, facilitators, and initial recommendations.* Retrieved from https://donaghue.org/wp-content/uploads/Final-Scaling-Up-Report.pdf

Oldenburg, B., Sallis, J., French, M., & Owen, N. (1999). Health promotion research and the diffusion and institutionalization of interventions. *Health education research, 14*(1), 121–130.

Olstad, D. L., Campbell, E. J., Raine, K. D., & Nykiforuk, C. I. (2015). A multiple case history and systematic review of adoption, diffusion, implementation and impact of provincial daily physical activity policies in Canadian schools. *BMC Public Health, 15*(1), 385.

Pawson, R., Tilley, N., & Tilley, N. (1997). *Realistic evaluation.* London, UK: Sage.

Pérez, D., Van der Stuyft, P., del Carmen Zabala, M., Castro, M., & Lefèvre, P. (2015). A modified theoretical framework to assess implementation fidelity of adaptive public health interventions. *Implementation Science, 11*(1), 91.

Proctor, E. K., Landsverk, J., Aarons, G., Chambers, D., Glisson, C., & Mittman, B. (2009). Implementation research in mental health services: An emerging science with conceptual, methodological, and training challenges. *Administration and Policy in Mental Health and Mental Health Services Research, 36*(1), 24–34.

Proctor, E. K., Silmere, H., Raghavan, R., Hovmand, P., Aarons, G., Bunger, A., . . . Hensley, M. (2011). Outcomes for implementation research: Conceptual distinctions, measurement challenges, and research agenda. *Administration and Policy in Mental Health and Mental Health Services Research, 38*(2), 65–76.

Ransford, C. R., Greenberg, M. T., Domitrovich, C. E., Small, M., & Jacobson, L. (2009). The role of teachers' psychological experiences and perceptions of curriculum supports on the implementation of a social and emotional learning curriculum. *School Psychology Review, 38*(4), 510–532.

Reis, R. S., Salvo, D., Ogilvie, D., Lambert, E. V., Goenka, S., Brownson, R. C., & Lancet Physical Activity Series 2 Executive (2016). Scaling up physical activity interventions worldwide: Stepping up to larger and smarter approaches to get people moving. *The Lancet, 388*(10051), 1337–1348.

Rogers, E. M. (2003). *The diffusion of innovation* (5th ed.). New York, NY: Free Press.

Rohrbach, L. A., Graham, J. W., & Hansen, W. B. (1993). Diffusion of a school-based substance abuse prevention program: Predictors of program implementation. *Preventive Medicine, 22*(2), 237–260.

Rush, E., Reed, P., McLennan, S., Coppinger, T., Simmons, D., & Graham, D. (2012). A school-based obesity control programme: Project energize. Two-year outcomes. *British Journal of Nutrition, 107*(4), 581–587.

Saldana, L., Chamberlain, P., Wang, W., & Brown, C. H. (2012). Predicting program start-up using the stages of implementation measure. *Administration and Policy in Mental Health and Mental Health Services Research, 39*(6), 419–425.

Sallis, J. F. (2018). Needs and challenges related to multilevel interventions: Physical activity examples. *Health Education & Behavior.* doi:10.1177/1090198118796458

Sallis, J. F., McKenzie, T. L., Alcaraz, J. E., Kolody, B., Faucette, N., & Hovell, M. F. (1997). The effects of a 2-year physical education program (SPARK) on physical activity and fitness in elementary school students. Sports, play and active recreation for kids. *American Journal of Public Health, 87*(8), 1328–1334.

Sallis, J. F., McKenzie, T. L., Alcaraz, J. E., Kolody, B., Hovell, M. F., & Nader, P. R. (1993). Project SPARK: Effects of physical education on adiposity in children. *Annals of the New York Academy of Sciences, 699*(1), 127–136.

Sallis, J. F., Owen, N., & Fisher, E. (2015). Ecological models of health behavior. *Health Behavior: Theory, Research, and Practice, 5*, 43–64.

Sanetti, L. M. H., & Kratochwill, T. R. (2009). Toward developing a science of treatment integrity: Introduction to the special series. *School Psychology Review, 38*(4), 476–495.

Simmons, R., Fajans, P., & Ghiron, L. (2007). *Scaling up health service delivery: From pilot innovations to policies and programmes.* Geneva, Switzerland: World Health Organization.

Simmons, R., & Shiffman, J. (2007). Scaling up health service innovations: A framework for action. *Scaling Up Health Service Delivery, 1*, 30.

Society for Implementation Research Collaboration. (2018). *SIRC website.* Retrieved from https://society-forimplementationresearchcollaboration.org/

Spence, J. C., Faulkner, G., Bradstreet, C. C., Duggan, M., & Tremblay, M. S. (2015). Active Canada 20/20: A physical activity plan for Canada. *Canadian Journal of Public Health, 106*(8), e470–e473.

Stirman, S. W., Miller, C. J., Toder, K., & Calloway, A. (2013). Development of a framework and coding system for modifications and adaptations of evidence-based interventions. *Implementation Science, 8*(1), 65.

Straus, S. E., Tetroe, J., & Graham, I. (2009). Defining knowledge translation. *Canadian Medical Association Journal, 181*(3–4), 165–168.

Syed, M. A. (2018). Knowledge translation facilitating co-creation of evidence in public health. *BMJ Evidence-Based Medicine.* doi:10.1136/bmjebm-2018-111017

Tabak, R. G., Khoong, E. C., Chambers, D. A., & Brownson, R. C. (2012). Bridging research and practice: Models for dissemination and implementation research. *American Journal of Preventive Medicine, 43*(3), 337–350.

United States National Institutes of Health. (2016). *Dissemination and implementation research in health.* Retrieved from https://grants.nih.gov/grants/guide/pa-files/par-16-238.html

Wandersman, A., Duffy, J., Flaspohler, P., Noonan, R., Lubell, K., Stillman, L., . . . Saul, J. (2008). Bridging the gap between prevention research and practice: The interactive systems framework for dissemination and implementation. *American Journal of Community Psychology, 41*(3–4), 171–181.

Wenger, E. (1999). *Communities of practice: Learning, meaning, and identity.* Cambridge, UK: Cambridge University Press.

Wilson, P. M., Petticrew, M., Calnan, M. W., & Nazareth, I. (2010). Disseminating research findings: What should researchers do? A systematic scoping review of conceptual frameworks. *Implementation Science, 5*(1), 91.

World Health Organization. (2010a). *ExpandNet: Scaling up health innovations.* Retrieved from http://www.expandnet.net/about.htm

World Health Organization. (2010b). *Nine steps for developing a scaling-up strategy.* Retrieved from https://www.who.int/immunization/hpv/deliver/nine_steps_for_developing_a_scalingup_strategy_who_2010.pdf

World Health Organization. (2018a). *Effective school health programmes.* Retrieved from https://www.who.int/school_youth_health/en/

World Health Organization. (2018b). *Global action plan on physical activity 2018–2030: More active people for a healthier world* (9241514183). Retrieved from https://www.who.int/ncds/prevention/physical-activity/global-action-plan-2018-2030/en/

Yamey, G. (2011). Scaling up global health interventions: A proposed framework for success. *PLoS medicine, 8*(6), e1001049.

22

EVALUATION OF PHYSICAL ACTIVITY INTERVENTIONS

Tara N. McGoey

Introduction

This chapter will cover the main concepts and methods relevant to the evaluation of physical activity (PA) interventions in child and adolescent populations (youth). The iterative phases of an intervention's development, testing, implementation, and dissemination will be explored and used to categorize evaluation questions relating to the concepts of feasibility, efficacy/effectiveness, process, reach, and generalizability. Theoretical underpinnings of behavior change and the influence of mediating factors will be explored when establishing the causal role of a given intervention, and principles of study design and scientific inference will be applied to the task of evaluating PA as a behavioral outcome. Finally, the complexity of translating evidence-based results into sustainable health promotion practice will be discussed using a framework that considers process evaluation and program dissemination. The phases of the research process and the synergy between evaluations of experimental outcome and intervention development will be highlighted throughout.

Overview of the Literature

Regular PA is associated with numerous health benefits in school-age youth (Poitras et al., 2016); however, globally, there is growing concern about low levels of PA in this population (Hallal et al., 2012). Although a wide variety of PA interventions have been shown to be effective, they have not been widely implemented (Reis et al., 2016), as evidenced by the persistent suboptimal PA levels of children and adolescents worldwide (Sallis et al., 2016). This discrepancy reflects a gap in the translation of research findings to real-world settings (Loef & Walach, 2015). Identifying the characteristics of effective and translatable PA-promotion strategies has therefore become a major concern for national governments and public health organizations (Waters et al., 2011). This endeavor is not straightforward, however, because interventions designed to change health-related behaviors are comprised of many components that are often interacting (Craig et al., 2008).

From the perspective of PA promotion research, interventions are considered 'complex' and as such, their effects are largely dependent upon the contexts in which they were conducted (Michie et al., 2011). For youth, relevant settings include (pre)school, community, family/home, and primary-care and, depending on the setting, PA intervention strategies may target one or operate across many levels of influence (Messing et al., 2019). At the individual (proximal) level, there are demographic and psychosocial factors underlying choice to engage in PA, while at the interpersonal and more distal environmental levels, PA-related choice is shaped by the social and physical environments, and by the geo-political and economic factors that impact neighborhoods and communities (Bauman et al., 2012; King, Stokols, Talen, Brassington, & Killingsworth, 2002; Rhodes, Janssen, Bredin, Warburton, & Bauman, 2017; van Sluijs & Kriemler, 2016). For example, within the school setting, intervention strategies may target individuals using curricular and/or extra-curricular activities, and may also involve parents and/or the community (McKenzie, 2019). Community-based contexts can include involvement with sports teams, use of sports facilities and parks, or engagement with other groups (e.g. clubs, church groups), and often have a link to the family/home setting (e.g. Welsby et al., 2014). Within these settings, PA opportunities can occur via the use of active video games and Smartphone apps, engagement in active play, and the use of active transport (e.g. Direito, Jiang, Whittaker, & Maddison, 2015; Larouche, Mammen, Rowe, & Faulkner, 2018), and there are also family physician-led strategies involving prescribed PA participation (e.g. James, Hess, Perkins, Taveras, & Scirica, 2017; Ortega-Sanchez et al., 2004). Compounding the variability associated with PA contexts are the multiple dimensions of the behavior itself, which produce a wide range of measurable outcomes and include frequency, intensity, duration, and type. Frequency is often measured as a participation rate and reported as number of hours or days spent in PA for a given time period (e.g. per week). Duration refers to the amount of time engaged in PA, and can also specify intensity. For example, PA may be reported as the number of minutes engaged in exercise per day, or as the percentage of daily minutes spent in a specific intensity of PA such as moderate-to-vigorous PA (MVPA). Alternatively, many studies measure specific types of PA, such as participation in active transportation, or daily number of steps taken based on pedometer data (Sylvia, Bernstein, Hubbard, Keating, & Anderson, 2014). Therefore, the complexities associated with PA interventions are numerous and stem from their variety of settings, strategies, levels of influence, and experimental outcomes.

Key Issues

Evaluations of PA interventions attempt to address their complex nature by identifying what works, and delineating where, when, how, why, and for whom the interventions are (un)successful. To that end, key considerations of an intervention evaluation should be built into the life cycle of the research process, which represents an iterative continuum of increasing evidence organized in four major phases (Campbell et al., 2000; Craig et al., 2008; Moore et al., 2015):

1   The development phase, which draws from the existing evidence base and appropriate theory;
2   The testing phase, which starts with exploratory feasibility studies and progresses to definitive efficacy and effectiveness trials;
3   The implementation phase, which uses process evaluations to inform how the intervention can be translated from research to practice; and
4   The scale-up and dissemination phase, which evaluates the intervention's translatability across different contexts.

Using the main phases of the research process as a framework (see Figure 22.1), this chapter further explores the concepts of theory application, internal versus external validity, study design, implementation fidelity, and applicability of findings to different settings, with reference to youth PA interventions as examples.

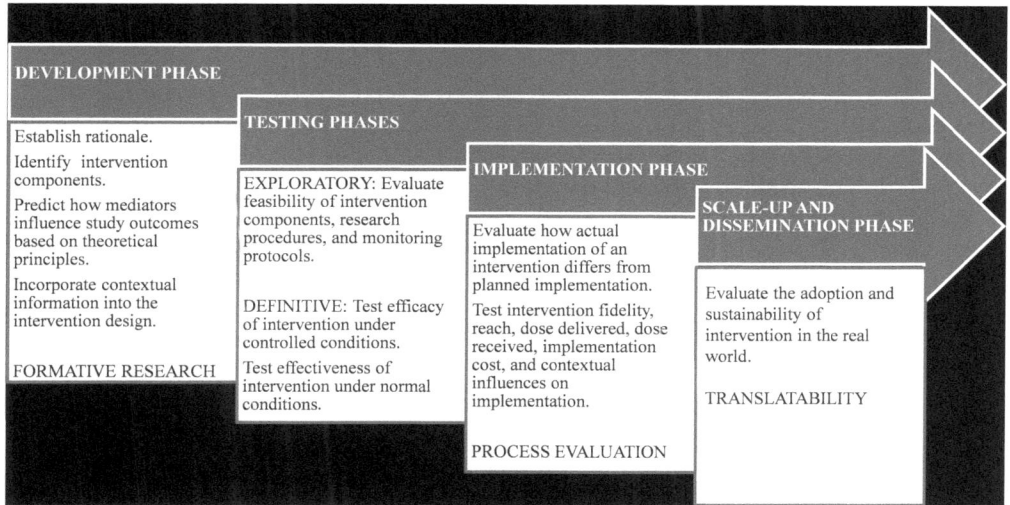

Figure 22.1 Iterative phases of the research process for complex health promotion interventions (as informed by Craig et al., 2008)

The Development Phase: Evaluating Evidence, Context, and Theory

Evaluating what works and why is informed by an intervention's rationale, core components, and predicted causal pathways (Lloyd, Logan, Greaves, & Wyatt, 2011; Wells, Williams, Treweek, Coyle, & Taylor, 2012). Because this foundational information provides a basis for understanding the impact of interventions, the 2008 Medical Research Council (MRC) framework for developing and evaluating complex interventions recommends that the first steps in designing an intervention be: a review of the evidence base, the preliminary collection of qualitative data to help understand context, and the identification of appropriate theory (Craig et al., 2018). Together, this information allows for studies to be planned prospectively so that the possible links between intervention components, context, and outcomes can be examined (Campbell et al., 2007; Craig et al., 2018).

Review of the Evidence Base

The development of an intervention typically begins with the identification of a problem and a review of what is already known about similar interventions (Campbell et al., 2000). The relevant literature to review when developing a PA intervention for children or adolescents includes that which reports on the relative successes and failures of different PA intervention strategies in these populations (Wight, Wimbush, Jepson, & Doi, 2016). For example, an intervention promoting the healthy behavior of second- and third-grade children (Lynch et al., 2016) was developed based on evidence of its strategic successes in the clinical setting (Polacsek et al., 2009) and with older elementary school children (Tucker et al., 2011). Similarly, the development of an intervention examining the impact of a teacher-facilitated High-Intensity Interval Training (HIIT) program on adolescent fitness levels (Leahy et al., 2019) was guided by published data supporting the effectiveness, safety, and acceptability of the techniques when delivered by external research teams (Bond, Weston, Williams, & Barker, 2017).

Preliminary Data Collection

While the evidence base informs the selection of strategic intervention techniques, incorporating qualitative research methods in the development phase enables a deeper understanding of the context in which the intervention is to be delivered (Campbell et al., 2000). The West Midlands ActiVe lifestyle and healthy Eating in School children (WAVES) (Griffin, Clarke, Lancashire, Pallan, & Adab, 2017) and the Healthy Lifestyles Programme (HeLP) (Wyatt et al., 2013) studies are school-based health promotion interventions that include PA components. During their development phases, each study conducted focus groups with key stakeholders (e.g. parents, children, teachers, and local education and health authorities) to prioritize intervention strategies (Adab et al., 2015; Lloyd & Wyatt, 2015; Lloyd et al., 2011; Pallan, Parry, & Adab, 2012). The WAVES study targeted South Asian children and, based on information collected during focus groups, considered the central role of religious practices in its design by avoiding the use of after-school clubs for PA promotion because that's when the majority of children are attending mosque (Pallan et al., 2012). The HeLP study was aimed at low-income children and, in response to feedback from stakeholder workshops (Lloyd et al., 2011), included an interactive drama component to encourage parental engagement in the program at school (Wyatt, Lloyd, Creanor, & Logan, 2011). As evidenced by these two studies, co-developing interventions with stakeholders who have an intimate knowledge of the targeted system (e.g. school) represents an important means of ensuring compatibility of intervention content with context (Hawkins et al., 2017; Moore & Evans, 2017).

The Role of Theory

The information collected from systematic literature reviews and preliminary qualitative methods can be organized using theoretical frameworks (Pallan, Parry, Cheng, & Adab, 2013). The MRC framework highlights the importance of having a theoretical basis for intervention development because theory facilitates an understanding of the mediating variables that influence the causal pathways between intervention components and outcomes (Craig et al., 2008; Hardeman et al., 2005; MacKinnon, 2011; Sallis et al., 2016; Wight et al., 2016). The evidence base for youth PA interventions indicates that changes in the following variables can mediate changes in PA behavior: attitudes, self-efficacy, enjoyment, outcome expectancies, perceived benefits, perceived barriers, social support, intention, and access to facilities (Brown, Hume, Pearson, & Salmon, 2013; van Stralen et al., 2011). Variables that have been shown to mediate intervention effects on PA behavior are fewer, and include self-efficacy and intention (Lubans, Foster, & Biddle, 2008; van Stralen et al., 2011). Conceptually, all of these variables link to various formalized theories or behavior change models, the most relevant of which is dependent upon the intervention's purpose and strategies.

When an intervention is targeting proximal influences on PA behavior, theories that focus on psychosocial factors are most applicable. For example, the Social Cognitive Theory (SCT) (Bandura, 1997), the Theory of Planned Behavior (TPB) (Ajzen, 1991), and the Self-Determination Theory (SDT) (Ryan & Deci, 2000) typically guide interventions that target the intra- (e.g. self-efficacy, intention) and inter- (e.g. parent- and teacher-support) personal processes mediating youth PA behaviors (Quested, Ntoumanis, Thøgersen-Ntoumani, Hagger, & Hancox, 2017). Alternatively, a social–ecological (SE) approach is well suited when the interactions of proximal and distal influences on health outcomes are being considered. SE frameworks highlight the plurality of potential influences on PA within a given context, including individual factors, interpersonal influences, environmental conditions (e.g. accessibility of recreational and park facilities), and the policies that create them (Atkin, van Sluijs, Dollman, Taylor, &

Stanley, 2016; Booth et al., 2001; Spence & Lee, 2003). The Youth Physical Activity Promotion Model (YPAPM), developed by Welk (1999), categorizes various mediators of PA as factors that predispose (e.g. enjoyment, outcome expectancies), reinforce (e.g. PA models, social support), or enable (e.g. availability of resources) PA behavior in youth. The YPAPM model is consistent with the SE perspective in that it includes multiple levels of influence, and postulates interactions among the multi-leveled constructs that can directly and indirectly influence behavior. Further, it allows for various constructs from different theories, such as the SCT and TPB, to be included in the framework (Welk, 1999). The Theory of Expanded, Extended, and Enhanced Opportunities (TEO) (Beets et al., 2016) recognizes the importance of these behavioral theories and models while incorporating the provision of PA opportunities into its formalized framework that links three broad mechanisms to behavioral change. These mechanisms include adding new PA opportunities (expansion), allocating additional time for existing PA opportunities (extension), and augmenting existing opportunities to increase the amount of PA accumulated during an allotted period of time (enhancement) (Beets et al., 2016). The use of each of these theories is exemplified following a brief discussion of the varying degrees of theory application in behavior change interventions.

When evaluating an intervention, an important theory-related consideration is the extent to which the theory was used during the intervention's development and design, because the degree to which theory promotes success of an intervention depends on how well the theory was used (Hendrie et al., 2012). Many PA interventions are atheoretical (i.e. have no theoretical underpinning), and among those that do use theory, the manner in which it is applied varies considerably (Prestwich et al., 2014). Therefore, it is important to differentiate amongst those studies that used theory to *inform* the development of the intervention without applying specific constructs in the study design, those that *applied* the theory by including measurements of one or more of the theory constructs, and those that *tested* the theory by statistically measuring the mediation effects of the theory constructs on PA behavior. To that end, Michie and Prestwich (2010) have developed a systematic method of assessing the degree to which theory has been applied to interventions. This coding scheme facilitates an understanding of the theoretical constructs that are relevant to an intervention by addressing the following six questions:

1   Is theory mentioned?
2   Are the relevant theoretical constructs targeted?
3   Is theory used to select recipients or tailor interventions?
4   Are the relevant theoretical constructs measured?
5   Is theory tested?
6   Were the results used to refine theory?

Examples of interventions that were explicitly designed and evaluated based on theory (i.e. affirmative answers to the first four items of the coding scheme) include the Active Schools: Skelmersdale and Great Live and Move Challenge (GLMC) studies. The former included measures of self-efficacy, and each of its intervention components aligned with elements of the SE model, the YPAPM, and the TEO (Taylor et al., 2018). Among the components were 30-second teacher-delivered active breaks designed for use within the restricted space of a classroom. These active breaks added new PA opportunities (TEO) that were reinforced and modeled by teachers (YPAPM), while considering the environmental conditions in which the activities were being delivered (SE). Similarly, the GLMC study measured constructs from the TPB and selected intervention techniques relating thereto; namely, persuasive messages were selected to address intention and attitudes, and self-monitoring and family engagement were selected to influence subjective norm and perceived behavioral control (Gourlan et al., 2018).

Identifying mediating links between intervention strategies and PA outcomes (i.e. addressing the last two items of the coding scheme) is vital for maximizing contributions to a broader evidence base (van Stralen et al., 2011). However, despite their increasing number (e.g. Chatzisarantis & Hagger, 2009; Dishman et al., 2004, 2005; Hortz & Petosa, 2008; Taymoori & Lubans, 2008), there are still relatively few analyses of mediating mechanisms of youth PA behavior change (Brown et al., 2013; Larouche et al., 2018; van Stralen et al., 2011). In response to this paucity, Demetriou and Bachner (2019) designed a physical education intervention based on the YPAPM, SDT and SCT that will measure the mediating effects of relevant theoretical constructs (autonomy, competence, relatedness, self-efficacy, and social support) on the PA of elementary school-aged girls. Likewise, the design protocol for a follow-up study of the GLMC program includes analyses of the mediating effects of the TPB constructs (intention, attitudes, subjective norm, perceived behavioral control) on children's PA (Cousson-Gélie et al., 2019).

The advantage of explicit theory use in an intervention over an atheoretical approach is its provision of a framework for identifying constructs that are hypothesized to be causally related to, and thus targets for, desired behavior change (Michie & Prestwich, 2010). However, the evidence comparing the effectiveness of theory-based versus atheoretical PA interventions is inconclusive (Rhodes et al., 2017). These equivocal effects further highlight a need for youth PA interventions to specify mediating links between constructs and outcomes, and to elucidate the conditions under which certain mediators are more (or less) influential on study outcomes. Taking an iterative approach, this information should be considered during the development phase, and refined based on evidence and data collected throughout the rest of the research process (i.e. during feasibility and efficacy/effectiveness studies and process evaluations) (Bonell, Fletcher, Morton, Lorenc, & Moore, 2012; Campbell et al., 2007; Linnan & Steckler, 2002; Prestwich, Webb, & Conner, 2015).

The Exploratory Testing Phase: Evaluating Feasibility

By the end of the development phase, intervention strategies and research procedures are selected. The feasibility of these selections is then evaluated in the next phase of the research process, which is also referred to as an exploratory phase (Campbell et al., 2000; Hallingberg et al., 2018). Any study conducted in preparation for full-scale implementation of a main study (i.e. a definitive trial) is categorized as a feasibility study, which, defined as such, includes pilot studies as a subset (Eldridge et al., 2016; O'Cathain et al., 2015). Considering feasibility as an overarching concept, pilot studies are those that implement the intervention on a scale smaller than that planned for the definitive trial, while non-pilot feasibility studies focus on select elements of the intervention to address questions about how and whether or not they can be conducted (e.g. modifications to better suit the context) (Eldridge et al., 2016; Fletcher et al., 2016). Although not all interventions are preceded by a feasibility study, when they are, the main purposes are to refine the intervention by addressing uncertainties and/or to assess the potential impact of an intervention using pilot data (Hallingberg et al., 2018). For example, the Move for Well-being in Schools (MVS) intervention included a feasibility phase that assessed the acceptability of the program and piloted its implementation at selected elementary schools (Smedegaard, Brondeel, Christiansen, & Skovgaard, 2017). Feedback from teacher surveys informed adjustments to the final trial's procedure, which included a reduction in the length of the program's exposure in order to maintain student engagement. In addition, baseline data from the pilot study were used to assess the validity of the survey tools used for measuring the study's PA-related outcomes.

The adequacy and applicability of PA measures are often assessed using feasibility studies since there is no single validated tool to measure all types of PA, in all settings, for all ages

(Atkin et al., 2016). Pilot work conducted prior to the wide-scale implementation of the Virtual Traveler intervention indicated a need for additional PA measures to complement the data collected from accelerometers, which alone under-estimated children's time spent in PA (Norris, Shelton, Dunsmuir, Duke-Williams, & Stamatakis, 2015). Although accelerometers have been shown to be a valid and reliable method for measuring PA in children (Rowlands, 2007), they have weaker sensitivity to the type of PA that was elicited by the Virtual Traveler intervention, namely non-ambulatory, on-the-spot movement (Trost, 2001). Therefore, in response to the pilot data, the researchers added a PA observation method to the larger trial (Norris, Dunsmuir, Duke-Williams, Stamatakis, & Shelton, 2016), which can assess these types of activities more reliably (Sirard & Pate, 2001). The accuracy of accelerometers is also dependent on wear-time compliance (Lewis, Napolitano, Buman, Williams, & Nigg, 2017), which is an important consideration when evaluating the feasibility of school-based PA interventions for adolescents, for whom higher compliance rates are associated with larger effects on total PA (Borde, Smith, Sutherland, Nathan, & Lubans, 2017).

An additional reason for including a feasibility phase in the research process is to perform sample size calculations using pilot data (Lancaster, Dodd, & Williamson, 2004). Sample size calculations determine the number of participants (or units of analysis) necessary for evaluating whether or not the intervention has an observable, significant effect based on statistical analyses (Kistin & Silverstein, 2015). For example, the GoActive pilot trial determined that adequate power to detect a meaningful group difference in MVPA of 5 minutes/day required recruitment of 16 schools and 150 participants per school for the full trial (Corder, Brown, Schiff, & van Sluijs, 2016).

Obtaining and maintaining the necessary sample size require efficient recruitment and adequate retention. While both can be challenging, particularly when working with young people (Schoeppe, Oliver, Badland, Burke, & Duncan, 2013), strategies can be evaluated using feasibility studies. For example, the recruitment approach used for the large-scale implementation of the Virtual Traveler intervention was changed from individual school email invitations to social media participant calls after pilot testing of the former technique resulted in a very low follow-up rate (Norris et al., 2015, 2016). Similarly, findings from the first iteration of a community-based PA intervention indicated that verbal presentations and communication with community partners failed to connect with the population of interest (13–18 year olds), thus prompting modifications to the program's future recruitment strategies (Jung, Bourne, & Gainforth, 2018).

Together, the information collected during the feasibility phase proactively addresses challenges related to key study logistics (e.g. procedure, outcome assessment, sample size, and recruitment), with pilot studies often generating preliminary data regarding efficacy/effectiveness (Campbell et al., 2007; Craig et al., 2008; Fletcher et al., 2016). However, limitations inherent to a pilot evaluation, such as relatively small sample size and no long-term follow-up, can significantly compromise the internal validity of these exploratory studies (Karczewski, Carter, & DeCator, 2016; Kistin & Silverstein, 2015).

The Definitive Testing Phase: Evaluating Efficacy/Effectiveness

The definitive testing phase of the research process emphasizes questions of efficacy/effectiveness and internal validity to assess whether or not there is evidence of a causal relationship between the intervention and its desired outcome. *Efficacy* is determined by studies that test the impact of an intervention under optimum conditions, whereas *effectiveness* is determined by those that test the impact of an intervention delivered under typical real-world conditions (Flay, 1986; Glasgow, Lichtenstein, & Marcus, 2003; Green & Glasgow, 2006). A region-specific, school-based PA program delivered by expert staff following a standardized research protocol for a defined length of time is an example of an efficacy trial (e.g. Schofield, Mummer, & Schofield, 2005). Comparatively, an effectiveness trial may follow a flexible protocol, use existing school resources and/or procedures, and rely on regular staff (e.g. teachers) across multiple schools to implement the PA intervention (e.g. Coleman et al., 2005).

A study's *internal validity* refers to its ability to measure what it intends to measure (Steckler & McLeroy, 2008). Internal validity is the focus of efficacy studies, which typically use experimental and quasi-experimental research designs (Victora, Habicht, & Bryce, 2004). The defining characteristic of these designs is the use of a parallel control group, participant assignment to which is either randomized (experimental) or non-randomized (quasi-experimental). In contrast, non-experimental studies draw inferences about the effect of an intervention on participants without comparison to a control group. Although the internal validity of non-experimental studies is compromised, they typically involve the observation of study participants in their natural setting, and thus consider the *external validity* of the intervention (Carlson & Morrison, 2009). External validity allows for generalizability of the results to different measures, populations, settings, and times, and is thus an important consideration for effectiveness studies (Calder, Phillps, & Tybout, 1982).

Depending on its research goal, a given study will employ a specific research design that emphasizes either internal or external validity and, in turn, introduces potential limitations (Higgins et al., 2011). For example, threats to a study's internal validity include *biases* that distort the planned comparison between intervention and outcome (Fewtrell et al., 2008). The different study designs are briefly summarized below, with reference to their respective issues of validity (biases), and insight into how to critically evaluate their outcomes.

Experimental Designs: Randomized Controlled Trials

Whenever randomization is practical, randomized controlled trials (RCTs) are recommended to evaluate the efficacy/effectiveness of interventions (Craig et al., 2008). Randomization offers a participant or cluster of participants (e.g. a school) an equal probability of being assigned to the experimental group (those exposed to the intervention) or to the control group (those not exposed to the intervention), thereby distributing unmeasured extraneous variables randomly and reducing the risk of selection bias (DeMets & Cook, 2019; Victora et al., 2004; Viswanathan, Berkman, Dryden, & Harling, 2013). Selection bias occurs when there are differences in the baseline characteristics of participants, and together with randomization, it can be minimized by recruiting participants based on eligibility criteria and ensuring their continued participation (Grimes & Schulz, 2002). However, if the rate of attrition is high (i.e. high drop-out rate), the risk of bias increases, particularly if those lost to follow-up differ from those retained in the study or if there is differential attrition between the intervention and control groups (Fewtrell et al., 2008). Another type of bias can be introduced if recruitment strategies result in samples that are comprised of only those willing to participate (i.e. volunteers). For youth, school is a common setting within which to target PA behavior (Hills, Dengel, & Lubans, 2015); however, school-based PA interventions require a multi-level recruitment process that involves the school district, school administrators, teachers, and students/parents (e.g. Edwardson et al., 2015). At the institution level, principals and teachers may decline invitations to participate in research due to scheduling issues, role overload, and/or student behavior issues (Lamb, Puskar, & Tusaie-Mumford, 2001), and at the participant level, parental consent and student assent are required (Schoeppe et al., 2013). For non-school-based PA interventions, recruiting youth typically involves parent-targeted media advertisements using traditional and/or social platforms, and announcements posted within the community such as in health-care centers, schools, recreational centers, daycares, and pediatric agencies (e.g. Shapiro et al., 2008). Each of these sampling techniques is susceptible to volunteer bias due to the likely presence of differences between consenters and non-consenters (Hernán, Hernández-Díaz, & Robins, 2004). For example, consenting parents are more likely to be conscious of health issues and their child's engagement in PA than are non-consenting parents (Harrington et al., 1997). Therefore, selection and volunteer bias are important considerations when evaluating the validity of (cluster-)RCTs (Carlson & Morrison, 2009).

Quasi-Experimental Designs: Non-Randomized Controlled Trials

When a randomized approach is not feasible, a quasi- or non-experimental design may be considered. Quasi-experimental designs include an external comparison group to assess whether trends in outcomes differ in exposed and non-exposed areas, but the intervention and control groups are included in the study as pre-existing, intact units (Speroff & O'Connor, 2004). This type of design may be employed when researchers want to examine the impact of an existing school playing environment (e.g. Wood, Gladwell, & Barton, 2014), implemented school policy (e.g. Cradock et al., 2014), or ongoing program (e.g. Haapala et al., 2017) on children's PA. In these scenarios, the intervention groups are pre-determined (students attending the exposed schools), and the comparison groups are drawn from separate schools that are as similar as possible to the intervention schools in terms of baseline characteristics, but that do not offer the examined PA opportunities.

Findings from non-randomized controlled trials provide evidence of a plausible causal effect; however, they cannot be relied upon to yield unbiased estimates of the effects of the intervention (Stoto & Cosler, 2008). The absence of randomization can produce groups that differ in important ways, thereby introducing selection bias due to extraneous factors such as confounders or moderators (Grimes & Schulz, 2002; Tooth, Ware, Bain, Purdie, & Dobson, 2005). For PA interventions, confounding factors include imbalances in baseline PA levels and fixed demographic factors such as age, sex, and socio-economic status (SES) (Bauman, Sallis, Dzewaltowski, & Owen, 2002; Rhodes et al., 2017). Because confounding variables can influence a study's results without being directly involved in the causal pathway, they should be controlled for in the study's design (Bauman et al., 2002). For example, in a quasi-experimental study conducted with two elementary schools (one intervention and one comparison) that differed significantly with respect to baseline SES, statistical analyses included SES as a covariate to minimize its potential confounding effect on children's PA (Nathan et al., 2017).

Moderating variables are those that affect the strength of the relationship between intervention and outcome (Bauman et al., 2002). For PA interventions among youth, an increasing body of evidence is indicating that programs appear to work better for girls than for boys, and for younger children than for older children (Gourlan et al., 2018; Yildirim et al., 2011). A better understanding of moderators can help tailor interventions to the needs of specific subgroups and/or places. For example, allowing only females to participate (e.g. Owen et al., 2018), specifying an age-range (e.g. Byun, Lau, & Brusseau, 2018) or focusing on low-income areas (e.g. Chuang, Sharma, Perry, & Diamond, 2018) can elucidate how different levels of the moderator variable can influence the impact of the intervention. While this strategy increases internal validity, it limits generalizability of the findings.

Non-Experimental Designs

Non-experimental designs do not include a control or comparison group; rather, they measure within-person or within-organization changes to evaluate the impact of an intervention, exposure, or program (Speroff & O'Connor, 2004). The major limitation of non-experimental designs

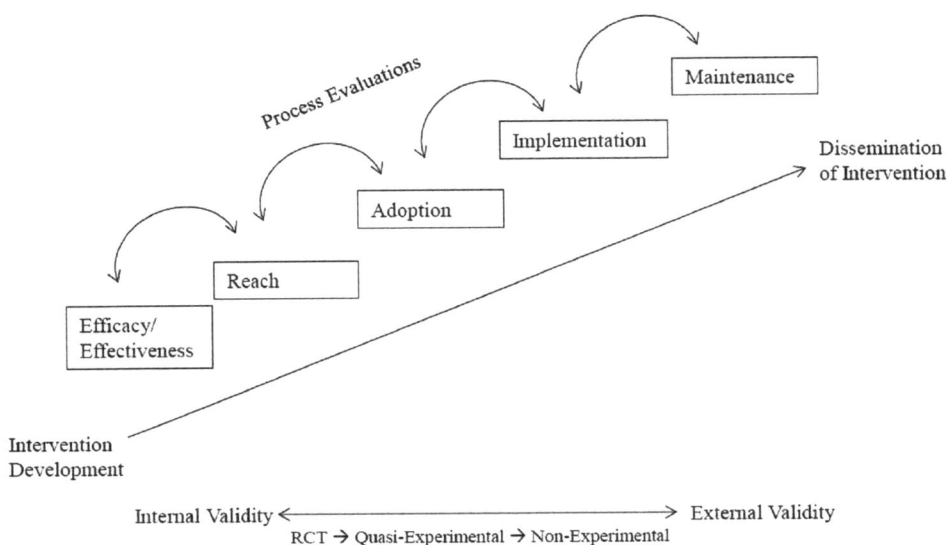

Figure 22.2   Using RE-AIM framework to evaluate implementation and dissemination of PA interventions (as informed by Reis et al., 2016). RCT: randomized controlled trial

is that, without a control group, there is no way to evaluate whether changes are attributable to the intervention or to other factors. For example, uncontrolled PA interventions conducted with youth cannot differentiate between exposure effects and the trajectories in PA change that are associated with age (Beltran-Valls et al., 2019) or seasonal variations (Ridgers, Salmon, & Timperio, 2015). Because they cannot support inference, non-experimental studies provide the lowest level of evidence when evaluating efficacy/effectiveness (Stoto & Cosler, 2008). Despite their low hierarchical position for evidence quality, these designs can provide useful information surrounding issues of external validity, and for this reason, are often used during other phases of the research process (e.g. feasibility, implementation) (see Figure 22.2).

Examples of non-experimental research designs employed in the field of PA promotion include the pre/post-intervention comparison method (e.g. Tomlin et al., 2012) and the case study method (e.g. Bowles, Ní Chróinín, & Murtagh, 2019). Pre/post studies measure baseline PA levels and compare them to PA levels after exposure to the intervention. The goal of this type of study is to attribute any differences across the two single time points (before and after) to the intervention. For example, the Dance 4 Your Life intervention could not include a control group due to timetabling challenges and the availability of students; however, measures collected prior to and following the 6-week contemporary dance program showed that the intervention significantly improved components of female adolescents' physical fitness and psychological well-being (Connolly, Quin, & Redding, 2011). While the design was not robust enough to unequivocally rule out extraneous factors associated with time, chance fluctuation, or placebo effect (Pellegrin, Carek, & Edwards, 1995), the findings contributed to the evidence base by supporting the use of dance as a strategy for PA promotion in this population.

For PA case studies, there is no comparison measure; rather, they provide detail about a specific case (e.g. school policy to promote PA) and imply a comparison between measured outcomes and those that would have been had the intervention not occurred (Campbell & Stanley, 1966). Case studies are typically conducted to obtain qualitative data, and may occur in the development and/or feasibility phases to understand how context might influence outcomes, to explore potential intervention delivery, or to hypothesize mechanisms of action (Fletcher et al., 2016; O'Cathain et al., 2015). Case studies may also be conducted after intervention testing to generate insight into factors that influenced the interpretation of the intervention program, its different components, and its implementation within a variety of contexts (Simovska & Carlsson, 2012). Following the collection of pilot data for Action Schools! BC, a whole-school PA intervention, a descriptive case study was conducted to evaluate the context and impact of the ecological partnership-based model at the provincial/systems level, and to identify facilitators and barriers associated with its delivery (Naylor, Macdonald, Reed, & McKay, 2006). The focus group data from this case study were used to inform the iterative phases of the intervention's evolution, which spanned 6 years and included assessments of feasibility (Naylor, Macdonald, Zebedee, Reed, & McKay, 2006), efficacy (Naylor, Macdonald, Warburton, Reed, & McKay, 2008) and effectiveness (Nettlefold et al., 2012), and implementation after scale-up across the province of British Columbia (McKay et al., 2015; Mâsse, McKay, Valente, Brant, & Naylor, 2012; Naylor et al., 2010).

The Implementation Phase: Evaluating Process

Understanding how *actual* implementation of an intervention differs from *planned* implementation helps to explain null findings and to identify issues important for the transferability of effective strategies outside of experimental conditions (O'Cathain, Thomas, Drabble, Rudolph, & Hewison, 2013). To that end, process evaluations (i.e. evaluations of an intervention's implementation) consider both internal and external validity of an intervention (Durlak & DuPre, 2008; Fletcher et al., 2016). The MRC developed a process evaluation framework (Moore et al., 2015) that functions to inform why an intervention was or was not successful by distinguishing between experimental outcomes and implementation-related outcomes (i.e. process evaluation components), and emphasizing their interactions with context (Durlak & DuPre, 2008; Saunders, Evans, & Joshi, 2005).

Although there is no consensus on the key implementation-related outcomes of a process evaluation (Moore et al., 2015), those that are conducted for complex health promotion interventions typically include measures of intervention fidelity, reach, dose delivered, dose received, implementation cost, and contextual influences on implementation (Durlak & DuPre, 2008; Hasson, 2010; Linnan & Steckler, 2002; Proctor et al., 2011; Saunders et al., 2005) (see Table 22.1). Implementation-related outcomes that are most often evaluated in youth PA interventions (Naylor et al., 2015) include participation/adherence to the intervention by the target population (i.e. dose received) (e.g. Pate et al., 2003) and implementer's adherence to protocol (i.e. dose delivered) (e.g. Huberty, Beets, Beighle, Saint-Maurice, & Welk, 2014). Contextual factors (i.e. facilitators and barriers) associated with variations in implementation of school-based PA interventions are increasingly being reported, and include scheduling issues, resource availability, and social influences (teacher motivation/engagement, student enjoyment, school board support) (Naylor et al., 2015; Nathan et al., 2018; Weatherson, McKay, Gainforth, & Jung, 2017). Less well reported in the field of PA promotion include evaluations of reach, fidelity, and costs (Langford et al., 2017; McGoey, Root, Bruner, & Law, 2015, 2016). Assessments of reach and fidelity are critical for interpreting and understanding results because participant engagement is essential for targeted behavior change (Lloyd, McHugh, Minton, Eke, & Wyatt, 2017), and adherence to protocol can influence the relationship between intervention and outcome (Quested et al., 2017). Similarly, cost-effectiveness evidence is important for policy makers and health system payers when making decisions about program investment and allocation of resources (Michie, Yardley, West, Patrick, & Greaves, 2017). Therefore, as expanded upon below in the Emerging Issues section, there is a growing need within the field of PA promotion for process evaluations to include these measures.

Table 22.1 Process evaluation components: implementation outcomes

Implementation-related outcome	Description
Intervention fidelity	The extent to which the intervention was delivered as intended with respect to its hypothesized mechanism of change (function). Compliance with intervention's purpose and core principles/intervention components.
Reach	The extent to which the intended audience comes into contact with the intervention.
Dose delivered	The extent to which all of the intended intervention features and materials were incorporated in delivery. Adherence to protocols and degree to which modifications were made.
Dose received	The extent to which participants engaged in the intervention activities Participant attendance, engagement, and compliance.
Implementation cost	The identification of specific costs associated with implementation, assessment of financial feasibility (i.e. cost is not a barrier to repeat and/or to transfer), and calculations of cost-effectiveness.
Context	The identification of factors external to the intervention (e.g. issues related to organization, community, and/or social/political/economic climate) that acted as barriers or facilitators to its implementation.

Note: Outcomes and descriptions were compiled from Durlak and DuPre (2008), Hasson (2010), Linnan and Steckler (2002), Proctor et al. (2011), and Saunders et al. (2005).

Process evaluations can precede, run parallel to, be embedded within, or follow intervention studies (Linnan & Steckler, 2002), often employing a combination of quantitative and qualitative research methods (i.e. mixed methods) (Grant, Treweek, Dreischulte, Foy, & Guthrie, 2013) and a variety of data collection methods, including checklists completed by intervention providers; surveys, interviews and focus groups with participants and providers; behavioral observations by researchers; and use of archival records and administrative data (Griffin et al., 2014; Shah et al., 2017). Evaluating implementation-related outcomes proactively (e.g. during the pilot phase) can influence future intervention delivery, while retroactive evaluations (e.g. after the testing phase) can examine unanticipated problems that occurred during implementation (see Figure 22.2) (Grant et al., 2013). To that end, several strategies for process evaluations have been employed, such as embedding them within the pilot or efficacy/effectiveness trial, integrating research and practice personnel within a participatory model, or employing more than one study design via the conductance of a companion study. The balance of this section uses select PA interventions to expand on and exemplify each of these strategies.

The process evaluation for Active Schools: Skelmersdale was embedded within the cluster-RCT and collected data from multiple sources using various methods, including teacher interviews, children focus groups with drawing, and researcher observations of students (Taylor, Noonan, Knowles, Owen, & Fairclough, 2018). Together, the data identified implementation barriers (time and space) and facilitators (flexibility of delivery), and highlighted how different school contexts influenced protocol adaptations, which, in turn, impacted the dose that was delivered to the participants.

The participatory model involves partnerships between the researchers and relevant stakeholders to address potential barriers related to cost-effectiveness and organizational structure, and to facilitate implementation and adoption of the intervention within its intended delivery system (Harden, Johnson, Almeida, & Estabrooks, 2017; Wandersman et al., 2008). For example, in their study examining whether a professional development workshop for teachers could increase student PA levels, Weaver et al. (2018) used a participatory-based approach that included teachers as key stakeholders. Both experimental outcomes (student PA levels) and implementation outcomes (fidelity) were measured, and statistical modeling techniques provided evidence that intervention strategies were implemented by participating teachers, and that implementation was related to increased student PA levels (Weaver et al., 2018).

Process evaluations in the form of companion studies often employ the use of a framework such as RE-AIM, the five dimensions of which (reach, efficacy/effectiveness, adoption, implementation, and maintenance) overlap to some extent with key implementation-related outcomes of a process evaluation (see Table 22.2) (Glasgow, Klesges, Dzewaltowski, Bull, & Estabrooks, 2004; Grant et al., 2013; Griffin et al., 2014). As defined in Table 22.2, the dimensions of the RE-AIM framework collectively operationalize factors related to the representativeness of the participants, implementers and settings, and consider the real-world applicability of an intervention (Glasgow, Vogt, & Boles, 1999). The JUMP-in program provides an example of how a RE-AIM process evaluation has been proactively applied to the design and implementation of a school-based, multi-level PA intervention aimed at the promotion of PA behavior in children. Using the RE-AIM framework, the researchers identified challenges in a pilot study (Jurg, Kremers, Candel, & de Meij, 2006), which were then addressed in the design and delivery of an adapted program (de Meij et al., 2010). The adaptations addressed key internal and external validity issues, as conceptualized by the five RE-AIM dimensions (italicized and illustrated as follows). Regarding internal validity, the *efficacy* of the revised intervention was evaluated using objective measures of PA and included mediation and moderation analyses to assess the effects of social environmental influences on PA behavior, and to determine whether effects were more prominent among or restricted to certain subgroups. Specific to external validity issues, the generalizability of the pilot study was compromised due to inadequate *reach* for at-risk individuals and because of barriers impeding *adoption* by all school staff. In response, the researchers incorporated intervention components that were tailored to the needs of at-risk children (i.e. those who were overweight, inactive, or who had motor disabilities), and increased participation among implementers by allowing for sufficient preparation time and providing clear expectations about tasks and responsibilities. To enhance translatability,

Table 22.2 RE-AIM dimensions and their application to process evaluations

Dimension	Description	Overlap with process evaluation components
Reach	The extent to which the sample of participants reflects the entirety of the potentially eligible population.	Reach
Efficacy/ Effectiveness	The impact of an intervention on important outcomes when tested under optimum conditions (efficacy) or in real-world settings by individuals who are not part of the research team (effectiveness).	Fidelity (impact of deviations from intervention processes on behavioral outcomes)
Adoption	The potential influences of the intervention's site characteristics on the intervention's delivery.	Dose Delivered, Context
Implementation	The fidelity of the intervention's delivery, and the costs associated therewith.	Fidelity, Dose Received, Dose Delivered
Maintenance	The sustainability of the intervention and the costs associated with its institutionalization.	Context

Note: RE-AIM dimensions and descriptions obtained from Glasgow et al. (2004).

the revised intervention was accompanied by continuous collection of *implementation*-related measures to gain further insight into which program components were used and how many children participated, and to gauge the level of parental engagement (de Meij, van de Wal, van Machelen, & Paw, 2013). Policies that support the adoption of evidence-based PA interventions are required to ensure their ongoing maintenance (Austin, Bell, Caperchione, & Mummery, 2011); therefore, to promote long-term *maintenance* of the JUMP-in program, its organization and management were modified to promote participation in local and national public health policy debate (de Meij et al., 2010). Together, these ongoing process evaluations maximized the adoption and implementation of the program, which has been successfully embedded within the Amsterdam municipal policy, and in the organizational structure and daily practices of the schools involved (de Meij et al., 2010).

The Scale-Up and Dissemination Phase: Evaluating Translatability

Once an evidence base of efficacy has been established, the ultimate goal of PA interventions should be their eventual dissemination into real-world settings, where they will be maintained and institutionalized (e.g. the Action Schools! BC and JUMP-in programs). Scale-up and dissemination involve the conversion of scientific knowledge into user-friendly products in a dynamic process called translation (Koorts et al., 2018; Lewis et al., 2017). Successful translation of a PA intervention implies the sustainability of its health benefits, meaning that it has become embedded within a system (Reis et al., 2016). For example, in a follow-up process evaluation conducted 2–5 years post-implementation of a healthy lifestyle school program, interviews with senior school staff revealed that it had become integrated into the elementary school's day-to-day organization and practices, thus confirming its sustainability and successful translation (Passmore & Jones, 2018).

Most evaluation efforts pertaining to translation of PA interventions focus on whether the program is reaching the specified target population and whether the intervention is being properly implemented (Reis et al., 2016). Additional considerations include effectiveness over time and compatibility in diverse practice systems (Milat et al., 2016). To that end, important features to consider when evaluating the scalability of health promotion interventions include program fidelity and the counter-acting pressure of program adaptation, as well as the cost-effectiveness of alternative approaches to intervention delivery (Milat, King, Bauman, & Redman, 2012).

As interventions increase further in scale (i.e. reach a greater proportion of the eligible population) and are disseminated widely into policy and practice, quality control and performance monitoring systems replace individual intervention evaluations (Milat et al., 2012). Another example of a widely disseminated health promotion initiative is New South Wales' government-funded state-wide Healthy Children Initiative, the organizational reach of which includes early childhood settings and primary schools (Innes-Hughes et al., 2017). Performance monitoring of programs associated with this initiative involved measures of service delivery (reach, local government follow-up and support, program participation by individual sites) and indicators of adoption of specific organizational practices (adoption of key practices, policy, training and information, planning and monitoring), which served as a feedback process to support improvements in delivery and impact, and as a mechanism to ensure that program goals were being met (Farrell et al., 2014). These key underlying concepts are addressed by the RE-AIM framework, expanding its use as an evaluative model to include considerations of the scalability and dissemination of PA interventions (see Figure 22.2) (Glasgow et al., 2003; Lewis et al., 2017; Reis et al., 2016).

Emerging Issues

Historically, researchers and the scientific community have prioritized internal validity, crediting it as a prerequisite for external validity since extrapolation of invalid results to the broader population is pointless (Grimes & Schulz, 2002). As a result, there is a relative dearth of external validity data, which, in turn, has resulted in poor translatability of research findings in areas of prevention, intervention, and education (Wandersman et al., 2008). The field of PA promotion is no exception to this phenomenon; systematic reviews of interventions conducted with both children (McGoey et al., 2016) and adolescents (McGoey et al., 2015) have reported a focus on establishing causal relationships between intervention strategies and PA outcomes, with minimal considerations of reach, adoption, and cost. While many PA interventions evaluate some process data, most use simplistic quantitative assessments of outcomes (Langford et al., 2017) with nominal input from qualitative research that could increase understanding of generalizability (Michie et al., 2017). Addressing these considerations in the design phase and across the continuum of intervention research would facilitate widespread adoption and maintenance of PA promotion programs (Milat et al., 2012).

To that end, PA interventions are increasingly being designed to accommodate adaptations based on contextual needs (e.g. Blaine et al., 2017; Cheung et al., 2019; Egan et al., 2018; Fairclough et al., 2013). However, the impacts of context-based modifications made to the intervention's form are rarely evaluated (Sutherland et al., 2017), which highlights a need to improve and standardize approaches to measuring implementation-related outcomes. Defining fidelity as evidence-of-fit with the principles of the hypothesized mechanisms of change (Hawe, Shiell, & Riley, 2004), this construct can be evaluated based on whether or not the intervention performed the same function (mechanism of change) while its form (less central components) was tailored to local contexts (Hawe, Shiell, & Riley, 2009). This would facilitate the demarcation of adaptations made to achieve a good ecological fit, and those that undermine intervention fidelity (i.e. those made to core program components). To that end, combining evaluation of process with intervention outcomes would allow researchers to elucidate the linkage between degree of fidelity achieved and impact on measured PA behavior, and ultimately, to more reliably compare results across studies (Koorts et al., 2018; Moore et al., 2015; Naylor et al., 2015; Schaapp, Bessems, Otten, Kremers, & van Nassau, 2018).

Recommendations for Researchers/Practitioners

In summary, the purpose of PA intervention evaluations is to disentangle the factors that influence the success of intervention strategies, thus informing their transition from research to practice. This can be challenging due to context sensitivity of the findings, variability in outcome measures, problems obtaining statistically sufficient numbers of participants who are representative of the target population, fidelity in terms of delivery of the intervention, and varying levels of engagement with the intervention. Further, multiple perspectives need to be considered, including those from national governments, policy makers, research funders, academic researchers, the staff delivering the intervention, and the participants. Addressing research questions targeting what works, and delineating where, when, how, why, and for whom an intervention strategy is effective involve assimilating data from a broad range of study designs. To facilitate this assimilation, a systematic method for capturing the different types of reported relationships in the cumulative body of evidence is required. To that end, Table 22.3 serves as a framework that organizes evaluation questions relating to the concepts of an intervention's efficacy/effectiveness and translatability.

Table 22.3 PA intervention evaluation questions: assessing what works, for whom, and under which conditions

What works: Establishing a link between intervention and outcome	For Whom: Defining the population exposed to the intervention	Under what conditions		How	Why
		When	Where		
What was the intervention's aim/objective?	What was the age range of the targeted sample?	What was the context of the measured PA?	What was the setting for the intervention?	What, if any, was the extent to which theory was used?	Was a process evaluation conducted to examine implementation and dissemination?
• Specific strategies employed such as the use of playground markings, or a computer-based delivery • Length of intervention	• Preschoolers • Children • Adolescents	• Overall (weekdays and weekends) • In-school (class-based and/or recess)	• School-based • Day care • Community-based • Family-based • Primary-care based • Combination	• Identification of theory and theoretical constructs • Measurement of theoretical constructs • Measurement of the mediating effects of theoretical constructs	• Implementation fidelity • Implementation costs • Attendance rates (Dose) • Implementers' evaluation of the program (e.g. teacher willingness and ability to deliver) • Participants' assessment of the program (e.g. student feedback) • Stakeholder's engagement with the program (e.g. parent feedback)
Which level(s) of influence was/were targeted?	Was a specific sub-population targeted?	• Leisure time (after-school) • Organized sports	Was a specific region targeted for delivery of the intervention?	Were there resources dedicated to or consumed by the intervention?	
• Individual • Interpersonal • Environmental • Political	• Female or male • Low SES • Minority population • At-risk population (e.g. for obesity)	How many times were measures collected?	• Rural or urban areas • Low-income or high-income • Use of a built environment (e.g. park, sidewalks, recreational facility)	• Money • Staff time • Facilities and equipment	How was the implementation data collected?
How was PA measured?	What was the recruitment method?	• Baseline • Mid-intervention • Post-intervention • Follow-up		Who delivered the intervention?	• Teacher interviews • Parent Focus groups • Questionnaires • Participant journals
• Observation • Self-report • Parental report • Accelerometer • Pedometer • Combination	• Invitation sent to school or school district • Parent-and/or adolescent-targeted announcements posted in the community, on social media, or mailed as fliers			• Researchers • Practice personnel (e.g. teachers) • Combination	Is the current status of the program/intervention known?
Which PA dimension was measured?	What was the reach of the intervention?			Was training and/or technical assistance/coaching/on-site assistance offered?	• Long-term follow-up data • Adoption of the program within a system
• Frequency • Duration • Intensity • Type	• Participation rate (number participating/number eligible) • Comparisons between the characteristics of the consenters and non-consenters				
How was the PA outcome reported?	Was the sample size reduced during the intervention?				
• Counts per minute • Steps per day • Minutes of MVPA/day • Percentage of time spent in MVPA • Participation in organized sports activities • Energy expenditure in METS • Active transportation	• Attrition • Issues with monitor refusal, non-return, non-wear or insufficient wear time (when using objective measure) • Were the characteristics of those lost to follow-up compared to those who remained in the study?				

Note: PA: physical activity, MVPA: moderate-to-vigorous physical activity, METS: metabolic equivalents, SES: socioeconomic status.

References

Adab, P., Pallan, M. J., Lancashire, E. R., Hemming, K., Frew, E., Griffin, T., . . . Deeks, J. (2015). A cluster-randomised controlled trial to assess the effectiveness and cost-effectiveness of a childhood obesity prevention programme delivered through schools, targeting 6–7 year old children: The WAVES study protocol. *BMC Public Health, 15*(1), 488.

Ajzen, I. (1991). The theory of planned behavior. *Organizational Behavior and Human Decision Processes, 50*(2), 179–211. doi:10.1016/0749-5978(91)90020-T

Atkin, A. J., van Sluijs, E. M. F., Dollman, J., Taylor, W. C., & Stanley, R. M. (2016). Identifying correlates and determinants of physical activity in youth: How can we advance the field? *Preventive Medicine, 87*, 167–169.

Austin, G., Bell, T., Caperchione, C., & Mummery, W. K. (2011). Translating research to practice: Using the RE-AIM framework to examine an evidence-based physical activity intervention in primary school settings. *Health Promotion Practice, 12*(6), 932–941.

Bandura, A. (1997). *Self-efficacy: The exercise of control.* New York: W.H. Freeman and Company.

Bauman, A. E., Reis, R. S., Sallis, J. F., Wells, J. C., Loos, R. J., & Martin, B. W. (2012). Correlates of physical activity: Why are some people physically active and others not? *The Lancet, 380*(9838), 258–271.

Bauman, A. E., Sallis, J. F., Dzewaltowski, D. A., & Owen, N. (2002). Toward a better understanding of the influences on physical activity: The role of determinants, correlates, causal variables, mediators, moderators, and confounders. *American Journal of Preventive Medicine, 23*(2), 5–14. doi:10.1016/S0749-3797(02)00469-5

Beets, M. W., Okely, A., Weaver, R. G., Webster, C., Lubans, D., Brusseau, T., . . . Cliff, D. P. (2016). The theory of expanded, extended, and enhanced opportunities for youth physical activity promotion. *International Journal of Behavioral Nutrition and Physical Activity, 13*(1), 120.

Beltran-Valls, M. R., Janssen, X., Farooq, A., Adamson, A. J., Pearce, M. S., Reilly, J. K., . . . Reilly, J. J. (2019). Longitudinal changes in vigorous intensity physical activity from childhood to adolescence: Gateshead Millennium Study. *Journal of Science and Medicine in Sport, 22*(4), 450–455.

Blaine, R. E., Franckle, R. L., Ganter, C., Falbe, J., Giles, C., Criss, S., . . . Davison, K. K. (2017). Using school staff members to implement a childhood obesity prevention intervention in low-income school districts: The Massachusetts Childhood Obesity Research Demonstration (MA-CORD Project), 2012–2014. *Preventing Chronic Disease, 14*, E03.

Bond, B., Weston, K. L., Williams, C. A., & Barker, A. R. (2017). Perspectives on high-intensity interval exercise for health promotion in children and adolescents. *Open Access Journal of Sports Medicine, 8*, 243–265.

Bonell, C., Fletcher, A., Morton, M., Lorenc, T., & Moore, L. (2012). Realist randomised controlled trials: A new approach to evaluating complex public health interventions. *Social Science & Medicine, 75*(12), 2299–2306.

Booth, S. L., Sallis, J. F., Ritenbaugh, C., Hill, J. O., Birch, L. L., Frank, L. D., . . . Hays, N. P. (2001). Environmental and societal factors affect food choice and physical activity: Rationale, influences, and leverage points. *Nutrition reviews, 59*(3), S21–S36. doi:10.1111/j.1753-4887.2001.tb06983.x

Borde, R., Smith, J. S., Sutherland, R., Nathan, N., & Lubans, D. R. (2017). Methodological considerations and impact of school-based interventions on objectively measured physical activity in adolescents: A systematic review and meta-analysis. *Obesity Reviews, 18*(4), 476–490. doi:10.1111/obr.12517

Bowles, R., Ní Chróinín, D., & Murtagh, E. (2019). Attaining the Active School Flag: How physical activity provision can be enhanced in Irish primary schools. *European Physical Education Review, 25*(1), 76–88.

Brown, H., Hume, C., Pearson, N., & Salmon, J. (2013). A systematic review of intervention effects on potential mediators of children's physical activity. *BMC Public Health, 13*(1), 165. doi:10.1186/1471-2458-13-165

Byun, W., Lau, E., & Brusseau, T. (2018). Feasibility and Effectiveness of a Wearable Technology-Based Physical Activity Intervention in Preschoolers: A Pilot Study. *International Journal of Environmental Research and Public Health, 15*(9), 1821.

Calder, B. J., Phillips, L. W. & Tybout, A. M. (1982). The concept of external validity. *Journal of Consumer Research, 9*, 240–244.

Campbell, D. T., & Stanley, J. C. (1966). *Experimental and quasi-experimental designs for research.* Chicago, IL: Rand McNally College Pub Co.

Campbell, M., Fitzpatrick, R., Haines, A., Kinmonth, A. L., Sandercock, P., Spiegelhalter, D., & Tyrer, P. (2000). Framework for design and evaluation of complex interventions to improve health. *BMJ, 321*(7262), 694–696.

Campbell, N. C., Murray, E., Darbyshire, J., Emery, J., Farmer, A., Griffiths, F., . . . Kinmonth, A. L. (2007). Designing and evaluating complex interventions to improve health care. *BMJ, 334*(7591), 455–459.

Carlson, M. D. A., & Morrison, R. S. (2009). Study design, precision, and validity in observational studies. *Journal of Palliative Medicine, 12*(1), 77–82.

Chatzisarantis, N. L., & Hagger, M. S. (2009). Effects of an intervention based on self-determination theory on self-reported leisure-time physical activity participation. *Psychology and Health, 24*(1), 29–48.

Cheung, P., Franks, P., Kramer, M., Drews-Botsch, C., Welsh, J., Kay, C., . . . Gazmararian, J. (2019). Impact of a Georgia elementary school-based intervention on physical activity opportunities: A quasi-experimental study. *Journal of Science and Medicine in Sport, 22*(2), 191–195.

Chuang, R. J., Sharma, S. V., Perry, C., & Diamond, P. (2018). Does the CATCH early childhood program increase physical activity among low-income preschoolers?—Results from a pilot study. *American Journal of Health Promotion, 32*(2), 344–348.

Coleman, K. J., Tiller, C. L., Sanchez, J., Heath, E. M., Sy, O., Milliken, G., & Dzewaltowski, D. A. (2005). Prevention of the epidemic increase in child risk of overweight in low-income schools: The El Paso co-ordinated approach to child health. *Archives of Pediatrics and Adolescent Medicine, 159*, 217–224.

Connolly, M. K., Quin, E., & Redding, E. (2011). Dance 4 your life: Exploring the health and well-being implications of a contemporary dance intervention for female adolescents. *Research in Dance Education, 12*(1), 53–66.

Corder, K., Brown, H. E., Schiff, A., & van Sluijs, E. M. (2016). Feasibility study and pilot cluster-randomised controlled trial of the GoActive intervention aiming to promote physical activity among adolescents: Outcomes and lessons learnt. *BMJ Open, 6*(11), e012335.

Cousson-Gélie, F., Carayol, M., Fregeac, B., Mora, L., Jeanleboeuf, F., Coste, O., . . . Gourlan, M. (2019). The "great live and move challenge": A program to promote physical activity among children aged 7–11 years. Design and implementation of a cluster-randomized controlled trial. *BMC Public Health, 19*(1), 367.

Cradock, A. L., Barrett, J. L., Carter, J., McHugh, A., Sproul, J., Russo, E. T., . . . Gortmaker, S. L. (2014). Impact of the Boston Active School Day Policy to Promote Physical Activity among Children. *American Journal of Health Promotion, 28*(3_suppl), S54–S64.

Craig, P., Di Ruggiero, E., Frolich, K. L., Mykhalovskiy, E., & White, M. on behalf of the Canadian Institutes of Health Research (CIHR) – National Institute for Health Research (NIHR) Context Guidance Authors Group. (2018). Taking account of context in population health intervention research: Guidance for producers, users and funders of research. Southampton: NIHR Evaluation, Trials and Studies Coordinating Centre.

Craig, P., Dieppe, P., Macintyre, S., Michie, S., Nazareth, I., & Petticrew, M. (2008). Developing and evaluating complex interventions: The new medical research council guidance. *British Medical Journal (Clinical Research Ed.), 337*, a1655.

de Meij, J. S. B., Paw, M. J. M, Kremers, S. P. J., van der Wal, M. F., Jurg, M. E., & van Machelen, W. (2010). Promoting physical activity in children: The stepwise development of the primary school-based JUMP-in intervention applying the RE-AIM evaluation framework. *British Journal of Sports Medicine, 44*(12), 879–887.

de Meij, J. S., van der Wal, M. F., van Mechelen, W., & Paw, M. J. (2013). A mixed methods process evaluation of the implementation of JUMP-in, a multilevel school-based intervention aimed at physical activity promotion. *Health Promotion Practice, 14*(5), 777–790.

Demetriou, Y., & Bachner, J. (2019). A school-based intervention based on self-determination theory to promote girls' physical activity: Study protocol of the CReActivity cluster randomised controlled trial. *BMC Public Health, 19*(1), 519.

DeMets, D. L. & Cook, T. (2019). Challenges of non-intention-to-treat analyses. *Journal of the American Medical Association, 321*(2), 145–146.

Direito, A., Jiang, Y., Whittaker, R., & Maddison, R. (2015). Smartphone apps to improve fitness and increase physical activity among young people: Protocol of the Apps for IMproving FITness (AIMFIT) randomized controlled trial. *BMC Public Health, 15*(1), 635.

Dishman, R. K., Motl, R. W., Saunders, R., Felton, G., Ward, D. S., Dowda, M., & Pate, R. R. (2004). Self-efficacy partially mediates the effect of a school-based physical-activity intervention among adolescent girls. *Preventive Medicine, 38*(5), 628–636.

Dishman, R. K., Motl, R. W., Saunders, R., Felton, G., Ward, D. S., Dowda, M., & Pate, R. R. (2005). Enjoyment mediates effects of a school-based physical-activity intervention. *Medicine and Science in Sports and Exercise, 37*(3), 478–487.

Durlak, J. A., & DuPre, E. P. (2008). Implementation matters: A review of research on the influence of implementation on program outcomes and the factors affecting implementation. *American Journal of Community Psychology, 41*(3–4), 327–350.

Edwardson, C. L., Harrington, D. M., Yates, T., Bodicoat, D. H., Khunti, K., Gorely, T., . . . Davies, M. J. (2015). A cluster randomised controlled trial to investigate the effectiveness and cost effectiveness of the 'Girls Active' intervention: A study protocol. *BMC Public Health, 15*(1), 526.

Egan, C. A., Webster, C., Weaver, R. G., Brian, A., Stodden, D., Russ, L., . . . Vazou, S. (2018). Partnerships for Active Children in Elementary Schools (PACES): First year process evaluation. *Evaluation and Program Planning, 67,* 61–69.

Eldridge, S. M., Lancaster, G. A., Campbell, M. J., Thabane, L., Hopewell, S., Coleman, C. L., & Bond, C. M. (2016). Defining feasibility and pilot studies in preparation for randomised controlled trials: Development of a conceptual framework. *PloS One, 11*(3), e0150205.

Fairclough, S. J., Hackett, A. F., Davies, I. G., Gobbi, R., Mackintosh, K. A., Warburton, G. L., . . . Boddy, L. M. (2013). Promoting healthy weight in primary school children through physical activity and nutrition education: A pragmatic evaluation of the CHANGE! randomised intervention study. *BMC Public Health, 13*(1), 626.

Farrell, L., Lloyd, B., Matthews, R., Bravo, A., Wiggers, J., & Rissel, C. (2014). Applying a performance monitoring framework to increase reach and adoption of children's healthy eating and physical activity programs. *Public Health Research & Practice, 25*(1), e2511408.

Fewtrell, M. S., Kennedy, K., Singhal, A., Martin, R. M., Ness, A., Hadders-Algra, . . . Lucas, A. (2008). How much loss to follow-up is acceptable in long-term randomized trials and prospective studies? *Archives of Disease in Childhood, 93*(6), 458–461.

Flay, B. R. (1986). Efficacy and effectiveness trials (and other phases of research) in the development of health promotion programs. *Preventive Medicine, 15,* 451–474.

Fletcher, A., Jamal, F., Moore, G., Evans, R. E., Murphy, S., & Bonell, C. (2016). Realist complex intervention science: Applying realist principles across all phases of the Medical Research Council framework for developing and evaluating complex interventions. *Evaluation, 22*(3), 286–303.

Glasgow, R. E., Lichtenstein, E., & Marcus, A. (2003). Why don't we see more translation of health promotion research to practice? Rethinking the efficacy to effectiveness transition. *American Journal of Public Health, 93,* 1261–1267.

Glasgow, R. E., Klesges, L. M., Dzewaltowski, D. A., Bull, S. S., & Estabrooks, P. (2004). The future of health behavior change research: What is needed to improve translation of research into health promotion practice? *Annals of Behavioral Medicine, 27,* 3–12.

Glasgow, R. E., Vogt, T. M., & Boles, S. M. (1999). Evaluating the public health impact of health promotion interventions: The RE-AIM framework. *American Journal of Public Health, 89,* 1322–1327.

Gourlan, M., Takito, M., Lambert, C., Fregeac, B., Alméras, N., Coste, O., . . . Cousson-Gélie, F. (2018). Impact and moderating variables of an intervention promoting physical activity among children: Results from a pilot study. *International Quarterly of Community Health Education, 38*(3), 195–203.

Grant, A., Treweek, S., Dreischulte, T., Foy, R., & Guthrie, B. (2013). Process evaluations for cluster-randomised trials of complex interventions: A proposed framework for design and reporting. *Trials, 14,* 15.

Green, L. W., & Glasgow, R. E. (2006). Evaluating the relevance, generalization, and applicability of research: Issues in external validation and translation methodology. *Evaluation & the Health Professions, 29*(1), 126–153.

Griffin, T. L., Clarke, J. L., Lancashire, E. R., Pallan, M. J., & Adab, P. (2017). Process evaluation results of a cluster randomised controlled childhood obesity prevention trial: The WAVES study. *BMC Public Health, 17*(1), 681.

Griffin, T. L., Pallan, M. J., Clarke, J. L., Lancashire, E. R., Lyon, A., Parry, J. M., & Adab, P. (2014). Process evaluation design in a cluster randomised controlled childhood obesity prevention trial: The WAVES study. *International Journal of Behavioral Nutrition and Physical Activity, 11*(1), 112.

Grimes, D. A. & Schulz, K. F. (2002). Bias and causal associations in observational research. *The Lancet, 359,* 248–252.

Haapala, H. L., Hirvensalo, M. H., Kulmala, J., Hakonen, H., Kankaanpää, A., Laine, K., . . . Tammelin, T. H. (2017). Changes in physical activity and sedentary time in the Finnish Schools on the move program: A quasi-experimental study. *Scandinavian Journal of Medicine & Science in Sports, 27*(11), 1442–1453.

Hallal, P. C., Andersen, L. B., Bull, F. C., Guthold, R., Haskell, W., & Ekelund, U. (2012). Global physical activity levels: Surveillance progress, pitfalls, and prospects. *Lancet, 380,* 247–257. doi:10.1016/S0140-6736(12)60646-1

Hallingberg, B., Turley, R., Segrott, J., Wight, D., Craig, P., Moore, L., . . . Moore, G. (2018). Exploratory studies to decide whether and how to proceed with full-scale evaluations of public health interventions: A systematic review of guidance. *Pilot and Feasibility Studies, 4*(1), 104.

Hardeman, W., Sutton, S., Griffin, S., Johnston, M., White, A., Wareham, N. J., & Kinmonth, A. L. (2005). A causal modelling approach to the development of theory-based behaviour change programmes for trial evaluation. *Health Education Research, 20*(6), 676–687.

Harden, S. M., Johnson, S. B., Almeida, F. A., & Estabrooks, P. A. (2017). Improving physical activity program adoption using integrated research–practice partnerships: An effectiveness-implementation trial. *Translational Behavioral Medicine, 7*, 28–38.

Harrington, K. F., Binkley, D., Reynolds, K. D., Duvall, R. C., Copeland, J. R., Franklin, F., & Raczynski, J. (1997). Recruitment issues in school-based research: Lessons learned from the High 5 Alabama Project. *The Journal of School Health, 67*(10), 415–421.

Hasson, H. (2010). Systematic evaluation of implementation fidelity of complex interventions in health and social care. *Implementation Science, 5*(1), 67.

Hawe, P., Shiell, A., & Riley, T. (2004). Complex interventions: How "out of control" can a randomised controlled trial be?. *BMJ, 328*(7455), 1561–1563.

Hawe, P., Shiell, A., & Riley, T. (2009). Theorising interventions as events in systems. *American Journal of Community Psychology, 43*(3–4), 267–276.

Hawkins, J., Madden, K., Fletcher, A., Midgley, L., Grant, A., Cox, G., . . . White, J. (2017). Development of a framework for the co-production and prototyping of public health interventions. *BMC Public Health, 17*(1), 689.

Hendrie, G. A., Brindal, E., Corsini, N., Gardner, C., Baird, D., & Golley, R. K. (2012). Combined home and school obesity prevention interventions for children: What behavior change strategies and intervention characteristics are associated with effectiveness?. *Health Education & Behavior, 39*(2), 159–171.

Hernán, M. A., Hernández-Díaz, S., & Robins, J. M. (2004). A structural approach to selection bias. *Epidemiology, 15*(5), 615–625.

Higgins, J. P. T., Altman, D. G., Gøtzshe, P. C., Jüni, P., Moher, D., Oxman, A. D., . . . Sterne, J. A. C. (2011). The Cochrane Collaboration's tool for assessing risk of bias in randomized trials. *BMJ, 343*. doi:10.1136/bmj.d5928

Hills, A. P., Dengel, D. R., & Lubans, D. R. (2015). Supporting public health priorities: Recommendations for physical education and physical activity promotion in schools. *Progress in Cardiovascular Diseases, 57*(4), 368–374.

Hortz, B., & Petosa, R. L. (2008). Social cognitive theory variables mediation of moderate exercise. *American Journal of Health Behavior, 32*(3), 305–314.

Huberty, J. L., Beets, M. W., Beighle, A., Saint-Maurice, P. F., & Welk, G. (2014). Effects of ready for recess, an environmental intervention, on physical activity in third-through sixth-grade children. *Journal of Physical Activity and Health, 11*, 384–395.

Innes-Hughes, C., Bravo, A., Buffett, K., Henderson, L., Lockeridge, A., Pimenta, N., . . . Rissel, C. 2017. *NSW healthy children initiative: The first five years July 2011 – June 2016.* Sydney, Australia: NSW Ministry of Health.

James, A. K., Hess, P., Perkins, M. E., Taveras, E. M., & Scirica, C. S. (2017). Prescribing outdoor play: Outdoors Rx. *Clinical Pediatrics, 56*(6), 519–524.

Jung, M. E., Bourne, J. E., & Gainforth, H. L. (2018). Evaluation of a community-based, family focused healthy weights initiative using the RE-AIM framework. *International Journal of Behavioral Nutrition and Physical Activity, 15*(1), 13.

Jurg, M. E., Kremers, S., Candel, M., & de Meij, J. (2006). A controlled trial of a school-based environmental intervention to improve physical activity in Dutch children: JUMP-in, kids in motion. *Health Promotion International, 21*(4), 320–330.

Karczewski, S. A., Carter, J. S., & DeCator, D. D. (2016). The role of ethnicity in school-based obesity intervention for school-aged children: A pilot evaluation. *Journal of School Health, 86*(11), 778–786.

King, A. C., Stokols, D., Talen, E., Brassington, G. S., & Killingsworth, R. (2002). Theoretical approaches to the promotion of physical activity: Forging a transdisciplinary paradigm. *American Journal of Preventive Medicine, 23*(2), 15–25.

Kistin, C., & Silverstein, M. (2015). Pilot studies: A critical but potentially misused component of interventional research. *JAMA, 314*(15), 1561–1562.

Koorts, H., Eakin, E., Estabrooks, P., Timperio, A., Salmon, J., & Bauman, A. (2018). Implementation and scale up of population physical activity interventions for clinical and community settings: The PRACTIS guide. *International Journal of Behavioral Nutrition and Physical Activity, 15*(1), 51.

Lamb, J., Puskar, K. R., & Tusaie-Mumford, K. (2001). Adolescent research recruitment issues and strategies: Application in a rural school setting. *Journal of Pediatric Nursing, 16*(1), 43–52.

Lancaster, G. A., Dodd, S., & Williamson, P. R. (2004). Design and analysis of pilot studies: Recommendations for good practice. *Journal of Evaluation in Clinical Practice, 10*(2), 307–312.

Langford, R., Bonell, C., Komro, K., Murphy, S., Magnus, D., Waters, E., . . . Campbell, R. (2017). The health promoting schools framework: Known unknowns and an agenda for future research. *Health Education & Behavior, 44*(3), 463–475.

Larouche, R., Mammen, G., Rowe, D. A., & Faulkner, G. (2018). Effectiveness of active school transport interventions: A systematic review and update. *BMC Public Health, 18*(1), 206.

Leahy, A. A., Eather, N., Smith, J. J., Hillman, C. H., Morgan, P. J., Plotnikoff, R. C., . . . Lubans, D. R. (2019). Feasibility and preliminary efficacy of a teacher-facilitated high-intensity interval training intervention for older adolescents. *Pediatric Exercise Science, 31*(1), 107–117.

Lewis, B. A., Napolitano, M. A., Buman, M. P., Williams, D. M., & Nigg, C. R. (2017). Future directions in physical activity intervention research: Expanding our focus to sedentary behaviors, technology, and dissemination. *Journal of Behavioral Medicine, 40*(1), 112–126.

Linnan, L., & Steckler, A. (2002). *Process evaluation for public health interventions and research* (pp. 1–23). San Francisco, CA: Jossey-Bass.

Lloyd, J. J., Logan, S., Greaves, C. J., & Wyatt, K. M. (2011). Evidence, theory and context – Using intervention mapping to develop a school-based intervention to prevent obesity in children. *International Journal of Behavioural Nutrition and Physical Activity, 8*, 73.

Lloyd, J., McHugh, C., Minton, J., Eke, H., & Wyatt, K. (2017). The impact of active stakeholder involvement on recruitment, retention and engagement of schools, children and their families in the cluster randomised controlled trial of the Healthy Lifestyles Programme (HeLP): A school-based intervention to prevent obesity. *Trials, 18*(1), 378.

Lloyd, J., & Wyatt, K. (2015). The Healthy Lifestyles Programme (HeLP) – An overview of and recommendations arising from the conceptualization and development of an innovative approach to promoting healthy lifestyles for children and their families. *International Journal of Environmental Research and Public Health, 12*, 1003–1019.

Loef, M., & Walach, H. (2015). How applicable are results of systematic reviews and meta-analyses of health behaviour maintenance? A critical evaluation. *Public Health, 129*, 377–384. doi:10.1016/j.puhe.2015.01.014

Lubans, D. R., Foster, C., & Biddle, S. J. (2008). A review of mediators of behavior in interventions to promote physical activity among children and adolescents. *Preventive Medicine, 47*(5), 463–470.

Lynch, B. A., Gentile, N., Maxson, J., Quigg, S., Swenson, L., & Kaufman, T. (2016). Elementary school–Based obesity intervention using an educational curriculum. *Journal of Primary Care & Community Health, 7*(4), 265–271.

MacKinnon, D. P. (2011). Integrating mediators and moderators in research design. *Research on Social Work and Practice, 21*(6), 675–681.

Mâsse, L. C., McKay, H., Valente, M., Brant, R., & Naylor, P. J. (2012). Physical activity implementation in schools: A 4-year follow-up. *American Journal of Preventive Medicine, 43*(4), 369–377.

McGoey, T., Root, Z., Bruner, M. W., & Law, B. (2015). Evaluation of physical activity interventions in youth via the reach, efficacy/effectiveness, adoption, implementation, and maintenance (RE-AIM) framework: A systematic review of randomised and non-randomised trials. *Preventive Medicine, 76*, 58–67.

McGoey, T., Root, Z., Bruner, M. W., & Law, B. (2016). Evaluation of physical activity interventions in children via the reach, efficacy/effectiveness, adoption, implementation, and maintenance (RE-AIM) framework: A systematic review of randomized and non-randomized trials. *Preventive Medicine, 82*, 8–19.

McKay, H. A., Macdonald, H. M., Nettlefold, L., Masse, L. C., Day, M., & Naylor, P. J. (2015). Action schools! BC implementation: From efficacy to effectiveness to scale-up. *British Journal of Sports Medicine, 49*(4), 210–218.

McKenzie, T. L. (2019). Physical activity within school contexts: The bigger bang theory. *Kinesiology Review, 8*(1), 48–53.

Messing, S., Rütten, A., Abu-Omar, K., Ungerer-Röhrich, U., Goodwin, L., Burlacu, I., & Gediga, G. (2019). How can physical activity be promoted among children and adolescents? A systematic review of reviews across settings. *Frontiers in Public Health, 7*, 55.

Michie, S., Ashford, S., Sniehotta, F. F., Dombrowski, S. U., Bishop, A., & French, D. P. (2011). A refined taxonomy of behaviour change techniques to help people change their physical activity and healthy eating behaviours: The CALO-RE taxonomy. *Psychology & Health, 26*(11): 1479–1498.

Michie, S., & Prestwich, A. (2010). Are interventions theory-based? Development of a theory coding scheme. *Health Psychology, 29*(1), 1–8.

Michie, S., Yardley, L., West, R., Patrick, K., & Greaves, F. (2017). Developing and evaluating digital interventions to promote behavior change in health and health care: Recommendations resulting from an international workshop. *Journal of Medical Internet Research, 19*(6), e232.

Milat, A. J., King, L., Bauman, A. E., & Redman, S. (2012). The concept of scalability: Increasing the scale and potential adoption of health promotion interventions into policy and practice. *Health Promotion International, 28*(3), 285–298.

Milat, A. J., Newson, R., King, L., Rissel, C., Wolfenden, L., Bauman, A., . . . Giffin, M. (2016). A guide to scaling up population health interventions. *Public Health Research & Practice, 26*(1), e2611604.

Moore, G. F., Audrey, S., Barker M., Bond, L., Bonell, C., Hardeman, W., Moore, L., . . . Baird, J. (2015). Process evaluation of complex interventions: Medical Research Council guidance. *BMJ, 350*, h1258.

Moore, G. F., & Evans, R. E. (2017). What theory, for whom and in which context? Reflections on the application of theory in the development and evaluation of complex population health interventions. *SSM-Population Health, 3*, 132–135.

Nathan, N., Elton, B., Babic, M., McCarthy, N., Sutherland, R., Presseau, J., . . . Wolfenden, L. (2018). Barriers and facilitators to the implementation of physical activity policies in schools: A systematic review. *Preventive Medicine, 107*, 45–53.

Nathan, N., Sutherland, R., Beauchamp, M. R., Cohen, K., Hulteen, R. M., Babic, M., . . . Lubans, D. R. (2017). Feasibility and efficacy of the Great Leaders Active StudentS (GLASS) program on children's physical activity and object control skill competency: A non-randomised trial. *Journal of Science and Medicine in Sport, 20*(12), 1081–1086.

Naylor, P. J., Macdonald, H. M., Reed, K. E., & McKay, H. A. (2006). Action Schools! BC: A socioecological approach to modifying chronic disease risk factors in elementary school children. *Preventing Chronic Disease, 3*(2), A60.

Naylor, P. J., Macdonald, H. M., Warburton, D. E., Reed, K. E., & McKay, H. A. (2008). An active school model to promote physical activity in elementary schools: Action schools! BC. *British Journal of Sports Medicine, 42*(5), 338–343.

Naylor, P. J., Macdonald, H. M., Zebedee, J. A., Reed, K. E., & McKay, H. A. (2006). Lessons learned from Action Schools! BC—an 'active school' model to promote physical activity in elementary schools. *Journal of Science and Medicine in Sport, 9*(5), 413–423.

Naylor, P. J., Nettlefold, L., Race, D., Hoy, C., Ashe, M. C., Higgins, J. W., & McKay, H. A. (2015). Implementation of school based physical activity interventions: A systematic review. *Preventive Medicine, 72*, 95–115.

Naylor, P. J., Scott, J., Drummond, J., Bridgewater, L., McKay, H. A., & Panagiotopoulos, C. (2010). Implementing a whole school physical activity and healthy eating model in rural and remote First Nations schools: A process evaluation of Action Schools! BC. *Rural and Remote Health, 10*(2), 1296.

Nettlefold, L., McKay, H., McGuire, A., Warburton, D., Bredin, S., & Naylor, P. (2012). Action Schools! BC: A whole-school physical activity model to increase children's physical activity. *Journal of Science and Medicine in Sport, 15*, S114.

Norris, E., Dunsmuir, S., Duke-Williams, O., Stamatakis, E., & Shelton, N. (2016). Protocol for the 'Virtual Traveller' cluster-randomised controlled trial: A behaviour change intervention to increase physical activity in primary-school Maths and English lessons. *BMJ Open, 6*(6), e011982.

Norris, E., Shelton, N., Dunsmuir, S., Duke-Williams, O., & Stamatakis, E. (2015). Virtual field trips as physically active lessons for children: A pilot study. *BMC Public Health, 15*(1), 366.

O'Cathain, A., Hoddinott, P., Lewin, S., Thomas, K. J., Young, B., Adamson, J., . . . Donovan, J. L. (2015). Maximising the impact of qualitative research in feasibility studies for randomised controlled trials: Guidance for researchers. *Pilot and Feasibility Studies, 1*(1), 32.

O'Cathain, A., Thomas, K. J., Drabble, S. J., Rudolph, A., & Hewison, J. (2013). What can qualitative research do for randomised controlled trials? A systematic mapping review. *BMJ Open, 3*(6), e002889.

Ortega-Sanchez, R., Jimenez-Mena, C., Cordoba-Garcia, R., Muñoz-Lopez, J., Garcia-Machado, M., & Vilaseca-Canals, J. (2004). The effect of office-based physician's advice on adolescent exercise behavior. *Preventive Medicine, 38*(2), 219–226.

Owen, M., Kerner, C., Taylor, S., Noonan, R., Newson, L., Kosteli, M. C., . . . Fairclough, S. (2018). The feasibility of a novel school peer-led mentoring model to improve the physical activity levels and sedentary time of adolescent girls: The Girls Peer Activity (G-PACT) project. *Children, 5*(6), 67.

Pallan, M., Parry, J., & Adab, P. (2012). Contextual influences on the development of obesity in children: A case study of UK South Asian communities. *Preventive Medicine, 54*(3–4), 205–211.

Pallan, M., Parry, J., Cheng, K. K., & Adab, P. (2013). Development of a childhood obesity prevention programme with a focus on UK South Asian communities. *Preventive Medicine, 57*, 948–954.

Passmore, S., & Jones, L. (2018). A review of the sustainability and impact of a healthy lifestyles programme in primary schools 2–5 years after the intervention phase. *Health Education Research, 34*(1), 72–83.

Pate, R. R., Saunders, R. P., Ward, D. S., Felton, G., Trost, S. G., & Dowda, M. (2003). Evaluation of a community-based intervention to promote physical activity in youth: Lessons from active winners. *American Journal of Health Promotion, 17*, 171–182.

Pellegrin, K. L., Carek, D., & Edwards, J. (1995). Use of experimental and quasi-experimental methods for data-based decisions in QI. *The Joint Commission Journal on Quality Improvement, 21*(12), 683–691.

Poitras, V. J., Gray, C. E., Borghese, M. M., Carson, V., Chaput, J. P., Janssen, I., . . . Sampson, M. (2016). Systematic review of the relationships between objectively measured physical activity and health indicators in school-aged children and youth. *Applied Physiology, Nutrition, and Metabolism, 41*(6), S197–S239. doi:10.1139/apnm-2015-0663

Polacsek, M., Orr, J., Letourneau, L., Rogers, V., Holmberg, R., O'Rourke, K., . . . Gortmaker, S. L. (2009). Impact of a primary care intervention on physician practice and patient and family behavior: Keep ME Healthy—The Maine youth overweight collaborative. *Pediatrics, 123*(Supplement 5), S258–S266.

Prestwich, A., Sniehotta, F. F., Whittington, C., Dombrowski, S. U., Rogers, L., & Michie, S. (2014). Does theory influence the effectiveness of health behavior interventions? Meta-analysis. *Health Psychology, 33*(5), 465.

Prestwich, A., Webb, T. L., & Conner, M. (2015). Using theory to develop and test interventions to promote changes in health behavior: Evidence, issues, and recommendations. *Current Opinion in Psychology, 5*, 1–5.

Proctor, E., Silmere, H., Raghavan, R., Hovmand, P., Aarons, G., Bunger, A., . . . Hensley, M. (2011). Outcomes for implementation research: Conceptual distinctions, measurement challenges, and research agenda. *Administration and Policy in Mental Health and Mental Health Services Research, 38*(2), 65–76.

Quested, E., Ntoumanis, N., Thøgersen-Ntoumani, C., Hagger, M. S., & Hancox, J. E. (2017). Evaluating quality of implementation in physical activity interventions based on theories of motivation: Current challenges and future directions. *International Review of Sport and Exercise Psychology, 10*(1), 252–269.

Reis, R. S., Salvo, D., Ogilvie, D., Lambert, E. V., Goenka, S., & Brownson, R. C. (2016). Scaling up physical activity interventions worldwide: Stepping up to larger and smarter approaches to get people moving. *The Lancet, 388*, 1337–1348.

Rhodes, R. E., Janssen, I., Bredin, S. S. D., Warburton, D. E. R., & Bauman, A. (2017). Physical activity: Health impact, prevalence, correlates and interventions. *Psychology & Health, 32*(8), 942–975.

Ridgers, N. D., Salmon, J., & Timperio, A. (2015). Too hot to move? Objectively assessed seasonal changes in Australian children's physical activity. *International Journal of Behavioral Nutrition and Physical Activity, 12*(1), 77.

Rowlands, A. V. (2007). Accelerometer assessment of physical activity in children: An update. *Pediatric Exercise Science, 19*(3), 252–266.

Ryan, R. M., & Deci, E. L. (2000). Self-determination theory and the facilitation of intrinsic motivation, social development, and well-being. *American Psychologist, 55*(1), 68.

Sallis, J. F., Bull, F., Guthold, R., Heath, G. W., Inoue, S., Kelly, P., . . . Lancet Physical Activity Series 2 Executive Committee. (2016). Progress in physical activity over the Olympic quadrennium. *The Lancet, 388*(10051), 1325–1336.

Saunders, R. P., Evans, M. H., & Joshi, P. (2005). Developing a process-evaluation plan for assessing health promotion program implementation: A how-to guide. *Health Promotion Practice, 6*(2), 134–147.

Schaapp, R., Bessems, K., Otten, R., Kremers, S., & van Nassau, F. (2018). Measuring implementation fidelity of school-based obesity prevention programmes: A systematic review. *International Journal of Behavioral Nutrition and Physical Activity, 15*, 75.

Schoeppe, S., Oliver, M., Badland, H. M., Burke, M., & Duncan, M. J. (2013). Recruitment and retention of children in behavioral health risk factor studies: REACH strategies. *International Journal of Behavioral Medicine, 21*(5), 794–803.

Schofield, L., Mummery, W. K., & Schofield, G. (2005). Effects of a controlled pedometer-intervention trial for low-active adolescent girls. *Medicine & Science in Sports & Exercise, 37*, 1414–1420.

Shah, S., Allison, K. R., Schoueri-Mychasiw, N., Pach, B., Manson, H., & Vu-Nguyen, K. (2017). A review of implementation outcome measures of school-based physical activity interventions. *Journal of School Health, 87*(6), 474–486.

Shapiro, J. R., Bauer, S., Hamer, R. M., Kordy, H., Ward, D., & Bulik, C. M. (2008). Use of text messaging for monitoring sugar-sweetened beverages, physical activity, and screen time in children: A pilot study. *Journal of Nutrition Education and Behavior, 40*(6), 385–391.

Simovska, V., & Carlsson, M. (2012). Health-promoting changes with children as agents: Findings from a multiple case study research. *Health Education, 112*(3), 292–304.

Sirard, J. R., & Pate, R. R. (2001). Physical activity assessment in children and adolescents. *Sports Medicine, 31*(6), 439–454.

Smedegaard, S., Brondeel, R., Christiansen, L. B., & Skovgaard, T. (2017). What happened in the 'Move for Well-being in School': A process evaluation of a cluster randomized physical activity intervention using the RE-AIM framework. *International Journal of Behavioral Nutrition and Physical Activity, 14*(1), 159.

Spence, J. C., & Lee, R. E. (2003). Toward a comprehensive model of physical activity. *Psychology of Sport and Exercise, 4*(1), 7–24. doi:10.1016/S1469-0292(02)00014-6

Speroff, T. & O'Connor, G. T. (2004). Study designs for PDSA quality improvement research. *Quality Management in Health Care, 13*(1), 17–32.

Steckler, A., & McLeroy, K. R. (2008). The importance of external validity. *American Journal of Public Health, 98*(1), 9–10.

Stoto, M. A., & Cosler, L. E. (2008). Evaluation of public health interventions. In L. F. Novick, C. B. Morrow, & G. P. Mays (Eds.), *Public health administration: Principles for population-based management* (pp. 495–544). Sudbury, MA: Jones and Bartlett.

Sutherland, R. L., Nathan, N. K., Lubans, D. R., Cohen, K., Davies, L. J., Desmet, C., . . . Wolfenden, L. (2017). An RCT to facilitate implementation of school practices known to increase physical activity. *American Journal of Preventive Medicine, 53*(6), 818–828.

Sylvia, L. G., Bersntein, E. E., Hubbard, J. L., Keating, L., & Anderson, E. J. (2014). A practical guide to measuring physical activity. *Journal of the Academy of Nutrition and Dietetics, 114*(2), 199–2018.

Taylor, S. L., Noonan, R. J., Knowles, Z. R., Owen, M. B., & Fairclough, S. J. (2018). Process evaluation of a pilot multi-component physical activity intervention–active schools: Skelmersdale. *BMC Public Health, 18*(1), 1383.

Taylor, S., Noonan, R., Knowles, Z., Owen, M., McGrane, B., Curry, W., & Fairclough, S. (2018). Evaluation of a pilot school-based physical activity clustered randomised controlled trial—Active Schools: Skelmersdale. *International Journal of Environmental Research and Public Health, 15*(5), 1011.

Taymoori, P., & Lubans, D. R. (2008). Mediators of behavior change in two tailored physical activity interventions for adolescent girls. *Psychology of Sport and Exercise, 9*(5), 605–619.

Tomlin, D., Naylor, P. J., McKay, H., Zorzi, A., Mitchell, M., & Panagiotopoulos, C. (2012). The impact of Action Schools! BC on the health of Aboriginal children and youth living in rural and remote communities in British Columbia. *International Journal of Circumpolar Health, 71*(1), 17999.

Tooth, L., Ware, R., Bain, C., Purdie, D. M., & Dobson, A. (2005). Quality of reporting of observational longitudinal research. *American Journal of Epidemiology, 161*(3), 208–288.

Trost, S. G. (2001). Objective measurement of physical activity in youth: Current issues, future directions. *Exercise and Sport Sciences Reviews, 29*(1), 32–36.

Tucker, S., Lanningham-Foster, L., Murphy, J., Olsen, G., Orth, K., Voss, J., . . . Lohse, C. (2011). A school based community partnership for promoting healthy habits for life. *Journal of Community Health, 36*(3), 414–422.

van Sluijs, E. M. F., & Kriemler, S. (2016). Reflections on physical activity intervention research in young people – Dos, don'ts, and critical thoughts. *International Journal of Behavioral Nutrition and Physical Activity, 13*, 25.

van Stralen, M. M., Yildirim, M., te Velde, S. J., Brug, J., van Mechelen, W., & Chinapaw, M. J. (2011). What works in school-based energy balance behaviour interventions and what does not? A systematic review of mediating mechanisms. *International Journal of Obesity, 35*(10), 1251.

Victora, C. G., Habicht, J.-P., & Bryce, J. (2004). Evidence-based public health: Moving beyond randomized trials. *American Journal of Public Health, 94*(3), 400–405.

Viswanathan, M., Berkman, N. D., Dryden, D. M., & Hartling, L. (2013). Assessing risk of bias and confounding in observational studies of interventions or exposures: Further development of the RTI Item Bank. Methods Research Report. Agency for Healthcare Research and Quality Publication No. 13-EHC106-EF. Rockville, MD.

Wandersman, A., Duffy, J., Flaspohler, P., Noonan, R., Lubell, K., Stillman, L., . . . Saul, J. (2008). Bridging the gap between prevention research and practice: The interactive systems framework for dissemination and implementation. *American Journal of Community Psychology, 41*, 171–181.

Waters, E., de Silva-Sanigorski, A., Burford, B. J., Brown, T., Campbell, K. J., Gao, Y., . . . Summerbell, C. D. (2011). Interventions for preventing obesity in children. *Cochrane Database of Systematic Reviews, 12*, Art. No.: CD001871. doi:10.1002/14651858.CD001871.pub3

Weatherson, K. A., McKay, R., Gainforth, H. L., & Jung, M. E. (2017). Barriers and facilitators to the implementation of a school-based physical activity policy in Canada: Application of the theoretical domains framework. *BMC Public Health, 17*(1), 835.

Weaver, R. G., Webster, C. A., Beets, M. W., Brazendale, K., Chandler, J., Schisler, L., & Aziz, M. (2018). Initial outcomes of a participatory-based, competency-building approach to increasing physical education teachers' physical activity promotion and students' physical activity: A pilot study. *Health Education & Behavior, 45*(3), 359–370.

Welk, G. J. (1999). The youth physical activity promotion model: A conceptual bridge between theory and practice. *Quest, 51*(1), 5–23.

Wells, M., Williams, B., Treweek, S., Coyle, J., & Taylor, J. (2012). Intervention description is not enough: Evidence from an in-depth multiple case study on the untold role and impact of context in randomised controlled trials of seven complex interventions. *Trials, 13*(1), 95.

Welsby, D., Nguyen, B., O'Hara, B. J., Innes-Hughes, C., Bauman, A., & Hardy, L. L. (2014). Process evaluation of an up-scaled community based child obesity treatment program: NSW Go4Fun®. *BMC Public Health, 14*(1), 140.

Wight, D., Wimbush, E., Jepson, R., & Doi, L. (2016). Six steps in quality intervention development (6SQuID). *Journal of Epidemiology and Community Health, 70*, 520–525.

Wood, C., Gladwell, V., & Barton, J. (2014). A repeated measures experiment of school playing environment to increase physical activity and enhance self-esteem in UK school children. *PloS One, 9*, e108701.

Wyatt, K. M., Lloyd, J. J., Abraham, C., Creanor, S., Dean, S., Densham, E., . . . Taylor, R. S. (2013). The healthy lifestyles programme (HeLP), a novel school-based intervention to prevent obesity in school children: Study protocol for a randomised controlled trial. *Trials, 14*(1), 95.

Wyatt, K. M., Lloyd, J. J., Creanor, S., & Logan, S. (2011). The development, feasibility and acceptability of a school-based obesity prevention programme: Results from three phases of piloting. *BMJ Open, 1*, e000026.

Yildirim, M., Van Stralen, M. M., Chinapaw, M. J., Brug, J., Van Mechelen, W., Twisk, J. W., . . . Energy-Consortium. (2011). For whom and under what circumstances do school-based energy balance behavior interventions work? Systematic review on moderators. *International Journal of Pediatric Obesity, 6*(sup3), e46–e57.

PART 7

School-Based Interventions

23

PHYSICAL EDUCATION-BASED PHYSICAL ACTIVITY INTERVENTIONS

Dean Dudley, Aaron Beighle, Heather Erwin, John Cairney,
Lee Schaefer, and Kenneth Murfay

Introduction

For more than two decades the field of physical education (PE) has been called to play a role in the public health battle against youth physical inactivity and associated non-communicable diseases. In 1991, Sallis and McKenzie (1991) advocated for an approach to PE that acknowledged the mounting evidence of health benefits associated with regular physical activity (PA) for youth. This chapter provides a focus for PE, which throughout its rich history had struggled with a 'muddled mission' (Pate & Hohn, 1994). That is, PE lacked, and continues to lack, a true identity that resonated with both the public and education sectors. Examination of the field shows a shifting focus that began with a heavy emphasis on gymnastics-based skills and fitness. Post-World Wars the focus shifted toward game-based models that progressed to perceptual motor skills, fitness outcomes, and then to academic integration. Currently, a health-promotion or public health approach to PA focusing on PA promotion is advocated by many (Sallis et al., 2012). This ever-changing emphasis has contributed to the continued marginalization of the field in both public and education sectors (Siedentop, 2009).

Perhaps as a result of this lack of consistency, and the content of specific foci such as fitness and sport, pedagogical approaches in different epochs have served to alienate large numbers of children and youth – the effects of which appear to last far beyond the immediate experiences of the class. According to Cardinal, Yan, and Cardinal (2013), an individual's feelings toward PA can be influenced by negative memories of their childhood experiences in PE. They conclude that the long-term effects of using poor pedagogical and assessment practices in PE may result in many adults remembering negative experiences, which may affect their desire to maintain a physically active lifestyle as they age. In the same light, Ladwig, Vazou, and Ekkekakis (2018) found that while positive memories of PE in childhood were associated with higher levels of PA in adulthood, negative memories correlated with increased sedentary behavior. Negative memories include remembering feelings of embarrassment, lack of enjoyment, being bullied, social-physique anxiety, and being punished by the PE teacher. Recently, international consortiums have sought to define Quality Physical Education (QPE) as a means of alleviating this phenomenon. Therefore, prior to an in-depth examination of the PA outcomes of interventions in PE, it is essential to first define QPE (PA has been defined elsewhere in this book). QPE by contrast to PA is a:

> planned, progressive, inclusive learning experience that forms part of the curriculum in early years, primary and secondary education. In this respect, quality physical education (QPE) acts as the foundation for a lifelong engagement in physical activity and sport. The learning

experience offered to children and young people through physical education lessons should be developmentally appropriate to help them acquire the psychomotor skills, cognitive understanding and social and emotional skills they need to lead a physically active life.

(UNESCO, 2015, p. 9)

The United Nations expanded this definition to detail that QPE is an experience for youth that promotes movement competence to structure thinking, the expression of feelings, and enriched understanding. It does this through competition and cooperation, appreciation of rule structures, conventions, values, performance criteria and fair play, celebrating each student's varying contributions, as well as appreciating the demands and benefits of teamwork (UNESCO, 2015).

In short, this international definition suggests that the role of QPE is to provide students with the skills, knowledge, and attitudes requisite for a lifetime of health enhancing PA. In addition, it clearly states that QPE is educative, part of a curriculum, and based on the needs of youth. Often PE is confused with PA. That is, PE is used synonymously with recess, sports, and play. It is important to be clear that the impact of PE interventions on PA discussed here is focused on PE as outlined by these definitions. For instance, students are provided the opportunity and instruction needed to develop physical skills needed for a lifetime of diverse activity opportunities. Learning experiences that translate knowledge such as game tactics, goal-setting, and PA principles are provided in PE. In addition, the PE environment includes PA experiences in a healthy, meaningful setting to meet the needs of the individual student in developing positive attitudes and dispositions toward PA.

Given the earlier definitions and a public health imperative that places increased strain on education generally and PE specifically to address the inactivity crisis, PE has been increasingly challenged to increase youth PA during PE and promote PA beyond PE lessons. More recently, PE has been identified as the centerpiece of comprehensive school-based efforts to promote PA for youth. There are many examples around the world of these types of approaches such as the World Health Organization's Heath Promoting Schools Framework and the Centers for Disease Control Comprehensive School Physical Activity Program that are rolled out in the United States.

In short, schools and PE are uniquely positioned and have great potential for influencing the PA levels of youth. Specific components of this comprehensive approach (e.g. recess, classroom PA) are discussed in other chapters of this book. To this end, based on an examination of curricula from countries across the world, Dudley, Okely, Pearson, and Cotton (2011) suggest PE instructional time to be dedicated to high levels of PA, movement skill instruction and practice, as well as learning strategies associated with PA in an enjoyable and active environment.

Overview of the Literature

Despite the well-defined charge and clearly articulated importance of PA in PE and youth health, the field of PE has been slow to align itself with PA as an outcome. In two separate reviews, Fairclough and Stratton (2005, 2006) found students were active in 37% of elementary lesson time and 27–47% of secondary school lesson time. Furthermore, the most recent review of 25 studies across seven countries reports that the average proportion of PE spent in moderate-to-vigorous physical activity (MVPA) is 40% (Hollis et al., 2017). While there are variables that may contribute to low PA levels, this finding may suggest teachers are focused on other learning outcomes and not placing a priority on PA levels. It may also suggest, however, that teachers do not value the importance of PA, or do not have the skill requisite to engage students in high levels of PA during lessons. It is important to be mindful of the multiple outcomes that can be met through quality PE instruction.

In 2012, Sallis and colleagues provided a follow-up to their heavily cited 1991 paper referenced earlier. This paper highlighted the many advances in research over 20 years including support for PE coming from professionals in fields such as medicine, exercise science, and public health, as well as the emergence of evidence-based PE programs, and the mounting data connecting PA and learning. The paper appeals to the field of PE to further define and measure PE quality, provide more evidence of the impact of PE on PA, and disseminate evidence associated with these findings. Unfortunately, the field has been slow to take on the responsibility of PA as an outcome of PE and even slower to prioritize investing in research to support this notion. Much of this resistance stems from fears that PE could become recess with PE teachers simply supervising free play. However, adopting PA as an outcome need not come at the expense of other learning imperatives. Here, we advocate that the educational component of PE be rigorously maintained while maximizing PA during lessons. That is, it is not one or the other, PE is optimized when both exist.

While some in the field are resistant to this push for focusing on PA outcomes in PE, some researchers within the field, and many outside of the field, are examining its impact. In the past decade several reviews and meta-analyses have been conducted examining the potential impact of PE as an intervention strategy to increase PA levels in youth (Dudley et al., 2011; Kriemler et al., 2011; Lonsdale, Rosenkranz, Peralta, Bennie, Fahey, & Lubans, 2013). Based on outcomes of these investigations, the authors of all three reviews/meta-analyses were cautiously optimistic about the potential for PE interventions to impact youth PA. The primary reason for the caution was the limited number of studies examining the impact of PE-based interventions on a variety of variables, which included increasing PA. Although the body of evidence that exists is small, there is a common belief in the research to date that in order to increase PA levels in PE lessons, there needs to be significant teacher professional development with an emphasis on lesson efficiency before this will occur. For instance, providing training on how to efficiently organize and manage students to maximize movement was a necessity. Also, teacher training that focused on appropriate and best practices for instruction were required. Finally, a recommended strategy was to supplement some low activity PE lessons with some of higher intensity. This could mean trading a traditional target games lesson, which typically involves less intense activity, with an invasion games lesson that would typically involve higher intensity.

While the topic has been understudied, a few studies on the impact PA accrued during PE on overall PA have been published. Morgan, Beighle, and Pangrazi (2007) found that students were significantly more active on days in which they had PE class, supporting the contributory relationship between PE and daily PA. In addition, a quality, 30-minute PE class accounted for approximately 20% of daily PA for the least active children. Another segmented day PA study indicated that PE accounted for 8–11% of children's total daily PA (Tudor-Locke, Lee, Morgan, Beighle, & Pangrazi, 2006). While at first glance, these figures may seem low or insignificant, when considering that the PE classes measured were 30 minutes in length, this becomes a very valuable and significant source of PA for youth. So much so is that a 2017 study conducted in Europe reported that while students spent on average 29% of PE time in MVPA and 29% in more sedentary activities, each additional MVPA minute in PE was associated with 1.4 more daily MVPA minutes. On days with PE, students had 18 more minutes of MVPA and 10 minutes less sedentary time compared with days without PE (Mooses et al., 2017).

In concordance with the information on time spent in PA during PE from an earlier section, focusing on making PA levels a priority during PE, making teachers aware of the importance of PA, or providing teachers with proper skills to engage students in high levels of PA during lessons becomes particularly substantive. However, PA levels cannot be the only target of PE-based intervention and research.

The role of PE in lifelong PA is of utmost importance to the fields of health and education. Fairclough, Stratton, and Baldwin (2002) surveyed PE teachers across England regarding the secondary school PE curriculum and its contribution to lifetime PA. They found that most secondary PE teachers focused on team games over lifetime PA activities. The female teachers were more likely than the male teachers to offer lifetime PA activities in their curriculum. Kirk (2005) echoed the findings that secondary PE programs have not been successful in promoting lifelong physical activities. Wallhead and Buckworth (2004) reviewed large-scale PE-based PA interventions and summarized the most effective were those that utilized a pedagogical framework targeting variables associated with motivation related to PA (i.e. perceived competence, enjoyment, and self-determination).

The discipline of PE has great potential for impacting the PA levels of youth and, in turn, a population in general. However, this at the simplest level requires maximizing the levels of PA students experience during PE. Another is teaching PE in a manner as to make PA meaningful for all students that, in turn, promote PA participation beyond the curriculum. Unfortunately, thus far the literature on these two areas is limited, and to some extent, is hostile toward each other (Tinning, 2015). For PE to reach its potential as an agent of change in the health of populations around the world by increasing PA, strategies to maximize meaningful PA opportunities during PE and beyond are warranted.

Key Issues

It is clear that the role PE plays in society has been evolving for generations. This has led to not only to a 'muddled mission', but also a lack of empirical evidence supporting the need for the field and a clear body of literature supporting a unified direction that most stakeholders can agree on. This section will provide key issues associated with the utility of PE as a PA intervention.

Calls for the enactment of QPE since 2015 by the United Nations as a necessary first step to affect consistent changes in the pedagogical and assessment practices of this discipline now seem well supported. In July 2017, over 200 ministers, senior officials, intergovernmental, and non-governmental organizations from around the world responsible for PE, sports, and PA met under the auspices of UNESCO to debate the *Kazan Action Plan*. The preamble of the plan states that there is a

> broad consensus amongst these stakeholders that the UNESCO 2030 Agenda, the Declaration of Berlin, as well as the International Charter of Physical Education, Physical Activity and Sport constitute an interconnected, solid foundation for policy development and that, based on this foundation, policy development should henceforth focus on translating policy intent into measurable implementation.
>
> *(UNESCO, 2017, p. 1)*

Specifically, 20 action items across sports, public health, and education sectors are identified. Most relevant to this chapter, Action Area 1.6 of the plan articulates the need to *Foster QPE and active schools* (UNESCO, 2017, p. 6).

In conjunction with the definitions of QPE discussed earlier in this chapter, the member states of UNESCO unanimously supported this enactment of the Kazan Action Plan, which requires 'Fostering quality physical education and active schools needs provision that is varied, frequent, challenging, meaningful and inclusive' (UNESCO, 2017, pp. 7–8). This allows for physical educators to focus on immediate provision goals rather than outcomes that may be nebulous and distant from the immediate pedagogical context.

To place this in context of PA promotion, a QPE initiative promotes PA whereby movement is the learning medium through which students learn and experience the joys of PA. Therefore, QPE engages students in PA for as long as possible to sustain quality-learning experiences. However, to receive the known health benefits of PA and to develop the skills, knowledge, and attitudes to be active for a lifetime, the time allocated during PE is not sufficient as a public health strategy. That is, with the time allotted to PE, content must be such that it promotes PA beyond the PE learning experience. With this approach as the backdrop, we identify the following key issues for the field of PE if it is to embrace its role as a learning and PA intervention initiative: curriculum, policy, inclusivity, and meaningful movement experiences.

A Varied PE Curriculum

As outlined in the Kazan Action Plan (2017), evidence supports an approach to offering a PE curriculum with a variety of activities that impact youth PA throughout life. Youth who engage in more varied PA and movement opportunities experience greater well-being, have better peer relationships, demonstrate better psychological regulation, and feel more of a sense of school belonging (Busseri, Rose-Krasnor, Willoughby, & Chalmers, 2006; Fredricks & Eccles, 2006). Cleland, Schmidt, Salmon Dwyer, and Venn (2011) suggest that exposure to a variety of PA experiences in childhood predicts adult PA. Wright and Côté (2003) showed that varied sporting and PA experiences during childhood promoted university level athletes with better peer relationships and leadership skills. In the last decade, some longitudinal studies have also found that youth who are involved in a varied and diverse range of physical activities score more favorably on personal and social outcome measures when compared to those youth who specialize early (Strachan, Côté, & Deakin, 2009).

It is apparent that different types of activities and activity environments offer different opportunities for socialization and different social contexts for discovery. For example, swimming and many net/wall games may see students spending a greater amount of time one-on-one with a teacher than a student participating in a team sport such as soccer or ultimate Frisbee. On the other hand, involvement in activities with larger teams/groups may provide learning experiences that are not available in an individual activity such as archery or running. Therefore, it is suggested that variety in a PE curriculum has the potential to promote a broader spectrum of developmental experiences and outcomes than a narrow or specialized PE curricula. Further, an important aspect of providing varied movement opportunities is to help students' movement and PA transition into adulthood, and it has been shown that diverse experiences enable this (McKenzie & Lounsbery, 2014).

Impact of Policy

Many PE programs fall short of best practice and policy recommendations in terms of curricula, time, active teaching and learning time, and intensity (UNESCO, 2015). An increasing body of literature showing the efficacy of improving physical, behavioral, and relationship outcomes with improved cognitive performance of students in these schools supports the call for more frequent and even daily PE classes (Dudley & Burden, 2019; Kohl III & Cook, 2013; Trudeau, Laurencelle, Tremblay, Rajic, & Shephard, 1999). A recent Swedish intervention study concluded that daily implementation of QPE in the school curriculum and one hour per week of motor skills training in students with specific needs garnered improvements in motor skills, academic results, and the proportion of pupils who qualify for upper secondary school (Ericsson & Karlsson, 2014).

Dudley and Burden's (2019) most recent meta-analysis on the effect of increasing the proportion of curriculum time allocated to PE on learning concluded that if schools increase the proportion of curriculum time allocated to PE, they could significantly improve student learning by over 0.4 of a standard deviation. Moreover, this move would see learning improve by as much as 0.83 (psychomotor learning) and as little as 0.14 (cognitive learning) of a standard deviation indicating no detrimental effect on student learning by doing so.

In a period of increased standardized testing regimes and crowded curricula, PE can often be seen as 'taking away' from 'real' learning time. While we argue there is important academic learning happening in PE, researchers have also shown, more PE is not detrimental to other areas of academic performance (Dudley & Burden, 2019; Shephard, 1997).

Focused Inclusivity

Evidence suggests that PA at school is most effective if these activities include a supportive policy on how to enable the participation of all students (Stewart-Brown, 2005). However, inclusion in PE has traditionally been very challenging because of the active nature of the learning environment. In general, 'inclusivity' in education should be started at pre-school or elementary school since educational objectives are most often referenced to cognitive, social, motor development, or adaptive behavior (Fisher & Meyer, 2002; Hundert, Hahoney, Mundy, & Vernon, 1998). It is these developmental skills that lay the foundation for later learning required in secondary school. Accepted instructional strategies for both young children with and without disabilities encourage child-initiated learning and children's active physical engagement with each other and with the environment (Wolery et al., 1994; Wolery & Sainato, 1996).

The evidence-based positive outcomes of inclusive PE are numerous but are even more significant given that youth with a disability are particularly at risk of disease associated with sedentary living (Carroll et al., 2014). Interestingly, youth in this demographic are less likely than their comparative peers to exhibit harmful health behaviors (i.e. alcohol, tobacco, and illicit drug consumption), but are more likely to have unhealthy eating habits and engage more in sedentary leisure activities (Kalnins et al.,1999; Steele et al., 1996). In addition to the numerous physiological benefits of participation in PA, being active with peers is a socially normalizing experience for children with and without a disability (Taub & Greer, 2000).

The inclusive aspects of QPE also support the contention for inclusive right of access to QPE across all the schooling years. Data from the landmark Cardiovascular Risk in Young Finns Study suggested that high levels of PA in late adolescence are a significant predictor of adult PA levels (Telama et al., 2005). The authors of the study were clear that while the correlations are moderate, PA levels during this age are associated with adult PA and ultimately have long-term public health implications. Telama (2009) in a later review of more than 40 studies concluded that efforts to increase PA during childhood and adolescence are a public health concern and therefore warranted. Specifically, he suggests that PA appears to track 'reasonably well' from adolescence into adulthood. Thus, ensuring youth are active into 'late adolescence' is empirically supported and of great importance.

Interestingly though, in 2008, 86 participants in the landmark 1970–1977 Trois-Rivières Study completed a questionnaire examining their current PA level and different correlates of PA (i.e. individual's intention to engage in PA, perceived enjoyment, usefulness and ease in engaging in PA, perceived social support, and social norms). Participants had initially been assigned to either an experimental program (5 hours per week of specialist-taught PE) or a control group (40 minutes per week of home-room teacher-taught PE) from grades 1 to 6. Nearly 40 years later, there were no differences between the experimental and control groups neither in the frequency, duration nor volume of PA being undertaken in the captured follow-up cohort ($n = 86$). Furthermore, no differences between groups were found for any of the PA correlates examined. The authors of this follow-up study conclude that providing daily PE throughout primary school seems insufficient to ensure that individuals will remain active in midlife and that the development of a life-course approach to PA promotion is thus warranted (Larouche, Laurencelle, Shephard, & Trudeau, 2015).

Meaningful Movement Experiences

An often-overlooked component of PE experiences is notions of motivation. That is, are the lessons motivating to students and are they inspiring youth to be active beyond the lesson? Standage, Duda, and Ntoumanis (2005), using self-determination theory, found that when tasks are challenging but attainable and supported by the teacher, students found greater satisfaction in the activity. Challenge in activity can also be used to provide a sense of risk, which contributes to the natural urge for children to engage in risky play (Sandseter, 2009). While less research has focused on the need for PE to be challenging, activities that present challenge could add an element of excitement and enjoyment to PE. Appropriately challenging activities, referred to by Weiss and Ebbeck (1996) as 'Optimal Challenges', are those that are within reach of a given student's ability but require effort and persistence to reach the goal. This notion is grounded in the importance of perceived competence, that is, a student's judgment on their ability within the PA context (Stodden et al., 2008). Activities that are not challenging enough are likely to yield boredom, resulting in low motivation. Activities that are too difficult are likely to result in angst, anxiety, frustration, and potentially off-task behavior or refusal to participate. According to Stodden et al. (2008), youth use goal attainment, effort, and improvement as the criteria for determining their competency. Thus, the optimal challenges in PE could provide a context to establish perceptions of competency within the student's ability range. To exemplify this point, a recent longitudinal study of children from grades 4 to 8 (ages 9 to 14) in the Canadian public school system noted the importance of considering the association between perceived competence and enjoyment in PE to be variable over time and by gender. The study by Cairney and colleagues (2012) found a three-way interaction between time, gender (sex), and perceived competence on enjoyment: girls with low competence had the fastest (steepest) overall rates of decline in enjoyment of PE over the time period. When considering the appropriate level of challenge, we must be mindful of the influences of gender (and other factors) on perceptions of competence. The differences are undoubtedly linked to social and socializing influences that disadvantage some children, and privilege others.

Linked to motivation is the notion that for PE experiences to impact student PA they must be personally relevant to the student (Kretchmar, 2008). Students who have repeated negative experiences in PE result in an increased likelihood of developing a negative association with PA over their life span (Cardinal et al., 2013; Strean, 2010). This also complicates conversations similar to earlier ones regarding PE frequency, as we know that more negative experiences may simply enhance the disdain for movement. For these reasons, one strategy in QPE is to assist students in finding personal or intrinsic meaning, for PA. The notion has been supported by Kretchmar (2008) in his research and advocacy for having students find the 'joy' in their PA experiences. Furthermore, numerous pedagogical scholars of PE, such as Bunker and Thorpe (1982), Siedentop (1994), and Hellison (1995), have spent their careers advocating for PE curricula and practices that attune to the broader cognitive, social, and affective domains of learning whereby 'enjoyment' or 'joy' become a legitimate by-products. All these scholars identified inherent limitations with mere PA or sports-based models of PE and make compelling cases for PE classes with enriched learning experiences to enact both learning and behavior change in students.

Beni, Fletcher, and Ní Chróinín (2017), in a review of meaningful experiences in PE, identified the importance of social interaction, fun, challenge, motor competence, and personally relevant learning in creating meaningful experiences for participants. The review also suggests the importance of a balanced approach where criteria are considered in combination rather than the prioritization of any one criterion (Beni et al., 2017) lending more weight to the diversity in PE position being made in this chapter.

From a PA perspective, we know that 'play' is a personally meaningful experience for an individual (Barab, Gresalfi, & Ingram-Goble, 2010). Deliberate and diverse play therefore serves as a way for youth to explore their physical capacities in various contexts and potentially enhance their motor competence. This kind of meaningful play activity involves an engagement of time that is hard to match with more structured practice sessions. Qualitative analyses of children's early involvement in activities such as tennis (Carlson, 1988; Côté, 1999), rowing (Côté, 1999), and baseball (Hill, 1993) showed that meaningful play-like activities were important in the first few years of engagement in sports. Soberlak and Côté (2003) showed that before age 20, elite players in certain sports actually spent more time in play-type activities than deliberate practice sessions.

Recommendations for Researchers and Practitioners

Along with the key issues pertaining to PE-based PA, there is more to develop in terms of research and practice. We know this is a complicated conversation given the variety of outcomes that can be met through a quality PE program; however, we also know that on average, students do not engage in MVPA for most of any given PE lesson. Therefore, effective strategies for increasing PA while maintaining other outcomes in PE are warranted. Focus around pedagogical training that emphasizes lesson efficiency is important. However, increasing PA in a quality PE program is not as simple as having well trained PE professionals. We also know that a varied curriculum, effective policy support, inclusivity and meaningful, joyful, movement experiences are key factors in increasing PA not only in PE, but in a lifelong manner. The following section addresses some points to consider for future research and practice.

Future Research

As noted previously, Beni and colleagues (2017) suggest that social interaction, fun, challenge, motor competence, and personally relevant learning are essential for meaningful QPE experiences that, in turn, will promote PA participation beyond the schooling years. These notions are captured by the statement in UNESCO's Kazan Action Plan (2017) that was formulated from an international audience with a diverse range of backgrounds. While future scholars and practitioners may debate this definition and the purpose of QPE, we believe research investigating the empirical weight of frequent, varied, inclusive, challenging, and meaningful PE is essential in determining what we expect of PE curricula and PE practice. Such research may result in something we can all 'hang our hat on' and detangle our 'muddled mission'. This requires the following: First, there must be intentional planning around curriculum and pedagogical approaches to specifically target each domain. Students simply engaging in an activity cannot be simply assumed as providing challenge or meaning. The experience must be structured to emphasize these factors. Second, each domain must be measured and tracked to evaluate outcomes of the intervention. This need not simplify to just pre- and post-evaluation. Ongoing tracking of competence, challenge, enjoyment, can guide the practitioner to make course corrections throughout the duration of the class. This is consistent with a response to intervention paradigm where measurement is used to guide practice.

Another area that requires far more research before PE practices shift markedly is the influence PA has on different areas of academic performance. In the last decade, a growing interest has emerged in studying the influence of PA on cognitive functioning in youth (Fedewa & Ahn, 2011). Meta-analyses conducted by Álvarez-Bueno et al. (2017) concluded that if schools appropriately implement PA interventions, they can significantly improve academic achievement of youth by between $d = 0.14–0.28$. It is important to note though that many of the studies included in this analysis suffered from poor research designs and a high degree of publication bias. Nonetheless, these small increases in standardized testing scores have unfairly led to a tsunami of journalists and popular media advocating that the 'new' role of PE is to engage youth in sufficient PA in efforts to drive up student test scores. Recent newspaper articles have splayed headline such as 'Teach physical education every day because it boosts the brain, say scientists' (https://www.telegraph.co.uk/science/2017/11/24/teach-physical-education-everyday-boosts-brain-say-scienitsts/) and 'More physical education in schools leads to better grades, study suggests' (https://www.sciencedaily.

com/releases/2012/05/120523114728.htm). Not only does this type of thinking undermine the broader educative purpose and lifelong learning inculcated by a QPE initiative, it does not constitute a worthwhile schooling investment in student achievement (Hattie, 2009).

Rather, we support future research addressing how PE contributes to the holistic learning of youth. A recent meta-analysis by Dudley and Burden (2019) shows that simply increasing the frequency of PE students become exposed to had pooled effect sizes of $d = 0.41$ on student learning across cognitive, affective, and psychomotor learning outcomes. However, the larger effect sizes were observed in the affective ($d = 0.66$) and psychomotor ($d = 0.83$) learning domains. Cognitive learning only equated for around $d = 0.14$ of the pooled effect size. So, while the benefits of increasing PA to health and learning are well known, the effects to the cognitive domain of learning are often overstated.

Examining the impact of PE on other learning outcomes makes it clear that there is more to PE than PA there is a value-added component that is likely connected directly to the pedagogy associated with the discipline. From a public health perspective, the education sector is often viewed opportunistically for intervention because of its reach (lots of children) and capture (all in the same place at the same time). However, the mission of public health and education is complementary but also distinct. For PE to be meaningful in the context of education, it cannot be reduced to simply a conduit to increasing PA – it must be connected to both health and learning. Future research should seek to ascertain the degree of causality between PA and learning AND learning and PA.

Future Practice

Students must be provided a diversity of PA opportunities in the context of PE that provide various social, physical, and cognitive experiences. Thus, a balanced curriculum exposing students to individual activities, fitness activities, cooperative experiences, team sports, outdoor/adventure pursuits, rhythmic activities, and gymnastics is advocated (Pangrazi & Beighle, 2015). This added variety, in turn, should increase enjoyment of PA through novelty and therefore has the potential to reach a diverse student population. Enjoyment of PE is known to be a strong predictor of PA in children and youth (Cairney et al., 2012).

Given the limited time allocated to PE, one could argue that including a variety of activities prevents students from having the time to gain the skills they need for a lifetime of activity. While this is a point well taken, we would suggest that QPE addresses skills and concepts with a high degree of transferability throughout the program. For example, a concept like weight transfer can be included in gymnastics, or in throwing activities, or locomotion activities. Each of these activities, while diverse, offers opportunities to both experience weight transfer during diverse movement patterns and understand its importance in a variety of contexts. Movement skills such as sending are taught in a variety of settings throughout the year and throughout the scope of the QPE program. For instance, students are taught the foundations of sending with hands, feet, and the body in elementary years and apply those foundational tenants in more complex ways with short-handed and long-handed implements in activities such as softball, cricket, tennis, hockey, and lacrosse to name a few. In high school programs, focusing on coordinated limb movement, range of motion, and the generation of velocity while taking a shot in hockey, shooting a soccer ball, making a lay-up in basketball, or a slam in tennis offers ample opportunity to teach motor capacity while engaged in a variety of diverse activities. This type of structured diversity could be compared to deliberate play experiences that are particularly important in childhood, as they provide children the opportunities to develop competencies, increase motivation, and enhance participation experiences (Kirk, 2010), in a variety of movements and activities.

Practitioners can often feel the weight of curriculum and assessment demands upon them (whether perceived or not) which can interfere with their ability to be more open and receptive to restructuring their teaching environment and their overall program to ensure that they allow for more diverse PA and movement experiences. However, it is essential for the practitioner to consider how they might diversify not only the movement and PA experiences in their programs but also how they might diversify the opportunities for social engagement and interaction with both peers and the teacher. This requires the practitioner to become much more cognizant of how they construct their social space to ensure a genuine culture of support and growth is in place. Practitioners can sometimes be sidetracked to believe that it is only the development of physical skills that is of paramount importance in our programs. QPE is as much about the social interactions within the PE programs that students experience as it is about the social policies that constrain or enhance them.

While few could argue that more QPE would hinder our students' physical and social development, as mentioned earlier, there seems to be concern with taking time from other more academic subjects to put toward PE. To combat this, a growing body of research linking academic success and PA is being generated (Álvarez-Bueno et al., 2017; Kreider, 2019). While some schools may see an increase in PE time due to the merits of increasing academic achievement, this approach seems to position QPE as a primer for other areas, as a means to an end. PE is important because of its unique contribution to educating the entire student, but unfortunately, many educators do not read it, thus the decrease in prevalence of required QPE.

The marginal nature of PE in both schools and the public also plays a role in fighting for more time in a subject that is often times positioned as a non-learning space within and outside of schools (Kirk, 2010). The struggle for more frequent time often lies outside of the PE teachers' hands except in terms of advocacy at all levels of influence. A tactic best employed is that teachers seek equal share of total curricula time rather than minimum minutes which often is seen to impede on other subject areas.

Policy to Practice Perspectives

From a policy and practice perspective, increasing the frequency of PE alone (while effective) will underestimate the true potential of PE unless what occurs during this time significantly changes. Dudley, Okely, Pearson, Cotton, and Caputi (2012) argue that a substantial proportion of lesson time is spent in management type activities like having students change into sporting attire, setting up learning spaces, and organizing students into groups. In the early years of secondary school, this can average as much as 31% of allocated curricula time for PE in some disadvantaged schools. Other studies in Australian (Brown & Holland, 2005), Asian (Chow, McKenzie, & Louie, 2009), and early secondary years schooling in the United States (McKenzie et al., 2004) reported average management times being between 10% and 20% of allocated PE time. This level of disruption to learning time in PE needs to be addressed at both policy and practice levels of schools (Dudley, Pearson, Okely, & Cotton, 2015).

The ability to practice inclusive QPE appears achievable if teachers have access to appropriate and ongoing support structures. According to Simpson and Mandich (2012), these supports need to include providing necessary staffing to support teachers in PE (both in the primary and secondary years). This may include providing opportunities for educational assistants to assist students with their PE classes or appointing PE and special education specialists for consultation and coaching of teachers. Furthermore, teachers require having access to adapted and specialized equipment but even this is not always necessary if teachers are given opportunities and training to adapt curriculum expectations to suit the individual student's needs. Schools' and classes' infrastructures also need to ensure that students can physically navigate the learning space and that resources and lack of teacher training do not add additional barriers to their capacity to learn and participate. It is encouraging nonetheless that there is an overall sense among teachers and schools that all students deserve equal opportunity to have QPE experiences (Simpson & Mandich, 2012).

The practice of providing challenging movement experiences in PE to students may indeed be the most difficult to implement, but perhaps one of the most important as it seems that students often associate challenge with enjoyment (Beni et al., 2017; Linda Rikard & Banville, 2006). When we think about the diversity of developmental levels in our classrooms, it becomes easy to understand how complex a task it may be to provide developmentally challenging experiences for each student.

A key strategy for providing challenge is to provide some degree of structured student choice during lessons. This choice must be within a structured program or lesson as 'student choice' (e.g. students have complete control of activity choices) alone does not track well with achievement outcomes in the empirical evidence (Hattie, 2009). A PE teacher may, however, structure choice by allowing students to choose the type of object they use to engage in a kicking type activity, or a preferred catching challenge (e.g. with one hand, two hands, or behind the back). Within a secondary program, teachers can generate 'modules' (e.g. team sports, outdoor pursuits, and fitness) for students to select from during the program or semester (Darst, Pangrazi, Brusseau, & Erwin, 2014). Students then select their preferred module based on how they would like to be challenged. Keeping in mind that students will often choose what they are comfortable with, so need to be pushed outside of their comfort zones. Teachers can also utilize alternative environments like the outdoors to introduce risky, challenging play that allows students to set their own challenge level, test their limits, and explore their own boundaries through movement (Sandseter, 2009).

Determining an appropriate level of challenge for each student also requires an environment that allows for exploration and failure. Students who do not feel safe, physically or emotionally, will be unlikely to open themselves up to failure for fear of ridicule from their peers or negative judgment from their teacher. The practitioner has much to consider when striving to create a culture of learning that embraces risk-taking and trust amongst their students. Constructing opportunities that allow each student to find their entry point to learning requires the teacher being in tune with the mindset that each student brings with them to the PE space. This becomes possible when teachers work on establishing positive relationships with each student which draws attention back to the need to ensure that the social structure of the teaching space is highly considered during the planning process. Actively constructing opportunities for more one-to-one or small group time with students should be a high priority for practitioners when designing the learning activities in the lessons and units taught in their PE programs.

When it comes to thinking about meaningful PE, in a culminating way, each of these areas plays an important role in providing meaningful experiences for students. If experiences are diverse, provide challenges, and are frequent enough to both build skill and create a motivation to move then perhaps we have, at least in some form, criteria to adhere to as we consider the creation of meaningful experiences through PE. It is hoped that this meaning making goes beyond sports, movement patterns, or academic achievement to instill a disposition to move that becomes a part of who students are, a way of being.

Just as the forms of knowledge 'make sense' of aspects of our existence, our mobile ability or physical adeptness enables us to come to terms with and giving meaning to the world. Where the thorough grasp of a form of knowledge opens up new avenues of experience and a corresponding enrichment of our interaction with the world, the development of our physical capacities opens up new possibilities of experience and offers an extension of our understanding of a particular aspect of the world (Whitehead, 1990, p. 11). Often lost is the desire to provide meaningful experiences, given the focus on utilitarian discourses that position PE as a means to an end. Many aspects of quality are lost in this utilitarian quest, including the joy of movement (Kretchmar, 2008).

Students must find joy not only in PE experiences but also in the transfer of these experiences into their lives outside of PE and outside of school. This does not mean that all experiences will be, or need to be, enjoyable for students, but more often than not when students find PE to be personally meaningful they will find joy in it.

Drawing further on Whitehead (1990), finding joy in movement creates a disposition to move that goes beyond sculpting the body, fitness, academic achievement, and even health. A personally meaningful experience in PE requires opportunities for students to reflect upon their learning and to draw out real life connections to the relevancy of the experiences themselves. If they find little or no relevancy in the experience, there is a greater likelihood that disengagement will rise or that they will be participating purely for compliance reasons. It therefore requires practitioners to embed time for reflective discussions with their students as part of the balanced approach to the delivery of the curriculum. Through the vehicle of student reflection, practitioners can gain valuable insight into just how personally meaningful the PE experiences are to each of their students and to consider this qualitative data when formulating and designing best ways to move teaching and learning forward.

Physical educators are encouraged to teach students how to set goals, evaluate progress toward goals, and make goal adjustments accordingly as a means of making experiences personally meaningful. This is not only a valuable skill, but it also fosters a growth mindset where not meeting a goal is simply part of the process, not failure. Finally, in order to make PE and PA meaningful for all students, it is imperative that physical educators know their students as individuals. This takes time, energy, and persistence to get to know some students. Nonetheless, it is impossible to make PA meaningful for an individual, without knowing the individual.

References

Álvarez-Bueno, C., Pesce, C., Cavero-Redondo, I., Sánchez-López, M., Garrido-Miguel, M., & Martínez-Vizcaíno, V. (2017). Academic achievement and physical activity: A meta-analysis. *Pediatrics, 140*(6), e20171498.

Barab, S. A., Gresalfi, M., & Ingram-Goble, A. (2010). Transformational play: Using games to position person, content, and context. *Educational Researcher, 39*(7), 525–536.

Beni, S., Fletcher, T., & Ní Chróinín, D. (2017). Meaningful experiences in physical education and youth sport: A review of the literature. *Quest, 69*(3), 291–312.

Brown, T. D., & Holland, B. V. (2005). Student physical activity and lesson context during physical education. *ACHPER Healthy Lifestyles Journal, 52*(3/4), 17–23.

Bunker, D., & Thorpe, R., (1982). A model for the teaching of games in the secondary school. *The Bulletin of Physical Education, 18*(1), 5–8.

Busseri, M. A., Rose-Krasnor, L., Willoughby, T., & Chalmers, H. (2006). A longitudinal examination of breadth and intensity of youth activity involvement and successful development. *Developmental Psychology, 42*(6), 1313.

Cairney, J., Kwan, M. Y., Velduizen, S., Hay, J., Bray, S. R., & Faught, B. E. (2012). Gender, perceived competence and the enjoyment of physical education in children: A longitudinal examination. *International Journal of Behavioral Nutrition and Physical Activity, 9*(1), 26.

Cardinal, B. J., Yan, Z., & Cardinal, M. K. (2013). Negative experiences in physical education and sport: How much do they affect physical activity participation later in life?. *Journal of Physical Education, Recreation & Dance, 84*(3), 49–53.

Carlson, R. (1988). The socialization of elite tennis players in Sweden: An analysis of the players' backgrounds and development. *Sociology of Sport Journal, 5*(3), 241–256.

Carroll, D. D., Courtney-Long, E. A., Stevens, A. C., Sloan, M. L., Lullo, C., Visser, S. N., . . . Dorn, J. M. (2014). Vital signs: Disability and physical activity – United States, 2009–2012. *MMWR. Morbidity and Mortality Weekly Report, 63*(18), 407–413.

Chow, B. C., McKenzie, T. L., & Louie, L. (2009). Physical activity and environmental influences during secondary school physical education. *Journal of Teaching in Physical Education, 28*(1), 21–37.

Cleland, V. J., Schmidt, M. D., Salmon, J., Dwyer, T., & Venn, A. (2011). Correlates of pedometer-measured and self-reported physical activity among young Australian adults. *Journal of Science and Medicine in Sport, 14*(6), 496–503.

Côté, J. (1999). The influence of the family in the development of talent in sport. *The Sport Psychologist, 13*(4), 395–417.

Darst, P., Pangrazi, R., Brusseau, T., & Erwin, H. (2014). *Dynamic physical education for secondary school students* (8th ed.). San Francisco, CA: Pearson.

Dudley, D., & Burden, R. (2019). What effect does increasing the proportion of curriculum time allocation to physical education have on learning? A systematic review and meta-analysis. *European Physical Education Review, 26*(1), 85–100.

Dudley, D., Okely, A., Pearson, P., & Cotton, W. (2011). A systematic review of the effectiveness of physical education and school sport interventions targeting physical activity, movement skills and enjoyment of physical activity. *European Physical Education Review, 17*(3), 353–378.

Dudley, D. A., Okely, A. D., Pearson, P., Cotton, W. G., & Caputi, P. (2012). Changes in physical activity levels, lesson context, and teacher interaction during physical education in culturally and linguistically diverse Australian schools. *International Journal of Behavioral Nutrition and Physical Activity, 9*(1), 114.

Dudley, D. A., Pearson, P., Okely, A. D., & Cotton, W. G. (2015). Recommendations for policy and practice of physical education in culturally and linguistically diverse Australian secondary schools based on a two-year prospective cohort study. *School Psychology International, 36*(2), 172–188.

Ericsson, I., & Karlsson, M. K. (2014). Motor skills and school performance in children with daily physical education in school–a 9-year intervention study. *Scandinavian Journal of Medicine & Science in Sports, 24*(2), 273–278.

Fairclough, S.J., & Stratton, G. (2005). Physical activity levels in middle and high school physical education: A review. *Pediatric Exercise Science, 17*(3), 217–236.

Fairclough, S. J., & Stratton, G. (2006). A review of physical activity levels during elementary school physical education. *Journal of Teaching in Physical Education, 25*(2), 240–258.

Fairclough, S.J., Stratton, G., & Baldwin, G. (2002). The contribution of secondary school physical education to lifetime physical activity. *European Physical Education Review, 8*(1), 69–84.

Fedewa, A. L., & Ahn, S. (2011). The effects of physical activity and physical fitness on children's achievement and cognitive outcomes: A meta-analysis. *Research Quarterly for Exercise and Sport, 82*(3), 521–535.

Fisher, M., & Meyer, L. H. (2002). Development and social competence after two years for students enrolled in inclusive and self-contained educational programs. *Research and Practice for Persons with Severe Disabilities, 27*(3), 165–174.

Fredricks, J. A., & Eccles, J. S. (2006). Extracurricular involvement and adolescent adjustment: Impact of duration, number of activities, and breadth of participation. *Applied Developmental Science, 10*(3), 132–146.

Hattie, J. A. (2009). *Visible learning: A synthesis of 800+ meta-analyses on achievement.* Abingdon, UK: Routledge.

Hellison, D. (1995). *Teaching personal and social responsibility through physical activity.* Champaign, IL: Human Kinetics.

Hill, G. M. (1993). Youth sport participation of professional baseball players. *Sociology of Sport Journal, 10*(1), 107–114.

Hollis, J. L., Sutherland, R., Williams, A. J., Campbell, E., Nathan, N., Wolfenden, L., . . . Wiggers, J. (2017). A systematic review and meta-analysis of moderate-to-vigorous physical activity levels in secondary school physical education lessons. *International Journal of Behavioral Nutrition and Physical Activity, 14*(1), 52.

Hundert, J., Mahoney, B., Mundy, F., & Vernon, M. L. (1998). A descriptive analysis of developmental and social gains of children with severe disabilities in segregated and inclusive preschools in southern Ontario. *Early Childhood Research Quarterly, 13*(1), 49–65.

Kalnins, I. V., Steele, C., Stevens, E., Rossen, B., Biggar, D., Jutai, J., & Bortolussi, J. (1999). Health survey research on children with physical disabilities in Canada. *Health Promotion International, 14*(3), 251–260.

Kirk, D. (2005). Physical education, youth sport and lifelong participation: The importance of early learning experiences. *European Physical Education Review, 11*(3), 239–255.

Kirk, D. (2010). *Physical Education Futures.* London, UK: Routledge.

Kohl III, H. W., & Cook, H. D. (Eds.). (2013). *Educating the student body: Taking physical activity and physical education to school.* Washington, DC: National Academies Press.

Kreider, C. (2019). Physically active students learn better: Finding new ways to implement movement in the elementary classroom. *Childhood Education, 95*(3), 63–71.

Kretchmar, R. S. (2008). The increasing utility of elementary school physical education: A mixed blessing and unique challenge. *The Elementary School Journal, 108*(3), 161–170.

Kriemler, S., Meyer, U., Martin, E., van Sluijs, E. M., Andersen, L. B., & Martin, B. W. (2011). Effect of school-based interventions on physical activity and fitness in children and adolescents: A review of reviews and systematic update. *British Journal of Sports Medicine, 45*(11), 923–930.

Ladwig, M. A., Vazou, S., & Ekkekakis, P. (2018). "My best memory is when I was done with it": PE memories are associated with adult sedentary behavior. *Translational Journal of the American College of Sports Medicine, 3*(16), 119–129.

Larouche, R., Laurencelle, L., Shephard, R. J., & Trudeau, F. (2015). Daily physical education in primary school and physical activity in midlife: The Trois-Rivières study. *The Journal of Sports Medicine and Physical Fitness, 55*(5), 527–534.

Linda Rikard, G., & Banville, D. (2006). High school student attitudes about physical education. *Sport, Education and Society, 11*(4), 385–400.

Lonsdale, C., Rosenkranz, R. R., Peralta, L. R., Bennie, A., Fahey, P., & Lubans, D. R. (2013). A systematic review and meta-analysis of interventions designed to increase moderate-to-vigorous physical activity in school physical education lessons. *Preventive Medicine, 56*(2), 152–161.

McKenzie, T. L., & Lounsbery, M. A. (2014). The pill not taken: Revisiting physical education teacher effectiveness in a public health context. *Research Quarterly for Exercise and Sport, 85*(3), 287–292.

McKenzie, T. L., Sallis, J. F., Prochaska, J. J., Conway, T. L., Marshall, S. J., & Rosengard, P. (2004). Evaluation of a two-year middle-school physical education intervention: M-SPAN. *Medicine & Science in Sports & Exercise, 36*(8), 1382–1388.

Mooses, K., Pihu, M., Riso, E. M., Hannus, A., Kaasik, P., & Kull, M. (2017). Physical education increases daily moderate to vigorous physical activity and reduces sedentary time. *Journal of School Health, 87*(8), 602–607.

Morgan, C. F., Beighle, A., & Pangrazi, R. P. (2007). What are the contributory and compensatory relationships between physical education and physical activity in children?. *Research Quarterly for Exercise and Sport, 78*(5), 407–412.

Pangrazi, R., & Beighle, A., (2015). *Dynamic physical education for elementary school children* (18th ed.).San Francisco, CA: Pearson.

Pate, R. R., & Hohn, R. C. (1994). Introduction: A contemporary mission for physical education. In R. R. Pate & R. C. Hohn (Eds.), *Health and fitness through physical education* (pp. 1–8). Champaign, IL: Human Kinetics.

Sallis, J. F., & McKenzie, T. L. (1991). Physical education's role in public health. *Research Quarterly for Exercise and Sport, 62*(2), 124–137.

Sallis, J. F., McKenzie, T. L., Beets, M. W., Beighle, A., Erwin, H., & Lee, S. (2012). Physical education's role in public health: Steps forward and backward over 20 years and HOPE for the future. *Research Quarterly for Exercise and Sport, 83*(2), 125–135.

Sandseter, E. B. H. (2009). Affordances for risky play in preschool: The importance of features in the play environment. *Early Childhood Education Journal, 36*(5), 439–446.

Shephard, R. J. (1997). Curricular physical activity and academic performance. *Pediatric Exercise Science, 9*(2), 113–126.

Siedentop, D. (1994). *Sport education: Quality PE through positive sport experiences.* Champaign, IL: Human Kinetics.

Siedentop, D. (2009). *Introduction to physical education, fitness, and sport* (7th ed.). New York, NY: McGraw-Hill.

Simpson, K., & Mandich, A. (2012). Creating inclusive physical education opportunities in elementary physical education. *Physical & Health Education Journal, 77*(4), 18.

Soberlak, P., & Côté, J. (2003). The developmental activities of elite ice hockey players. *Journal of Applied Sport Psychology, 15*(1), 41–49.

Standage, M., Duda, J. L., & Ntoumanis, N. (2005). A test of self-determination theory in school physical education. *British Journal of Educational Psychology, 75*(3), 411–433.

Steele, C. A., Kalnins, I. V., Jutai, J. W., Stevens, S. E., Bortolussi, J. A., & Biggar, W. D. (1996). Lifestyle health behaviours of 11-to 16-year-old youth with physical disabilities. *Health Education Research, 11*(2), 173–186.

Stewart-Brown, S. (2005). Promoting health in children and young people: Identifying priorities. *Perspectives in Public Health, 125*(2), 61.

Stodden, D. F., Goodway, J. D., Langendorfer, S. J., Roberton, M. A., Rudisill, M. E., Garcia, C., & Garcia, L. E. (2008). A developmental perspective on the role of motor skill competence in physical activity: An emergent relationship. *Quest, 60*(2), 290–306.

Strachan, L., Côté, J., & Deakin, J. (2009). "Specializers" versus "samplers" in youth sport: Comparing experiences and outcomes. *The Sport Psychologist, 23*(1), 77–92.

Strean, W. B. (2010). Moving (literally) to engage students: Putting the (physically) active in active learning. *Collected Essays on Learning and Teaching, 3*, 33–37.

Taub, D. E., & Greer, K. R. (2000). Physical activity as a normalizing experience for school-age children with physical disabilities: Implications for legitimation of social identity and enhancement of social ties. *Journal of Sport and Social Issues, 24*(4), 395–414.

Telama, R. (2009). Tracking of physical activity from childhood to adulthood: A review. *Obesity Facts*, *2*(3), 187–195.

Telama, R., Yang, X., Viikari, J., Välimäki, I., Wanne, O., & Raitakari, O. (2005). Physical activity from childhood to adulthood: A 21-year tracking study. *American Journal of Preventive Medicine*, *28*(3), 267–273.

Tinning, R. (2015). 'I don't read fiction': Academic discourse and the relationship between health and physical education. *Sport, Education and Society*, *20*(6), 710–721.

Trudeau, F., Laurencelle, L., Tremblay, J. A., Rajic, M., & Shephard, R. J. (1999). Daily primary school physical education: Effects on physical activity during adult life. *Medicine and Science in Sports and Exercise*, *31*(1), 111–117.

Tudor-Locke, C., Lee, S. M., Morgan, C. F., Beighle, A., & Pangrazi, R. P. (2006). Children's pedometer-determined physical activity during the segmented school day. *Medicine & Science in Sports & Exercise*, *38*(10), 1732–1738.

United Nations Educational, Scientific, and Cultural Organization. (2015). *Quality physical education (QPE): Guidelines for policy makers*. Paris: UNESCO Publishing.

United Nations Educational, Scientific, and Cultural Organization. (2017). *Kazan action plan*. Paris: UNESCO Publishing.

Wallhead, T. L., & Buckworth, J. (2004). The role of physical education in the promotion of youth physical activity. *Quest*, *56*(3), 285–301.

Weiss, M. R., & Ebbeck, V. (1996). Self-esteem and perceptions of competence in youth sport: Theory, research, and enhancement strategies. In O. Bar-Or (Ed.), *The encyclopedia of sports medicine: The child and adolescent athlete* (pp. 364–382). Oxford, UK: Blackwell Science, Ltd.

Whitehead, M. (1990). Meaningful existence, embodiment and physical education. *Journal of Philosophy of Education*, *24*(1), 3–14.

Wolery, M., Martin, C. G., Schroeder, C., Huffman, K., Venn, M. L., Holcombe, A., . . . Fleming, L. A. (1994). Employment of educators in preschool mainstreaming: A survey of general early educators. *Journal of Early Intervention*, *18*(1), 64–77.

Wolery, M., & Sainato, D. M. (1996). General curriculum and intervention strategies. In S. L. Odom & M. E. McLean (Eds.), *Early intervention/early childhood special education: Recommended Practices* (pp. 125–158). Austin, TX: PRO-ED.

Wright, A., & Côté, J. (2003). A retrospective analysis of leadership development through sport. *The Sport Psychologist*, *17*(3), 268–291.

24

SCHOOL RECESS PHYSICAL ACTIVITY INTERVENTIONS

Nicola D. Ridgers, Anne-Maree Parrish, Jo Salmon,
and Anna Timperio

School Recess Context

Derived from the Latin word 'recessus' (a going back, retreat), recess refers to a break during the school day for children to play that typically takes place outside within the school grounds. Recess has been a part of the school day for as long as schools have outdoors existed (Pellegrini, 2005). Little information has documented the origins of school recess, though records from the 1800s have reported the requirement for formal provision of recess periods during the school day (Education Department of Western Australia, 1898; Kahan, 2008). The rationale for recess periods is simple; after a period of work, there needs to be a period of rest (Kahan, 2008; Pellegrini, 2005). For example, regulations from the Education Department of Western Australia (1898) highlight the importance of such periods, stating that '*[morning recess]* is intended solely for the benefit of their *[children's]* health, and to enable the rest of the morning's lessons to be carried out more easily by them' (p. 4). Similarly, Harris stated that '*[recess]* seems to meet certain physiological requirements of the young and growing individuals… in a better manner than any other device yet proposed can do' (National Education Association of the United States, 1884, p. 337).

School recess is a unique context that plays an important role in a child's growth and development (Pellegrini & Smith, 1993; Ramstetter, Murray, & Garner, 2010). It provides children and adolescents with up to 390 opportunities per school year (based on two times a day, 5 days a week, 39 weeks per school year) to engage in freely chosen leisure activities with their peers, which are relatively free from adult control (Pellegrini & Bohn, 2005; Ridgers, Carter, Stratton, & McKenzie, 2011). Furthermore, school recess has numerous academic, physical, cognitive, social, and emotional benefits (Pellegrini & Bohn, 2005; Ramstetter et al., 2010). For example, children learn key social skills such as sharing, cooperating, taking turns, negotiating, conflict management, and problem solving (Bjorklund & Brown, 1998; Pellegrini, Blatchford, Kato, & Baines, 2004; Ramstetter et al., 2010). There are opportunities to practice motor skills, gain confidence in their movements, and to be physically active (Evans, 1996; Ridgers, Stratton, & Fairclough, 2006). Benefits to classroom behavior have also been reported, with children more attentive and productive following recess (Jarrett et al., 1998; Pellegrini, 2005; Pellegrini, Huberty, & Jones, 1995).

Despite this, however, the role and value of recess in the school day have been extensively debated. Over the past 25 years, research has documented the trend of reducing the frequency and duration of school recess, or even removing it altogether (Blatchford & Baines, 2006; Blatchford & Sumpner, 1998; Pellegrini & Bohn, 2005; Ramstetter et al., 2010). Reasons for this include academic pressures, with recess taking up valuable academic instruction time, or behavioral problems occurring during recess (Blatchford & Baines, 2006; Blatchford & Sumpner, 1998; Ginsburg, 2007; Pellegrini, 2005). In fact, these concerns are not new. In one of the earliest documented debates in the United States, Ellis outlined key reasons for adopting a 'no recess' plan to counter concerns that included the health and safety of the children, poor playground behavior, and the negative impact of recess on concentration and learning time (National Education Association of the United States, 1884). From a physical activity perspective, the reduction or removal of recess from the school day has potentially wide reaching and long-term implications, particularly as school recess provides an important and salient contribution to both children's and adolescents' daily physical activity and recommended activity levels (Ridgers et al., 2006; Ridgers, Timperio, Crawford, & Salmon, 2012).

Definition of School Recess

The definition, delivery, and composition of recess varies between countries (Pellegrini & Smith, 1993), which can cause confusion within the literature as to what this term is referring to (Escalante, Garcia-Hermoso, Backx, & Saavedra, 2014). As an example, the terms 'school recess', 'recess', 'break time', and 'playtime' have also been used to refer to specific periods of the day and/ or the sum of all recess periods on one day (e.g. morning, lunchtime, and afternoon; Huberty et al., 2011; Mota et al., 2005; Ridgers, Timperio, Crawford, & Salmon, 2013), depending on the age of the children. For the purpose of this chapter, school recess is considered to be the non-curriculum time regularly allocated by schools between lessons for children and adolescents to engage in discretionary leisure activities (Pellegrini & Smith, 1993; Ridgers et al., 2006). Unless otherwise specified, school recess is considered to be the sum of all of these periods (e.g. morning recess and lunchtime). Finally, it is acknowledged that in recent years, schools have begun to offer structured recess periods where games and activities are organized and led by facilitators. Debates currently exist as to whether such approaches can be truly considered recess given the general lack of truly discretionary activities (Ramstetter et al., 2010), but literature concerning structured recess is included in this chapter for information (see *Structured Recess* below).

School Recess Interventions

As noted, recess provides a regular opportunity for children in many countries to engage in physical activity on a daily basis (Parrish, Okely, Stanley, & Ridgers, 2013). However, until recently, recess could claim to be the forgotten part of the school day, with few physical activity interventions targeting this setting (Ridgers et al., 2006). In recent years, more and more recess interventions have emerged as it has been recognized that recess may provide the greatest opportunity for daily physical activity promotion in schools (Ridgers, Salmon, Parrish, Stanley, & Okely, 2012). Broadly speaking, recess interventions can be described as structured or unstructured strategies (Hyndman, 2015), though which strategies fall into these categories can be debated. Some of the more common intervention strategies are discussed in this chapter, but it is acknowledged that this is not an exhaustive list.

Playground Modifications

Arguably the main intervention approach implemented within recess settings to date is physical changes to the playground environment, which typically involve the introduction of multicolor playground markings (hopscotch, sports zones, targets, mazes; Blaes et al., 2013; Stratton, 2000; Stratton & Leonard, 2002; Stratton & Mullan, 2005) and/or physical structures (fencing, soccer goals, basketball hoops; Ridgers, Fairclough, & Stratton, 2010a; Ridgers, Stratton, Fairclough, &

Twisk, 2007a, 2007b), and major school playground renovations (e.g. outdoor gyms, climbing frames, stages, shade areas (Anthamatten et al., 2011; Brink et al., 2010; Hamer et al., 2017)). While it has been suggested that playground modifications are an example of structured recess interventions (Hyndman, 2015), it should be noted that such approaches can be used to enable children to engage in active, discretionary behaviors in an unstructured way with their peers, which is important for physical activity accumulation (Pate, Baranowski, Dowda, & Trost, 1996; Welk, 1999). The important distinction is that while playground modifications provide physical structure to the available space (e.g. activity zones; Janssen, Toussaint, Van Mechelen, & Verhagen, 2011), children are free to choose the games they wish to play using the markings and/or physical structures during recess, rather than being required to engage in set activities (see *Structured Recess* section). Indeed, such games and activities using markings and/or physical structures may be both active and inactive; the key point is children can freely choose.

In one of the earliest studies, Stratton (2000) examined the short-term effects of painting playground markings such as a castle, pirate ship, dragon, and snakes and ladders on children's recess physical activity. Significant increases in children's moderate- to vigorous-intensity physical activity were observed (18 minutes per day), suggesting that simple markings can stimulate and support physical activity and play behaviors (Stratton, 2000). A number of other studies have also shown that playground markings increase children's physical activity within a 2–4-week period post-redesign compared to control schools (Blaes et al., 2013; Stratton & Leonard, 2002; Stratton & Mullan, 2005), though concerns have been raised that such findings may be attributable to novelty effects. In contrast, Ridgers and colleagues (2007a) found no significant changes in recess physical activity 6 weeks after a playground redesign that used a zonal design (Figure 24.1) compared to children attending control schools after accounting for factors that may confound effects (e.g. age, sex). Despite this, stronger effects were observed for younger children. It was suggested that the introduction of playground markings and physical structures decreased the dominance of older children on playground space (Epstein, Kehily, Mac an Ghaill, & Redman, 2001) and provided more opportunities for younger children to be physically active (Ridgers et al., 2007a).

Until recently, scant research had examined the longer-term impacts of playground modifications on children's physical activity levels during recess (Escalante et al., 2014; Parrish et al., 2013). Such information is important for identifying the effectiveness of these strategies over time and the development of physical activity programming and policies in schools (Escalante et al., 2014; Ridgers, Salmon, et al., 2012). Evaluating a combination of playground markings and physical structures, Ridgers and colleagues (2007b, 2010a) examined the effect of the intervention at

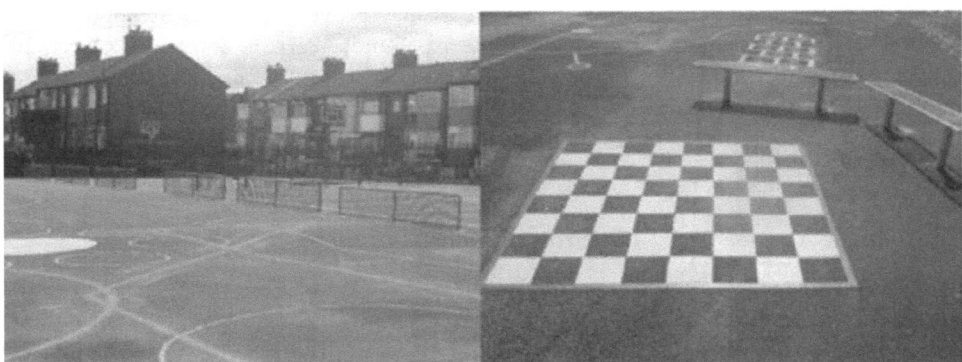

Figure 24.1 Example of playground redesign using playground markings and physical structures (Photograph courtesy of N. Ridgers)

6-month and 12-month post-modification on children's recess physical activity. It was found that adding playground markings and physical structures into the playground were effective in increasing children's physical activity levels at 6-month post-modification, and the strongest intervention effects were observed at this time point (Ridgers et al., 2007b, 2010a). While the intervention still had positive effects on activity levels at 12-month post-modification, these were no longer significant (Ridgers et al., 2010a). It was suggested that additional strategies may be needed in the longer-term to maintain initial increases observed in activity levels (Ridgers et al., 2010a).

A number of studies have examined the impact of major school playground renovations on children's activity levels over time. Such changes included introducing age appropriate play equipment, shaded areas, landscaped areas (e.g. seated areas, vegetable gardens; Anthamatten et al., 2011; Brink et al., 2010) through the Learning Landscapes Program, and outdoor gyms, climbing frames, and games pitches (Hamer et al., 2017). However, only one study specifically examined children's recess activity levels, finding that there were no differences in activity levels compared to children attending control schools, despite more children in the intervention schools accessing the school playground at this time (access during lunchtime was optional (Anthamatten et al., 2011)). In contrast, children were more active in redesigned school playgrounds compared to control schools, but data collected in and out of school time were combined (Brink et al., 2010). Finally, Hamer and colleagues (2017) also reported no significant differences in school-day activity levels 12-month post-modification; yet this time frame included both recess and class time. Consequently, little is known as to the short- and longer-term effects of major redesigns on children's activity levels during school recess.

Loose Equipment

Interventions examining the effects of loose equipment on children's recess activity levels can typically be categorized as games equipment (e.g. balls, bats, skipping ropes, circus equipment) and recycled materials (e.g. car tires, milk crates, buckets). Interestingly, few studies to date have been conducted using loose equipment (Parrish et al., 2013). In one of the first studies, Verstraete and colleagues examined the effects of games equipment on children's physical activity levels during recess and lunchtime (Verstraete, Cardon, DeClercq, & De Bourdeaudhuij, 2006). Three months after the introduction of the games equipment, intervention children's vigorous and moderate-to-vigorous-intensity physical activity actually decreased during morning recess, while increases were observed at lunchtime (Verstraete et al., 2006). It should be noted that intervention schools were asked to regularly rotate equipment to prevent children losing interest. While no information was reported about the frequency with which equipment were rotated, if at all (Verstraete et al., 2006), these findings suggest that such an approach may not necessarily negate potential novelty effects for having access to new equipment. However, it is also possible that during the shorter recess periods the collection of equipment and organization of activities accounted for a greater proportion of time, therefore resulting in decreased activity levels during morning recess. In contrast, Lopes and colleagues found that the use of games equipment significantly increased children's vigorous-intensity physical activity during recess, but decreases were observed for moderate-intensity physical activity (Lopes, Lopes, & Pereira, 2009). These results suggest that games equipment was effective at increasing time spent engaged in higher intensities, but may not have replaced time spent in lower activity intensities.

The impact of introducing recycled loose materials on children's physical activity during recess has also been examined. The underlying premise is that active, imaginative play is stimulated because these materials (e.g. milk crates, empty containers, hay-bales) have no immediate or obvious use (Bundy et al., 2011; Engelen et al., 2013; Hyndman et al., 2014). Such materials are typically low-cost and often readily available, providing a viable alternative to more commonly implemented recess interventions. In 2009, Bundy and colleagues reported that after an 11-week period where children from one school were provided with recycled materials, children were significantly more active during lunchtime compared to baseline. However, as only an indication of activity volume was reported, it is not known whether moderate- to vigorous-intensity physical activity increased (Bundy et al., 2009). In a follow-up study involving 12 schools, significant increases in moderate- to vigorous-intensity physical activity were reported after a 13-week intervention period, which equated to a 1.8 minute change (Engelen et al., 2013). Hyndman and colleagues (2014) also examined the impact of loose recycled materials on children's lunchtime activity at the end of the intervention (7 weeks) and at 8-month follow-up. Intervention children took more steps than control children after 7 weeks (13 steps per minute) and were observed to engage in more vigorous-intensity physical activity (6% of observations). Smaller but significant effects also persisted after 8 months for these outcomes (six steps per minute; 6% of observations; Hyndman et al., 2014). The results suggest that recycled materials can increase activity levels in the short-term, but further research is needed to establish the longer-term effects.

Active Video Games

One study investigated the effects of active video game play during lunchtime on children's physical activity levels. In this study, children were asked to play the Nintendo Wii twice a week for 6 weeks. Duncan and Staples (2010) found that during the first week of the study, children took more steps per minute during active video game play compared to children taking part in usual lunchtime activities (control group). However, by the end of the study, children playing active video games were less active than their peers who were engaging in free-play (Duncan & Staples, 2010). These results suggest that active video gaming should not replace traditional free-play opportunities in school settings (Parrish et al., 2013). Active video gaming (or similar activity promoting technology) may have an impact on activity levels during recess periods when outdoor play is not possible (e.g. during inclement weather), though no research to date has investigated this.

Structured Recess

The emergence of structured recess as an intervention strategy is predicated on two points, namely children require assistance and encouragement to be active during recess, and children must be physically active in order to address rising obesity levels (Murray & Ramstetter, 2013; Ramstetter et al., 2010). During a structured recess, games and activities are planned, led, and supervised by trained adults such as teachers, coaches, and research staff to increase time spent in physical activity (Beyler, Bleeker, James-Burdumy, Fortson, & Benjamin, 2014; Ramstetter et al., 2010). The primary focus is to engage more children in activities during recess and at higher activity intensities (Murray & Ramstetter, 2013). Examples of structured recess interventions include obstacle courses (Scruggs, Beveridge, & Watson, 2003), recess activity of the week (Stellino, Sinclair, Partridge, & King, 2010), modeling active games (Efrat, 2013), and organized games, often within specified activity zones (Beyler et al., 2014; Bleeker, Beyler, James-Burdumy, & Fortson, 2015; Chin & Ludwig, 2013; Howe, Freedson, Alhassan, Feldman, & Osganian, 2012; Huberty et al., 2011). Such interventions may require all children to engage in a specific activity (e.g. Scruggs et al., 2003), while others may provide a range of organized activities for children to undertake (e.g. Bleeker et al., 2015).

Structured recess interventions have been found to increase time spent in moderate- to vigorous-intensity physical activity (Huberty et al., 2011; Scruggs et al., 2003) and elicit higher energy expenditure during recess (Howe et al., 2012). However, others have reported no significant changes compared to control schools (Beyler et al., 2014; Bleeker et al., 2015) or activity accumulated during usual recess periods (Stellino et al., 2010), while Efrat (2013) reported decreased engagement in moderate- to vigorous-intensity physical activity. It should be noted that there may be differential benefits of structured recess for some children. For example, studies have indicated that girls' recess activity levels may benefit from structured activities (Bleeker et al., 2015; Scruggs et al., 2003; Stellino et al., 2010) as on average their overall activity levels are generally lower (Ridgers, Salmon, et al., 2012) and boys tend to dominate play spaces during recess (Knowles, Parnell, Stratton, & Ridgers, 2013; Thomson, 2005). However, contrasting findings have been noted regarding children's liking and enjoyment of structured recess breaks. Scruggs and colleagues (2003) noted that girls liked fitness breaks less than boys, and less than 'usual' recess periods. In comparison, Howe and colleagues (2012) reported that teachers perceived their students to have a high level of enjoyment during structured recess though no data were collected from children themselves. These results suggest that while structured recess periods may benefit children's activity levels, children's enjoyment of such approaches must also be considered as this may influence engagement over time.

Multicomponent Strategies

Given the range of potential factors (correlates) that may influence children's physical activity levels during school recess (Ridgers, Salmon, et al., 2012), it is unsurprising that an increasing number of studies are examining the effects of multicomponent interventions that target these factors (Parrish et al., 2013). In the context of this discussion, multicomponent interventions are considered those that have combined strategies across multiple levels of influence (Parrish et al., 2013; Ridgers, Salmon, et al., 2012). Several studies have combined environmental changes (e.g. playground modifications, games equipment) with social support strategies (e.g. teacher encouragement, activity coaches; Elder, McKenzie, Arredondo, Crespo, & Ayala, 2011; Janssen et al., 2011; Van Kann et al., 2017), while others have combined environmental changes with policy changes such as increasing access to playground areas during recess, reduced rules (Farmer et al., 2017; Parrish, Okely, Batterham, Cliff, & Magee, 2016), and staff training (Huberty, Beets, Beighle, Saint-Maurice, & Welk, 2014; Huberty et al., 2011).

In general, mixed effects of multicomponent recess interventions on physical activity have been reported in the short- and longer-term. Some studies have found that children attending intervention schools engage in significantly more recess physical activity than children attending control schools, though different effects were observed across activity intensities (Huberty et al., 2011, 2014; Janssen, Twisk, Toussaint, van Mechelen, & Verhagen, 2015; Van Kann et al., 2017). In contrast, others have reported non-significant changes (Farmer et al., 2017; Parrish et al., 2016) or decreases in moderate-to-vigorous physical activity (Elder et al., 2011; Huberty et al., 2014). While little research has examined whether targeting multiple components is more effective than targeting single components (Parrish et al., 2013), some studies have investigated whether intervention implementation may provide insights into the findings. For example, Elder and colleagues (2011) reported difficulties in delivering the intervention in schools, while Huberty et al. (2014) found that school staff tended to focus on children's safety rather than actively promote or encourage physical activity. When Van Kann and colleagues (2017) considered the number of intervention components implemented in different schools (dose), significantly greater changes in moderate-to-vigorous-intensity physical activity were observed in schools that provided more physical changes targeting higher activity intensities. Interestingly, intervention effects did not vary by level of school commitment (Van Kann et al., 2017). Overall, these results highlight the importance of process evaluations that may help to explain why interventions were, or were not, effective to inform the development and delivery of future recess-based strategies in schools.

Key Issues for School Recess Interventions

Over the past 10 years there has clearly been an increase in a range of interventions conducted during school recess with the aim of increasing children's physical activity levels. There are, however, a number of key issues that require further consideration and investigation during the planning and evaluation of such interventions. The following issues highlight some of the main considerations and knowledge gaps.

Structured Versus Unstructured Recess

In recent years there has been some debate about the role of adults within recess and, in particular, how they can support children to be physically active during this period of time. As previously noted, recess arguably provides one of the last daily play opportunities for children that is relatively free from adult control (Pellegrini & Bohn, 2005). As already discussed, recess periods where adults (e.g. volunteers, coaches, teachers) plan, lead, and teach activities may increase activity levels, but threaten the main role of recess and can detract from the numerous benefits of recess that have been observed. That is, recess is an unstructured time for children to choose to engage in self-directed and often spontaneous activities (Blatchford, 1996; Murray & Ramstetter, 2013; Pellegrini & Bohn, 2005; Ramstetter et al., 2010). While these could be physically active in nature, they can also include creative, imaginative, rough and tumble social behaviors that may be constrained during structured activities (Murray & Ramstetter, 2013; Ramstetter et al., 2010).

Perceived encouragement from peers, parents, and teachers has been found to be positively associated with physical activity levels during recess in adolescents (Hohepa, Scragg, Schofield, Kolt, & Schaaf, 2007). For example, school staff can be trained to encourage and support physical activity through demonstrating traditional playground games and providing instruction on how to play games (Blatchford & Sumpner, 1998) though this may be more appealing to primary school–aged children. Demonstrating games can be ad hoc rather than formally structured, but importantly they can help pass on knowledge across generations, and contribute to the active playground culture (Blatchford, 1996). The challenge for schools and teachers moving forward is to provide a safe, fun, and enjoyable supportive environment for physical activity that meets the needs of children during recess. Given that children are the recess experts (Blatchford & Sumpner, 1998), researchers and educators should consider participatory approaches to identify strategies to implement within schools (Blatchford & Sharp, 1994).

Effectiveness of Interventions in Different Populations

When evaluating the effects of an intervention, it is useful to know how, why, and for which population group the intervention worked (Fairchild & McQuillin, 2010). Such information is critical for identifying who and what to target in future physical activity interventions. To achieve this, researchers can examine which factors explain how an intervention increased activity levels (i.e. mediator analyses) or modify the strength and/or direction of a relationship (i.e. moderator analyses; Fairchild & McQuillin, 2010; Wu & Zumbo, 2008). However, few studies have specifically examined moderators of recess interventions, and only one study to date has examined mediators of the impact of a whole school intervention approach on recess physical activity (Yildrim et al., 2014). In a meta-analysis of 13 studies undertaken by Erwin, Ickes, Ahn, and Fedewa (2014), moderation according to age, sex, and intervention length was examined. It was reported that interventions were more effective for younger children and during longer recess periods (Erwin et al., 2014). This may be because interventions reduce the dominance of older children on the playground and longer recess periods provide more time for children to engage in different activities during this time (Ridgers et al., 2007b; Zask, van Beurden, Barnett, Brooks, & Dietrich, 2001).

Other studies have reported that interventions were more effective for less active children (Ridgers et al., 2007a), older children (Janssen et al., 2015), committed schools (Van Kann et al., 2017), girls (Janssen et al., 2015), and in summer/autumn (Janssen et al., 2015). In contrast, some studies have reported no differences in intervention effects by sex (Engelen et al., 2013; Ridgers et al., 2007a, 2007b; Verstraete et al., 2006), baseline activity (Ridgers et al., 2007a; Verstraete et al., 2006), or body mass index (Ridgers, Fairclough, & Stratton, 2010b). Given that these moderators have been examined across a wide range of intervention types (e.g. playground markings, games equipment, recycled materials, multicomponent strategies), more research is needed to determine which interventions are effective for each of these groups. There is also a critical need for more research focusing on mediators in order to understand the key factors that facilitate intervention effectiveness.

Time Allocated to School Recess

New international guidelines for children's physical activity, sedentary behavior, and sleep incorporate the 24-hour period (Canadian Society for Exercise Physiology, 2019), drawing attention to the need to optimize opportunities to be physically active and reduce sitting time throughout the day. With increasing rates of sedentary behavior, every minute of recess is a precious opportunity to allow children to be physically active, often providing the opportunity for half or more of the 60 minutes of physical activity recommended per day (US Department of Health and Human Services, 2018; Hidding, Altenburg, van Ekris, & Chinapaw, 2017).

Time allocated to recess varies between and within countries by the number of recess periods, the form of the break, total time allocated to the recess period, and the level of schooling (Beresin, 2016). An example of the variability in recess time varies from 'no time' allocated to recess in mainland China to 90 minutes per day in Finland with 6 breaks of 15 minutes (Beresin, 2016). In the United Kingdom there are usually two recess periods per day, with a total average time of 75 minutes (Baines & Blatchford, 2019). In the United States, the Centers for Disease Control and Prevention (2011) recommends at least 20 minutes of recess per day for elementary school students. However, state laws vary with recess time ranging between no recess and a minimum of 30 minutes of recess per day (National Institutes of Health, 2015). Further, schools in lower socioeconomic or urban regions were less likely to allocate time to recess (Ramstetter et al., 2010). In some states in Australia recess is mandated and traditionally consists of one longer and one shorter break each day (e.g. 15 minute and 60 minute (lunch break) recess; New South Wales Department of Education, 2016). However, in 1991 individual school principals were afforded the right to vary 'standard' school hours (this included variations on school start and finish times), which resulted in shorter periods of recess (New South Wales Department of Education, 2016; Victorian State Government, 2019). In many instances recess duration often decreases as children age, particularly as they move into secondary school (Ramstetter et al., 2010; Zavacky & Michael, 2017). The length of the break can be reflective of the opportunity for play, for instance, shorter recess breaks often only afford enough time for children visit the bathroom or consume food, while longer breaks can allow opportunities for more active play (Beresin, 2016).

The length of recess is a contentious issue. Principals and teachers are pressured to meet academic targets and may replace recess time with classroom learning. Such initiatives can be counterproductive, with literature indicating that regular breaks from concentration are required for cognitive processing and academic performance (Ramstetter et al., 2010). Recess should afford students sufficient time to participate in physical activity and play which also assists their social and emotional development (Pellegrini, 2008). It is one of the few opportunities in the school day where students engage with their peers and socialize. It is important for policy makers to optimize professional development opportunities for executive staff and teachers to understand the links between recess and positive social, health, and cognitive outcomes (Beard, 2018). Moreover, from a workplace perspective, teachers have the right to a break during the school day for their own health and well-being (National Education Union UK, 2018; The Fair Work Commission Australia, 2010).

The timing of recess in relation to meal times is an important yet understudied area to date. Research has examined the impact of the timing of recess on food consumption and waste; yet little is known about the relationship between recess timing and physical activity. A recent study found that there was no effect on moderate-to-vigorous physical activity regardless of whether food was eaten immediately prior to or following recess, though there was greater residual energy when food was consumed after recess (McLoughlin et al., 2019). Further research is needed to understand whether the timing of recess around meal times may influence physical activity levels.

Recess Policies

Policies relating to recess vary considerably within and between countries. While under researched, organizational policy may impact children's physical activity levels (Ridgers, Salmon, et al., 2012). Some policies are implemented by National, State, or District education authorities, while others are formed at the school level. In some instances, federal policies unrelated to recess can impact time allocated for recess. In the United States (US), the introduction of the 'no child left behind policy' resulted in a reduction of time allocated to recess and personal development, health, and physical education in elementary schools in order to spend more time on curriculum targets (van der Mars, 2018). In 2016 the US 'State of the nation report' indicated that only eight states had policies relating to recess in elementary schools and no record of policies in middle and high schools (Society of Health and Physical Educators America, 2016). Internationally, it is not uncommon for teachers to restrict children from having recess as punishment for poor academic performance or poor classroom behavior (Turner, Chriqui, & Chaloupka, 2013). In the United States, more than 70% of elementary schools in one study withheld recess as a form of punishment for poor behavior or academic reasons (Turner et al., 2013). A variation of this policy exists in Victoria, Australia, where teachers are not permitted to use more than half of the recess period as punishment (Victorian State Government, 2019). Such policies seem counterintuitive when cognitive processing and academic performance rely on regular breaks from concentrated work (Ramstetter et al., 2010).

While such policies can have a marked impact on recess time, 'within school policies' evoke similar outcomes. Some examples include no running on concrete, no games that involved tackling, no climbing trees, no ball games near school buildings, compulsory restrictive school uniforms, having access to non-fixed equipment, 'no hat not play', and limiting access to play areas (Evans, 2003; Parrish, Yeatman, Iverson, & Russell, 2011). Many of these rules are the result of increasing awareness of teachers' duty of care, resulting in policing rather than supervising the playground (Evans, 2003). However, well-structured and supervised recess with supportive environmental conditions and well-maintained equipment is a means of reducing such concerns (Ramstetter et al., 2010).

In some instances, school health policy can be conflicting. For example, in Australian primary schools the 'no hat – no play' policy can result in children spending recess indoors. This policy is the result of the high levels of melanoma in Australia (Parrish et al., 2011). Unfortunately, this well-meaning policy while aiming to improve one health outcome impacts another. Policies can be modified to meet the health needs of children, with some schools adopting a 'no hat - play in the shade' policy which restricts but does not prevent physical activity at recess (Parrish et al., 2011).

Several other policy-related factors can also inhibit physical activity during recess, even when recess is mandated. In primary (elementary) schools in particular, school policies often warrant that children sit for a period of time within the recess period to consume their food prior to playing (Evans, 2003). Some schools mandate a time frame that all children must remain seated while other schools allow students to play once their food is consumed (Parrish et al., 2011). This policy can also vary by year group (e.g. younger children may take longer to eat their food; Evans, 2003). In addition, some schools allow access to indoor environments during recess which typically promote more sedentary activities (e.g. access to computer labs or the library; Pawlowski, Andersen, Troelsen, & Schipperijn, 2016). Identifying strategies to promote physically active indoor recess periods is needed, particularly when required due to weather conditions. This is an area of research anticipated to develop in the future. Arguably one of the biggest challenges that schools will have to overcome is children's free access to electronic devices during recess, which can compromise opportunities for active play (New South Wales Department of Education, 2019).

In a more positive light, some school policies support children's activity during recess; examples include exclusive areas for younger children to play, access to non-fixed equipment and play areas and rules to prevent bullying (Parrish et al., 2011). Importantly recess policies should be evaluated for their effectiveness and regularly updated to reflect the literature at both organizational and school level (Beard, 2018). Professional development is key to providing both executive staff and teachers with updated evidence encouraging the optimization of recess policies (Beard, 2018).

Intervention Sustainability

Ensuring that recess interventions are sustained over time is often challenging. While teachers may acknowledge the importance of intervention outcomes, competing priorities and time limitations can take precedence (Parrish et al., 2011). Changes in school executive or teaching staff can also influence the sustainability of an intervention, particularly when teachers' priorities do not align with intervention aims or there is no ongoing training and support to sustain the intervention (Bundy et al., 2011). Teacher training may assist the sustainability of physical activity interventions in relation to risk aversion in the school setting (Bundy et al., 2011; Sutherland et al., 2016).

Few studies have investigated the long-term sustainability of interventions in the recess setting. A 12-month follow-up of a physical activity intervention delivered twice each week during recess demonstrated poor reach with many students showing low levels of intervention awareness and girls less likely to be aware than boys (Sutherland et al., 2016). Interventions utilizing physical environmental variables (such as loose equipment) can also be impacted by budgetary constraints associated with ongoing equipment maintenance (Parrish et al., 2011). Interventions that are solely delivered by a research team are more likely to desist when these outside resources are removed (Lewis, Napolitano, Buman, Williams, & Nigg, 2017). While many recess interventions to date have focused on physical environmental changes to the school environment, the sustainability of these interventions is equally reliant on conducive social environments during recess, enforced safety and behavioral expectations, supportive teachers and executive, supportive recess policies, and ongoing budgetary allocation (Centers for Disease Control and Prevention and Society of Health and Physical Educators America, 2017; Parrish et al., 2011; Parrish et al., 2013).

Emerging Issues for School Recess Intervention Research

Adolescent Recess Interventions

Physical activity levels decline as children progress toward adolescence, which is mirrored in the recess period (Ridgers, Timperio, et al., 2012). However, recess interventions targeting adolescents are few and far between, which may reflect the limited or non-existent time allocated to recess in some countries (Reilly, Johnston, McIntosh, & Martin, 2016). A recess intervention for adolescents in Finland found that recess physical activity levels were positively influenced by organized activities, the provision of equipment and sporting facilities, and student recess activators (Haapala et al., 2014).

An Australian intervention introduced organized physical activity during recess for 2 days each week, supported by loose equipment such as balls and ropes (as part of a larger study); however changes in physical activity levels were not reported for the recess period (Sutherland et al., 2016). The provision of equipment or allowing adolescents to bring their own equipment to school has been found to have positive effects on recess physical activity levels both cross-sectionally and over time (Ridgers et al., 2013). It was suggested that such provisions may continue to facilitate activity in adolescents who choose to be active during recess (Ridgers et al., 2013), but other strategies such as organized social activities may be required. Given that qualitative data have shown that peers can influence recess moderate-to-vigorous physical activity, identifying strategies where adolescents can provide social support may be important for increasing activity and engaging in game play (Hohepa, Scragg, Schofield, Kolt, & Schaaf, 2009; Leggett, Irwin, Griffith, Xue, & Fradette, 2012). In New Zealand, a study among adolescents indicated that lower levels of peer support were associated with lower odds of being active during school recess (Hohepa et al., 2007), while the absence of friends is a barrier for recess physical activity (Hohepa et al., 2009; Leggett et al., 2012).

An ever increasing barrier to recess physical activity is the continual updating of modern technology. A recent Australian government review indicated that the growing number of mobile devices used for non-educational purposes in school playgrounds is an increasing problem and is thought to negatively impact adolescents' physical activity levels (New South Wales Department of Education, 2019). The document supported the restriction of smart phones during school recess.

Overall, few recess interventions have targeted adolescents. Based on the limited research to date, it appears that loose equipment has the potential to increase physical activity in these settings; however some differences in preferences for activity types by gender may exist (Klinker et al., 2014). Social support and the influence of peers are important factors for intervention development (Hohepa et al., 2009), and must be considered in the design of strategies targeting this age group. Interventions must also consider contemporary technologies and their impact on the behaviors that adolescents engage in during recess (New South Wales Department of Education, 2019).

Playground Design

The physical environment is a key facilitator of children's physical activity during recess. Children have been shown to like playgrounds that have a mix of areas with different surfaces (Willenberg et al., 2010), have suitable spaces to play different games (Pawlowski et al., 2016; Stanley, Boshoff, & Dollman, 2012), and are not overcrowded (Knowles et al., 2013; Pawlowski et al., 2016; Stanley et al., 2012). However, this is often in direct contrast to the types of conventional play spaces provided to children that comprise of asphalt playground and small open fields (Dyment, Bell, & Lucas, 2009). In order to design diverse play spaces that meet the needs of children while optimizing activity opportunities during recess, there is a need for more research to examine what playground features facilitate physical activity.

A range of measurement tools can be used to examine playgrounds designs and physical activity levels. For example, global positioning system (GPS) devices and direct observation methods can provide rich contextual data about the spaces and/or equipment that children access during school recess, how active they are, and how long they spend in these spaces (Clevenger, Sinha, & Howe, 2019; Pawlowski et al., 2016; Saint-Maurice, Welk, Silva, Siahpush, & Huberty, 2011; Van Kann et al., 2016). While it is recognized that such information may be school specific and possibly influenced by children's experiences of existing play spaces and the playground culture (i.e. what are acceptable play behaviors), consistent findings can provide key considerations for future intervention development. Several studies have shown that higher levels of physical activity occur in areas where fixed equipment (e.g. soccer goals, high bars) is provided (Dyment et al., 2009; Van Kann et al., 2016), while others have found that open green spaces are active areas (Dyment et al., 2009;

Pawlowski et al., 2016). Spaces such as paved sporting areas where children can engage in basketball, soccer, and four-square have also been shown to be popular, but activity levels tended to be lower as children had to wait in turn for their opportunities to play games (Dyment et al., 2009; Pawlowski et al., 2016). This highlights the need to activate the spaces provided so that there is sufficient equipment and markings (for example) to increase the numbers of children being active. Moreover, boys are more active than girls in the majority of school play spaces, especially when more boys were present and sports games were played (Saint-Maurice et al., 2011). This demonstrates the need to design spaces that enable girls to be active (Dyment et al., 2009). Overall, it is clear that to increase our understanding of how playground designs facilitate physical activity, researchers and practitioners should consider using combined methodological approaches. By focusing on where (and why) children choose to spend their recess and how active they are in these spaces, this has the potential to inform the development and/or redesign of school playgrounds in the future.

Seasonal Differences

One factor that may need to be considered in the development and implementation of recess interventions is whether children's physical activity levels differ across seasons. While recognizing that school policies relating to weather conditions are likely to differ, schools typically require children to access the school grounds during recess in most weather conditions and when it is considered safe to do so (Thomson, 2004). Thus, it is possible that physical activity during recess varies across seasons. However, inconsistent findings have been reported. Several studies have reported no differences in recess physical activity levels between seasons (Ridgers & Stratton, 2005; Ridgers, Stratton, Clark, Fairclough, & Richardson, 2006) while others have reported children are more active in spring compared to autumn or winter (Saint-Maurice et al., 2011), or in cooler compared to warmer months (Ridgers, Salmon, & Timperio, 2018). A limitation of most of these studies is that season is used as a proxy for meteorological conditions (e.g. rainfall, maximum temperature) at certain times of the year; yet the actual conditions during data collection are not reported. For example, negative associations have been reported between temperature and physical activity, particularly for higher intensities (Fairclough, Beighle, Erwin, & Ridgers, 2012; Ridgers, Fairclough, & Stratton, 2010b). It has been suggested that children are more active in colder temperatures due to a thermoregulatory need to keep warm, while in warmer temperatures children are less inclined to be active, possibly due to heat stress (Fairclough et al., 2012; Ridgers et al., 2006; Stanley et al., 2012). Associations between rainfall and physical activity are less consistent, with some studies reporting that activity levels are lower during heavy rainfall (Harrison et al., 2011) and others reporting no effects (Fairclough et al., 2012). Interestingly, rain has been more commonly cited as a barrier to physical activity than cold weather as it prevents access to some areas (e.g. grass pitches) and equipment that could make them dirty (Pawlowski et al., 2016; Willenberg et al., 2010) and only small sheltered areas may be present (if at all; Harrison et al., 2011). This highlights the need for more research to understand the underlying reasons behind differences in children's activity levels between seasons and across a range of meteorological influences to identify when and under what conditions strategies may be needed to increase activity levels.

Recommendations for Future Research and Practice

Requirement of Recess Policies

In many countries globally (e.g. Australia, United Kingdom, Denmark) recess is a mandated part of the school day and typically consists of a morning recess and a lunch break, though some notable exceptions have been reported (Ridgers, Toth, & Uvacsek, 2009). However, few schools provide afternoon recess. Afternoon recess has often been removed from the school day without a concomitant increase in time allocated to the remaining recess periods (Blatchford & Baines, 2006; Blatchford & Sumpner, 1998). Recess duration aside, this has also impacted the number of recess opportunities available to children (e.g. removal of 195 recess periods per year based on 39 weeks of school). In the United States, there is little consistency in the way that recess is implemented (Pellegrini & Bohn, 2005). Few states have policies requiring schools to provide recess on a daily basis (Piekarz et al., 2016). Of greater concern, it has been reported that children attending schools in cities or with a higher proportion of students living in disadvantage are less likely to have daily recess (Center for Education Statistics, 2005). Taken together, there is a need for policies to require and/or protect daily recess provisions and for research to examine the impact of such policies on children's activity over time. This is to ensure that future generations of children have the opportunity to be physically active and gain the developmental benefits obtained from recess. As Blatchford and Sumpner (1998) noted, to fail to protect recess may mean that '... we may recognise the value of breaktime [recess] to pupils long after changes have severely altered or reduced it' (p. 93).

Risky and Challenging Play

A child's safety during school recess is a major consideration for parents, teachers, and principals (Murray & Ramstetter, 2013). It has been acknowledged that in the societal drive for safety and to minimize risk, schools are often reported to have developed recess policies (written and/or ad hoc) that restrict behaviors (e.g. no contact games) and ban games (e.g. 'British bulldog', 'Red Rover') that children can engage in on the playground (Knowles et al., 2013). It is ironic that such efforts to improve safety can lead to children engaging in the types of behaviors that are restricted or banned in the first place (Thomson, 2003). Of greater concern, some schools shorten or remove recess altogether, which, in turn, has major implications on the health, development, and well-being of youth (Blatchford & Sumpner, 1998; Ginsburg, 2007).

Children learn through play and games. A key part of this is trial and error, where children learn how to solve problems and address personal limitations (Bundy et al., 2009). A number of researchers have examined interventions that involved risky and challenging play, either through introducing recycled material with no fixed purpose, relaxing school policies (e.g. access to sports fields), and playing outdoors in inclement weather (Bundy et al., 2009; Engelen et al., 2013; Farmer et al., 2017; Hyndman et al., 2014; Parrish et al., 2016). While changes in physical activity levels were generally small, which may be attributable to the methods used to measure activity, the introduction of risky and challenging play was generally well received at participating schools. In addition, there were improvements in children's play behaviors (Bundy et al., 2009; Farmer et al., 2017) and no increase in injuries (Bundy et al., 2009). Moving forward, schools should consider how to increase opportunities for risky and challenging play in the playground. It is important to note that risky activities are not necessarily unsafe, and agreed rules and boundaries and staff training can help manage and address perceptions of acceptable and unacceptable risky play during recess (Ramstetter et al., 2010).

Summary

This chapter focused on the promotion of physical activity during school recess, which provides an important and valuable opportunity for children and adolescents to be active on a regular basis. In recent years there has been an increase in both structured and unstructured physical activity interventions in this context, with promising findings concerning playground modifications, multicomponent strategies, and loose equipment observed. There are, however, a number of gaps in the current literature base, including recess interventions targeting adolescent populations, and the impact of recess policies on activity. More research focusing on the longer-term sustainability of recess interventions is also required. Overall, recess is a critical component of the school day. The challenge moving forward is to ensure this time is protected and that future generations of children and adolescents have access to supportive school environments where they have the option to be active.

References

Anthamatten, P., Brink, L., Lampe, S., Greenwood, E., Kingston, B., & Nigg, C. (2011). An assessment of schoolyard renovation strategies to encourage children's physical activity. *International Journal of Behavioral Nutrition and Physical Activity, 8*, 27. doi:10.1186/1479-5868-8-27

Baines, E., & Blatchford, P. (2019). *School break and lunch times and young people's social lives: A follow-up national study*. Retrieved from http://www.breaktime.org.uk/.

Beard, V. (2018). *A study of the purpose and value of recess in elementary schools as perceived by teachers and administrators* (Doctoral dissertation). East Tennessee State University, Johnson City, TN. Retrieved from https://dc.etsu.edu/etd/3433.

Beresin, A. (2016). Playing with time: Towards a global survey of recess practices. *International Journal of Play, 5*(2), 159–165. doi:10.1080/21594937.2016.1203920

Beyler, N., Bleeker, M., James-Burdumy, S., Fortson, J., & Benjamin, M. (2014). The impact of Playworks on students' physical activity during recess: Findings from a randomized controlled trial. *Preventive Medicine, 69*, S20–S26. doi:10.1016/j.ypmed.2014.10.011

Bjorklund, D. F., & Brown, R. D. (1998). Physical play and cognitive development: Integrating activity, cognition, and education. *Child Development, 69*(3), 604–606.

Blaes, A., Ridgers, N. D., Aucouturier, J., Van Praagh, E., Berthoin, S., & Baquet, G. (2013). Effects of a playground markings intervention on school recess physical activity in French children. *Preventive Medicine, 57*, 580–584.

Blatchford, P. (1996). "We did more then": Changes in pupils' perceptions of breaktime (recess) from 7 to 16 years. *Journal of Research in Childhood Education, 11*(1), 14–24.

Blatchford, P., & Baines, E. (2006). *A follow up national survey of breaktimes in primary and secondary schools*. Retrieved from https://www.nuffieldfoundation.org/sites/default/files/Breaktimes_Final%20report_Blatchford.pdf

Blatchford, P., & Sharp, S. (1994). Introduction: Why understand and why change school breaktime behaviour? In P. Blatchford & S. Sharp (Eds.), *Breaktime and the school: Understanding and changing playground behaviour* (pp. 1–10). London, UK: Routledge.

Blatchford, P., & Sumpner, C. (1998). What do we know about breaktime? Results from a national survey of breaktime and lunchtime in primary and secondary schools. *British Educational Research Journal, 24*, 79–94.

Bleeker, M., Beyler, N., James-Burdumy, S., & Fortson, J. (2015). The impact of Playworks on boys' and girls' physical activity during recess. *Journal of School Health, 85*(3), 171–178.

Brink, L. A., Nigg, C. R., Lampe, S. M. R., Kingston, B. A., Mootz, A. L., & van Vliet, W. (2010). Influence of schoolyard renovations on children's physical activity: The Learning Landscapes Program. *American Journal of Public Health, 100*(9), 1672–1678.

Bundy, A. C., Luckett, T., Tranter, P. J., Naughton, G. A., Wyver, S. R., Ragen, J., & Spies, G. (2009). The risk is that there is 'no risk': A simple, innovative intervention to increase children's activity levels. *International Journal of Early Years Education, 17*(1), 33–45.

Bundy, A. C., Naughton, G., Tranter, P., Wyver, S., Baur, L., Schiller, W., . . . Brentnall, J. (2011). The Sydney playground project: Popping the bubblewrap – Unleashing the power of play: A cluster randomized controlled trial of a primary school playground-based intervention aiming to increase children's physical activity and social skills. *BMC Public Health, 11*, 680.

Canadian Society for Exercise Physiology. (2019). Canadian 24-hour movement guidelines for children and youth: An integration of physical activity, sedentary behaviour, and sleep. Retrieved from https://csepguidelines.ca/

Centers for Disease Control and Prevention. (2011). School health guidelines to promote healthy eating and physical activity. *MMWR Recommendations and Reports, 60*(RR-5), 1–76.

Centers for Disease Control and Prevention and Society of Health and Physical Educators America. (2017). *Strategies for recess in schools*. Retrieved from https://www.cdc.gov/healthyschools/physicalactivity/pdf/2016_12_16_schoolrecessstrategies_508.pdf

Center for Education Statistics. (2005). *Fast response survey system.* Washington, DC: United States Department of Education.

Chin, J. J., & Ludwig, D. (2013). Increasing children's physical activity during school recess periods. *American Journal of Public Health, 103*(7), 1229–1234.

Clevenger, K. A., Sinha, G., & Howe, C. A. (2019). Comparison of methods for analyzing Global Positioning System and accelerometer data during school recess. *Measurement in Physical Education and Exercise Science, 23*(1), 58–68. doi:10.1080/1091367X.2018.1512495

Duncan, M. J., & Staples, V. (2010). The impact of a school-based active video game play intervention on children's physical activity during recess. *Human Movement, 11*(1), 95–99. doi:10.2478/v10038-009-0023-1

Dyment, J. E., Bell, A. C., & Lucas, A. J. (2009). The relationship between school ground design and intensity of physical activity. *Children's Geographies, 7*(3), 261–276.

Education Department of Western Australia. (1898). Morning recess. In *The Education Circular Western Australia* (Vol. 1, No. 5, pp. 4). East Perth, WA: Education Department Western Australia.

Efrat, M. W. (2013). Exploring effective strategies for increasing the amount of moderate-to-vigorous physical activity children accumulate during recess: A quasi-experimental intervention study. *Journal of School Health, 83*(4), 265–272.

Elder, J. P., McKenzie, T. L., Arredondo, E. M., Crespo, N. C., & Ayala, G. X. (2011). Effects of a multipronged intervention on children's activity levels at recess: The Aventuras para Niños Study. *Advances in Nutrition, 2*(2), 171S–176S. doi:10.3945/an.111.000380

Engelen, L., Bundy, A. C., Naughton, G., Simpson, J. M., Bauman, A., Ragen, J., …van der Ploeg, H. P. (2013). Increasing physical activity in young primary school children – It's child's play: A cluster randomised controlled trial. *Preventive Medicine, 56*(5), 319–325.

Epstein, D., Kehily, M., Mac an Ghaill, M., & Redman, P. (2001). Boys and girls come out to play. *Men and Masculinities, 4*(2), 158–172.

Erwin, H., Ickes, M., Ahn, S., & Fedewa, A. (2014). Impact of recess interventions on children's physical activity – A meta-analysis. *American Journal Health Promotion, 28*(3), 159–167.

Escalante, Y., Garcia-Hermoso, A., Backx, K., & Saavedra, J. M. (2014). Playground designs to increase physical activity levels during school recess: A systematic review. *Health Education and Behavior, 41*(2), 138–144.

Evans, J. (1996). Children's attitudes to recess and changes taking place in Australian primary schools. *Research in Education, 56*, 49–61.

Evans, J. (2003). Changes to (primary) school recess and their effect on children's physical activity: An Australian perspective. *Journal of Physical Education New Zealand, 36*(1), 53–62.

Fairchild, A. J., & McQuillin, S. D. (2010). Evaluating mediation and moderation effects in school psychology: A presentation of methods and review of current practice. *Journal of School Psychology, 48*(1), 53–84.

Fairclough, S. J., Beighle, A., Erwin, H., & Ridgers, N. D. (2012). School day segmented physical activity patterns of high and low active children. *BMC Public Health, 12*, 406. doi:10.1186/1471-2458-12-406.

Farmer, V. L., Williams, S. M., Mann, J. I., Schofield, G., McPhee, J. C., & Taylor, R. W. (2017). The effect of increasing risk and challenge in the school playground on physical activity and weight in children: A cluster randomised controlled trial (PLAY). *International Journal of Obesity, 41*, 793–800.

Ginsburg, K. R. (2007). The importance of play in promoting health child development and maintaining strong parent-child bonds. *Pediatrics, 119*, 182–191.

Haapala, H. L., Hirvensalo, M. H., Laine, K., Laakso, L., Hakonen, H., Lintunen, T., & Tammelin, T. H. (2014). Adolescents' physical activity at recess and actions to promote a physically active school day in four Finnish schools. *Health Education Research, 29*(5), 840–852. doi:10.1093/her/cyu030

Hamer, M., Aggio, D., Knock, G., Kipps, C., Shankar, A., & Smith, L. (2017). Effect of major school playground reconstruction on physical activity and sedentary behaviour: Camden active spaces. *BMC Public Health, 17*, 522. doi:10.1186/s12889-017-4483-5

Harrison, F., Jones, A. P., Bentham, G., van Sluijs, E. M. F., Cassidy, A., & Griffin, S. J. (2011). The impact of rainfall and school break time policies on physical activity in 9–10 year old British children: A repeated measures study. *International Journal of Behavioral Nutrition and Physical Activity, 8*, 47. doi:10.1186/1479-5868-8-47

Hidding, L. M., Altenburg, T. M., van Ekris, E., & Chinapaw, M. J. M. (2017). Why do children engage in sedentary behavior? Child- and parent-perceived determinants. *International Journal of Environmental Research and Public Health, 14*(7), 671. doi:10.3390/ijerph14070671

Hohepa, M., Scragg, R., Schofield, G., Kolt, G. S., & Schaaf, D. (2007). Social support for youth physical activity: Importance of siblings, parents, friends and school support across a segmented school day. *International Journal of Behavioral Nutrition and Physical Activity, 4*, 54. doi:10.1186/1479-5868-4-54

Hohepa, M., Scragg, R., Schofield, G., Kolt, G. S., & Schaaf, D. (2009). Self-reported physical activity levels during a segmented school day in a large multiethnic sample of high school students. *Journal of Science and Medicine in Sport, 12*(2), 284–292. doi:10.1016/j.jsams.2007.11.005

Howe, C. A., Freedson, P. S., Alhassan, S., Feldman, H. A., & Osganian, S. K. (2012). A recess intervention to promote moderate-to-vigorous physical activity. *Pediatric Obesity, 7*(1), 82–88.

Huberty, J. L., Beets, M. W., Beighle, A., Saint-Maurice, P., & Welk, G. (2014). Effects of Ready for Recess, an environmental intervention, on physical activity in third-through sixth-grade children. *Journal of Physical Activity and Health, 11*(2), 384–395. doi:10.1123/jpah.2012-0061

Huberty, J. L., Siahpush, M., Beighle, A., Fuhrmeister, E., Silva, P., & Welk, G. J. (2011). Ready for Recess: A pilot study to increase physical activity in elementary school children. *Journal of School Health, 81*, 251–257.

Hyndman, B. (2015). Where to next for school playground interventions to encourage active play? An exploration of structured and unstructured school playground strategies. *Journal of Occupational Therapy, Schools, and Early Intervention, 8*, 55–67.

Hyndman, B. P., Benson, A. C., Ullah, S., & Telford, A. (2014). Evaluating the effects of the Lunchtime Enjoyment Activity and Play (LEAP) school playground intervention on children's quality of life, enjoyment and participation in physical activity. *BMC Public Health, 14*, 164. doi:10.1186/1471-2458-14-164

Janssen, M., Toussaint, H. M., Van Mechelen, W., & Verhagen, E. A. L. M. (2011). Playgrounds: Effect of a PE playground program in primary schools on PA levels during recess in 6 to 12 year old children. Design of a prospective controlled trial. *BMC Public Health, 11*, 282. doi:10.1186/1471-2458-11-282.

Janssen, M., Twisk, T. W. R., Toussaint, H. M., van Mechelen, W., & Verhagen, E. A. L. M. (2015). Effectiveness of the Playgrounds programme on PA levels during recess in 6-year-old to 12-year-old children. *British Journal of Sports Medicine, 49*(4), 259–264. doi:10.1136/bjsports-2012-091517

Jarrett, O. S., Maxwell, D. M., Dickerson, C., Hoge, P., Davies, G., & Yetley, A. (1998). Impact of recess on classroom behavior: Group effects and individual differences. *Journal of Educational Research, 92*(2), 121–126.

Kahan, D. (2008). Recess, extracurricular activities, and active classrooms. *Journal of Physical Education, Recreation and Dance, 79*(2), 26–39. doi:10.1080/07303084.2008.10598131

Klinker, C. D., Schipperijn, J., Christian, H., Kerr, J., Ersbøll, A. K., & Troelsen, J. (2014). Using accelerometers and global positioning system devices to assess gender and age differences in children's school, transport, leisure and home based physical activity. *International Journal of Behavioral Nutrition and Physical Activity, 11*, 8. doi:10.1186/1479-5868-11-8

Knowles, Z. R., Parnell, D., Stratton, G., & Ridgers, N. D. (2013). Learning from the experts: Exploring playground experience and activities using a write and draw technique. *Journal of Physical Activity and Health, 10*, 406–415.

Leggett, C., Irwin, M., Griffith, J., Xue, L., & Fradette, K. (2012). Factors associated with physical activity among Canadian high school students. *International Journal of Public Health, 57*(2), 315–324. doi:10.1007/s00038-011-0306-0

Lewis, B. A., Napolitano, M. A., Buman, M. P., Williams, D. M., & Nigg, C. R. (2017). Future directions in physical activity intervention research: Expanding our focus to sedentary behaviors, technology, and dissemination. *Journal of Behavioral Medicine, 40*(1), 112–126. doi:10.1007/s10865-016-9797-8

Lopes, L., Lopes, V., & Pereira, B. (2009). Physical activity levels in normal weight and overweight Portuguese children: An intervention study during an elementary school recess. *International Electronic Journal of Health Education, 12*, 175–184.

McLoughlin, G. M., Edwards, C. G., Jones, A., Chojnacki, M. R., Baumgartner, N. W., Walk, A. D., . . . Khan, N. A. (2019). School lunch timing and children's physical activity during recess: An exploratory study. *Journal of Nutrition Education and Behavior, 51*(5), 616–622.

Mota, J., Silva, P., Santos, M. P., Ribeiro, J. C., Oliveira, J., & Duarte, J. A. (2005). Physical activity and school recess time: Differences between the sexes and the relationship between children's playground physical activity and habitual physical activity. *Journal of Sports Sciences, 23*(3), 269–275. doi:10.1080/02640410410001730124

Murray, R., & Ramstetter, C. (2013). The crucial role of recess in school. *Pediatrics, 131*(1), 183–188.

National Education Association of the United States. (1884). *Proceedings of the department of superintendent of the national educational association (1882–1884)* (pp. 279–448). New York, NY: J.J. Little & Co.

National Education Union UK. (2018). *Work load and working time*. Retrieved from https://neu.org.uk/advice/workload-and-working-time

National Institutes of Health. (2015). *Classification of laws associated with school students*. Retrieved from https://class.cancer.gov/download.aspx

New South Wales Department of Education. (2019). *Review into the non-educational use of mobile devices in NSW schools.* Retrieved from https://education.nsw.gov.au/about-us/strategies-and-reports/our-reports-and-reviews/mobile-devices-in-schools.

New South Wales Government Education. (2016). *The school day fact sheet.* Retrieved from https://beta.dec.nsw.gov.au/__data/assets/pdf_file/0006/264795/The-School-Day-Fact-Sheet-October-2016.pdf

Parrish, A.-M., Okely, A. D., Batterham, M., Cliff, D., & Magee, C. (2016). PACE: A group randomised controlled trial to increase children's break-time playground physical activity. *Journal of Science and Medicine in Sport, 19*, 413–518.

Parrish, A.-M., Okely, A. D., Stanley, R. M., & Ridgers, N. D. (2013). The effect of school recess interventions on physical activity: A systematic review. *Sports Medicine, 43*, 287–299.

Parrish, A.-M, Yeatman, H., Iverson, D., & Russell, K. (2011). Using interviews and peer pairs to better understand how school environments affect young children's playground physical activity levels: A qualitative study. *Health Education Research, 27*(2), 269–280. doi:10.1093/her/cyr049

Pate, R. R., Baranowski, T., Dowda, M., & Trost, S. G. (1996). Tracking of physical activity in young children. *Medicine and Science in Sports and Exercise, 28*(1), 92–96.

Pawlowski, C. S., Andersen, H. B., Troelsen, J., & Schipperijn, J. (2016). Children's physical activity behavior during school recess: A pilot study using GPS, accelerometer, participant observation, and go-along interview. *PLoS ONE, 11*(2), e0148786.

Pellegrini, A. D. (2005). *Recess: Its role in education and development.* Mahwah, NJ: Lawrence Erlbaum Associates, Inc.

Pellegrini, A. D. (2008). The recess debate; a disjuncture between educational policy and scientific research. *American Journal of Play, 1*(2), 181–191.

Pellegrini, A. D., Blatchford, P., Kato, K., & Baines, E. (2004). A short-term longitudinal study of children's playground games in primary school: Implications for adjustment to school and social adjustment in the USA and the UK. *Social Development, 13*(1), 107–123.

Pellegrini, A. D., & Bohn, C. (2005). The role of recess in children's cognitive performance and school adjustment. *Educational Researcher, 34*(1), 13–19.

Pellegrini, A. D., Huberty, P. D., & Jones, I. (1995). The effects of recess timing on children's playground and classroom behaviors. *American Educational Research Journal, 32*(4), 845–864.

Pellegrini, A. D., & Smith, P. K. (1993). School recess: Implications for education and development. *Review of Educational Research, 63*(1), 51–67.

Piekarz, E., Schermbeck, R., Young, S. K., Leider, J., Ziemann, M., & Chriqui, J. F. (2016). *School district wellness policies: Evaluating progress and potential for improving children's health eight years after the Federal Mandate. School Years 2006–07 through 2013–14 (Volume 4).* Chicago, IL: Bridging the Gap Program and the National Wellness Policy Study, Institute for Health Research and Policy, University of Illinois at Chicago.

Ramstetter, C. L., Murray, R., & Garner, A. S. (2010). The crucial role of recess in schools. *Journal of School Health, 80*(11), 517–526. doi: 10.1111/j.1746-1561.2010.00537.x

Reilly, J. J., Johnston, G., McIntosh, S., & Martin, A. (2016). Contribution of school recess to daily physical activity: Systematic review and evidence appraisal. *Health Behavior and Policy Review, 3*(6), 581–589. doi:10.14485/HBPR.3.6.7

Ridgers, N. D., Carter, L. M., Stratton, G., & McKenzie, T. L. (2011). Examining children's physical activity and play behaviors during school playtime over time. *Health Education Research, 26*, 586–595.

Ridgers, N. D., Fairclough, S. J., & Stratton, G. (2010a). Variables associated with children's physical activity levels during recess: The A-CLASS project. *International Journal of Behavioral Nutrition and Physical Activity, 7*(1), 74.

Ridgers, N. D., Fairclough, S. J., & Stratton, G. (2010b). Twelve-month effects of a playground intervention on children's morning and lunchtime recess physical activity levels. *Journal of Physical Activity and Health, 7*(2), 167–175.

Ridgers, N. D., Salmon, J., Parrish, A.-M., Stanley, R. M., & Okely, A. D. (2012). Physical activity during school recess: A systematic review. *American Journal of Preventive Medicine, 43*(3), 320–328. doi:10.1016/j.amepre.2012.05.019

Ridgers, N. D., Salmon, J., & Timperio, A. (2018). Seasonal changes in physical activity during school recess and lunchtime among Australian children. *Journal of Sports Sciences, 36*, 1508–1514.

Ridgers, N. D., & Stratton, G. (2005). Physical activity during school recess – The Liverpool Sporting Playgrounds Project. *Pediatric Exercise Science, 17*, 281–290.

Ridgers, N. D., Stratton, G., & Fairclough, S. J. (2006). Physical activity levels of children during school playtime. *Sports Medicine, 36*(4), 359–371. doi:3645 [pii]

Ridgers, N. D., Stratton, G., Fairclough, S. J., & Twisk, J. W. R. (2007a). Children's physical activity levels during school recess: A quasi-experimental intervention study. *International Journal of Behavioral Nutrition and Physical Activity, 4*(1), 19.

Ridgers, N. D., Stratton, G., Fairclough, S. J., & Twisk, J. W. R. (2007b). Long-term effects of a playground markings and physical structures on children's recess physical activity levels. *Preventive Medicine, 44*(5), 393–397.

Ridgers, N. D., Timperio, A., Crawford, D., & Salmon, J. (2012). Five-year changes in school recess and lunchtime and the contribution to children's daily physical activity. *British Journal of Sports Medicine, 46*(10), 741–746. doi:10.1136/bjsm.2011.084921

Ridgers, N. D., Timperio, A., Crawford, D., & Salmon, J. (2013). What factors are associated with adolescents' school break time physical activity and sedentary time? *PLoS ONE, 8*(2), e56838. doi:10.1371/journal.pone.0056838

Ridgers, N. D., Toth, M., & Uvacsek, M. (2009). Physical activity levels of Hungarian children during school recess. *Preventive Medicine, 49*(5), 410–412. doi:10.1016/j.ypmed.2009.08.008

Saint-Maurice, P., Welk, G. J., Silva, P., Siahpush, M., & Huberty, J. (2011). Assessing children's physical activity behaviors at recess: A multi-method approach. *Pediatric Exercise Science, 23*, 585–599.

Scruggs, P. W., Beveridge, S. K., & Watson, D. L. (2003). Increasing children's school time physical activity using structured fitness breaks. *Pediatric Exercise Science, 15*, 156–169.

Society of Health and Physical Educators America. (2016). *Shape of the nation; Status of physical education in the USA.* Retrieved from https://www.shapeamerica.org//advocacy/son/2016/upload/Shape-of-the-Nation-2016_web.pdf

Stanley, R. M., Boshoff, K., & Dollman, J. (2012). Voices in the playground: A qualitative exploration of the barriers and facilitators of lunchtime play. *Journal of Science and Medicine in Sport, 15*(1), 44–51.

Stellino, M. B., Sinclair, C. D., Partridge, J. A., & King, K. M. (2010). Differences in children's recess physical activity: Recess activity of the week intervention. *Journal of School Health, 80*(9), 436–444.

Stratton, G. (2000). Promoting children's physical activity in primary school: An intervention study using playground markings. *Ergonomics, 43*, 1538–1546.

Stratton, G., & Leonard, J. (2002). The effects of playground markings on the energy expenditure of 5–7-year-old school children. *Pediatric Exercise Science, 14*(2), 170–180.

Stratton, G., & Mullan, E. (2005). The effect of multicolor playground markings on children's physical activity level during recess. *Preventive Medicine, 41*, 828–833.

Sutherland, R., Campbell, E., Lubans, D. R., Morgan, P. J., Okely, A. D., Nathan, N., . . . Wiggers, J. (2016). 'Physical Activity 4 Everyone' school-based intervention to prevent decline in adolescent physical activity levels: 12 month (mid-intervention) report on a cluster randomised trial. *British Journal of Sports Medicine, 50*(8), 488–495. doi:10.1136/bjsports-2014-094523

The Fair Work Commission Australia. (2010). *Educational services (teachers) award 2010.* Retrieved from http://awardviewer.fwo.gov.au/award/show/MA000077#P63_2371

Thomson, S. (2003). A well equipped hamster cage: The rationalisation of primary school playtime. *Education 3–13, 31*, 54–59.

Thomson, S. (2004). Just another classroom? Observations of primary school playgrounds. In P. Vertinsky & J. Bale (Eds.), *Sites of sport: Space, place, experience* (pp. 73–82). London: Routledge.

Thomson, S. (2005). 'Territorialising' the primary school playground: Deconstructing the geography of playtime. *Children's Geographies, 1*, 63–78.

Turner, L., Chriqui, J. F., & Chaloupka, F. J. (2013). Withholding recess from elementary school students: Policies matter. *Journal of School Health, 83*(8), 533–541. doi:doi:10.1111/josh.12062

US Department of Health and Human Services. (2018). *Physical activity guidelines for Americans* (2nd ed.). Washington, DC: US Department of Health and Human Services.

van der Mars, H. (2018). Policy development in Physical Education … The last best chance? *Quest, 70*(2), 169–190. doi:10.1080/00336297.2018.1439391

Van Kann, D. H. H., de Vries, S. I., Schipperijn, J., de Vries, N. K., Jansen, M. W. J., & Kremers, S. P. J. (2016). Schoolyard characteristics, physical activity, and sedentary behavior: Combining GPS and accelerometry. *Journal of School Health, 86*(12), 913–921.

Van Kann, D. H. H., de Vries, S. I., Schipperijn, J., de Vries, N. K., Jansen, M. W. J., & Kremers, S. P. J. (2017). A multicomponent schoolyard intervention targeting children's recess physical activity and sedentary behavior: Effects after 1 year. *Journal of Physical Activity and Health, 14*, 866–875.

Verstraete, S. J., Cardon, G. M., DeClercq, D. L., & De Bourdeaudhuij, I. M. (2006). Increasing children's physical activity levels during recess periods in elementary schools: The effects of providing game equipment. *European Journal of Public Health, 16*, 415–419.

Victorian State Government. (2019). *School policy school hours.* Retrieved from https://www.education.vic. gov.au/school/principals/spag/management/Pages/hours.aspx#link37

Welk, G. (1999). The youth physical activity promotion model: A conceptual bridge between theory and practice. *Quest, 51*, 5–23.

Willenberg, L., Ashbolt, R., Holland, D., Gibbs, L., MacDougall, C., Garrard, J., . . . Waters, E. (2010). Increasing school playground physical activity: A mixed methods study combining environmental measures and children's perspectives. *Journal of Science and Medicine in Sport, 13*, 210–216.

Wu, A. D., & Zumbo, B. D. (2008). Understanding and using mediators and moderators. *Social Indicators Research, 87*, 367–392.

Yildrim, M., Arundell, L., Cerin, E., Carson, V., Brown, H., Crawford, D., . . . Salmon, J. (2014). What helps children to move more at school recess and lunchtime? Mid-intervention results from Transform-Us! cluster-randomised controlled trial. *British Journal of Sports Medicine, 48*(3), 271–277.

Zask, A., van Beurden, E., Barnett, L., Brooks, L. O., & Dietrich, U. C. (2001). Active school playgrounds – Myth or reality? Results of the "Move It Groove It" Project. *Preventive Medicine, 33*, 402–408.

Zavacky, F., & Michael, S. L. (2017). Keeping recess in schools. *Journal of Physical Education, Recreation & Dance, 88*(5), 46–53. doi:10.1080/07303084.2017.1295763

25

CLASSROOM-BASED PHYSICAL ACTIVITY INTERVENTIONS

Jo Salmon, Emiliano Mazzoli, Natalie Lander,
Ana María Contardo Ayala, Lauren Sherar, and Nicola D. Ridgers

Introduction to Classroom-Based Physical Activity

Although it varies by country, children and adolescents spend approximately 6.5 hours a day at school. Research from the United Kingdom and Australia shows that up to 70% of the school day is spent sedentary, with only 10% and 14% of the school day spent stepping in these two samples, respectively (Clemes et al., 2016). Not surprisingly, much of the time spent in class is highly sedentary. Therefore, embedding physical activity within classroom time has the potential to not only reduce time children spend sitting but also contribute to daily physical activity of children and adolescents. With governments of many countries publishing daily physical activity targets for schools (e.g. in the United States, 30 minutes of physical activity per school day is recommended), classroom-based physical activity has never been more topical.

The purpose of this chapter is to describe the different types of classroom-based physical activity strategies that have been developed and tested in schools. These strategies exclude physical education and school sport. We will provide a critical overview of the evidence of the impact of active classrooms on child and adolescent physical activity, sedentary behavior, physical and mental health, classroom behaviors, and cognitive and academic outcomes. Finally, the key challenges in implementation, emerging issues, and future directions will be discussed.

Defining Classroom-Based Physical Activity

Table 25.1 provides an overview of definitions of classroom-based physical activity. There are no universally accepted definitions, so this table defines what we mean by classroom-based physical activity strategies for the purpose of this chapter. The various strategies include: active lessons (sometimes referred to active academics); active breaks (e.g. <10 minutes); and active classroom environments.

The distinction between an 'active lesson' and an 'active break linked to the curriculum' presented in Table 25.1 is mainly in terms of duration. If a teacher asks students to *hop on one leg* to give their answer to a math equation, but the students sit for the majority of the lesson, this would be an 'active break linked to the curriculum'. On the other hand, if teachers have children moving throughout the math lesson, this would be an active lesson. 'Active classroom environments' may directly or indirectly support active lessons and active breaks. For example, the provision of an interactive whiteboard to display physical activities to students can be used to support delivery of active lessons or breaks (Norris, Shelton, Dunsmuir, Duke-Williams, & Stamatakis, 2015), whereas availability of height-adjustable desks in the classroom need not be linked to active learning pedagogy.

Table 25.1 Defining classroom-based physical activity

Strategy	Definition
Active lessons	Integrating movement into a class lesson for a learning outcome. For example, students engaging in physical activity for most of their mathematics, science, or language lessons
Active breaks	
Non-curriculum linked	Interrupting a seated academic lesson to take short physical activity break(s) (e.g. ≤10 minutes) that are not linked to the curriculum. For example, students might do jumping jacks or dance on the spot without any alignment to the curriculum
Curriculum linked	Interrupting a seated academic lesson to take short physical activity break(s) that are linked to the curriculum. For example, a teacher might ask students to hop on one leg in response to a math equation
Cognitively challenging	Interrupting a seated academic lesson to take a short physical activity break that is cognitively challenging. For example, playing a physical activity mirror game with increasingly complex choreography
Active classroom environments	
Classroom layout or setting	Height-adjustable or stand-biased desks, active stations (e.g. art easels in one corner of the classroom), outdoor classrooms
Equipment in the classroom	Screens (e.g. projector, interactive whiteboard, or large computer monitor to display physical activities to students), sport or circus equipment, music player
Combined strategies	May include a combination of the earlier strategies and also connect to other settings (e.g. links to the family setting)

History of Active Lessons Used in Pedagogy

Teachers have for many years used active learning and teaching in their class lessons. The active learning and teaching phenomenon originates in *natural history*, and is embedded in human psychology and biology (Corrigan, 2013). Indeed, active learning can be mapped as far back as anthropology and archaeology study will allow, with the learnings of hunting, farming, crafting, building and medicine all delivered 'actively'. Therefore, even if 'active learning and teaching' or 'active pedagogy' has only been labeled so recently, it has been practiced for as long as teaching and learning have existed. The term 'active learning' usually refers to how students engage in learning as active participants (*plan*, *do* and *review*) (Sylva, 1994, p. 142), rather than passively taking in information. Therefore, as the contemporary pedagogies of active learning are offering new insights, practices, and evidence, they are providing renewed attention to the oldest and deepest ways of teaching and learning. In this chapter the term 'active learning' refers to physically active learning; however, that does not mean that the student is not also actively engaged in the lesson cognitively and experientially.

Impact of Active Learning on Children's Physical Activity, Sedentary Behavior, Cognition, and Health

Table 25.2 summarizes the findings from eight systematic reviews on the effects of classroom-based physical activity interventions on children's physical activity, sedentary behavior, classroom behavior (i.e. on-/off-task behaviors, referred to as active or passive engagement in class lessons appropriate to the learning situation), cognition or cognitive function (i.e. all the processes that allow children to perceive, interpret, and manipulate information in order to understand, be aware

Table 25.2 Summary of conclusions from systematic reviews of active classrooms

Author	Focus (n = studies)	Outcomes	Comments
Barr-Anderson et al. (2011)	Short bouts of physical activity (n = 23)	+ PA	Also reviewed studies from workplaces (not included in the 23 studies here) Short bouts of PA during PE lessons were also included in the review Bouts ranged from <10 minutes up to 20 minutes
Daly-Smith et al. (2018)	Active lessons (n = 10) Active breaks (n = 8)	+ LPA + MVPA − SB + classroom behavior/time-on-task ? cognition ? academic outcomes	Quality of studies low-medium Longer MVPA bouts >10 minutes or shorter VPA bouts linked to improved classroom behavior
Martin and Murtagh (2017)	Active lessons (n = 15)	+ PA + learning outcomes + on-task behavior + feasibility and enjoyment − student BMI	Medium to large effect sizes for PA outcomes
Minges et al. (2016)	Classroom environment (height-adjustable desks) (n = 8)	+ standing time − sitting time + PA + EE + classroom behavior 0 musculoskeletal pain 0 adiposity/BMI	Standing time: moderate effect size Sitting time: small to moderate effect
Norris et al. (2015)	Active lessons (n = 11)	+ PA +/0 educational outcomes	Active lesson freq. varied from 1 to 2 lessons/day to 1 lesson/day × 3 days/week
Owen et al. (2016)	Classroom breaks (n = 5) Classroom integration (n = 4)	+ school engagement 0 school disengagement	School engagement related to classroom breaks only
Rasberry et al. (2011)	Classroom-based physical activity (n = 9)	+ classroom behavior/time-on-task + academic achievement + cognitive functioning	Did not differentiate between effectiveness of classroom-based physical activity strategies
Watson et al. (2017)	Active lessons (n = 13) Active breaks (n = 19) Curriculum-linked active breaks (n = 7)	+ MVPA (during lessons, and across school day) + on-task classroom behavior − off-task classroom behavior + selective attention ? executive function ? fluid intelligence + academic achievement (if using progress monitoring tool) 0 academic achievement (if using national standardized tests)	Review did not always separate effects of the different active classroom strategies Dose-response evidence for academic and cognitive outcomes: • 10-minute breaks • MVPA intensity • MVPA breaks twice a day optimal

PA: physical activity; LPA: light-intensity physical activity; MVPA: moderate-to-vigorous physical activity; SB: sedentary behavior; EE: energy expenditure; BMI: body mass index; PE: physical education; + overall positive associations; − overall negative associations; 0: overall null associations; ?: overall associations mixed.

of, and interact effectively with what surrounds them), academic outcomes (i.e. evidence of the knowledge, skills, and abilities children have acquired through the school curriculum), and health (Barr-Anderson, AuYoung, Whitt-Glover, Glenn, & Yancey, 2011; Daly-Smith et al., 2018; Martin & Murtagh, 2017; Minges et al., 2016; Norris et al., 2015; Owen et al., 2016; Rasberry et al., 2011; Watson, Timperio, Brown, Best, & Hesketh, 2017). There has been a substantial increase in classroom-based physical activity interventions in the last 10 years as reflected by the more recent reviews. While the majority of reviews identify that there remains significant limitations in the evidence with respect to study design, study duration, and sample size, there is an emerging consistency in findings.

Most reviews concluded that classroom-based physical activity interventions lead to a significant increase in children's physical activity (Barr-Anderson et al., 2011; Daly-Smith et al., 2018; Martin & Murtagh, 2017; Minges et al., 2016; Norris et al., 2015; Watson et al., 2017). More recent reviews have identified reductions in children's sedentary behavior and increases in standing (Minges et al., 2016), light-intensity physical activity (Daly-Smith et al., 2018), and moderate-to-vigorous physical activity (MVPA) during lesson time and across the school day (Watson et al., 2017). Martin and Murtagh (2017) found that most studies reported medium to large effect sizes for physical activity outcomes.

The majority of reviews identified positive effects on children's classroom behaviors. Effects on cognition such as core executive function (i.e. inhibition (also including selective attention), working memory and task shifting), and high-order executive functions (e.g. fluid intelligence) were mixed. Some reviews reported favorable effects on learning and academic outcomes (e.g. Martin & Murtagh, 2017; Rasberry et al. 2011), and on school engagement (for active breaks only) (Owen et al., 2016). However, other reviews reported mixed evidence (Daly-Smith et al., 2018; Norris et al., 2015). Watson and colleagues (2017) identified different associations with academic outcomes depending on the measure used. For example, studies that used an academic progress monitoring tool tended to report a positive association with physical activity classroom-based interventions, whereas most studies that assessed academic outcomes using national standardized test results reported null associations.

At the time of these reviews, few studies had reported the effects of physical activity classroom-based interventions on children's physical health. Only two reviews reported on the physical health effects of these types of interventions (Martin & Murtagh, 2017; Minges et al., 2016). Minges et al. (2016) reported no effects on children's musculoskeletal discomfort or body mass index (BMI) from using height-adjustable desks in the classroom. However, Martin and Murtagh (2017) reported a significant reduction in children's BMI from active lessons.

The following sections provide more detail on outcomes and strategies used in the selection of classroom-based physical activity intervention studies.

Active Lessons

There is consensus between systematic reviews that active lessons can positively impact children's physical activity (Daly-Smith et al., 2018; Martin & Murtagh, 2017; Norris et al., 2015; Watson et al., 2017); however, evidence on education outcomes is mixed. Some studies have explored the effects of active lessons on cognitive outcomes. For example, Reed and colleagues (2010) developed active lessons that embedded physical activity (e.g. walking, hopping, fundamental movement skills) into core curricula (e.g. math, social studies, language). Teachers were asked to deliver these active lessons for at least 30 minutes, three times a week. It was found that children who completed active lessons for three times a week over 3 months performed better on a test of fluid intelligence (the ability to reason quickly and abstractly) than the control group. However, a major limitation of this study was that fluid intelligence was not assessed at baseline.

The Texas I-CAN! program (Bartholomew & Jowers, 2011) described some interesting implementation learnings from working with teachers to deliver active lessons. They first offered teachers professional development sessions to integrate physical activity into their class lessons. However, fewer than 25% of teachers delivered these strategies in their lessons. The researchers then tested implementation of the Take10 program, but teachers did not feel the program adequately aligned with the school curriculum. Finally, the researchers worked with a committee of teachers to develop a new set of curriculum-linked active lessons for teachers to implement. Although dose fidelity is not provided and the duration and frequency of delivery of these lessons are unclear, significant increases in children's physical activity (with approximately 20% of lesson time spent in accelerometer-assessed moderate-to-vigorous activity) were reported. Significant improvements in time-on-task and academic achievement were also noted (Bartholomew & Jowers, 2011). This is consistent with the 'Encouraging Activity to Stimulate Young Minds' study with Australian children, which observed in a pilot study delivered by researchers a 20% difference in time-on-task in favor of the intervention group compared with usual practice (Riley, Lubans, Morgan, & Young, 2015). However, there was a 14% difference in the subsequent randomized controlled trial (RCT) when delivered by trained teachers (Riley, Lubans, Holmes, & Morgan, 2016). A recent Australian pilot study also reported significant improvements in spelling and on-task behavior among Grade 4 children who received integrated physical activity into English lessons three times a week (40 minute lessons) over 4 weeks (Mavilidi, Lubans, Eather, Morgan, & Riley, 2018).

Conversely, an active language and math program that was delivered to children in the Netherlands for 20–30 minutes, three times a week over 2 years reported no improvements in executive function (de Greeff et al., 2016). There were significant improvements in speed-coordination fitness, but no effects on other fitness parameters (e.g. cardiovascular and muscular fitness) were found. The program was delivered in the first year by external teachers trained by the research team, and Year 2 was delivered by the children's own classroom teacher. This may have influenced outcomes of the program. A sample of math and English teachers at three secondary schools in East England were trained in delivering physically active lessons (Gammon et al., 2019). While the lessons were considered acceptable by teachers and students, there were no significant effects on students' sitting time. More research in the secondary/senior school setting is needed.

Most of the studies that have incorporated active lessons into the curriculum have focused on math, science, language arts, and social studies (Norris et al., 2015). In Texas I-Can!, an example of integration with a science lesson is the *Cardiac Relay* where children learnt about the structure and function of the cardiovascular system by pretending they were oxygenated (holding a red disc) or unoxygenated (holding a blue disc) red-blood cells circulating through the body to deliver oxygen from the lungs to the heart to the muscles and back (Bartholomew & Jowers, 2011). Commonly, active lessons integrate movement with math. For example, Martin and Murtagh (2017) describe *Jump the Deck* in which children were presented with two randomly selected playing cards and performed a specific MVPA (e.g. jumping jacks) corresponding to the card suit and number while adding the total. It is apparent from previous research that it is important that teachers feel the lessons align with curriculum (Bartholomew & Jowers, 2011). While active lessons can increase children's physical activity, more research is needed to identify the impacts on children's cognitive function and academic outcomes.

Few studies have integrated physical activity in preschool classrooms. Trost, Fees, and Dzewaltowski (2008) examined the feasibility and effectiveness of active lessons in preschool children (3–5 years old) over a period of 8 weeks. In the last 4 weeks of the intervention, children in the intervention group showed significantly increased MVPA and vigorous-intensity physical activity compared with the control group. More research to test the impact of active lessons on preschool children's physical activity, cognition, and learning outcomes is needed.

Active Breaks

In this chapter we have differentiated between curriculum- and non-curriculum-linked and cognitively challenging active breaks (see Table 25.1 for definitions). A key reason for this is to identify the specific strategies employed by these interventions, and to also consider (where available) issues regarding implementation fidelity. The systematic review and meta-analysis by Watson et al. (2017) distinguished between curriculum-linked and non-curriculum-linked breaks. The curriculum-linked active breaks generally had more consistency in strategies between studies, mainly because they integrated movement with a key subject such as math or science. Conversely, active breaks unrelated to the curriculum included a variety of simple activities (e.g. jogging or marching on the spot) which require no equipment, or games involving the use of online activities (e.g. GoNoodle.com), music, or equipment (e.g. balls). Cognitively challenging breaks involve physical exertion as well as cognitive demand, which are often built around the core cognitive functions of working memory, inhibition, and task shifting. Examples of cognitively demanding breaks include physical games which involve reasoning, problem solving or complex movement coordination. In this chapter, cognitively demanding forms of active breaks have been grouped in a dedicated subsection.

Non-Curriculum-Linked Active Breaks

The limited available evidence suggests that non-curriculum-linked active breaks can increase children's physical activity (Ahamed et al., 2007; Carlson et al., 2015) and improve other health-related physical outcomes such as physical fitness (Katz et al., 2010) and bone mass (McKay et al., 2005). For example, Ahamed and colleagues (2007) found that children in the intervention group increased their MVPA by 47 minutes per week, significantly more than the control group. Also, Carlson et al. (2015) reported that children whose teachers regularly implemented active breaks increased the time spent in MVPA by more than 3 minutes during school hours, and were 75% more likely to achieve 30 minutes of physical activity during school hours, compared to children whose teachers who did not implement active breaks regularly.

Beyond the physical benefits, studies have shown that active breaks can help children improve their focus during school time. According to Daly-Smith et al. (2018), who reviewed studies focusing on the acute (i.e. immediate) effects of active breaks, children's behavior appears positively affected when the physical activity intensity was moderate-to-vigorous and sustained for more than 10 minutes or when the physical activity bouts were shorter (~5 minutes) and more intense. Unlike evidence for active lessons, there is agreement between previous studies that children's time on-task improves following non-curriculum-linked active breaks, compared to traditional class time activity (Carlson et al., 2015; Howie, Beets, & Pate, 2014; Ma, Le Mare, & Gurd, 2014; Whitt-Glover, Ham, & Yancey, 2011).

Daly-Smith et al. (2018) also highlighted positive acute effects of active breaks on children's cognitive functions and/or academic achievement. Various studies have demonstrated that active breaks can improve children's attention (Altenburg, Chinapaw, & Singh, 2016; Hill et al., 2010; Janssen et al., 2014; Ma, Le Mare, & Gurd, 2015). Exploring what activity intensity is likely to produce the best cognitive outcomes, Janssen et al. (2014) found that MVPA showed the biggest improvements in children's selective attention, although improvements were observed across all intensities. Improvements in children's executive functions (Hill et al., 2010), and academic achievement (Howie, Schatz, & Pate, 2015) have also been reported after active breaks. While there is no evidence suggesting that active breaks have a negative effect on academic achievement (Ahamed et al., 2007; Watson, Timperio, Brown, & Hesketh, 2019), more evidence is needed to clarify the effects of non-curriculum-linked active breaks on cognition and academic outcomes.

Curriculum-Linked Active Breaks

Active breaks related to curricular content have been found to increase children's physical activity levels (Bailey & DiPerna, 2015; Erwin, Beighle, Morgan, & Noland, 2011; Liu et al., 2008), as well as physical activity intensity and energy expenditure (Stewart, Dennison, Kohl, & Doyle, 2004). For example, Bailey and DiPerna (2015) found that the active breaks program *Energizers* significantly increased children's steps during the school day. Erwin et al. (2011) compared the effects of active breaks with educational content in an 8-month non-randomized trial between one intervention and one control school. While there were no significant effects on children's overall physical activity, compared to controls, children's steps increased by 33% more in the intervention group if their teacher delivered at least one active break a day.

The active breaks program TAKE10! has been disseminated globally since 2002. The program was developed in 1999 by the International Life Sciences Institute Center for Health Promotion (ILSI CHP), a not-for-profit organization funded primarily by the food industry (Kibbe et al., 2011). With input from education and health experts, the program's purpose was to increase classroom-based physical activity without detracting from the academic curriculum and was therefore aligned with subjects such as math, language, science, and reading. The 10-minute duration was based on adult guidelines from 1996 that recommended physical activity be accumulated in bouts of at least 10 minutes (US Department of Health and Human Services, 1996). Take10! was adapted for schools in China (called the Happy 10 program) and resulted in greater positive changes in children's average daily self-reported physical activity time and energy expenditure (also from the self-report measure) in the intervention compared to control group (Liu et al., 2008).

A paper from the ILSI CHP provided a 10-year overview of ten studies that had evaluated the Take10! program (Kibbe et al., 2011), and concluded that teachers were able to deliver the program on an average of 4.2 days per week, and that the active breaks resulted in significant increases in children's physical activity (>13%), energy expenditure, and time-on-task, and also improvements in reading, math, and spelling. There were inconsistencies in the effects of Take10! on children's BMI. While this overview paper reported positive effects on children's BMI in an obesity prevention study by Hollar and colleagues (2010), Take10! was only delivered in the second year of that trial which also included dietary and several other obesity-prevention strategies making it difficult to attribute the effects to active breaks. The Physical Activity Across the Curriculum (PAAC) study by Donnelly and colleagues (2009) found no significant effects on children's BMI after a 3-year RCT implementing Take10!; however, there were some favorable effects among children whose teachers delivered >75 minutes/week.

As already observed with the non-curriculum-linked active breaks, children's time-on-task often improved following curriculum-linked active breaks compared to traditional uninterrupted lessons (Goh, Hannon, Webster, Podlog, & Newton, 2016; Grieco, Jowers, & Bartholomew, 2009; Mahar et al., 2006). Studies have also shown benefits to children's academic-related outcomes. For example, Vazou, Gavrilou, Mamalaki, Papanastasiou, and Sioumala (2012) found that 10-minute active breaks linked with curricular subjects for 2 weeks significantly increased children's academic motivation (perceived academic competence), compared with the normal practice. Also, other studies (Erwin, Fedewa, & Ahn, 2012; Fedewa, Ahn, Erwin, & Davis, 2015) found that curriculum-linked active breaks had positive effects on children's academic achievement, especially math, although there was no evidence of the effects of active breaks on fluid intelligence.

Cognitively Challenging Active Breaks

More recently, research has begun to explore the possible impact of physically active breaks that combine physical exertion and cognitive engagement, that is the cognitive effort involved in the performance of a task. This approach is hypothesized to produce greater cognitive outcomes than physical activity breaks without a cognitively challenging component (Best, 2010), due to its inherent cognitive stimulation. It has been proposed that this type of physical activity activates the prefrontal cortex, which is the same region of the brain involved in higher-order thinking, thus resulting in improvements in the neural connectivity in that specific brain region (Pesce & Ben-Soussan, 2016).

To our knowledge, just four studies have investigated the effects of cognitively challenging active breaks. Schmidt, Benzing, and Kamer (2016) used a four-arm study design to determine effects of breaks on children's attention before and immediately after each of the following conditions: (i) sedentary break; (ii) sedentary and cognitively engaging break; (iii) active break; and (iv) active and cognitively engaging break. Only the conditions that involved cognitive engagement were positively associated with children's attention. Using a similar study design, Egger, Conzelmann, and Schmidt (2018) examined the effects of cognitively challenging active breaks on children's executive functions. Interestingly, that study revealed that after delivery of the cognitively engaging active breaks, children's cognitive flexibility (one type of executive function) was poorer than the non-cognitively engaging types of breaks. No effects were found for inhibition and working memory. The authors speculated that perhaps the breaks were too cognitive demanding. Adjusting the dose of cognitive demand may be necessary in order to meet children's optimal challenge point (Pesce et al., 2013).

A further three-arm study by Egger, Benzing, Conzelmann, and Schmidt (2019) implemented 200 cognitively engaging active breaks in the classroom over a period of 20 weeks. It was found that long-term cognitively engaging classroom-based active breaks improved children's cognitive flexibility, but not their inhibition or working memory. In addition, cognitively engaging activities (both active breaks and sedentary engaging activities) improved children's mathematic skills more than physically active breaks with low cognitive engagement (Egger et al., 2019).

A recent proof-of-concept study conducted among teachers in mainstream and special primary schools in Australia explored the feasibility of delivering 4-minute cognitively challenging active breaks to children during class lessons (Mazzoli et al., 2019). Teachers in mainstream schools found the breaks feasible to deliver and perceived they were of potential benefit to children's concentration and health. Most children thought it was enjoyable and fun, and reported that many of the children were laughing during the cognitively challenging active breaks. While teachers in special schools thought that these types of breaks would be beneficial for children in their class prior to delivery, once they had experienced implementing the breaks, their perceptions were not so favorable. In particular, teachers felt that the breaks would need to be tailored for children with different needs and the cognitively challenging breaks did not suit all of their children. These findings highlight some of the challenges with classroom-based physical activity initiatives and the need for active breaks to be tailored for children with varying abilities and needs in the population.

A list of freely available resources for active breaks in the classroom is provided in Table 25.3.

Table 25.3 Some available resources for schools to use to support active breaks in the classroom

- The 'Colorado Education Initiative' provides a series of active breaks for secondary classrooms: http://www.coloradoedinitiative.org/wp-content/uploads/2014/08/CEI-Take-a-Break-Teacher-Toolbox.pdf
- *Energizers* is a freely available manual of curriculum-linked active breaks provided by 'Eat Smart Move More, North Carolina': https://www.eatsmartmovemorenc.com/Energizers/EnergizersForSchools.html
- *GoNoodle* provides educators with over 300 free physical activity and mindfulness videos that can be used in the classroom: https://www.gonoodle.com/
- *Super Movers* involves a partnership between the Premier League (the English football league system) and the BBC, which provides free literacy and numeracy activities for children to do in primary school and at home: https://www.bbc.com/sport/supermovers/43560951

Active Classroom Environments

When American psychologist Roger Barker developed the behavior setting theory, he identified four major influences on behavior: (1) the behavior setting exists independent of individuals' perceptions of it and their behavior conforms to that setting; (2) behavior settings are 'synomorphic' which means they are consistent across physical environments that 'surround' behaviors; (3) the setting self-regulates (i.e. has purpose); and (4) individuals are both 'responders' to the behavioral setting and are also part of the setting themselves, providing cues for the behaviors of others (Scott, 2005). In consideration of the classroom as a behavioral setting, it is easy to understand what an important influence it can be on children's behavior.

There are a lot of consistencies in classroom environments across the world, and it could be argued that this setting has remained unchanged for many decades. However, this was not always the case as classrooms have changed over time in line with education methods and purposes. For example, in Ancient Greece, there was no distinct classroom boundary and students gathered around the teacher as permitted by the surrounding physical space (Park & Choi, 2014). In the middle ages, the classroom layout was more formal, often presented as two rows facing each other in the style of pews in a church. By the industrial revolution, many rows of desks facing the front of the room were squeezed into school classrooms as the number of young people in the population accessing free education increased (Park & Choi, 2014). In the 1960s, open-plan classrooms became popular; however, research showed there was a negative impact of noise on children's concentration and learning (Shield, Greenland, & Dockrell, 2010) and this type of layout declined in popularity.

In spite of a lack of rigorous research on effective physical learning environments (Higgins, Hall, Wall, Woolner, & McCaughey, 2005), open-plan classrooms are again experiencing a revival (Shield et al., 2010), and in some schools the type and placement of classroom furniture are moving away from rows of desks facing the front of the room. 'Active learning' principles are increasingly being adopted, with students sitting around tables in small groups (Park & Choi, 2014). These modified physical learning environments can be beneficial to students' physical, emotional, and social outcomes as well as their learning (Kariippanon, Cliff, Lancaster, Okely, & Parrish, 2018). However, many of these classrooms contain primarily seated furniture and few standing options. Evidence of the impact of the classroom layout, including the type and placement of school furniture, on children's physical activity and educational outcomes will be presented in the following section.

Classroom Layout

As summarized in Table 25.2, a systematic review by Minges et al. (2016) on the impact of standing or height-adjustable desks in mainly primary school classrooms found overall positive effects on students' standing time, physical activity, energy expenditure, and classroom behavior, as well as reductions in sitting time. Few studies reported significant effects on musculoskeletal health or BMI. A recent Australian study by Contardo Ayala and colleagues (2018) examined the effects of height-adjustable desks in a secondary school classroom (used by students ranging in age from 12 to 17 years) over a 17-week period on students' energy expenditure, waist circumference, musculoskeletal health, and BMI compared with students who used traditional classrooms over this period. At 17 weeks, the 49 students who used the height-adjustable desks expended 37.7 kcal/ lesson more, and had an average 2.64 cm lower waist circumference than the 39 adolescents (matched by year level and subject) that used traditional classrooms. There were no intervention effects on BMI or musculoskeletal discomfort at the end of the trial. These findings are consistent with those from previous studies with primary school-aged children (Aminian, Hinckson, &

Stewart, 2015; Cardon, De Clercq, De Bourdeaudhuij, & Breithecker, 2004; Contardo Ayala et al., 2016; Koepp et al., 2012).

In addition to changes to classroom furniture, Lanningham-Foster and colleagues (2008) compared physical activity levels of the same group of 24 children when they were in a traditional classroom to when they were in a classroom with height-adjustable desks ('Standing classroom') or when they were in an 'activity permissive' environment ('The Neighborhood'). 'The Neighborhood' was designed to resemble a village square and was constructed inside an indoor athletic club (35,000 feet²). In addition to housing a standing classroom, there were also basketball hoops, indoor soccer, climbing mazes, and other opportunities for children to be active. A separate group of 16 children had their physical activity monitored during summer break as a comparison group. Three to four days of objective activity data were collected in each of these settings. After 12 weeks, there were no differences in activity levels (m/s²) between the traditional classroom and the standing classroom. This is unsurprising given the activity monitor was assessing movement in m/s² and did not capture energy expenditure or postural transitions. Children's physical activity while in 'The Neighborhood' was significantly greater than the traditional classroom, but no different from activity levels of children during their summer vacation. Clearly, redesigning classrooms in this way is not feasible, but it does highlight the importance of design and providing opportunities to move within the classroom.

While few of these studies have reported the impact of the classroom layout on learning and cognition, research shows it is possible to increase children's physical activity and energy expenditure in the short term through environmental changes. However, how these changes affect children's learning and health and well-being in the longer term is unknown. Few studies have focused on older age groups in the secondary/senior school setting or on children with special needs.

Equipment in the Classroom

Equipment such as screens, sport or physical activity equipment has been used in the classroom to promote children's physical activity (Watson et al., 2017; Salmon et al., 2011). Screens such as computer monitors, projectors or whiteboards, and music players have been used to support the implementation of active breaks in the classroom. For example, in delivery of the Brain Break program, a study with over 280 primary school children in Macedonia required schools to have a computer, a projector, and 'good' internet connection (Popeska et al., 2018). The materials for the Instant Recess program, a 10-minute active breaks initiative for children in the classroom, were made available for schools on DVD and CD formats and required the users to have access to devices to play them (Whitt-Glover et al., 2011). These two programs reported favorable outcomes in relation to feasibility and acceptability of the breaks (Popeska et al., 2018) and increases in children's physical activity (Whitt-Glover et al., 2011). The Transform-Us! program provided school classrooms with tubs of sports and novel physical activity equipment (e.g. circus apparatus) to help teachers deliver active breaks during class lessons (Salmon et al., 2011). Although it is not possible to separate additional effects of access to equipment from the effects of the teacher doing the activity breaks, providing support for teachers in this way will likely facilitate implementation in the classroom.

Key and Emerging Issues

Implementation Challenges

Some of the key issues with active classrooms relate to challenges of implementation. For example, several studies reported the impact of implementing active breaks in class, but also the difficulties for some teachers in doing so (e.g. Bartholomew & Jowers, 2011; Carlson et al., 2015). There is emerging recognition that demonstration of efficacy or effectiveness may not reflect how well a school-based physical activity program is adopted, adapted, and implemented at scale (Koorts et al., 2018; Mâsse, McKay, Valente, Brant, & Naylor, 2012; Naylor et al., 2006). Factors such as alignment with state-, national-, and school-level policies; organizational buy-in; barriers to adoption; and economic costs of changing environments to support physical activity (to name a few) are all critical components that influence successful implementation of active classrooms. Some of the approaches discussed in this chapter are targeting educational systems and cultures that are very difficult to change (Carlson et al., 2015).

Research has shown that teachers tend to perceive physical activity in the classroom as competing with their need to deliver the set curriculum (Naylor et al., 2006). Yet contrary to the assumption that implementing physical activity in the classroom might detract from curricular activities, as noted earlier in this chapter, few studies have shown that classroom-based physical activity has detrimental effects on learning or academic outcomes (Daly-Smith et al., 2018; Martin & Murtagh, 2017; Norris et al., 2015; Rasberry et al., 2011; Watson et al., 2017). Indeed, a growing body of evidence suggests that physical activity in the classroom enhances children's learning and improves their focus and attention in class.

Lack of time is a common barrier to the implementation of classroom-based physical activity reported by teachers (e.g. Dinkel, Lee, & Schaffer, 2016; Mazzoli et al., 2019). A further barrier for 26% of n = 346 elementary teachers from the Midwest in the United States was issues with behavior management (Dinkel et al., 2016). This is in spite of approximately three-quarters of teachers believing that their students' behavior improved when they incorporated physical activity breaks into class lessons. Lack of available training and administrative support were also raised as barriers for 45% of teachers in that study. While ongoing professional development or continuing education credits for in-service teachers is a requirement of the profession, there are also many competing priorities in the education space. Two-thirds of teachers in the study by Dinkel et al. (2016) reported a preference for learning about classroom-based physical activity through training at their school. The next most preferred method (42%) was via a website or online training videos. A further challenge with offering professional development to in-service teachers is that most initiatives go out of vogue quickly, can be expensive to deliver, and it is difficult to reach in-service teachers at scale. Ideally, the next generation of teachers will learn about active lessons and breaks as pre-service teachers so that these techniques become part of routine practice and not something 'extra' that teachers need to take on in the classroom.

Pre-Service Teacher Education

Pre-service teacher education provides an integral platform for scaffolding critical pedagogical skills, strategies, knowledge, and capabilities (Darling-Hammond & Baratz-Snowden, 2005). In recent years, there has been a surge of research interest in the connection between quality teaching and successful student outcomes. Pre-service teacher education is a crucial link in producing quality teachers, and more positive student outcomes. Indeed, the impact of pre-service teacher education on teacher effectiveness and student outcomes is internationally recognized as pivotal (Caires & Almeida, 2005), but it is an under-studied, and perhaps under-utilized, setting for physical activity and sedentary behavior intervention research.

Pre-service teachers bring with them a set of beliefs and biographies that constitutes their emerging sense of teacher identity, and this is directly influenced, and molded, by their prior experiences as students, as well as their observations of their own teachers. Specifically, pre-service teachers' prevailing negative experiences of physical activity at school are of particular concern, given that the personal school experiences of classroom teachers are significant predictors of their confidence, competence, and willingness to teach (Morgan & Hansen, 2008; Webster, Monsma, & Erwin, 2010). This highlights the importance of pre-service teacher education in regards to disrupting pre-conceived notions of classroom-based physical activity. Teachers' beliefs about their ability to teach effectively and form meaningful connections with their students continue to be formed early in their teaching career, particularly in initial teacher education (Woolfolk Hoy & Burke-Spero, 2005). Pre-service teachers who are comprehensively and positively immersed in active pedagogy early in their teacher training are potentially more likely to develop a better commitment to active teaching, possibly resulting in improved teaching and learning outcomes (Webster et al., 2010).

Teachers are expected to alter curricula on the basis of new knowledge and ways of knowing, to change styles of teaching depending on needs of the student population, and to change methods when research indicates more effective practice. To enable this, we need skilled academic educators who can proactively model, educate, and inform our future teachers around these facets of teaching (Mergler & Tangen, 2010), in particular active learning and teaching strategies. However, negotiating the heavily prescribed pre-service teacher curriculum, governance, and regulation, in conjunction with disrupting the 'status quo' in regards to pre-service teacher education models, may present a set of perceived challenges in regards to 'change' in pre-service teacher education (Mayer, 2014; Richardson, 1998).

Literature suggests that teachers and academic educators resist doing whatever is being proposed, as they want to cling to their 'old ways' (Mayer, 2014). Indeed, the view of the academic educator as reluctant to change is strong and widespread, particularly when the change is suggested or mandated by those who are external to the setting in which the teaching is taking place: administrators, policy-makers, and staff developers. Indeed our own research experience with incorporating active learning strategies into the undergraduate curriculum for pre-service teachers has highlighted the challenges, as illustrated by the following quote from a primary education academic who participated in this research:

> Change is hard, and there is so often resistance to change, but I think the evidence behind, and the results from this type of [physical activity] program will drive the much needed change in regards to initial teacher education …
>
> *(Interview with primary education academic)*

However, what is also known is that teachers and academic educators do undertake change voluntarily, following their own sense of what their students need and what is working. These changes, while often minor adjustments to teaching styles, methods, and/or instructional models, can have substantial effects (Richardson, 1990). This autonomous change often leads to a more embedded and sustained approach, as the teacher action is linked directly to improved student outcomes. If the academic educator is empowered with the knowledge, skills, and strategies in regards to active teaching, and subsequently experiences more positive student (pre-service teacher) outcomes within their own teaching, this may lead to both individual and organizational change. Therefore, more 'upstream' approaches to increasing children's physical activity via integrating active teaching pedagogy and practice into pre-service teacher education may provide a more effective and potentially sustainable approach. What is unknown, however, is how feasible and effective this approach is.

Recommendations for Research

- Surprisingly few studies of active classrooms have reported on longer-term health effects, cognitive or academic performance. Prolonged interventions with long-term follow-up are needed.
- In addition to the earlier point, further clarity on the physical activity intensity, frequency, duration, and type during active breaks and active lessons is needed.

- Research is needed to explore the feasibility and impact of embedding active pedagogy into pre-service teacher education on children's physical activity, and academic (i.e. on-task time and executive function) and health-related outcomes.
- There is currently a lack of evidence of the feasibility and impact of physical activity classrooms in secondary/senior school and preschool settings. Although some research in Australian secondary schools is emerging (Leahy, Eather, Smith, Hillman, Morgan, Nilsson et al., 2019; Leahy, Eather, Smith, Hillman, Morgan, Plotnikoff et al., 2019), further research is required to determine whether this approach is feasible and effective in these settings.
- Mazzoli et al. (2019) found that teachers in special schools reported the need to tailor cognitively challenging active breaks for children with special needs. More research is needed with special populations and inclusive education settings.
- While active classroom environments and equipment in the classroom have been shown to be effective for increasing children's physical activity, there is potential for future research to use new technologies such as robotics (e.g. bot-led active breaks) or artificial intelligence (e.g. technology that detects when children's concentration is waning and they 'need' to move).

Conclusions and Recommendations

Evidence suggests that active breaks and active lessons have the potential to increase children's physical activity, and improve classroom behaviors, and concentration and attention. Effects on executive function and fluid intelligence, and learning or academic outcomes have been mixed. Changing the classroom environment through the addition of standing or height-adjustable desks can increase children's standing time, physical activity, energy expenditure and improve classroom behavior, as well as reduce time spent sitting and not adversely affect musculoskeletal health.

While this chapter explored the impact of the classroom environment on children's physical activity, the research reviewed was limited to indoor classrooms. There is emerging evidence of the effects of outdoor lessons and education programs on children's learning, social engagement, and physical activity. A systematic review of 13 studies (eight primary and six secondary school studies) found most reported beneficial academic and social outcomes from outdoor classes; however, only two case studies reported (positive) effects on children's physical activity (Becker, Lauterbach, Spengler, Dettweiler, & Mess, 2017). That review concluded that more research on the impact of outdoor learning environments on child and adolescent physical activity is needed. Given that time spent outdoors is an important predictor of children's overall physical activity (Cleland et al., 2008), this would seem a valuable consideration for children's learning environments.

With the implementation of active classrooms being a major challenge identified by various studies, it is critical to make sure that any classroom-based physical activity initiative aligns with the school's priorities and curriculum, and that the training for the program is informed by teachers and meets their expectations. Ensuring that the program can be delivered 'at scale' is also important. See for example the CLASS Physically Active Learning (PAL) initiative, a UK implementation study designed to investigate the degree and process of implementation of integrating movement into lessons (Routen et al., 2017). Using tools and guides such as the World Health Organization's (WHO) pragmatic guide for successful scaling up interventions, or Koorts et al.'s (2018) PRACTical planning for Implementation and Scale-up (PRACTIS guide) may assist in navigating the parameters of the setting, identifying key stakeholders to engage, and anticipating and working through barriers and facilitators.

Based on the earlier conclusions about active classrooms, we recommend schools and teachers deliver daily curriculum-aligned active breaks and active lessons to children in their class, and that this is undertaken in a supportive environment that helps teachers and children achieve higher levels of physical activity, better classroom behavior and concentration, and greater learning outcomes.

References

Ahamed, Y., Macdonald, H., Reed, K., Naylor, P.-J., Liu-Ambrose, T., & Mckay, H. (2007). School-based physical activity does not compromise children's academic performance. *Medicine and Science in Sports and Exercise, 39*, 371. doi:10.1249/01.mss.0000241654.45500.8e

Altenburg, T. M., Chinapaw, M. J., & Singh, A. S. (2016). Effects of one versus two bouts of moderate intensity physical activity on selective attention during a school morning in Dutch primary schoolchildren: A randomized controlled trial. *Journal of Science & Medicine in Sport, 19*, 820–824. doi:10.1016/j.jsams.2015.12.003.

Aminian, S., Hinckson, E. A., & Stewart, T. (2015). Modifying the classroom environment to increase standing and reduce sitting. *Building Research & Information, 43*, 631–645. doi:10.1080/09613218.2015.1058093

Bailey, C. G., & DiPerna, J. C. (2015). Effects of classroom-based energizers on primary grade students' physical activity levels. *Physical Educator, 72*, 480–495.

Barr-Anderson, D. J., AuYoung, M., Whitt-Glover, M. C., Glenn, B. A., & Yancey, A. K. (2011). Integration of short bouts of physical activity into organizational routine. A systematic review of the literature. *American Journal of Preventive Medicine, 40*, 76–93. doi:10.1016/j.amepre.2010.09.033

Bartholomew, J. B., & Jowers, E. M. (2011). Physically active academic lessons in elementary children. *Preventive Medicine, 52*, S51–S54. doi:10.1016/j.ypmed.2011.01.017

Becker, C., Lauterbach, G., Spengler, S., Dettweiler, U., & Mess, F. (2017). Effects of regular classes in outdoor education settings: A systematic review on students' learning, social and health dimensions. *International Journal of Environmental Research and Public Health, 14*, 485. doi:10.3390/ijerph14050485

Best, J. R. (2010). Effects of physical activity on children's executive function: Contributions of experimental research on aerobic exercise. *Developmental Review, 30*, 331–351. doi:10.1016/j.dr.2010.08.001

Caires, S., & Almeida, L. (2005). Teaching practice in Initial Teacher Education: Its impact on student teachers' professional skills and development. *Journal of Education for Teaching, 31*, 111–120. doi:10.1080/02607470500127236

Cardon, G., De Clercq, D., De Bourdeaudhuij, I., & Breithecker, D. (2004). Sitting habits in elementary schoolchildren: A traditional versus a "moving school." *Patient Education and Counseling, 54*, 133–142. doi:10.1016/S0738-3991(03)00215-5

Carlson, J. A., Engelberg, J. K., Cain, K. L., Conway, T. L., Mignano, A. M., Bonilla, E. A., . . . Sallis, J. F. (2015). Implementing classroom physical activity breaks: Associations with student physical activity and classroom behavior. *Preventive Medicine, 81*, 67–72. doi:10.1016/j.ypmed.2015.08.006

Cleland, V., Crawford, D., Baur, L., Hume, C., Timperio, A., & Salmon, J. (2008). A prospective examination of children's time spent outdoors, objectively measured physical activity and overweight. *International Journal of Obesity, 32*, 1685–1693. doi:10.1038/ijo.2008.171

Clemes, S., Barber, S., Bingham, D., Ridgers, N., Fletcher, E., Pearson, N., . . . Dunstan, D. W. (2016). Reducing children's classroom sitting time using sit-to-stand desks: Findings from pilot studies in UK and Australian primary schools. *Journal of Public Health, 38*, 526–533. doi:10.1093/pubmed/fdv084

Contardo Ayala, A. M., Salmon, J., Timperio, A., Sudholz, B., Ridgers, N. D., Sethi, P., . . . Dunstan, D. W. (2016). Impact of an 8-month trial using height-adjustable desks on children's classroom sitting patterns and markers of cardio-metabolic and musculoskeletal health. *International Journal of Environmental Research and Public Health, 13*, 1227. doi:10.3390/ijerph13121227

Contardo Ayala, A. M., Sudholz, B., Salmon, J., Dunstan, D., Ridgers, N., Arundell, L., & Timperio, A. (2018). The impact of height-adjustable desks and prompts to break-up classroom sitting on adolescents' energy expenditure, adiposity markers and perceived musculoskeletal discomfort. *PLoS One, 13*, e0203938. doi:10.1371/journal.pone.0203938

Corrigan, T. (2013). *Active learning has an ancient history. Teaching and learning in higher education.* Retrieved from https://teachingandlearninginhighered.org/2013/11/30/active-learning-has-an-ancient-history/

Daly-Smith, A. J., Zwolinsky, S., McKenna, J., Tomporowski, P. D., Defeyter, M. A., & Manley, A. (2018). Systematic review of acute physically active learning and classroom movement breaks on children's physical activity, cognition, academic performance and classroom behaviour: Understanding critical design features. *BMJ Open Sport and Exercise Medicine, 4*(1), e000341. doi:10.1136/bmjsem-2018-000341

Darling-Hammond, L., & Baratz-Snowden, J. (2005). *A good teacher in every classroom: Preparing the highly qualified teachers our children deserve.* San Francisco, CA: John Wiley & Sons.

de Greeff, J., Hartman, E., Mullender-Wijnsma, M., Bosker, R., Doolaard, S., & Visscher, C. (2016). Long-term effects of physically active academic lessons on physical fitness and executive functions in primary school children. *Health Education Research, 31*, 185–194. doi:10.1093/her/cyv102

Dinkel, D. M., Lee, J. M., & Schaffer, C. (2016). Examining the knowledge and capacity of elementary teachers to implement classroom physical activity breaks. *International Electronic Journal of Elementary Education, 9*, 182–196.

Donnelly, J. E., Greene, J. L., Gibson, C. A., Smith, B. K., Washburn, R. A., Sullivan, D. K., . . . Williams, S. L. (2009). Physical activity across the curriculum (PAAC): A randomized controlled trial to promote physical activity and diminish overweight and obesity in elementary school children. *Preventive Medicine, 49*, 336–341. doi:10.1016/j.ypmed.2009.07.022

Egger, F., Benzing, V., Conzelmann, A., & Schmidt, M. (2019). Boost your brain, while having a break! The effects of long-term cognitively engaging physical activity breaks on children's executive functions and academic achievement. *PLoS One, 14*, e0212482. doi:10.1371/journal.pone.0212482

Egger, F., Conzelmann, A., & Schmidt, M. (2018). The effect of acute cognitively engaging physical activity breaks on children's executive functions: Too much of a good thing? *Psychology of Sport and Exercise, 36*, 178–186. doi:10.1016/j.psychsport.2018.02.014

Erwin, H., Beighle, A., Morgan, C. F., & Noland, M. (2011). Effect of a low-cost, teacher-directed classroom intervention on elementary students' physical activity. *Journal of School Health, 81*, 455–461. doi:10.1111/j.1746-1561.2011.00614.x

Erwin, H., Fedewa, A., & Ahn, S. (2012). Student academic performance outcomes of a classroom physical activity intervention: A pilot study. *International Electronic Journal of Elementary Education, 4*(3), 473.

Fedewa, A. L., Ahn, S., Erwin, H., & Davis, M. C. (2015). A randomized controlled design investigating the effects of classroom-based physical activity on children's fluid intelligence and achievement. *School Psychology International, 36*, 135–153. doi:10.1177/0143034314565424

Gammon, C., Morton, K., Atkin, A., Corder, K., Daly-Smith, A., Quarmby, T., . . . van Sluijs, E. (2019). Introducing physically active lessons in UK secondary schools: Feasibility study and pilot cluster-randomised controlled trial. *BMJ Open, 9*, e025080. doi:10.1136/bmjopen-2018-025080

Goh, T., Hannon, J., Webster, C., Podlog, L., & Newton, M. (2016). Effects of a TAKE 10! classroom-based physical activity intervention on 3rd to 5th grades children's on-task behavior. *Journal of Physical Activity & Health, 13*, 712–718. doi:10.1123/jpah.2015-0238

Grieco, L. A., Jowers, E. M., & Bartholomew, J. B. (2009). Physically active academic lessons and time on task: The moderating effect of body mass index. *Medicine and Science in Sports and Exercise, 41*, 1921–1926. doi:10.1249/MSS.0b013e3181a61495

Higgins, S., Hall, E., Wall, K., Woolner, P., & McCaughey, C. (2005). *The impact of school environments: A literature review.* London, UK: Design Council, sponsored by CfBT Research and Development. Retrieved from http://www.ncef.org/content/impact-school-environments-literature-review

Hill, L. J., Williams, J. H., Aucott, L., Milne, J., Thomson, J., Greig, J., . . . Mon-Williams, M. (2010). Exercising attention within the classroom. *Developmental Medicine and Child Neurology, 52*, 929–934. doi:10.1111/j.1469-8749.2010.03661.x

Hollar, D., Messiah, S. E., Lopez-Mitnik, G., Hollar, T. L., Almon, M., & Agatston, A. S. (2010). Healthier options for public schoolchildren program improves weight and blood pressure in 6- to 13-year-olds. *Journal of the American Dietetic Association, 110*, 261–267. doi:10.1016/j.jada.2009.10.029

Howie, E. K., Beets, M. W., & Pate, R. R. (2014). Acute classroom exercise breaks improve on-task behavior in 4th and 5th grade students: A dose-response. *Mental Health and Physical Activity, 7*, 65–71. doi:10.1016/j.mhpa.2014.05.002

Howie, E. K., Schatz, J., & Pate, R. R. (2015). Acute effects of classroom exercise breaks on executive function and math performance: A dose-response study. *Research Quarterly for Exercise and Sport, 86*, 217–224. doi:10.1080/02701367.2015.1039892

Janssen, M., Chinapaw, M. J. M., Rauh, S. P., Toussaint, H. M., Van Mechelen, W., & Verhagen, E. A. L. M. (2014). A short physical activity break from cognitive tasks increases selective attention in primary school children aged 10–11. *Mental Health and Physical Activity, 7*, 129–134. doi:10.1016/j.mhpa.2014.07.001

Kariippanon, K. E., Cliff, D. P., Lancaster, S. L., Okely, A. D., & Parrish, A. M. (2018). Perceived interplay between flexible learning spaces and teaching, learning and student wellbeing. *Learning Environments Research, 21*, 301–320. doi:10.1007/s10984-017-9254-9

Katz, D. L., Cushman, D., Reynolds, J., Njike, V., Treu, J. A., Walker, J., . . . Katz, C. (2010). Putting physical activity where it fits in the school day: Preliminary results of the ABC (activity bursts in the classroom) for fitness program. *Preventing Chronic Disease, 7*, A82. PMC2901580

Kibbe, D. L., Hackett, J., Hurley, M., McFarland, A., Godburn Schubert, K., Schultz, A., & Harris, S. (2011). Ten years of TAKE 10!: Integrating physical activity with academic concepts in elementary school classrooms. *Preventive Medicine, 52*, S43–S50. doi:10.1016/j.ypmed.2011.01.025

Koepp, G. A., Snedden, B. J., Flynn, L., Puccinelli, D., Huntsman, B., & Levine, J. A. (2012). Feasibility analysis of standing desks for sixth graders. *Child Obesity and Nutrition, 4*, 89–92. doi:10.1177/1941406412439414

Koorts, H., Eakin, E., Estabrooks, P., Timperio, A., Salmon, J., & Bauman, A. (2018). Implementation and scale up of population physical activity interventions for clinical and community settings: The PRACTIS guide. *International Journal of Behavioral Nutrition and Physical Activity, 15*(1), 51. doi:10.1186/s12966-018-0678-0

Lanningham-Foster, L., Foster, R. C., McCrady, S. K., Manohar, C. U., Jensen, T. B., Mitre, N. G., . . . Levine, J. A. (2008). Changing the school environment to increase physical activity in children. *Obesity, 16*, 1849–1853. doi:10.1038/oby.2008.282

Leahy, A., Eather, N., Smith, J. J., Hillman, C. H., Morgan, P. J., Nilsson, M., . . . Lubans, D. R. (2019). A school-based physical activity intervention for older adolescents: Rationale and study protocol for the Burn 2 Learn cluster randomised controlled trial. *British Medical Journal Open, 9*, e026029. doi:10.1136/bmjopen-2018-026029

Leahy, A. A., Eather, N., Smith, J. J., Hillman, C. H., Morgan, P. J., Plotnikoff, R. C., . . . Lubans, D. R. (2019). Feasibility and preliminary efficacy of a teacher-facilitated high-intensity interval training intervention for older adolescents. *Pediatric Exercise Science, 31*, 107–117. doi:10.1123/pes.2018-0039

Liu, A., Hu, X., Ma, G., Cui, Z., Pan, Y., Chang, S., . . . Chen, C. (2008). Evaluation of a classroom-based physical activity promoting programme. *Obesity Reviews, 9*(Suppl 1), 130–134. doi:10.1111/j.1467-789X.2007.00454.x

Ma, J. K., Le Mare, L., & Gurd, B. J. (2014). Classroom-based high-intensity interval activity improves off-task behaviour in primary school students. *Applied Physiology, Nutrition & Metabolism, 39*, 1332–1337. doi:10.1139/apnm-2014-0125

Ma, J. K., Le Mare, L., & Gurd, B. J. (2015). Four minutes of in-class high-intensity interval activity improves selective attention in 9- to 11-year olds. *Applied Physiology, Nutrition & Metabolism, 40*, 238–244. doi:10.1139/apnm-2014-0309

Mahar, M. T., Murphy, S. K., Rowe, D. A., Golden, J., Shields, A. T., & Raedeke, T. D. (2006). Effects of a classroom-based program on physical activity and on-task behavior. *Medicine and Science in Sports and Exercise, 38*, 2086. doi:10.1249/01.mss.0000235359.16685.a3

Martin, R., & Murtagh, E. M. (2017). Effect of active lessons on physical activity, academic, and health outcomes: A systematic review. *Research Quarterly for Exercise and Sport*, 1–20. doi:10.1080/02701367.2017.1294244

Mâsse, L. C., McKay, H., Valente, M., Brant, R., & Naylor, P. J. (2012). Physical activity implementation in schools: A 4-year follow-up. *American Journal of Preventive Medicine, 43*, 369–377. doi:10.1016/j.amepre.2012.06.010

Mavilidi, M., Lubans, D., Eather, N., Morgan, P., & Riley, N. (2018). Preliminary efficacy and feasibility of "thinking while moving in English": A program with physical activity integrated into primary school English lessons. *Children, 5*, 109. doi:10.3390/children5080109

Mayer, D. (2014). Forty years of teacher education in Australia: 1974–2014. *Journal of Education for Teaching, 40*, 461–473. doi:10.1080/02607476.2014.956536

Mazzoli, E., Koorts, H., Salmon, J., Pesce, C., May, T., Teo, W.-P., & Barnett, L. M. (2019). Feasibility of breaking up sitting time in mainstream and special schools with a cognitively challenging motor task. *Journal of Sport and Health Science, 8*, 137–148. doi:10.1016/j.jshs.2019.01.002

McKay, H., MacLean, L., Petit, M., MacKelvie-O'Brien, K., Janssen, P., Beck, T., & Khan, K. (2005). "Bounce at the bell": A novel program of short bouts of exercise improves proximal femur bone mass in early pubertal children. *British Journal of Sports Medicine, 39*, 521–526. doi:10.1136/bjsm.2004.014266

Mergler, A. & Tangen, D. (2010). Using microteaching to enhance teacher efficacy in pre-service teachers. *Teaching Education, 21*, 199–210. doi:10.1080/10476210902998466

Minges, K., Chao, A., Irwin, M., Owen, N., Park, C., Whittemore, R., . . . Salmon, J. (2016). Classroom standing desks and sedentary behaviour: A systematic review. *Pediatrics, 137*, e20153087. doi:10.1542/peds.2015-3087

Morgan, P., & Hansen, V. (2008). Physical education in primary schools: Classroom teachers' perceptions of benefits and outcomes *Health Education Journal, 67*, 196–207. doi:10.1177/0017896908094637

Naylor, P.-J., Macdonald, H. M., Zebedee, J. A., Reed, K. E., & McKay, H. A. (2006). Lessons learned from action schools! BC – An 'active school' model to promote physical activity in elementary schools. *Journal of Science and Medicine in Sport, 9*, 413–423. doi:10.1016/j.jsams.2006.06.013

Norris, E., Shelton, N., Dunsmuir, S., Duke-Williams, O., & Stamatakis, E. (2015). Physically active lessons as physical activity and educational interventions: A systematic review of methods and results. *Preventive Medicine, 72*, 116–125. doi:10.1016/j.ypmed.2014.12.027

Owen, K. B., Parker, P. D., Van Zanden, B., MacMillan, F., Astell-Burt, T., & Lonsdale, C. (2016) Physical activity and school engagement in youth: A systematic review and meta-analysis. *Educational Psychologist, 51*, 129–145. doi:10.1080/00461520.2016.1151793

Park, E. L. & Choi, B. K. (2014). Transformation of classroom spaces: Traditional versus active learning classroom in colleges. *Higher Education, 68*, 749–771.

Pesce, C., & Ben-Soussan, T. D. (2016). "Cogito ergo sum" or "ambulo ergo sum"? New perspectives in developmental exercise and cognition research. In T. McMorris (Ed.), *Exercise-cognition interaction: A neuroscience perspective* (pp. 251–281). Amsterdam, Netherlands: Elsevier.

Pesce, C., Crova, C., Marchetti, R., Struzzolino, I., Masci, I., Vannozzi, G., . . . Forte, R. (2013). Searching for cognitively optimal challenge point in physical activity for children with typical and atypical motor development. *Mental Health and Physical Activity, 6*, 172–180. doi:10.1016/j.mhpa.2013.07.001

Popeska, B., Jovanova-Mitkovska, S., Chin, M. K., Edginton, C. R., Ching Mok, M. M., & Gontarev, S. (2018). Implementation of Brain Breaks in the classroom and effects on attitudes toward physical activity in a Macedonian school setting. *International Journal of Environmental Research and Public Health, 15*, 1127. doi:10.3390/ijerph15061127

Rasberry, C. N., Lee, S. M., Robin, L., Laris, B. A., Russell, L. A., Coyle, K. K., & Nihiser, A. J. (2011). The association between school-based physical activity, including physical education, and academic performance: A systematic review of the literature. *Preventive Medicine, 52*, S10–S20. doi:10.1016/j.ypmed.2011.01.027

Reed, J. A., Einstein, G., Hahn, E., Hooker, S. P., Gross, V. P., & Kravitz, J. (2010). Examining the impact of integrating physical activity on fluid intelligence and academic performance in an elementary school setting: A preliminary investigation. *Journal of Physical Activity & Health, 7*, 343. doi:10.1123/jpah.7.3.343

Richardson, V. (1990). Significant and worthwhile change in teaching practice. *Educational Researcher, 19*, 10–18. doi:10.3102/0013189X019007010

Richardson, V. (1998). How teachers change. What will lead to change that benefits student learning? *Focus on Basics. Connecting Research and Practice, 2* (Issue C). Retrieved from http://ncsall.net/index.html@id=395.html

Riley, N., Lubans, D. R., Holmes, K., & Morgan, P. J. (2016). Findings from the EASY Minds cluster randomized controlled trial: Evaluation of a physical activity integration program for mathematics in primary schools. *Journal of Physical Activity and Health, 13*, 198–206. doi:10.1123/jpah.2015-0046

Riley, N., Lubans, D. R., Morgan, P. J., & Young, M. (2015). Outcomes and process evaluation of a programme integrating physical activity into the primary school mathematics curriculum: The EASY Minds pilot randomised controlled trial. *Journal of Science and Medicine in Sport, 18*, 656–661. doi:10.1016/j.jsams.2014.09.005

Routen, A., Biddle, S., Bodicoat, D. H., Cale, L. A., Clemes, S., Edwardson, C. L., . . . Sherar, L. B. (2017). Study design and protocol for a mixed methods evaluation of an intervention to reduce and break-up sitting time in primary school classrooms in the UK: The CLASS PAL (physically active learning) programme. *BMJ Open, 7*, e019428. doi:10.1136/bmjopen-2017-019428

Salmon, J., Arundell, L., Hume, C., Brown, H., Hesketh, K., Dunstan, D. W., . . . Crawford, D. (2011). A cluster-randomized controlled trial to reduce sedentary behavior and promote physical activity and health of 8-9 year olds: The Transform-Us! study. *BMC Public Health, 11*, 1. doi:10.1186/1471-2458-11-759

Schmidt, M., Benzing, V., & Kamer, M. (2016). Classroom-based physical activity breaks and children's attention: Cognitive engagement works! *Frontiers in Psychology, 7*, 1474. doi:10.3389/fpsyg.2016.01474

Scott, M. M. (2005). A powerful theory and a paradox. Ecological psychologists after Barker. *Environment and Behavior, 37*, 295–329. doi:10.1177/0013916504270696

Shield, B., Greenland, E., & Dockrell, J. (2010). Noise in open plan classrooms in primary schools: A review. *Applied Aspects of Auditory Distraction, 12*, 225–234. doi:10.4103/1463-1741.70501

Stewart, J. A., Dennison, D. A., Kohl, H. W., & Doyle, J. A. (2004). Exercise level and energy expenditure in the TAKE 10! in-class physical activity program. *Journal of School Health, 74*, 397–400. doi:10.1111/j.1746-1561.2004.tb06605.x

Sylva, K. (1994). School influences on children's development. *Journal of Child Psychology and Psychiatry, 35*, 135–170. doi:10.1111/j.1469-7610.1994.tb01135.x

Trost, S. G., Fees, B., & Dzewaltowski, D. (2008). Feasibility and efficacy of a "move and learn" physical activity curriculum in preschool children. *Journal of Physical Activity & Health, 5*, 88. doi:10.1123/jpah.5.1.88

US Department of Health and Human Services. (1996). *Physical activity and health: A report of the surgeon general*. Atlanta, GA: US Department of Health and Human Services, Public Health Service, CDC, National Center for Chronic Disease Prevention and Health Promotion.

Vazou, S., Gavrilou, P., Mamalaki, E., Papanastasiou, A., & Sioumala, N. (2012). Does integrating physical activity in the elementary school classroom influence academic motivation? *International Journal of Sport & Exercise Psychology, 10*, 251–263. doi:10.1080/1612197x.2012.682368

Watson, A., Timperio, A., Brown, H., Best, K., & Hesketh, K. D. (2017). Effect of classroom-based physical activity interventions on academic and physical activity outcomes: A systematic review and meta-analysis. *International Journal of Behavioral Nutrition and Physical Activity, 14*, 114. doi:10.1186/s12966-017-0569-9

Webster, C. A., Monsma, E., & Erwin, H. (2010). The role of biographical characteristics in preservice classroom teachers' physical activity promotion attitudes. *Journal of Teaching in Physical Education, 29*, 358–377. doi:10.1123/jtpe.29.4.358

Whitt-Glover, M. C., Ham, S. A., & Yancey, A. K. (2011). Instant recess: A practical tool for increasing physical activity during the school day. *Progress in Community Health Partnerships: Research, Education, and Action, 5*, 289–297.

Woolfolk Hoy, A. & Burke Spero, R. (2005). Changes in teacher efficacy during the early years of teaching: A comparison of four measures. *Teaching and Teacher Education, 21*, 343–356. doi:10.1016/j.tate.2005.01.007

26

SCHOOL-BASED RUNNING PROGRAMS

Lauren B. Sherar, Anna E. Chalkley, Trish Gorely,
and Lorraine A. Cale

Introduction

A recently popularized, practical and cost-effective approach to providing additional school-based physical activity which falls outside of Physical Education (PE) time is school-based running programs. Upon hearing this concept for the first time, one might assume that this is an after-school training program for young cross country or track/athletics enthusiasts. However, these programs encourage children to be more active during the school day through providing opportunities for students to walk/run around a marked route for approximately 15 minutes. This new genre of program has a number of attractive features for schools making it a potentially useful public health initiative.

Daily running programs have gained significant momentum in the United Kingdom over the past 5 years. While many may be under the impression that the concept of daily running within the school day was invented by a head teacher in Scotland (who has been responsible for cementing The Daily Mile concept), there is prior evidence of running programs having been implemented in schools, although perhaps not at scale. For example, GreatFun2Run, the Golden Mile and Marathon Kids UK (formally known as Kids Marathon) were officially established in 2008, 2012 and 2013, respectively. Furthermore, school-based running programs have long been part of comprehensive school health programs in the United States. These have ranged from programs delivered as part of breakfast clubs, during the curriculum, e.g. Just Run (http://www.justrun.org) and/or after school, e.g. Marathon Kids in the United States (http://www.marathonkids.org).

This chapter provides an overview of the benefits and typical features of some popular school-based running programs. It then critiques the evidence-base for these programs before concluding with some proposed future directions and implications for practice.

Why Running?

Locomotor skills, including running, is one of the three skill domains that categorize fundamental movement skills (FMS). These skills are considered the foundation for developing more specialized and refined movement patterns necessary for participation in physical activity (Gallahue & Ozmun, 2011). Promoting running can embrace a child's natural desire to move. Although most children develop a basic level of natural physical competence, proficiency in FMS is more likely if they are provided with the opportunity to practise their skills and receive encouragement and support (Clarke & Metcalfe, 2002). Researchers have suggested that FMS development should be included in school-based interventions given that children with such skills are more likely to participate in physical activity and possess better fitness in later life (Barnett, Van Beurden, Morgan, Brooks, & Beard, 2008; Jaakkola, Yli-Piipari, Huotari, Watt, & Liukkonen, 2016). Indeed, high levels of FMS competence in childhood have been found to be related to a number of health and physical activity outcomes (Borde, Smith, Sutherland, Nathan, & Lubans, 2017; Lubans, Morgan, Cliff, Barnett, & Okely, 2010).

Another key driving force behind running programs is the known benefits that running has on children's cardiorespiratory fitness (CRF) (Brown, Harrower, & Deeter, 1972; Ekblom, 1969). There is robust evidence to suggest that better CRF is associated with a variety of positive health indicators that range from lower adiposity levels to favorable cardiometabolic biomarker profiles and physical self-perception among children (Lang et al., 2018). Further, adolescents with low CRF have an increased risk of developing cardiovascular disease in later life (Högström, Nordström, & Nordström, 2014) and experiencing premature mortality (Högström, Nordström, & Nordström, 2016). There is also evidence of a secular decline in children's CRF worldwide (Lamoureux et al., 2018), which is largely thought to be attributed to an erosion of habitual physical activity. Because of the confounding effects of variation in biological maturation on physical function (Baxter-Jones, Eisenmann, & Sherar, 2005) and the varied nature of children's activities, it is difficult to elucidate the specific relationship between running and CRF in children. However, a study over 30 years ago showed boys who participated in a running program (three 30-minute sessions per week for 12 weeks in lieu of attendance in regular PE classes) performed better on an 800-metre run and had lower pulse rates than boys in a control group (who attended regular PE). Despite this, improvements only lasted for 5 months after the trial (Tuckman & Hinkle, 1986).

Other pragmatic reasons why running programs are appealing as a school-based intervention are because they can be conducted with minimal cost, with no specialized equipment or resource, and can be implemented by teachers/staff with little training. All of these factors have been listed as barriers to the uptake of interventions in schools (Naylor et al., 2015). As a FMS, running also demands relatively limited initial skill levels from children. Running programs could therefore be considered more inclusive than other types of interventions. Finally, the simplicity of running programs means that they can be replicated, with ease, between schools.

Political Interest and Commitment

Traditionally schools have been viewed as key settings within which to address a range of public health issues (Inman, van Bakergem, LaRosa, & Garr, 2011). The political focus on schools as vehicles for the promotion of healthy active lifestyles was most recently driven by the hosting of the London 2012 Olympics and promise of an Olympic legacy which would use sports to inspire a generation and create healthy habits for life ("Beyond 2012: The London 2012 legacy story – GOV.UK", 2012). Consequently, the United Kingdom has seen a renewed emphasis on health-related policy goals for PE and school sport in recent years, an observation mirrored in other countries. This shift has recognized the need to offer not only a broader range of physical activities but also for these to be made available across the school day in order to engage students in leading healthy active lifestyles (Lindsey, 2020). Similarly, England's Childhood Obesity Strategy ("Childhood obesity: A plan for action – GOV.UK", 2016) provided some very clear and decisive actions for schools relating to physical activity, including the ambition for all primary schools to ensure that every child engages in at least 30 minutes of moderate-to-vigorous physical activity (MVPA) every school day. The strategy furthermore identified active mile programs (school-based programs where children are encouraged to walk or run daily for approximately one mile or 15 minutes), as an approach schools could adopt to provide additional physical activity time. This political commitment toward active mile programs was reinforced by the second chapter of the United Kingdom (UK) government's Childhood Obesity Plan, which promoted a "national ambition for every primary school to adopt an active mile initiative" ("Childhood obesity: A plan for action, chapter 2 – GOV.UK", 2018) and subsequently by the cross-government School Sport and Physical Activity Action Plan which endorsed the use of active mile programs to establish physical activity as an integral part of children's routines (School Sport and Activity Action Plan, 2019).

A year earlier, the Scottish Government had already issued their commitment to such a national ambition. In 2015 all schools in Scotland were encouraged "to consider implementing The Daily Mile scheme (an initiative whereby children leave the classroom for approximately 15 minutes every day to walk, jog or run at their own pace) or develop their own physical activity initiatives" and in their 2016 manifesto Ministers supported the idea of a Daily Mile Nation, with every school being "offered help to become a Daily Mile school" ("How is the SNP encouraging people to be more active? – Scottish National Party", 2017). Similarly, the Welsh Government followed suit in 2017 and issued a joint letter to all head teachers in primary schools in Wales to "encourage them to consider simple and innovative approaches to improve the health and well-being of children during the school day – including adopting the Daily Mile initiative" ("Welsh Government|Written statement – Encouraging the use of the Daily Mile Scheme by primary schools", 2017).

In addition to the political cross-sector commitment for running programs, the doubling of the PE and Sport Premium funding in England (Department for Education, 2017) represented a significant opportunity to upskill staff and embed running programs as part of longer-term school strategies for inspiring daily physical activity. The Premium funding (now £320 million per year) was introduced in 2013 to support the delivery of PE and sports in primary schools with the vision of all students leaving primary education physically literate and with the knowledge, skills and motivation necessary to equip them for a healthy lifestyle and lifelong participation in physical activity and sports. The PE and Sport Premium is paid directly to English primary schools and is ring-fenced to spend on improving the quality of PE and sport provision for the benefit of all students so that they develop healthy lifestyles. While there was intuitive and case study evidence that running programs would be an appealing investment for schools and teachers within the earlier context, efficacy and implementation evidence was lacking. The key factors underlying the successful implementation of initiatives such as running programs, including how to maximize and sustain school engagement and which features of the program were successful in influencing physical activity, were not known at that time.

Running Programs

The interest in school-based running programs may certainly have been helped by the growth in popularity of other grass roots initiatives taking place beyond school such as Parkrun which provide organized, free events for communities to participate in (Reece, Quirk, Wellington, Haake, & Wilson, 2018). Since 2013, children and young people have been specifically targeted via the Junior Parkrun series and there are now more than 200 2 km such events for 4- to 14-year olds and their families across the United Kingdom (Iacobucci, 2018).

Undeniably, in the United Kingdom and perhaps globally, the grass roots support for running programs has increased exponentially from relatively humble beginnings with the broadcasting and subsequent launch and national advertising of The Daily Mile initiative. Other programs with a similar concept to The Daily Mile include the "1 km a day" (Brustio et al., 2018), Marathon Kids (Chalkley et al., 2018b) and "The 100 Mile Club" (Wright et al., 2019). Common to most programs is that students regularly walk/run, while in school uniform/regular school clothing, along a marked route in the school grounds (field and/or playground) for approximately 15 minutes. Running programs have been created, most often, by practitioners (teachers or physical activity providers) rather than researchers and are introduced as a pragmatic solution to concerns over childhood inactivity. Because of this, few have been developed using psychological theories of motivation or behavior change and/or implementation frameworks, although many can be/ have been retrofitted in this regard.

To illustrate the similarities and differences between running programs, two indicative programs, The Daily Mile, a curriculum-based initiative, and Marathon Kids UK, an extra-curricular program, both of which have been independently evaluated, are described below.

The Daily Mile

The Daily Mile is a well-known example of a running initiative implemented during curricular time. The Daily Mile was conceived by Elaine Wylie, a head teacher of a primary school in Scotland in 2012 in response to concerns over obesity and overweight, and a lack of fitness in her students. As noted earlier, the premise behind The Daily Mile is that during class time all children leave the classroom and are encouraged to walk, jog or run around the playground for approximately 15 minutes every day. Continuously running during this time would equate to approximately 1 mile a day for most children, hence the name. National (and later international) media picked up on this head teacher-led initiative, giving it much publicity, which led to a grass roots explosion in the interest in running programs from teachers, parents, school governors and local authorities in the United Kingdom. Subsequently, The Daily Mile Foundation (http:// www.thedailymile.co.uk) was established and received substantial donor funding. It is now safe to say that The Daily Mile has become a household name and has raised the status and visibility of running programs in the United Kingdom, Europe and more recently globally. The Daily Mile Foundation has reported huge numbers in scaling up the program. For example, as of April 2019, 9090 schools from 65 countries and 1,865,429 children were registered for The Daily Mile ("Global Map|The Daily Mile UK", 2019) and based on these figures it has been suggested that the program is an implementation success.

Despite the limited information on the impact the initiative has had, and the extent to which participating schools have achieved and sustained high-quality delivery, The Daily Mile continues to evolve at pace and scale. In what is its biggest expansion to date, The Daily Mile Foundation has recently received £1.5 million of National Lottery funding from Sport England to help support English primary schools to deliver the initiative ("Funding to help children get active|Sport England", 2018). This investment has funded the recruitment of national and local coordinators to support and encourage more schools in England to sign-up for the initiative and marks their shared vision to bring daily physical activity to all 20,000 primary schools in England. Furthermore, the potential for The Daily Mile to be transferable across different settings has recently been recognized. Inspired by the Scottish Government's pledge to become the first "Daily Mile Nation", The Daily Mile Foundation has launched its Fit for Life program (http://www.the-dailymilefitforlife.com) to encourage all childminders, nurseries, primary and secondary (high) schools, colleges, universities and workplaces to take up the initiative.

Marathon Kids UK

With a distinct but overlapping philosophy, there are a number of school-based programs that focus on running during students' discretionary time (i.e. lunch, break and/or before/after school). Marathon Kids UK is one such example. The Marathon Kids UK program is managed and delivered by a UK charity, Kids Run Free, and provides primary school students with the challenge of walking/running up to four marathons per school year. The program encourages students to complete laps of a predefined course on the school grounds once or twice a week during lunch break.

For every lap completed, students receive an elastic band, and these are subsequently recorded by the school using an online tracking system. Distance is accumulated and monitored over time and rewards are given at key milestones (e.g. quarter, half, three quarter and full marathon). A number of tools and resources support the program (e.g. certificates, posters, how to guide and checklist) and optional on-site support is provided during a school launch by a member of staff from the charity. On the school's request, this member of staff delivers an assembly to school staff and students, demarcates the running route(s) and provides training on how to administer the program to a staff member ("Marathon Champion") and a selection of peer leaders or students ("Marathon Ambassadors"). Marathon Kids UK is also partnered with Marathon Kids US and both share a number of core principles of practice including: goal setting, tracking, role modeling, celebrating and rewards.

Although the characteristics of the aforementioned running programs are similar (i.e. they all draw on the simplicity and replicability of running to engage and include all students), important distinctions center around implementation, goal setting, tracking and rewards. All are nonetheless focused, or started off focusing on primary-aged children. That said, following more recent promotional efforts such as from The Daily Mile Foundation, we are now seeing evidence of some programs being implemented with older students (such as secondary/high school) as well as younger children at nurseries and other early years settings.

Overview of the Literature

Evidence of Effectiveness of Running Programs

Despite the growing popularity of running programs, evidence for their success is currently only anecdotal and there is a relative dearth of literature and published research on their effectiveness. Notably, high-quality randomized controlled trials (RCTs) of daily running programs are lacking; however, results are soon to be released from a large RCT examining the clinical and cost-effectiveness of The Daily Mile for the purpose of improving health and well-being (Breheny et al., 2018). The study has involved 40 primary schools located in Birmingham, UK, which were randomized to either the intervention (The Daily Mile) or control (usual practice in relation to health and well-being) arm. Measures of body composition, fitness, quality of life, well-being and academic attainment were collected from children at baseline, 4 months and 12 months following the initiation of the intervention. In addition, semi-structured interviews with teaching staff in participating schools were conducted to ascertain information on barriers and facilitators to and strategies of implementation, appropriateness of outcome measures (process evaluation) and opportunity cost (economic evaluation) of The Daily Mile. It is hoped that, once published, the Birmingham Daily Mile research will provide a robust evaluation and comprehensive assessment of its impact on a wide variety of outcomes which include children's physical and psychological health and academic attainment.

A quasi-experimental pilot study in two primary schools in Scotland is the first published evidence on the effectiveness of The Daily Mile (Chesham et al., 2018). Nearly 400 children (n=391) aged 4–12 years from two schools participated in the research. One school (intervention) was about to introduce The Daily Mile and one (control) had no intention of doing so. Students in the control school followed their usual curriculum. Results showed significant improvements in children's accelerometer assessed MVPA (increase of ~9 minutes/day), sedentary time (decrease in ~18 minutes/day), fitness and body composition (skinfolds) in the Daily Mile School. Although the results are promising, the small sample size (i.e. two schools), low numbers of students providing valid accelerometer data at both time points, bias in school recruitment and the lack of randomization are just a few of the limitations of this study.

Previous research on Marathon Kids US provides some foundation for its potential effectiveness. Two separate studies were conducted to evaluate the impact of the program on elementary school students' physical activity behavior. The first study was a quasi-experimental study involving 4th and 5th grade children (n= 1595) in seven elementary schools in Houston, Texas (four Marathon Kids schools and three comparison schools) and eight elementary schools in Round Rock, Texas. Data were collected at four time points during the school year: in October/November 2008 (preceding and immediately following a Kick-Off event), in December 2008 and February 2009 (interim measures) and in April 2009 (post-test). The second study was a cross-sectional study with a larger and ethnically and socio-economically diverse sample of elementary school children in central Texas which used a self-administered physical activity questionnaire with 4th and 5th grade students in 32 schools (n = 1,084 students). As an additional measure, a subsample of 5th grade students in four schools (two Marathon Kids schools and two comparison schools) were asked to wear a pedometer for four consecutive days during two time periods. While there were no significant differences found in any of the pedometer-based physical activity indicators by student participation in Marathon Kids, those who enrolled in the program were found to engage in a higher mean number of times of running for the three pooled post-Kick-Off event measurement periods compared to their peers who did not enroll (mean = 4.22 vs. 3.97 times, respectively; p = 0.035). In addition, positive effects were found on running and psycho-social-related factors such as athletic identity, parent social support for physical activity, outcome expectations for physical activity and physical activity self-efficacy (Springer et al., 2012). Clearly further high-quality research is required to establish the optimum implementation and scale-up of running programs but the findings from these initial studies are nonetheless promising.

Implementation of Running Programs

Research on the implementation of running programs in schools is similarly relatively underdeveloped. Schools are complex social structures with unique qualities which can influence the quantity and quality of implementation, meaning it is not always possible for programs to be transferred from one school to another with predictable results (Naylor & McKay, 2009). Indeed, sub-optimal implementation is likely a driving factor for small effect sizes in many school-based interventions (Borde et al., 2017; Naylor & McKay, 2009). However, only a few studies have specifically looked at barriers and facilitators to the implementation of running programs in schools. A study conducted in Italy which gathered questionnaire data from students (N = 140; aged 12 years) and teachers who had implemented a walk/run program for 4 months reported high feasibility (i.e. adherence, costs, safety) and acceptability (i.e. satisfaction, intent to continue use, perceived appropriateness) of the initiative (Brustio et al., 2018).

Chalkley and colleagues (2018a) examined the barriers and facilitators to the implementation of Marathon Kids within primary schools in England. Their study examined the perspectives of several different stakeholders including the program developers and the Marathon Kids Champion from a selection of 20 schools which had implemented the program and a sample of students who had participated. Despite there being a suggested delivery model for the program, there was variability in implementation across the different schools and as such, multiple factors were reported as being influential. These included features of the program (e.g. ethos and resources), the school climate (e.g. school culture; whole school engagement; school PE and physical activity policies and goals; and the physical environment) and program implementation decisions (e.g. aspirations for the school and its use of the program and planning and sustainability). Many factors were described as acting as both facilitators and barriers to implementation (e.g. the school environment; student choice and control over participation; peer influence; and interrelationships) and were frequently described as being interrelated. However, lack of staff "buy in" was consistently identified as the main barrier for schools when implementing Marathon Kids.

In a similar manner, Ryde and colleagues (2018) examined the factors associated with successful implementation of The Daily Mile in four schools in Scotland. Of significance in this study is that one of the four schools had sustained implementation of The Daily Mile over a long period (6 years). Based on interviews with teaching staff with a significant role for implementing The Daily Mile within their school, the researchers found that having simple core intervention components, flexible delivery that supports teacher autonomy and being adaptable to suit the specific primary school context were key aspects associated with implementation success. Other factors identified as contributing toward its successful implementation related to how The Daily Mile was developed, trialed and rolled out. Another study on The Daily Mile with teachers from eight primary schools in Scotland reported inadequate all-weather running surfaces and time constraints as barriers to implementation. Teacher reported benefits of the program however included increased teacher–child rapport and perceived enhanced fitness and concentration levels of the students (Malden & Doi, 2019).

Meanwhile, in Massachusetts, United States, of seven schools from lower-income communities randomized to a daily walk-run program (100 Mile Club), over a quarter did not implement the program at all, and of those that did, many stopped delivering it over a 2-year period. Monitoring (displaying children's mileage progress) and parent volunteers to aid tracking and encouragement appeared to be intervention ingredients that were associated with maintained student enthusiasm and participation in the walk/run program (Wright et al., 2019).

All studies support the findings from previous literature on the implementation of school-based physical activity programs suggesting that program, organizational and system level factors are important. In summary, in order to maximize the potential of running programs, there is a need to understand how they can best be delivered and the factors that influence their implementation, in order to ensure they are being employed effectively and appropriately and engaging all children, including the least active. Clearly though there is no "one size fits all" approach when it comes to implementation.

Key Issues

Choice: Mandating vs. Non-Mandating

Mandating increased physical activity in schools has become popular due to the belief that it will lead to enhanced adherence to physical activity and thereby be more effective in combatting obesity and overweight, as opposed to relying on students' voluntary compliance to lifestyle change. However, the effectiveness of school policy that makes physical activity compulsory as a strategy for increasing children's physical activity is unknown. It is also arguably at odds with a key desired outcome of physical activity/health promotion in schools which should be to empower young people to make informed and independent choices about their physical activity/health behaviors (Cale, Harris, & Hooper, 2020). Activity choice has furthermore been identified as a positive feature of school-based physical activity programs (Cale, 2017).

Critics of daily school-based running programs have suggested that such policies may fail to address what children value in terms of participation in physical activity (Fairhurst & Hotham, 2017). Running may also not be appropriate for or appealing to many young people and enforcing the activity may therefore be counterproductive. For example, it has been reported that negative experiences of primary school sport and physical activity are associated with low levels of physical activity in adults, particularly in girls (Ladwig, Vazou, & Ekkekakis, 2018). Some of the potential reasons cited for these negative experiences relate to injury, lack of enjoyment and social-physique anxiety, which could all be valid and relevant issues with running programs, especially if the quality of delivery varies within and/or between schools. Sustained running is also by nature, repetitive and could therefore be deemed to be dull, boring and not in keeping with young people's natural physical activity patterns which are more sporadic and spontaneous in nature (Bailey et al., 1995). Indeed, the potential limitations of school-based physical activity programs which focus heavily on vigorous activity, endurance training/exercise and/or repetitive activities have been highlighted (Cale, 2017). Cale has argued that while such activities may positively influence short-term fitness gains, they are narrow in focus, may be inappropriate and unappealing to many young people and are therefore unlikely to be successful in promoting lifetime physical activity. At the same time running, as an activity, can be presented in varied, fun and challenging ways and it could be claimed that key to a program's success may be the way in which physical activity is delivered rather than its specific focus or content per se (Lubans et al., 2017). Many countries have however seen changes in the traditional activity offerings in schools in recent years to better accommodate the broad definition of physical activity and realize the known health benefits, as well as better meet the varied needs and interests of their students. For instance, it is not uncommon for schools to now offer yoga, street dancing, parkour and Wii Fit to name just a few. While running undoubtedly has health benefits, overemphasis on this one activity, particularly if this is at the expense of time spent on other activities, could be perceived as a retrograde step and as simply reverting to traditional, narrow and more restricted physical activity provision. Rather, the need for schools to offer a broad and balanced range of activities both within and beyond the curriculum is recognized as good practice (Harris & Cale, 2018). It is thus argued that running programs can make a useful and valuable contribution to schools' activity offerings, but that they should not become the sole focus.

Replacing Physical Education

Although the majority of running programs state that the activity should not replace high-quality PE, whether this is or is not happening in practice has yet to be established. It is conceivable that in certain circumstances (for example, when a supply/substitute teacher is required to cover PE or when an indoor facility or hall is out of use), schools may opt to deliver an activity that all students are familiar with and which requires little planning and specialized instruction. In such cases, a running program may become an attractive, easy and safe option. Certainly, a large barrier to implementing activity programs in schools is a lack of time in the curriculum (Naylor et al., 2015). Previous evidence has further suggested that PE is often the subject most at risk of being displaced during busy times and due to other academic pressures during the year (Cale & Harris, 2005; Marshall & Hardman, 2000; Youth Sport Trust, 2018). However, running programs are neither equivalent to nor should be seen or used as a substitute for PE. While both physical activity and PE can contribute meaningfully to the development of healthy, active children, they and their goals are quite different (Association for Physical Education, 2015). Physical activity programs tend to have a behavioral focus with the goal of increasing the amount of time children spend engaged in MVPA. By comparison, PE is an instructional program with more broad ranging goals which span from the development of physical and social skills, moral values, spirituality, intellectual ability, to fitness, recreation and health (Kirk, 2010). The Association for Physical Education in the United Kingdom explicitly highlights the differences in their Health Position Paper describing PE as the planned, progressive learning that takes place in school curriculum timetabled time and which is delivered to all students. This involves both "learning to move" (i.e. becoming more physically competent) and "moving to learn" (e.g. learning through movement, a range of skills and understandings beyond physical activity such as co-operating with others). The context for the learning is physical activity, (but) with children experiencing a broad range of activities, including sport and dance (Association for Physical Education, 2015, p. 3). This distinction is discussed in detail in Chapter 23.

Compensation

An issue related to school-based running programs is the potential for physical activity compensation, that is, children engaging in less school day or after-school physical activity on days where they have participated in organized, structured running. The concept of compensation is based on the biological basis of physical activity (Rowland, 1998) which suggests that compensatory changes occur to maintain a stable level of physical activity or energy expenditure. Research on physical activity compensation during the school day is limited. However, given that school lunch and break times are active periods of free play for some children (Erwin et al., 2012), particularly for boys (Dudley, Cotton, Peralta, & Winslade, 2018), and are a significant contributor to students' school day and daily physical activity, it is conceivable that running programs implemented during this time may replace free play. Children who are sedentary during this time are already assumed to be disengaged from physical activity and evidence is lacking as to whether this group would choose to engage in an optional running activity program. Indeed, evidence from a mixed studies systematic review and meta-analysis of school-based interventions to promote physical activity and/or reduce sedentary time in children found that the interventions had a moderate effect on physical activity but that this was not replicated across the school day, suggesting compensatory behaviors (Jones, Defever, Letsinger, Steele, & Mackintosh, 2019). When studies measured changes in physical activity during the actual intervention there was moderate evidence of effect, whereas those that measured changes in physical activity during the school day presented inconclusive evidence of effect, and those that measured changes in physical activity over a whole day yielded no evidence of effect.

A Sole Focus on Running

As alluded to earlier, focusing on running programs in isolation and at the expense of a broader range of activities could be criticized as not fostering or developing a range of physical and social skills. Physical literacy is a term used to describe the motivation, confidence, physical competence, knowledge and understanding to value and take responsibility for engagement in physical activities for life ("International Physical Literacy Association", 2016) and fundamental to this is children being able to confidently participate in a variety of sports and activities in later life. Running is clearly only one component necessary for the promotion of children's physically literacy, alongside others such as agility, object interception and the development of additional motor skills. Schools clearly need to develop these broader competences both within and beyond the curriculum and through activities such as dance, gymnastics, games, outdoor and adventurous activities, swimming and so on, in addition to running. Finally, evidence is lacking as to whether participation in running programs during the formative years will lead to positive active behaviors during adolescence and adulthood. Running programs should not therefore be seen as the whole solution to physical inactivity among youth but as a promising part of the solution.

Parents and the Home Environment

The majority of running programs that have been developed to date involve no participation of family or caregivers, despite evidence suggesting that programs involving both the home and school setting have the most success in preventing childhood obesity (Wang et al., 2015). Parents have a major influence on children's lives with the potential to either reinforce or undermine health promotion efforts. Thus, engaging them would instinctively appear to be important for consolidating the beliefs, attitudes and behaviors underpinning activity programs (Boddy,

Hackett, & Stratton, 2010; Cohen et al., 2011; Sandercock, Voss, McConnell, & Rayner, 2010; Van Lippevelde et al., 2012). Of particular concern in recent years is the recognition that children's fitness is in decline (Lamoureux et al., 2018) and, despite the best efforts of schools, children's fitness may decrease during the summer holiday months to the point where any gains made during the academic year are lost by the time children return to school in the Autumn term (Mann et al., 2019). Furthermore, children from the poorest areas are likely to be the most affected (Fu, Brusseau, Hannon, & Burns, 2017) in that inequalities are more pronounced when children are outside of school time (Bastian, Maximova, McGavock, & Veugelers, 2015). This brings into question the feasibility of school-based running programs for making any significant or lasting contributions to children's health without a concerted effort to extend these to develop an out of school/term hours community element. Thus, caution is needed against over-relying on running programs as the "silver bullet" to the alleged inactivity crisis.

Emerging Issues

Alignment with Whole School Approaches to Promoting Physical Activity

One suggestion as to why schools are effective settings to promote health enhancing behaviors relates to the Structured Days Hypothesis (Brazendale et al., 2017), that is that school days are fundamentally different from less structured days at weekends and during school holiday due to the daily structure and routine afforded by formal and informal physical activity opportunities. Indeed, the utility of running programs in contributing to children's short-term physical activity levels has been supported (Chesham et al., 2018; Powell, Woodfield, Powell, Nevill, & Myers, 2018); however, there have been suggestions that for meaningful change, such programs would be better placed as part of a broader framework of health promotion such as a whole school approach to physical activity (Chalkley et al., 2018a). Whole school approaches to the promotion of physical activity are reportedly the most effective way of maximizing physical activity opportunities in schools and embedding cultural change (Global Advocacy for Physical Activity (GAPA) the Advocacy Council of the International Society for Physical Activity and Health (ISPAH), 2012) yet are still relatively underdeveloped. There is therefore real potential to explore the use of these programs as a context for learning within and beyond the curriculum. Doing so would help to raise awareness and promote knowledge and understanding of the importance of and relationship between physical activity and health alongside other health/physical activity-related learning outcomes, and, in turn, contribute to meeting specific curriculum expectations. For example, such learning can be readily reinforced within assemblies, whole school events and/or in subjects such as Personal, Social, Health and Economic Education and Science. Other cross-curricular learning opportunities include collecting and analyzing running data as part of Numeracy or Science, or planning/mapping out running routes in Geography. Embedding learning more explicitly within and through running programs should help to raise their status and thereby secure buy-in across the whole school.

Special Populations and Inclusive Education Settings

Inclusive education is enshrined in national and international legislation and schools have not only a moral and social obligation but also a legal one to promote inclusion, meet the needs of all students, remove barriers and ensure an inclusive environment and curriculum. This obligation equally applies to the context of school physical activity (Harris & Cale, 2018) and thus should apply to school-based running programs.

Many of the challenges to physical activity participation are a consequence of the environment in which the activity takes place and its organization and delivery rather than an individual's ability to participate. The external environment is not just a physical activity or sport setting but rather encompasses many factors that influence the way in which activity is delivered. Most children can do most activities most of the time but there may be specific reasons which may preclude some youngsters from physically participating. For running programs to be truly inclusive there is a need to define participation more broadly (for example, a child who cannot physically walk/run should be still be able to participate such as by monitoring distances covered and awarding lap bands). Running programs are promoted as fully inclusive and suitable for every child regardless of age, ability or circumstance. It is advocated that the focus for participation should be on time spent being active and promoting regular physical activity rather than on performance (for example, on distance or speed). Regardless, any activities that are offered to children should provide an appropriate and safe level of challenge based on individual abilities. Further, the activities and practices employed should be developmentally appropriate (physically, psychologically, cognitively, socially) and account for and recognize children and young people's different capacities, needs, interests and preferences for physical activity. Indeed, while participating in physical activity is important and beneficial for all young people it may be particularly so for some such as those with low self-esteem, physical competence or confidence, those who are overweight or obese and those with other common medical conditions (Harris & Cale, 2018). In addition to the obvious physical health and psychological benefits associated with physical activity, there are opportunities for these young people to develop social skills and friendships, experience decreased isolation, develop higher expectations, meet more demanding challenges and enhance their appreciation of difference and equity (Fitzgerald & Stride, 2012).

Use of Technology

Goal setting may enhance participation in and sustainability of running programs and, as highlighted earlier, is an intervention component of some programs. Goal setting theory suggests that individuals improve their performance when they recognize the need for change, set a challenging goal, monitor progress toward that goal, and reward themselves for goal achievement (Locke & Latham, 2006). Providing rewards and/or incentives may also support the aforementioned as these can help provide immediate gratification/satisfaction. Certainly, goal setting and rewards have been documented as positive components by students and teachers in Marathon Kids UK (Chalkley et al., 2018a). However, the "clunky" system of handing out elastic bands has also been cited as a barrier to participation, with this hampering smooth delivery of the program and allegedly leading to cheating and subsequently discontent amongst some students (Chalkley et al., 2018a). A tracking system based on radio-frequency identification (RFiD) technology can be used in combination with goal setting and incentives may provide necessary ongoing support to schools. Indeed, there are a growing number of off-the-shelf technologies that could be utilized by schools to accurately and objectively track children's running participation and performance (distance, speed) and deliver timely feedback with minimal burden. The majority of schools organize running as a whole class, as several classes, or even as a whole school at the same time. Therefore, any technology used needs to be able to track a large number of children simultaneously. For a system to be used daily it needs to be user friendly, time efficient and for collected data to be easily accessible. Playgrounds, especially in primary schools, serve many purposes and are used at break and lunch times as well as for PE; therefore any timing system must also take up minimal space or be easily portable. All of these factors must be considered when deciding if a technology will be useful within this context. However, recent technological developments should be able to alleviate these issues.

Extending the Program to Secondary/High Schools

Key life periods, such as the transition from primary to secondary school, have been associated with changes in children and young people's physical activity. Specifically, Brooke and colleagues have observed a stronger decline in MVPA at these ages during times where school grounds are key locations for physical activity (Brooke, Atkin, Corder, Ekelund, & van Sluijs, 2016). Thus, running programs could provide an appropriate intervention at key points in the school day potentially helping to offset some of this decline. There are considerable differences in the nature of the school environment between primary and secondary schools (Harrison, van Sluijs, Corder, & Jones, 2016). Secondary schools are larger overall and typically have more available space and facilities than primary schools. Daily running programs could therefore be an attractive and effective strategy to encourage physical activity amongst secondary-aged children. However, there are many unique contextual factors and timetable constraints which often prevent physical activity programs from being trialed or implemented in secondary schools (Harris & Cale, 2018). Furthermore, it is not known if these programs hold the same value for adolescents as they do for younger children. Given this, for programs to be sustainable in the longer term complementary and/or adapted strategies may be needed to take into account the different context and to develop and maintain the interest and enthusiasm in running amongst the secondary age group.

Recommendations for Research/Practitioners

Given the small evidence base surrounding school-based running programs, there are a number of possible areas for future research. Longitudinally following children from schools who are committed to daily running is essential to elucidate the physical, mental and social benefits of programs, student experiences, compensation and any potential limitations. For example, with regard to the former whether there are any risks to children of (over-use) injury from regular running on concrete or other hard surfaces has yet to be determined. Essential to this research would be establishing a precise measure of dose (i.e. duration, frequency and intensity) of running. From an educational perspective, there is a need to extend our knowledge regarding the extent to which programs achieve their aims of being inclusive and appropriate to all, whether and which students are disengaged or excluded and to investigate and develop strategies which might enhance inclusion. Longitudinally tracking the implementation of running programs is also important to ascertain their sustainability and/or effects on physical activity behavior beyond the first (honeymoon) year. Related to this is the need to explore what approaches specifically might be used and contribute most to ensuring or enhancing participation and sustainability perhaps, building on previous work (Chalkley et al., 2018a). Finally, frequent measures in varied sites should be employed in future evaluation projects to understand the impact of season and weather on participation.

From a practical perspective, if governments wish to endorse school-based running programs it is important to evaluate the variation in the size, condition and suitability of school grounds and environments (e.g. considering pollution/weather) in the specific county/country/jurisdiction. If daily running programs cannot be implemented in all school sites, then the program could just contribute to an ever-widening deprivation gap in organized sports (Vander Ploeg, Maximova, McGavock, Davis, & Veugelers, 2014).

Political interest, increased investment and perceived public health necessity have supported a dramatic increase in the attention and support for running programs. The evidence behind the effectiveness and implementation of these programs is sparse but growing. However, if schools are to be successful in ensuring all students engage in the 15 minutes of extra physical activity afforded by these initiatives, it is feasible that this will increase the amount of physical activity that children accumulate throughout a school day. Although running programs are not the silver bullet for increasing school-based physical activity, they could be an effective component of a whole school approach. As evaluation activities increase, we should be able to learn more about the intervention components that are behind the wide appeal of running programs and how these can be transferred to other school-based interventions.

References

Association for Physical Education. (2015). Retrieved from http://www.afpe.org.uk/physical-education/wp-content/uploads/afPE_Health_Position_Paper_Web_Version2015.pdf

Bailey, R. C., Olson, J., Pepper, S. L., Porszasz, J., Barstow, T. J., & Cooper, D. M. (1995). The level and tempo of children's physical activities: An observational study. *Medicine and Science in Sports and Exercise, 27*(7), 1033–1041.

Barnett, L. M., Van Beurden, E., Morgan, P. J., Brooks, L. O., & Beard, J. R. (2008). Does childhood motor skill proficiency predict adolescent fitness? *Medicine and Science in Sports and Exercise, 40*(12), 2137–2144.

Bastian, K. A., Maximova, K., McGavock, J., & Veugelers, P. (2015). Does school-based health promotion affect physical activity on weekends? And, does it reach those students most in need of health promotion? *PloS One, 10*(10), e0137987.

Baxter-Jones, A. D. G., Eisenmann, J. C., & Sherar, L. B. (2005). Controlling for maturation in pediatric exercise science. *Pediatric Exercise Science, 17*(1), 18–30.

Beyond 2012: The London 2012 legacy story – GOV.UK. (2012). Retrieved January 6, 2019, from https://www.gov.uk/government/publications/beyond-2012-the-london-2012-legacy-story

Boddy, L. M., Hackett, A. F., & Stratton, G. (2010). Changes in fitness, body mass index and obesity in 9–10 year olds. *Journal of Human Nutrition and Dietetics : The Official Journal of the British Dietetic Association, 23*(3), 254–259.

Borde, R., Smith, J. J., Sutherland, R., Nathan, N., & Lubans, D. R. (2017). Methodological considerations and impact of school-based interventions on objectively measured physical activity in adolescents: A systematic review and meta-analysis. *Obesity Reviews : An Official Journal of the International Association for the Study of Obesity, 18*(4), 476–490.

Brazendale, K., Beets, M. W., Weaver, R. G., Pate, R. R., Turner-McGrievy, G. M., Kaczynski, A. T., . . . von Hippel, P. T. (2017). Understanding differences between summer vs. school obesogenic behaviors of children: The structured days hypothesis. *International Journal of Behavioral Nutrition and Physical Activity, 14*(1), 100.

Breheny, K., Adab, P., Passmore, S., Martin, J., Lancashire, E., Hemming, K., & Frew, E. (2018). A cluster randomised controlled trial evaluating the effectiveness and cost-effectiveness of the daily mile on childhood obesity and wellbeing: The Birmingham Daily Mile protocol. *BMC Public Health, 18*(1), 126.

Brooke, H. L., Atkin, A. J., Corder, K., Ekelund, U., & van Sluijs, E. M. F. (2016). Changes in time-segment specific physical activity between ages 10 and 14 years: A longitudinal observational study. *Journal of Science and Medicine in Sport, 19*(1), 29–34.

Brown, C. H., Harrower, J. R., & Deeter, M. F. (1972). The effects of cross-country running on pre-adolescent girls. *Medicine and Science in Sports, 4*(1), 1–5.

Brustio, P. R., Moisè, P., Marasso, D., Miglio, F., Rainoldi, A., & Boccia, G. (2018). Feasibility of implementing an outdoor walking break in Italian middle schools. *PLoS One, 13*(8), e0202091.

Cale, L. (2017). Teaching about healthy active lifestyles. In C. D. Ennis (Ed.), *Routledge handbook of physical education pedagogies* (pp. 399–411). Oxon, UK: Routledge.

Cale, L., & Harris, J. (2005). *Exercise and young people : Issues, implications and initiatives.* Basingstoke, UK: Palgrave Macmillan.

Cale, L., Harris, J., & Hooper, O. (2020). Debating health knowledge and health pedagogies in physical education. In S. Capel & R. Blair (Eds.), *Debates in physical education* (pp. 256–277). Oxon, UK: Routledge.

Chalkley, A. E., Routen, A. C., Harris, J. P., Cale, L. A., Gorely, T., & Sherar, L. B. (2018a). A retrospective qualitative evaluation of barriers and facilitators to the implementation of a school-based running program. *BMC Public Health, 18*(1), 1189.

Chalkley, A. E., Routen, A. C., Harris, J. P., Cale, L. A., Gorely, T., & Sherar, L. B. (2018b). Marathon Kids UK: Study design and protocol for a mixed methods evaluation of a school-based running program introduction school-based physical activity programs have rapidly grown in within the public health policy agenda over recent years. *BMJ Open, 8*, e022176.

Chesham, R. A., Booth, J. N., Sweeney, E. L., Ryde, G. C., Gorely, T., Brooks, N. E., & Moran, C. N. (2018). The Daily Mile makes primary school children more active, less sedentary and improves their fitness and body composition: A quasi-experimental pilot study. *BMC Medicine, 16*(1), 64.

Childhood obesity: A plan for action, chapter 2 – GOV.UK. (2018). Retrieved December 10, 2018, from https://www.gov.uk/government/publications/childhood-obesity-a-plan-for-action-chapter-2

Childhood obesity: A plan for action – GOV.UK. (2016). Retrieved January 10, 2019, from https://www.gov.uk/government/publications/childhood-obesity-a-plan-for-action

Clarke, J., & Metcalfe, J. (2002). The mountain of motor development: A metaphor. In J. Clarke & J. Humprehy (Eds.), *Motor development: Research and reviews* (2nd ed., pp. 163–190). Reston, VA: NASPE Publications.

Cohen, D., Voss, C., Taylor, M., Delextrat, A., Ogunleye, A., & Sandercock, G. (2011). Ten-year secular changes in muscular fitness in English children. *Acta Paediatrica, 100*(10), e175–e177.

Department for Education. (2017). PE and Sports Premium doubles to £320 million - GOV.UK. *Gov.Uk*. Retrieved from https://www.gov.uk/government/news/pe-and-sports-premium-doubles-to-320-million

Dudley, D. A., Cotton, W. G., Peralta, L. R., & Winslade, M. (2018). Playground activities and gender variation in objectively measured physical activity intensity in Australian primary school children: A repeated measures study. *BMC Public Health, 18*(1), 1101.

Ekblom, B. (1969). Effect of physical training in adolescent boys. *Journal of Applied Physiology, 27*(3), 350–355.

Erwin, H., Abel, M., Beighle, A., Noland, M. P., Worley, B., & Riggs, R. (2012). The contribution of recess to children's school-day physical activity. *Journal of Physical Activity & Health, 9*(3), 442–448.

Fairhurst, A., & Hotham, S. (2017). Going further than the "Daily Mile". *Perspectives in Public Health, 137*(2), 83–84.

Fitzgerald, H., & Stride, A. (2012). Stories about physical education from young people with disabilities. *International Journal of Disability, Development and Education, 59*(3), 283–293.

Fu, Y., Brusseau, T. A., Hannon, J. C., & Burns, R. D. (2017). Effect of a 12-week summer break on school day physical activity and health-related fitness in low-income children from CSPAP schools. *Journal of Environmental and Public Health, 2017*, 1–7.

Funding to help children get active|Sport England. (2018). Retrieved January 10, 2019, from https://www.sportengland.org/news-and-features/news/2018/december/17/the-daily-mile-receives-15-million-investment-of-national-lottery-funding/

Gallahue, D., & Ozmun, J. (Eds.). (2011). *Understanding motor development : Infants, children, adolescents, adults* (6th ed.). Boston, MA: McGraw-Hill.

Global Advocacy for Physical Activity (GAPA) the Advocacy Council of the International Society for Physical Activity and Health (ISPAH). (2012). Investments that work for physical activity. *British Journal of Sports Medicine, 46*(10), 709–712.

Global Map|The Daily Mile UK. (n.d.). Retrieved November 29, 2018, from https://thedailymile.co.uk/participation-map/

Harris, J., & Cale, L. (2018). *Promoting active lifestyles in schools*. Champaign, IL: Human Kinetics.

Harrison, F., van Sluijs, E. M. F., Corder, K., & Jones, A. (2016). School grounds and physical activity: Associations at secondary schools, and over the transition from primary to secondary schools. *Health & Place, 39*, 34–42.

Högström, G., Nordström, A., & Nordström, P. (2014). High aerobic fitness in late adolescence is associated with a reduced risk of myocardial infarction later in life: A nationwide cohort study in men. *European Heart Journal, 35*(44), 3133–3140.

Högström, G., Nordström, A., & Nordström, P. (2016). Aerobic fitness in late adolescence and the risk of early death: A prospective cohort study of 1.3 million Swedish men. *International Journal of Epidemiology, 45*(4), 1159–1168.

How is the SNP encouraging people to be more active? – Scottish National Party. (2017). Retrieved November 29, 2018, from https://www.snp.org/policies/pb-how-is-the-snp-encouraging-people-to-be-more-active/

Iacobucci, G. (2018). Sixty seconds on . . . parkrun. *BMJ, 361*, k2767. doi:10.1136/bmj.k2767

Inman, D. D., van Bakergem, K. M., LaRosa, A. C., & Garr, D. R. (2011). Evidence-based health promotion programs for schools and communities. *American Journal of Preventive Medicine, 40*(2), 207–219.

International Physical Literacy Association. (2016). Retrieved December 5, 2018, from https://www.physical-literacy.org.uk/

Jaakkola, T., Yli-Piipari, S., Huotari, P., Watt, A., & Liukkonen, J. (2016). Fundamental movement skills and physical fitness as predictors of physical activity: A 6-year follow-up study. *Scandinavian Journal of Medicine & Science in Sports, 26*(1), 74–81.

Jones, M., Defever, E., Letsinger, A., Steele, J., & Mackintosh, K. A. (2019). A mixed studies systematic review and meta-analysis of school-based interventions to promote physical activity and/or reduce sedentary time in children. *Journal of Sport and Health Science, 9*(1), 3–17.

Kirk, D. (2010). *Physical education futures*. Routledge. Retrieved from https://books.google.co.uk/books/about/Physical_Education_Futures.html?id=kubH8748fC4C&redir_esc=y

Ladwig, M., Vazou, S., & Ekkekakis, P. (2018). "My best memory is when I was done with it": PE memories are associated with adult sedentary behavior. *Translational Journal of the American College of Sports Medicine, 3*(16), 119–129.

Lamoureux, N. R., Fitzgerald, J. S., Norton, K. I., Sabato, T., Tremblay, M. S., & Tomkinson, G. R. (2018). Temporal trends in the cardiorespiratory fitness of 2,525,827 adults between 1967 and 2016: A systematic review. *Sports Medicine, 49*(1), 41–55.

Lang, J. J., Belanger, K., Poitras, V., Janssen, I., Tomkinson, G. R., & Tremblay, M. S. (2018). Systematic review of the relationship between 20 m shuttle run performance and health indicators among children and youth. *Journal of Science and Medicine in Sport, 21*(4), 383–397.

Lindsey, I. (2020). Analysing policy change and continuity: Physical education and school sport policy in England since 2010. *Sport, Education and Society, 25*(1), 27–42.

Locke, E. A., & Latham, G. P. (2006). New directions in goal-setting theory. *Current Directions in Psychological Science, 15*(1), 265–268.

Lubans, D. R., Lonsdale, C., Cohen, K., Eather, N., Beauchamp, M. R., Morgan, P. J., . . . Smith, J. J. (2017). Framework for the design and delivery of organized physical activity sessions for children and adolescents: Rationale and description of the "SAAFE" teaching principles. *The International Journal of Behavioral Nutrition and Physical Activity, 14*(1), 24.

Lubans, D. R., Morgan, P. J., Cliff, D. P., Barnett, L. M., & Okely, A. D. (2010). Fundamental movement skills in children and adolescents. *Sports Medicine, 40*(12), 1019–1035.

Malden, S., & Doi, L. (2019). The Daily Mile: Teachers' perspectives of the barriers and facilitators to the delivery of a school-based physical activity intervention. *BMJ Open, 9*(3), e027169.

Mann, S., Wade, M., Jones, M., Sandercock, G., Beedie, C., & Steele, J. (2019). One-year surveillance of body mass index and cardiorespiratory fitness in UK primary school children in North West England and the impact of school deprivation level. *Archives of Disease in Childhood*. doi:10.1136/archdischild-2018-315567.

Marshall, J., & Hardman, K. (2000). The state and status of physical education in schools in international context. *European Physical Education Review, 6*(3), 203–229.

Naylor, P.-J., & McKay, H. A. (2009). Prevention in the first place: Schools a setting for action on physical inactivity. *British Journal of Sports Medicine, 43*(1), 10–13.

Naylor, P.-J., Nettlefold, L., Race, D., Hoy, C., Ashe, M. C., Wharf Higgins, J., & McKay, H. A. (2015). Implementation of school based physical activity interventions: A systematic review. *Preventive Medicine, 72*, 95–115.

Powell, E., Woodfield, L. A., Powell, A. J., Nevill, A. M., & Myers, T. D. (2018). Evaluation of a walking-track intervention to increase children's physical activity during primary school break times. *Children (Basel, Switzerland), 5*(10), 135.

Reece, L. J., Quirk, H., Wellington, C., Haake, S. J., & Wilson, F. (2018). Bright spots, physical activity investments that work: Parkrun; A global initiative striving for healthier and happier communities. *British Journal of Sports Medicine*. doi:10.1136/bjsports-2018-100041

Rowland, T. W. (1998). The biological basis of physical activity. *Medicine and Science in Sports and Exercise, 30*(3), 392–399.

Ryde, G. C., Booth, J. N., Brooks, N. E., Chesham, R. A., Moran, C. N., & Gorely, T. (2018). The Daily Mile: What factors are associated with its implementation success? *PLoS One, 13*(10), e0204988.

Sandercock, G., Voss, C., McConnell, D., & Rayner, P. (2010). Ten year secular declines in the cardiorespiratory fitness of affluent English children are largely independent of changes in body mass index. *Archives of Disease in Childhood, 95*(1), 46–47.

School Sport and Activity Action Plan. (2019). Retrieved from https://assets.publishing.service.gov.uk/government/uploads/system/uploads/attachment_data/fil

Springer, A. E., Kelder, S. H., Ranjit, N., Hochberg-Garrett, H., Crow, S., & Delk, J. (2012). Promoting physical activity and fruit and vegetable consumption through a community-school partnership: The effects of Marathon Kids on low-income elementary school children in Texas. *Journal of Physical Activity & Health, 9*(5), 739–753.

Tuckman, B. W., & Hinkle, J. S. (1986). An experimental study of the physical and psychological effects of aerobic exercise on schoolchildren. *Health Psychology : Official Journal of the Division of Health Psychology, American Psychological Association, 5*(3), 197–207.

Van Lippevelde, W., Verloigne, M., De Bourdeaudhuij, I., Brug, J., Bjelland, M., Lien, N., & Maes, L. (2012). Does parental involvement make a difference in school-based nutrition and physical activity interventions? A systematic review of randomized controlled trials. *International Journal of Public Health, 57*(4), 673–678.

Vander Ploeg, K. A., Maximova, K., McGavock, J., Davis, W., & Veugelers, P. (2014). Do school-based physical activity interventions increase or reduce inequalities in health? *Social Science & Medicine, 112*, 80–87.

Wang, Y., Cai, L., Wu, Y., Wilson, R. F., Weston, C., Fawole, O., . . . Segal, J. (2015). What childhood obesity prevention programs work? A systematic review and meta-analysis. *Obesity Reviews : An Official Journal of the International Association for the Study of Obesity, 16*(7), 547–565.

Welsh Government|Written statement – Encouraging the use of the Daily Mile Scheme by primary schools. (2017). Retrieved December 10, 2018, from https://gov.wales/about/cabinet/cabinetstatements/2017/dailymile/?lang=en

Wright, C. M., Chomitz, V. R., Duquesnay, P. J., Amin, S. A., Economos, C. D., & Sacheck, J. M. (2019). The FLEX study school-based physical activity programs – Measurement and evaluation of implementation. *BMC Public Health, 19*(1), 73.

Youth Sport Trust. (2018). *Re-imagining the future of secondary PE|Youth Sport Trust.* Retrieved December 21, 2018, from https://youthsporttrust.org/resource/re-imagining-future-secondary-pe

27

INTRODUCTION TO MULTICOMPONENT SCHOOL-BASED PHYSICAL ACTIVITY PROGRAMS

Timothy A. Brusseau and Ryan D. Burns

Schools are increasingly being asked to do more to help with the cognitive, physical, social, and emotional development of children. In fact, the United States Centers for Disease Control and Prevention (CDC) has developed the Whole School, Whole Community, Whole Child Model centered around ten components. The model calls for greater alignment, integration, and collaboration between education (learning) and health (Lewallen, Hunt, Potts-Datema, Zaza, & Giles, 2015). One of the primary components of the model includes physical education and physical activity. Researchers continue to find that physical activity can be added to school curriculum without negative academic consequences (Story, Nanney, & Schwartz, 2009) and actually improve academic performance. In the United States, the CDC developed a stand-alone physical activity model called a Comprehensive School Physical Activity Program (CSPAP; Figure 27.1).

A CSPAP is a multicomponent school physical activity model designed to ensure that youth have access to 60 minutes of physical activity opportunities each day. Multicomponent school-based programming has many names and is a priority in numerous countries. Ireland (Active School Flag), Poland (PE with Class), and Finland (Finnish Schools on the Move) are just a few

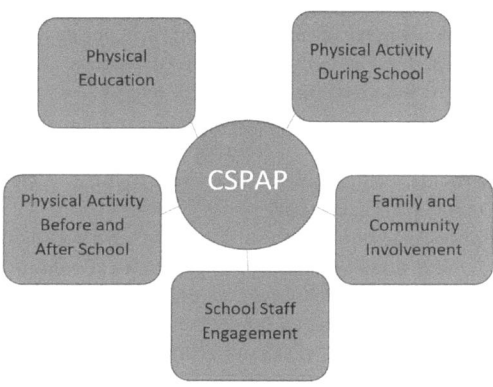

Figure 27.1 CSPAP components

examples of nationally recognized multicomponent programs (McMullen, Choinin, Tammelin, Pogorselska, & van der Mars, 2015). Beyond national initiatives, many other examples of multi-component programs are highlighted in the research literature from around the world. Some early examples include CATCH (United States; Luepker at al., 1996), APPLES (United Kingdom; Sahota et al., 2001), and Move It Groove It (Australia; van Beurden et al., 2003). More recent examples include the Active Living program (Netherlands; Van Kann, Kremers, De Vries, De Vries, & Jansen, 2016), Y-PATH (Ireland; Belton, O'Brien, McGann, & Issartel, 2018), and a CSPAP (United States; Brusseau et al., 2018). The key to multicomponent programming is they combine numerous physical activity opportunities across settings within the school. Individual components are discussed in earlier chapters and may include (but are not limited to) before- and after-school physical activity (including active transport; Chapters 31 and 33), school-day physical activity (including classroom and recess; Chapters 24 and 25), physical education (Chapter 23), family and community engagement (Chapters 29 and 30), as well as other programming and opportunities (Chapter 26). Table 27.1 highlights examples of what may be included in a multicomponent program. For the purpose of this chapter, for a study to be considered a multicomponent program it must have included at least two different physical activity opportunities and be school-based.

Erwin, Beighle, Carson, and Castelli (2013) highlighted the strengths of the research done to examine the effectiveness of physical education, recess, and after-school programming individually but also noted the limited scope of research that has examined multicomponent interventions.

Table 27.1 Multicomponent program recommendations

Component	Example recommendation
Quality physical education	Provide 150 minutes/week and 225 minutes/week of PE for elementary schools and secondary schools, respectively
	Students are physically active for at least 50% of PE
	Provide quality PE that is enjoyable and teaches students movement and behavioral skills in PE
Physical activity during school (recess and classroom)	Provide students with opportunities to be active during recess
	Provide playground markings, access to equipment, and organized activities during break-times
	Integrate physical activity into the classroom to assist learning in other curriculum areas (e.g. mathematics and science) and to break up sitting time (e.g. energizers)
Before- and after-school physical activity	Offer a variety of intramural activities before and after school that are both competitive and non-competitive in nature
	Promote active transportation to school (i.e. walking and riding to school)
School staff involvement	Provide appropriate and on-going professional learning in physical activity instruction for staff members
	Provide wellness programs for staff members that encourage them to role model physical activity
	Encourage staff members to be active with students in PE and school sport
Family and community involvement	Involve family members and guardians as volunteers in PE and school sport
	Involve family members and guardians in evening and weekend special events
	Establish joint-use and shared-use agreements with community organizations to encourage use of school facilities before and after school

Adapted from Hills, Dengel, and Lubans (2015).

In their systematic review of controlled trials, van Sluijs, McMinn, and Griffin (2007) identified 16 multicomponent physical activity interventions for children and adolescents. Ten of these interventions were conducted with children of which three would be considered large high quality randomized control studies (Reilly et al., 2006; Sahota et al., 2001; McKenzie et al., 1996) with only one showing a significant positive effect on physical activity (McKenzie et al., 1996). Overall, these studies taken together were inconclusive in overall effectiveness. Six studies were conducted in an adolescent population with three being considered high quality controlled trials (Pate et al., 2005; Simon et al., 2004; Webber et al., 2008) which all showed positive results. A common theme of these interventions was the inclusion of family and community components. More recently, Love, Adams, and van Sluijs (2019) have highlighted the lack of impact of school-based interventions on overall physical activity.

De Meester, van Lenthe, Spittaels, Lien, and De Bourdeaudhuij (2009) in their review of physical activity studies targeting European teenagers found that multicomponent programming was more effective than single component programs for changing physical activity behavior. This is supported by Salmon, Booth, Phongsavan, Murphy, and Timperio (2007) who noted a number of methodological and evaluation issues with school-based interventions but found that multicomponent studies were the most effective. Similarly, Kriemler and colleagues (2011) suggested in their review of school-based interventions that multicomponent intervention strategies were the most consistent and promising approach. More specifically, they found that multicomponent interventions with family involvement were the most effective. Russ, Webster, Beets, and Phillips (2015) examined US-based multicomponent interventions that targeted changes in total daily physical activity in their meta-analysis. They identified 14 total studies with 12 including physical education as a component. Three studies targeted physical activity in the academic classroom, four studies had a recess component, and one study had a lunchtime activity drop-in program. Only one study included a before- or after-school component, two had a staff wellness component, while all 14 studies had some kind of family and/or community involvement. The primary ways of family involvement came from regular communication about physical activity or homework that engaged the entire family in physical activity. Their analysis indicated limited effectiveness of multicomponent interventions on total daily physical activity. Of interest, the interventions that specifically targeted physical activity during the school day (e.g. recess and classroom-based physical activity) as one of their components were more effective (e.g. Springer et al., 2012; Williamson et al., 2007). Although the research was limited in nature, staff wellness programming was also associated with greater program effectiveness (e.g. Gortmaker et al., 1999; Seo et al., 2013). Importantly, as the number of components increased, so did the intervention effectiveness. More recent studies have illustrated greater successes on increasing overall physical activity of youth participating in a multicomponent intervention (e.g. Sutherland, Campbell, Lubans, Morgan, Okely, et al. (2016). Multicomponent interventions have had success impacting other outcomes beyond total day activity. Burns, Brusseau, and Hannon (2015) and Centeio et al. (2014) found their programs significantly increased school-day physical activity. Metzler, Barrett-Williams, Hunt, Marquis, and Trent (2015) found significant improvements in the number of students in the FitnessGram Healthy Fitness Zone and overall physical activity knowledge. McGrane, Belton, Fairclough, Powell, & Issartel (2018) and Burns, Fu, Hannon, & Brusseau (2017) indicated a positive impact on gross motor skills. Other studies have indicated some potential to improve enjoyment (Fu, Burns, Brusseau, & Hannon, 2016), classroom on task behavior (Burns, Brusseau, Fu, Myer, & Hannon, 2016), waist circumference (Leme et al., 2016), and metabolic health (Burns, Brusseau, & Hannon, 2017). Table 27.2 shows a number of recent multicomponent interventions.

Table 27.2 Recent multicomponent school-based studies

Author (YR)	Sample	Intervention	Components	Outcomes	Results
Christiansen et al. (2018)	2797 Danish 4th–6th graders	Cluster RCT	PE, classroom, recess	Self-perception, self-worth, body attractiveness, social competence	Increases in control and intervention groups
Sutherland (2016)	1150 Australian 7th graders	PA 4 everyone cluster RCT (YR1)	PE, recess, parents, and community	MVPA	Significant intervention increases in MVPA/week
Cohen, Morgan, Plotnikoff, Callister, & Lubans (2015)	460 Australian 3rd–4th graders	SCORES cluster RCT	PE, family involvement	PA, cardiorespiratory fitness and fundamental motor skills	Significant intervention increases in MVPA, FMS, and cardiorespiratory fitness
Van Kann et al. (2016)	520 Netherlands 8–11 year olds	The Active Living quasi-experimental study	Physical and social environments impacting recess, active commuting, community activity	Sedentary time and PA	No significant differences in PA and SB compared to matched schools
Sutherland (2016)	1150 Australian 7th graders	PA 4 everyone cluster RCT (YR2)	PE, recess, parents and community	MVPA	Significant increases in intervention MVPA
Braun, Kay, Cheung, Weiss, & Gazmararian (2017)	3479 US 4th graders	CSPAP pre/post design	PE, recess, classroom PA, before school, family and staff involvement	Estimated PA and cardiorespiratory fitness	Increases in estimated physical activity and increases in cardiorespiratory fitness
Burns et al. (2015)	327 US 4th and 5th graders	CSPAP pre/post design	PE, recess, classroom PA	School-day step counts	Significant increase in school step counts
Brusseau et al. (2016)	1390 US k–6th graders	CSPAP pre/post design	PE, recess, classroom PA, before/after-school PA	Step counts and PACER laps	Significant increases in school step counts and PACER laps
McGrane et al. (2018)	482 Irish 12–13 year olds	Y-PATH RCT	PE, parent involvement, teacher training	FMS	Significant increases in FMS
Leme et al. (2016)	253 Brazilian adolescents	Healthy habits, healthy girls – Brazil RCT	PE, school breaks	BMI, waist circumference, leisure time PA, sedentary behavior	Significant decrease in waist circumference in the intervention group
Haapala et al. (2017)	319 Finnish 7–15 years old	Finnish schools on the move quasi-experimental study	Bottom up approach that increases changes to PE, recess, and classroom PA	MVPA and sedentary time	Significant increases in MVPA and decreases in sedentary time compared to matched schools
Taylor et al. (2018)	289 UK children 9–10 years old	Pilot active schools: Skelmersdale – RCT	Active breaks, bounce at the bell, born to move videos, Daily Mile, playground activity challenge cards, PE teacher training, newsletters, activity homework	School-day MVPA, school-day sedentary time, fitness, BMI z-score	Significant decreases in school-day sedentary time

Keys to Successful Implementation

Program Leadership

When designing a multicomponent physical activity program it is important to establish a committee that is invested in the health of youth (CDC, 2013). The committee should be made up of members that are also involved in school health or wellness committees. Members might include health and physical education teachers, classroom teachers, school staff, administrators, parents, students, and community members. Table 27.3 highlights some of the roles and responsibilities of committee members. Ideally, a physical activity leader (PAL) is identified from this group who will be responsible for coordinating school physical activity efforts. This person should organize meetings, work with community partners, manage any resources available and work to sustain the program. Carson, Castelli, Beighle, and Erwin (2014) have highlighted that a quality leader is a necessity in order to influence school-based physical activity programming. More specifically, Beighle, Erwin, Castelli, and Ernst (2009) identified the physical education teacher as the person who should be this leader in schools. It is important that these leaders have organization and administration skills, public health knowledge, advocacy tools and physical activity backgrounds. Carson (2012) suggests that physical activity leaders need training and also highlights that this person should ideally be the physical education teacher. Heidorn and Centeio (2012) identify the role of the PAL to train school personnel to develop and integrate physical activity into academic curricula, provide encouragement, and create opportunities for school personnel to participate in activities themselves. Jones and colleagues (2014) found that classroom teachers and school staff in addition to the physical education teacher all provide leadership in multicomponent physical activity efforts suggesting that a group effort is needed to be successful. In addition, Goh, Hannon, Webster, and Brusseau (2019) found that the physical education teacher has limited time to provide the necessary leadership alone to successfully implement CSPAP. While little is known about the impact of the PAL on program effectiveness, Brusseau and Burns (2018) suggested that a stand-alone PAL might have the time and availability to help produce greater improvements in

Table 27.3 Multicomponent committee members and possible roles

Committee member	Role
School administrators	Gain teacher and staff support and commitment
	Allocate resources for program implementation, evaluation, and sustainability
	Serve as a model for school teachers and staff
School teachers and staff	Plan, teach, and infuse more physical activity in lessons and activities
	Promote the importance of physical activity throughout the school day
	Include more physical activity opportunities before, during, and after school
Students	Identify activities that are enjoyable
	Promote physical activity in school
Parents and parent organizations	Serve as a role model for their children and encourage them to be active
	Help to raise funds and find resources to help with implementation
	Encourage administrators and teachers to support and implement physical activity
	Volunteer time to assist with and promote physical activity
School health or wellness committee	Serve on committee
	Promote importance of physical activity to decision makers, leaders, and other members of school community
	Develop, implement, enforce school health and physical activity policy/programs

Adapted from CDC (2013).

physical activity by working directly with physical education teachers, recess supervisors, classroom teachers, and before- or after-school program leaders. They also noted, however, that there is an increased cost with a stand-alone position. When physical activity leaders set goals for students, research has shown greater increases in physical activity (Burns, Brusseau, & Fu, 2017). It has also been noted previously that teachers need on-going professional development and this has been linked to CSPAP effectiveness (Carson, Castelli, Pulling et al., 2014). It has also been highlighted that quality leadership and a point person are important for the success of multicomponent programming; however, there is limited research examining the role these leaders play in program effectiveness highlighting a potential future line of inquiry.

Training Quality

Maintaining a strong program training quality is an important, and often overlooked, aspect to successful program implementation. Teachers and physical activity leaders should be considered key facilitators in the implementation and sustainability of school-based programs such as CSPAP (Castelli, Carson, & Kulinna, 2017). In addition, strong leadership is needed to enforce systems change in the school setting (Chen & Gu, 2017). Training for most CSPAPs usually involves a physical education director or research investigator training graduate students, physical educators, and/or physical activity leaders on implementing student-centered and enjoyable programming. Quality instructional elements. including good task design, task presentation, class management, and adequate instructional response, are all contributors of children's physical activity levels (Chen & Gu, 2017) and thus should be of focus during training sessions. It is possible that many professionals in the field have familiarity with developing student-centered and enjoyable school programs. Regardless, these trainings should be held regularly to ensure the most up-to-date strategies are being implemented and to help maintain program fidelity. Trainings should also be held regularly to account for possible staff turnover that may occur over multi-year programs. Trainings should give teachers and physical activity leaders choice in the type of programming that could be implemented across a given time period. This will keep curricula flexible and allow a trial-and-error approach to be followed, given varying student likes and dislikes, weather, school scheduling, which may preclude less flexible physical activity curricula.

There is evidence that quality trained personnel may enhance physical activity opportunities throughout the day. Carson, Castelli, Beighle, et al. (2014). found that teachers who were trained on CSPAP provided more physical activity opportunities than non-intervention trained teachers. Teachers and physical activity leaders should work together to develop achievable action plans to provide expanded, extended, and/or enhanced physical activity opportunities (Beets et al., 2016; Carson et al., 2017). Specifically, CSPAP training should focus on providing additional, enhanced, or expanded physical activity across its five components: before and after school, during school, in the classroom, staff involvement, and family/community engagement (Centers for Disease Control and Prevention, 2013). It is helpful to provide these trainings on-site, within the same environment where teachers or physical activity leaders will implement across components. Information regarding program implementation should also be placed within an online format in the form of progressive modules for easy access. During physical education, training should align with goals for children to meet at least 50% of class time in moderate-to-vigorous physical activity (MVPA) (Brusseau, Hannon, & Burns, 2016). If training teachers, training should align with validated programs such as "TAKE 10!" or "Energizers" and should be implemented optimally at least two to three times per day (Goh, Hannon, Webster, Podlog, & Newton, 2016; Mahar et al., 2006). A significant portion of success of CSPAPs hinges on quality training of teachers and physical activity leaders. Therefore, planning comprehensive and quality training sessions should be of the highest priorities for researchers and practitioners wishing to implement school-based health programming.

Program Fidelity

Sustaining a high level of program fidelity is another aspect of school-based physical activity programming that contributes to successful physical activity programming implementation. Fidelity is a function of the interventionists and is the quality of the delivery of an intervention or the extent to which an intervention was implemented and in the manner to which it was intended (Linnan & Steckler, 2002). Evaluating program fidelity can be accomplished by collecting process information throughout the duration of a respective program. Other process information that may correlate with fidelity is program reach, or the proportion of intended participants that actually do participate, and dose, or what actually was delivered during an intervention and what actually was received during an intervention (Robbins, Pfeiffer, Wesolek, & Lo, 2014). Efficacy or effectiveness of school-based physical activity programs may correlate with maintained program fidelity; however this relationship is made unclear by the limited amount of process evaluation information reported in most research manuscripts (Moore et al., 2015). Unfortunately, many studies that evaluate the efficacy or effectiveness of school-based physical activity programs fail to collect and/or report process information, and if they do, the methodology is often considered weak (McGraw et al., 1996; Schaap, Bessems, Otten, Kremers, & van Nassau, 2018).

For programs like CSPAP, process evaluation data should be collected across all five components and use a variety of assessment methods. For example, fidelity can be assessed by randomly selecting days to which a process evaluator will record program delivery information using validated methodology (Robbins et al., 2014). Often times direct observational methods are used to assess delivery of the program during respective components of an intervention (e.g. physical education, classroom, recess). Because fidelity is a function of the interventionists, much of the information pertaining to program fidelity should align with teacher or PAL characteristics or behavior, although information collected on the student level or even on the level of the program director can be collected to support fidelity, which will enhance the quality of the assessment. Characteristics of the interventionists that maintain program fidelity may include appearing positive, enthusiastic, and well prepared for the delivered activity and/or lessons. Behaviors of the interventionists that may maintain program fidelity may include giving clear activity instructions, maintaining physical activity enjoyment throughout the duration of a lesson, providing activity modality choice, and emphasizing the health and wellness benefits of physical activity outside of school.

The number of fidelity components is numerous, as there are many ways to assess fidelity linking to varying frameworks within the field of health promotion, but often the components of dose, responsiveness, adherence, and quality of delivery are targeted (Schaap et al., 2018). Quality of fidelity assessment is determined by whether there was a model or framework used in the evaluation, whether or not the evaluation was conducted on multiple intervention levels (e.g. program director, teacher, and student), and the use of multiple validated instruments to collect fidelity information, among others (Schaap et al., 2018). That being said, the extent to which process evaluation is to be collected should correlate with the characteristics of each physical activity program; therefore inherently, there is no consensus on the proper methodology used to assess school-based physical activity interventions (Nilsen, 2015). Researchers and practitioners are advised to emphasize the importance of program fidelity through their respective programs and collect and report on process information when possible to determine the link with observed program efficacy or effectiveness.

Interest and Enjoyment

Psychosocial aspects of school-based physical activity programming may also play an important role in program efficacy or effectiveness. One construct that has been shown to mediate effects of school-based physical activity programs on specific behavioral and health outcomes is physical activity enjoyment (Dishman et al., 2005). Physical activity enjoyment is a motivational construct that has found to be a significant contributor to children's and adolescents' physical activity behaviors (Gao, Podlog, & Huang, 2013). Enjoyment is characterized by fun, liking, and pleasure and may be influenced by how a child or adolescent perceives success and failure in addition to the child or adolescent's emotional state prior to engaging in physical activity (Smith & St. Pierre, 2009; Wankel, 1993). Indeed, children and adolescents are more likely to participate in and have sustained physical activity if they find it to be enjoyable (Cairney et al, 2012; Prochaska, Sallis, Slyman, & McKenzie, 2003). For some school-based physical activity interventions, novelty of school-based programs may initially improve physical activity behaviors; however, physical activity behaviors may return to baseline levels due to decreases in enjoyment if program novelty is attenuated.

Some established school-based physical activity interventions have been shown to elicit improvements in physical activity enjoyment (Burns, Fu, & Podlog, 2017). Fairclough et al. (2016) examined the effect of a program called "Born to Move" in a sample of children. The "Born to Move" activities were designed to increase enjoyment and student inclusiveness, providing all students the opportunity to participate regardless of skill level. Classes also taught age-appropriate motor skills for the intent of increasing health and skill-related fitness. The study reported a relatively large increase in physical activity enjoyment over a 6-week period, which changed concurrently with increases in physical activity levels. Age-appropriateness of the employed physical activity and exercises in this program may have sustained higher levels of enjoyment during the intervention period. A study by Huberty, Dinkel, and Beets (2014) also displayed a relatively large increase in physical activity enjoyment using a program called "GoGirlGo!". This intervention focused on improving health in elementary school-aged girls. Half of the program focused on life skills and the other half focused on physical activity using cooperative games to increase enjoyment and inclusiveness. The authors reported significantly increased physical activity enjoyment over a 5-month period, which concurrently changed with a 3-minute increase in MVPA. The use of inclusiveness may have been a major contributor for this program's ability to increase physical activity enjoyment across the 5-month intervention period. Inclusiveness is a construct that may be especially effective for behavior change in girls and was inherently enhanced by the girls-only nature of the intervention via removal or lowering potential physical activity participation barriers such as body image concerns, lower levels of perceived competence and self-efficacy (when comparing ability to boys), and fears of bullying.

Programs often promote physical activity enjoyment using a student-centered and inclusive approach. However, other key factors may impact physical activity enjoyment. For instance, variables related to the nature of the physical activity itself (e.g. type of activity, the variety of physical activity forms), social support, or intra-individual factors (e.g. efficacy beliefs, attitudes toward physical activity) may all influence physical activity enjoyment levels (Dimmock, Jackson, Podlog, & Magaraggia, 2013). Motivational constructs such as self-efficacy, perceived competence, and enjoyment have complex but significant inter-relationships that may be affected by age-appropriate physical activity opportunities (Cairney et al., 2012). Perceptions of competence and perceived success have been shown to correlate with physical activity enjoyment in children (Cairney et al., 2012). Although developmentally appropriate activities are often incorporated into successful interventions, with longer multi-year interventions, developmentally appropriate is inherently variable at the student level and needs to be addressed via accounting for physical development and the development of gross motor skills in order to maintain enjoyment of physical activity.

Physical activity enjoyment is certainly an important consideration when attempting to maximize the efficacy or effectiveness of school-based physical activity programs. Fortunately, many programs have shown that there can be an increase in enjoyment after program implementation (Burns, Fu, & Podlog, 2017). Multicomponent CSPAPs have also been shown to increase levels of physical activity enjoyment (Fu, Burns, Brusseau, & Hannon, 2016). Increasing enjoyment seems to be a function of administering age-appropriate activities, providing a sense of inclusiveness, and maintaining program novelty. Building in mechanisms to sustain these constructs are recommended when trying to improve enjoyment and program efficacy or effectiveness.

Challenges and Barriers to Implementation

Cost

Physical inactivity directly contributes to 1.5–3.0% of global health care costs (Oldridge, 2008); however, cost is also an important consideration when implementing school-based physical activity interventions. This is especially important when programs target adolescents from disadvantaged backgrounds, where need for effective physical activity programming is high but dispensable resources (including income) are low. Barrett et al. (2015), using a simulated cohort of the US population, estimated that it would cost $70.1 million nationally in the first year to implement a nation-wide "active PE" policy for children to meet at least 50% of physical education time in MVPA, which would increase physical activity at a cost of $0.34 per MET-hour per person per day (e.g. 1 MET-hour = being physically active at an intensity of 4 METs for 15 minutes per day). However, these estimates are confounded by a number of factors at both the program and school level.

Unfortunately, it is unclear what the approximate costs of implementing a single intervention are, given the varying lengths of programs, the number of components involved in a respective program, the number of physical activity leaders used, and needed new equipment and personnel training, among others. In addition, a distinction has to be made regarding whether an intervention is a research-based program under highly controlled conditions (an efficacy intervention) or if an intervention is implemented and disseminated under a real-world setting (effectiveness interventions; Courneya, 2010). Therefore, cost of intervention implementation can vary widely. For example, it was found that the total cost for schools implementing classroom break physical activity intervention was only approximated at $180 per school for implementation materials (Erwin, Beighle, Morgan, & Noland, 2011). Conversely, a larger multi-year comprehensive school-based intervention was found to be implemented at a cost of $394 per student (Sutherland, Reeves et al., 2016). Cost-effectiveness across the 2-year program was found to be at approximately $56 per additional minute of MVPA per person per day (Sutherland et al., 2016). These estimates are certainly cost-effective; however, for some lower-income schools, implementing large multicomponent school interventions in order to elicit meaningful increases in health behaviors and health outcomes may be prohibitive. This could be circumvented by tailoring interventions to be time-efficient, training staff and personnel who are already employed at a respective school to implement programming, efficient use of equipment and play space, and overall time organization. Nevertheless, maximizing intervention cost-effectiveness is an ongoing area of research given that many of the schools that could benefit greatly from physical activity programming are low-income, and thus, this is an important consideration when designing school-based health programs.

Time Restrictions

Time is an important commodity for teachers, intervention personnel, and students during the school day (National Center for Education Statistics, 2009). Many schools have strict time schedules that adhere to academic classes and other required programs (Wilkins et al., 2003). Schools also may have bell schedules in flux due to assemblies, special programs, testing days. Therefore, an important consideration when designing school-based physical activity programs is the use of time. Just like program cost, time use across school-based physical activity interventions is highly variable. Single component interventions may not have as significant time constraints as multicomponent programs. Many classroom-based interventions only require 10–20 minutes of the school day (Goh et al., 2016; Mahar et al., 2006). Likewise, if an intervention is solely focused during physical education, time has already been allocated for physical activity; therefore there are no additional time use issues in regard to scheduling or rescheduling. Indeed, many efficient programs make use of already allotted time for physical activity and improve physical activity behaviors by forgoing expanding time duration or lesson frequency, and focusing on merely enhancing the quality of the programming via novel and validated pedagogical strategies (Institute of Medicine, 2013).

Unlike single component physical activity interventions, time may be a liability when attempting to implement multicomponent interventions (Greaney et al., 2014). Multicomponent interventions need various designated time slots throughout the school day to implement programming to increase physical activity behaviors, which may be restricted because of school scheduling. Therefore, with multicomponent programs, intervention personnel must remain flexible. Successful implementation of interventions requires team work between school staff and intervention staff, and successful programs foster empowerment of members of the school community (Murillo Pardo et al., 2013). A "give-and-take" approach may be a successful strategy when attempting to reach objectives from both the school academic perspective and the intervention program perspective. That being said, from commencement of school-based physical activity program everyone involved in the program must be on board with implementation scheduling: from the school principal, physical activity director, physical education teachers, physical activity leaders, and other personnel involved in a respective program (Murillo Pardo et al., 2013). Careful planning must take place months before commencement of a program. Ideally, intervention personnel should arrange group and individual meetings with school staff to plan use of time throughout an entire academic year, making provisional plans if unexpected school schedule changes arise. This will attenuate and/or circumvent any issues that arise over school-day time use and make the overall physical activity intervention more efficient and effective.

Program Burden on Teachers

In conjunction with time use, program burden on teachers plays a significant role in developing and implementing school-based physical activity programs (van Sluijs & Kriemler, 2016). Teachers, along with the physical activity leaders, are agents of change within school-based physical activity programs. However, if time use is not effectively organized, there is a possibility that physical activity programming, especially in the academic classroom, will place a significant burden on academic teachers. This may especially be the case during classroom-based physical activity interventions. Programs may not align with school professionals' needs and feasibility of implementation may be initially questionable from the perspective of teachers (Christian et al., 2015). Despite the fact these programs aim to ease burden on teachers by improving classroom behavior and academic achievement through health-enhancing physical activity, the stress of implementing something new in the form of classroom activity breaks may not be well received (van den Berg et al., 2017). Indeed, prior beliefs on child health and the role of school staff in the responsibility of improving health behaviors play an important role on the perceptions of implementing school-based programming (Todd et al. 2015).

Fortunately, however, research has shown that on average this is not the case during school-based physical activity programming, as most programs are well received by both teachers and administrators, especially if the programs are easy to manage, academically orientated, and enjoyable (Goh et al., 2016; McMullen, Kulinna, & Cothran, 2014). As long as there is collaborative support for teachers among physical education teachers, physical activity leaders, or other intervention staff, and time use has been well planned before commencement of programming, the risk of significant burden placed on the classroom teachers should be attenuated (Dinkel, Schaffer, Snyder, & Lee, 2017; Webster, Russ, Vazou, Goh, & Erwin, 2015). Providing teachers flexibility to implement classroom activity breaks is necessary if schedule changes do arise. Regular meetings with teachers during programs will facilitate and attenuate potential for future logistical issues. Intervention staff should also help the classroom teachers when possible as a "payback" for helping implement physical activity program and improve social relations. Aiding teachers in organizing lessons, transporting students around school, or helping teachers deal with off-task students all ease burden on the teachers during their academic pursuits and also provide a sense of team work. Acknowledging is burden potential, realizing the importance of teachers as agents of change within school-based health programming, and treating the intervention staff-teachers social relation with care and respect will improve collaborative social relations and increase program efficiency and quality.

Gaps, Emerging Issues, and Future Directions

Program Length

Intervention length plays a role on program design, cost, and feasibility; unfortunately, there is no consensus regarding the optimal program length to elicit health behavior and/or health outcome benefits. Most research-based school physical activity interventions range in duration from 6 weeks to 2 years (Minatto, Barbosa Filho, Berria, & Petroski, 2016; van Sluijs, McMinn, & Griffin, 2008). In research, programs usually focus on implementing an efficacy intervention rather than effectiveness intervention. Efficacy interventions aim to explore whether a program produces the intended effect within ideal circumstances while effectiveness interventions explore whether a program yields significant effects under "real world" conditions (Cochrane, 1972; Courneya, 2010). That being said, interventions can incorporate both aspects of efficacy and effectiveness methodology, to varying degrees, that may influence intervention length. Because of limited resources, highly controlled and manipulated programs that use efficacy methodology tend to be of short duration. Conversely, interventions that use effectiveness methodology in natural settings tend to be longer and reflect a sustained "real world" program. Program length may affect novelty over time and affect a child's interest and enjoyment in the program if mechanisms are not built in to maintain these psychosocial constructs (Burns, Fu, & Podlog, 2017). A decrease in interest and enjoyment in participating in physical activity programming may decrease physical activity behavior and ultimately targeted health outcomes. Because of its potential mediating effect on health behavior, physical activity enjoyment should be of importance in the research design stage to promote sustained physical activity adherence, especially within longer, effectiveness school-based interventions (Coulter & Woods, 2011).

There have been a few published systematic reviews that have specifically looked at the effect of intervention length on targeted health outcomes during school-based physical activity interventions. In a systematic review with meta-analysis conducted by Minatto et al. (2016), examining the effect of school-based interventions on cardiorespiratory endurance in older adolescents, it was found that interventions ranging from 13 to 24 weeks in duration yielded greater improvements in cardiorespiratory endurance compared to interventions of shorter and longer durations. There could be an optimal intervention length to elicit improvements in health outcomes. The findings from Minatto et al. (2016) support this possibility; however the mechanisms for variation in effect due to length are unknown. In another review with meta-regression, Burns, Brusseau, and Fu (2018) found no relationship between intervention length and cardiorespiratory endurance in a younger pooled sample of primary school-aged children. As stated previously, longer interventions may attenuate novelty and interest in younger children, which may affect motivational constructs such as physical activity enjoyment (Burns, Fu, & Podlog, 2017). Because habitual physical activity is needed to improve health outcomes such as cardiorespiratory endurance, decreases in the latter construct may be found with longer interventions. Conversely, very short duration interventions may not be long enough to elicit the physiological responses needed to improve health outcomes in children or adolescents. Despite these theoretical mechanisms, current literature suggests that intervention length may not relate to specific observed health outcomes in younger children. Therefore, other intervention characteristics may play a role in eliciting favorable health outcomes. Besides intervention length, other moderators that may influence outcomes are physical activity intensity and the duration of specific physical activity bouts within each respective school-based intervention. Interestingly, in adolescents, Minatto et al. (2016) did observe trends among the intensity of physical activity, weekly frequency of physical activity sessions, and the observed standardized effects on cardiorespiratory endurance; however these moderators were not tested statistically and there are many studies that do not report these specific characteristics when communicating the intervention; therefore, it is difficult to conclude whether these variables would play a significant role in eliciting favorable outcomes.

These inconclusive findings regarding appropriate intervention length are important for both researchers and practitioners who are planning and implementing physical activity programming in schools. With the limited physical activity opportunities in schools and the challenge and cost of long duration interventions, even short single component interventions may have positive benefits if structured appropriately. Specifically, the enhancement of physical education or the expansion of classroom-based physical activity may have the ability to positively impact health outcomes in primary school-aged children. There may be positive changes in a short period of time (e.g. 6 weeks), thus making programming appear more feasible for teachers and/or school staff. If physical education teachers know that they can make meaningful change over the course of a unit, instead of an entire year, they may be more likely to implement programming and there may be less of a burden placed on them as well. Similarly, if research paraprofessionals or a classroom teacher realizes that a shorter intervention can have a meaningful impact, they may be more likely to try something new and once they try it, have success, perhaps they are more likely to continue with the program for the long term. Indeed, tailoring of interventions to elicit the most favorable outcomes is inherently complex and identifying appropriate program lengths and other moderators that may optimize effects should be a consideration for future research and practice.

Number of Implemented Components

School-based physical activity interventions focus on providing extended, enhanced, or expanded physical activity opportunities during specific school components such as during physical education or by incorporating activity breaks within the academic classroom (Beets et al., 2016; Mears & Jago, 2016; Watson, Timperio, Brown, Best, & Hesketh, 2017). Increasingly, interventions have been incorporating a multicomponent approach, such as CSPAP, which uses all available resources throughout the school day to improve physical activity behaviors and decrease sedentary times in children and adolescents (Carson, Castelli, Beighle et al., 2014). Both single and multicomponent interventions have been shown to be successful in being implemented within schools. These implemented interventions most often align with various established theoretical frameworks such as the social cognitive theory, self-determination theory, or ecological models (Brusseau et al., 2016; Mahar et al., 2006; Vander Ploeg, McGavock, Maximova, & Veugelers, 2014). However, it is unclear if multicomponent intervention approaches significantly yield greater efficacy or effectiveness compared to single component intervention approaches and if other characteristics of said interventions modify program efficacy. Therefore, given the relatively large pool of published work in this area, much can be learned by further testing these physical activity intervention characteristics as potential moderators. Within the current literature, there have been a few studies examining effects of and differences in outcomes between single and multicomponent programs. Russ et al. (2015) found overall small pooled effects of multicomponent interventions and Burns et al. (2018) found no impact on component number (single versus multicomponent) on cardiorespiratory endurance in children. However, systematic reviews and meta-analysis support the multicomponent recommendation in older adolescents, as interventions using the multicomponent paradigm have yielded greater effects compared to single components programs for increasing physical activity levels (van Sluijs et al., 2008). Specific components of programs such as CSPAP include promotion of physical activity during school, before and after school, staff wellness, and family and community engagement (Centers for Disease Control and Prevention, 2013). Multicomponent programs have also been recommended across the globe in countries such as Ireland, Finland, France, Germany, the United States, and Switzerland (Tannehill, Van der Mars, & McPhail, 2014). Although these types of physical activity programs have been recommended, adoption and evaluation have been sparse because of limited resources including cost, time, and availability of quality trained staff to implement the programming (Russ et al., 2015).

Despite recommendations and evidence supporting multicomponent versus single component interventions, there is also evidence that both types of physical activity programming can be effective. For example, Reed et al. (2008) implemented a multicomponent intervention called "Action Schools! BC" where six "Action Zones" were targeted across a 1-year intervention. These "Action Zones" are similar to those incorporated into CSPAP but also include novel components such as "School Spirit" (i.e. school challenges). Cardiorespiratory endurance was the outcome with the greatest change at the end of the intervention, with the authors reporting 20.4% unadjusted difference (increase) in change in shuttle run laps. Conversely, Sollerhed and Ejlertsson (2008) reported similar strong effects on cardiorespiratory endurance; however this particular program employed a single component approach by merely expanding the frequency of physical education lessons from two to four lessons per week across a 3-year intervention. Given the drastically different methodological paradigms from the two aforementioned interventions, it can be suggested that single component interventions, such as merely increasing the time or frequency of physical education, can be just as effective as implementing large-scale multicomponent programs. What may be of greater influence is the quality of the staff training and the degree of intervention program fidelity (Carson et al., 2014). In addition, specific programming characteristics such as the specific intensity of physical activity and frequency may also be potential moderators, as examined in Minatto et al. (2016). These potential effects should be explored with additional research.

Inclusion of Resistance Training

Most school-based physical activity programs usually focus on increasing ambulatory MVPA. However, an exercise modality that may also have an impact on health in youth and can be implemented within school-based physical activity programs is resistance training (Faigenbaum, 2017; Sigal et al., 2014). Resistance training is any exercise that causes the muscles to contract against an external resistance with the expectation of increases in strength, tone, mass, and/or endurance. The history of resistance training guidelines and the benefits in its application across all areas of health and performance have been well described (Kraemer et al., 2017). The health-related fitness domains of muscular strength and endurance, which are directly impacted by resistance training, have been independently associated with cardio-metabolic health profiles in the pediatric population (Peterson, Saltarelli, Visich, & Gordon, 2014). Resistance training may also be an enjoyable modality for children and adolescents with overweight or obesity, because the modality does not require musculoskeletal support to move bodyweight during long and sustained bouts of repetitive ambulatory movement (Van Der Heijden et al., 2010).

Despite observational studies correlating muscular strength and endurance levels to specific health markers in youth, what is unknown is whether resistance-training interventions can be effective in improving health behaviors and health outcomes within the context of school-based physical activity interventions. The feasibility of incorporating resistance-training programs within school settings and how well received these types of programs will be in both children and adolescents are also unknown. If resistance-training programs can be shown to be effective in improving markers of health, and they can be implemented with strong fidelity, then this would provide support that this exercise modality as a viable complement to aerobic exercise within school-based interventions to objectively improve health behaviors, health outcomes, and improve disease risk in the pediatric population.

There have been a few randomized controlled trials that have shown the benefits of resistance training in the pediatric population. At the end of the employed periodized program, Shaibi et al. (2006) reported significant improvements in fasting insulin and insulin sensitivity in a sample of overweight Latino adolescent males. Interestingly, Shaibi et al. (2006) reported administering a high resistance training intensity between 92% and 97% 1-repetition maximum (RM). Many other studies showing lack of effects on metabolic health implement programs characterized by much lower resistance intensity (60%–70% 1-RM; Fedewa, Gist, Evans, & Dishman, 2014). Another study conducted by Hansen, Landstad, Gundersen, Torjesen, and Svebak (2012) compared a maximal resistance-training program (five sets, 3–4 repetitions at 60%–85% of 1-RM) to that of an endurance resistance-training program (three sets, 12–15 repetitions, at 45%–65% of 1-RM) and found that both programs improved insulin resistance, albeit from different mechanisms. The maximal resistance-training program increased muscular glucose uptake capacity while the endurance resistance-training program increased the insulin sensitivity of the muscles. Most other successful programs use resistance training in conjunction with aerobic training or with a complementary nutrition education program (Fedewa et al., 2014). Examination of resistance-training programs within the context of school-based physical activity programs has not been extensively examined and remains a priority for future research. It is also unknown whether these programs can significant increase MVPA and its psychosocial mediators (e.g. enjoyment) within the context of school-based interventions (Cox, Fairclough, Kosteli, & Noonan, 2019).

Because of the small number of quality studies examining the impact of resistance training on health outcomes in youth, much more research needs to be conducted using resistance training as a primary or complementary exercise modality and to explore how this exercise modality can be better tailored to the pediatric population to elicit favorable health improvements. Resistance training is a complement to aerobic exercise; however evidence is sparse showing how this exercise modality can be effectively implemented in school-based settings.

In conclusion, multicomponent interventions have shown some effectiveness for improving health behaviors such as physical activity and health outcomes such as health-related fitness. However, their sustainability over time is questionable. Implementation of these programs can be cost-effective; however great care must be made in the proper training of personnel and efficient use of equipment and space. Numerous areas of research regarding multicomponent school-based programming need to be undertaken to advance the field and to discover novel and effective methods to improve physical activity and health in children and adolescents.

References

Barrett, J. L., Gortmaker, S. L., Long, M. W., Ward, Z. J., Resch, S. C., Moodie, M. L., . . . Cradock, A. L. (2015). Cost effectiveness of an elementary school activity physical education policy. *American Journal of Preventive Medicine, 49*, 148–159.

Beets, M. W., Okely, A., Weaver, R. G., Webster, C., Lubans, D., Brusseau, T. A., . . . Cliff, D. P. (2016). The theory of expanded, extended, and enhanced opportunities for youth physical activity promotion. *International Journal of Behavioral Nutrition and Physical Activity, 16*, 120.

Beighle, A., Erwin, H., Castelli, D., & Ernst, M. (2009). Preparing physical educators for the role of physical activity director. *Journal of Physical Education, Recreation & Dance, 80*, 24–29.

Belton, S., O'Brien, W., McGann, J., & Issartel, J. (2018). Bright spots physical activity investments that work: Youth-physical activity towards health (Y-PATH). *British Journal of Sports Medicine.* doi:10.1136/bjsports-2018-099745

Braun, H. A., Kay, C. M., Cheung, P., Weiss, P. S., & Gazmararian, J. A. (2017). Impact of an elementary school-based intervention on physical activity time and aerobic capacity, Georgia, 2013–2014. *Public Health Reports, 132*(2 Suppl), 24S–32S.

Brusseau, T. A., & Burns, R. D. (2018). The physical activity leader and comprehensive school physical activity program effectiveness. *Biomedical Human Kinetics, 10*(1), 127–133. doi:10.1515/bhk-2018-0019

Brusseau, T. A., Hannon, J. C., & Burns, R. D. (2016). Effect of a comprehensive school physical activity program on physical activity and health-related fitness in children from low-income families. *Journal of Physical Activity and Health, 13*, 888–894.

Brusseau, T. A., Hannon, J. C., Fu, Y., Fang, Y., Nam, K., Goodrum, S., & Burns, R. D. (2018). Trends in physical activity, health-related fitness, and gross motor skills in children during a two-year comprehensive school physical activity program. *Journal of Science and Medicine in Sport, 21*, 828–832.

Burns, R. D., & Brusseau, T. A., & Fu Y. (2017). Influence of goal setting on physical activity and cardiorespiratory endurance in low-income children enrolled in CSPAP schools. *American Journal Health Education, 48*, 32–40.

Burns, R. D., Brusseau, T. A., & Fu, Y. (2018). Moderators of school-based physical activity interventions on cardiorespiratory endurance in primary school-aged children: A meta-regression. *International Journal of Environmental Research and Public Health, 15*, 1764. doi:10.3390/ijerph15081764

Burns, R. D., Brusseau, T. A., Fu, Y., Myrer, R. S., & Hannon, J. C. (2016). Comprehensive school physical activity programming and classroom behavior. *American Journal of Health Behavior, 40*(1), 100–107.

Burns, R. D., Brusseau, T. A., & Hannon, J. C. (2015). Effect of a comprehensive school physical activity program on school day step counts in children. *Journal of Physical Activity and Health, 12*(12), 1536–1542.

Burns, R. D., Brusseau, T. A., & Hannon, J. C. (2017). Effect of comprehensive school physical activity programming on cardiometabolic health markers in children from low-income schools. *Journal of Physical Activity and Health, 14*(9), 671–676.

Burns, R. D., Fu, Y., Hannon, J. C., & Brusseau, T. A. (2017). School physical activity programming and gross motor skills in children. *American Journal of Health Behavior, 41*(5), 591–598.

Burns, R. D., Fu, Y., & Podlog, L. W. (2017). School-based physical activity interventions and physical activity enjoyment: A meta-analysis. *Preventive Medicine, 103*, 84–90.

Cairney, J., Kwan, M. Y. W., Velduizen, S., Hay, J., Bray, S. R., & Faught, B. E. (2012). Gender, perceived competence and the enjoyment of physical education in children: A longitudinal examination. *International Journal of Behavioral Nutrition and Physical Activity, 9*, 26.

Carson, R. L. (2012). Certification and duties of a director of physical activity. *Journal of Physical Education, Recreation & Dance, 83*, 16–29.

Carson, R. L., Castelli, D. M., Beighle, A., & Erwin, H. (2014). School-based physical activity promotion: A conceptual framework for research and practice. *Childhood Obesity, 10*, 100–116.

Carson, R. L., Castelli, D. M., Pulling Kuhn, A. C, Moore, J. B., Beets, M. W., Beighle, A., . . . Glowacki, E. M. (2014). Impact of trained champions of comprehensive school and sedentary behaviors. *Preventive Medicine, 69*, S12–S19.

Castelli, D. M., Carson, R. L., & Kulinna, P. H. (2017). PETE programs creating teacher leaders to integrate comprehensive school physical activity programs. *Journal of Physical Education, Recreation, and Dance, 88*, 8–10.

Centeio, E. E., McCaughtry, N., Gutuskey, L., Garn, A. C., Somers, C., Shen, B., . . . Kulik, N. L. (2014). Chapter 8: Physical activity change through comprehensive school physical activity programs in urban elementary schools. *Journal of Teaching in Physical Education, 33*(4), 573–591.

Centers for Disease Control and Prevention. (2013). *Comprehensive school physical activity programs: A guide for schools.* Atlanta, GA: U.S. Department of Health and Human Services.

Chen, S., & Gu, X. (2017). Toward active living: Comprehensive school physical activity program research and implications. *Quest, 70,* 191–212.

Christian, D., Todd, C., Davies, H., Rance, J., Stratton, G., Rapport, F., & Brophy S. (2015). Community led active schools programme (CLASP) exploring the implementation of health interventions in primary schools: Headteachers' perspectives. *BMC Public Health, 15,* 238.

Christiansen, L. B., Lund-Cramer, P., Brondeel, R., Smedegaard, S., Holt, A. D., & Skovgaard, T. (2018). Improving children's physical self-perception through a school-based physical activity intervention: The move for well-being in school study. *Mental Health and Physical Activity, 14,* 31–38.

Cochrane, A. L. (1972). *Effectiveness and efficiency: Random reflection on health services.* London, UK: Nuffield Provincial Hospitals Trust.

Cohen, K. E., Morgan, P. J., Plotnikoff, R. C., Callister, R., & Lubans, D. R. (2015). Physical activity and skills intervention: SCORES cluster randomized controlled trial. *Medicine and Science in Sports and Exercise, 47*(4), 765–774.

Coulter, M., & Woods, C. B. (2011). An exploration of children's perceptions and enjoyment of school-based physical activity and physical education. *Journal of Physical Activity and Health, 8,* 645–654.

Courneya, K. S. (2010). Efficacy, effectiveness, and behavior change trials in exercise research. *International Journal of Behavioral Nutrition and Physical Activity, 7,* 81.

Cox, A., Fairclough, S. J., Kosteli, M., & Noonan, R. J. (2019). The efficacy of school-based interventions to increase MVPA and MBSE outcomes in adolescent males. A systematic review and meta-analysis. doi:10.31236/osf.io/95snr

De Meester, F., van Lenthe, F. J., Spittaels, H., Lien, N., & De Bourdeaudhuij, I. (2009). Interventions for promoting physical activity among European teenagers: A systematic review. *International Journal of Behavioral Nutrition and Physical Activity, 6*(1), 82.

Dimmock, J., Jackson, B., Podlog, L., & Magaraggia, C. (2013). The effect of variety expectations on interest, enjoyment, and locus of causality in exercise. *Motivation and Emotion, 37,* 146–153.

Dinkel, S., Schaffer, C., Snyder, K., & Lee, J. M. (2017). They just need to move: Teacher's perception of classroom physical activity breaks. *Teaching and Teacher Education, 63,* 186–195.

Dishman, R. K., Motl, R. W., Saunders, R., Felton, G., Ward, D. S., Dowda, M., & Pate, R. R. (2005). Enjoyment mediates effects of a school-based physical activity intervention. *Medicine and Science in Sports and Exercise, 37,* 478–487.

Erwin, H., Beighle, A., Carson, R. L., & Castelli, D. M. (2013). Comprehensive school-based physical activity promotion: A review. *Quest, 65*(4), 412–428.

Erwin, H. E., Beighle, A., Morgan, C. F., & Noland, M. (2011). Effect of a low-cost, teacher-directed classroom intervention on elementary students' physical activity. *Journal of School Health, 81,* 455–461.

Faigenbaum, A. (2017). Resistance exercise and youth: Survival of the strongest. *Pediatric Exercise Science, 29,* 14–18.

Fairclough, S. J., McGrane, B., Sanders, G., Taylor, S., Owen, M., & Curry, W. (2016). A non-equivalent group pilot trial of a school-based physical activity and fitness intervention for 10–11-year-old English children: Born to move. *BMC Public Health, 16,* 861.

Fedewa, M. V., Gist, N. H., Evans, E. M., & Dishman, R. K. (2014). Exercise and insulin resistance in youth: A meta-analysis. *Pediatrics, 133,* 3163–3174.

Fu, Y., Burns, R. D., Brusseau, T. A., & Hannon, J. C. (2016). Comprehensive school physical activity programming and activity enjoyment. *American Journal of Health Behavior, 40,* 496–502.

Gao, Z., Podlog, L., & Huang, C. (2013). Associations among children's situational motivation, physical activity participation, and enjoyment in an active dance video game. *Journal of Sport and Health Science, 2*(2), 122–128.

Goh, T. L., Webster, C., Brusseau, T, & Hannon, J. (2019). Infusing physical activity leadership training in PETE programs through university-school partnership: Principals' and graduate students' experiences. *Physical Educator, 76*(1), 238–257.

Goh, T. L., Hannon, J. C., Webster, C., Podlog, L., & Newton, M. (2016). Effects of a TAKE10! Classroom-based physical activity intervention on third- to fifth-grade children's on-task behavior. *Journal of Physical Activity and Health, 13,* 712–718.

Gortmaker, S. L., Cheung, L. W., Peterson, K. E., Chomitz, G., Cradle, J. H., Dart, H., . . . Field, A. E. (1999). Impact of a school-based interdisciplinary intervention on diet and physical activity among urban primary school children: Eat well and keep moving. *Archives of Pediatrics & Adolescent Medicine, 153*(9), 975–983.

Greaney, M. L., Hardwick, C. K., Spadano-Gasbarro, J. L., Mezgebu, S., Horan, C. M., Schlotterbeck, S., . . . Peterson, K. E. (2014). Implementing a multicomponent school-based obesity prevention intervention: A qualitative study. *Journal of Nutrition Education and Behavior, 46,* 576–582.

Haapala, H. L., Hirvensalo, M. H., Kulmala, J., Hakonen, H., Kankaanpää, A., Laine, K., . . . Tammelin, T. H. (2017). Changes in physical activity and sedentary time in the Finnish schools on the move program: A quasi-experimental study. *Scandinavian Journal of Medicine & Science in Sports, 27*(11), 1442–1453.

Hansen, E., Landstad, B. J., Gundersen, K. T., Torjesen, P. A., & Svebak, S. (2012). Insulin sensitivity after maximal and endurance resistance training. *Journal of Strength and Conditioning Research, 26*, 327–334.

Heidorn, B., & Centeio, E. (2012). The director of physical activity and staff involvement. *Journal of Physical Education, Recreation & Dance, 83*, 13–26.

Hills, A. P., Dengel, D. R., & Lubans, D. R. (2015). Supporting public health priorities: Recommendations for physical education and physical activity promotion in schools. *Progress in Cardiovascular Diseases, 57*(4), 368–374.

Huberty, J. L., Dinkel, D. M., & Beets, M. W. (2014). Evaluation of GoGirlGo!; A practitioner based program to improve physical activity. *BMC Public Health, 14*, 118.

Institute of Medicine. (2013). *Educating the student body: Taking physical activity and physical education to school.* Washington, DC: The National Academies Press.

Jones, E. M., Taliaferro, A. R., Elliott, E. M., Bulger, S. M., Kristjansson, A. L., Neal, W., & Allar, I. (2014). Chapter 3: Feasibility study of comprehensive school physical activity programs in Appalachian communities: The McDowell CHOICES project. *Journal of Teaching in Physical Education, 33*, 467–491.

Kraemer, W. J., Ratamess, N. A., Flanagan, S. D, Shurley, J. P., Todd, J. S., & Todd, T. C. (2017). Understanding the science of resistance training: An evolutionary perspective. *Sports Medicine, 47*, 2415–2435.

Kriemler, S., Meyer, U., Martin, E., van Sluijs, E. M., Andersen, L. B., & Martin, B. W. (2011). Effect of school-based interventions on physical activity and fitness in children and adolescents: A review of reviews and systematic update. *British Journal of Sports Medicine, 45*(11), 923–930.

Leme, A. C. B., Lubans, D. R., Guerra, P. H., Dewar, D., Toassa, E. C., & Philippi, S. T. (2016). Preventing obesity among Brazilian adolescent girls: Six-month outcomes of the healthy habits, healthy girls–Brazil school-based randomized controlled trial. *Preventive Medicine, 86*, 77–83.

Lewallen, T. C., Hunt, H., Potts-Datema, W., Zaza, S., & Giles, W. (2015). The whole school, whole community, whole child model: A new approach for improving educational attainment and healthy development for students. *Journal of School Health, 85*(11), 729–739.

Linnan, L., & Steckler, A. (2002). Process evaluation for public health interventions and research. In A. Steckler & L. Linnan (Eds.), *Process evaluation for public health interventions and research* (1st ed., pp. 1–23). San Francisco, CA: Jossey-Bass.

Love, R., Adams, J., & van Sluijs, E. M. (2019). Are school-based physical activity interventions effective and equitable? A meta-analysis of cluster randomized controlled trials with accelerometer-assessed activity. *Obesity Reviews, 20*, 859–870.

Luepker, R. V., Perry, C. L., McKinlay, S. M., Nader, P. R., Parcel, G. S., Stone, E. J., . . . Kelder, S. H. (1996). Outcomes of a field trial to improve children's dietary patterns and physical activity: The child and adolescent trial for cardiovascular health (CATCH). *JAMA, 275*(10), 768–776.

Mahar, M. T., Murphy, S. K., Rowe, D. A., Golden, J., Shileds, A. T., & Taedeke, T. D. (2006). Effects of a classroom-based program on physical activity and on-task behavior. *Medicine and Science in Sports and Exercise, 38*, 2086–2094.

McGrane, B., Belton, S., Fairclough, S. J., Powell, D., & Issartel, J. (2018). Outcomes of the Y-PATH randomized controlled trial: Can a school-based intervention improve fundamental movement skill proficiency in adolescent youth? *Journal of Physical Activity and Health, 15*(2), 89–98.

McGraw, S. A., Sellers, D. E., Stone, E. J., Bebchuck, J., Edmundson, E. W., Johnson, C. C., . . . Luepker, R. V. (1996). Using process data to explain outcomes: An illustration from the child and adolescent trial for cardiovascular health (CATCH). *Evaluation Review, 20*, 291–312.

McKenzie, T. L., Nader, P. R., Strikmiller, P. K., Yang, M., Stone, E. J., Perry, C. L., . . . Kelder, S. H. (1996). School physical education: Effect of the child and adolescent trial for cardiovascular health. *Preventive Medicine, 25*(4), 423–431.

McMullen, J., Kulinna, P., & Cothran, D. (2014). Physical activity opportunities during the school day: Classroom teachers' perceptions of using activity breaks in the classroom. *Journal of Teaching Physical Education, 33*, 51–527.

McMullen, J., Ní Chróinín, D., Tammelin, T., Pogorzelska, M., & van der Mars, H. (2015). International approaches to whole-of-school physical activity promotion. *Quest, 67*(4), 384–399.

Mears, R., & Jago, R. (2016). Effectiveness of after-school interventions at increasing moderate-to-vigorous physical activity levels in 5- to 18-year olds: A systematic review and meta-analysis. *British Journal of Sports Medicine.* doi:10.1136/bjsports-2015-094976

Metzler, M., Barrett-Williams, S., Hunt, K., Marquis, J., & Trent, M. (2015). *Final report: Establishing a comprehensive school physical activity program*. Atlanta, GA: Centers for Disease Control and Prevention & Georgia State University Seed Award Program for Social and Behavioral Science Research.

Minatto, G., Barbosa Filho, V. C., Berria, J., & Petroski, E. L. (2016). School-based interventions to improve cardiorespiratory fitness in adolescents: Systematic review with meta-analysis. *Sports Medicine, 46,* 1273–1292.

Moore, G. F., Audrey, S., Barker, M., Bond, L., Bonell, C., Hardeman, W., . . . Baird, J. (2015). Process information of complex interventions: Medical research council guidance. *British Medical Journal, 35,* h1258.

Murillo Pardo, B., Garcia Bengoechea, E., Generelo Lanaspa, E., Bush, P. L., Zaragoza Casterad, J., Julian Clemente, J. A., . . . Garcia Gonzalez, L. (2013). Promising school-based strategies and intervention guidelines to increase physical activity of adolescents. *Health Education Research, 28,* 523–538.

National Center for Education Statistics. (2009). *Digest of education statistics: 2008*. Washington, DC: National Center for Education Statistics.

Nilsen, P. (2015). Making sense of implementation theories, models, and frameworks. *Implementation Science, 10,* 53.

Oldridge, N. B. (2008). Economic burden of physical inactivity: Healthcare costs associated with cardiovascular disease. *European Journal of Cardiovascular Prevention and Rehabilitation, 15,* 130–139.

Pate, R. R., Ward, D. S., Saunders, R. P., Felton, G., Dishman, R. K., & Dowda, M. (2005). Promotion of physical activity among high-school girls: A randomized controlled trial. *American Journal of Public Health, 95*(9), 1582–1587.

Peterson, M. D., Saltarelli, W. A., Visich, P. S., & Gordon P. M. (2014). Strength capacity and cardiometabolic risk clustering in adolescents. *Pediatrics, 133,* e896–e903.

Prochaska, J. J., Sallis, J. F., Slymen, D. J., & McKenzie, T. L. (2003). A longitudinal study of children's enjoyment of physical education. *Pediatric Exercise Science, 15,* 170–178.

Reilly, J. J., Kelly, L., Montgomery, C., Williamson, A., Fisher, A., McColl, J. H., . . . Grant, S. (2006). Physical activity to prevent obesity in young children: Cluster randomised controlled trial. *British Medical Journal, 333*(7577), 1041.

Robbins, L. B., Pfeiffer, K. A., Wesolek, S. M., & Lo, Y. J. (2014). Process evaluation for a school-based physical activity intervention for 6th and 7th grade boys: Reach, dose, and fidelity. *Evaluation and Program Planning, 42,* 21–31.

Russ, L. B., Webster, C. A., Beets, M. W., & Phillips, D. S. (2015). Systematic review and meta-analysis of multi-component interventions through schools to increase physical activity. *Journal of Physical Activity and Health, 12*(10), 1436–1446.

Sahota, P., Rudolf, M. C., Dixey, R., Hill, A. J., Barth, J. H., & Cade, J. (2001). Randomised controlled trial of primary school based intervention to reduce risk factors for obesity. *British Medical Journal, 323*(7320), 1029.

Salmon, J., Booth, M. L., Phongsavan, P., Murphy, N., & Timperio, A. (2007). Promoting physical activity participation among children and adolescents. *Epidemiologic Reviews, 29*(1), 144–159.

Schaap, R., Bessems, K., Otten, R., Kremers, S., & van Nassau, F. (2018). Measuring implementation fidelity of school-based obesity prevention programmes: A systematic review. *International Journal of Behavioral Nutrition and Physical Activity, 15,* 75.

Seo, D. C., King, M. H., Kim, N., Sovinski, D., Meade, R., & Lederer, A. M. (2013). Predictors for moderate-and vigorous-intensity physical activity during an 18-month coordinated school health intervention. *Preventive Medicine, 57*(5), 466–470.

Shaibi, G. Q., Ball, G. D. C., Cruz, M. L., Weigensberg, M. J., Salem, G. J., & Goran, M. I. (2006). Cardiovascular fitness and physical activity in children with and without impaired glucose tolerance. *International Journal of Obesity, 30*(1), 45–49.

Sigal, R. J., Alberga, A. S., Goldfield, G. S, Prud'homme, D., Hadjiyannakis, S., Gougeon, R., . . . Kenny, G. P. (2014). Effects of aerobic training, resistance training, or both on percentage body fat and cardio-metabolic risk markers in obese adolescents: The healthy eating aerobic and resistance training in youth randomized clinical trial. *JAMA Pediatrics, 168,* 1006–1014.

Simon, C., Wagner, A., DiVita, C., Rauscher, E., Klein-Platat, C., Arveiler, D., . . . Triby, E. (2004). Intervention centred on adolescents' physical activity and sedentary behaviour (ICAPS): Concept and 6-month results. *International Journal of Obesity, 28*(S3), S96.

Smith, M. A., & St. Pierre, P. E. (2009). Secondary students' perceptions of enjoyment in physical education: An American and English perspective. *Physical Educator, 66,* 209–221.

Sollerhed, A. C., & Ejlertsson, G. (2008). Physical benefits of expanded physical education in primary school: Findings from a 3-year intervention study in Sweden. *Scandinavian Journal of Medicine and Science in Sports, 18,* 102–107.

Springer, A. E., Kelder, S. H., Ranjit, N., Hochberg-Garrett, H., Crow, S., & Delk, J. (2012). Promoting physical activity and fruit and vegetable consumption through a community-school partnership: The effects of Marathon Kids® on low-income elementary school children in Texas. *Journal of Physical Activity and Health, 9*(5), 739–753.

Story, M., Nanney, M. S., & Schwartz, M. B. (2009). Schools and obesity prevention: Creating school environments and policies to promote healthy eating and physical activity. *The Milbank Quarterly, 87*(1), 71–100.

Sutherland, R. L., Campbell, E. M., Lubans, D. R., Morgan, P. J., Nathan, N. K., Wolfenden, L., . . . Williams, A. J. (2016). The physical activity 4 everyone cluster randomized trial: 2-year outcomes of a school physical activity intervention among adolescents. *American Journal of Preventive Medicine, 51*(2), 195–205.

Sutherland, R. L., Campbell, E. M., Lubans, D. R., Morgan, P. J., Okely, A. D., Nathan, N., . . . Wiggers, J. (2016). 'Physical activity 4 everyone' school-based intervention to prevent decline in adolescent physical activity levels: 12 month (mid-intervention) report on a cluster randomised trial. *British Journal of Sports Medicine, 50*(8), 488–495.

Sutherland, R., Reeves, P., Campbell, E., Lubans, D. R., Morgan, P. J., Nathan, N., . . . Wiggers, J. (2016). Cost effectiveness of a multi-component school-based physical activity intervention targeting adolescents: The 'physical activity 4 everyone' cluster randomized trial. *International Journal of Behavioral Nutrition and Physical Activity, 13*, 94.

Tannehill, D., Van der Mars, H., & McPhail, A. (2014). Comprehensive school physical activity programs. In D. Tannehill, H. Van der Mars, & A. McPhail (Eds.). *Building effective physical education programs* (pp. 27–54). Burlington, MA: Jones and Bartlett Learning.

Taylor, S., Noonan, R., Knowles, Z., Owen, M., McGrane, B., Curry, W., & Fairclough, S. J. (2018). Evaluation of a pilot school-based physical activity clustered randomised controlled trial – Active schools: Skelmersdale. *International Journal of Environmental Research and Public Health, 15*, 1011. doi:10.3390/ijerph15051011

Todd, C., Christian, D., Davies, H., Rance, J., Stratton, G., Rapport, F., & Brophy, S. (2015). Headteachers: Prior beliefs on child health and their engagement in school-based health interventions: A qualitative study. *BMC Research Notes, 8*, 161.

van Beurden, E., Barnett, L. M., Zask, A., Dietrich, U. C., Brooks, L. O., & Beard, J. (2003). Can we skill and activate children through primary school physical education lessons? "Move it groove it" – A collaborative health promotion intervention. *Preventive Medicine, 36*(4), 493–501.

Van den Ber, V., Salimi, R., de Groot, R. H. M., Jolles, J., Chinapaw, M. J. M., & Singh, A. S. (2017). "It's a battle…You want to do it, but how will you get it done?": Teachers' and principals' perceptions of implementing additional physical activity in school for academic performance. *International Journal of Environmental Research and Public Health, 14*, 1160.

Van Der Heijden, G. J., Wang, Z. J., Chu, Z., Toffolo, G., Manesso, E., Sauer, P. J., & Sunehag, A. L. (2010). Strength exercise improves muscle mass and hepatic insulin sensitivity in obese youth. *Medicine and Science in Sports and Exercise, 42*, 1973–1980.

Van Kann, D. H. H., Kremers, S. P. J., De Vries, N. K., De Vries, S. I., & Jansen, M. W. J. (2016). The effect of a school-centered multicomponent intervention on daily physical activity and sedentary behavior in primary school children: The active living study. *Preventive Medicine, 89*, 64–69.

van Sluijs, E. M., & Kriemler, S. (2016). Reflections of physical activity intervention research in young people – Do's, don'ts and critical thoughts. *International Journal of Behavioral Nutrition and Physical Activity, 13*, 25.

van Sluijs, E. M., McMinn, A. M., & Griffin, S. J. (2007). Effectiveness of interventions to promote physical activity in children and adolescents: Systematic review of controlled trials. *British Medical Journal, 335*(7622), 703.

van Sluijs, E. M., McMinn, A. M., & Griffin, S. J. (2008). Effectiveness of interventions to promote physical activity in children and adolescents: A systematic review of controlled trials. *British Journal of Sports Medicine, 42*, 653–657.

Vander Ploeg, K. A., McGavock, J., Maximova, K., & Veugelers, P. J. (2014). School-based health promotion and physical activity during and after school hours. *Pediatrics, 133*, e371–e378.

Wankel, L. M. (1993). The importance of enjoyment to adherence and psychological benefits from physical activity. *International Journal of Sport Psychology, 24*, 151–169.

Watson, A., Timperio, A., Brown, H., Best, K., & Hesketh, K. D. (2017). Effect of classroom-based physical activity interventions on academic and physical activity outcomes: A systematic review and meta-analysis. *International Journal of Behavioral Nutrition and Physical Activity, 14*, 114. doi:10.1186/s12966-017-0569-9

Webber, L. S., Catellier, D. J., Lytle, L. A., Murray, D. M., Pratt, C. A., Young, D. R., . . . Pate, R. R. (2008). Promoting physical activity in middle school girls: Trial of activity for adolescent girls. *American Journal of Preventive Medicine, 34*(3), 173–184.

Webster, C. A., Russ, L., Vazou, S., Goh, T. L., & Erwin, H. (2015). Integrating movement in academic classrooms: Understanding, applying and advancing the knowledge base. *Obesity Reviews, 16*, 691–701.

Wilkins, J. L. M., Graham, G., Parker, S., Westfall, S., Fraser, R. G., & Tembo, M. (2003). Time in the arts and physical education and school achievement. *Journal of Curriculum Studies, 35*, 721–734.

Williamson, D. A., Copeland, A. L., Anton, S. D., Champagne, C., Han, H., Lewis, L., . . . Ryan, D. (2007). Wise Mind project: A school-based environmental approach for preventing weight gain in children. *Obesity, 15*(4), 906–917.

28

PRESCHOOL AND CHILDCARE CENTER PHYSICAL ACTIVITY INTERVENTIONS

Rachel A. Jones, Eduarda Sousa-Sá, Michele Peden,
and Anthony D. Okely

Introduction

Early childhood education and care (ECEC) environments are unique settings that offer educa-tion and care for children. In this chapter, we use ECEC to refer to all types of early childhood settings, including preschool, day or family childcare, long day care, kindergarten or Pre-K (pre-kindergarten) and nursery. Children who attend some ECEC centers can be as young as 6 months of age, up to the age of seven in some countries. In high-income countries, such settings are typically informed by standard regulatory frameworks; high-quality ECEC environments have profound influence on children health and behavioral outcomes in the short- and long-term, with higher quality ECEC environments influencing children's outcomes more significantly (Melhuish, Belsky, Leyland, Barnes, & Team, 2008).

Attendance rates in ECEC settings are increasing globally. Data from the Organisation for Economic Co-operation and Development (OECD) show that 35% of children aged 0-to-2 years old participate in some form of childcare and this percentage increases to 84% for children aged 3-to-5 years old (OECD, 2018). While much of this increase has been in high-income countries, more recently increases have also been reported in many low- and middle-income countries. The time children spend in these settings is not insignificant, as high as 40–50 hours per week in some countries. Given the reach of ECECs, this setting has been suggested as an ideal environment for the promotion of many health behavior-related outcomes, including physical activity. Further-more, ECEC settings generally have the space and equipment to promote physical activity and it is a key part of ECEC curricula in many countries such as Australia (AUGov, 2017), United Kingdom (UKGov, 2018), New Zealand (NZGov, 2017) and United States (USAGov, 2018).

Healthy levels of physical activity are associated with a number of short- and long-term health benefits including improved cardio-metabolic outcomes, more positive self-efficacy/self-image, better executive functioning and healthier weight status (Carson et al., 2017). Given these out-comes, physical activity should be promoted from a young age. Furthermore, physical activity levels track from early childhood to childhood and from childhood to adolescence and into adult-hood (Jones, Hinkley, Okely, & Salmon, 2013). Establishing healthy physical activity habits from a young age is critically important for children's cognitive and social development, as well as their physical development.

The US Health and Medicine Division (previously known as the Institute of Medicine) recommends that children should spend at least 15 minutes of each hour in ECEC settings in physical activity and no more than 30 minutes being sedentary at any one time (Institute of Medicine, 2011).

International data (almost exclusively from high-income countries) show that while attending ECEC settings, many children are not meeting the current physical activity recommendations (Ellis et al., 2017; O'Brien, Vanderloo, Bruijns, Truelove, & Tucker, 2018). The low prevalence of physical activity in ECEC settings, along with the high number of children who attend ECEC, reinforces the need to develop and test interventions to increase physical activity levels and to scale up those that are effective to ensure as many children as possible can benefit. Unfortunately, the physical domain of child development is often deemed as less important compared with cognitive, social, and emotional domains. It is often perceived that young children are already highly active and don't need to be supported to improve their physical and motor development.

This chapter will first provide an overview of the literature on effective interventions to promote physical activity in ECEC settings. Components that may contribute to more successful interventions will be evaluated. Finally, the chapter will address some of the key issues, emerging themes and key recommendations pertaining to ECEC-based physical activity interventions.

Brief Overview of the Literature

This umbrella review has been informed by 10 systematic reviews, published between 2009 and 2018 (Engel, Broderick, van Doorn, Hardy, & Parmenter, 2018; Finch, Jones, Yoong, Wiggers, & Wolfenden, 2016; Gordon, Tucker, Burke, & Carron, 2013; Mehtälä, Sääkslahti, Inkinen, & Poskiparta, 2014; Morris, Skouteris, Edwards, & Rutherford, 2015; Temple & Robinson, 2014; Timmons et al., 2012; Ward, Vaughn, McWilliams, & Hales, 2009; Ward, Bélanger, Donovan, & Carrier, 2015; Zhou, Emerson, Levine, Kihlberg, & Hull, 2014). The review highlights ECEC-based interventions that focus on physical activity or are inclusive of a physical activity component (for example, those with a focus on obesity prevention). Included is a summary of the outcomes, with emphasis on those that have reported significant changes in physical activity outcomes and the potential intervention components that may have facilitated these changes.

To provide a summary of the best evidence, this umbrella review focused on controlled trials – inclusive of randomized controlled trials (RCTs) and pilot RCTs –, cluster RCTs and quasi-experimental trials. Observational studies or those without a control group were not included in this review.

All studies had physical activity as the primary or secondary outcome. The studies that had physical activity as the primary outcome evaluated a physical activity-specific intervention. For example, Trost, Fees, and Dzewaltowski (2008) assessed the potential efficacy of the Move and Learn program, which involved integrating physical activity into other key learning areas such as numeracy and literacy learning experiences. Jones, Riethmuller, et al.'s (2011), Bonvin et al.'s (2013) and Meghan Finch et al.'s (2014) interventions focused on providing additional physical activity opportunities through structured physical activity sessions, several times a week. Razak and colleagues' intervention involved scheduling three separate periods of outdoor free play. Jones, Riethmuller, et al. (2011), Bonvin et al. (2013) and Razak et al. (2018) measured physical activity using accelerometers while Finch et al. (2014) measured changes in physical activity using pedometers.

The studies where physical activity was a secondary outcome typically evaluated obesity prevention targeted interventions. In these studies, the primary outcome was an adiposity-related outcome. These studies usually had a number of secondary outcomes, one of which included physical activity. Other outcomes in these studies included nutrition, media use and parental knowledge. For example, Annesi, Smith, and Tennant (2013) assessed the effect of the 9-month Start for Life trial on physical activity and body mass index (BMI). The primary outcome was changes in BMI, and physical activity measured using accelerometers was a secondary outcome. Reilly et al. (2006) implemented an obesity prevention intervention in 26 nurseries in Scotland

(United Kingdom). For this study the primary outcome was changes in BMI and secondary outcomes included proficiency of fundamental movement skills, sedentary behavior and physical activity (Reilly et al., 2006).

Evaluation of Studies

The majority of interventions were US-based and targeted children aged between 3 and 5 years from general populations. Inclusion criteria for most studies were generally broad with participants only being excluded if they had a developmental or medical condition. A few studies did target specialized groups. Fitzgibbon et al.'s (2005) and Fitzgibbon et al.'s (2006) obesity prevention interventions recruited African-American and Latino preschool children, respectively. In both studies, the intervention period was 14 weeks and outcomes, inclusive of physical activity (measured by parent-proxy report), were assessed at 1- and 2-year follow-up. Both interventions were well received and the intervention targeting African-American children was effective in reducing subsequent increases in BMI. Annesi et al. (2013) recruited predominately African-American preschool-aged children into their 8-week ECEC-based intervention. The intervention group participated in 30 minutes of additional physical activity per day, which resulted in a significant increase (approximately 40 minutes per day) in time spent in moderate-to-vigorous physical activity (MVPA) for the intervention group when compared to the control group.

The average sample size for most studies was several hundred children. Of the studies included in the systematic reviews, several had a sample size greater than 500 at baseline (Annesi et al., 2013; Bürgi et al., 2012; Cardon, Labarque, Smits, & De Bourdeaudhuij, 2009; De Bock, Fischer, Hoffmann, & Renz-Polster, 2010; Nemet, Geva, & Eliakim, 2011; Reilly et al., 2006; Roth et al., 2015). Fewer studies had a sample size of less than 100 at baseline (Alhassan et al., 2012; Alhassan, Nwaokelemeh, Lyden, Goldsby, & Mendoza, 2013; Alhassan, Sirard, & Robinson, 2007; Jones, Riethmuller, et al., 2011; Trost et al., 2008).

Most ECEC-based physical activity interventions or inclusive of a physical activity component were implemented for less than 1 year, with the majority measured in months. Of the studies reviewed, only a handful investigated the longer-term impact of the interventions. Fitzgibbon et al. (2005) and Fitzgibbon et al. (2006) assessed physical activity outcomes at 1 and 2 years, following a 14-week intervention and Reilly et al.'s (2006) study had a 6-month intervention phase and physical activity outcome data were collected at 6- and 12-months. De Craemer et al. (2014) objectively measured and assessed the effect of the Toy-Box intervention on preschoolers' (4–6 years) physical activity levels in Belgium. The length of the intervention was 24 weeks, and follow-up physical activity data were collected 1 year later. Puder et al.'s (2011) study was a 1-year multidimensional lifestyle intervention in preschool children in Switzerland. Follow-up data were collected 12 months after baseline data.

In the majority of interventions, educators were encouraged to provide additional time for children to spend in physical activity (either structured or unstructured physical activity learning experiences). In most studies, children were encouraged to spend between 20 and 45 minutes of additional physical activity, 2 or 3 times a week. For example, Fitzgibbon et al.'s (2005) and Fitzgibbon et al.'s (2006) interventions involved children participating in 20 minutes of aerobic physical activity 3 days a week. Reilly et al.'s (2006) intervention involved children participating in 30 minutes of additional physical activity 3 days per week and Alhassan et al.'s (2012) intervention involved children participating in an additional 30 minutes of structured physical activity (focusing on locomotor and movement skills), twice a week. In the interventions conducted by Nemet, Geva, Pantanowitz, et al. (2011) and Razak et al. (2018) children participated in an additional 45 minutes of physical activity each day of the week; however this time was divided in three 15-minute sessions spread throughout the day. O'dwyer et al.'s (2013) and De Craemer et al.'s (2014) interventions both included 1 hour of structured active play sessions, once a week, in addition to what was routinely offered.

A small number of studies involved modifications to the indoor environment only (De Craemer et al., 2014), the indoor and outdoor environments (Bonvin et al., 2013; Finch et al., 2014) or the outdoor environment only (Cardon et al., 2009). Bonvin et al. (2013) provided funding to the intervention centers for the purchase of the mobile equipment and for the rearrangement of the environments to make them more activity-friendly (no further details provided). The aim was to complement the physical activity component of the intervention which included participating in additional physical activity sessions several times a week. Cardon et al.'s (2009) 6-week intervention did not prescribe additional physical activity opportunities; rather it investigated the impact of additional play equipment and/or outdoor ground markings. This intervention involved four interventions arms: (1) additional play equipment; (2) ground markings; (3) additional play equipment and ground markings and (4) control group (no additional play equipment or ground markings). Physical activity was measured using accelerometers. Counts per minutes and time spent in sedentary behavior, light-intensity physical activity and MVPA were assessed. No significant differences between groups for all intensities of physical activities were reported.

Parent involvement in ECEC-based physical activity interventions is recommended as parents and the family environment are recognized as the main influences on young children's behaviors. Less than half of the studies reviewed included a parental component and where a parental component was included, it was only detailed briefly. Parents either participated in two or three workshop/educational sessions (Bürgi et al., 2012; Eliakim, Nemet, Balakirski, & Epstein, 2007; Nemet, Geva, & Eliakim, 2011) or were provided with newsletters (Fitzgibbon et al., 2005, 2006, 2011; Yin et al., 2012) or printed information (Reilly et al., 2006). Interventions evaluated by Bonvin et al. (2013) and De Craemer et al. (2014) reported that parents received some education but no further details were provided. Additional information about the content of the workshops or the newsletters was not provided for any study.

Most interventions were facilitated by educators who had received training from the research team. In the reviews summarized, a small number of interventions were co-led by researchers and educators. Eliakim et al.'s (2007) intervention was led by a professional youth coach for 2 days and then by the educators for the other days. Similarly, Nemet, Geva, and Eliakim's (2011) study was led by a professional youth coach once a week and the educator on the other days. Alhassan et al.'s (2013) intervention was exclusively facilitated by researchers, although it was helped by the educators and De Bock et al.'s (2010) study was led exclusively by external gym trainers.

In general, educators received training/professional development to deliver the intervention from members of the research team. All training/professional development was facilitated face-to-face; however there was variability in the intensity and frequency of the training and in the resources provided. Some studies incorporated many hours of training/professional development. For example, Annesi et al. (2013) provided 4 hours of educator training, Finch et al. (2014) offered 6 hours of training for educators; Bonvin et al. (2013) provided five training workshops and interventions conducted by Alhassan et al. (2013) included 8 hours of educator training. Others provided minimal training, for example in Eliakim et al.'s (2007) study educators were trained to deliver the intervention in three 15 minute in-class sessions. Various resources were provided as part of the training. Examples included prepared lesson plans or resources (e.g. newsletters, posters, music CD, stickers, child achievement cards) (Alhassan et al., 2013; Annesi et al., 2013; Bellows, Davies, Anderson, & Kennedy, 2013; De Craemer et al., 2014) equipment (Alhassan et al., 2012, 2013; De Craemer et al., 2014; Puder et al., 2011), additional face-to-face support (Bonvin et al., 2013; Finch et al., 2014; Puder et al., 2011).

In the studies reviewed, the majority used accelerometers to measure physical activity. These were all attached to the waist and worn for a number of hours or days. Accelerometers are the most valid and reliable instrument for the collection of physical activity data in field-based studies among young children (Cliff, Reilly, & Okely, 2009). The different intensities of physical activities were assessed using either 'Pate et al' cut-points (e.g. Annesi et al., 2013; Bonvin et al., 2013; Fitzgibbon et al., 2011) or 'Sirard et al' cut-points (e.g. Alhassan et al., 2012; Cardon et al., 2009; O'dwyer et al., 2013). Wear time of accelerometers varied from 1 day (e.g. Annesi et al., 2013; Bonvin et al., 2013) to 7 consecutive days (e.g. Alhassan et al., 2012). Other instruments used to measure physical activity included pedometers (steps/day) (Bellows et al., 2013; Eliakim et al., 2007; Finch et al., 2014; Yin et al., 2012), heart rate monitors (Parish, Rudisill, & Onge, 2007), parent-proxy report (Fitzgibbon et al., 2005, 2006) and observational tools such as NAPSACC (Ward et al., 2008).

Changes in Physical Activity

ECEC-based interventions that focused on physical activity or were inclusive of physical activity outcomes reported mixed success in modifying the time and intensity of physical activity among children.

In studies with physical activity as the main outcome, few reported significant changes in physical activity outcomes at the end of the intervention. Trost et al.'s (2008) intervention, Move and Learn, involved integrating physical activity in normal curricula activities. Teachers were required to include two Move and Learn activities, lasting 10 minutes or longer into each 2.5-hour session. Objectively measured physical activity (accelerometer) levels were assessed biweekly throughout the intervention period. Significant changes between the intervention group and the control group in MVPA and vigorous-intensity physical activity during classroom time were reported during the last 4 weeks of the intervention (weeks 5, 6, 7 and 8, all $p < 0.05$). Razak et al.'s (2018) intervention involved ECEC services scheduling three separate period of outdoor play, eat at least 15 minutes in duration. Physical activity was objectively measured using accelerometers over a 5-day period. Children in the intervention group participated in significantly more MVPA (mean daily minutes, adjusted difference between groups 5.21 minutes, 95% CI 0.59–9.83, $p = 0.03$) compared to children in the control group.

Similarly, few studies where physical activity was a secondary outcome (i.e. in the obesity prevention interventions) reported significant behavior change. One notable exception was Fitzgibbon's et al. (2011) Hip-Hop to Health Jr trial, which involved nine intervention ECECs and nine control ECECs. Children in the intervention ECECs participated in a 14-week educator-led program. Physical activity was measured objectively using accelerometers. Children from the intervention group spent significantly more time in MVPA compared with children from the control group (differences between adjusted group means = 7.46 minutes/day, $p = 0.02$) (Fitzgibbon et al., 2011). Annesi et al. (2013) reported an increase of 9.3% ($p = 0.05$) in time spent in vigorous-intensity physical activity and 8.7% ($p = 0.02$) in time spent in MVPA among the intervention group compared to the control group.

Given modest number of ECEC-based interventions that have reported significant changes in physical activity outcomes as well as the variability in the studies reviewed, it is difficult to identify the influence of specific intervention components on children's physical activity outcomes. Intervention efficacy seemed to vary and does not seem to be particularly dependent on the intervention or trial design characteristics. Although it is difficult to identify key components of ECEC-based physical activity interventions that make them effective, the reviews consistently mention two components worth noting. These are staff behavior and training/professional development and the provision of educator-facilitated intentional physical activity opportunities several times a week (Finch et al., 2014). The authors of the reviews suggest that further research needs long-term follow-up, multi-strategy interventions that include changes in the physical activity environment, reporting of cost data, and consideration of sustainability (Finch et al., 2014; Zhou et al., 2014). As Finch et al. (2016) described 'evidence gaps remain for policymakers and practitioners regarding the effectiveness and feasibility of childcare-based physical activity interventions'.

Key Issues

This umbrella review has highlighted a number of the key findings from ECEC-based interventions that focused on physical activity or had a physical activity outcome. Four main gaps are apparent in the following areas: (1) the lack of interventions in infants and toddlers; (2) the mode and duration of training/professional development and support; (3) the need for longer-term assessments and (4) the lack of parental involvement.

Despite physical activity being an important component of holistic child development and a behavior that should be encouraged from birth (Carson et al., 2017; Janssen & LeBlanc, 2010) the majority of interventions targeted preschool-aged children (i.e. ages 3–5 years). There were a few exceptions to this; for example, Bonvin et al. (2013) included children aged between 2 and 4 years and Nemet, Geva, Pantanowitz, et al. (2011) included children up to 6.5 years of age. Even though these studies included slightly younger or older children, the mean age of the children was between 3 and 5 years. The consistent focus on preschool children is not discussed within the literature; however this may be due to the large number of 3–5-year-old children attending ECEC settings or it may be that educators and researchers feel that physical activity learning experiences are more relevant for older children as these children have increased movement and cognitive abilities (compared to children aged 0–3 years). Despite this, it is still critically important to provide intentional physical activity opportunities for children in the younger age groups. The format of such interventions will obviously need to be considered to ensure that they are age appropriate.

Most interventions were facilitated by educators which is understandable given that educators have established rapport with the children in their centers and know the needs of each child. Educators are well versed in their center's routines and community needs and have the capacity to be trained to facilitate physical activity interventions (Jones, Gowers, Stanley, & Okely, 2017). Training/professional development received by educators in all ECEC-based interventions reviewed was facilitated via face-to-face channels. The duration and content of the training varied for each study; however the delivery mode was consistent. Face-to-face professional development is widely used within the ECEC sector; however it is associated with a number of limitations. For example, on completion of the workshop the attending educators are expected to transfer the 'new' information to other educators in their centers, which rarely occurs (Yoong et al., 2015). Furthermore, such traditional professional development may not meet the needs of educators. Educators want training/professional development that is contextually relevant and content-specific (Buysse, Winton, & Rous, 2009), offering opportunities to reflect on practices and providing ongoing support guidance and mentoring (from educators and professionals (Nuttall, 2013; Pianta, 2006) and a place for ongoing professional conversations (Wood & Bennett, 2000). Alternate methods of training/professional development such as blended delivery may be more viable for the ECEC sector.

A recent study from Australia trialed delivering training/professional development using a blended medium (i.e. a combination of face-to-face training and online training) (Peden, 2019, under review). The training comprised one full day face-to-face workshop and 12 weeks of synchronous and asynchronous online training. Significant, albeit small, changes for the percentage of time children spent in light-intensity physical activity were reported at the end of the intervention period (adjusted difference = 0.01%, 95% CI (0.00,0.01), $p = 0.02$) as well as at the end of the maintenance period (adjusted difference = 0.01%, 95% CI (0.00,0.02), $p = 0.04$). When assessing the quality of environment in relation to physical activity (measured using the Environmental and Policy Assessment and Observation (EPAO)), significant differences were observed for the total physical activity EPAO score between the intervention and control groups. Significant differences were reported at the end of the intervention period (adjusted difference = 5.33, 95% CI (−0.30,10.37), $p = 0.04$), which were further increased at the end of the maintenance period (adjusted difference = 8.54, 95% CI (1.61,15.48), $p = 0.02$) (Peden, 2019).

Few studies have assessed physical activity outcomes beyond 1 year. Assessment of intervention outcomes over a longer period is recommended as adequate 'soak time' is needed for change to become part of the ECEC routine and for behaviors to change and new norms to be re-established (Jones, Sinn, et al., 2011). This is true for both educators and children. Educators need the time to process new information offered in training/professional development sessions. They need time to discuss and reflect on the new information and to strategize sustainable methods of change within their center, with their staff and consistent with their pedagogical practices. The children also need time to adapt to new routines and learning experiences and to become comfortable with these experiences. Change within the ECEC sector is no different from other educational sectors; it is typically met with resistance and considerable effort and support is needed to ensure that long-term changes are implemented and sustained. The best method of support to enable long-term change in ECEC settings remains unknown; however, a recent study suggested that telephone support may be the most preferred and successful option for the ECEC sector, at least in high-income countries like Australia (Strooband, Stanley, Okely, & Jones, 2018). Additional research is needed as to determine the best support mechanisms for the ECEC sector which will ensure that changes in children's physical activity behaviors are maintained.

Few of the reviewed studies included a parental component. For optimal outcomes in children's behaviors, consistent messaging from the ECEC environment and the home environment is needed. Furthermore, most ECEC curricula strongly promote communication and interaction between the ECEC environment and the home environment. Although critically important, involving parents in ECEC-based physical activity interventions is extremely challenging, at least in high-income countries where most parents have limited time at drop-off and pick-up for discussions and show limited interest in attending additional sessions or workshops pertaining to activities that occur within ECEC settings. Communication and meaningful interaction between the ECEC environment and the home environment remain a challenge and the best methods of engagement and interaction are not clear. Despite this, consistency between the ECEC environment and the home environment is critical for optimal child health and well-being outcomes, including physical activity.

Emerging Issues and Developments

The ECEC environment has changed significantly since 2000, as new national and international regulations have been introduced, making it a complex environment for the implementation of interventions. As new regulations have been enforced, the demands on educators have exponentially increased and this has coincided with the increased number of children attending ECEC settings as well as the renewed emphasis on school readiness and academic achievement.

Children's physical activity in ECEC settings is influenced by myriad factors, which include the age and sex of the child, their gross motor skill proficiency, time spent outside, their interaction and engagement with educators and the ECEC quality and routine (Tonge, Jones, & Okely, 2016). Boys are typically more active than girls and those with high levels of gross motor proficiency are consistently more active than those with lower proficiency (Tonge et al., 2016). Children who spend more than 4 hours per day outside are consistently more active than those that spend less than 4 hours outside (Tonge, 2019). Recent data from Australia have also shown that children who attend free flowing routines (i.e. are able to move freely between the indoor ECEC environment and the outdoor ECEC environment) spend significantly more time in MVPA than those that attend ECEC settings with more structured routines (i.e. children have designated times for indoor learning experiences and outdoor learning experiences) (Tonge, 2019). The numbers of studies that report on such relationships, specifically those related to the time spent outdoors and the ECEC routines, are relatively small; however what is consistently reported is that children's physical activity is suboptimal in ECEC settings and that this environment is an ideal setting for the promotion of physical activity.

ECEC-based physical activity interventions that are high in methodological quality are needed to enhance physical activity levels of young children while attending ECEC settings. As highlighted in the umbrella review, such interventions to date have varied in approach, training/professional development and intervention components and changes in physical activity outcomes have been mixed.

Given the complexity and uniqueness of the ECEC environment several additional emerging issues and trends may need to be considered in the formative stages of such interventions. ECEC environments today have an exceptionally high turn-over of staff which makes the transfer of knowledge and consistent pedagogical practices difficult (Siraj et al., 2017). Staff turn-over largely occurs as a result of educators moving between rooms (interacting with different children) within one center or moving between centers when centers are managed by an overarching organization. ECEC-based interventions that focus on physical activity need to consider how to maximize knowledge transfer during the implementation period (and beyond) of an intervention. Ongoing or online training/professional development may be one viable method of ensuring consistent high-quality pedagogical practice.

There is convincing evidence to suggest that educators who engage in continuous or ongoing training/professional development offer higher quality care and education than those who never participate in training or attend one-off training (Elliott, 2006; Norris, 2001; Snell, Forston, Stanton-Chapman, & Walker, 2013). Ongoing training enhances positive changes in children health and learning, continuity and stability of the quality of ECEC programs (Melhuish et al., 2016). Ongoing training/professional development provides an opportunity for educators to be continually reminded of the key messages of the intervention and be accountable for the changes in their centers. Ongoing training/professional development also offers educators opportunities for professional collaborations and conversations – both of which are key factors of training/professional development that educators are seeking (Linder, Rembert, Simpson, & Ramey, 2016). Furthermore, ongoing training/professional development offers an opportunity for more diverse content to be explored or the content to be explored and discussed in more depth. Given the large number of factors that influence physical activity and the high turn-over of staff, additional and continuous training/professional development is likely to be beneficial.

Shaping or reshaping educators' perceptions in relation to physical activity may also be an important area to investigate in future interventions. It is well established that educators have a critical role in shaping the behaviors and patterns of the children in their care (Siraj-Blatchford, 2009). Some studies have shown that educator's behaviors positively influence physical activity behaviors of children (Bower et al., 2008; Vanderloo et al., 2014; D. Ward et al., 2008). That is, where educators provide positive prompts in relation to physical activity or role model positive physical activity behaviors, children are consistently more active. In contrast, and perhaps what is more common, other studies suggest that the main role of educators in relation to physical activity is a passive supervisory role and that young children are sufficiently active during ECEC hours and do not need intentional physical activity learning experiences (Ellis et al., 2017; Strauss, 1999). Educators also shy away from providing intentional physical activity experiences due to their own low levels of self-efficacy in this area. Several studies have highlighted that educators do not feel comfortable or knowledgeable enough about physical activity or know what experiences to offer the children; therefore educators tend not to offer any (Dyment & Coleman, 2012; Jones et al., 2017). Ensuring that educator training programs include content and experiences to build pre-service teachers' skills and confidence is needed. Addressing these areas through continuous professional development for staff is also important. Incorporating into such training the link between child physical activity and areas that are particularly salient for educators, such as self-regulation and cognitive development, may help educators prioritize the promotion of physical activity within their setting.

Allocating time to inform educators of the vital importance of physical activity in children's development and discussing examples of successful and engaging physical activity learning experiences may be a critical component of ECEC-based interventions that focus on physical activity or are inclusive of a physical activity component. Physical activity for young children is often (mis) conceptualized by educators as structured activities or activities that just involve running or jumping at high intensity. However, for preschool children, physical activity is a broad term that should be inclusive of risky play, fine and gross motor skills, social interactions, movement vocabulary, engagement and communication between children, and their families and educators. It is much more than traditional perceptions of physical activity.

Although physical activity continues to be recognized as an important component of national and international ECEC curriculums, it is often underrepresented in current practice. Other key learning domains such as the cognitive and social/emotional domains seem to take higher priority. This may be attributed to the greater diagnosed or undiagnosed needs of children with ECEC settings, where children with higher social and emotional needs require more attention from educators and thus more time is spent specifically on enhancing the social and emotional needs of children. The reduced emphasis on the physical learning domain may also be consequence of the requirements for educators to provide holistic comprehensive programs. For example educators are required to integrate Science, Technology, Engineering and Mathematics (STEM) learning experiences, as well as learning experiences that are inclusive of sustainability and cultural competence components, health and hygiene and child protection. In some countries, the overarching push for children to become 'school ready' well before they enter school may also influence the time spent in high-quality physical activity learning experiences. In such countries, the emphasis is on learning to read and write to ensure that children are adeptly prepared to transition to formal schooling. However, school readiness is actually about the ability for children to develop independence, follow instructions, form friendships and socialize, listen, complete an experience or task, communicate, engage and interact with their peers and educators. It is also about appropriate development of fine and gross motor skills and strong core muscle development. Many of these attributes are developed through the participation of age-appropriate physical activity inclusive intentional learning experiences rather than academic-based skills. Helping educators see the links between physical activity and other domains of a child's development promotes more holistic approaches to children's learning and development. This results in educators realizing that it is possible to plan experiences for children that can be physically active as well as enhancing their cognitive, social and emotional, and language development.

The administration burden of educators has exponentially increased in the past decade. While educators have always been required to provide documentation on their educational programs and developmental outcomes of children, they are now also required to adhere to comprehensive assessment and compliance requirements. For example, in Australia ECECs must gather evidence and complete documentation across seven quality areas outlined under the National Quality Standards (DEEWR, 2009) which involves completing an ongoing Quality Improvement Plan and provides evidence of how educators are critically reflecting on policies and practices across seven quality areas. Furthermore, in many countries, educators are required to be in constant communication with parents throughout the day via daily electronic notice boards (e.g. Story Park [www.storypark.com/au], Kinderloop (https://kinderloop.com)) so that parents can view the learning experiences their children participate in throughout the day. While communication with families is highly encouraged within the ECEC sector and a critical component of the curriculum and the education and care that is offered, these added responsibilities now have the potential to deter educators away from their core business.

These emerging issues and developments within the ECEC sector are likely to continue and thus need to be considered as new interventions that focus on physical activity or are inclusive of a physical activity component introduced and implemented. ECEC-based interventions need to be thoughtfully planned and considered to ensure that the emerging ECEC cultural trends are acknowledged and addressed.

Recommendations

The ECEC sector continues to be a key environment for the promotion of physical activity. Equipping educators with new knowledge and skills pertaining to physical activity is key to changing children's physical activity behaviors. Well-designed and implemented interventions that are educator-facilitated and perhaps are multi-faceted seem to be more favorable.

In light of the umbrella review, the key issues and the emerging trends within the international ECEC sector, future ECEC-based physical activity interventions should consider:

1   The provision of ongoing high-quality training/professional development for educators prior, during and beyond the intervention phase (i.e. ongoing support). Given the low competence and confidence levels of most educators in the area of physical activity, explicit ongoing training/professional development should be a priority. The training should be delivered by experts with experience working within the ECEC sector. Educators are more likely to respond to those who understand the needs of educators. Ongoing training should include information on the critical role of the physical domain in child development as well as the provision of examples of indoor and outdoor physical activity learning experiences. Given the influential role educators have, the role of the educator and the importance of meaningful interactions between educators and children in physical activity learning experiences should also be discussed in future training.

2   Interventions that are 'outside the box'. The majority of ECEC-based physical activity interventions have been standard in intervention design and delivery; they have involved a face-to-face training/professional development, a prescriptive physical activity component for the children and a few suggestions of additional resources. Given the modest changes in physical activity outcomes, future interventions should start to think 'outside the box' in regard to intervention components and delivery. The following questions might be helpful as future interventions are planned: can blended training/professional development be used? To date, only one study has trialed the use of blended professional development (Peden, 2019). This study was successful in modifying physical activity outcomes.

What role can technology play in physical activity interventions? Technology is an important component of most ECEC curricula and is encouraged in different formats in different ECEC settings (DEEWR, 2009). Given the diversity of apps and technology-related programs that are currently available, can they be used to enhance physical activity learning experiences? Is it important to consider the health, well-being and physical activity levels of the educators? Recent data show that in ECEC settings where educators are more active, the children in their care are also more active compared to those where educators are less active (Tonge, 2019). Can interventions target educators' physical activity? Very few studies have investigated the well-being of educators in relation to physical activity experiences provided by children (Linnan et al., 2017). Can interventions incorporate a combination of intervention components, for example, structured physical activity learning experiences, outdoor markings and energy breaks? Are other types of physical activity interventions that don't add to the overcrowded day possible? Are specific intervention needed for specific groups (i.e. those from lower socioeconomic groups)? Finally, can interventions take a 'stealth' approach? That is, target outcomes that are highly salient to educators such as school readiness; and cognitive, social and emotional, and language development while at the same time resulting in increased physical activity levels (as a by-product of the intervention)?

3   High methodological quality interventions. Factors such as selection bias, appropriately powered samples (i.e. ensuring that the sample sizes are large enough to be able to report statistically significant differences between groups), potential confounders, blinding of data collectors to group allocation, appropriate attrition and retention rates and intervention integrity need to be considered a priori. Furthermore, a well-planned data analysis procedure, which accounts for potential clustering effects, missing/incomplete data sets, needs to be considered. Transparent reporting of such factors should also be of paramount concern in future interventions.

4   Meaningful and trustworthy collaborations between educators and researchers. Developing collaborative professional relationships between researchers and educators can help maximize children's physical activity outcomes. A recent paper suggests successful collaboration involves researchers spending time learning about the ECEC environment and presenting research finding in an easily interpretable manner to educators (Jones et al., 2017). Furthermore, the importance of researchers understanding the profound place of relationships within the ECEC sector and the importance of including educators in the research process were also highlighted as being critical (Jones et al., 2017). Trustworthy and meaningful relationships between educators and researchers are particularly paramount for the success of intervention studies that often require additional responsibilities from educators and change within their centers (Jones et al., 2017).

5   The influence of the quality of the ECEC environment. It is well established that the quality of the ECEC environment has a significant influence on children's outcomes both in the short- and long-term. Several key studies, such as the Effective Pre-school, Primary and Secondary Education Project (Sylva, Melhuish, Sammons, Siraj-Blatchford, & Taggart, 2012), have shown that higher quality ECEC environments result in better cognitive, social and behavioral outcomes immediately (ages 3–5 years) and several years later (e.g. at ages 11 and 16) (Siraj-Blatchford, 2009). In fact, literacy outcomes at age 11 are influenced more by the quality of the ECEC environment rather than the family's income or father's education or the quality of the primary school (Siraj-Blatchford, 2009). Thus, future interventions should consider assessment of the quality of the environment in relation to physical activity and consider how this could be improved through the intervention components. To date, there are relatively few reliable and valid instruments available that assess the quality of the ECEC environment in relation to physical activity. The MOVERS Scale (Archer & Siraj, 2017), which was published in 2017, was the first instrument to assess the product and process quality of the ECEC environment in relation to physical activity. It has four subscales: (i) Curriculum, environment and resources for physical development; (ii) pedagogy for physical development; (iii) supporting physical activity and critical thinking and (iv) parents/carers and staff. It focuses on the influence of the educators in regard to physical activity as well as physical activity learning experiences offered to the children. High-quality instruments that measure the quality of the ECEC environment in relation to physical activity should be considered as a measure in future interventions.

This chapter provides a broad summary of ECEC interventions that focus on physical activity or have a physical activity component. A number of key issues were highlighted as well as emerging trends that need to be considered in future interventions. Five broad recommendations were also offered. The information presented in this chapter should be considered in light of the interventions reviewed. Lessons and recommendations can also be ascertained from smaller pilot studies or pre-test, post-test design studies; however these were not reviewed in this chapter. The ECEC sector is also inclusive of family day care which is where care is provided for children in a home environment; however, to date, no reviews of family day care-based physical activity interventions have been evaluated and published and thus were not included. Physical activity interventions that focused on adherence to policies were not included in the review. A number of such interventions have been evaluated and may also offer important advice for future interventions (Wolfenden et al., 2011). The majority of ECECs may not have written comprehensive physical activity-related policies, an area that could also be investigated in future.

ECEC-based interventions that focus on physical activity or have a physical activity component continue to be evaluated. In more recent years, more studies in low- and middle-income countries have been completed. Although these are currently few in number, it is anticipated that this will increase in due course. Comparisons between interventions implemented in low- and middle-income countries and those in high-income countries (which form the overwhelming majority included in this chapter) are needed to determine if interventions may need to be different in such countries. For example, a study conducted by Tomaz (2018) from South Africa suggests that preschool-aged children exceed the recommended levels of physical activity during ECEC hours; however the ECEC environment is of extremely poor quality.

With the release of recent physical activity guidelines for the early years from a number of countries (including Australia, Canada, United Kingdom, South Africa) as well as those released from the World Health Organization, it is clear that the promotion of physical activity must continue to be a global priority to ensure the health and well-being of young children now and in the future. The ECEC environment, although a challenging and complex environment, needs to continue to be a key environment for the promotion of physical activity.

References

Alhassan, S., Nwaokelemeh, O., Ghazarian, M., Roberts, J., Mendoza, A., & Shitole, S. (2012). Effects of locomotor skill program on minority preschoolers' physical activity levels. *Pediatric Exercise Science, 24*(3), 435–449.

Alhassan, S., Nwaokelemeh, O., Lyden, K., Goldsby, T., & Mendoza, A. (2013). A pilot study to examine the effect of additional structured outdoor playtime on preschoolers' physical activity levels. *Child Care in Practice, 19*(1), 23–35.

Alhassan, S., Sirard, J. R., & Robinson, T. N. (2007). The effects of increasing outdoor play time on physical activity in Latino preschool children. *International Journal of Pediatric Obesity, 2*(3), 153–158.

Annesi, J. J., Smith, A. E., & Tennant, G. A. (2013). Effects of the start for life treatment on physical activity in primarily African American preschool children of ages 3–5 years. *Psychology, Health & Medicine, 18*(3), 300–309.

Archer, C., & Siraj, I. (2017). *Movement environment rating ccale (MOVERS) for 2–6-year-olds provision: Improving physical development through movement and physical activity.* London, UK: Institute of Education Press.

AUGov. (2017). *Australian 24-Hour Movement Guidelines for the Early Years (Birth to 5 years): An Integration of Physical Activity, Sedentary Behaviour, and Sleep.* Canberra: Commonwealth of Australia. Retrieved from http://www.health.gov.au/internet/main/publishing.nsf/content/npra-0-5yrs-brochure

Bellows, L. L., Davies, P. L., Anderson, J., & Kennedy, C. (2013). Effectiveness of a physical activity intervention for Head Start preschoolers: A randomized intervention study. *American Journal of Occupational Therapy, 67*(1), 28–36.

Bonvin, A., Barral, J., Kakebeeke, T. H., Kriemler, S., Longchamp, A., Schindler, C., . . . Puder, J. J. (2013). Effect of a governmentally-led physical activity program on motor skills in young children attending child care centers: A cluster randomized controlled trial. *International Journal of Behavioral Nutrition and Physical Activity, 10*(1), 90.

Bower, J. K., Hales, D. P., Tate, D. F., Rubin, D. A., Benjamin, S. E., & Ward, D. S. (2008). The child-care environment and children's physical activity. *American Journal of Preventive Medicine, 34*(1), 23–29. doi:10.1016/j.amepre.2007.09.022

Bürgi, F., Niederer, I., Schindler, C., Bodenmann, P., Marques-Vidal, P., Kriemler, S., & Puder, J. J. (2012). Effect of a lifestyle intervention on adiposity and fitness in socially disadvantaged subgroups of preschool-ers: A cluster-randomized trial (Ballabeina). *Preventive Medicine, 54*(5), 335–340.

Buysse, V., Winton, P. J., & Rous, B. (2009). Reaching consensus on a definition of professional develop-ment in the early childhood field. *Topics in Early Childhood Special Education, 28*(4), 235–243.

Cardon, G., Labarque, V., Smits, D., & De Bourdeaudhuij, I. (2009). Promoting physical activity at the pre-school playground: The effects of providing markings and play equipment. *Preventive Medicine, 48*(4), 335–340.

Carson, V., Lee, E.-Y., Hewitt, L., Jennings, C., Hunter, S., Kuzik, N., . . . Gray, C. (2017). Systematic review of the relationships between physical activity and health indicators in the early years (0–4 years). *BMC Public Health, 17*(5), 854.

Cliff, D. P., Reilly, J. J., & Okely, A. D. (2009). Methodological considerations in using accelerometers to assess habitual physical activity in children aged 0–5 years. *Journal of Science and Medicine in Sport, 12*(5), 557–567.

De Bock, F., Fischer, J. E., Hoffmann, K., & Renz-Polster, H. (2010). A participatory parent-focused in-tervention promoting physical activity in preschools: Design of a cluster-randomized trial. *BMC Public Health, 10*(1), 49.

De Craemer, M., De Decker, E., Verloigne, M., De Bourdeaudhuij, I., Manios, Y., & Cardon, G. (2014). The effect of a kindergarten-based, family-involved intervention on objectively measured physical ac-tivity in Belgian preschool boys and girls of high and low SES: The ToyBox-study. *International Journal of Behavioral Nutrition and Physical Activity, 11*(1), 38.

DEEWR. (2009). *Belonging, being and becoming: The early years learning framework for Australia.* Retrieved from https://www.education.gov.au/

Dyment, J., & Coleman, B. (2012). The intersection of physical activity opportunities and the role of early childhood educators during outdoor play: Perceptions and reality. *Australasian Journal of Early Childhood, 37*(1), 90.

Eliakim, A., Nemet, D., Balakirski, Y., & Epstein, Y. (2007). The effects of nutritional-physical activity school-based intervention on fatness and fitness in preschool children. *Journal of Pediatric Endocrinology and Metabolism, 20*(6), 711–718.

Elliott, A. (2006). Early childhood education: *Pathways to quality and equity for all children.* Australian Council for Educational Research, Camberwell, Victoria, Australia.

Ellis, Y. G., Cliff, D. P., Janssen, X., Jones, R. A., Reilly, J. J., & Okely, A. D. (2017). Sedentary time, physical activity and compliance with IOM recommendations in young children at childcare. *Preventive Medicine Reports, 7*, 221–226.

Engel, A. C., Broderick, C. R., van Doorn, N., Hardy, L. L., & Parmenter, B. J. (2018). Exploring the relationship between fundamental motor skill interventions and physical activity levels in children: A systematic review and meta-analysis. *Sports Medicine, 48*, 1845–1857.

Finch, M., Jones, J., Yoong, S., Wiggers, J., & Wolfenden, L. (2016). Effectiveness of centre-based childcare interventions in increasing child physical activity: A systematic review and meta-analysis for policymak-ers and practitioners. *Obesity Reviews, 17*(5), 412–428.

Finch, M., Wolfenden, L., Morgan, P. J., Freund, M., Jones, J., & Wiggers, J. (2014). A cluster randomized trial of a multi-level intervention, delivered by service staff, to increase physical activity of children at-tending center-based childcare. *Preventive Medicine, 58*, 9–16.

Fitzgibbon, M. L., Stolley, M. R., Schiffer, L. A., Braunschweig, C. L., Gomez, S. L., Van Horn, L., & Dyer, A. R. (2011). Hip-hop to health Jr. obesity prevention effectiveness trial: Postintervention results. *Obesity, 19*(5), 994–1003.

Fitzgibbon, M. L., Stolley, M. R., Schiffer, L., Van Horn, L., KauferChristoffel, K., & Dyer, A. (2005). Two-year follow-up results for Hip-Hop to Health Jr.: A randomized controlled trial for overweight prevention in preschool minority children. *The Journal of Pediatrics, 146*(5), 618–625.

Fitzgibbon, M. L., Stolley, M. R., Schiffer, L., Van Horn, L., KauferChristoffel, K., & Dyer, A. (2006). Hip-hop to health Jr. for Latino preschool children. *Obesity, 14*(9), 1616–1625.

Gordon, E. S., Tucker, P., Burke, S. M., & Carron, A. V. (2013). Effectiveness of physical activity interven-tions for preschoolers: A meta-analysis. *Research Quarterly for Exercise and Sport, 84*(3), 287–294.

Institute of Medicine. (2011). *Early childhood obesity prevention policies: Goals, recommendations, and potential actions* (Vol. Recommendations June 2011). Washington, DC: Institute of Medicine.

Janssen, I., & LeBlanc, A. G. (2010). Systematic review of the health benefits of physical activity and fitness in school-aged children and youth. *International Journal of Behavioral Nutrition and Physical Activity, 7*(1), 40.

Jones, R. A., Gowers, F. L., Stanley, R. M., & Okely, A. D. (2017). Enhancing the effectiveness of early childhood educators and researchers working together to achieve common aims. *The Australasian Journal of Early Childhood, 42*, 81–84.

Jones, R. A., Hinkley, T., Okely, A. D., & Salmon, J. (2013). Tracking physical activity and sedentary behavior in childhood: A systematic review. *American Journal of Preventive Medicine, 44*(6), 651–658.

Jones, R. A., Riethmuller, A., Hesketh, K., Trezise, J., Batterham, M., & Okely, A. D. (2011). Promoting fundamental movement skill development and physical activity in early childhood settings: A cluster randomized controlled trial. *Pediatric Exercise Science, 23*(4), 600–615.

Jones, R. A., Sinn, N., Campbell, K. J., Hesketh, K., Denney-Wilson, E., Morgan, P. J., . . . Magarey, A. (2011). The importance of long-term follow-up in child and adolescent obesity prevention interventions. *International Journal of Pediatric Obesity, 6*(3–4), 178–181.

Linder, S. M., Rembert, K., Simpson, A., & Ramey, M. D. (2016). A mixed-methods investigation of early childhood professional development for providers and recipients in the United States. *Professional Development in Education, 42*(1), 123–149.

Linnan, L., Arandia, G., Bateman, L. A., Vaughn, A., Smith, N., & Ward, D. (2017). The health and working conditions of women employed in child care. *International Journal of Environmental Research and Public Health, 14*(3). doi:10.3390/ijerph14030283

Mehtälä, M. A. K., Sääkslahti, A. K., Inkinen, M. E., & Poskiparta, M. E. H. (2014). A socio-ecological approach to physical activity interventions in childcare: A systematic review. *International Journal of Behavioral Nutrition and Physical Activity, 11*(1), 22.

Melhuish, E., Belsky, J., Leyland, A. H., Barnes, J., & Team, N. E. o. S. S. R. (2008). Effects of fully-established Sure Start Local Programmes on 3-year-old children and their families living in England: A quasi-experimental observational study. *The Lancet, 372*(9650), 1641–1647.

Melhuish, E., Howard, S. J., Siraj, I., Neilsen-Hewett, C., Kingston, D., de Rosnay, M., . . . Luu, B. (2016). Fostering Effective Early Learning (FEEL) through a professional development programme for early childhood educators to improve professional practice and child outcomes in the year before formal schooling: study protocol for a cluster randomised controlled trial. *Trials, 17*(1), 602.

Morris, H., Skouteris, H., Edwards, S., & Rutherford, L. (2015). Obesity prevention interventions in early childhood education and care settings with parental involvement: A systematic review. *Early Child Development and Care, 185*(8), 1283–1313.

Nemet, D., Geva, D., & Eliakim, A. (2011). Health promotion intervention in low socioeconomic kindergarten children. *The Journal of Pediatrics, 158*(5), 796–801. e791.

Nemet, D., Geva, D., Pantanowitz, M., Igbaria, N., Meckel, Y., & Eliakim, A. (2011). Health promotion intervention in Arab-Israeli kindergarten children. *Journal of Pediatric Endocrinology and Metabolism, 24*(11–12), 1001–1007.

Norris, D. J. (2001). Quality of care offered by providers with differential patterns of workshop participation. *Child and Youth Care Forum, 30*(2), 111–121.

Nuttall, J. (2013). The potential of developmental work research as a professional learning methodology in early childhood education. *Contemporary Issues in Early Childhood, 14*(3), 201–211.

NZGov. (2017). *What your child learns at ECE.* Retrieved from https://parents.education.govt.nz/early-learning/learning-at-an-ece-service/what-your-child-learns-at-ece/

O'Brien, K. T., Vanderloo, L. M., Bruijns, B. A., Truelove, S., & Tucker, P. (2018). Physical activity and sedentary time among preschoolers in centre-based childcare: A systematic review. *International Journal of Behavioral Nutrition and Physical Activity, 15*(1), 117. doi:10.1186/s12966-018-0745-6

O'dwyer, M., Fairclough, S., Ridgers, N., Knowles, Z., Foweather, L., & Stratton, G. (2013). Effect of a school-based active play intervention on sedentary time and physical activity in preschool children. *Health Education Research, 28*(6), 931–942.

OECD. (2018). *PF3.2: Enrolment in childcare and pre-schools. 2014.* Retrieved January 31, 2020 from https://www.oecd.org/els/soc/PF3_2_Enrolment_childcare_preschool.pdf

Parish, L. E., Rudisill, M. E., & Onge, P. M. S. (2007). Mastery motivational climate: Influence on physical play and heart rate in African American toddlers. *Research Quarterly for Exercise and Sport, 78*(3), 171–178.

Pate, R. R., Almeida, M. J., McIver, K. L., Pfeiffer, K. A., & Dowda, M. (2006). Validation and calibration of an accelerometer in preschool children. *Obesity, 14*(11), 2000–2006.

Peden, M. (2019) Evidence-based mediated professional learning program for Early Childhood Education and Care addressing physical activity and healthy eating. (Doctor of Philosophy Thesis). University of Wollongong, Wollongong, Australia.

Pianta, R. C. (2006). Standardized observation and professional development: A focus on individualized implementation and practices. In M. Zaslow & I. Martinez-Beck (Eds.), *Critical Issues in Early Childhood Professional Development* (pp. 231–254). Baltimore, MD: Brookes.

Puder, J. J., Marques-Vidal, P., Schindler, C., Zahner, L., Niederer, I., Bürgi, F., . . . Kriemler, S. (2011). Effect of multidimensional lifestyle intervention on fitness and adiposity in predominantly migrant pre-school children (Ballabeina): Cluster randomised controlled trial. *BMJ, 343*, d6195.

Razak, L. A., Yoong, S. L., Wiggers, J., Morgan, P. J., Jones, J., Finch, M., . . . Clinton-McHarg, T. (2018). Impact of scheduling multiple outdoor free-play periods in childcare on child moderate-to-vigorous physical activity: A cluster randomised trial. *International Journal of Behavioral Nutrition and Physical Activity, 15*(1), 34.

Reilly, K. L., Montgomery, C., Williamson, A., Fisher, A., McColl, J. H., . . . Grant, S. (2006). Physical activity to prevent obesity in young children: Cluster randomised controlled trial. *BMJ, 333*(7577), 1041.

Roth, K., Kriemler, S., Lehmacher, W., Ruf, K. C., Graf, C., & Hebestreit, H. (2015). Effects of a physical activity intervention in preschool children. *Medicine and Science in Sports and Exercise, 47*(12), 2542–2551.

Siraj, I., Kingston, D., Neilsen-Hewett, C., Howard, S., Melhuish, E., de Rosnay, M., & Luu, B. (2017). *Fostering effective early learning study*. University of Wollongong, Wollongong, Australia. Retrieved 13, 2018, from https://education.nsw.gov.au/media/ecec/pdfdocuments/FEEL-Study-Literature-Review-Final.pdf

Siraj-Blatchford, I. (2009). Conceptualising progression in the pedagogy of play and sustained shared thinking in early childhood education: A Vygotskian perspective. *Education and Child Psychology, 26*(2), 77–89.

Sirard, J. R., Trost, S. G., Pfeiffer, K. A., Dowda, M., & Pate, R. R. (2005). Calibration and evaluation of an objective measure of physical activity in preschool children. *Journal of Physical Activity and Health, 2*(3), 345–357.

Snell, M. E., Forston, L. D., Stanton-Chapman, T. L., & Walker, V. L. (2013). A review of 20 years of research on professional development interventions for preschool teachers and staff. *Early Child Development and Care, 183*(7), 857–873.

Strauss, R. (1999). Childhood obesity. *Current Problems in Pediatrics, 29*(1), 1–29.

Strooband, K. F., Stanley, R. M., Okely, A. D., & Jones, R. A. (2018). Support to enhance level of implementation in physical activity interventions: An observational study. *Australasian Journal of Early Childhood, 43*(1), 25.

Sylva, K., Melhuish, E., Sammons, P., Siraj-Blatchford, I., & Taggart, B. (2012). The effective pre-school, primary and secondary education 3 – 14 project (EPSSE 3–14) final report for the key stage 3 phase, influences on students' development from age 11 to 14. *Research Report DfE-RR202*. London: Department for Education.

Temple, M., & Robinson, J. C. (2014). A systematic review of interventions to promote physical activity in the preschool setting. *Journal for Specialists in Pediatric Nursing, 19*(4), 274–284.

Timmons, B. W., LeBlanc, A. G., Carson, V., Connor Gorber, S., Dillman, C., Janssen, I.,. . . Tremblay, M. S. (2012). Systematic review of physical activity and health in the early years (aged 0–4 years). *Applied Physiology, Nutrition, and Metabolism, 37*(4), 773–792.

Tomaz, S. (2018) Physical activity and gross motor skills in rural South African preschool children. (Doctor of Philosophy Thesis) University of Cape Town, Cape Town, South Africa.

Tonge, K. (2019) The Relationship between Educator Engagement and Interaction and Children's Physical Activity in Early Childhood Education and Care Services. (Doctor of Philosophy Thesis, University of Wollongong, Wollongong, Australia).

Tonge, K. L., Jones, R. A., & Okely, A. D. (2016). Correlates of children's objectively measured physical activity and sedentary behavior in early childhood education and care services: A systematic review. *Preventive Medicine, 89*, 129–139.

Trost, S. G., Fees, B., & Dzewaltowski, D. (2008). Feasibility and efficacy of a "move and learn" physical activity curriculum in preschool children. *Journal of Physical Activity and Health, 5*(1), 88–103.

UKGov. (2018). *Statutory framework for the early years foundation stage – Setting the standards for learning, development and care for children from birth to five*. Retrieved from https://www.gov.uk/government/publications/early-years-foundation-stage-framework--2.

USAGov. (2018). *Child care aware*. Retrieved from http://childcareaware.org/

Vanderloo, L. M., Tucker, P., Johnson, A. M., van Zandvoort, M. M., Burke, S. M., & Irwin, J. D. (2014). The influence of centre-based childcare on preschoolers' physical activity levels: A cross-sectional study. *International Journal of Environmental Research and Public Health, 11*(2), 1794–1802. doi:10.3390/ijerph110201794

Ward, D., Hales, D., Haverly, K., Marks, J., Benjamin, S., Ball, S., & Trost, S. (2008). An instrument to assess the obesogenic environment of child care centers. *American Journal of Health Behavior, 32*(4), 380–386. doi:10.5555/ajhb.2008.32.4.380

Ward, D. S., Benjamin, S. E., Ammerman, A. S., Ball, S. C., Neelon, B. H., & Bangdiwala, S. I. (2008). Nutrition and physical activity in child care: Results from an environmental intervention. *American Journal of Preventive Medicine, 35*(4), 352–356.

Ward, D. S., Vaughn, A., McWilliams, C., & Hales, D. (2009). Physical activity at child care settings: Review and research recommendations. *American Journal of Lifestyle Medicine, 3*(6), 474–488.

Ward, S., Bélanger, M., Donovan, D., & Carrier, N. (2015). Systematic review of the relationship between childcare educators' practices and preschoolers' physical activity and eating behaviours. *Obesity Reviews, 16*(12), 1055–1070.

Wolfenden, L., Neve, M., Farrell, L., Lecathelinais, C., Bell, C., Milat, A., . . . Sutherland, R. (2011). Physical activity policies and practices of childcare centres in Australia. *Journal of Paediatrics and Child Health, 47*(3), 73–76. doi:10.1111/j.1440-1754.2010.01738.x

Wood, E., & Bennett, N. (2000). Changing theories, changing practice: Exploring early childhood teachers' professional learning. *Teaching and Teacher Education, 16*(5–6), 635–647.

Yin, Z., Parra-Medina, D., Cordova, A., He, M., Trummer, V., Sosa, E., . . . Wu, X. (2012). Miranos! Look at us, we are healthy! An environmental approach to early childhood obesity prevention. *Childhood Obesity (Formerly Obesity and Weight Management), 8*(5), 429–439.

Yoong, S. L., Williams, C. M., Finch, M., Wyse, R., Jones, J., Freund, M., . . . Wolfenden, L. (2015). Childcare service centers' preferences and intentions to use a web-based program to implement healthy eating and physical activity policies and practices: A cross-sectional study. *Journal of Medical Internet Research, 17*(5), e108.

Zhou, Y. E., Emerson, J. S., Levine, R. S., Kihlberg, C. J., & Hull, P. C. (2014). Childhood obesity prevention interventions in childcare settings: Systematic review of randomized and nonrandomized controlled trials. *American Journal of Health Promotion, 28*(4), e92–e103.

29

SCHOOL PHYSICAL ACTIVITY FOR CHILDREN WITH DISABILITIES

Cindy H. P. Sit and Thomas L. McKenzie

Introduction

This chapter provides an overview of school physical activity (PA) for children with disabilities and emphasizes how school environments influence their PA levels. It also examines the challenges of PA measurements and intervention outcomes, and how we learn from the past and move forward to meet the health recommendations derived from PA in this special needs population.

For optimal health benefits, international authorities recommend that all children aged 5–17 years accumulate at least 60 minutes of moderate-to-vigorous-physical activity (MVPA) daily (World Health Organization [WHO], 2018). There are also recommendations for children, regardless of having a disability or not, to spend no more than 2 hours per day in recreational screen time behavior (Canadian 24-Hour Movement Guidelines for Children and Youth, 2016). Relative to these guidelines, children with disabilities generally have sedentary lifestyles and low levels of PA – factors which are related to increased risk for obesity, obesity-related chronic diseases, and other health problems (Rimmer & Marques, 2012). Numerous studies also show that children with disabilities, compared to their typically developing (TD) peers, are much less physically active, engage in sedentary pursuits more frequently, and can be three to six times more at risk for obesity (e.g., Jung, Leung, Schram, & Yun, 2018; Lobenius-Palmér, Sjöqvist, Hurtig-Wennlöf, & Lundqvist, 2018; National Centre on Health, Physical Activity and Disability [NCHPAD], 2018; Neter et al., 2011; Stanish et al., 2019).

Approximately 15% of the world's population lives with some form of disability, and about 5.1% of children aged 0–14 years (95 million) have a disabling condition (WHO, 2011b). The International Classification of Functioning, Disability and Health (ICF) has identified disability as an umbrella term that includes impairments (problems in body function and structure), activity limitations (difficulties in executing activities), and participation restrictions (problems engaging in life situations) (WHO, 2018). These conditions include some forms of functional disability such as a mobility, cognition, hearing, vision, independent living, or self-care challenge (Okoro, Hollis, Cyrus, & Griffin-Blake, 2018).

The ICF model includes a focus on PA engagement as an important part of the functioning and well-being of persons with disability as it has been used widely in research (WHO, 2018). The model recognizes the prominence that both personal and environmental factors play in influencing the PA of those with disabilities (Imms et al., 2016). Personal factors (e.g., age, gender, health status) interact with both physical and social environmental factors that exist in settings where children with disabilities live and interact, such as schools (Li et al., 2016, 2017).

An ICF for Children and Youth (ICF–CY) was developed specifically for working with young people with disabilities. It recognizes the salient characteristics of children and their surrounding environment plus the person-environment interactions that influence physical, social, and psychological development (WHO, 2001). A review using ICF framework has identified that environmental factors (e.g., location, equipment, peer social support) significantly influence both the extent and the intensity of PA in children with disabilities (Fekete, & Rauch, 2012).

Studies have found that PA levels vary as a function of disability type, gender, and age. For example, children with physical and severe intellectual disabilities (compared to mild intellectual disabilities) (Sit et al., 2017) and girls and older children have been found to be less active than their male and younger counterparts (Lobenius-Palmér et al., 2018; Sit et al., 2017). Meanwhile, a recent meta-analysis reported that youths with disabilities (and in younger ages) engaged in less MVPA than their peers without disabilities (Jung et al., 2018).

The Report Card on Children and Adolescents that was developed and released by the Active Healthy Kids Global Alliance in Canada (Tremblay et al., 2016) identified PA as a top priority for doing research. Despite a call for more Report Cards to include data on children with disabilities, only 2 of 49 countries or regions with Report Cards included a section for children with disabilities – the Netherlands and Finland (Aubert et al., 2018).

The first country to release a Report Card for children with a chronic condition or disability was the Netherlands in 2017. Among 11 indicators that followed pre-determined benchmarks, the average PA indicator grade was D, indicative of only 26% of children were meeting the 60 minutes MVPA daily recommendation. Younger girls (i.e., 4–11 years vs. 12–17 years) and younger children (i.e., 6–12 years vs. 16–19 years) that had a mental, motor, visual, or auditory disability were reported to be more active than their older counterparts. On their 2018 Report Card, the PA grade for those with a chronic medical condition in the Netherlands was lower than that of TD peers (i.e., D+ vs. C−). In Finland, fewer children with functional limitations met PA recommendations than their same age peers without disabilities (e.g., 35% vs. 41% of children aged 11 years). Overall, fewer girls and fewer children with more severe functional limitations met the PA recommendation than boys and children with less severe limitations. Another recent study also showed that children with disabilities were less likely to meet the PA recommendation than peers without disabilities (i.e., 6% vs. 29%; Stanish et al., 2019). As overall PA is important for reducing the prevalence of obesity and a number of secondary conditions in children with disabilities, the development of effective PA interventions is seen as a public health priority (Rimmer & Marques, 2012).

Overview of the Literature

School Environments and Physical Activity

As children with disabilities generally have low levels of PA, especially compared to their TD peers, interventions specifically targeting them are needed. In this regard, schools have been identified as an important setting where children can accumulate health-enhancing PA (CDCP, 2013; Healthy People, 2020; McKenzie, 2010). Healthy People 2020, for example, provides public health objectives for promoting children's PA at school, and these include the provision of mandated, structured physical education (PE) programs in which students engage in MVPA during at least 50% of lesson time.

In addition to active PE, health authorities also recommend that schools provide diverse leisure time PA opportunities such as recess and before- and after-school programs (CDC, 2013; Institute of Medicine [IOM], 2013). The National Association for Sport and Physical Education [NASPE] (2016), for example, suggested that all children be provided with at least 20 minutes recess daily. Meanwhile, the Convention on the Rights of Persons with Disabilities (CRPD, 2019) has advocated that children with disabilities have equal rights, including access to participation in recreation, leisure, and sport in different settings, including schools. Along this line, the United Nations Educational, Scientific and Cultural Organization (UNESCO, 2015) has called for global action that promotes quality PE consisting of providing flexible curricula, adapted facilities and equipment, and teaching and learning materials for children with disabilities.

Children with disabilities, however, have been found to spend 70% of their day at school being sedentary and accruing little MVPA (e.g., 17 minutes) (Sit et al., 2017). Other studies have reported that only 29% of children with disabilities had PE classes 5 days a week (NCHPAD, 2018). In addition, even when a PE classes were conducted in special schools, only 7.9 MVPA minutes were accrued by students. This was 41.9% of total lesson time and short of the 50% activity intensity recommendation (Sit, McManus, McKenzie, & Lian, 2007). Similar findings were also reported in a study by Pan, Liu, Ching, and Hsu (2015), which showed that children with intellectual disabilities failed to achieve the recommended 50% MVPA during PE and 40% MVPA during recess. These findings of low levels of MVPA during PE are not similar to those found for TD children in the U.S. (McKenzie & Smith, 2017) and other countries (Smith, McKenzie, & Hammons, 2019).

In addition, children's PA during PE are influenced by teacher behavior and lesson context, with their PA accrual greater when teachers emphasize fitness-related activities (Pan, Tsai, & Hsieh, 2011; Sit et al., 2007) and in schools which provide more support for PA (Sit, McKenzie, Lian, & McManus, 2008). It is also noteworthy to consider that children's PA during PE is related to where lessons are taught (e.g., outdoor classes may be more active) and the level of social interaction with peers (Pan et al., 2011). In addition, children with disabilities may be more active during recess than during PE (Sit et al., 2007; Sit, McKenzie, Cerin, McManus, & Lian 2013; Pan et al., 2015).

There is a particular need that teachers conduct PE and PA programs at schools for children with disabilities to have specialized training (Pan et al., 2015). Teachers especially should understand the importance of children with disabilities being encouraged to participate in diverse forms of PA so they can gain health benefits from it. Although the concept of mainstreaming in regular schools is typically promoted, children with disabilities are often at a disadvantage related to PA engagement in classes where TD peers are typically more physically fit and physically skilled. Employing PE teachers and activity programers who have had specialized training can help alleviate this problem (Bredahl, 2013).

In summary, children with disabilities are not sufficiently active in general, but peer involvement, access to facilities, and convenient PA locations help facilitate their PA (Shields, Synnot, & Barr, 2012). In this regard, schools are convenient locations for PA and the provision of PE, organized activities, and playground supervision have been shown to be positively related to activity accrual (e.g., Sit et al., 2013). A recent study also confirmed that children with physical disabilities accrued more PA at school than at home, and they were more active during recess and lunchtime than before and after school, and that prompts to be active from peers contributed to their activity accrual (Sit, Yu, Wong, Capio, & Masters, 2019). Studies such as these not only indicate the importance of schools in contributing to the PA of children with disabilities but begin to identify salient features within school environments that are particularly more influential.

Measures of PA and Associated Variables

Assessing the PA of children with disabilities is challenging due to complexities (e.g., severity) both within and among disability types (Strath, Pfeiffer, & Whitt-Glover, 2012). A systematic review of instruments for measuring the PA of children with physical disabilities indicated that only a few had established reliability and validity and that a combination of subjective and objective instruments was recommended (Capio, Sit, & Abernethy, 2010). Another systematic review indicated that subjective measures, including self-reports, were commonly used to assess the PA of children with different types of disabilities and that accelerometry offered promise (Ross et al., 2016). Recent studies using accelerometers have confirmed that children with disabilities are insufficiently active (e.g., Brian et al., 2019; Lobenius-Palmér et al., 2018; Sit et al., 2017; Stanish et al., 2019; Wouters, Evenhuis, & Hilgenkamp, 2019). Accelerometers have the advantage of providing accurate, precise objective PA data; however, their use is limited to ambulatory children (Nooijen et al., 2015) and compliance to wearing them by children with disabilities may be low (McGarty, Penpraze, & Melville, 2014). In addition, accelerometers provide information only on PA without assessing the important contextual factors with the environment that may be influencing it (McKenzie, 2016).

In view of the importance of simultaneously assessing children's PA and associated environmental characteristics in settings, a series of reliable and valid observation methods have been developed and been used with children having disabilities. Direct observation methods are particularly important for assessing children's PA because they allow contextual variables to be studied objectively without placing a response burden on a child (McKenzie, 2016; Van der Mars & McKenzie, 2019 – Chapter 14 in this book). The System for Observing Fitness Instruction Time [SOFIT] (McKenzie, Sallis, Nader, 1992), for example, is a comprehensive tool that not only documents children's PA but also assesses associated lesson contexts (i.e., how PE is being delivered) and teacher behavior (e.g., promotes or demonstrates fitness, and instructs generally). It has been used to effectively study these factors during PE in special schools (Sit et al., 2007, 2008). In addition, Behaviors of Eating and Activity for Child Health: Evaluation System [BEACHES] (McKenzie et al., 1992) has been used to examine children's PA and eating behavior while documenting associated environmental characteristics and events (e.g., location, people present, motivator, viewing media) in both home and school settings (Li et al., 2017; Sit et al., 2019). Additionally, the System for Observing Play and Recreation in Community [SOPARC] (McKenzie, Cohen, Sehgal, Williamson, & Golinelli, 2006) has been used to assess children's PA and associated environmental characteristics in specific target areas at school in terms of their accessibility (e.g., not locked), usability (e.g., not excessively wet or roped off for repair), presence of equipment (e.g., balls and jump ropes provided by the school), supervision (i.e., closely monitored by school staff), and organized activities (e.g., scheduled events or PA classes led by school staff). The PA codes for these observational tools have been validated for use in children with physical disabilities. For example, moderate-to-strong associations and high levels of agreement have been shown between observed SOFIT data and accelerometer-measured PA in both PE and free play periods in special schools (Capio, Sit, Abernethy, & Rotor, 2010).

Findings using these direct observation instruments have been useful in identifying how environmental factors affect the PA of children with disabilities. SOFIT studies, for example, have shown that children with disabilities accrue little PA during both recess and PE and that their PA is attributable to PE lesson context and teacher behavior (Sit et al., 2007, 2008). SOPARC has been to assess children's PA during both PE and free play periods, and children with disabilities were found to be sedentary during about 50% of their leisure time and their PA to be associated with the provision of playground supervision and organized activities (Sit et al., 2013). A study using BEACHES also showed that children with physical disabilities spent little time in MVPA (range from 6.3% to 17%) at home (before dinner) and during four school settings (before classes, recess, lunch breaks, after classes) (Sit et al., 2019). At school, prompts to be active contributed to children's MVPA% before classes and during recess and lunch breaks. MVPA was also associated with the presence of a child's mother before classes at school and with the presence of peers during recess and lunch breaks.

School-Based Interventions: Key Issues in
Design and Outcomes

In general, children with disabilities accrue small amounts of MVPA during school time and there are differences among disability types, with children having physical and severe intellectual disabilities being less physically active than those with sensory impairments and mild/moderate intellectual disabilities (Sit et al., 2007, 2017). Given the important role of schools in promoting health-enhancing PA of this population, there is a pressing need to design and implement effective school-based interventions that consider both contextual and personal factors.

Appropriate interventions should begin early in order for children to enjoy the health benefits that are derived from regular participation in PA. Little is known, however, about how effective interventions in schools are on various specific health or behavioral outcomes. Studies that have examined PA or exercise interventions for children with disabilities have been conducted primarily in clinical/community/home settings. Reviews have been published relative to physical disabilities (Bloemen, Van Wely, Mollema, Dallmeijer, & Groot, 2017; Reedman, Boyd, & Sakzewski, 2017; Ryan, Cassidy, Noorduyn, & O'Connell, 2017), intellectual disabilities (Frey, Temple, & Stanish, 2017; Maïano et al., 2019; McGarty, Downs, Melville, & Harris, 2018), visual impairments (Haegele & Porretta, 2015), autism spectrum disorder/attention-deficit hyperactivity disorder [ASD/ADHD] (Bremer, Crozier, & Lloyd, 2016, Cerrillo-Urbina et al., 2015; Tan, Pooley, & Speelman, 2016), and behavioral challenges (Ash, Bowling, Davison, & Garcia, 2017) with a focus on promoting PA and/or health outcomes including motor, social, and cognitive functioning. In general, most of the intervention studies were limited in their research design and conceptualization (Frey et al., 2017) and the overall findings are inconclusive. Overall small or no significant effects were found for objectively measured PA after the intervention or during follow-up measures (Ross et al., 2016). Unfortunately, many studies do not include stringent process measures (e.g., assessment of program implementation, adherence to protocols, instructor behavior) so the reasons for limited maintenance and generalizability are unknown.

Very few studies in the reviews were conducted at schools or used a guiding framework such as ICF. Nonetheless, intervention studies have been implemented at schools. For example, studies using accelerometry have shown increased PA in children with visual impairments (e.g., Cervantes & Porretta, 2013), physical disabilities (e.g., Cleary, Taylor, Dodd, & Shields, 2017; Zwinkels et al., 2018), and developmental coordinator disorders (Sit et al., 2019). Cleary et al.'s (2017) study used aerobic exercise with a long intervention period and found that children's PA was sustained at least up to 10-week post-intervention.

The content of school-based interventions has typically focused on aerobics or physical fitness and has included children with developmental coordination disorders (e.g., Bonney, Rameckers, Ferguson, & Smits-Engelsman, 2018), physical disabilities (e.g., Cleary et al., 2017; Zwinkels et al., 2018), and intellectual disabilities (e.g., Giagazoglou et al., 2013; Wallén, Müllersdorf, Christensson, & Marcus, 2012; Wu et al., 2017). Other outcome variables have included balance (Giagazoglou et al., 2013; Wu et al., 2017), body composition (Wu et al., 2017; Zwinkels et al., 2018), psychological affects such as enjoyment (Bonney et al., 2018; Cleary et al., 2017), and behavioral components such as social functioning (Bowling et al., 2017).

The interventions were typically implemented by teachers in the schools; however, study protocols varied widely. Program length ranged from 7 weeks to 2 years, session length ranged from 20 to 60 minutes, and session frequency ranged from 1 to 5 times weekly. As examples of diversity, Wu et al. (2017) used cross-circuit training to improve both the physical fitness and weight of children with intellectual disabilities, and Giagazoglou et al. (2013) used trampolines with children having similar challenges. Giagazoglou et al. (2013) stated the trampoline activities required children to adapt to moving on unstable surfaces, thus facilitating their movement and sensory and spatial responses. They reported not only the children found the activities to be interesting and enjoyable but they also improved in their balance and other motor tasks.

It is important to note that these interventions were conducted in special schools and that the program results were generally positive. This suggests that special schools are promising settings for promoting health and well-being in this special population, especially with well-trained teachers. Rosso (2016), for example, found that instructors with prior knowledge of the needs of children with disabilities and having a low instructor-to-participant ratio were two factors that were crucial to the delivery of school-based programs that motivated children to participate in PA. Meanwhile, a recent study by Najafabadi et al. (2018) also showed that using the SPARK (Sports, Play and Active Recreation for Kids), an evidence-based program with a 30-year (McKenzie, Sallis, Rosengard, & Ballard, 2016), resulted in significant positive outcomes in the physical health, balance, bilateral coordination, and social interactions of children with disabilities such as ASD. This kind of PE program could be a viable choice for promoting PA and in the development of physical fitness, motor skills, and social interactions for children with disabilities. Nonetheless, to embed high-quality adapted PE programs into standard school policies requires substantial initial and ongoing support from teachers, administrators, and school boards.

Recommendations for Researchers/Practitioners

With research on PA being a high priority (Tremblay et al., 2016) and only 2 of 49 countries including a section for children with disabilities in their national PA Report Cards (Aubert et al., 2018), it is clear that additional research, including national surveillance studies, needs to be done. Meanwhile, general findings indicate that children with disabilities are overall insufficiently active and that schools, which have been identified as primary settings for children to engage in ample amounts of PA and become physically fit and motorically skilled, are not meeting the challenge and that interventions are needed.

With "disability" being a complex social construct (Barg, Armstrong, Hetz, & Latimer, 2010), the one golden standard/rule for school-based PA interventions for children with disabilities is that programs be tailored to meet the needs and interests of specific children. Only in this way will the health, functioning, and quality of life of those with disabilities be maximized.

For school-based PA interventions for children with disabilities to be successful, schools will need to work close with parents and caretakers and ensure they become directly involved in decision-making and program implementation. From a research view, there is need for school-based PA interventions to be grounded within a sound theoretical framework and that programs be examined using standardized scientific practices (e.g., sufficient sample sizes, control groups, randomization). Only in this way can the effectiveness of interventions in different locations and with children facing different disabling conditions be compared appropriately so that those programs that work be scaled up and disseminated widely.

Currently there is limited research on improving the MVPA engagement of children with special needs, and those studies that have been conducted in schools have typically focused on PE settings only. Meanwhile, "whole-of-school approaches," often referred to as "Comprehensive School Physical Activity Programs" or "CSPAPs," toward increasing PA on school campuses are now being advanced (CDC, 2013; IOM, 2013). How this model affects accrual of PA by children with various types of disabilities and in diverse school settings is unknown and should be examined.

McKenzie (2019) has suggested that the "biggest bang" for promoting PA in schools would result from the development and implementation of school PA policies. To date, there have been few investigations relative to policies and the PA of children with disabilities at school. This includes a lack of studies on policy development, policy implementation, policy adoption, and outcomes (see Chapter 11, Lounsbery, McKenzie, & Smith, 2019). Given that successful policy implementations can bring about total school environmental changes that affect all children and over extended time periods, an increase in school policy research on the PA of children with disabilities is warranted.

References

Ash, T., Bowling, A., Davison, K., & Garcia, J. (2017). Physical activity interventions for children with social, emotional, and behavioral disabilities: A systematic review. *Journal of Developmental and Behavioral Pediatrics, 38*, 431–445.

Aubert, S., Barnes, J. D., Abdeta, C., Nader, P. A., Adeniyi, A. F., Aguilar-Farias, N., . . . Tremblay, M. S. (2018). Global Matrix 3.0 physical activity report card grades for children and youth: Results and analysis from 49 countries. *Journal of Physical Activity and Health, 15*, S251–S273.

Barg, C. J., Armstrong, B. D., Hetz, S. P., & Latimer, A. E. (2010). Physical disability, stigma, and physical activity in children. *International Journal of Disability, Development and Education, 57*, 378.

Bloemen, M., Van Wely, L., Mollema, J., Dallmeijer, A., & Groot, J. (2017). Evidence for increasing physical activity in children with physical disabilities: A systematic review. *Developmental Medicine and Child Neurology, 59*, 1004–1010.

Bonney, E., Rameckers, E., Ferguson, G., & Smits-Engelsman, B. (2018). "Not just another Wii training": A graded Wii protocol to increase physical fitness in adolescent girls with probable developmental coordination disorder – A pilot study. *BMC Pediatrics, 18*, 78.

Bowling, A., Slavet, J., Miller, D. P., Haneuse, S., Beardslee, W., & Davison, K. (2017). Cybercycling effects on classroom behavior in children with behavioral health disorders: An RCT. *Pediatrics, 139*, e20161985

Bredahl, A. (2013). Sitting and watching the others being active: The experienced difficulties in PE when having a disability. *Adapted Physical Activity Quarterly, 30*, 40–58.

Bremer, E., Crozier, M., & Lloyd, M. (2016). A systematic review of the behavioural outcomes following exercise interventions for children and youth with autism spectrum disorder. *Autism, 20*, 899–915.

Brian, A., Pennell, A., Haibach-Beach, P., Foley, J., Taunton, S., & Lieberman, L. J. (2019). Correlates of physical activity among children with visual impairments. *Disability and Health Journal, 12*, 328–333.

Canadian Society for Exercise Physiology (CSEP). (2016). *Canadian 24-hour movement guidelines for children and youth: An integration of physical activity, sedentary behaviour, and sleep guideline development report.* Ottawa, ON: 24-Hour Movement Guidelines Leadership Group.

Capio, C. M., Sit, C. H. P., & Abernethy, B. A. (2010). Physical activity measurement using MTI (actigraph) among children with cerebral palsy. *Archives of Physical Medicine and Rehabilitation, 91*, 1283–1290.

Capio, C. M., Sit, C. H. P., Abernethy, B. A., & Rotor, E. (2010). Physical activity measurement instruments for children with cerebral palsy: A systematic review. *Developmental Medicine and Child Neurology, 52*, 908–916.

Centers for Disease Control and Prevention [CDC]. (2013). *Comprehensive school physical activity programs: A guide for schools.* Atlanta, GA: CDC.

Cerrillo-Urbina, A. J., García-Hermoso, A., Sánchez-López, M., Pardo-Guijarro, M. J., Santos Gómez, J. L., & Martínez-Vizcaíno, V. (2015). The effects of physical exercise in children with attention deficit hyperactivity disorder: A systematic review and meta-analysis of randomized control trials. *Child, Health and Development, 41*, 779–788.

Cervantes, C. M., & Porretta, D. L. (2013). Impact of after school programming on physical activity among adolescents with visual impairments. *Adapted Physical Activity Quarterly, 29*, 127–146.

Cleary, S. L., Taylor, N. F., Dodd, K. J., & Shields, N. (2017). An aerobic exercise program for young people with cerebral palsy in specialist schools: A phase I randomized controlled trial. *Developmental Neurorehabilitation, 20*, 331–338.

Convention on the Rights of Persons with Disabilities [CRPD]. (2019). Articles. Department of Economic and Social Affairs. United Nations. Retrieved June 30, 2019 from https://www.un.org/development/desa/disabilities/convention-on-the-rights-of-persons-with-disabilities/convention-on-the-rights-of-persons-with-disabilities-2.html

Fekete, C., & Rauch, A. (2012). Correlates and determinants of physical activity in persons with spinal cord injury: A review using the international classification of functioning, disability and health as reference framework. *Disability and Health Journal, 5*, 140–150.

Frey, G. C., Temple, V. A., & Stanish, H. I. (2017). Interventions to promote physical activity for youth with intellectual disabilities. *Salud Publica de Mexico, 59*, 437–445.

Giagazoglou, P., Kokaridas, D., Sidiropoulou, M., Patsiaouras, A., Karra, C., & Neofotistou, K. (2013). Effects of a trampoline exercise intervention on motor performance and balance ability of children with intellectual disabilities. *Research in Developmental Disabilities, 34*, 2701–2707.

Haegele, J. A., & Porretta, D. (2015). Physical activity and school-age individuals with visual impairments: A literature review. *Adapted Physical Activity Quarterly, 32*, 68–82.

Imms, C., Adair, B., Keen, D., Ullenhag, A., Rosenbaum, P., & Granlund, M. (2016). Participation: A systematic review of language, definitions, and constructs used in intervention research with children with disabilities. *Developmental Medicine and Child Neurology, 58*, 29–38.

Institute of Medicine [IOM]. (2013). *Educating the student body: Taking physical activity and physical education to school*. Washington, DC: The National Academies Press.

Jung, J., Leung, W., Schram, B. M., & Yun, J. (2018). Meta-analysis of physical activity levels in youth with and without disabilities. *Adapted Physical Activity Quarterly, 35*, 381–402.

Li, R., Sit, C. H. P., Yu, J. J., Duan, J. Z. J., Fan, T. C. M., McKenzie, T. L., & Wong, S. H. S. (2016). Correlates of physical activity in children and adolescents with physical disabilities: A systematic review. *Preventive Medicine, 89*, 184–193.

Li, R., Sit, C. H. P., Yu J. J., Sum, R. K. W., Wong, S. H. S., Cheng, K. C. C., & McKenzie, T. L. (2017). Children with physical disabilities at school and home: Physical activity and contextual characteristics. *International Journal of Environmental Research and Public Health, 14*, 687.

Lobenius-Palmér, K., Sjöqvist, B., Hurtig-Wennlöf, A., & Lundqvist, L. O. (2018). Accelerometer-assessed physical activity and sedentary time in youth with disabilities. *Adapted Physical Activity Quarterly, 35*, 1–19.

Lounsbery, M. A. F., McKenzie, T. L., & Smith, N. J. (2019). School and community policies: Implications for youth physical activity and research. *The Routledge Handbook of Youth Physical Activity. Chapter 11*.

Maïano, C., Hue, O., Morin, A. J. S., Lepage, G., Tracey, D., & Moullec, G. (2019). Exercise interventions to improve balance for young people with intellectual disabilities: A systematic review and meta-analysis. *Developmental Medicine & Child Neurology, 61*, 406–418.

McGarty, A. M., Penpraze, V., & Melville, C. A. (2014). Accelerometer use during field-based physical activity research in children and adolescents with intellectual disabilities: A systematic review. *Research in Developmental Disabilities, 35*, 973–981.

McGarty, A. M., Downs, S., Melville, C. A., & Harris, L. (2018). A systematic review and meta-analysis of interventions to increase physical activity in children and adolescents with intellectual disabilities: Effect of interventions on physical activity. *Journal of Intellectual Disability Research, 62*, 312–329.

McKenzie, T. L. (2010). 2009 C. H. McCloy lecture: Seeing is believing: Observing physical activity and its contexts. *Research Quarterly for Exercise and Sport, 81*, 113–122.

McKenzie, T. L. (2016). Context matters: Systematic observation of place-based physical activity. *Research Quarterly for Exercise and Sport, 87*, 334–341.

McKenzie, T. L. (2019). Physical activity within school contexts: The bigger bang theory. *Kinesiology Review, 8*, 48–53.

McKenzie, T. L., Cohen, D. A., Sehgal, A., Williamson, S., & Golinelli, D. (2006). System for observing play and leisure activity in communities (SOPARC): Reliability and feasibility measures. *Journal of Physical Activity and Health, 1*, S203–S217.

McKenzie, T. L., Sallis, J. F., & Nader, P. R. (1992). SOFIT: System for observing fitness instruction time. *Journal of Teaching in Physical Education, 11*(2), 195–205.

McKenzie, T. L., Sallis, J. F., Rosengard, P. R., & Ballard, K. (2016). The SPARK programs: A public health model of physical education research and dissemination. *Journal of Teaching in Physical Education, 35*, 381–389.

McKenzie, T. L., & Smith, N. J. (2017). Studies of physical education in the United States using SOFIT: A Review. *Research Quarterly for Exercise and Sport, 88*, 492–502.

Najafabadi, M. G., Sheikh, M., Hemayattalab, R., Memari, A.-H., Aderyani, M. R., & Hafizi, S. (2018). The effect of SPARK on social and motor skills of children with autism. *Pediatrics and Neonatology, 59*, 481–487.

National Association for Sport and Physical Education. (2016). *Guide for recess policy*. Reston, VA: National Association for Sport and Physical Education. Retrieved June 30, 2019 from https://www.shapeamerica.org/advocacy/upload/Guide-for-Recess-Policy.pdf

National Centre on Health, Physical Activity and Disability [NCHPAD]. (2018). *Physical activity and sport in youth with a disability*. Retrieved June 30, 2019 from https://www.nchpad.org/fppics/Physical%20Activity%20and%20Sport%20in%20Youth%20with%20Disability_Info%20Brief.pdf

Neter, J. E., Schokker, D. F., de Jong, E., Renders, C. M., Seidell, J. C., & Visscher, T. L. (2011). The prevalence of overweight and obesity and its determinants in children with and without disabilities. *Journal of Pediatrics, 158*, 73599.

Nooijen, C. F. J., de Groot, J. F., Stam, H. J., van den Berg-Emons, R. J. G., Bussmann, H. B. J., & Fit for the Future Consortium. (2014). Validation of an activity monitor for children who are partly or completely wheelchair-dependent. *Journal of Neuroengineering and Rehabilitation, 12*, 11.

Okoro, C. A., Hollis, N. D., Cyrus, A. C., & Griffin-Blake, S. (2018). Prevalence of disabilities and health care access by disability status and type among adults – United States, 2016. *Morbidity and Mortality Weekly Report, 67*, 882–887.

Pan, C. Y., Liu, C. W., Ching, I. C., & Hsu, P. J. (2015). Physical activity levels of adolescents with and without intellectual disabilities during physical education and recess. *Research in Developmental Disabilities, 36*, 579–586.

Pan, C. Y., Tsai, C. L., & Hsieh, K. W. (2011). Physical activity correlates for children with autism spectrum disorders in middle school physical education. *Research Quarterly for Exercise and Sport, 82*, 491–498.

Reedman, S., Boyd, R. N., & Sakzewski, L. (2017). The efficacy of interventions to increase physical activity participation of children with cerebral palsy: A systematic review and meta-analysis. *Developmental Medicine and Child Neurology, 59*, 1011–1018.

Rimmer, J. H., & Marques, A. C. (2012). Physical activity for people with disabilities. *Lancet, 380*, 193–195.

Ross, S. M., Bogart, K. R., Logan, S. W., Case, L., Fine, J., & Thompson, H. (2016). Physical activity participation of disabled children: A systematic review of conceptual and methodological approaches in health research. *Frontiers in Public Health, 4*, 187.

Rosso, E. G. F. (2016). Brief report: Coaching adolescents with autism spectrum disorder in a school-based multi-sport program. *Journal of Autism and Developmental Disorders, 46*, 2526–2531.

Ryan, J. M., Cassidy, E. E., Noorduyn, S. G., & O'Connell, N. E. (2017). Exercise interventions for cerebral palsy. *Cochrane Database Systematic Review, 6*, CD011660.

Shields, N., Synnot, A. J., & Barr, M. (2012). Perceived barriers and facilitators to physical activity for children with disability: A systematic review. *British Journal of Sports Medicine, 46*, 989–997.

Sit, C. H. P., Li, R., McKenzie, T. L., Cerin, E., Wong, S. H. S., Sum, R. K. W., & Leung, F. L. (2019). Physical activity of children with physical disabilities: Associations with environmental and behavioral variables at home and school. *International Journal of Environmental Research and Public Health, 16*, 1394.

Sit, C. H. P., McKenzie, T. L., Cerin, E., Chow, B. C., Huang, W. Y. J., & Yu, J. J. (2017). Physical activity and sedentary time among children with different disabilities at school. *Medicine and Science in Sports and Exercise, 49*, 292–297.

Sit, C. H. P., McKenzie, T. L., Cerin, E., McManus, A. M., & Lian, J. (2013). Physical activity for children in special school environment. *Hong Kong Medical Journal, 19*(4), S42–S44.

Sit, C. H. P., McKenzie, T. L., Lian, J., & McManus, A. (2008). Activity levels during physical education and recess in two special schools for children with mild intellectual disabilities. *Adapted Physical Activity Quarterly, 25*, 249–261.

Sit, C. H. P., McManus, A., McKenzie, T. L., & Lian, J. (2007). Physical activity levels of children in special schools. *Preventive Medicine, 45*, 424–431.

Sit, C. H. P., Yu, J. J., Wong, S. H. S., Capio, C. M., & Masters, R. (2019). A school-based physical activity intervention for children with developmental coordination disorder: A randomized controlled trial. *Research in Developmental Disabilities, 89*, 1–9.

Smith, N. J., McKenzie, T. L., & Hammons, A. J. (2019). International studies of physical education using SOFIT: A review. *Advances in Physical Education, 9*, 53–74.

Stanish, H. I., Curtin, C., Must, A., Phillips, S., Maslin, M., & Bandini, L. G. (2019). Does physical activity differ between youth with and without intellectual disabilities? *Disability and Health Journal, 12*, 503–508.

Strath, S. J., Pfeiffer, K. A., & Whitt-Glover, M. C. (2012). Accelerometer use with children, older adults, and adults with functional limitations. *Medicine and Science in Sports and Exercise, 44*, S77–S85.

Tan, B. W., Pooley, J. A., & Speelman, C. P. (2016). A meta-analytic review of the efficacy of physical exercise interventions on cognition in individuals with autism spectrum disorder and ADHD. *Journal of Autism and Developmental Disorders, 46*, 3126–3143.

Tremblay, M. S., Carson, V., Chaput, J. P., Conner, Gorber, S., Dinh, T., Duggan, M., . . . Janssen, I. (2016). Canadian 24-hour movement guidelines for children and youth: An integration of physical activity, sedentary behaviour, and sleep. *Applied Physiology, Nutrition, and Metabolism, 41*, S311–S327.

Van der Mars, H., & McKenzie, T. L. (2019). Direct observation: Assessing youth physical Activity and its contexts. *The Routledge Handbook of Youth Physical Activity. Chapter 14.*

Wallén, E. F., Müllersdorf, M., Christensson, K., & Marcus, C. (2012). A school-based intervention associated with improvements in cardiometabolic risk profiles in young people with intellectual disabilities. *Journal of Intellectual Disabilities, 17*, 38–50.

World Health Organization [WHO]. (2001). *International classification of functioning, disability and health: ICF.* Geneva, Switzerland: World Health Organization.

World Health Organization [WHO]. (2011b). *World report on disability.* Geneva, Switzerland: World Health Organization. Retrieved January 30, 2019 from http://whqlibdoc.who.int/publications/2011/9789240685215_eng.pdf

World Health Organization [WHO]. (2018). *Global action plan on physical activity 2018–2030: More active people for a healthier world.* Geneva, Switzerland: World Health Organization.

Wouters, M., Evenhuis, H. M., & Hilgenkamp, T. I. M. (2019). Physical activity levels of children and adolescents with moderate-to-severe intellectual disability. *Journal of Applied Research in Intellectual Disabilities, 32*, 131–142.

Wu, W. L., Yang, Y. F., Chu, I. H., Hsu, H. T., Tsai, F. H., & Liang, J. M. (2017). Effectiveness of a cross-circuit exercise training program in improving the fitness of overweight or obese adolescents with intellectual disability enrolled in special education schools. *Research in Developmental Disabilities, 60*, 83–95.

Zwinkels, M., Verschuren, O., Balemans, A., Lankhorst, K., Te Velde, S., van Gaalen, L., . . . Takken, T. (2018). Effects of a school-based sports program on physical fitness, physical activity, and cardiometabolic health in youth with physical disabilities: Data from the Sport-2-Stay-Fit study. *Frontiers in Paediatrics, 6*, 75.

PART 8

Family and Community Interventions

30

PHYSICAL ACTIVITY INTERVENTIONS FOR YOUNG PEOPLE AND THEIR PARENTS

Amy S. Ha, Johan Y. Y. Ng, Joni H. Zhang, and Wai Chan

Introduction

Parents are an important agent of behavior change for young children. They could promote or inhibit physical activity (PA) participation of their children. Positive parental behaviors may be conducive to children's PA behaviors (e.g., parental socialization, role modeling, parental support; Mitchell et al., 2012; Pugliese & Tinsley, 2007; Yao & Rhodes, 2015). For example, parental support was found to explain more than 25% variance of child's light or moderate-to-virgorous PA (MVPA) (Rhodes, Stearns et al., 2019). On the contrary, a parent's own barriers to PA could also translate to their children (Wiseman, Patel, Dwyer, & Nebeling, 2018), such as lack of time or motivation in parents, or low availability of facilities (Bellows-Riecken & Rhodes, 2008; Ha, Chan, & Ng, Under Review; Mailey, Huberty, Dinkel, & McAuley, 2014; Rhodes & Lim, 2018). These barriers also discouraged parents to provide more support to children (Jarvis, Harrington, & Manson, 2017). Parental perception of PA facilities weighted even more to child PA outcomes than child's perception (Horodyska et al., 2018). Recent studies using accelerometer devices demonstrated that mothers and their young children shared similarly low PA and high sedentary levels (Barkin et al., 2017; Dlugonski, DuBose, & Rider, 2017; Hnatiuk, DeDecker, Hesketh, & Cardon, 2017).

To counteract low activity levels, family- or home-based intervention programs were designed with an intended goal of increasing children's PA. Nonetheless, these interventions were not as well represented in literature as compared to those programs based on school or childcare settings (e.g., 3 reviews on family/home setting versus 32 reviews on school/childcare setting; Messing et al., 2019). Indeed, most PA intervention programs for young children aged 0–5 were implemented in preschool/childcare settings instead of others (Hnatiuk et al., 2019). Nevertheless, family-based intervention seemed promising with 66% of 47 reviewed studies finding a positive impact on PA levels of children (Brown et al., 2016). For obesity prevention programs in preschool, both parents and children participants should be actively involved for higher effectiveness (Ling, Robbins, & Wen, 2016). Given the importance of parent involvements in PA intervention to young children or adolescents, this chapter serves to provide an additional overview of recent relevant studies, including intervention programs with evidence-supported efficacy and effectiveness, as well as ongoing and promising ones with innovative features that deserved to be highlighted. A few recommendations will hence be presented.

Overview of the Literature

For interventions that have targeted both parents or did not specify a parent, it is frequently observed that mothers tend to be the contact person (Rhodes, Naylor, & McKay, 2010) and participation rates of mothers tend to be higher (Chen, Weiss, Heyman, & Lustig, 2009; Nyberg, Norman, Sundblom, Zeebari, & Elinder, 2016). For interventions designed to include only the primary caregiver, mothers are also often assumed to be the program target (Chen et al., 2009). Despite the dominance of mothers in PA interventions, there were only a few intervention programs targeted specifically at mothers and their children. Furthermore, findings on sex relations (e.g., mother-based versus father-based) in the area of PA interventions have been inconsistent and speculative. The examination of whether sex is a factor in parent-child PA behaviors can be separated into two broad categories: (1) difference by parent sex and (2) differences by child sex. The differences between the categories should be understood and treated cautiously when researchers want to better understand how child sex, parent sex, and the interaction between the two may impact children's PA levels and intervention effectiveness.

A thorough examination of sex relations in parent-child relationships is beyond the scope of this chapter. More details on this topic can be found in Gustafson and Rhodes (2006). In this chapter, we are especially interested in looking at research-based interventions that have specifically targeted mother-child relationships, with an overarching aim to elicit what might be some effective strategies to conducting mother-based PA interventions.

The literature for parent-child PA interventions is dominated by either *mother-daughter* or *father-son* interventions. It is not yet known whether or not targeting specifically mother-daughter relationships would be more beneficial than targeting other relationships. Therefore, in this chapter, we reviewed the literature on all mother-based PA interventions. Eventually, this chapter also calls into question: are mother-based interventions really effective for increasing PA in children?

Parent-Based PA Interventions

It has been argued that mothers, women, and girls are at higher risk to be inactive when compared to fathers, men, and boys (Bellows-Riecken & Rhodes, 2008; Scharff, Homan, Kreuter, & Brennan, 1999). Example reasons for mothers' and women's inactivity include conflict with child-care responsibilities, role conflict (e.g., working female and housewife), and lack of confidence or knowledge in performing PA (Lewis & Ridge, 2005). Moreover, from a slightly more social perspective, there is evidence that mothers' and women's decision-making about PA is heavily influenced and shaped by their multiple roles (Lewis & Ridge, 2005; Reczek, Beth Thomeer, Lodge, Umberson, & Underhill, 2014). Even so, no consistent evidence was showed for differences on mother's versus father's influences on child's PA levels (Neshteruk, Nezami, Nino-Tapias, Davison, & Ward, 2017).

Studies have documented that children's PA levels decrease as they move through adolescence, and this trend was found to be particularly alarming in girls (Kimm et al., 2002; McKenzie et al., 2006; Sallis, Prochaska, & Taylor, 2000). For example, data from the 2010 to 2011 Youth Risk Behavior Surveillance System recorded that the percentage of girls that had not participated in at least 60 minutes of PA within a 7-day period steadily increased from 9th grade (13.9%) to 12th grade (20.6%), whereas the percentage of boys only increased from 8.7% to 10.8% during the same period of time (Eaton et al., 2012). In terms of the prevalence of meeting PA guidelines (i.e., 60 minutes MVPA per day), the percentage of girls decreased steadily from 9th grade (44.5%) to 12th grade (32.0%), whereas the percentage of boys only decreased from 52.9% to 44.8% during the same period of time. Moreover, it has been repeatedly reported that girls exhibit lower levels of fitness than boys (Sallis et al., 2000; World Health Organization, 2014).

It is worth noting that physical education (PE) is believed to be a venue to conduct evidence-based interventions to address the dramatic decline in PA among youth. However, PE-related research has consistently reported that female students are significantly less active and engaged during PE lesson time than their male counterparts (McKenzie et al., 2006; Troiano et al., 2008). Although these interventions can be effective in terms of in-lesson PA, there is insufficient evidence that such effects can extend beyond school PE.

Taken together, the evidence presented in this section suggests that there are definitely compelling reasons why we need to pay more attention to mothers-based programs, and population-specific interventions designed exclusively for them may be impactful.

Mother-Daughter Interventions

We begin this section by first reviewing existing mother-daughter interventions. Although there are several such studies, this area of research is still at its infancy. Unanimous conclusions cannot be drawn due to the lack of high-quality randomized controlled trials (RCTs; Barnes et al., 2018), but we believe it is still useful to unite existing studies so that we can elicit useful elements to aid the design of future studies. In this section, we take on a narrative approach with an aim to identify common elements and strategies that appear to be effective. The section will be further divided into three parts: (1) the Physical Activity and Nutrition in Children (PANIC; Venäläinen et al., 2016; Viitasalo et al., 2016; N = 506 children at baseline) study; (2) Iranian Mother/Daughter Dyadic Study in the Childhood and Adolescence Surveillance and Prevention of Adult Non-communicable disease (CASPIAN I; Ahadi et al., 2014; Kargarfard et al., 2012; N = 206 children) study; and (3) other parent- or mother-based PA interventions. The PANIC program was first selected for discussion because it gives insight into the process of integrating PA components to a larger public health intervention program with a very large reach of participants. On the other hand, the CASPIAN was selected for discussion because it is one of the most recent successful mother-daughter PA studies, and it reported excellent participation and retention rates. Lastly, other mother-based PA interventions are discussed to provide a general panorama on the topic.

PANIC study (Venäläinen et al., 2016; Viitasalo et al., 2016)

The PANIC study program was a two-arm controlled, parallel matched group intervention study conducted in the city of Kuopio, Finland. It ran for 2 years. It was designed for children aged 6–8 years. Recruitment was based on 16 out of all 26 primary schools in the region. Over the course of 1.5 years, the children and parent participants in the experiment group received a total of 6 individualized PA counseling and 6 dietary counseling sessions (on 0.5, 1.5, 3, 6, 12, 18 months after baseline). Each session was 30–45 minutes long with a specific topic of PA or nutrition (e.g., how to raise total PA with a great variety of exercises, and how to reduce sedentary behaviors). One of the program highlights was financial support for PA, e.g., sport equipment and tickets for indoor sports. Fact sheets were also provided to parents and their children about exercise opportunities in the region. Parents and their children from the control group received advice on verbal and written information on health.

PA of children was assessed by a questionnaire validated with a monitor integrating both heart rate and accelerometry measures (i.e., Actiheart monitor; Väistö et al., 2014). Types, duration, levels of PA, and sedentary behaviors were extensively documented (e.g., organized sport, unsupervised PA, PA during recess). Based on linear mixed modeling results, an increase in total PA and unsupervised PA from the treatment group was significant, and a decrease in screen-based sedentary behaviors in the treatment group was also observed. The program succeeded in promoting PA levels in children.

Multiple program features are noteworthy in this intervention. First, it had a longer treatment duration (i.e., approximately18 months) than most intervention programs which ran only for several weeks, but its dosage was relatively mild with only six sessions on PA-related topics throughout the treatment. The interval of each session was sparsely spread out, e.g., with up to 6 months at most in between. The effectiveness was still noticeable at follow-up measurement, 6 months after the last session. This suggests that sessions at an irregular interval might be effective, being more flexible or less demanding on participants. Then, the program allowed room for choices of PA participation by offering sport equipment and tickets for sports instead of requiring attendances on regular PA sessions at a specified location. These may somehow help maintain the treatment effect and avoid program aversion, a backfire issue usually observed in programs in school setting (e.g., Demetriou & Höner, 2012). More importantly, individualized advice was offered to parents and their children at each PA counseling, even though the session was just 45 minutes at most. These techniques may be particularly meaningful to those families who were in need for personalized help with health management or PA development.

Iranian Mother/Daughter Dyadic Study (CASPIAN I; Kargarfard et al., 2012)

This study employed a two-arm, parallel non-randomized controlled design, and was part of a national program in Iran. Its subsample was specified to target physical co-activity among mother-daughter dyads, like after-school PA program (Kargarfard et al., 2012). It was designed for adolescent girls from grades 7 to 10, and their mothers. In order to be eligible for the treatment, participants should have engaged in not more than two PA sessions each week or have any health conditions preventing them from PA. The program consisted of 24 sessions on a school site, each for 90 minutes and twice a week. Each session offered the fitness-focused activity (lasted for 60 minutes) and nutrition education or counseling (approximately 30 minutes). The activity sessions included sport play (e.g., basketball) and structured group aerobic (e.g., Salsa dance). All sessions were delivered by female coaches. Effort was maximized to keep participants from modifying their diets by monitoring their dietary records so that the treatment effect could be mostly attributed to the PA components. The same protocol applied to the control group in which no mothers were recruited (i.e., daughters only).

Outcome measures included multiple indicators for fitness performance, e.g., cardiorespiratory fitness (1-minute walk), upper and abdominal muscular strength and endurance, and hamstring flexibility. Other physiological data was also collected, e.g., body mass index (BMI). Using ANOVA with the baseline scores as covariates, the mother and daughter treatment group demonstrated a larger improvement in flexibility, aerobic capacity and fitness, and abdominal muscle strength and endurance than the daughters-only control group. However, there was no significant improvement in the BMI outcome in daughters. For the mothers from the treatment group, they demonstrated significant improvement in all outcomes at posttreatment, e.g., BMI, 1-minute walk, upper and abdominal muscle strength, and endurance. To note, Kargarfard et al.'s study (2012) demonstrated evidence for a parent-based PA program. The PA sessions were served as one of the core components of CASPIAN I study and paved a foundation of subsequent stages of the larger CASPIAN study.

Various program characteristics provided us with insights. First, the program was well designed by being culturally sensitive to the study participants. Kargarfard et al. (2012) acknowledged the social norms in the Middle East where outdoor exercises were not common to females so the PA intervention program was arranged at school sites and only female coaches were allowed in the activity sessions. That might account for the full attendance rates in the first month of the program and higher than 96% in the second month for both treatment and control groups. Then,

Kargarfard et al. (2012) was one of the first studies that yielded empirical support for the improvement of parents in which the PA intervention program primarily targeted at children. Those findings on mothers suggested a varying degree of feasibility and benefits of physical co-activity intervention program between parents and children.

Other Mother-Based PA Interventions

A recent systematic review on mother and daughter PA interventions documented 14 studies and focused on 4 outcome measures (e.g., PA, fitness, nutrition, and adiposity; Barnes et al., 2018). Only a half of these studies were RCTs ($n = 7$). Most programs were delivered in the community setting (e.g., after-school activity sessions, summer camp, home-based program). The findings suggested that no more than one fifth of theses intervention programs were effective, leaving the success of mother and daughter interventions in doubt. This was partly due to lack of consistently valid and objective measures or high-quality RCTs (Barnes et al., 2018). Therefore, the following sections would start a discussion on more recent (2018 or onward) parent- or mother-based intervention programs using RCT and objective valid measures (e.g., accelerometers) in order to gain more insights for future studies.

Mothers And dauGhters daNcing togEther Trial (MAGNET; Alhassan et al., 2018; Burkart, Laurent, & Alhassan, 2017)

Alhassan and colleagues (2018) reported a culturally tailored mother-daughter PA activity intervention for African Americans ($n = 76$ dyads). Daughters aged between 7 and 10 years were eligible for the study. It was a three-arm parallel group RCT (i.e., daughters and mothers, daughter only, control comparison). It was primarily a dance intervention program, given that the focus group data revealed that dance was a format of PA appealing to this ethnic minority in Springfield, Massachusetts (Alhassan, Greever, Nwaokelemeh, Mendoza, & Barr-Anderson, 2014). The program ran for 12 weeks, with 3 weekly sessions. Each session consisted of an hour of dance activity lesson and 2 hours of nutrition educational session. Participants across groups received a weekly newsletter. Daughters from the wait list control group were required to attend the nutrition educational session and to receive the dance curriculum after the daughters and mothers group. The daughters-only group was also offered the curriculum after the treatment group.

The outcome measures were based on ActiGraph accelerometers. Activities at all intensities and sedentary behaviors were recorded with the device. Percent time spent on each of these activities were modeled as outcomes. BMI data was also collected. Based on the linear mixed model analyses supplement by ANOVA, the program demonstrated some effectiveness. Daughters from the treatment group demonstrated a larger increase in MVPA than those girls in the daughters-only group during the period of dance intervention time. They also had a greater rise in vigorous PA during after-school intervention time. However, no similar pattern was observed in the total daily PA. Besides, mothers from the treatment group displayed a larger increase in total daily PA than those mothers from the daughters-only group.

The MAGNET study demonstrated several program features worthwhile our attention. First, the dance curriculum was developed as culturally sensitive to African-American culture and the self-efficacy development (i.e., interests in cultural dance). Then, this intervention exemplified the dance curriculum as an intergenerational activity shared by daughters and mothers in the form of PA (Burkart et al., 2017). Even though the mothers' well-being were not systematically measured, their enjoyment of the dance with the daughters was reported in the process evaluation (Burkart et al., 2017). In other words, these mothers and daughter PA intervention might yield both physical and psychological benefits to participants.

Family PA Planning Study (Rhodes, Blanchard, Quinian, Naylor, & Warburton, 2019; Rhodes et al., 2010; Quinlan, Rhodes, Blanchard, Naylor, & Warburton, 2015)

It was a two-arm parallel RCT. aiming at children aged 6–12 years and being physically inactive during the past 3 months. Eligible children and their parents were randomized to either a standard information condition with planning curriculum or the control comparison group which had the standard information only. The standard information included Canadian PA guidelines (e.g., a recommendation of 60 minutes of PA every day), while an adapted information booklet was added to the intervention, which underscored PA benefits and practical advices for staying physically active. Also, a set of family PA planning materials and workbook was provided to the intervention group, for example, instructions on "what", "when", "where", and "how" PA could be engaged. Post-intervention measurement was conducted at 6 weeks, 3 months, and 6 months after the delivery of program materials.

Child outcome measures included MVPA and fitness performance (e.g., aerobic fitness, flexibility, and muscular strength). Based on the accelerometry data, MVPA of children from the treatment group (i.e., information and family PA planning) improved more than the control group only at 6 weeks and 3 months. However, such treatment effect was diminished 6 months after the intervention (Rhodes, Blanchard et al., 2019).

Even though this intervention program produced a short-term efficacy in child outcomes, its program design was noteworthy. First, unlike most PA interventions, it was merely a provision of educational and planning materials, suggesting that parental cognition and belief may serve as a feasible starting point with regard to PA behavioral changes. Then, the findings posed an implication to policy making with the information distribution related to health benefits accrued by PA that family planning was indispensable to result in an improvement in PA. In other words, pure PA information dissemination was merely a necessary but not yet a sufficient condition for an increase in PA.

Guiding Theories

In this section, common theoretical frameworks are listed and a brief discussion is provided for the two most popular theories in PA interventions. It is well known that PA interventions are more effective when constructed based on theoretical frameworks. Frequently cited theoretical frameworks in PA interventions include the Health Belief Model (HBM; Rosenstock, 1974), Social Cognitive Theory (SCT; Bandura, 1998, 2004), Transtheoretical Model (TTM; Prochaska, Johnson, & Lee, 2009), Theory of Planned Behavior (TPB; Ajzen, 1991), Self-Determination Theory (SDT; Deci & Ryan, 2000), Protection Motivation Theory (PMT; Rogers, 1983), and Health Action Process Approach (HAPA; Schwarzer, 2016).

Bandura's SCT has been extensively used to aid the development, implementation, and evaluation of family-based intervention. The SCT is well suited for explaining behaviors and behavior change in a family setting because its constructs cover individual, social, and environmental factors in a holistic manner. According to SCT, individual (e.g., self-efficacy), social (e.g., parent and child interaction), and environmental factors (e.g., availability of sport equipment) interact with each other and may mediate behavior change (Bandura, 1986; Baranowski, Cullen, Nicklas, Thompson & Baranowski, 2003). The theory points out that when one of these factors change, it is likely that the others will change, and therefore when interventions target all three factors, it is more likely that the intended change in behavior (e.g., increased PA level) will occur.

The MAGNET program designed its intervention components based on the SCT. It has thoroughly attempted to operationalize the three major constructs of the theory including self-efficacy, social support, and outcome expectations. For example, the program provided participants with skill-based exercise sessions to help them increase self-efficacy for performing exercise-related activities, and incorporated positive role modeling (e.g., by parents, instructors). However as mentioned, the program was not successful in changing children's PA levels. On the other hand, it has been highlighted that SCT-framed school-based interventions have demonstrated consistent success in increasing children's PA in the context of PE lessons (Wilson et al., 2008). Further research in increasing children's PA outside of school contexts is therefore warranted.

Another frequently cited theoretical framework in PA interventions is self-determination theory (SDT; Ryan & Deci, 2002). SDT argues that human will act effectively and become motivated when the three inherent basic psychological needs (i.e., competence, autonomy, and relatedness) are fulfilled (Ryan & Deci, 2002). Competence refers to the sense of having the opportunities and also the ability to perform a task effectively. Autonomy refers to a sense of volition and willingness, and perceived choice towards the behavior. Relatedness refers to a sense of belongingness and support within a social group. Basic need satisfaction plays an important role in supporting individuals' adaptive motivation, as well as their physical and psychological well-being (Ng et al., 2012). It is well supported that interventions designed based on SDT constructs have a positive effect on autonomous motivation for PA (Ryan & Deci, 2017; Teixeira, Carraça, Markland, Silva, & Ryan, 2012). For example, in the study by Ha, Ng, Lonsdale, Lubans, and Ng (2019), intervention components were specifically designed to support participants' competence by strengthening children's and parents' fundamental movement skills in a need supportive manner. Autonomy was supported through fun games and guiding participants to create new games. Intervention activities were also designed to increase parent-child interaction, and participants were also constantly reminded to provide encouragements to one another. These behaviors were likely to support participants' need for relatedness. It is worth noting that this intervention was not designed specifically for mother-based interventions, but generally for parents of any roles. Nonetheless, the principles or techniques should be equally effective for mother-specific programs.

Recently, researchers have also applied the behavior change wheel (Michie, van Stralen, & West, 2011) framework on mother-based PA interventions. The framework was proposed by Michie et al. (2011), stating that when designing interventions, the capability (physical and psychological), opportunity (social and physical), and motivation (automatic and reflective) regarding the behavior should be considered. The framework also includes nine specific intervention functions (e.g., education and persuasion) and seven policy categories (e.g., guidelines and environmental/social planning) to guide intervention design. Recently, a study by Murtagh, Barnes, McMulen, and Morgan (2018) applied the framework in designing a mother-daughter intervention, by selecting specific functions (e.g., education and incentivization) and applying behavior change techniques (e.g., goals and planning, and feedback and monitoring). Despite the results of the intervention are not yet available, this framework had been applied to other behavior change programs and may serve as a systematic structure for family-based PA intervention design.

Key Issues

Who?

The quality of program facilitators can have a direct and large impact on adherence rates. This section aims to summarize the recommended attributes that a program facilitator should possess, especially facilitators be directly responsible for the delivery of lessons and activity sessions. Who should deliver the lessons or activity sessions? In reality, it is possible that individuals of different backgrounds would be involved, such as school teachers, PE teachers, researchers, and coaches. Therefore, rather than restricting the discussion to the type of persons (e.g., qualified coaches), we wish to list out the recommended attributes that we believe these individuals should have.

What?

What might be the most effective program components? Common components of interventions include tutoring, after-school classes, activity classes, counseling services, and some interventions were delivered online. It has been reported that activities such as dancing and yoga were more popular among mothers and daughters (Barnes et al., 2018). However, this does not imply researchers should naturally assume these activities are always preferred by mothers and children. In fact, the key constructs within the theories applied may be operationalized differently for specific target groups. One relevant grouping in this context would be the sex and ages of the children. The preference in terms of activity choice or the approaches being used may differ greatly between boys and girls, or children of different ages. Co-design approaches (e.g., Ha et al., 2019; Thabrew, Fleming, Hetrick, & Merry, 2018), such as the inclusion of focus groups interviews during intervention design phases, may be considered to ensure the designed interventions are relevant and appropriate.

Researchers should also make an effort to ensure the fidelity of the interventions, or at least have methods to capture whether, or to what extent, intervention components were delivered or adhered to as intended. This will not be an easy feat as many of the intervention activities take place outside the direct observation of researchers. The use of technology in intervention provision can be seen as a double-sided sword. When used well, technology could help researchers accurate track the dosage (e.g., time spent on viewing videos) and contents of the interactions. By contrast, the ease of self-initiation could also mean that the actual intervention received for each participant would become more diversified. This heterogeneity may reduce the power to detect real changes that were brought about by the intervention. Therefore, process evaluation should become a necessity in future intervention research. This is particularly important considering the infancy of this line of research.

Where?

Interventions targeting specifically mothers and children were mostly delivered using face-to-face interactions in small groups and group sessions. Common settings include community-based, school-based, home-based, or a combination of these settings. More interventions have combined mothers and children during delivery; for example, mothers and children would attend group activity classes together. However, it should be noted that mothers and their children may have different preferences. For example, an intervention process evaluation study reported that girls preferred activity lessons to be held at schools, while mothers reported that they did not mind as long as it was convenient (Barnes et al., 2018). We therefore strongly advise researchers to conduct focus groups to collect mothers' and children's opinions and account for potential differences between mothers and daughters. It is generally assumed that school-based interventions should be delivered in schools, or community-based interventions should be delivered at community centers. However, researchers should not feel restricted to such approaches, it is certainly worthwhile for researchers to take a step back and consider what might be some other venues or settings that would be appropriate and favorable for mothers and daughters. In our current and previous projects, we learnt that mothers preferred to take part in lessons, activities, and events at schools because it was convenient for them to do so after dropping off or picking up their child.

Conclusions

Although there exist limited numbers of mother-based intervention studies and the topic has not been extensively studied, it appears that at least findings on recruitment strategies and strategies to achieve favorable participation and adherence rates are reasonably well supported by unanimous evidence (e.g., the importance of having high-quality female facilitators). However, it is intriguing that the existing programs seem to be more successful in changing mothers' PA and maternal beliefs than daughters. Future studies on the current topic are therefore required to elucidate what needs to be done to improve the situation with daughters (or girls in general). We acknowledge that the prospect of being able to improve mothers' conditions with mother-based interventions serves as a continuous stimulus for further development in this regard. However, this current trend has thrown up at least one important question: are mother-based interventions really the way to go for increasing PA in children?

In conclusion, we discussed the current status quo of mother-based PA interventions in this chapter. Although the number of studies are limited, we united a number of studies to elicit the good practices and areas where further research is warranted. Topics such as challenges in implementation and scalability issues have not been discussed for mother-based PA intervention in this chapter because we feel that mother-based PA interventions have not been extensively studied. More sex-specific studies (e.g., mother-daughter and mother-son) may also be needed to elicit the different dynamics and interactions between such designs. Nonetheless, the main research question should still be the following: are mother-based interventions really effective for increasing PA in children? This is a vital issue for future research.

References

Ahadi, Z., Shafiee, G., Qorbani, M., Sajedinejad, S., Kelishadi, R., Arzaghi, S. M., . . . Heshmat, R. (2014). An overview on the successes, challenges and future perspective of a national school-based surveillance program: The CASPIAN study. *Journal of Diabetes & Metabolic Disorders, 13*, 120. doi:10.1186/s40200-014-0120-3

Alhassan, S., Greever, C., Nwaokelemeh, O., Mendoza, A., & Barr-Anderson, D. J. (2014). Facilitators, barriers, and components of a culturally-tailored afterschool physical activity program in preadolescent African-American girls and their mothers. *Ethnicity & Disease, 24*(1), 8.

Alhassan, S., Nwaokelemeh, O., Greever, C. J., Burkart, S., Ahmadi, M., St. Laurent, C. W., & Barr-Anderson, D. J. (2018). Effect of a culturally-tailored mother-daughter physical activity intervention on pre-adolescent African-American girls' physical activity levels. *Preventive Medicine Reports, 11*, 7–14. doi:10.1016/j.pmedr.2018.05.009

Baranowski, T., Cullen, K. W., Nicklas, T., Thompson, D., & Baranowski, J. (2003). Are current health behavioral change models helpful in guiding prevention of weight gain efforts? *Obesity Research, 11*(S10), 23S–43S.

Barkin, S. L., Lamichhane, A. P., Banda, J. A., JaKa, M. M., Buchowski, M. S., Evenson, K. R., . . . Stevens, J. (2017). Parent's physical activity associated with preschooler activity in underserved populations. *American Journal of Preventive Medicine, 52*, 424–432. doi:10.1016/j.amepre.2016.11.017

Bandura, A. (1986). The explanatory and predictive scope of self-efficacy theory. *Journal of Social and Clinical Psychology, 4*(3), 359–373.

Bandura, A. (1998). Health promotion from the perspective of social cognitive theory. *Psychology and Health, 13*(4), 623–649.

Bandura, A. (2004). Health promotion by social cognitive means. *Health Education & Behavior, 31*, 143–164.

Barnes, A. T., Young, M. D., Murtagh, E. M., Collins, C. E., Plotnikoff, R. C., & Morgan, P. J. (2018). Effectiveness of mother and daughter interventions targeting physical activity, fitness, nutrition and adiposity: A systematic review. *Preventive Medicine, 111*, 55–66. doi:10.1016/j.ypmed.2017.12.033

Bellows-Riecken, K. H., & Rhodes, R. E. (2008). A birth of inactivity? A review of physical activity and parenthood. *Preventive Medicine, 46*, 99–110. doi:10.1016/j.ypmed.2007.08.003

Brown, H. E., Atkin, A. J., Panter, J., Wong, G., Chinapaw, M. J. M., & van Sluijs, E. M. F. (2016). Family-based interventions to increase physical activity in children: A systematic review, meta-analysis and realist synthesis. *Obesity Reviews, 17*, 345–360. doi:10.1111/obr.12362

Burkart, S., St. Laurent, C. W., & Alhassan, S. (2017). Process evaluation of a culturally-tailored physical activity intervention in African-American mother-daughter dyads. *Preventive Medicine Reports, 8*, 88–32. doi:10.1016/j.pmedr.2017.08.002

Chen, J.-L., Weiss, S., Heyman, M. B., & Lustig, R. H. (2009). Efficacy of a child-centred and family-based program in promoting healthy weight and healthy behaviors in Chinese American children: A randomized controlled study. *Journal of Public Health, 32*(2), 219–229.

Demetriou, Y., & Höner, O. (2012). Physical activity interventions in the school setting: A systematic review. *Psychology of Sport and Exercise, 13*(2), 186–196.

Dlugonski, D., DuBose, K. D., & Rider, P. (2017). Accelerometer-measured patterns of shared physical activity among mother-young child dyads. *Journal of Physical Activity and Health, 14*, 808–814. doi:10.1123/jpah.2017-0028

Eaton, D. K., Kann, L., Kinchen, S., Shanklin, S., Flint, K. H., Hawkins, J., . . . Chyen, D. (2012). Youth risk behavior surveillance – United States, 2011. *Morbidity and Mortality Weekly Report: Surveillance Summaries, 61*(4), 1–162.

Gustafson, S. L., & Rhodes, R. E. (2006). Parental correlates of physical activity in children and early adolescents. *Sports Medicine, 36*(1), 79–97.

Ha, A. S., Chan, W., & Ng, Y. (Under Review). *Barriers to physical activity of parents and its correlates: A latent profile analysis.*

Ha, A. S., Ng, J. Y. Y., Lonsdale, C., Lubans, D., & Ng, F. F. (2019). Promoting physical activity in children through family-based intervention: Protocol of the "Active 1+FUN" randomized controlled trial. *BMC Public Health, 19*, 218. doi:10.1186/s12889-019-6537-3

Hnatiuk, J. A., Brown, H. E., Downing, K. L., Hinkley, T., Salmon, J., & Hesketh, K. D. (2019). Interventions to increase physical activity in children 0–5 years old: A systematic review, meta-analysis and realist synthesis. *Obesity Reviews, 20*, 75–87. doi:10.1111/obr.12763

Hnatiuk, J. A., DeDecker, E., Hesketh, K. D., & Cardon, G. (2017). Maternal-child co-participation in physical activity-related behaviours: Prevalence and cross-sectional associations with mothers and children's objectively assessed physical activity levels. *BMC Public Health, 17*, 506. doi:10.1186/s12889-017-4418-1

Horodyska, K., Boberska, M., Knoll, N., Scholz, U., Radtke, T., Liszewska, N., & Luszczynska, A. (2018). What matters, parental or child perceptions of physical activity facilities? A prospective parent-child study explaining physical activity and body fat among children. *Psychology of Sport and Exercise, 34*, 39–46.

Jarvis, J. W., Harrington, D. W., & Manson, H. (2017). Exploring parent-reported barriers to supporting their child's health behaviors: A cross-sectional study. *International Journal of Behavioral Nutrition and Physical Activity, 14*, 77–87. doi:10.1186/s12966-017-0508-9

Kargarfard, M., Kelishadi, R., Ziaee, V., Ardalan, G., Halabchi, F., Mazaheri, R., . . . Hayatbakhsh, M. R. (2012). The impact of an after-school physical activity program on health-related fitness of mother/daughter pairs: CASPIAN study. *Preventive Medicine, 54*(3–4), 219–223.

Kimm, S. Y., Glynn, N. W., Kriska, A. M., Barton, B. A., Kronsberg, S. S., Daniels, S. R., . . . Liu, K. (2002). Decline in physical activity in black girls and white girls during adolescence. *New England Journal of Medicine, 347*(10), 709–715.

Lewis, B., & Ridge, D. (2005). Mothers reframing physical activity: Family oriented politicism, transgression and contested expertise in Australia. *Social Science & Medicine, 60*(10), 2295–2306.

Ling, J., Robbins, L. B., & Wen, F. (2016). Interventions to prevent and manage overweight or obesity in preschool children: A systematic review. *International Journal of Nursing Studies, 53*, 270–289. doi:10.1016/j.ijnurstu.2015.10.017

Mailey, E. L., Huberty, J., Dinkel, D., & McAuley, E. (2014). Physical activity barriers and facilitators among working mothers and fathers. *BMC Public Health, 14*, 657. doi:10.1186/1471-2458-14-657

Mckenzie, T. L., Catellier, D. J., Conway, T., Lytle, L. A., Grieser, M., Webber, L. A., . . . Elder, J. P. (2006). Girls' activity levels and lesson contexts in middle school PE: TAAG baseline. *Medicine and Science in Sports and Exercise, 38*(7), 1229–1235.

Messing, S., Rütten, A., Abu-Omar, K., Ungerer-Röhrich, U., Goodwin, L., Burlacu, I., & Gediga, G. (2019). How can physical activity be promoted among children and adolescents? A systematic review of reviews across settings. *Frontiers in Public Health, 7*, 55. doi:10.3389/fpubh.2019.00055

Michie, S., van Stralen, M. M., & West, R. (2011). The behaviour change wheel: A new method for characterising and designing behaviour change interventions. *Implementation Science, 6*, 42. doi:10.1186/1748-5908-6-42

Mitchell, J., Skouteris, H., McCabe, M., Ricciardelli, L. A., Milgrom, J., Baur, L. A., . . . Dwyer, G. (2012). Physical activity in young children: A systematic review of parental influences. *Early Child Development and Care, 182*, 1411–1437. doi:10.1080/03004430.2011.619658

Murtagh, E. M., Barnes, A. T., McMullen, J., & Morgan, P. J. (2018). Mothers and teenage daughters walking to health: Using the behaviour change wheel to develop an intervention to improve adolescent girls' physical activity. *Public Health, 158*, 37–46. doi:10.1016/j.puhe.2018.01.012

Neshteruk, C. D., Nezami, B. T., Nino-Tapias, G., Davison, K. K., & Ward, D. S. (2017). The influence of fathers on children's physical activity: A review of the literature from 2009–2015. *Preventive Medicine, 102*, 12–19. doi:10.1016/j.ypmed.2017.06.027

Ng, J. Y. Y., Ntoumanis, N., Thøgersen-Ntoumani, C., Deci, E. L., Ryan, R. M., Duda, J., & Williams, G. C. (2012). Self-determination theory applied to health contexts: A meta-analysis. *Perspectives on Psychological Science, 7*(4), 325–340. doi:10.1177/1745691612447309

Nyberg, G., Norman, Å., Sundblom, E., Zeebari, Z., & Elinder, L. S. (2016). Effectiveness of a universal parental support programme to promote health behaviours and prevent overweight and obesity in 6-year-old children in disadvantaged areas, the Healthy School Start Study II, a cluster-randomised controlled trial. *International Journal of Behavioral Nutrition and Physical Activity, 13*(1), 4.

Prochaska, J. O., Johnson, S., & Lee, P. (2009). The transtheoretical model of behavior change. In S. A. Shumaker, J. K. Ockene & K. A. Riekert (Eds), *The handbook of health behavior change* (pp. 59–83). New York: Springer Publishing Company.

Pugliese, J.& Tinsley, B. (2007). Parental socialization of child and adolescent physical activity: A meta-analysis. *Journal of Family Psychology, 21*, 331–343. doi: 10.1037/0893-3200.21.3.331

Quinlan, A., Rhodes, R. E., Blanchard, C. M., Naylor, P.-J., & Warburton, D. E. R. (2015). Family planning to promote physical activity: A randomized controlled trial protocal. *BMC Public Health, 15*, 1011. doi:10.1186/s12889-015-2309-x

Reczek, C., Beth Thomeer, M., Lodge, A. C., Umberson, D., & Underhill, M. (2014). Diet and exercise in parenthood: A social control perspective. *Journal of Marriage and Family, 76*(5), 1047–1062.

Rhodes, R. E., Blanchard, C. M., Quinlan, A., Naylor, P.-J., & Warburton, D. E. R. (2019). Family physical activity planning and child physical activity outcomes: A randomized trial. *American Journal of Preventive Medicine.* Advance online publication. doi:10.1016/j.amepre.2019.03.007

Rhodes, R. E., & Lim, C. (2018). Promoting parent and child physical activity together: Elicitation of potential intervention targets and preferences. *Health Education & Behavior, 45*, 112–123. doi:10.1177/1090198117704266 10.1177/10

Rhodes, R. E., Naylor, P.-J., & McKay, H. A. (2010). Pilot study of a family physical activity planning intervention among parents and their children. *Journal of Behavioral Medicine, 33*(2), 91–100.

Rhodes, R. E., Stearns, J., Berry, T., Faulkner, G., Latimer-Cheung, A., O'Reilly, N., . . . Spence, J. C. (2019). Predicting parental support and parental perceptions of child and youth movement behaviors. *Psychology of Sport & Exercise, 41*, 80–90. doi:10.1016/j.psychsport.2018.11.016

Rogers, R. W. (1983). Cognitive and psychological processes in fear appeals and attitude change: A revised theory of protection motivation. In J. T. Cacioppo & E. P. Richard (Eds), *Social Psychophysiology: A Sourcebook* (pp. 153–176). New York: Guilford Press

Rosenstock, I. M. (1974). The health belief model and preventive health behavior. *Health Education Monographs, 2*(4), 354–386.

Ryan, R. M., & Deci, E. L. (2002). Overview of self-determination theory: An organismic-dialectical perspective. In E. L. Deci & R. M. Ryan (Eds.), *Handbook of self-determination research*. Rochester, NY: The University of Rochester Press.

Ryan, R. M., & Deci, E. L. (2017). *Self-determination theory: Basic psychological needs in motivation, development, and wellness.* New York, NY: Guilford Publications.

Sallis, J. F., Prochaska, J. J., & Taylor, W. C. (2000). A review of correlates of physical activity of children and adolescents. *Medicine and Science in Sports and Exercise, 32*(5), 963–975.

Scharff, D. P., Homan, S., Kreuter, M., & Brennan, L. (1999). Factors associated with physical activity in women across the life span: Implications for program development. *Women & Health, 29*(2), 115–134.

Schwarzer, R. (2016). Health Action Process Approach (HAPA) as a theoretical framework to understand behavior change. *Actualidades en Psicología, 30*(121), 119–130.

Teixeira, P. J., Carraça, E. V., Markland, D., Silva, M. N., & Ryan, R. M. (2012). Exercise, physical activity, and self-determination theory: A systematic review. *International Journal of Behavioral Nutrition and Physical Activity, 9*(1), 78.

Thabrew, H., Fleming, T., Hetrick, S., & Merry, S. (2018). Co-design of eHealth interventions with children and young people. *Frontiers in Psychiatry, 9*, 481. doi:10.3389/fpsyt.2018.00481

Troiano, R. P., Berrigan, D., Dodd, K. W., Masse, L. C., Tilert, T., & McDowell, M. (2008). Physical activity in the United States measured by accelerometer. *Medicine & Science in Sports & Exercise, 40*(1), 181–188.

Väistö, J., Eloranta, A. M., Viitasalo, A., Tompuri, T., Lintu, N., Karjalainen, P., . . . Lindi, V. (2014). Physical activity and sedentary behaviour in relation to cardiometabolic risk in children: cross-sectional findings from the Physical Activity and Nutrition in Children (PANIC) Study. *International Journal of Behavioral Nutrition and Physical Activity, 11*(1), 55.

Venäläinen, T. M., Viitasalo, A. M., Schwab, U. S., Eloranta, A.-M., Haapala, E. A., Jalkanen, H. P., . . . Lakka, T. A. (2016). Effect of a 2-y dietary and physical activity intervention on plasma fatty acid composition and estimated desaturase and elongase activities in children: The physical activity and nurition in children study. *American Journal of Clinical Nutrition, 104*, 964–972. doi:10.3945/ ajcn.116.136580

Viitasalo, A., Eloranta, A.-M., Lintu, N., Väistö, J., Venäläinen, T., Kiiskinen, S., . . . Lakka, T. A. (2016). The effects of a 2-year individualized and family-based lifestyle intervention on physical activity, sedentary behavior and diet in children. *Preventive Medicine, 87*, 81–88. doi:10.1016/j.ypmed.2016.02.027

Wilson, D. K., Kitzman-Ulrich, H., Williams, J. E., Saunders, R., Griffin, S., Pate, R., . . . Addy, C. L. (2008). An overview of "the active by choice today" (ACT) trial for increasing physical activity. *Contemporary Clinical Trials, 29*(1), 21–31.

Wiseman, K. P., Patel, M., Dwyer, L. A., & Nebeling, L. C. (2018). Perceived weight and barriers to physical activity in parent–adolescent dyads. *Health Psychology, 37*, 767–774. doi:10.1037/hea0000635

World Health Organization. (2014). *Global status report on noncommunicable diseases 2014.* Retrieved from https://apps.who.int/iris/bitstream/handle/10665/148114/9789241564854_eng.pdf

Yao, C. A., & Rhodes, R. E. (2015). Parental correlates in child and adolescent physical activity: A meta-analysis. *International Journal of Behavioral Nutrition and Physical Activity, 12*(1), 10. doi:10.1186/ s12966-015-0163-y

31

THE ROLE OF FATHERS IN OPTIMIZING CHILDREN'S PHYSICAL ACTIVITY

Philip J. Morgan, Myles D. Young, and Emma R. Pollock

Introduction

Parents have a major influence on the physical activity levels of their children. This influence operates through a host of mechanisms, including their own behaviors (e.g. physical activity modelling), attitudinal disposition (e.g. attitudes toward physical activity), and parenting practices (e.g. logistic support) (Edwardson & Gorely, 2010). In this sense, parents are not just role models, but 'gatekeepers' to their children's physical activity opportunities and experiences (Gustafson & Rhodes, 2006).

Given the global issue of physical inactivity in both children and adults, the number of studies evaluating the impact of family-based interventions to improve children's physical activity levels has been increasing significantly (Brown et al., 2016). However, the impact of these programs has been modest and the quality of studies has been questionable (Brown et al, 2016). While it is widely acknowledged that parents should be involved in interventions to improve children's physical activity levels, there is a lack of agreement regarding the most effective strategies to use and the optimal nature of parental involvement.

Although both parents play a key role in promoting their children's physical activity levels, a growing body of evidence indicates that the role of fathers may be particularly important (Morgan & Young, 2017). Despite this, there has been a pervasive lack of father engagement in family-based physical activity studies (Davison et al., 2016; Morgan et al., 2017). A review of 667 observational studies on parenting and childhood obesity-related behaviors (including physical activity) found that fathers represented only 17% of parents (Davison et al., 2016). Further, only 10% of studies reported any father-specific data (Davison et al., 2016). In a systematic review examining 213 randomized controlled trials (RCTs) of family-based programs targeting children's lifestyle behaviors, fathers represented only 6% of parents (Morgan et al., 2017). Moreover, only two trials (1%) reported using strategies to increase father engagement and only four (2%) acknowledged lack of fathers as a study limitation. Father representation was not moderated by any study factors (e.g. targeted behavior, program mode or setting, child age group).

The challenge of engaging fathers has also been reported in other fields of pediatric research including psychology (Phares, Fields, & Binitie, 2006), chronic illness treatment (Taylor, Fredericks, Janisse, & Cousino, 2019), adolescent drug prevention (Thornton et al., 2018), and parenting programs in general (Panter-Brick et al., 2014). This is likely due to the historical nature of mothers as primary caretakers with fathers spending greater time in paid employment and less time in child care (Baxter & Smart, 2011). However, as the labor force has changed, there has been a corresponding shift in traditional parenting roles. Fathers now spend more time with their children than ever before (Yogman, Garfield, & the Committee on Psychosocial Aspects of Child and Family Health, 2016). As such, it is an opportune time for researchers to specifically target fathers in the next wave of family-based physical activity research.

Overview of the Literature

The Important Role of Fathers

To better understand how fathers contribute to their children's physical activity behavior, it is important to appreciate the varied roles that fathers may assume within families. As parents, providers, and partners, fathers play multiple social, economic and/or emotional roles in families (Lamb, 2010). In addition to the amount of father-child interaction, the nature of father involvement also includes their degree of warmth-responsiveness and control (e.g. in terms of monitoring and decision-making affecting their children) (Pleck, 2010b). There is strong longitudinal evidence for the positive influence of engaged fathers on children's social, behavioral, emotional, and cognitive outcomes (Sarkadi, Kristiansson, Oberklaid, & Bremberg, 2008; Yogman et al., 2016). Indeed, father involvement and father-child closeness are strong predictors of children's long-term psychosocial health (Lamb & Lewis, 2010).

Positive father involvement enhances children's growth and development through both direct and indirect mechanisms (Lamb & Lewis, 2010). Fathers influence their children directly through their own behavior and attitudes, which are particularly important when different to mothers. Fathers also indirectly influence their children through family dynamics and how they affect other family members (e.g. the level of emotional and instrumental support they provide to mothers) (Lamb & Lewis, 2010). In a seminal text book on the role of fathers, Lamb (2010) proposed that this indirect pattern of influence is as important, if not more important, than any direct effect. This understanding is based on the premise that fathers and their children are components of complex social systems. In this instance, the social system is the family, and each family member influences the other reciprocally, directly, and indirectly. Fathers thereby influence their children by engaging with them, but they also influence mothers' behaviors and involvement (as do mothers influence fathers) and children influence their parents (Lamb & Lewis, 2010). This concept is well-illustrated in the Family Systems Theory, which postulates that the family is a complex and interactive social system where all members' needs and experiences affect the others (Golan & Weizman, 2001).

Of note, recent fathering research purports that many 'established' behavioral differences between mothers and fathers may not be as widespread as previous thought (Pleck, 2010a). In essence, the evidence for an independent influence of fathers has been debated. For example, while Jeynes (2016) meta-analysis indicated that fathers do have an independent impact on their children's social, psychological, and academic outcomes, Pleck (2010a) argued gender differences between parents are of little significance to children and that children are no better off psychologically if they have more 'masculine' fathers. While acknowledging the complexity of concepts of fatherhood and masculinity, Pleck argued that good fathering is one of a number of aspects that optimizes child development, but is not "essential, unique or specifically masculine" (p. 13).

However, children do seem to benefit from having parents with different personalities, particularly in family contexts where parents are satisfied with their marriage and caretaking arrangements (Lamb, 2010). Exposing children to greater diversity and more stimulating involvement from two parents also prevents them from developing sex-stereotyped attitudes about male and female roles (Lamb, 2010). This evidence suggests that having 'differentiated' parents may be the key to stimulating child development in most areas, rather than a specific and unique father influence. Indeed, Bourçois (1997) showed that, in dual-parent families, children from involved and differentiated parents (with distinct functions such as caregiver versus playmate) often have better social skills and are better prepared for competition and cooperation than those with involved but undifferentiated parents (Paquette, 2004). This indicates that children may develop relationships with their parents through different dimensions of parenting, and that mothers and fathers may interact with their children in different, but complementary ways.

Importantly, the suggestion that positive fathering and masculinity are independent constructs does not minimize the reality that fathers have a major influence on their children (Lamb, 2010). Fathers' influences on children are often statistically independent of mothers' and account for unique variance beyond that explained by mothers. However, the nature of fathers' effects appear to be the same as mothers, rather than distinct from them (Pleck, 2010a). Indeed, Lamb (2010) suggests that fathers and mothers appear to impact on their children in similar (as opposed to dissimilar) ways. That is, warmth, closeness, and nurturance are keys for children's development, and these parental characteristics may be more important than gender-related characteristics. Notably, one exception to this argument may be physical activity parenting, where behavioral differences between mothers and fathers are more clear-cut and may represent a unique and independent feature of the father-child relationship.

The Importance of Father-Child Co-Physical Activity

While parental support is a consistent correlate of child physical activity (Trost & Loprinzi, 2011), research suggests that mothers are more often involved in logistic support (e.g. providing transport to sporting practice), whereas fathers are much more likely to offer verbal encouragement and co-participate in physical activity with their children (Lamb, 2010; Zahra, Sebire, & Jago, 2015). While fathers generally spend less time with their children than mothers, they are much more likely to spend this time engaged in physical play (Craig, 2006; Lindsey, Mize, & Pettit, 1997). The nature of this physical play is another common difference between fathers and mothers. Fathers typically engage in a type of play described as physical, vigorous, stimulating, risky, boisterous, emotionally arousing, competitive, unpredictable, and fun compared to mothers who prefer quiet activities that permit calmness (Paquette, 2004). Examples of common father-child play include rough and tumble play (RTP; e.g. play wrestling), practicing sports skills together, and participating in imaginary play and physical challenges.

Of interest, this form of play begins very early in a child's life (Fletcher, May, St George, Morgan, & Lubans, 2011; Lamb & Lewis, 2010). Fathers typically play more often with their infants than mothers and in a far more vigorous and physical manner (Pleck, 2010a). They are also more likely to demonstrate more energetic touch and movement of infants' limbs and do more bouncing and lifting (Power & Parke, 1983). These patterns of engagement have also been observed in preschool and primary school populations. For example, in a study of preschoolers which examined the difference between child-mother and child-father play interactions, mothers tended to structure, guide, and engage in empathetic conversations, while fathers engaged in physical play, acted like they were the same age as their children, followed the child's lead, and challenged the children (John, Halliburton, & Humphrey, 2013).

Paquette (2004) described the tendency for fathers to 'excite, surprise and momentarily destabilize children' (p. 193) as a key ingredient for nurturing an emotional bond he called the father-child 'activation relationship'. This relationship develops primarily through physical play (Paquette, 2004) and has been acknowledged as a core context where fathers bond with their children (Harrington, 2006). In this way, father-child co-physical activity may lead to a whole range of holistic benefits for children. Other than the obvious physical health benefits, father-child co-physical activity has been reported to enhance the quality of the father-child relationship (Lamb, 2010) and children's social-emotional well-being (Fletcher et al., 2011; Lindsey, Cremeens, & Caldera, 2010; Paquette, 2004). Studies have also shown strong associations with play and attachment security (Newland, Coyl, & Freeman, 2008).

These findings are quite robust and demonstrate that it is not just that fathers and mothers tend to play differently, but that play is a very important aspect to the father-child relationship. This appears to be an international phenonmena and common across cultures and countries (Lamb & Lewis, 2010). Indeed, father playfulness may make them seem particularly salient to children, which may enhance fathers' influence relative to the time they spend with children (Lamb, 2010). As this type of play leads to positive responses from children, studies have shown they may prefer to play with fathers when they have the choice (Lamb & Lewis, 2010). Fathers also tend to report greater satisfaction in more active pursuits with their young children, thus, it is mutually gratifying. Importantly, while this style of play can also be actioned by mothers, it is generally more likely to be initiated, enjoyed, repeated, and sustained by fathers. As such, mothers have described fathers as the family's 'physical activity leaders' who are generally responsible for engaging children in sports and physical activities at home and in the community, and are more likely to initiate and facilitate co-physical activity at home (Zahra et al., 2015).

Overall, the evidence suggests that co-participation in physical activity is very influential and salient as it enables fathers and their children to enjoy activities together, foster more meaningful relationships, and increase enjoyment of relatively small amounts of time spent together. These bonds that are forged during these interactions are likely to yield significant physical and psychological impacts for the entirety of their children's lives. While clearly this is an area in need of further investigation (Kwon, Janz, Letuchy, Burns, & Levy, 2016), the potential effect mechanisms regarding father-child co-participation in physical activity may be explained by this 'activation relationship'.

Paternal Influences on Children's Physical Activity Levels

Emerging observational and longitudinal data suggest that fathers' behaviors, beliefs, and parenting practices play an important role in promoting children's physical activity. However, due to low father response rates and a predominance of small, cross-sectional studies with ungeneralizable samples, scholars have been unable to answer the important questions of how this influence operates and in which subgroups, contexts, and conditions it is most important (Davison et al., 2016; Neshteruk, Nezami, Nino-Tapias, Davison, & Ward, 2017). For example, a recent review of the influence of fathers on child physical activity (Neshteruk et al., 2017) found that only 52% of father-child physical activity associations were significant and positive. Given the lack of high-quality studies and the significant variation in the way physical activity was measured, the authors highlighted the need for further studies to elucidate the specific ways in which fathers influence children's physical activity.

A major limitation of the field is most studies combine data from both parents. Without considering the potential independent influence of fathers and mothers, it may be that unique associations between father and child physical activity levels have been suppressed. To illustrate the point, a review of environmental correlates of child physical activity highlighted that, while no associations in parent-child activity were found in studies with combined parental data, father physical activity was significantly associated with child physical activity in 52% of cases where maternal/paternal data were separated (Ferreira et al., 2007). In contrast, maternal physical activity levels were largely unrelated to child physical activity.

Although the understanding of paternal influence on child physical activity is somewhat limited, strong data are available to suggest that father-child co-physical activity is an important factor. For example, a large study including more than 10,000 children identified that the amount of time fathers spent playing with their children significantly predicted child physical activity levels (Beets & Foley, 2008). Further, the influence of fathers has also been found to be longitudinally associated with sporting participation in young people from low socio-economic areas (Kwon et al., 2016).

A potential mechanism explaining this effect could be the vigorous and stimulating playstyle that fathers often exhibit, which may be more likely to increase children's physical fitness and strength. Active play is an important aspect of child development and challenges children to use their bodies in a way that expends energy and/or utilizes their strength (Paquette, Bolté, Turcotte, Dubeau, & Bouchard, 2000). When fathers engage with their children in active play, this also provides opportunities for physical activity modeling and health-enhancing levels of moderate-to-vigorous intensity physical activity. This higher intensity physical activity provides an opportunity for children to develop both aerobic and muscular fitness.

Another potential mechanism for improved child physical activity levels from father-child play is that fathers often seek to help or teach children fundamental movement skills (FMS) and other sports-specific skills and tactics. That is, father-child co-physical activity becomes a context for educational and coaching opportunities (Rhodes & Lim, 2018). Of interest, a recent review identified a positive association between parent motor skill confidence and child motor skill ability (Barnett et al., 2016). While it was unclear whether this effect was moderated by parent sex, it is likely that fathers would report greater motor skill confidence than mothers due to the increased opportunities and reinforcement boys and men receive to practice these skills throughout life (Hallal et al., 2012; Telford, Telford, Olive, Cochrane, & Davey, 2016; Trost et al., 2002). The important role that fathers play in improving their children's sporting ability is noteworthy given the strong association between FMS proficiency and physical activity (Lubans, Morgan, Cliff, Barnett, & Okely, 2010).

A much loved and unique type of father-child play that has both physical and psycho-social health benefits in children is RTP. Pellegrini and Smith (1998) described RTP as a variant of physical activity play involving vigorous "wrestling, grappling, kicking, and tumbling that would appear to be aggressive except for the playful context" (p. 579). Smith (2010) described the characteristics of RTP to include positive facial expressions (play face, laughter, smile), self-restraint, role-reversal, invitation as initiation, and togetherness at the end of play. RTP is one of the most frequent forms of physical play between father and child (Paquette, 2004). High-quality father-child RTP is characterized by being highly enjoyable for the child, and should involve the use of moderate control on the father's part to allow a reciprocal exchange of 'dominant' and 'subordinate' roles during the physical play (Paquette, 2004).

Extensive animal research, particularly in rats and monkeys, has laid the foundation for the study of RTP in humans. It has provided a model to understand the organization, development, and neural controls that regulate this form of play. Noteworthy components of animal play fighting that have been identified as similar to human RTP include self-handicapping against smaller opponents and alternating between offensive and defensive roles (Boulton, 1991; Boulton & Smith, 1992). These unique patterns of play require independence, tactics, and varying bodily configurations, and have been linked to different neural mechanisms that influence cognitive, emotional, and social competency in animals (Von Frijtag, Schot, van den Bos, & Spruijt, 2002). Rodent studies have found that depriving rats from play fighting impairs the ability to coordinate bodily movements against an opponent (Pellis, Field, & Whishaw, 1999) and can lead to deficiencies in parts of the lower brain stem which are associated with social interaction (e.g. rule learning, recognizing social partners) (Bell, McCaffrey, Forgie, Kolb, & Pellis, 2009; Van den Berg et al., 1999). Given the parallels between RTP in humans and animals, an emerging area of research has been how RTP may impact on child development.

Studies of father-child RTP have shown that participation begins in small amounts before 1 year, peaks in the preschool years, and reduces after 10 years of age (MacDonald & Parke, 1986). Boys typically receive more physical play from their fathers than girls (St George & Freeman, 2017), and fathers may do less RTP when the mother/partner is present (Goldberg, Clarke-Stewart, Rice, & Dellis, 2002). The excitement and arousal of the physical interaction (which may or may not include play fighting but also tickling, wrestling, swinging in the air) may be the mechanism for the social-emotional and physical benefits of RTP for children. For example, studies have demonstrated that affective touch can impact positively on heart rate, blood pressure, cortisol, and oxytocin (Field, 2010). A recent review and meta-analyses demonstrated that RTP is positively associated with several important child behavioral domains, including social competence, emotional skills, and self-regulation (St George & Freeman, 2017). Regardless of the type of assessment, child social competence, child self-regulation, and emotional skills (e.g. emotional encoding and decoding) were shown to be significantly positively associated with both quantity and quality attributes of father-child RTP. Along with the physical and social-emotional benefits, parents have also identified RTP as a key interaction strategy to strengthen the father-child relationship (St George, Goodwin, & Fletcher, 2018).

Co-Physical Activity with Sons and Daughters

Boys generally receive more parent support and physical activity facilitation than girls (Gustafson & Rhodes, 2006). From age 1, it has been found that fathers spend less time in co-physical activity with daughters than sons (Lee et al., 2010; Zahra et al., 2015). For example, Lindsey and Mize (2001) have demonstrated that mothers spend more time in pretend play with their daughters, whereas fathers specialize in physical play with their sons and this predicts that type of play with peers. This may in fact explain recent findings from two cross-sectional studies that demonstrated positive associations between fathers' moderate-to-vigorous physical activity and that of their sons but not with their daughters (Bringolf-Isler, Schindler, Kayser, Suggs, & Probst-Hensch, 2018; Brouwer et al., 2018). There has been limited studies examining the potential moderating effect of child sex on fathers' physical activity parenting practices (Neshteruk et al., 2017) and thus should be explored further in future research.

Fathers also struggle to motivate daughters to participate in co-physical activity with them (Rhodes & Lim, 2018). This also minimizes girls' opportunities for physical activity, sports skill development, and bonding with their fathers, a gap which only widens in adolescence (Lamb & Lewis, 2010). However, an interesting qualitative study demonstrated that when fathers do engage in co-physical activity with their daughters, these experiences are often cherished by both parties for life (Barrett & Morman, 2013).

Physical Activity and the Transition to Fatherhood

Becoming a father is commonly described as joyful and fulfilling, but it also is associated with a number of new challenges, which can have an adverse impact on men's physical and psychological health (Durette, Marrs, & Gray, 2011; Garfield, Clark-Kauffman, & Davis, 2006). In particular, researchers have observed a distinct decline in the activity levels of men during early fatherhood. Low levels of physical activity are common among parents (Bellows-Reicken & Rhodes, 2008) and are largely attributed to numerous barriers including family responsibilities busy schedules, guilt, lack of social support, and work commitments (Mailey, Huberty, Dinkel, & McAuley, 2014). While these barriers may affect both mothers and fathers, fathers tend to experience a greater decrease in physical activity.

This greater decrease has been explained by the sex differences in leisure-time physical activity between men and women before children are born (Hallal et al., 2012). Compared to men without children, fathers participate in significantly fewer minutes of moderate-to-vigorous physical activity per week, are less likely to meet physical activity recommendations, and are less likely to play sport (Hull et al., 2010; Pot & Keizer, 2016). These lower physical activity levels are of concern given the powerful protective effect of physical activity on physical and mental health (Lee et al., 2012; Mammen & Faulkner, 2013) and the potential flow-on effects for their children's well-being. Those fathers who maintain physical activity levels report newfound enjoyment from family-based physical activity and a greater desire to be a positive role model for their families (Mailey et al., 2014).

Father-Focused Physical Activity Interventions

Fathers face multiple unique barriers to maintaining or increasing their physical activity levels. In this context, targeted interventions for fathers may be particularly timely and important because (i) both fathers and children are not sufficiently active (Kohl et al., 2012), (ii) fathers are more naturally inclined to participate in and enjoy physical activity with their children, and (iii) the influential relationship between father and child physical activity is likely bi-directional (Neshteruk et al., 2017). Thus, interventions targeting father-child co-physical activity may be particularly beneficial for both groups and may have the potential to improve broader family health outcomes (Pot & Keizer, 2016).

A recent systematic review of father involvement in family-based lifestyle programs (Morgan et al., 2017) revealed 19 interventions that explicitly targeted mothers only. While it is possible that these interventions could have a ripple effect on fathers' behavior, there is little evidence to support this notion, suggesting more direct targeting is required (Walsh et al., 2014). In contrast, the review identified only one intervention that specifically targeted fathers – the *Healthy Dads Healthy Kids (HDHK)* program (Morgan et al., 2011), which was published by our research group at the University of Newcastle. Since this review, we have also published results from the *Dads And Daughters Exercising and Empowered (DADEE)* study (Morgan, Young, Barnes, et al., 2019; Young et al., 2019), which appears to be the only RCT that has tested a father-daughter intervention in any field. Evidence for the programs has been demonstrated in pilot RCTs (Morgan et al., 2011; Morgan, Young, Barnes, et al., 2019), community RCTs (Morgan et al., 2014), and dissemination trials (Morgan et al., 2019). Importantly, positive intervention outcomes were sustained beyond post-intervention assessments for most key outcomes, and program satisfaction, retention, and attendance have been very high across all trials.

At the time of writing, we are unaware of other published RCTs that have targeted physical activity behavior specifically in fathers and children. As such, the following section will feature an overview of key insights gained from our work, which may have utility for researchers and practitioners. The following discussion will focus on the physical activity components of the interventions.

Overview of 'Healthy Dads, Healthy Kids' and 'Dads And Daughters Exercising and Empowered'

The HDHK and DADEE programs started as 8-week interventions and have since increased to include 9×90 min weekly sessions. The programs include both educational and practical sessions each week plus home tasks that target the behavior change constructs from Social Cognitive Theory (e.g. self-efficacy, goals, social support) (Bandura, 1986). DADEE also operationalizes Self-Determination Theory variables (i.e., autonomy, competence, relatedness) (Deci & Ryan, 1985). Both programs are based on extensive formative work including quantitative (e.g. process evaluation) and qualitative (e.g. focus groups and interviews) studies with both fathers and mothers (Barnes, Plotnikoff, Collins, & Morgan, 2015; Morgan, Young, Smith, & Lubans, 2016). For a summary of key program details for the HDHK and DADEE programs, see Tables 31.1 and 31.2, respectively.

Table 31.1 Characteristics of the Healthy Dads Healthy Kids trials

Characteristics	HDHK pilot RCT	HDHK community RCT	HDHK dissemination trial
Study characteristics			
Year	2008–2009	2010–2011	2011–2012
Study design	Randomized controlled trial	Randomized controlled trial	Non-randomized, prospective trial
Number of programs	1 × intervention group, 1 × wait-list	2 × intervention groups, 2 × wait-list	10 × intervention groups
Study location(s)	Callaghan, NSW	Maitland and Singleton, NSW	Maitland, Singleton, Muswellbrook, and Cessnock, NSW
Father exclusion criteria			
BMI outside range (25–40 kg/m²)	✓	✓	✓ (≥25 kg/m² only)
Outside age range (18–65 years)	✓	✓	–
Did not live with children	✓	✓	–
Fail pre-exercise screener	✓	✓[a]	✓[a]
Recent weight loss (≥4.5 kg)	✓	✓	–
Involved in other weight loss program	✓	✓	–
No internet access	✓	✓	–
Major health issue (e.g. diabetes)	✓	✓[a]	✓[a]
Child exclusion criteria			
Outside age range (5–12 years)	✓	✓	✓ (4–12 years)
Extreme obesity (BMI-z > 4)	✓	–	–
Assessments	Baseline, 3 and 6 months	Baseline and 3 months	Baseline, 3, 6 and 12 months
Publications			
Primary outcomes	Morgan et al. (2011)	Morgan et al. (2014)	Morgan et al. (2019)
Secondary outcomes	Burrows et al. (2012), Lubans et al. (2012)	Lloyd, Lubans, Plotnikoff, and Morgan (2014), Lloyd et al. (2015), Williams et al. (2018)	–
Program characteristics			
Facilitators	Research team	Trained, local facilitators	Trained, local facilitators
Number and duration of sessions			
Fathers only	5 × 75 minutes	4 × 90 minutes	4 × 90 minutes
Fathers and children	3 × 75 minutes	3 × 90 minutes	4 × 90 minutes
Total	8 × 75 minutes	7 × 90 minutes	8 × 90 minutes
Program delivery site	University of Newcastle	Local schools	Local schools
Sample characteristics			
Participants	53 fathers, 71 children	93 fathers, 132 children	189 fathers, 306 children

Characteristics	HDHK pilot RCT	HDHK community RCT	HDHK dissemination trial
Socio-economic status (quintiles)[b]			
1 (Most disadvantaged)	2%	0%	19%
2	9%	3%	17%
3	42%	35%	57%
4	36%	61%	7%
5 (Most advantaged)	11%	0%	0%

Notes

a These exclusion criteria could be bypassed if the participant provided a doctor's clearance to participate.

b Socio-economic status was determined by cross-referencing postcodes of residence with the Australian Socio-Economic Index For Areas (SEIFA) database (Relative Socio-Economic Advantage and Disadvantage). Percentages may not sum to 100 due to rounding.

Table 31.2 Characteristics of the 'Dads And Daughters Exercising and Empowered' (DADEE) trials

Characteristics	DADEE pilot RCT	DADEE community RCT	DADEE dissemination trial
Study characteristics			
Year	2015	2016	2017–2019
Study design	Randomized controlled trial	Randomized controlled trial	Non-randomized, prospective trial
Number of programs	4 (2 × intervention groups, 2 × wait-list)	7 (4 × intervention groups, 3 × wait-list)	Trial ongoing
Study location(s)	Callaghan, NSW	Carrington, Mayfield East, and Stockton, NSW	Carrington, Mayfield East, Hamilton, and Hamilton South, NSW
Father exclusion criteria			
Outside age range (18–65 years)	✓	✓	✓
Did not live with children ≥3 days/week	✓	✓	–
Fail pre-exercise screener	✓[a]	✓[a]	✓[a]
Major health issue (e.g. diabetes)	✓[a]	✓[a]	✓[a]
Did not have a daughter (4–12 years)	✓	✓	✓
Child exclusion criteria			
Outside age range (4–12 years)	✓	✓	✓
Assessments	Baseline, 2 and 9 months	Baseline and 3 months	Baseline, 3 and 12 months
Publications			
Primary outcomes	Morgan, Young, Barnes, et al. (2019)	In preparation	Trial ongoing
Secondary outcomes	Young et al. (2019)	In preparation	Trial ongoing
Program characteristics			
Facilitators	Research team	Trained, local facilitators	Trained, local facilitators

(Continued)

Characteristics	*DADEE pilot RCT*	*DADEE community RCT*	*DADEE dissemination trial*
Number and duration of sessions			
Fathers and daughters	8 × 90 minutes	9 × 90 minutes	9 × 90 minutes
Program delivery site	University of Newcastle	Local schools	Local schools
Sample characteristics			
Participants	115 fathers, 153 daughters	158 fathers, 193 daughters	Trial ongoing
Socio-economic status (quintiles)[b]			
1 (Most disadvantaged)	0%	0%	Trial ongoing
2	24%	23%	
3	42%	40%	
4	17%	22%	
5 (Most advantaged)	17%	15%	

Notes

a These exclusion criteria could be bypassed if the participant provided a doctor's clearance to participate.

b Socio-economic status was determined by cross-referencing postcodes of residence with the Australian Socio-Economic Index For Areas (SEIFA) database (Relative Socio-Economic Advantage and Disadvantage).

While both programs have unique elements, they have similar goals to educate fathers and optimize children's lifestyle behaviors. Both are face-to-face group programs that engage fathers as agents of change to improve their own health and the health of their children through evidence-based parenting strategies. Importantly, the programs also engage children to become healthy role models to influence their fathers. Aside from physical activity promotion, the HDHK program also focuses on weight management and nutrition, and includes both sons and daughters. In contrast, the DADEE program only includes fathers and daughters and has a unique focus on optimizing girls' social-emotional well-being. The DADEE program also redefines gender norms in relation to physical activity, develops girls' critical thinking skills, and encourages fathers to become gender equity advocates.

The structure of both programs is the same (15-minute education session with fathers and children together; 30-minute education sessions for fathers and children separately, and then a combined 45-minute practical session). The education sessions for fathers include evidence-based parenting tips to increase children's physical activity, fitness, and sport skills, and provide fathers with strategies to optimize their own physical activity levels. Importantly, the sessions focus on 'how to teach' sports skills and strategies to make physical activity with their children more enjoyable, and reinforce the unique role of fathers in this parenting domain. The practical session is identical for both programs and engages fathers and children in fun, co-physical activities targeting RTP, FMS, and aerobic and muscular fitness. Co-physical activity and sport skills are also a core focus of the home-based tasks.

Of particular importance, both programs are socio-culturally tailored to appeal specifically to fathers, which is hypothesized to optimize their engagement in interventions. That is, the preferences, attributes, values, and motivators of fathers are integrated into the programs' recruitment methods, content, format (i.e., setting and mode of delivery), facilitator selection, and pedagogy (i.e., teaching strategies) (for a summary of this tailoring process, see Morgan et al., 2016). This is important as many men and fathers believe that personal- or family-based physical activity programs are designed for females and mothers (Morgan et al., 2017; Robertson et al., 2014).

Data from several RCTs indicate that both HDHK (Morgan et al., 2011, 2014) and DADEE (Morgan, Young, Barnes, et al., 2019) significantly improved objectively measured physical activity levels in fathers and children at post-intervention and longer-term follow-up assessments, represented by medium to large effect sizes. These effects were observed in the HDHK pilot RCT (delivered by the research team), the HDHK community RCT (delivered by trained facilitators in rural areas with high rates of mining and shift-work employment), and a 12-month dissemination trial, which included ten programs delivered by trained facilitators across a range of underserved communities.

In a pilot RCT, the 8-week DADEE program increased objectively measured physical activity levels at 9 months by approximately 1,000–2,000 steps/day in intervention daughters and fathers, respectively, compared to a control group. While modest, these improvements represent an important change from the usual decline in physical activity experienced at this age for girls (Hallal et al., 2012). There were sustained intervention effects for numerous associated outcomes including daughters' FMS proficiency, fathers' and daughters' screen-time, and several physical activity parenting constructs and co-physical activity (Morgan, Young, Barnes, et al., 2019). Significant intervention effects were also detected for the daughters' social-emotional well-being and the quality of the father-daughter relationship (Young et al., 2019). These findings are noteworthy given that most parent-child co-physical activity interventions have been unsuccessful (Rhodes & Lim, 2018). The program is now being evaluated in a community effectiveness RCT and a dissemination trial.

Potential Mechanisms of Effect

Although RCTs provide the highest level of evidence to establish whether a program has been effective, other forms of analyses are needed to provide insights into *how* a program has (or has not) worked. Of interest, a mediation analysis of the HDHK community RCT determined that, while the program impacted on both parental modeling of physical activity and co-physical activity, only co-physical activity acted as a substantive mediator of children's physical activity improvements (representing approximately 60% of the overall intervention effect) (Lloyd, Lubans, Plotnikoff, & Morgan, 2015). In addition to mediation analyses, qualitative data can also provide important insights. For example, in a qualitative study with families who participated in the HDHK program, two consistent themes that emerged from independent focus groups with fathers, mothers, and children were that participation in HDHK: (i) strengthened relationships between fathers and children, and (ii) improved family cohesiveness as a whole.

The DADEE studies have also examined the holistic benefits of father-daughter co-physical activity by investigating whether improvements in this outcome significantly mediated the intervention's positive effects on girls' well-being in several domains (Morgan, Young, Lubans, et al., 2018). This analysis indicated that, in addition to acting as a mediator of girls' physical activity behavior, father-daughter co-physical activity also mediated the program's impact on the girls' social-emotional well-being and the quality of the father-daughter relationship from both the fathers' and daughters' perspectives (Morgan, P.J., Young, M.D., Lubans, D.R., Barnes, A.T., Eather, N., & Pollock, E.R., 2018). These findings highlight the importance of fathers actively participating in physical activity with their daughters and the range of holistic benefits this can have for girls' physical, social, and emotional development.

Although this study only considered the quantity of father-daughter co-physical activity, emerging evidence also indicates that the quality of these interactions may play a key role. In HDHK and DADEE, the program activities maximize opportunities for moving, laughing, talking, and learning, and fathers are encouraged to participate in fun, novel, one-on-one co-physical activity experiences with their children, giving them their complete attention. These 'enhanced' co-physical activities may result in superior outcomes for some children compared to more basic co-physical activities (e.g. simply passing a ball back and forth) that may not be as enticing to participate in for some children. This hypothesis requires empirical validation in future research.

Recommendations for Researchers/Practitioners

Through working on the HDHK and DADEE studies, we have gained a number of experiential insights relating to recruiting and engaging fathers in family-based physical activity interventions. As such, the following section contains a series of recommendations for both researchers and practitioners looking to increase the representation of fathers in their research studies or programs. For interested readers, additional insights have also been published elsewhere alongside a conceptual model that highlights several strategies to enhance the socio-cultural relevance of physical activity interventions in both design and delivery (Morgan et al., 2016).

Recruiting Fathers

Recruitment for physical activity programs can be challenging, particularly when targeting men and fathers. To increase the response rate of fathers through recruitment materials, it is essential to explicitly highlight/mention fathers. Research shows that mothers and fathers commonly assume the term 'parent' is interchangeable with mother when viewing recruitment material (Burgess, 2006). It may also be important to focus on socio-culturally relevant 'hooks' of value to fathers. For example, emphasizing the 'activation relationship' between fathers and children in both text and images, and highlighting the opportunity to engage in fun, co-physical activity and enhance their children's sports skills. Other research has suggested that fathers prefer programs that allow them to spend time with their children, provide practical parenting tips, include opportunities for interaction with other fathers, maximize co-physical activity, and are delivered by credible facilitators (Morgan et al., 2016; Phares et al., 2006). Finally, programs should be held at convenient times for fathers (e.g. after work and on weekends).

Engaging Fathers

The quality of program facilitators may also have an important moderating influence on the effectiveness of father-focused programs (Morgan et al., 2016). This is particularly important in physical activity promotion programs, where facilitators are required to deliver safe, engaging, and effective practical sessions and need to have a strong 'presence'. In these environments, the skills and expertise of qualified Physical Education or primary teachers, or similar, have been highly valuable. During program delivery, it is also key for facilitators to adopt a strengths-based approach to fathering, where fathers' unique abilities and skills are championed. Finally, while these programs focus predominantly on fathers, it is still important to engage mothers in some capacity given they are commonly key decision-makers and social supports within families. To this end, mothers (and other family members) are invited to one session in the HDHK and DADEE programs and encouraged to participate in the home family activities.

Targeting Valued Outcomes

Importantly, both HDHK and DADEE have a focus on educating fathers about the holistic benefits of program engagement and feature outcomes that are highly valued by fathers. Both programs highlighted that physical activity participation can improve children's social-emotional well-being and the quality of the father-child relationship (Morgan et al., 2016). Indeed, the strategies used in HDHK and DADEE to target valued psychosocial outcomes and engage children as agents of change were recognized in a systematic review and realist synthesis of family-based interventions as effective strategies to increase child and family physical activity levels (Brown et al., 2016).

In response to feedback from fathers, the programs have also been adapted over time to ensure both fathers and children are invited to every session, as spending quality time together was often the fathers' most valued program outcome.

Reciprocal Reinforcement

It is likely that the improvements in physical activity for fathers in the HDHK and DADEE programs were due in part to the programs' encouragement of fathers to be positive role models for their children. In addition, the children were encouraged to motivate their fathers to be more active and given responsibility to drive some of the home-based tasks. This concept of 'reciprocal reinforcement' (Bandura, 1978; Golan & Weizman, 2001) has been described as key when individuals are attempting to change or even sustain new behaviors (Brown et al., 2016) and may be an important construct for researchers to target in future studies.

Further Research Targeting Fathers

Outside of the clear physical health benefits, physical activity plays a vital role in promoting the father-child relationship and fostering children's health and well-being. As such, studies that specifically engage fathers in both personal- and family-based physical activity interventions are a research priority. As fathers appear to have a particularly important influence on physical activity levels of their children and are spending more time with their children than ever before, much more high-quality research is warranted to identify the unique mechanisms of this effect. Understanding how differences in parenting roles and co-parenting affect children's physical activity behaviors is key.

As fathers have reported a preference for father-only programs, an interesting challenge for researchers will be to identify how to increase intervention effects through meaningful mother involvement, without compromising levels of father engagement. Engaging fathers and co-parenting couples successfully will be a key priority. In programs that target both mothers and fathers, researchers are encouraged to explore the unique influences of fathers, independent of mothers, which are often lost when parental data are combined. The potential moderating effect of parent sex is an area in need of further research, as is the exploration of paternal influence when maternal involvement and sibling relationships are controlled for. Reciprocal causation needs to be also taken into account as paternal involvement can influence children through indirect effects on mothers and on the child's sibling relationships.

Some other important questions to explore include the following:

* What is it specifically about father involvement that leads to improvements in children's physical activity; are these elements of parenting and engagement unique to fathers?
* How can fathers be best targeted to improve their children's physical activity levels?
* Is there a differential impact on children's physical activity by targeting fathers-only, mothers-only, or both mothers and fathers in interventions?

Given that co-physical activity may lead to a host of valued outcomes for parents, further work is also needed to determine the following:

* What is the optimal intensity, duration, purpose, and nature of co-physical activity from fathers to elicit improvements in children's physical activity attitudes and behaviors?
* How can the quality and quantity measurement of co-physical activity be improved using more advanced techniques (e.g. wearable cameras, digital recorders, observations, diaries, GPS, additional sensors)?

Researchers need to also distinguish whether parental physical activity is undertaken alone or with their children, and whether parent or child sex is influential. Importantly, mediation analyses are required to determine how parents may influence child physical activity and to help identify possible intervention targets.

Researchers should also consider expanding the definition of 'father' beyond 'biological father' and acknowledge the diversity of fathering. Most children have a father, but they may or may not be residing with them. This variation in fathering can be based on residential status, biological status, presence of a mother, and other blended families. A 'father' has been broadly defined as

> the male or males identified as most involved in caregiving and committed to the well-being of the children, regardless of living situation, marital status or biological relation. A father may be a biological, foster or adoptive father, a stepfather or a grandfather.
>
> *(Coleman, Garfield, & Committee on Psychosocial Aspects of Child and Family Health, 2004)*

The changing nature of relationships and roles of fathers requires a broadening of focus from scholars and researchers to include not just biological fathers from two-parent families but also married and not-married step fathers, resident and non-resident fathers. Indeed, it is particularly important to highlight that the positive involvement of non-traditional fathers has also been associated with a broad array of social-emotional and behavioral benefits for children (Adamsons & Johnson, 2013). Moreover, the role of parenting is dynamic and changes as children grow and develop, and thus, there is a strong rationale for age-specific programs at various child developmental stages.

Conclusion

Strong evidence highlights the important role that fathers play in optimizing the health of their families. As such, the lack of fathers in family-based lifestyle research is concerning, particularly as physical activity and sports have been considered the dominant cultural contexts where fathers leave an enduring legacy with their children (Harrington, 2006). While physical play has important benefits for both fathers and children, it has also led to a somewhat unidimensional misrepresentation that fathers are specialists in play and mothers are specialists in caretaking and nurturing (Lamb, 2010). With men increasingly involved in caretaking activities, the paternal role and proportion of time in play is changing. Fathers can and do engage with their children in many different ways, not just as playmates, and there is a great variation both within and between fathers (Lamb, 2010), although it is important to note that within-gender variation is substantial.

While fathers' own physical activity behaviors and parenting practices likely play an important role in promoting physical activity in their children, the evidence is mostly from observational studies. Indeed, the lack of meaningful father representation in physical activity research is a major evidence gap, which has likely reduced the effectiveness of family-based interventions. Some scholars have even argued that implementing parenting programs without engaging fathers is poor practice, wastes resources, provides incomplete data, and may undermine the duty of care that researchers and practitioners have to optimize child well-being (Panter-Brick et al., 2014).

Fathers have a profound influence on children (Yogman et al., 2016) but are the 'invisible parent' when considering their absence from both observational and experimental studies concerning child physical activity (Davison et al., 2016; Khandpur, Blaine, Fisher, & Davison, 2014; Morgan et al., 2017). Given the importance of physical activity for (i) maintaining optimal physical and mental health in fathers, (ii) enhancing the father-child relationship, and (iii) optimizing child health and well-being, family-based physical activity interventions that meaningfully engage fathers are urgently required.

References

Adamsons, K., & Johnson, S. K. (2013). An updated and expanded meta-analysis of nonresident fathering and child well-being. *Journal of Family Psychology, 27*(4), 589–599.

Bandura, A. (1978). The self system in reciprocal determinism. *The American Psychologist, 33*(4), 344–358.

Bandura, A. (1986). *Social foundations of thought and action: A social cognitive theory.* Englewood Cliffs, NJ: Prentice-Hall.

Barnes, A. T., Plotnikoff, R. C., Collins, C. E., & Morgan, P. J. (2015). Feasibility and preliminary efficacy of the M.A.D.E (Mothers And Daughters Exercising) 4 life program: A pilot randomized controlled trial. *Journal of Physical Activity and Health, 12*(10), 1378–1393. doi:10.1123/jpah.2014-0331

Barnett, L. M., Lai, S. K., Veldman, S. L., Hardy, L. L., Cliff, D. P., Morgan, P. J., . . . Okely, A. D. (2016). Correlates of gross motor competence in children and adolescents: A systematic review and meta-analysis. *Sports Medicine, 46,* 1663–1688. doi:10.1007/s40279-016-0495-z

Barrett, E. L., & Morman, M. T. (2013). Turning points of closeness in the father/daughter relationship. *Human Communication, 15*(4), 241–259.

Baxter, J., & Smart, D. (2011). Fathering in Australia among couple families with young children. *Family Matters, 88,* 15–26.

Beets, M. W., & Foley, J. T. (2008). Association of father involvement and neighborhood quality with kindergartners' physical activity: A multilevel structural equation model. *American Journal of Health Promotion, 22*(3), 195–203. doi:10.4278/ajhp.22.3.195

Bell, H. C., McCaffrey, D. R., Forgie, M. L., Kolb, B., & Pellis, S. M. (2009). The role of the medial prefrontal cortex in the play fighting of rats. *Behavioral Neuroscience, 123*(6), 1158.

Bellows-Reicken, K., & Rhodes, R. (2008). A birth of inactivity? A review of physical activity and parenthood. *Preventive Medicine, 46,* 99–110.

Boulton, M. J. (1991). A comparison of structural and contextual features of middle school children's playful and aggressive fighting. *Ethology and Sociobiology, 12*(2), 119–145.

Boulton, M. J., & Smith, P. K. (1992). The social nature of play fighting and play chasing: Mechanisms and strategies underlying cooperation and compromise. In J. H. Barkow, L. Cosmides, & J. Tooby (Eds.), *The adapted mind: Evolutionary psychology and the generation of culture* (pp. 429–444). New York, NY: Oxford University Press.

Bourçois, V. (1997). Modalités de présence du père et développement social de l'enfant d'âge préscolaire. *Enfance, 50*(3), 389–399.

Bringolf-Isler, B., Schindler, C., Kayser, B., Suggs, L. S., & Probst-Hensch, N. (2018). Objectively measured physical activity in population-representative parent-child pairs: Parental modelling matters and is context-specific. *BMC Public Health, 18*(1), 1024.

Brouwer, S. I., Küpers, L. K., Kors, L., Sijtsma, A., Sauer, P. J. J., Renders, C. M., & Corpeleijn, E. (2018). Parental physical activity is associated with objectively measured physical activity in young children in a sex-specific manner: The GECKO Drenthe cohort. *BMC Public Health, 18*(1), 1033.

Brown, H. E., Atkin, A. J., Panter, J., Wong, G., Chinapaw, M. J., & van Sluijs, E. M. (2016). Family-based interventions to increase physical activity in children: A systematic review, meta-analysis and realist synthesis. *Obesity Reviews, 17,* 345–360. doi:10.1111/obr.12362

Burgess, A. (2006). *Engaging fathers in their children's learning: Tips for practitioners.* Abergavenny, Wales: Fatherhood Institute.

Burrows, T., Morgan, P. J., Lubans, D. R., Callister, R., Okley, T., Bray, J., & Collins, C. E. (2012). Dietary outcomes of the Healthy Dads Healthy Kids randomised controlled trial. *Journal of Pediatric Gastroenterology and Nutrition, 55*(4), 408–411. doi:10.1097/MPG.0b013e318259aee6

Coleman, W. L., Garfield, C. F., & Committee on Psychosocial Aspects of Child and Family Health. (2004). Fathers and pediatricians: Enhancing men's roles in the care and development of their children. *Pediatrics, 113*(5), 1406–1411.

Craig, L. (2006). Does father care mean fathers share? A comparison of how mothers and fathers in intact families spend time with children. *Gender & Society, 20*(2), 259–281.

Davison, K. K., Gicevic, S., Aftosmes-Tobio, A., Ganter, C., Simon, C. L., Newlan, S., & Manganello, J. A. (2016). Fathers' representation in observational studies on parenting and childhood obesity: A systematic review and content analysis. *American Journal of Public Health, 106*(11), e14–e21. doi:10.2105/AJPH.2016.303391

Deci, E., & Ryan, R. (1985). *Intrinsic motivation and self-determination in human behavior.* New York, NY: Plenum.

Durette, R., Marrs, C., & Gray, P. B. (2011). Fathers faring poorly: Results of an Internet-based survey of fathers of young children. *American Journal of Men's Health, 5*(5), 395–401. doi:10.1177/1557988310378365

Edwardson, C. L., & Gorely, T. (2010). Parental influences on different types and intensities of physical activity in youth: A systematic review. *Psychology of Sport and Exercise, 11,* 522–535.

Ferreira, I., van der Horst, K., Wendel-Vos, W., Kremers, S., van Lenthe, F. J., & Brug, J. (2007). Environmental correlates of physical activity in youth – A review and update. *Obesity Reviews, 8*(2), 129–154. doi:10.1111/j.1467-789X.2006.00264.x

Field, T. (2010). Touch for socioemotional and physical well-being: A review. *Developmental Review, 30*(4), 367–383.

Fletcher, R., May, C., St George, J., Morgan, P. J., & Lubans, D. R. (2011). Fathers' perceptions of rough-and-tumble play: Implications for early childhood services. *Australasian Journal of Early Childhood, 36*(4), 131–138.

Garfield, C. F., Clark-Kauffman, E., & Davis, M. M. (2006). Fatherhood as a component of men's health. *JAMA – Journal of the American Medical Association, 296*(19), 2365–2368. doi:10.1001/jama.296.19.2365

Golan, M., & Weizman, A. (2001). Familial approach to the treatment of childhood obesity. A conceptual model. *Journal of Nutrition Education, 33,* 102–107.

Goldberg, W. A., Clarke-Stewart, K. A., Rice, J. A., & Dellis, E. (2002). Emotional energy as an explanatory construct for fathers' engagement with their infants. *Parenting: Science and Practice, 2*(4), 379–408.

Gustafson, S. L., & Rhodes, R. E. (2006). Parental correlates of physical activity in children and early adolescents. *Sports Medicine, 36*(1), 79–97.

Hallal, P. C., Andersen, L. B., Bull, F. C., Guthold, R., Haskell, W., & Ekelund, U. (2012). Global physical activity levels: Surveillance progress, pitfalls, and prospects. *Lancet, 380,* 247–257. doi:10.1016/S0140-6736(12)60646-1

Harrington, M. (2006). Sport and leisure as contexts for fathering in Australian families. *Leisure Studies, 25*(2), 165–183.

Hull, E. E., Rofey, D. L., Robertson, R. J., Nagle, E. F., Otto, A. D., & Aaron, D. J. (2010). Influence of marriage and parenthood on physical activity: A 2-year prospective analysis. *Journal of Physical Activity and Health, 7*(5), 577–583.

Jeynes, W. H. (2016). Meta-analysis on the roles of fathers in parenting: Are they unique. *Marriage & Family Reviews, 52*(7), 665–688.

John, A., Halliburton, A., & Humphrey, J. (2013). Child–mother and child–father play interaction patterns with preschoolers. *Early Child Development and Care, 183*(3–4), 483–497.

Khandpur, N., Blaine, R. E., Fisher, J. O., & Davison, K. K. (2014). Fathers' child feeding practices: A review of the evidence. *Appetite, 78,* 110–121. doi:10.1016/j.appet.2014.03.015

Kohl, H. W., 3rd, Craig, C. L., Lambert, E. V., Inoue, S., Alkandari, J. R., Leetongin, G., . . . Lancet Physical Activity Series Working Group. (2012). The pandemic of physical inactivity: Global action for public health. *Lancet, 380*(9838), 294–305. doi:10.1016/S0140-6736(12)60898-8

Kwon, S., Janz, K. F., Letuchy, E. M., Burns, T. L., & Levy, S. M. (2016). Parental characteristic patterns associated with maintaining healthy physical activity behavior during childhood and adolescence. *International Journal of Behavioral Nutrition and Physical Activity, 13*(1), 58. doi:10.1186/s12966-016-0383-9

Lamb, M. E. (2010). How do fathers influence children's development? Let me count the ways. In M. E. Lamb (Ed.), *The role of the father in child development* (5th ed., pp. 1–26). Hoboken, NJ: John Wiley & Sons.

Lamb, M. E., & Lewis, C. (2010). The development and significance of father-child relationships in two-parent families. In M. E. Lamb (Ed.), *The role of the father in child development* (5th ed., pp. 94–153). Chichester, UK: John Wiley & Sons.

Lee, I., Shiroma, E. J., Lobelo, F., Puska, P., Blair, S. N., Katzmarzyk, P. T., & Lancet Physical Activity Series Working Group. (2012). Effect of physical inactivity on major non-communicable diseases worldwide: An analysis of burden of disease and life expectancy. *Lancet, 380*(9838), 219–229. doi:10.1016/S0140-6736(12)61031-9

Lee, S., Nihiser, A., Strouse, D., Das, B., Michael, S., & Huhman, M. (2010). Correlates of children and parents being physically active together. *Journal of Physical Activity and Health, 7*(6), 776–783.

Lindsey, E. W., Cremeens, P. R., & Caldera, Y. M. (2010). Mother–child and father–child mutuality in two contexts: Consequences for young children's peer relationships. *Infant and Child Development: An International Journal of Research and Practice, 19*(2), 142–160.

Lindsey, E. W., & Mize, J. (2001). Contextual differences in parent–child play: Implications for children's gender role development. *Sex Roles, 44*(3–4), 155–176.

Lindsey, E. W., Mize, J., & Pettit, G. S. (1997). Mutuality in parent-child play: Consequences for children's peer competence. *Journal of Social and Personal Relationships, 14*(4), 523–538.

Lloyd, A. B., Lubans, D. R., Plotnikoff, R. C., & Morgan, P. J. (2014). Impact of the 'Healthy Dads, Healthy Kids' lifestyle programme on the activity- and diet-related parenting practices of fathers and mothers. *Pediatric Obesity, 9*(6), e149–e155. doi:10.1111/ijpo.248

Lloyd, A. B., Lubans, D. R., Plotnikoff, R. C., & Morgan, P. J. (2015). Paternal lifestyle-related parenting practices mediate changes in children's dietary and physical activity behaviors: Findings from the Healthy Dads, Healthy Kids community randomized controlled trial. *Journal of Physical Activity and Health, 12*(9), 1327–1335. doi:10.1123/jpah.2014-0367

Lubans, D., Morgan, P., Cliff, D., Barnett, L., & Okely, A. (2010). Fundamental movement skills in children and adolescents: Review of associated health benefits. *Sports Medicine, 40*(12), 1019–1035. doi:10.2165/11536850-000000000-00000

Lubans, D. R., Morgan, P. J., Collins, C. E., Okely, A. D., Burrows, T. L., & Callister, R. (2012). Mediators of weight loss in the 'healthy dads, healthy kids' pilot study for overweight fathers. *International Journal of Behavioral Nutrition and Physical Activity, 9*(45). doi:10.1186/1479-5868-9-45

MacDonald, K., & Parke, R. D. (1986). Parent-child physical play: The effects of sex and age of children and parents. *Sex Roles, 15*(7–8), 367–378.

Mailey, E. L., Huberty, J., Dinkel, D., & McAuley, E. (2014). Physical activity barriers and facilitators among working mothers and fathers. *BMC Public Health, 14,* 657. doi:10.1186/1471-2458-14-657

Mammen, G., & Faulkner, G. (2013). Physical activity and the prevention of depression: A systematic review of prospective studies. *American Journal of Preventive Medicine, 45*(5), 649–657. doi:10.1016/j.amepre.2013.08.001

Morgan, P. J., Collins, C. E., Lubans, D. R., Callister, R., Lloyd, A. B., Plotnikoff, R. C, . . . Young, M.D. (2019). Twelve-month outcomes of a father-child lifestyle intervention delivered by trained local facilitators in under-served communities: The Healthy Dads Healthy Kids dissemination trial. *Translational Behavioral Medicine, 9*(3), 560–569. doi:10.1093/tbm/ibz031

Morgan, P. J., Collins, C. E., Plotnikoff, R. C., Callister, R., Burrows, T., Fletcher, R., . . . Lubans, D. R. (2014). The 'Healthy Dads, Healthy Kids' community randomized controlled trial: A community-based healthy lifestyle program for fathers and their children. *Preventive Medicine, 61,* 90–99. doi:10.1016/j.ypmed.2013.12.019

Morgan, P. J., Lubans, D. R., Callister, R., Okely, A. D., Burrows, T. L., Fletcher, R., & Collins, C. E. (2011). The 'Healthy Dads, Healthy Kids' randomized controlled trial: Efficacy of a healthy lifestyle program for overweight fathers and their children. *International Journal of Obesity, 35*(3), 436–447. doi:10.1038/ijo.2010.151

Morgan, P. J., & Young, M. D. (2017). The influence of fathers on children's physical activity and dietary behaviors: Insights, recommendations and future directions. *Current Obesity Reports.* doi:10.1007/s13679-017-0275-6

Morgan, P. J., Young, M. D., Barnes, A. T., Eather, N., Pollock, E. R., & Lubans, D. R. (2019). Engaging fathers to increase physical activity in girls: The 'Dads and Daughters Exercising and Empowered' (DADEE) randomized controlled trial. *Annals of Behavioral Medicine, 53*(1), 39–52. doi:10.1093/abm/kay015

Morgan, P. J., Young, M. D., Lloyd, A. B., Wang, M. L., Eather, N., Miller, A., . . . Pagoto, S. L. (2017). Involvement of fathers in pediatric obesity treatment and prevention trials: A systematic review. *Pediatrics, 139*(2). doi:10.1542/peds.2016-2635

Morgan, P. J., Young, M. D., Lubans, D. R., Barnes, A. T., Eather, N., & Pollock, E. R. (2018). Better together: Investigating the holistic benefits of father–daughter co-physical activity with mediation analyses. *Journal of Science and Medicine in Sport, 21*(Supplement 1), S13.

Morgan, P. J., Young, M. D., Smith, J. J., & Lubans, D. R. (2016). Targeted health behavior interventions promoting physical activity: A conceptual model. *Exercise and Sport Sciences Reviews, 44*(2), 71–80. doi:10.1249/jes.0000000000000075

Neshteruk, C. D., Nezami, B. T., Nino-Tapias, G., Davison, K. K., & Ward, D. S. (2017). The influence of fathers on children's physical activity: A review of the literature from 2009 to 2015. *Preventive Medicine, 102,* 12–19. doi:10.1016/j.ypmed.2017.06.027

Newland, L., Coyl, D., & Freeman, H. (2008). Predicting preschoolers' attachment security from fathers' involvement, internal working models, and use of social support. *Early Child Development and Care, 178*(7 & 8), 785–801.

Panter-Brick, C., Burgess, A., Eggerman, M., McAllister, F., Pruett, K., & Leckman, J. F. (2014). Practitioner review: Engaging fathers – Recommendations for a game change in parenting interventions based on a systematic review of the global evidence. *Journal of Child Psychology and Psychiatry and Allied Disciplines, 55*(11), 1187–1212. doi:10.1111/jcpp.12280

Paquette, D. (2004). Theorizing the father-child relationship: Mechanisms and developmental outcomes. *Human Development, 47*(4), 193–219.

Paquette, D., Bolté, C., Turcotte, G., Dubeau, D., & Bouchard, C. (2000). A new typology of fathering: Defining and associated variables. *Infant and Child Development: An International Journal of Research and Practice, 9*(4), 213–230.

Pellegrini, A., & Smith, P. K. (1998). Physical activity play: Consensus and debate. *Child Development, 69*, 577–598.

Pellis, S. M., Field, E. F., & Whishaw, L. Q. (1999). The development of a sex-differentiated defensive motor pattern in rats: A possible role for juvenile experience. *Developmental Psychobiology: The Journal of the International Society for Developmental Psychobiology, 35*(2), 156–164.

Phares, V., Fields, S., & Binitie, I. (2006). Getting fathers involved in child-related therapy. *Cognitive and Behavioral Practice, 13*(1), 42–52. doi:10.1016/j.cbpra.2005.06.002

Pleck, J. H. (2010a). Fatherhood and masculinity. In M. E. Lamb (Ed.), *The role of the father in child development* (5th ed., pp. 27–57). Hoboken, NJ: John Wiley & Sons.

Pleck, J. H. (2010b). Paternal involvement: Revised conceptualization and theoretical linkages with child outcomes. In M. E. Lamb (Ed.), *The role of the father in child development* (5th ed., pp. 58–93). Hoboken, NJ: John Wiley & Sons.

Pot, N., & Keizer, R. (2016). Physical activity and sport participation: A systematic review of the impact of fatherhood. *Preventive Medicine Reports, 4*, 121–127. doi:10.1016/j.pmedr.2016.05.018

Power, T. G., & Parke, R. D. (1983). Patterns of mother and father play with their 8-month-old infant: A multiple analyses approach. *Infant Behavior and Development, 6*(4), 453–459.

Rhodes, R. E., & Lim, C. (2018). Promoting parent and child physical activity together: Elicitation of potential intervention targets and preferences. *Health Education and Behavior, 45*(1), 112–123.

Robertson, C., Archibald, D., Avenell, A., Douglas, F., Hoddinott, P., van Teijlingen, E., . . . Fowler, C. (2014). Systematic reviews of and integrated report on the quantitative, qualitative and economic evidence base for the management of obesity in men. *Health Technology Assessment, 18*(35), 1–424.

Sarkadi, A., Kristiansson, R., Oberklaid, F., & Bremberg, S. (2008). Fathers' involvement and children's developmental outcomes: A systematic review of longitudinal studies. *Acta Paediatrica, 97*, 153–158.

Smith, P. K. (2010). Physical activity play: Exercise play and rough-and-tumble. In P. K. Smith (Ed.), *Children and play: Understanding children's worlds* (pp. 99–123). Chichester, UK: Wiley-Blackwell.

St George, J., & Freeman, E. (2017). Measurement of father-child rough-and-tumble play and its relation to child behavior. *Infant Mental Health Journal, 38*(6), 709–725.

St George, J., Goodwin, J. C., & Fletcher, R. J. (2018). Parents' views of father–child rough-and-tumble play. *Journal of Child and Family Studies, 27*(5), 1502–1512.

Taylor, S. E., Fredericks, E. M., Janisse, H. C., & Cousino, M. K. (2019). Systematic review of father involvement and child outcomes in pediatric chronic illness populations. *Journal of Clinical Psychology in Medical Settings. Family-based interventions to increase physical activity in children: A systematic review, meta-analysis and realist synthesis, 27*, 89–106. doi:10.1007/s10880-019-09623-5

Telford, R. M., Telford, R. D., Olive, L. S., Cochrane, T., & Davey, R. (2016). Why are girls less physically active than boys? Findings from the LOOK longitudinal study. *PLoS One, 11*(3). doi:10.1371/journal.pone.0150041

Thornton, L. K., Chapman, C., Leidl, D., Conroy, C., Teesson, M., Slade, T., . . . Newton, N. (2018). Climate schools plus: An online, combined student and parent, universal drug prevention program. *Internet Interventions, 12*, 36–45. doi:10.1016/j.invent.2018.03.007

Trost, S. G., & Loprinzi, P. D. (2011). Parental influences on physical activity behavior in children and adolescents: A brief review. *American Journal of Lifestyle Medicine, 5*(2), 171–181.

Trost, S. G., Pate, R. R., Sallis, J. F., Freedson, P. S., Taylor, W. C., Dowda, M., & Sirard, J. (2002). Age and gender differences in objectively measured physical activity in youth. *Medicine and Science in Sports and Exercise, 34*(2), 350–355.

Van den Berg, C. L., Hol, T., Van Ree, J. M., Spruijt, B. M., Everts, H., & Koolhaas, J. M. (1999). Play is indispensable for an adequate development of coping with social challenges in the rat. *Developmental Psychobiology: The Journal of the International Society for Developmental Psychobiology, 34*(2), 129–138.

Von Frijtag, J. C., Schot, M., van den Bos, R., & Spruijt, B. M. (2002). Individual housing during the play period results in changed responses to and consequences of a psychosocial stress situation in rats. *Developmental Psychobiology: The Journal of the International Society for Developmental Psychobiology, 41*(1), 58–69.

Walsh, A. D., Lioret, S., Cameron, A. J., Hesketh, K. D., McNaughton, S. A., Crawford, D., & Campbell, K. J. (2014). The effect of an early childhood obesity intervention on father's obesity risk behaviors: The Melbourne InFANT program. *International Journal of Behavioral Nutrition and Physical Activity, 11*, 18. doi:10.1186/1479-5868-11-18

Williams, A., de Vlieger, N., Young, M., Jensen, M. E., Burrows, T. L., Morgan, P. J., & Collins, C. E. (2018). Dietary outcomes of overweight fathers and their children in the Healthy Dads, Healthy Kids community randomised controlled trial. *Journal of Human Nutrition and Dietetics, 31*, 523–532. doi:10.1111/jhn.12543

Yogman, M., Garfield, C. F., & the Committee on Psychosocial Aspects of Child and Family Health. (2016). Fathers' roles in the care and development of their children: The role of pediatricians. *Pediatrics, 138*(1). doi:10.1542/peds.2016-1128

Young, M. D., Lubans, D. R., Barnes, A. T., Eather, N., Pollock, E. R., & Morgan, P. J. (2019). Impact of a father-daughter physical activity program on girls' social-emotional well-being: A randomized controlled trial. *Journal of Consulting and Clinical Psychology, 87*(3), 294–307. doi:10.1037/ccp0000374

Zahra, J., Sebire, S. J., & Jago, R. (2015). 'He's probably more Mr. sport than me' – A qualitative exploration of mothers' perceptions of fathers' role in their children's physical activity. *BMC Pediatrics, 15*. doi:10.1186/s12887-015-0421-9

32

BEFORE- AND AFTER-SCHOOL INTERVENTIONS IN YOUTH PHYSICAL ACTIVITY
Current Situation and Future Directions

Sarahjane Belton and Wesley O'Brien

Introduction

Babey, Wu, and Cohen (2014) identified four types of school-based approaches aimed at increasing physical activity (PA) participation in youth: (1) extending the school day to provide 60 minutes of regular Physical Education provision, (2) short (10-minute) in-class PA breaks, (3) before-school programs, and (4) after-school programs. This chapter is concerned with the latter of these identified approaches, namely, before- and after-school interventions. Drawing on the work of other authors, the term 'extra-curricular PA' (ECPA) will be used in this chapter to encompass the provision of PA opportunities that are offered within the school setting, but outside of the formal Physical Education curriculum (Penney & Harris, 1997; Woods, Moyna, Quinlan, Tannehill, & Walsh, 2010). In this context, the before- and after-school periods are considered to be two of the key opportunities for the provision of ECPA opportunities. Atkin, Gorely, Biddle, Cavill, and Foster (2011) describe the period immediately after school as the critical hours of opportunity, for which young people can engage in a considerable proportion of their daily PA behavior.

The study of school-based PA participation for children and youth has received much attention in the literature (Belton, O'Brien, McGann, & Issartel, 2018; Dobbins, Husson, Decorby, & LaRocca, 2013; Kriemler et al., 2011; Mâsse, McKay, Valente, Brant, & Naylor, 2012; Strong et al., 2005), and embedding PA within the before-school and after-school periods represents promising strategies for promoting PA (Beets, 2012). School-based PA intervention programs are often considered cost-effective models because (1) transportation of children to the site is not needed, (2) equipment and facilities are readily available, and (3) quite often, school staff may be willing to act as facilitators of the programs (Mears & Jago, 2016). Empirically speaking, after-school PA programs have received considerably more evaluative research, when compared to before-school PA programs for children and youth (Babey et al., 2014). In order to heighten our understanding of the complexity associated with youth PA participation behaviors, the Theory of Expanded, Extended, and Enhanced Opportunities (TEO) (Beets et al., 2016) presents a common taxonomy, by which appropriate intervention targets in children and youth can be identified, across different settings and contexts. In the case of this chapter regarding before- and after-school programs, the proposed TEO model may contribute to the future design of intervention studies lead to a greater impact on youth PA behavior (Beets et al., 2016).

Overview of the Literature

Hesketh et al. (2014) suggest that targeted interventions focusing on periods when children are less active may result in larger increases in children's PA participation. As part of the need for targeted interventions, in 2008, the Scottish Government Schools Act for health promotion and nutrition identified that children and youth needed to understand that PA 'can be incorporated into all aspects of school life, and life beyond school, through such activities as walking to and from school or work, attending a dance class, playing outside with friends, rambling and cycling' (p. 16) (Scottish Government, 2008). Interestingly, Harris and Cale (2018) outline that a healthy school focusing on PA promotion depends on three key elements: (1) the curriculum, (2) the 'hidden' curriculum, and (3) the community. In addition to these three elements, however, the authors further outline that a healthy school for PA promotion is committed to curricular, extra-curricular, and organizational active school practices (Harris & Cale, 2018).

Before-School Periods

Babey et al. (2014) in their economic analysis of school-based programs outlined that a before-school activity program should include a volunteer or provide professional supervision '*available 30 minutes before school during regular school days for students to participate in physical activities, informal sports, or interscholastic sports*' (p. S56). While patterns of PA behavior in the before-school period are less researched than the after-school period, the evidence still suggests that this period may offer an opportunity for PA promotion, specifically for less active youth. Previous studies have investigated the patterns of PA participation of young people in various time periods of the day, and compared the levels of PA accumulated by highly active children, with those of low active children within these time periods. Garriguet and Colley (2012) found that the most active cohort of youth were significantly more active during the 7–9am period than the least active cohort. Findings of Belton, O'Brien, Issartel, McGrane, and Powell (2016) similarly suggest that the most active young people are again accumulating more minutes of moderate-to-vigorous PA (MVPA) during this before-school period, when compared to the least physically active groups. This evidence would suggest that before school is a period of time when more activity is possible; however, the least active youth do not avail of this opportunity – hence, before school is a potential time period for targeted PA interventions with youth. There are many benefits to participating in before-school PA programs, beyond the most identifiable target of improving levels of MVPA. Whooten, Perkins, Gerber, and Taveras (2018) highlighted that children who participated in a 12-week before-school PA program had improved their body mass index (BMI), prevented increases in child obesity, and increased their social-emotional wellness, when compared to the respective control groups.

After-School Periods

It is well understood that after-school programs, which do not detract from the school day, are a useful way to supplement PA time for youth (Beets, Beighle, Erwin, & Huberty, 2009). A previous study reported that such programs can provide up to 20 minutes of a child's daily 60 minutes requirement of MVPA (Trost, Rosenkranz, & Dzewaltowski, 2008). Furthermore, an analytic review by Beets (2012) titled 'Enhancing the translation of PA interventions in afterschool programs' found that these time periods can provide anywhere between 8 and 24 minutes of MVPA participation daily, with the possibility of children accumulating between 2,600 and 3,200 steps per day, specifically as part of these after-school programs.

Garriguet and Colley (2012) reported that when they considered their data according to the MVPA levels of the cohort (participants grouped into tertiles from least to most active), they found that the largest difference in PA accumulation between the 'most active' and the 'least active' tertile of children and youth was found in the block just after school from 3 to 5pm. Another study that considered the patterns of PA participation with early Irish adolescent youth, aged 12–14 years old (Belton et al., 2016), highlighted the after-school period as the time when the greatest difference was exhibited between the most and least active quartile of students, irrespective of gender. Again, similar to the before-school period, these results would suggest that the after-school period is a time when it is possible for youth to accumulate a significant amount of MVPA; however, the least active youth are not capitalizing on this time period for accruing minutes of PA. This highlights the after-school period as an important time zone to target PA promotion through interventions, and particularly so for those youth that are currently at most risk – the most physically inactive cohorts.

ECPA within the Before- and After-School Periods

When we consider the literature available around extra-curricular sport and ECPA provision, we may start to better understand the gap between the least and most active children during this period. The extent, quality, and variety of ECPA opportunities varies across schools, and can depend on a range of factors including facilities, funding, school ethos, and staff availability (Woods et al., 2010). The focus quite often in many schools is on competitive sports and frequently on a limited range of such competitive sports (Penney & Harris, 1997; Woods et al., 2010). As such, the ECPA opportunities available in many schools, both before and after school, may be more attractive to those young people that are already more physically active and quite possibly more physically able. Most recent research suggests that children with higher levels of motor competence have an increased likelihood of meeting the recommended MVPA guidelines, compared to their less competent peers (De Meester et al., 2018).

Penney and Harris (1997) highlighted the need for ECPA provision in schools to be broadened, so that rather than reinforcing the gap between less and more 'able' young people, opportunities for PA participation are provided for all abilities. In doing so, this supports Randsell, Dinger, Huberty, and Miller's (2009) work on using intervention activities that are based on appropriate behavior change theories for the target population, such as the example of the TEO (Beets et al., 2016), which offers new ways to understand youth PA behaviors across all settings where youth PA is intervened. The need for 'participation'-oriented ECPA programs is now apparent, specifically targeting the less active youth, who may shy away from the more traditional competitive sporting activities offered through ECPA provision (Penney & Harris, 1997; Woods et al., 2010). Mears and Jago (2016), in a review of after-school PA interventions, identify a range of program types offered as interventions in the after-school period; these include (1) structured or unstructured play, (2) planned MVPA, (3) multi-sport physical activities, and (4) single-sport PA. Though there may be a sound rationale justifying the before- and after-school time periods as opportunities for intervening to increase youth PA, there is a need to interrogate the available evidence as to whether or not such interventions are effective, efficient, and sustainable.

Key Issues

The Evidence behind Before- and After-School Interventions

Considering the reported decline in Physical Education provision (Harrington et al., 2016; Tremblay et al., 2015; Woods et al., 2010), many researchers and practitioners have focused their attention towards increasing school-based PA opportunities throughout the day and beyond formalized Physical Education classes (Babey et al., 2014; Beets, 2012; Beets et al., 2009; Whooten et al., 2018). In achieving this, McMullen, van der Mars, and Jahn (2014) discuss the implementation of a whole-school approach to PA promotion, with a plausible solution known as the Comprehensive School PA Program (CSPAP) (Carson, Castelli, Beighle, & Erwin, 2014). The CSPAP is a conceptual framework representing a system of influences that are interacting with one another, which impacts PA behaviors in schools. As discussed previously, one component of the CSPAP framework is before-/after-school programs (McMullen et al., 2014), which include additional PA opportunities in and around the school setting for students, teachers, and families. In the context of available research-informed evidence, the impact of before-school PA programs is sparsely dispersed within the literature (Babey et al., 2014). However, such programs are still considered a viable option for PA opportunities among children and youth (McMullen, Ní Chróinín, Tammelin, Pogorzelska, & van der Mars, 2015; McMullen et al., 2014; Whooten et al., 2018), with some positively reported case study examples present.

Impact of Before-School PA Interventions

A previous economic analysis comparing school-based PA programs (Babey et al., 2014) reported that there was an absence of published evidence available, which specifically examined before-school PA programs. While it is generally acknowledged that before-school PA programs are less reported in the literature, some empirical evidence for these program types do exist (Knight, 2015; Mahar, Vuchenich, Golden, DuBose, & Raedeke, 2011; Stylianou et al., 2016). A previous study (Mahar et al., 2011) examined the effects of a before-school PA program on elementary school-aged children's PA participation and on-task behavior. This study found that those who attended the 'First-Class Activity Program' (n = 27; mean age = 8.2 ± 0.5 years) spent an average of 46.4% of time in MVPA (9.3 ± 2.9 minutes), and obtained approximately one-third of the recommended time for school-based PA, which was acknowledged by Mahar et al. (2011), as 30 minutes MVPA participation per day for children within schools. Another study by Knight (2015) evaluated the effects of a simple, low-cost PA program before school on third-grade children's PA levels (n = 28). Objectively measured findings from this research using pedometers showed that children took an average of 987 (± 344) steps during this before-school PA program and were active at a rate of 58.6 (± 20.8) steps per minute. Furthermore, Knight (2015) observed through accelerometer-based measurements that participants spent 22.1% (± 8.5) of their time at the program in MVPA, and overall, participants spent more time in light, moderate, and vigorous PA during the school day, when compared to their participation on the days after the program was over. More recently, Stylianou et al. (2016) found that a before-school running/walking club for third- and fourth-grade children (n = 88) in two schools (1 public and 1 private) resulted in participants accumulating between 8 and 10 minutes of daily MVPA, as part of these program initiatives. This research provides preliminary evidence supporting the integration of short (15 to 20 minutes) sessions of running/walking before school as a means of positively contributing to elementary-aged children's PA participation levels.

It is, however, important to note the limitations in the data available for the studies above (Knight, 2015; Mahar et al., 2011; Stylianou et al., 2016). In each of these studies, there was a small sample size reported in all cases, and there was an absence of a matched control arm against which to compare PA levels (feasibility and efficacy studies only), and for these reasons it was difficult to determine whether MVPA accumulation for children was greater in these after-school time periods. Interestingly, as a comparative intervention study entitled 'Build Our Kids Success' (BOKS), Whooten et al. (2018) examined the effectiveness of a before-school PA program on obesity prevention and wellness in a much larger sample of children (n = 1,229 children, aged 5–14 years old) across 24 participating schools in three Massachusetts communities. It is important to note in this larger study that BMI was the primary outcome measurement (n = 707 with follow-up data) however, and the intervention dosage ranged from 3 days of 60 minutes per week (intervention group 1), to 2 days of 60 minutes per week (intervention group 2), in comparison with a respective control group arm, across a 12-week comparative cycle. Findings from this before-school PA program reveal that the higher intervention dosage had most effectiveness for positive BMI change; specifically, children who participated in the 3 days per week BOKS program had significantly higher odds of being in a lower BMI category at follow-up, when compared to baseline. This finding surrounding intervention effectiveness, however, was not seen in children who participated in BOKS 2 days per week or in the control group.

While sample size and control arm comparisons were identified as the study limitations above for measuring before-school intervention effectiveness for PA-related programs with children (Knight, 2015; Mahar et al., 2011; Stylianou et al., 2016), the larger comparative BOKS study (Whooten et al., 2018) suggests that intervention dosage and frequency are also key variables in examining the effectiveness of before-school PA programs in children, particularly when BMI is a primary outcome variable. For this reason, and despite the sparsely populated evidence surrounding before-school PA programs, the BOKS study is uniquely positioned as an evaluative trial for BMI outcome measurements in a before-school PA intervention setting. These case study findings open new avenues for PA interventions in youth, specifically that the before-school time period may now be considered as a promising strategy for increased PA promotion (Knight, 2015; Mahar et al., 2011; Stylianou et al., 2016) and healthier body composition (Whooten et al., 2018) in children.

Impact of After-School PA Interventions

A meta-analysis carried out by Beets et al. (2009), investigating the impact of after-school programs on PA participation and fitness, concluded that although the number of studies available for the analysis was limited, after-school programs that include a PA participatory component can improve overall PA levels in youth, along with other health-related aspects. Demetriou, Gillison, and McKenzie (2017) in a more recent review of reviews on after-school PA interventions highlighted very meaningful differences that existed across six published reviews in the area (Atkin et al., 2011; Beets et al., 2009 Branscum & Sharma, 2012; Mears & Jago, 2016; Pate & O'Neill, 2009; Vasques et al., 2014), and concluded that there is modest support for the effectiveness of after-school programs on children's PA levels. In another recent review carried out by Mears and Jago (2016), mixed effectiveness of after-school PA interventions on overall MVPA was reported. Fifteen papers met the inclusion criteria in this study. Of these, the study with the largest reported increase in PA was Barbeau et al. (2007), which used a self-report measure of MVPA and reported a mean of 22.2 minutes adjusted difference in MVPA at follow-up, between the control and intervention conditions.

Sub-group analyses carried out by Mears and Jago (2016) revealed benefits within specific groups of participants (overweight/obese in three studies and boys in two studies), highlighting the potential importance of adapting program content to meet the specific needs of particular groups of children. This would further suggest the need to move away from a 'one-size fits all' approach, to adapt program content to the needs of particular groups rather than a general program for all participants (Demetriou et al., 2017). These systematic review and meta-analyses findings are in line with the previously mentioned data in relation to before-school PA programs for children. Specifically, a 'one-size fits all' approach is less likely to be effective (Knight, 2015;

Mahar et al., 2011; Stylianou et al., 2016; Whooten et al., 2018), and particular variables, such as BMI (included the BOKS study) (Whooten et al., 2018), require uniquely tailored advances to before- and after-school PA intervention strategies.

Key Components of Effective Interventions

Generally, when developing any intervention program for PA promotion, it is accepted that framing the content on a relevant theory of behavior change adds strength and increases the chance of program success (Beets et al., 2016; Harris & Cale, 2019; Ryan & Deci, 2000; Standage, Duda, & Ntoumanis, 2005; Stokols, 1992). Previous research has suggested that it is critically important to influence childhood PA at different levels. This is often targeted through ecological model-based approaches, and by using these multi-level strategies, there is an increased likelihood of understanding and promoting positive PA participation (Ward, Saunders, & Pate, 2007). More recent evidence supports the development of a new theory, previously mentioned in this chapter as TEO (Beets et al., 2016), by outlining that the primary mechanisms for change in youth PA interventions can be sub-divided in to three categories, namely:

a   The expansion of opportunities for youth to be active by the inclusion of a new occasion to be active,
b   The extension of an existing PA opportunity by increasing the amount of time allocated for that opportunity, and/or
c   The enhancement of existing PA opportunities through strategies designed to increase PA above routine practice (p. 1).

In light of the data presented in this chapter to-date, TEO aligns itself robustly, alongside the theme of before-school and after-school PA interventions, particularly TEO (Beets et al., 2016) discusses how the behavioral change approaches for increasing youth PA can be met through: (1) new occasions for activity, (2) heightened time for PA participation, and (3) innovative approaches beyond typical routine practice.

Most recently, Demetriou et al. (2017) in their review of reviews identified that social cognitive theory was the most commonly applied behavior change theory for after-school PA intervention studies (n = 23), with self-determination theory (used in three studies) the second most commonly used. Mears and Jago (2016) in their systematic review and meta-analysis of after-school PA interventions highlighted that while many programs based on a theory of behavior change were effective, programs that had no theoretical basis also showed effect. These findings led the authors to conclude that there was no convincing evidence that interventions based on behavior change theories were any more effective than programs with no underlying theory (Mears & Jago, 2016).

Active Ingredients? Examples of Before-School Programs

The systematic review, meta-analyses, and economic analyses examining the effectiveness of after-school PA programs are more prevalent in the literature (Babey et al., 2014; Beets, 2012; Beets et al., 2009), when compared to before-school PA programs. Specifically, Babey et al. (2014) in their economic analysis reported finding no published evidence examining before-school PA programs. Since this reported data (Babey et al., 2014), some efficacy trials (Knight, 2015; Stylianou et al., 2016) and effectiveness trials (Whooten et al., 2018) have been published in the literature documenting their respective intervention components. As the before-school PA interventions are less populated in the literature, examples of three programs evaluated in effectiveness and efficacy trials are presented for quick reference below, so that readers can start to identify the common ingredients present in such programs.

Build Our Kids Success (BOKS)

Pojednic et al. (2016) in their study protocol outlining their evaluative strategies for the BOKS program reported that this before-school PA intervention was 12 weeks in duration, facilitated for 2–3 times per week, and this dosage and frequency was dependent on the school district. In terms of intervention structure, BOKS sessions lasted for approximately 60 minutes and comprised of a typical session structure of the following: (1) a fun warm-up game; (2) transition in to running, relay races, or obstacle courses; and (3) 'skill of the week' (such as plank, running, or jumping). While the age group ranged from 5 to 14 years (Pojednic et al., 2016; Whooten et al., 2018), the authors outlined that the unique selling point of this 'school-based' intervention was the volunteer component; this included parents and school staff (such as nurses or Physical Education teachers) to lead and facilitate all BOKS sessions. In terms of intervention training, it is important to note that all volunteers within the program were trained by the research team regarding program content and pedagogical methods surrounding each session (Pojednic et al., 2016). An important strength of note within this successful BMI-oriented before-school PA program relates to the fact that the curricula components of the interventions have been developed by an experienced educational leadership team at the BOKS organization (Pojednic et al., 2016) – with issues relating to the intervention fidelity from the BOKS curriculum (lesson plans and student attendance) being tracked throughout the participating schools.

The First-Class Activity Program (First-Class).
Evaluation Study 1

Vuchenich's (2010) thesis previously reported the effects of a before-school PA intervention in the US, known as 'The First-Class Activity Program' (First-Class). Specifically, as part of this study protocol, the selected participants from two-grade three classes were required to wear objective accelerometer devices during the entire school day (8:00am–14:00pm). Following the completion of baseline assessments, the intervention dosage comprised of the 'HOPSports' system being set up within the multi-purpose school room every day, for approximately 30 minutes prior to the commencement of the school day (7:30–8:00am). The First-Class intervention lasted 8 weeks, and all participants had the option of participating in the program from 5 to 30 minutes each day. Of particular note within this initial First-Class intervention evaluation was the inclusion of an interactive multi-media PA training system, which utilizes DVR technology for promoting large sample student PA participation. Vuchenich (2010) reports that the focus of the HoPSports system is the creation of a fun and motivational environment, with the objective of improving the health and wellness of youth. Similar to the educational components of the BOKS program (Pojednic et al., 2016; Whooten et al., 2018), the HOPSports system includes a wide variety of lesson-based activities, which are age appropriate for elementary, middle, and high school-aged students. From a youth PA promotion perspective, the activities and equipment included within the HOPSports system target basic motor skills, sports-specific skills, dance, circuit training, and others.

The First-Class Activity Program (First-Class). Evaluation Study 2

More recently, Knight's (2015) thesis reported the effects of the First-Class program on PA, musculoskeletal fitness, and cognitive function in third-grade children; however, within this study, the intervention lasted for 10-week, in comparison with Vuchenich's (2010) 8-week study evaluation. Some additional information and differences regarding the First-Class intervention were reported by Knight (2015), specifically that children were informed about the purpose of the program in terms of PA participation, prior to their commencement. In terms of intervention structure, Knight's (2015) research documents the breakdown of the First-Class program in terms of activity timing into two distinct phases. Interestingly, the initial 10- to 15- minute phase of the program comprised of 'free-play, in which participants were prompted to be physically active on their own, with the support of research assistants or their student peers (if needed). While there is no reference to the HOPSports system within Knight's (2015) evaluation of the First-Class intervention, the most commonly reported equipment used in phase one were jump ropes, sports balls, and hula-hoops. Phase two of the program 7:30–7:40am (prior to breakfast dismissal) moved beyond the free-play component and focused on the organized activity component, as led by a member of the research team. Aligned with the purpose of Knight's (2015) study, which sought to evaluate the effectiveness of the program towards musculoskeletal fitness, it is unsurprising that many of these organized activities within phase two comprised of muscle- and bone-strengthening components, on at least 3 days per week, and aerobic activities were included every day. In terms of the provision of equipment for phase two of the First-Class intervention (Knight, 2015), the researchers and the school provided jump ropes, sports balls, small and large exercise balls, resistance tubing, and hula-hoops, etc.

Before-School Running/Walking Club (Stylianou et al., 2016)

Most recently, Stylianou et al. (2016) in their efficacy study reported the volume of PA accumulated by third- and fourth-grade (age range: 8–10 years old) children during a 5-week before-school running/walking club. While the program components are documented, this study reports the specific conditions for the two selected intervention schools (Schools A and B). It was interesting that the criterion for this before-school PA program was for participants to accumulate at least 5 minutes of MVPA during the daily intervention sessions. In terms of the intervention structure for School A participants (n = 39), the duration of the program was 20 minutes in total, each weekday, for 5 weeks. Aligned with heightening participation rates within the intervention, the Physical Education teacher implemented a reinforcement, rewards-based system for student compliance with the program. Specifically, in this study (Stylianou et al., 2016), as part of School A:

> The teacher monitored the distance students covered in the program and the students received "shoe"-shaped tokens for their shoestrings or backpacks for every 8 kilometers (5 miles) they covered.
>
> *(p. 4)*

In terms of the intervention structure for School B participants (n = 56), the duration of the program was 15 minutes in total, each weekday, for 5 weeks. Similar to School A, and as aligned with heightening participation rates within the intervention, the Physical Education teacher implemented a reinforcement, rewards-based system for student compliance with the program. Specifically, in this study (Stylianou et al., 2016), as part of School B:

> Students received a pencil for every two laps completed as well as a "caught being good" ticket (part of the school accountability system) each time they participated in the program.
>
> *(p. 4)*

Active Ingredients? Examples of After-School Programs

Demetriou et al. (2017), in their review of after-school PA intervention reviews, identified several considerations needed for effective future after-school PA program implementations and research evaluations. The authors highlighted advantages for implementing programs in school (the subject of this chapter), rather than in community settings. They further highlighted the need to offer programs on 2 or more days per week, consistent with the findings of Whooten et al. (2018) in the BOKS before-school PA study, and preferably over a longer duration. Authors emphasized the importance of ensuring high program attendance rates (Demetriou et al., 2017), consistent with Beets et al. (2009), who had previously identified exposure to the program, or attendance rate, as a key aspect worth consideration. The limited evidence available in this meta-analysis leads authors to conclude that a dose-response effect was most readily seen with high attendance levels, specifically those students who attend 40% or more of the sessions showing the greatest improvements in PA (Beets et al., 2009). Similar to the before-school PA programs, examples of three separate case study after-school PA programs, specifically evaluating intervention effectiveness, are presented for quick reference below, so that readers can again identify the common ingredients present in such programs:

10-Month After-School PA Program

The 10-month after school intervention, reported by Barbeau et al. (2007), found a 22.2-minute adjusted mean difference in MVPA at follow-up, between control and intervention condition. This unnamed case study (Barbeau et al., 2007) involved 278 females, aged 8–12 years old, from 8 schools in Georgia, and employed a 7-day PA self-report to measure MVPA. The intervention itself involved the participants in the intervention group staying at their school at the end of the day to receive a 110-minute intervention. The intervention consisted of 30 minutes of homework time, followed by 80 minutes of PA. The PA component included 25 minutes of skill development (the example given by the authors is 'how to dribble a basketball'), 35 minutes of MVPA, and 20 minutes of toning and stretching. Of note is the strategy employed within this intervention of teaching students how to maintain their heart rate above 150 beats per minute (to reflect MVPA intensity) during the MVPA portion of the intervention each day, using heart rate monitors. The intervention was offered during the school year, every day that school was in session. The intervention was delivered by classroom teachers and teaching assistants, with a research assistant also on site every day.

Bristol Girls Dance Project

Also, worthy of mention, when we consider specific after-school programs, are those highlighted by Mears and Jago (2016) as having included retention test data in the trials carried out. The first of these was a feasibility trial consisting of a three-arm cluster randomized controlled trial (RCT) of the Bristol Girls Dance Project, involving three interventions and four control schools (in two conditions) (Jago et al., 2012). MVPA was measured using accelerometry at baseline (time 0), during the last week of the 9-week dance program (time 1), and again at 20 weeks after the study commenced (time 2). Participants were 11–12 years of age, and attendance at the dance sessions over the course of the study was 13.3 sessions (out of 18), representing an average attendance rate of 74%. The intervention consisted of participants receiving two 90-minute after-school dance classes each week for 9 weeks. The sessions were delivered by instructors who were given an outline of the program and had attended a half-day content familiarization session. Authors reported between 5 and 12 more weekday MVPA minutes at time 2 in the intervention group, when compared to the control group.

Action 3.30

The third after-school intervention which also included a retention measure, as highlighted by Mears and Jago (2016), is the 'Action 3.30' program which targeted 9–11-year-old children (Jago et al., 2014). This study involved a cluster randomized feasibility trial involving ten control and ten intervention schools. MVPA was again measured using accelerometry at baseline (time 0), during the last weeks of the intervention (time 1; T1), and 4 months after the intervention ended (time 2; T2). The intervention consisted of 40 intended 60-minute sessions over a 20-week period. Two teaching assistants at each school received a 5-day training program focused on delivering the Self-Determination Theory-based after-school PA program. Mean attendance at the sessions was reported as 53%, and sex-stratified analyses indicated that the boys in the intervention condition accumulated 8.6 more minutes of weekday MVPA than boys in the control condition at T1, but that no significant effect existed for females (Jago et al., 2014). This further supports the earlier emphasized point regarding the importance of tailoring interventions to suit the specific needs of the groups in question that a 'one-size fits all' approach will not likely have an impact on all participants, specifically when mixed gender is considered. Analysis at T2 showed no significant differences between groups, suggesting that the program did not have a lasting impact on MVPA. A revised version of Action 3:30 was evaluated more recently, and again overall daily MVPA did not increase significantly between intervention and control groups (Jago et al., 2019). The authors reported almost 9 minutes per day difference in MVPA when Action 3:30 days were compared to days when the intervention was not scheduled. (Jago et al., 2019). Moreover, the estimated cost of revised version of the program was £2.06 per student per session, which was cheaper than existing provision with the added benefit of developing school staff (Jago et al., 2019). The authors highlighted the feasibility of Action 3:30 and that the way children swapped between different after-school activities instead of adding new ones likely reduced the likelihood of the program demonstrating effectiveness (Jago et al., 2019).

Recommendations for Researchers/Practitioners

While the evidence may suggest that school-based interventions for PA promotion are cost-effective, some economic arguments (Babey et al., 2014) challenge the high costs per student associated with before- and after-school programs, as these types of interventions can offer a small reach and appear unfeasible. Nonetheless, there are many reviews which highlight the potential of these strategies for increasing MVPA levels of children and youth, and most particularly for after-school programs. Research and evidence supporting after-school programs are much more plentiful than before-school; hence, further research is needed for before-school program effectiveness before any definitive conclusions regarding this type of program can be drawn. One overarching recommendation for practice in this area, regardless of before- or after-school programing, is to carefully consider the contexts, preferences, and activity patterns of the group being targeted, and tailor the intervention components specifically to their needs. Further recommendations specific to each program type are given below.

Before School

- The timing of these interventions seems best placed to be implemented approximately 30 minutes prior to the start of the school day (Knight, 2015; Stylianou et al., 2016; Whooten et al., 2018).
- The measurement of PA as a primary outcome measurement as part of these program types seems important; however, the inclusion of additional measurements, such as BMI,

musculoskeletal fitness, and cognitive behaviors, may hold promising intervention evaluative strategies for the before-school time period (Knight, 2015; Whooten et al., 2018).

- Of the limited evidence available, research findings indicate that children can spend between 20% and 50% (approximately) of their participation time in before-school programs in MVPA.
- In terms of study robustness for before-school PA programs, typically, small sample size comparisons exist, which may be perceived as a limitation in terms of empirical evidence (with the exception of the BOKS trial evaluation).
- With a weight status outcome measurement for before-school PA programs, it appears that as more children participate in terms of attendance rates, the increased likelihood of having a better body composition exists (Whooten et al., 2018).
- Finally, providing a range of equipment and a variety of activities seems worthwhile for before-school PA programs. Furthermore, the inclusion of experienced educational leaders and volunteers holds promise.

After School

- When compared to before-school PA programs, after-school PA programs can provide a substantial portion of a child's daily PA and energy expenditure (Beets, 2012; Trost, Rosenkranz, & Dzewaltowski, 2008)
- If ECPA is to be considered a formal part of after-school programs, it is important that all abilities are catered for (Woods et al., 2010). A 'one-size fits all' approach is less likely to be effective.
- While some studies reported very meaningful PA differences for after-school PA programs (Babey et al., 2014; Barbeau et al., 2007; Beets, 2012; Jago et al., 2014; Mears & Jago, 2016), the measurement techniques of PA from self-reported and device-based perspectives may need further consistency to avoid discrepancies within the research interpretations.
- While theoretical considerations are quite common in terms of after-school PA program design (Mears & Jago, 2016), there appear to be very few differences in effectiveness between those that use and those that do not use theoretical justification within their approaches for evaluating after-school PA.
- Finally, a dose-response for effectiveness seems to be correlated with high attendance rates in after-school PA programs.

References

Atkin, A. J., Gorely, T., Biddle, S. J. H., Cavill, N., & Foster, C. (2011). Interventions to promote physical activity in young people conducted in the hours immediately after school: A systematic review. *International Journal of Behavioral Medicine, 18*(3), 176–187. doi:10.1007/s12529-010-9111-z

Babey, S. H., Wu, S., & Cohen, D. (2014). How can schools help youth increase physical activity? An economic analysis comparing school-based programs. *Preventive Medicine, 69*(S), S55–S60. doi:10.1016/j.ypmed.2014.10.013

Barbeau, P., Johnson, M. H., Howe, C. A., Allison, J., Davis, C. L., Gutin, B., & Lemmon, C. R. (2007). Ten months of exercise improves general and visceral adiposity, bone, and fitness in black girls. *Obesity, 15*(8), 2077–2085. doi:10.1038/oby.2007.247

Beets, M. W. (2012). Enhancing the translation of physical activity interventions in afterschool programs. *American Journal of Lifestyle Medicine, 6*(4), 328–341. doi:10.1177/1559827611433547

Beets, M. W., Beighle, A., Erwin, H. E., & Huberty, J. L. (2009). After-school program impact on physical activity and fitness. A meta-analysis. *American Journal of Preventive Medicine, 36*(6), 527–537. doi:10.1016/j.amepre.2009.01.033

Beets, M. W., Okely, A., Weaver, R. G., Webster, C., Lubans, D., Brusseau, T., . . . Cliff, D. P. (2016). The theory of expanded, extended, and enhanced opportunities for youth physical activity promotion. *International Journal of Behavioral Nutrition and Physical Activity, 13*(120), 1–15. doi:10.1186/s12966-016-0442-2

Belton, S., O'Brien, W., Issartel, J., McGrane, B., & Powell, D. (2016). Where does the time go? Patterns of physical activity in adolescent youth. *Journal of Science and Medicine in Sport, 19*(11), 921–925. doi:10.1016/j.jsams.2016.01.008

Belton, S., O'Brien, W., McGann, J., & Issartel, J. (2018). Bright spots physical activity investments that work: Youth-physical activity towards health (Y-PATH). *British Journal of Sports Medicine*, 1–5. doi:10.1136/bjsports-2018-099745

Branscum, P., & Sharma, M. (2012). After-school based obesity prevention interventions: A comprehensive review of the literature. *International Journal of Environmental Research and Public Health, 9*(4), 1438–1457. doi:10.3390/ijerph9041438

Carson, R. L., Castelli, D. M., Beighle, A. E., & Erwin, H. (2014). School-based physical activity promotion: A conceptual framework for research and practice. *Childhood Obesity, 10*(2), 100–106. doi:10.1089/chi.2013.0134

De Meester, A., Stodden, D., Goodway, J., True, L., Brian, A., Ferkel, R., & Haerens, L. (2018). Identifying a motor proficiency barrier for meeting physical activity guidelines in children. *Journal of Science and Medicine in Sport, 21*(1), 58–62. doi:10.1016/j.jsams.2017.05.007

Demetriou, Y., Gillison, F., & McKenzie, T. L. (2017). After-school physical activity interventions on child and adolescent physical activity and health: A review of reviews. *Advances in Physical Education, 7*(2), 191–215. doi:10.4236/ape.2017.72017

Dobbins, M., Husson, H., Decorby, K., & LaRocca, R. (2013). School-based physical activity programs for promoting physical activity and fitness in children and adolescents aged 6 to 18 (review). *Cochrane Database of Systematic Reviews, 2*, 1–260.

Garriguet, D., & Colley, R. (2012, June). Daily patterns of physical activity among Canadians. Statistics Canada, Catalogue no. 82-003-XPE. *Health Reports, 23*(2). Retrieved from http://www.statcan.gc.ca/pub/82-003-x/2012002/article/11649-eng.pdf

Harrington, D. M., Murphy, M., Carlin, A., Coppinger, T., Donnelly, A., Dowd, K. P., . . . Belton, S. (2016). Results from Ireland North and South's 2016 report card on physical activity for children and youth. *Journal of Physical Activity and Health, 13*(Suppl 2), 183–188.

Harris, J., & Cale, L. (2019). *Promoting active lifestyles in schools.* Champaign, IL: Human Kinetics.

Hesketh, K. R., McMinn, A. M., Ekelund, U., Sharp, S. J., Collings, P. J., Harvey, N. C., . . . van Sluijs, E. M. F. (2014). Objectively measured physical activity in four-year-old British children: A cross-sectional analysis of activity patterns segmented across the day. *The International Journal of Behavioral Nutrition and Physical Activity, 11*(1), 1. doi:10.1186/1479-5868-11-1

Jago, R., Sebire, S. J., Cooper, A. R., Haase, A. M., Powell, J., Davis, L., . . . Montgomery, A. A. (2012). Bristol girls dance project feasibility trial: Outcome and process evaluation results. *International Journal of Behavioral Nutrition and Physical Activity, 9*, 1–10. doi:10.1186/1479-5868-9-83

Jago, R., Sebire, S. J., Davies, B., Wood, L., Edwards, M. J., Banfield, K., . . . Montgomery, A. A. (2014). Randomised feasibility trial of a teaching assistant led extracurricular physical activity intervention for 9 to 11 year olds: Action 3:30. *International Journal of Behavioral Nutrition and Physical Activity, 11*(1), 1–14. doi:10.1186/s12966-014-0114-z

Jago, R., Tibbitts, B., Sanderson, E., Bird, E. L., Porter, A., Metcalfe, C., . . . Sebire, S. J. (2019). Action 3:30R: Results of a cluster randomised feasibility study of a revised teaching assistant-led extracurricular physical activity intervention for 8 to 10 year olds. *International Journal of Environmental Research and Public Health, 16*(1), 131. Retrieved from https://www.mdpi.com/1660-4601/16/1/131

Knight, N. A. (2015). *Effects of a before school physical activity program on physical activity, musculoskeletal fitness, and cognitive function in third-grade children.* Greenville, NC: Faculty of the Department of Kinesiology, East Carolina University.

Kriemler, S., Meyer, U., Martin, E., van Sluijs, E. M. F., Andersen, L. B., & Martin, B. W. (2011). Effect of school-based interventions on physical activity and fitness in children and adolescents: A review of reviews and systematic update. *British Journal of Sports Medicine, 45*(11), 923–930. doi:10.1136/bjsports-2011-090186

Mahar, M. T., Vuchenich, M. L., Golden, J., DuBose, K. D., & Raedeke, T. D. (2011). Effects of a before-school physical activity program on physical activity and on-task behavior. *Medicine & Science in Sports & Exercise, 43*(Suppl 1), 24. doi:10.1249/01.MSS.0000402740.12322.07

Mâsse, L. C., McKay, H., Valente, M., Brant, R., & Naylor, P.-J. (2012). Physical activity implementation in schools: A 4-year follow-up. *American Journal of Preventive Medicine, 43*(4), 369–377. doi:10.1016/j.amepre.2012.06.010

McMullen, J., Ní Chróinín, D., Tammelin, T., Pogorzelska, M., & van der Mars, H. (2015). International approaches to whole-of-school physical activity promotion. *Quest, 67*(4), 384–399. doi:10.1080/00336297.2015.1082920

McMullen, J., van der Mars, H., & Jahn, J. A. (2014). Chapter 2: Creating a before-school physical activity program: Pre-service physical educators' experiences and implications for PETE. *Journal of Teaching in Physical Education, 33*(4), 449–466. doi:10.1123/jtpe.2014-0063

Mears, R., & Jago, R. (2016). Effectiveness of after-school interventions at increasing moderate-to-vigorous physical activity levels in 5- to 18-year olds: A systematic review and meta-analysis. *British Journal of Sports Medicine, 50*(21), 1315–1324. doi:10.1136/bjsports-2015-094976

Pate, R. R., & O'Neill, J. R. (2009). After-school interventions to increase physical activity among youth. *British Journal of Sports Medicine, 43*(1), 14–18. doi:10.1136/bjsm.2008.055517

Penney, D., & Harris, J. (1997). Extra-curricular physical education: More of the same for the more able? *Sport, Education and Society, 2*(1), 41–54. doi:10.1080/1357332970020103

Pojednic, R., Peabody, S., Carson, S., Kennedy, M., Bevans, K., & Phillips, E. M. (2016). The effect of before school physical activity on child development: A study protocol to evaluate the build our kids success (BOKS) program. *Contemporary Clinical Trials, 49*, 103–108. doi:10.1016/j.cct.2016.06.009

Randsell, L., Dinger, M. K., Huberty, J., & Miller, K. (2009). *Developing effective physical activity programs.* Champaign, IL: Human Kinetics.

Ryan, R. M., & Deci, E. L. (2000). Intrinsic and extrinsic motivations: Classic definitions and new directions. *Contemporary Educational Psychology, 25*(1), 54–67. doi:10.1006/ceps.1999.1020

Scottish Government. (2008). *Schools (health promotion and nutrition) Scotland act: Health promotion guidance for local authorities and schools.* Edinburgh, Scotland: Scottish Government.

Standage, M., Duda, J. L., & Ntoumanis, N. (2005). A test of self-determination theory in school physical education. *The British Journal of Educational Psychology, 75*(3), 411–433. doi:10.1348/000709904X22359

Stokols, D. (1992). Establishing and maintaining healthy environments. Toward a social ecology of health promotion. *American Psychologist, 47*(1), 6–22.

Strong, W. B., Malina, R. M., Blimkie, C. J. R., Daniels, S. R., Dishman, R. K., Gutin, B., . . . Trudeau, F. (2005). Evidence based physical activity for school-age youth. *The Journal of Pediatrics, 146*(6), 732–737. doi:10.1016/j.jpeds.2005.01.055

Stylianou, M., van der Mars, H., Kulinna, P. H., Adams, M. A., Mahar, M., & Amazeen, E. (2016). Before-school running/walking club and student physical activity levels: An efficacy study. *Research Quarterly for Exercise and Sport, 87*(4), 342–353. doi:10.1080/02701367.2016.1214665

Tremblay, M. S., Gonzalez, S. A., Katzmarzyk, P. T., Onywera, V. O., Reilly, J. J., & Tomkinson, G. (2015). Physical activity report cards: Active healthy kids global alliance and the Lancet physical activity observatory. *Journal of Physical Activity and Health, 12*, 297–298. doi:10.1123/jpah.2015-0184

Trost, S. G., Rosenkranz, R. R., & Dzewaltowski, D. (2008). Physical activity levels among children attending after-school programs. *Medicine and Science in Sports and Exercise, 40*(4), 622–629. doi:10.1249/MSS.0b013e318161eaa5

Vasques, C., Magalhães, P., Cortinhas, A., Mota, P., Leitão, J., & Lopes, V. P. (2014). Effects of intervention programs on child and adolescent BMI: A meta-analysis study. *Journal of Physical Activity & Health, 11*(2), 426–444. doi:10.1123/jpah.2012-0035

Vuchenich, M. (2010). Effects of a before school physical activity program on physical activity and on-task behavior in elementary school-aged children. Dissertation. Retrieved from http://thescholarship.ecu.edu/handle/10342/2941

Ward, D. S., Saunders, R. P., & Pate, R. R. (2007). *Physical activity interventions in children and adolescents.* Champaign, IL: Human Kinetics.

Whooten, R. C., Perkins, M. E., Gerber, M. W., & Taveras, E. M. (2018). Effects of before-school physical activity on obesity prevention and wellness. *American Journal of Preventive Medicine, 54*(4), 510–518. doi:10.1016/j.amepre.2018.01.017

Woods, C., Moyna, N., Quinlan, A., Tannehill, D., & Walsh, J. (2010). *The children's sport participation and physical activity study (CSPPA study). Report 1.* Retrieved from https://www4.dcu.ie/shhp/downloads/CSPPA.pdf

33

KEEPING KIDS ACTIVE

Summertime Interventions to Address Physical Activity

*Elizabeth M. Rea, Amy M. Bohnert, Jennette P. Moreno,
and Allie Hardin*

Introduction

Obesity has reached unprecedented levels among children and adolescents in developed countries across the globe, with recent estimates of 23.8% of boys and 22.6% of girls being overweight or obese (Ng et al., 2014). Until recently, the contribution of youth's out-of-school time, including summertime, had largely been overlooked. However, several large-scale longitudinal studies provide convincing evidence that youth gain more weight during the summer break from school. Decreased physical activity (PA) and increased sedentary time are postulated to be important contributing factors. This chapter will (1) provide a brief overview of summertime weight gain and fitness loss as well as the role of PA as a contributing factor; (2) summarize the existing literature examining how PA fluctuates during the school year versus summertime; (3) describe four key inter-related contextual factors that may drive these fluctuations (e.g., climate/weather, structured days, family socioeconomic status (SES), and safety); (4) review the existing literature on summertime interventions to address PA with a focus on "what works" to guide researchers and practitioners; and (5) highlight key issues that should be addressed in future research.

Overview

Weight Gain & Fitness Loss over the Summertime

Increasingly, evidence identifies extended periods of time spent out of school, particularly summertime, as a period of risk for weight gain among youth. Several longitudinal studies have shown that school-age children gain more weight over the summertime as compared to the school year (Moreno, Johnston, & Woehler, 2013; von Hippel & Workman, 2016). Three recent reviews drawing on these studies conclude that accelerated weight gain during the summer months occurs for at least a portion of the study populations in both the US and international samples (Baranowski et al., 2014; Franckle, Adler, & Davison, 2014; Tanskey, Goldberg, Chui, Must, & Sacheck, 2018). Not only do children gain more weight over the summer break as compared to the school year, but fitness gains made during the school year are lost. In one of the first studies to address summertime fitness loss, researchers demonstrated that fitness gains made over the course of the school year in a sample of middle schoolers, as measured by a VO_{2max} treadmill test, returned to pre-intervention levels following summer vacation (Carrel, Clark, Peterson, Eickhoff, & Allen, 2007). Similarly, children enrolled in a 3-year PA intervention improved their fitness during the school year, as measured by heart rate response to a bench-stepping task, but fitness levels were comparable to control school levels following summer break (Gutin, Yin, Johnson, & Barbeau, 2008). More recently, researchers reported that children from schools receiving a school year PA intervention decreased in both steps measured via a pedometer as well as PACER laps upon returning to school after summer break as compared to the end of the previous spring semester (Fu, Brusseau, Hannon, & Burns, 2017). Thus, evidence of summertime weight gain and fitness loss is compelling, leading to the question: what is driving this weight gain?

PA During the Summertime (Versus School Year)

Low levels of PA and high rates of sedentary behavior are postulated to be important contributing factors to weight gain and fitness loss over the summer months (Baranowski et al., 2014; Franckle et al., 2014). Several reviews of international studies have shown that in general, children's patterns of PA vary over the course of the year, with more PA occurring during warmer summer months (Carson & Spence, 2010; Rich, Griffiths, & Dezateux, 2012). However, a more recent review provided evidence of mixed results regarding shifts in PA and sedentary levels between the school year and summer (Tanskey et al., 2018). Differences in methodology both in terms of design (i.e., longitudinal versus cross-sectional) and measurement (i.e., self-report versus accelerometers) may contribute to these equivocal findings. In the following paragraphs, we summarize the various studies that have addressed fluctuations in PA during the summertime versus school year.

Longitudinal studies comparing PA levels across school year to summertime are scant. One small study of school-age children residing in rural Minnesota compared school year versus summer PA found that time spent in light and moderate PA assessed via accelerometers decreased over the summer, while sedentary time significantly increased during summer as compared to the school year (McCue, Marlatt, & Sirard, 2013). Similarly, in another longitudinal study using accelerometers in the UK, a sample of 7-year olds engaged in less moderate-to-vigorous physical activity (MVPA) over the summer compared to the spring, in certain subgroups of their sample including boys, children of normal weight, those living in urban areas, and those from high-income families. However, the lowest levels of MVPA were found in autumn and winter across their sample (Atkin, Sharp, Harrison, Brage, & van Sluijs, 2016). In the most recent longitudinal study, researchers compared levels of accelerometer-measured PA for a 9-day period in a school-aged sample of low-income minority youth in May (school year) and July (summer break). During the summer, children engaged in significantly less light intensity PA (23% of wake time versus 25% of wake time in the school year) and significantly more sedentary/screen time (69% of wake time during the summer versus 67% of wake time during the school year) as compared to the school year (Brazendale et al., 2018).

Although less rigorous than longitudinal designs, cross-sectional studies provide valuable insight into how PA levels vary based on the time of year. One study measured total energy expenditure (TEE) in overweight and obese youth using the doubly labeled water technique, and found no significant differences in TEE when comparing youth who were in- versus out-of-school (Zinkel et al., 2013). Another cross-sectional study of youth, aged 5–18 in Louisiana, showed that self-reported PA and television viewing were both significantly higher over the summer than during the school year (Staiano, Broyles, & Katzmarzyk, 2015). Similarly, a large cross-sectional study of a similar age group (6–19 years) utilizing NHANES (National Health and Nutrition Examination Survey) data reported 4.6 minutes more of MVPA per day (measured via accelerometers) and 18 minutes more of television viewing per day among youth surveyed over the summer months as compared with those surveyed during the school year (Wang, Vine, Hsiao, Rundle, & Goldsmith, 2015). Collectively, these studies suggest moderate evidence of diminished PA over the summer months; however, more longitudinal studies are needed that track the same youth over the summer and school year to draw more definitive conclusions. Further, the clinical relevance of fluctuations in PA needs to be explored as current findings suggest that statistically significant differences may not be that clinically meaningful given their magnitude (e.g., less than 10 minutes per day).

What Contextual Factors Are Driving These Changes?

Research examining school year-summer variations in PA and ultimately, weight gain and fitness loss, needs to take into account four key inter-related contextual factors, including (1) climate and weather, (2) degree of structure, (3) family SES, and (4) safety concerns. We acknowledge, however, that these factors could influence health behaviors other than PA (e.g., sleep, dietary intake) contributing to weight gain over the summer, but given the scope of this chapter, we will focus on PA specifically.

Climate and Weather

Changes in levels of PA by season could be impacted by climate and weather (also see Chapter 10 for further discussion). For example, one cross-sectional study discussed above (Staiano et al., 2015) took place in Louisiana, a warm sub-tropical climate with very hot and humid summers. Though participants self-reported more PA over the summer, when heat index was included in the model, these associations weakened, indicating that when it felt hotter outside, participants reported less PA. Additionally, participants who were surveyed during periods of high precipitation were less likely to report meeting PA guidelines. These findings align with another study of 12–14-year olds in eastern Massachusetts. Adolescents engaged in less PA (measured via accelerometer) on very hot or very cold days, throughout the winter, and on rainy or dark days, indicating an impact of climate and weather on PA levels (Quante et al., 2019). Similarly, in Montreal, Canada, 12–13-year olds self-reported significantly less PA in the winter and on rainy days (Bélanger, Gray-Donald, O'loughlin, Paradis, & Hanley, 2009). Temperatures and weather vary by region, and this leads to changes in patterns of PA with heat being a limiting factor in warmer climates and cold influencing PA in cooler climates. Taking into account weather- and climate-related factors is important when considering differences in PA across summer months compared to the school year, and researchers need to account for these factors in their design and analyses.

Degree of Structure

Several recent reviews have suggested that lack of structure during the summer months may contribute significantly to decreased PA (Baranowski et al., 2014; Franckle et al., 2014; Tanskey et al., 2018). Brazendale et al. (2017) have proposed the "Structured Days Hypothesis," as a possible explanation for variations in PA over the course of the year. This hypothesis suggests that unstructured time and settings significantly contributes to weight gain due to an increase in obesogenic behaviors, including less PA. This increase in obesogenic behaviors occurs because in more structured settings, including school, these behaviors are better regulated. Indeed, Brazendale and colleagues (2017) review studies comparing weekday obesogenic behaviors (i.e., more structured time) to weekend obesogenic behaviors (i.e., less structured time), with children generally participating in more obesogenic behaviors, including less PA, during the weekend compared to weekday. For example, a study of fifth graders in Colorado found that children participated in more sedentary behavior (measured via accelerometer) during out-of-school hours compared to in-school hours, and on weekend days compared to weekdays. In addition, the children spent more time in light PA on weekdays compared to weekend days (Beck, Chard, Hilzendegen, Hill, & Stroebele-Benschop, 2016). Collectively, when applied to summertime, these findings suggest without the structure of school, youth are more likely to engage in sedentary behavior and less PA which combined with other obesogenic behaviors (e.g., dietary changes, compromised sleep) likely contributes to weight gain.

Further evidence of the value of structure for mitigating weight gain can be found in several recent studies of summertime programing (Mahoney, 2011; Parente, Sheppard, & Mahoney, 2012; Park & Lee, 2015). Drawing on a nationally representative data set, two longitudinal studies of youth aged 10–18 years indicated that routine involvement in structured care during the summertime, including organized sports or other extracurricular activities or summer programs, was associated with lower rates of obesity and lower BMIs at later time points even when accounting for prior BMI and demographic factors (Mahoney, 2011; Parente et al., 2012). Park and Lee (2015) compared two groups of high school students before and after summer break: freshmen who participated in a mandatory summer school program and sophomores who experienced summer as usual. The summer school program was held 5 days per week for 5 weeks and consisted of academic programing along with 1 hour of PA per day. At the end of summer break, the summer-as-usual group gained significantly more weight and lost significantly more fitness, as assessed via the Queens College step test, than the summer school group. Additionally, for those who did not attend the summer school, their weight and fitness were significantly influenced by their SES, i.e., those with higher SES having better outcomes than those with lower SES. These differences related to SES were not present for those who attended summer school. Providing opportunities for youth to engage in organized, structured activities over the summer, even if programing is not specifically related to health behaviors, could provide a number of benefits and possibly curb summertime weight gain. The structure and routine of organized activities may allow for increased access to PA opportunities, but it also likely limits the amount of sedentary time as well as influencing other obesogenic behaviors.

Research comparing year-round schooling to traditional schooling also provides support for the importance of structure for preventing weight gain and improving PA and fitness over the summer (Weaver, Hunt, et al., 2020). In a natural experiment, comparing one year-round school (45 days of school, followed by 15 days off, with a 5-week summer break) with two traditional schools (a 10-week summer break) over the course of 15 months (including two summers), children in the year-round school experienced smaller increases in BMI, but also gained less fitness over the entire course of the study compared to those children in the traditional schools. Looking specifically at summer, the year-round students gained more fitness (as measured by PACER laps) during only the first summer (not the second), and showed smaller increases in BMI over both summers, as compared to the traditional schools. However, during the school year, this pattern was reversed such that students in the traditional schools showed smaller increases in BMI and increased their fitness more than the year-round school group. In support of the Structured Days Hypothesis, the traditional school group performed better during the school year, as they had fewer break days (more structure) than the year-round school. However, over the summertime the year-round school had fewer break days than the traditional school, and showed improvements in fitness and BMI. Similarly, research comparing traditional schooling to year-round schooling on a 1-week (traditional school) versus a 3-week (year-round school) spring break found no significant differences in PA and sedentary time between school weekdays and spring break weekdays for students in the traditional 1-week spring break. However, for students at the year-round school with a 3-week spring break, researchers observed significant increases in sedentary time of about 30 minutes and significant decreases in PA of 12 minutes on spring break weekdays compared to school weekdays (Weaver et al., 2018). These results indicate that the structure that school provides does impact obesogenic behaviors including PA, and that longer periods without this structure likely influences BMI.

Family SES

Although family income level certainly plays a role in how much PA youth get regardless of time of year (Ferreira et al., 2007; Jin & Jones-Smith, 2015), it may be a factor that is particularly salient during the summertime. Youth in low-income families might not be able to afford access to summer camps and summer activities where they would have more opportunity to participate in PA. Weaver, Beets, Brazendale, and Brusseau (2019) propose that, partially due to this lack of access to organized activities over the summer, low-income youth are exposed to a "health gap." Each summer that low-income youth cannot participate in summer programing, it is posited that they are at a greater risk to gain weight than their higher-income peers, creating a health gap. This health gap continues to widen over time as these low-income youth are continually unable to access summer programing and are at a greater risk of becoming overweight or obese.

Safety

A related factor is a lack of access to safe places to play and hold summer camps or activities which could also impact on youth's levels of PA over the summer months (see Chapters 8–11 in this volume for further discussion). Parents might not allow their children to play outside because of busy streets, concern of kidnapping, or not knowing where their children are (Ergler, Kearns, & Witten, 2013). Parents might encourage their children to play inside, for which options are generally more sedentary (playing board games, watching television, playing video games, etc.). A study in Belgium created "Play Streets," during summer vacation as a way to offer safe spaces for children to play outdoors and to encourage PA (D'Haese, Van Dyck, De Bourdeaudhuij, Deforche, & Cardon, 2015). Play Streets are streets that are closed off from motorized traffic and reserved specifically for the use of children. Compared to the control group, children who utilized the Play Streets over the summer experienced significant increases in MVPA and decreases in sedentary time. Offering increased access to safe, outdoor spaces for children to play over the summer could significantly improve PA. A similar study conducted in the US evaluated a safe schoolyard initiative in a low-income neighborhood in Louisiana. This schoolyard was supervised by hired attendants, for children to play in after school, on the weekends, and during the summer. Compared to the control neighborhood, for the entire two-year intervention period, 84% more children were outside and physically active in the intervention neighborhood and schoolyard, and reported decreases in sedentary time during the school week. However, schoolyard attendance was lower during the summer than during the school year (i.e., average of 71.4 children on weekdays during the school year compared to 27.8 on weekdays during the summer) (Farley et al., 2007).

Collectively, these four factors provide important explanations for why PA may fluctuate during the school year as compared to the summer months. These factors are inter-related suggesting that for low-SES families, the role of structure in promoting PA may be particularly important given safety issues that may preclude youth from being physically active in their neighborhoods or getting to and from programing during the summer months which are the hottest of the year and the time when violence increases (Bushman, Wang, & Anderson, 2005). A more comprehensive understanding of how these factors work together to uniquely influence PA during the summer months is an important agenda item for future research in this area.

How Effective Are Summertime Interventions to Address PA?

A variety of summertime PA interventions have been studied. For this summary, studies published from 2000 to 2018 that evaluated interventions conducted over the summer only and assessed PA as outcome were included. Interventions have focused on promoting changes in PA at both the (1) individual level, through offering more structured opportunities to engage in PA, specifically, through summer day camps (SDCs) and the (2) community level, by encouraging PA opportunities more broadly through the use of marketing, improved access, and engagement of community partners. Interventions were implemented with community samples of youth, at-risk youth, and overweight and obese youth. Results are summarized in the following sections as well as in Table 33.1, and are presented from most to least efficacious/rigorous. The various methods that were employed to increase PA and measure its improvement are described.

Table 33.1 Summary of findings from summer day camps (SDCs)

Summer day camps

	Weaver et al., 2017	Olvera et al., 2012	Evans et al., 2018	Bohnert et al., 2017	Meucci et al., 2013	Graziano et al., 2017	Kilanowski & Gordon, 2015	Baranowski et al., 2003
Age group	5–12-year-olds	9–14-year-olds	6–12-year-olds	10–14 year-olds	8–12-year-olds	4–8-year-olds	6–14-year-olds	8-year-olds
Sample size	1,830	99	51	64	22	16	171	35
Target population	Youth at existing summer day camps	Hispanic and African American overweight girls	Low-income youth	Urban girls (majority African American and Latina/Hispanic)	Overweight youth	Overweight youth	Children of migrant workers	African American girls
Physical activities	Extended and enhanced existing PA opportunities at the summer day camps including games and field trips	Team activities, yoga, pilates, circuit training, spinning, step aerobics, games, dancing	Games including mini soccer, golf, capture the flag, and kickball. Additional community partner activities including karate, hip hop dance, and obstacle courses	Sports-based PA and pool time	Swinging, hanging, climbing, stretching, yoga, hiking, brisk walking, fun-runs, sports	Group-based aerobic exercises and games like dodgeball and soccer	Calisthenics and sport lessons, had access to physical education/playground equipment such as sport balls, jump ropes, and softball field equipment	Jump-rope, running/walking, sports including basketball and soccer, swimming, active field trips
Number of weeks	8 weeks minimum	4 weeks	8 weeks	4 weeks	4 weeks or 8 weeks	8 weeks	7 weeks	4 weeks in-person camp; 8 weeks at home online
Number of days per week	5 days	5 days	5 days	5 days	5 days	5 days	5 days	5 days
Number of hours per day	At least 8 hours	8 hours	4 hours	6 hours	6 hours	9 hours	8 hours	9.5 hours
Study design	Two-group pre-post quasi-experimental trial	One-group quasi-experimental trial	Two-group quasi-experimental trial	One group pre-post quasi-experimental trial	Three-group pre-post quasi-experimental* trial	One-group nonrandomized pilot trial	Two-group pre-post quasi-experimental trial	Two-arm parallel group randomized control pilot study

Time frame	• Pre: July of summer before intervention • Post: July of summer of the intervention • BMI measurements occurred during first 2 weeks of June and first 2 weeks of August each year • Actigraphy data was collected on four nonconsecutive unannounced days during the summer camps at both time points	• Pre: 1 week before intervention • Post: last 2 days of intervention • Accelerometer and attendance data collected daily during the intervention	• Pre: at the end of the school year • Midsummer: during weeks 4 and 5 (actigraph worn for 7 days) • Post: last week of summer	• Pre: during the first weeks of participants' summer vacation, prior to programming • Post: during the final week of the program, approximately 4 weeks after first time point	• Pre: within 4 days of the beginning of the intervention • Post: within 48 hours after the 4- or 8-week intervention was completed	• Pre: before the start of the intervention • Post: 1–2 weeks after the intervention ended • Follow-up: 6–8 months after the intervention ended	• Pre: before the start of the intervention in late June • Post: after the intervention in early August	• Pre: March to May before the intervention in June • Post: at the end of the 4-week camp (only BMI measured at this time point) • Follow-up: 12 weeks after the beginning of camp in August through September (after online portion was completed)
PA measurement	Accelerometer	Accelerometer	Accelerometer	Accelerometer	Heart rate monitor; VO$_2$ max treadmill protocol	Side to side jump test	Muscle strength and flexibility; self-report questionnaire	Accelerometer
Key BMI outcomes	• BMI was calculated, but no BMI outcomes reported	• % Body fat decreased by 2.49% body fat points from pre- to post-intervention • WC decreased by 5.27cm • BMI decreased by a mean difference of 0.410 kg/m2	• Intervention group lost 0.04 BMIz units, comparison condition lost 0.03 BMIz units ($p=0.07$) • Participants who attended the most days of camp (30–39 days) lost 0.16 BMIz units ($p = 0.01$)	• No significant BMI changes found	• Body fat % decreased by 7.3% in the 4-week group and 6.7% in the 8-week group, while the control group did not change	• BMIz decreased from 2.02 at baseline to 1.54 posttreatment	• Comparison group increased mean weight over the intervention time frame, while the intervention group did not	• No significant differences between intervention and control group on any BMI outcomes • A subgroup of girls who were heavier at baseline trended towards lower BMI compared to heavier counterparts in control group ($p<.08$)

(*Continued*)

Summer day camps

	Weaver et al., 2017	Olvera et al., 2012	Evans et al., 2018	Bohnert et al., 2017	Meucci et al., 2013	Graziano et al., 2017	Kilanowski & Gordon, 2015	Baranowski et al., 2003
Key PA outcomes	Boys: • 88.7% of boys in intervention condition met 60 min/day of MVPA compared to 82.6% in control condition • Intervention condition improved 11.8 minutes in MVPA Girls: • 82% of girls in the intervention condition met 60 min/day of MVPA compared to 70.6% in the control condition • Intervention condition improved 12.8 min in MVPA compared to previous summer	• Significant increase in MVPA from 61.8 ± 14.9 min in week 1 to 99.2 ± 29.3 min in week 4 • 78% of girls meeting daily MVPA guidelines on average over the course of the intervention • 1-mile run time significantly decreased from week 1 to week 4	• Intervention condition spent 4.6% less time being sedentary compared to controls • On days when youth attended camp, they engaged in 41 more minutes per day of MVPA and 8.5% less sedentary time compared to days they did not attend camp	• 28.18 additional minutes of MVPA per day compared to pre-camp • 20% of participants meeting recommended 60 min per day of MVPA during camp • 2 hours less sedentary time during camp compared to pre-camp	• Resting energy expenditure was higher in both the 4-week and 8-week group versus the control group • Resting heart rate decreased from pre-program versus post-program: 97 ± 22 versus 80 ± 8 beat/min in the 8-week group versus control group • VO$_2$ peak significantly increased pre-program versus post-program in the 8-week group compared to the control group	• Improvements in number of side jumps completed in a 30-second period	• Improvements in muscle flexibility as measured by Sit and Reach • Improvements in healthy behavior attitudes as measured by self-report questionnaire	• No significant differences between intervention and control group

* Three groups: 4-week, 8-week, control.

Summer Day Camps

Camps that are designed specifically to occur on the weekdays during the summer are one way of offering consistent opportunities for PA over the summer. Whether these camps are targeted towards all youth, low-income youth, or overweight or obese youth, SDCs provide structure and can encourage youth to be more physically active during the summer. One SDC PA intervention took advantage of 20 already existing SDCs operated by 9 different organizations (e.g., YMCA camps, Boys and Girls Clubs of America, National Recreation and Parks Association), and sought to expand PA opportunities to ensure that all children at the camps (aged 5 to 12) accumulated 60 minutes of MVPA per day (Weaver et al., 2017). In the intervention condition, research staff met with SDC staff to design PA schedules at the camps, with a goal of including at least 3 hours of PA opportunities each day. If schedules could not accommodate an increase in PA opportunities, staff were encouraged to find ways to adjust current schedules to maximize PA. Suggestions included the addition of short activity breaks, active field trips (i.e., choosing to go to a pool or park rather than a movie), and maximizing MVPA opportunities during already scheduled activities. The control group consisted of youth attending similar SDCs who received a healthy eating attention intervention instead of a PA intervention. Measurements of PA took place in July prior to the intervention, and one year later while the intervention was taking place. To measure PA, researchers visited each camp for four nonconsecutive, unannounced days and had campers wear accelerometers. Youth attending the intervention condition camps were 2.04 (boys) and 3.84 (girls) times more likely to meet the 60 minutes per day guideline of MVPA than the youth in the control condition. Significant improvements in proportion of youth meeting the MVPA daily requirement, and overall MVPA minutes compared to the previous summer were also demonstrated, with youth in the intervention condition improving more than youth in the control condition. These findings suggest that capitalizing on existing summer camp infrastructure could be an efficient and cost-effective way to increase PA during the summertime.

Another SDC, targeting 9–14-year-old overweight and obese Hispanic and African American girls, demonstrated increases in PA and fitness (Olvera, Leung, Kellam, & Liu, 2013). Girls attended the SDC Monday through Friday during the month of July, and participated in daily exercise, nutrition education, and counseling sessions for the 4 weeks. PA opportunities included three to four 1-hour exercise sessions over the course of the day. The girls' mothers also attended 2-hour weekly exercise, nutrition, and counseling sessions. There was a significant increase in daily MVPA over the course of camp, with girls accruing 99.2 minutes per day of MVPA during the final week of camp (as compared to 61.8 minutes per day during the first week of camp). Additionally, 78% of girls met their MVPA guidelines on average, and 1-mile run time significantly decreased from pre-intervention to the last two days of the intervention. Of note, this intervention included behavioral counseling and the use of motivational interviewing (MI) for both the girls and their mothers to address underlying problems including self-esteem and behavioral issues, which no other intervention reviewed here included.

Similarly, Evans et al. (2018) offered a summertime intervention to low-income youth (6–12-year olds) which provided daily opportunities for PA, which also increased MVPA, for those who attended camp. Participants attended camp every day for 8 weeks. At least 2 hours of PA programming were offered each day throughout camp, which included various games and team sports, as well as evidence-based PA curriculum. The intervention also partnered with local community organizations to offer additional activities such as karate, Lego building, obstacle courses, hip hop dance, and creative movement. At the midpoint (week 4–5), participants spent 4.6% less time being sedentary on weekdays compared to the control group, as measured by accelerometer. Additionally, on days that youth attended camp, they spent 41 more minutes in MVPA and 8.5% less time in sedentary activity compared to days they did not attend camp, indicating that the camp was effective in increasing PA while youth were there.

Bohnert et al. (2017) also examined changes in PA for low-income urban girls participating in a SDC. The researchers tracked PA in youth aged 10–14 who participated in a community-based summer day program created for girls who live in low-income Chicago neighborhoods. The program was four weeks long for six hours each day and included sports and team-based PA as well as swimming pool time. Using accelerometer data, the researchers compared PA levels during the first week of summer vacation (prior to the start of camp) to the final week of camp. The participants significantly increased their MVPA by 28.18 minutes per day compared to before the camp. Additionally, before camp, only 5% of participants met the recommended 60 minutes per day of MVPA, while during the last week of camp, 20% of participants met the recommended 60 minutes per day. Notably though, girls could not wear the accelerometers during the daily pool time, and as a result, girls at the camp were more active than could be captured. Participants also decreased their sedentary time by over 2 hours per day when comparing pre-camp to the last week of camp.

Unlike these other SDC studies, Meucci et al. (2013) measured changes in overall fitness through resting energy expenditure, resting heart rate, and VO_{2peak}. This SDC was specifically offered to overweight 8–12-year olds for either 4 or 8 weeks. The intervention included diverse daily PA offerings such as hiking, swinging, fun-runs, sports, and yoga. This summer camp focused on teaching youth lifetime sports and activities that they could continue to do after camp to remain active, with no emphasis on reducing body weight. At the end of the camp, participants in the 8-week group showed improvements in fitness including an increase in peak aerobic capacity (VO_{2peak}) and decrease in resting heart rate compared to a control group who followed their usual summer break routine. Both the 4-week and 8-week groups showed increases in resting energy expenditure.

Similarly, an 8-week daily camp offered to a younger overweight sample, 4–8-year olds, showed improvements in fitness; however, these improvements were measured by number of side jumps completed within a 30-second period. Additionally, this camp showed long-term maintenance of this fitness improvement, as at 6-month follow-up, these results had maintained or improved. At this camp, children participated in 1.5 hours per day of PA through games such as soccer and dodgeball, in addition to nutrition and healthy lifestyle educations. Parents also attended a once-weekly class covering healthy lifestyle topics including PA (Graziano, Garcia, & Lim, 2017).

Another SDC targeted first- to eighth-grade children of migrant workers, while they were in an already existing summer school program from June through August (Kilanowski & Gordon, 2015). This intervention added structured time for PA through calisthenics and sport lessons, as well as other healthy lifestyle learning opportunities, while the youth were in summer school. Children received classroom instruction about nutrition, decreasing screen time and increasing PA. They were also provided with increased access to playground equipment including sports balls, jump ropes, and softball field equipment. The comparison group was students in a different summer school for children of migrant workers, who received Centers for Disease Control (CDC) flyers about healthy eating, but did not receive any additional classroom instruction or access to additional playground equipment. At the end of the intervention, youth in the intervention condition showed significant improvements in muscle flexibility (as measured by the Sit and Reach Test Box) and healthy behavior attitudes as measured by self-report questionnaire. Additionally, body weight increased among the comparison group, but not among the intervention group.

Of the eight SDC interventions designed to address PA over the summer, only one was not successful in increasing PA. This SDC was offered to 8-year-old African American girls in Houston, TX (Baranowski et al., 2003). Girls attended a 4-week SDC, followed by 8 weeks of access to a home internet intervention for both the girls and their parents. The SDC portion of the camp provided PA opportunities including pool days, field trips to the park, basketball, jump rope, and more. The internet portion of the intervention was designed to encourage girls to engage in PA and make healthy eating choices after camp was over. Girls and their parents were encouraged to log on weekly to read about that week's healthy behavior focus, including doing a fun PA activity at home, choosing healthy snacks, or drinking more water instead of soft drinks. The control group also attended a more general SDC and had access to a website with general health and homework advice. At the end of the 12 weeks of intervention, there were no significant differences in PA compared to the control group as measured by accelerometer. However, there was low participation in the internet portion of the intervention, with less than half of the sample ever logging in. Additionally, the second measurement point was after the completion of the online portion of the intervention (8 weeks after the completion of the SDC), with no PA measurement point immediately upon the conclusion of the in-person portion of the intervention (except for BMI). This lack of participation in the online portion and delayed measurement after completion of the SDC could have impacted overall results.

To summarize, evidence suggests that SDCs are an efficient and effective way to increase PA in youth over the course of the summer. Overall, seven out of the eight SDCs evaluated here produced some improvement in a PA-related outcome. Three SDCs produced clinically meaningful increases in daily MVPA while youth were at camp, ranging from increases of 11.8 to 37.4 minutes per day (Bohnert et al., 2017; Olvera et al., 2013; Weaver et al., 2017). Additionally, two SDCs reported that more than three quarters of their participants met the 60 minutes per day MVPA guideline while at camp (Olvera et al., 2013; Weaver et al., 2017). Four camps reported improvements in fitness outcomes, including a significant decrease in mile run times from week 1 to week 4 of camp (Olvera et al., 2013); improvements in resting energy expenditure, resting heart rate, and VO_{2peak} (Meucci et al., 2013); improvements in number of side jumps in a 30-second period (Graziano et al., 2017); and improvements on a sit and reach tests (Kilanowski & Gordon, 2015). Elements of these successful camps included consistent daily, structured PA time with a wide range of activities from team sports-based PA to yoga, dance, obstacle courses, spin, and step aerobics. Offering a variety of different PA opportunities could be an important factor to keep youth engaged over the summer months. All SDCs were fairly intensive offering from 4 to 8 weeks of programing, for 5 days per week, for a minimum of 4 hours per day. In addition, findings from Weaver et al. (2017) suggest that PA opportunities can be improved at existing SDCs, for example, planning more active field trips (a pool rather than a movie) or adding in short activity breaks throughout the day. Additionally, the inclusion of mothers as well as MI techniques (see Olvera et al., 2012) could be used to address barriers to engaging in PA, but this requires further investigation.

Community-Level Interventions

Interventions have also been implemented at a broad, community-level over the summertime. One community-level intervention that has increased PA focused on marketing PA as something fun to do with friends, and partnered with local community organizations and businesses in the community to offer PA opportunities. VERB Summer Scorecard (VSS), a community extension of the "VERB It's What you do," campaign launched by the CDC in 2002 (Alfonso et al., 2013; Bryant et al., 2010; DeBate et al., 2009). The VSS intervention promoted PA by providing scorecards to youth aged 9–13 that allowed them to track their PA activities and provided them with free or reduced-price admissions to different sports/activity classes and games throughout their community. Examples of these activities included taekwondo, swimming, bowling, skating, laser tag, tennis lessons, whiffle ball, dance aerobics, relay races, and more. The scorecards could then be redeemed for prizes.

Bryant et al. (2010) specifically examined the marketing strategy used in VSS. The intervention promoted PA as a fun thing to do with friends, and a way to gain new skills, rather than focusing only on health benefits. The intervention ran for 4 years, and three waves of data were collected. Participation improved over the course of the 4 years from 25% to between 30% and 37% among those who received a scorecard. Additionally, those who participated were more likely to be physically active more days per week than their peers who had not heard about VSS or heard about it and chose not to participate, though there were some gender differences in total number of days of PA reported (Alfonso et al., 2013; Bryant et al., 2010). Researchers also examined factors that were associated with the intention to participate in VSS in the future (DeBate et al., 2009). In this study, participants were asked about past participation in VSS, and intention to participate in the following year's VSS. Results showed that being female, having tried a new PA, not currently participating in out-of-school activities but wanting to, and self-monitoring of PA were all associated with wanting to participate in VSS in the future. In future interventions, it will be important to consider the way that PA is marketed to youth. Suggesting that engaging in PA is a fun way to spend time with friends and try new activities, rather than as a way to be healthy or lose weight, seemed to enhance participation.

Key Issues

To summarize, both SDC and community-level interventions improve PA outcomes, but SDCs provide more structure over the summer for youth which should lead to more consistent participation in PA. SDCs are encouraged to consult the Healthy Eating and Physical Activity (HEPA) standards endorsed by summertime organizations (e.g., American Camp Association). However, in order to successfully implement these standards, SDCs need guidance, ongoing training, as well as financial support if they are to be successful (Bohnert et al., 2017).

These findings also suggest the way that PA interventions are pitched to youth is important. The successful community-level intervention discussed here (VERB) encouraged PA as a way to have fun with friends, rather than a way to lose weight (Bryant et al., 2010). Three successful SDCs also encouraged PA without a direct emphasis on weight loss to youth. Weaver et al. (2017) used camps where the focus was not necessarily specific to weight loss or PA but to increase opportunities for PA at existing camps by including more active field trips and activity breaks throughout the day. Similarly, Meucci et al. (2013) exposed youth to a wide range of activities to encourage PA, without a focus on weight loss, even though the camp was specifically designed for overweight youth. The SDC evaluated by Bohnert et al. (2017) was targeted towards low-income adolescent females as a camp to learn new sports and leadership skills rather than a weight loss or PA intervention. The way that PA is addressed with youth as part of a camp or any other type of intervention may be key to long-term engagement in PA over the lifespan, as youth who learn that PA is a fun way to be social and enjoy a range of activities might be more likely to consistently seek out those opportunities as they grow, though research is needed to support this idea.

Year-round schools also might provide an avenue for consistent access to PA opportunities over the course of the year. However, preliminary research has been somewhat inconclusive. Weaver and colleagues (2019) did find that students in year-round schools improved fitness more over one summer, but not the second summer that was measured. During the school year, fitness gains made over the first summer reversed, and those students in traditional schools improved their fitness more than those in the year-round school. Year-round students also gained less fitness than traditional school students over the entire 15-month study period. Researchers also found a decrease in PA and increase in sedentary activity over a year-round school's 3-week spring break compared to a traditional school's 1-week spring break (Weaver et al., 2018). More research is needed in this area to draw firm conclusions about the potential for year-round schools to increase PA and ultimately, prevent weight gain in youth.

Recommendations for Researchers and Practitioners

Although research evidence is building in support of SDC and community-level PA interventions for youth, there are several important directions for future research. First, there needs to be a clearer understanding of what barriers exist that keep youth from participating in SDCs. Many families need child care over the summer months, and SDCs can address this need. The relevance of various obstacles including availability, costs associated with SDCs, challenges related to enrolling, beliefs about summertime, as well as transportation to and from the SDC needs more careful consideration in order to better understand choices that families make about summertime. Second, research that considers enrollment and attendance of various summertime programs needs to take into account developmental factors as these influence PA as well as weight gain. Several studies have identified the period from kindergarten through second grade as a risk period for weight gain and transition into overweight or obesity over the summer (e.g., von Hippel & Workman, 2016). Additionally, adolescence has been shown to be a time when PA levels decline (Dumith, Gigante, Domingues, & Kohl, 2011). Thus, developmental fluctuations and considerations are important to take into account when evaluating as well as creating summertime programs. Third, future attempts to understand weight gain and fitness loss over the school year and summer need more precise measurement windows. Many studies measure youth only in the spring (at the end of the school year) and the fall (at the beginning of the school year). Relying on longitudinal data with several measurement points over the course of the summer and school year will lead to better triangulation of when PA drops allowing for greater precision and ultimately, more strategic science. Fourth, careful examination of PA levels among children enrolled in year-round schools versus traditional schools is warranted given the role of structure in promoting health. Comparison of weight gain and PA between these two school calendars with larger samples could shed light on the importance of structure versus season which could influence policy and practice. A related point is that more studies are needed to examine the association between PA and growth throughout the year (i.e., autumn, winter, and spring) and in the Northern and Southern hemispheres given that these variables may be affected by seasonal influences which can vary by climate (Bogin, 1999; Moreno et al., 2019; Rich et al., 2012). These types of studies could assess seasonal versus school year summer differences in growth and PA patterns.

Researchers also need to better understand how PA gains made in summertime interventions can be carried over after the intervention is complete. Few studies implement follow-up data collection to examine how well interventions set children up for long-term PA engagement once the camp is over, and bridging this gap could lead to the establishment of long-term healthy behaviors in youth. Reviews of maintenance of behavioral change following the interventions have found that strategies that included longer intervention periods (24 weeks), more intervention contacts, and follow-up prompts were more likely to lead to maintenance of behavioral changes. Additionally, strategies such as setting intentions and identifying barriers to behavior change were used in interventions that led to maintenance of changes (Fjeldsoe, Neuhaus, Winkler, & Eakin, 2011). Levels of self-efficacy, and motivation and goal-setting have also been shown to be important factors in the maintenance of PA, specifically (Amireault, Godin, & Vezina-Im, 2013). However, much of this research has been focused on adult populations. More longitudinal research is needed to understand factors that encourage youth to continue to engage in PA once they have completed any summer programing. In closing, it is important to note that although SDCs may be an effective method of increasing PA and improving fitness in children while they were at camp, improvements in BMI were less common. Further, although improvements in PA are statistically significant, it is important to pay attention to whether this translates into meaningful clinical outcomes. Finally, adoption of multi-etiological approaches (see Baranowski, Motil, & Moreno, 2019) may allow for consideration of other factors beyond behaviors as well as the interaction of these behaviors with biology to address the complex problem of childhood obesity.

Funding

This work has been funded in part with federal funds from the USDA/ARS under Cooperative Agreement No. 58-3092-5-001. JPM is supported by Eunice Kennedy Shriver National Institute of Child Health & Human Development of the National Institutes of Health under Award Number K99HD091396.

References

Alfonso, M. L., Thompson, Z., McDermott, R. J., Colquitt, G., Jones, J. A., Bryant, C. A., . . . Zhu, Y. (2013). VERB™ summer scorecard: Increasing tween girls' vigorous physical activity. *Journal of School Health, 83*(3), 164–170.

Amireault, S., Godin, G., & Vezina-Im, L.-A. (2013). Determinants of physical activity maintenance: A systematic review and meta-analyses. *Health Psychology Review, 7*(1), 55–91.

Atkin, A. J., Sharp, S. J., Harrison, F., Brage, S., & van Sluijs, E. M. (2016). Seasonal variation in children's physical activity and sedentary time. *Medicine and Science in Sports and Exercise, 48*(3), 449.

Baranowski, T., Baranowski, J. C., Cullen, K. W., Thompson, D. I., Nicklas, T., Zakeri, I. F., & Rochon, J. (2003). The fun, food, and fitness project (FFFP): The Baylor GEMS pilot study. *Ethnicity and Disease, 13*(1 Supp 1), S1–S30.

Baranowski, T., Motil, K. J., & Moreno, J. P. (2019). Multi-etiological perspective on child obesity prevention. *Current Nutrition Reports, 8*(1), 1–10.

Baranowski, T., O'Connor, T., Johnston, C., Hughes, S., Moreno, J., Chen, T.-A., . . . Baranowski, J. (2014). School year versus summer differences in child weight gain: A narrative review. *Childhood Obesity, 10*(1), 18–24.

Beck, J., Chard, C. A., Hilzendegen, C., Hill, J., & Stroebele-Benschop, N. (2016). In-school versus out-of-school sedentary behavior patterns in US children. *BMC Obesity, 3*(1), 34.

Bélanger, M., Gray-Donald, K., O'loughlin, J., Paradis, G., & Hanley, J. (2009). Influence of weather conditions and season on physical activity in adolescents. *Annals of Epidemiology, 19*(3), 180–186.

Bogin, B. (1999). *Patterns of human growth* (Vol. 23). Cambridge University Press. Cambridge, England

Bohnert, A. M., Bates, C. R., Heard, A. M., Burdette, K. A., Ward, A. K., Silton, R. L., & Dugas, L. R. (2017). Improving urban minority girls' health via community summer programming. *Journal of Racial and Ethnic Health Disparities, 4*(6), 1237–1245.

Brazendale, K., Beets, M. W., Turner-McGrievy, G. M., Kaczynski, A. T., Pate, R. R., & Weaver, R. G. (2018). Children's obesogenic behaviors during summer versus school: A within-person comparison. *Journal of School Health, 88*(12), 886–892.

Brazendale, K., Beets, M. W., Weaver, R. G., Pate, R. R., Turner-McGrievy, G. M., Kaczynski, A. T., . . . von Hippel, P. T. (2017). Understanding differences between summer vs. school obesogenic behaviors of children: The structured days hypothesis. *International Journal of Behavioral Nutrition and Physical Activity, 14*(1), 100.

Bryant, C. A., Courtney, A. H., McDermott, R. J., Alfonso, M. L., Baldwin, J. A., Nickelson, J., . . . Thompson, Z. (2010). Promoting physical activity among youth through community-based prevention marketing. *Journal of School Health, 80*(5), 214–224.

Bushman, B. J., Wang, M. C., & Anderson, C. A. (2005). Is the curve relating temperature to aggression linear or curvilinear? A response to Bell (2005) and to Cohn and Rotton (2005). *Journal of Personality and Social Psychology, 89*(1), 74–77.

Carrel, A. L., Clark, R. R., Peterson, S., Eickhoff, J., & Allen, D. B. (2007). School-based fitness changes are lost during the summer vacation. *Archives of Pediatrics & Adolescent Medicine, 161*(6), 561–564.

Carson, V., & Spence, J. C. (2010). Seasonal variation in physical activity among children and adolescents: A review. *Pediatric Exercise Science, 22*(1), 81–92.

DeBate, R. D., McDermott, R. J., Baldwin, J. A., Bryant, C. A., Courtney, A. H., Hogeboom, D. L., . . . Alfonso, M. L. (2009). Factors associated with tweens' intentions to sustain participation in an innovative community-based physical activity intervention. *American Journal of Health Education, 40*(3), 130–138.

D'Haese, S., Van Dyck, D., De Bourdeaudhuij, I., Deforche, B., & Cardon, G. (2015). Organizing 'play streets' during school vacations can increase physical activity and decrease sedentary time in children. *International Journal of Behavioral Nutrition and Physical Activity, 12*(1), 14.

Dumith, S. C., Gigante, D. P., Domingues, M. R., & Kohl III, H. W. (2011). Physical activity change during adolescence: a systematic review and a pooled analysis. *International Journal of Epidemiology, 40*(3), 685–698.

Ergler, C. R., Kearns, R. A., & Witten, K. (2013). Seasonal and locational variations in children's play: Implications for wellbeing. *Social Science & Medicine, 91*, 178–185.

Evans, E. W., Bond, D. S., Pierre, D. F., Howie, W. C., Wing, R. R., & Jelalian, E. (2018). Promoting health and activity in the summer trial: Implementation and outcomes of a pilot study. *Preventive Medicine Reports, 10*, 87–92.

Farley, T. A., Meriwether, R. A., Baker, E. T., Watkins, L. T., Johnson, C. C., & Webber, L. S. (2007). Safe play spaces to promote physical activity in inner-city children: Results from a pilot study of an environmental intervention. *American Journal of Public Health, 97*(9), 1625–1631.

Ferreira, I., Van Der Horst, K., Wendel-Vos, W., Kremers, S., Van Lenthe, F. J., & Brug, J. (2007). Environmental correlates of physical activity in youth – A review and update. *Obesity Reviews, 8*(2), 129–154.

Fjeldsoe, B., Neuhaus, M., Winkler, E., & Eakin, E. (2011). Systematic review of maintenance of behavior change following physical activity and dietary interventions. *Health Psychology, 30*(1), 99.

Franckle, R., Adler, R., & Davison, K. (2014). Peer reviewed: Accelerated weight gain among children during summer versus school year and related racial/ethnic disparities: A systematic review. *Preventing Chronic Disease, 11*, 130355.

Fu, Y., Brusseau, T. A., Hannon, J. C., & Burns, R. D. (2017). Effect of a 12-week summer break on school day physical activity and health-related fitness in low-income children from CSPAP schools. *Journal of Environmental and Public Health, 2017*, 1–7.

Graziano, P. A., Garcia, A., & Lim, C. S. (2017). Summer healthy-lifestyle intervention program for young children who are overweight: Results from a nonrandomized pilot trial. *Journal of Developmental & Behavioral Pediatrics, 38*(9), 723–727.

Gutin, B., Yin, Z., Johnson, M., & Barbeau, P. (2008). Preliminary findings of the effect of a 3-year after-school physical activity intervention on fitness and body fat: The Medical College of Georgia Fitkid project. *International Journal of Pediatric Obesity, 3*(Supp 1), 3–9.

Jin, Y., & Jones-Smith, J. C. (2015). Peer reviewed: Associations between family income and children's physical fitness and obesity in California, 2010–2012. *Preventing Chronic Disease, 12*, 140392.

Kilanowski, J. F., & Gordon, N. H. (2015). Making a difference in migrant summer school: Testing a healthy weight intervention. *Public Health Nursing, 32*(5), 421–429.

Mahoney, J. L. (2011). Adolescent summer care arrangements and risk for obesity the following school year. *Journal of Adolescence, 34*(4), 737–749.

McCue, M. C., Marlatt, K. L., & Sirard, J. (2013). Examination of changes in youth diet and physical activity over the summer vacation period. *Internet Journal of Allied Health Sciences and Practice, 11*(1), 8.

Meucci, M., Cook, C., Curry, C. D., Guidetti, L., Baldari, C., & Collier, S. R. (2013). Effects of supervised exercise program on metabolic function in overweight adolescents. *World Journal of Pediatrics, 9*(4), 307–311.

Moreno, J. P., Crowley, S. J., Alfano, C. A., Hannay, K. M., Thompson, D., & Baranowski, T. (2019). Potential circadian and circannual rhythm contributions to the obesity epidemic in elementary school age children. *The International Journal of Behavioral Nutrition and Physical Activity, 16*(1), 25. doi:10.1186/s12966-019-0784-7

Moreno, J. P., Johnston, C. A., & Woehler, D. (2013). Changes in weight over the school year and summer vacation: Results of a 5-year longitudinal study. *Journal of School Health, 83*(7), 473–477.

Ng, M., Fleming, T., Robinson, M., Thomson, B., Graetz, N., Margono, C., . . . Abera, S. F. (2014). Global, regional, and national prevalence of overweight and obesity in children and adults during 1980–2013: A systematic analysis for the global burden of disease study 2013. *The Lancet, 384*(9945), 766–781.

Olvera, N., Leung, P., Kellam, S. F., & Liu, J. (2013). Body fat and fitness improvements in Hispanic and African American girls. *Journal of Pediatric Psychology, 38*(9), 987–996.

Parente, M. E., Sheppard, A., & Mahoney, J. L. (2012). Parental knowledge as a mediator of the relation between adolescent summer care arrangement configurations and adjustment the following school year. *Applied Developmental Science, 16*(2), 84–97.

Park, K.-S., & Lee, M.-G. (2015). Effects of summer school participation and psychosocial outcomes on changes in body composition and physical fitness during summer break. *Journal of Exercise Nutrition & Biochemistry, 19*(2), 81.

Quante, M., Wang, R., Weng, J., Kaplan, E. R., Rueschman, M., Taveras, E. M., . . . Redline, S. (2019). Seasonal and weather variation of sleep and physical activity in 12–14-year-old children. *Behavioral Sleep Medicine, 17*(4), 398–410.

Rich, C., Griffiths, L. J., & Dezateux, C. (2012). Seasonal variation in accelerometer-determined sedentary behaviour and physical activity in children: A review. *International Journal of Behavioral Nutrition and Physical Activity, 9*(1), 49.

Staiano, A., Broyles, S., & Katzmarzyk, P. (2015). School term vs. school holiday: Associations with children's physical activity, screen-time, diet and sleep. *International Journal of Environmental Research and Public Health, 12*(8), 8861–8870.

Tanskey, L. A., Goldberg, J., Chui, K., Must, A., & Sacheck, J. (2018). The state of the summer: A review of child summer weight gain and efforts to prevent it. *Current Obesity Reports, 7*(2), 112–121.

von Hippel, P. T., & Workman, J. (2016). From kindergarten through second grade, US children's obesity prevalence grows only during summer vacations. *Obesity, 24*(11), 2296–2300.

Wang, Y. C., Vine, S., Hsiao, A., Rundle, A., & Goldsmith, J. (2015). Weight-related behaviors when children are in school versus on summer breaks: Does income matter? *Journal of School Health, 85*(7), 458–466.

Weaver, R. G., Beets, M. W., Brazendale, K., & Brusseau, T. A. (2019). Summer weight gain and fitness loss: Causes and potential solutions. *American Journal of Lifestyle Medicine, 13*(2), 116–128.

Weaver, R. G., Beets, M. W., Perry, M., Hunt, E., Brazendale, K., Decker, L., . . . Saelens, B. E. (2018). Changes in children's sleep and physical activity during a 1-week versus a 3-week break from school: A natural experiment. *Sleep, 42*(1), zsy205.

Weaver, R. G., Brazendale, K., Chandler, J. L., Turner-McGrievy, G. M., Moore, J. B., Huberty, J. L., . . . Beets, M. W. (2017). First year physical activity findings from turn up the HEAT (healthy eating and activity time) in summer day camps. *PLoS One, 12*(3), e0173791.

Weaver, R. G., Hunt, E., Rafferty, A., Beets, M. W., Brazendale, K., Turner-McGrievy, G., . . . Youngstedt, S. (2020). The potential of a year-round school calendar for maintaining children's weight status and fitness: Preliminary outcomes from a natural experiment. *Journal of Sport and Health Science, 9*(1), 18–27..

Zinkel, S. R., Moe III, M., Stern, E. A., Hubbard, V. S., Yanovski, S., Yanovski, J., & Schoeller, D. (2013). Comparison of total energy expenditure between school and summer months. *Pediatric Obesity, 8*(5), 404–410.

34

ACTIVE TRANSPORT

Erika Ikeda, Sandra Mandic, Melody Smith, Tom Stewart,
and Scott Duncan

Physical activity (i.e., any bodily movement produced by skeletal muscles that requires energy expenditure) is fundamental to child and youth health (Strong et al., 2005). Recommendations for children and youth (aged 5–17 years) are to accumulate at least 60 minutes per day of moderate-to-vigorous intensity physical activity (MVPA) at least three times per week (Ministry of Health, 2017; National Health Service, 2018; Piercy et al., 2018; World Health Organization, 2010). MVPA is defined as activities that require a moderate to large amount of effort (three or more metabolic equivalents (METs)) and noticeably accelerate heart rate, often characterized as activities that make individuals "huff and puff". MVPA involves mostly aerobic and vigorous activities, including those that strengthen muscle and bone.

Globally, rates of sufficient physical activity for health are low in children and youth. Results from the Health Behaviour in School Children study showed that 14% of girls and 23% of boys aged 11–15 years were classified as being sufficiently active for health in 2010 (Kalman et al., 2015). In the 2018 Global Matrix 3.0 Physical Activity Report Card, 48 out of 49 counties reported grades of C+ or less for overall physical activity, indicating that at least 40% of children and youth were insufficiently active for health (Aubert et al., 2018). The average grade for overall physical activity across the countries was D−, suggesting that between 27% and 33% of children and youth were sufficiently active for health (Aubert et al., 2018).

Children and youth can accumulate physical activity across a number of domains, including unstructured play, participation in organized sports, and active transport. Active transport is an activity domain of particular interest due to the demonstrated associations with physical activity, regularity with which trips are made (e.g., to local destinations such as schools, shops and friends'/family's houses, and parks), and multiple co-benefits of shifting from passive to active transport modes (Aubert et al., 2018; D'Haese et al., 2015) (Figure 34.1). In children and youth, active transport has been associated with higher levels of overall physical activity and MVPA (Faulkner, Buliung, Flora, & Fusco, 2009; Kek, García Bengoechea, Spence, & Mandic, in press; Larouche, Saunders, Faulkner, Colley, & Tremblay, 2014; Oliver et al., 2016; Schoeppe, Duncan, Badland, Oliver, & Curtis, 2013; Stewart, Duncan, & Schipperijn, 2017), maintenance of healthy body weight (although more research in this area is needed) (Faulkner et al., 2009; Larouche et al., 2014), improved cardiovascular fitness (especially among children and youth using cycling as a mode of transport) (Larouche et al., 2014), and better mental health (Sun, Liu, & Tao, 2015; Van Dijk, De Groot, Van Acker, Savelberg, & Kirschner, 2014). Independent mobility (e.g., active transport without adult supervision) provides additional benefits including opportunities

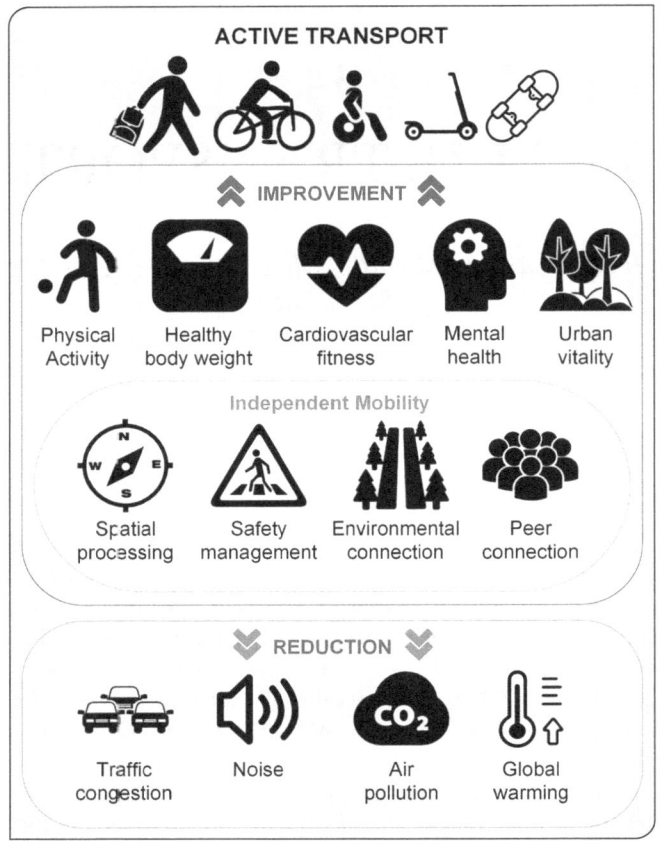

Figure 34.1   Benefits of active transport

to develop spatial processing skills and ability to manage safety around traffic and others, and can facilitate connections with peers and the natural/neighborhood environment (Brown, Mackett, Gong, Kitazawa, & Paskins, 2008; Mackett, Brown, Gong, Kitazawa, & Paskins, 2007; Marzi & Reimers, 2018; Mitchell, Kearns, & Collins, 2007; Morrow, 2003; Rissotto & Tonucci, 2002). Shifting motorized trips in favor of active transport modes can also reduce traffic congestion and associated noise and air pollution, ultimately contributing to urban vitality and climate change mitigation (Lindsay, Macmillan, & Woodward, 2011; Woodcock et al., 2009; Woodward & Lindsay, 2010). Furthermore, economic benefits of a motorized to active transport shift have been established (Grabow et al., 2012; Zapata-Diomedi et al., 2017).

Despite established and substantial benefits, active transport in children and youth has been declining in recent decades and is low internationally (Aubert et al., 2018; Fyhri, Hjorthol, Mackett, Fotel, & Kyttä, 2011; Ministry of Transport, 2015). Accordingly, encouraging active transport and providing built and social environments that support this behavior have become global priorities for human and environmental health (World Health Organization, 2018). For example, the World Health Organization Global Action Plan on Physical Activity 2018–2030 specifically notes the need for "policies that improve road safety, promote compact urban design, and prioritize access by pedestrians, cyclists and users of public transport to destinations and services …" with the aim of reducing the use of private vehicles (World Health Organization, 2018).

Definitions of active transport vary across studies depending on how active transport contributes to a certain outcome (e.g., health, physical activity, traffic congestion, carbon emissions) (Saunders, Green, Petticrew, Steinbach, & Roberts, 2013; Stevenson et al., 2016; Woodcock et al., 2009). However, generally active transport encompasses human-powered transport modes such as walking, cycling, wheeling, scootering, or skateboarding to travel between destinations, in contrast to passive (motorized) modes of transport. In some studies, public transport use is considered in combination with active transport (Stevenson et al., 2016), recognizing the demonstrated associations of public transport use with overall physical activity and walking in adults (Rissel, Curac, Greenaway, & Bauman, 2012; Saelens, Moudon, Kang, Hurvitz, & Zhou, 2014). Other studies have considered public transport as a motorized mode of transport (particularly where emissions are of interest) (Woodcock et al., 2009) or as a discrete mode of transport (Villanueva, Giles-Corti, & McCormack, 2008). The current chapter takes the latter approach, whereby public transport is considered a discrete transport mode from active or motorized transport.

Most extant evidence has focused on the school trip (Ikeda, Hinckson, Witten, & Smith, 2018, 2019; Mandic et al., 2015; Panter, Jones, & van Sluijs, 2008), likely due to the increased likelihood of trip-chaining during after-school trips (reducing sensitivity and specificity when determining associates or predictors of active school transport is the research aim). There is less knowledge regarding active transport to other neighborhood destinations such as parks, shops, recreational facilities, and friends' and family's houses (D'Haese et al., 2015; Larouche, Sarmiento, & Stewart, 2018; Oliver et al., 2016; Schoeppe et al., 2013; Stewart, Duncan et al., 2017). In school transport literature, differences in school transport behavior have been observed between the trip to and from school (Buliung, Larsen, Faulkner, & Ross, 2017; Larsen, Buliung, & Faulkner, 2016; Wilson, Clark, & Gilliland, 2018).

The techniques and tools used to quantify active transport also differ substantially in the literature. Common measurement approaches include self-reported or proxy-reported "usual" transport mode or frequency of active trips made over a specified time period; daily travel diaries to capture trip frequency, duration, and destinations; global positioning systems (GPS)-estimated trips to capture transport modes, destinations, and routes traveled; and hands-up surveys in classrooms and observations at school for transport mode on the survey/observation day (Ikeda, Hinckson et al., 2018; Stewart, Schipperijn, Snizek, & Duncan, 2017; Villa-González, Barranco-Ruiz, Evenson, & Chillón, 2018; Wong, Faulkner, & Buliung, 2011). Some studies collected data on each element of a multi-mode trip (e.g., walk-bus-walk) separately (Mandic et al., 2016; Stewart, Duncan et al., 2017; Stewart, Schipperijn et al., 2017). Other studies examined only the main modes of transport which can impact reports of prevalence as well as reducing ability to detect relationships with key variables of interest (e.g., Ikeda et al., 2019; Mandic et al., 2015). Accuracy of data is further problematic when assessing the main transport mode of multi-mode trip, as it can be challenging for participants to determine this with accuracy. For example, a child may be driven to a friend's house and walk from there to school. The distance of the car trip may be longer, but duration shorter; thus, it is difficult for the participant to identify the main transport mode with confidence or accuracy. These multi-mode trips could be accurately captured using GPS without relying on participants' memory (Larouche, Sarmiento et al., 2018; Stewart, Duncan et al., 2017), but the challenge of determining the main transport mode will remain in some cases. Furthermore, the design of surveys should be outlined cautiously to capture an individual's mode of transport. For example, non-motorized scooters and skateboards can be relevant to children and youth as one of the active transport modes (Ikeda et al., 2019). It is critical to design surveys that are customized to identify potential use of transport modes in children and youth.

Irrespective of the heterogeneity in destination and measurement approaches, the consistency in results reporting low levels of active transport in children and youth demonstrates the clear need for strategies to support active transport modes in this population. This chapter consists of three subsections. First, contemporary trends in active transport are explored to recognize the need for active transport in children and youth. In the following section, contributing factors that influence active transport are summarized from a socio-ecological perspective. Finally, existing interventions for active transport in children and youth are discussed, and recommendations for future interventions and research are provided.

Overview of Literature

Contemporary Trends in Active Transport

Active transport in children and youth has seen a decline over recent decades globally, but the extent of the decline varies by country. The highest level of evidence comes from national transport or health surveys examining transport mode to school within countries. In the US, there have been significant declines in walking and cycling to school (5–18 years) over 30 years, where 40.7% of students walked or cycled to school in 1969, and only 12.9% walked or cycled in 2001 (McDonald, 2007). Over the past 40 years, a sharp decline in the rate of active transport to school has particularly observed in students who lived within 1 mile of school, indicating distance to school has mattered more for the choice of school transport mode (National Centre for Safe Routes to School, 2011; U.S. Department of Transportation, 1972). Likewise, the proportion of Canadian children (11–13 years) walking to school declined from 53.0% to 42.5% between 1986 and 2006, and from 38.6% to 30.7% in older children (14–15 years) (Buliung, Mitra, & Faulkner, 2009). In Australia, the proportion of children who walked frequently to and from school (>6 trips per week) declined from 37.2% in 1985 to 25.7% in 2001, while the proportion of those who cycled to school (>1 trip per week) declined from 19.6% to 8.3% over the same period (Salmon, Timperio, Cleland, & Venn, 2005). New Zealand has one of the lowest rates of active transport to school internationally, with 28%–29% of children and youth (aged 5–17 years) walking and 2%–3% cycling to school in 2015 (Ministry of Transport, 2015). In comparison, in the late 1980s, 42% of New Zealand children (5–12 years) walked to school and 12% cycled, and 26% and 19% of youth (13–17 years) walked and cycled to school, respectively (Ministry of Transport, 2015). However, this trend of decline in the rates of active transport to school has not been as prominent in some countries. For example, in Switzerland, the proportion of children actively commuting to school decreased from 78.4% in 1994 to 71.4% in 2005 (Grize, Bringolf-Isler, Martin, & Braun-Fahrländer, 2010). In Denmark, approximately half of all children consistently cycle to school, and in Norway, the use of public transport (including school buses) holds the greatest mode share for transport to school (Fyhri et al., 2011).

The Global Matrix Physical Activity Report Cards, which consolidate nationally representative physical activity data (including active transport) to analyze global variations, were produced in 2014 (15 countries), 2016 (38 countries), and 2018 (49 countries) (Aubert et al., 2018; Tremblay et al., 2014, 2016). Country-specific rates of active transport from these reports are presented in Figure 34.2. The majority of countries showed similar or slightly improved rates of active transport during the 2014–2018 period. This trend can be, to some extent, due to the proliferation of active transport research and interventions in children and youth over the last decade (Ikeda, Hinckson et al., 2018; Rothman, Macpherson, Ross, & Buliung, 2018; Villa-González et al., 2018). In response to a growing number of studies and reviews on active transport in children and youth, there is a consensus that multiple factors can contribute to active transport in children and youth. The following section identifies and summarizes key factors which are associated with active transport in children and youth using a socio-ecological model.

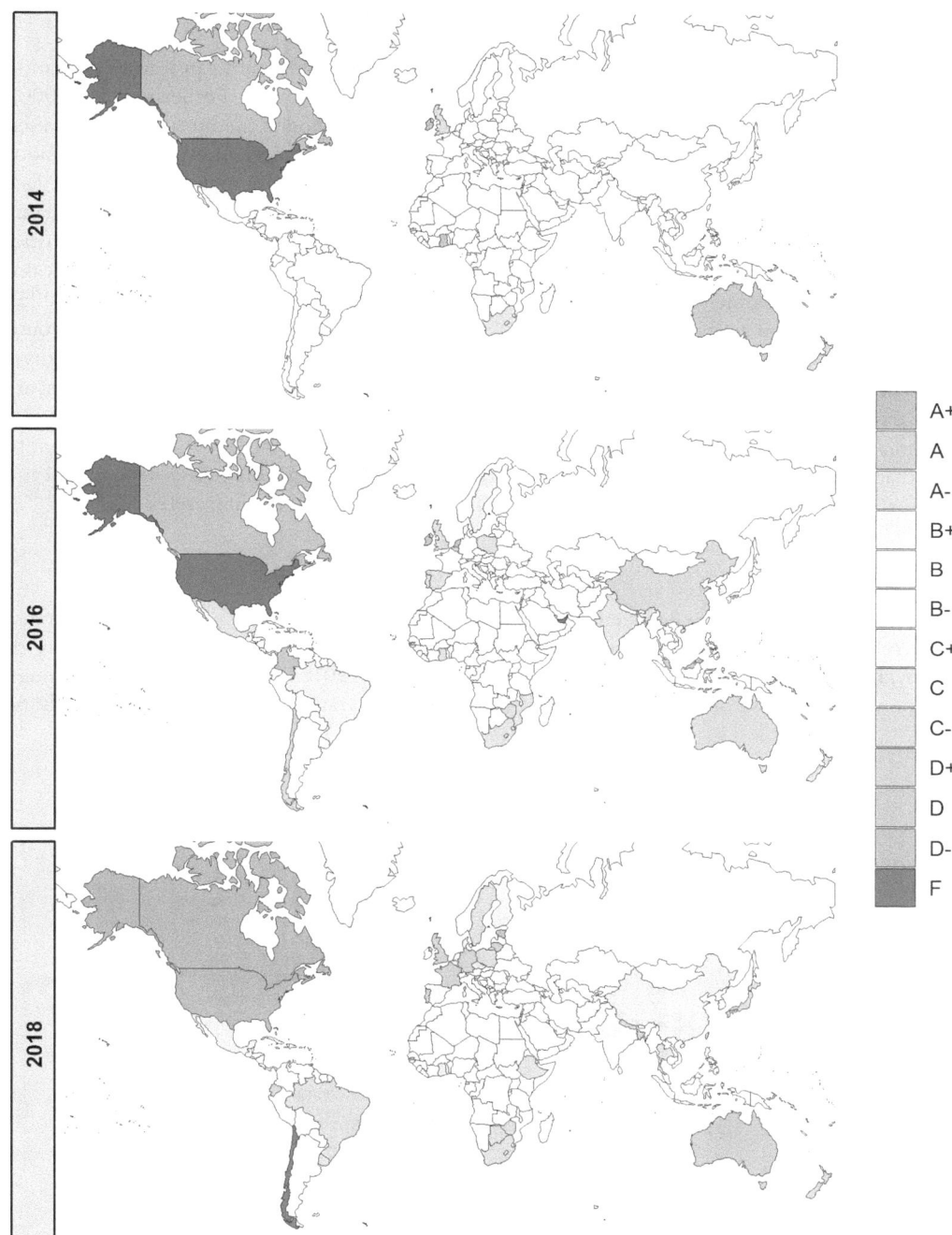

Figure 34.2   The grade of active transport in the 2014–2018 Global Matrix Physical Activity Report Cards
Note: A letter grade indicates the percentage of children and youth who utilized active transport. A+ = 94%–100%, A = 87%–93%, A– = 80%–86%; B+ = 74%–79%, B = 67%–73%, B– = 60%–66%; C+ = 54%–59%, C = 47%–53%, C– = 40%–46%; D+ = 34%–39%, D = 27%–33%, D– = 20%–26%; F = <20% (Aubert et al., 2018).

Factors that Influence Active Transport

Identifying factors that influence transport behavior in children and youth can lead to designing effective interventions for promoting active transport (Sallis, Owen, & Fotheringham, 2000). The application of theoretical models such as a socio-ecological model, the most commonly used model in active transport (Mitra, 2013; Panter et al., 2008; Pont, Ziviani, Wadley, & Abbott, 2011), may help to identify modifiable factors (such as policy, environmental, and social factors) that may encourage active transport. Transport behavior is influenced by personal and family factors, preferences, constraints, cost, environmental factors, and destination characteristics (McMillan, 2005). Choosing active transport is also influenced by enjoyment, perceived health benefits, built environment features, discomfort, and knowledge of safe routes (McMillan, 2005). Similarly, a choice of active transport to school and other destinations among children and youth is influenced by a multitude of factors including demographic characteristics, social and built environment factors, and policies (Adams et al., 2014; Davison, Werder, & Lawson, 2008; Panter et al., 2008; Pont, Ziviani, Wadley, Bennett, & Abbott, 2009; Wong et al., 2011). This section provides a summary of those factors (Figure 34.3) (Panter et al., 2008; Sallis et al., 2006). It is important to note that most of the information has been derived from studies examining transport to school and cross-sectional studies in which the causality of the evidence cannot be interpreted.

Individual Factors

Demographic factors such as age, gender, and socioeconomic status have effects on mode of transport in children and youth. Higher rates of active transport have been reported in boys versus girls (Babey, Hastert, Huang, & Brown, 2009; Ikeda, Stewart et al., 2018; Larsen et al., 2009), although variations exist across countries. Reduction in rates of active transport to school from childhood

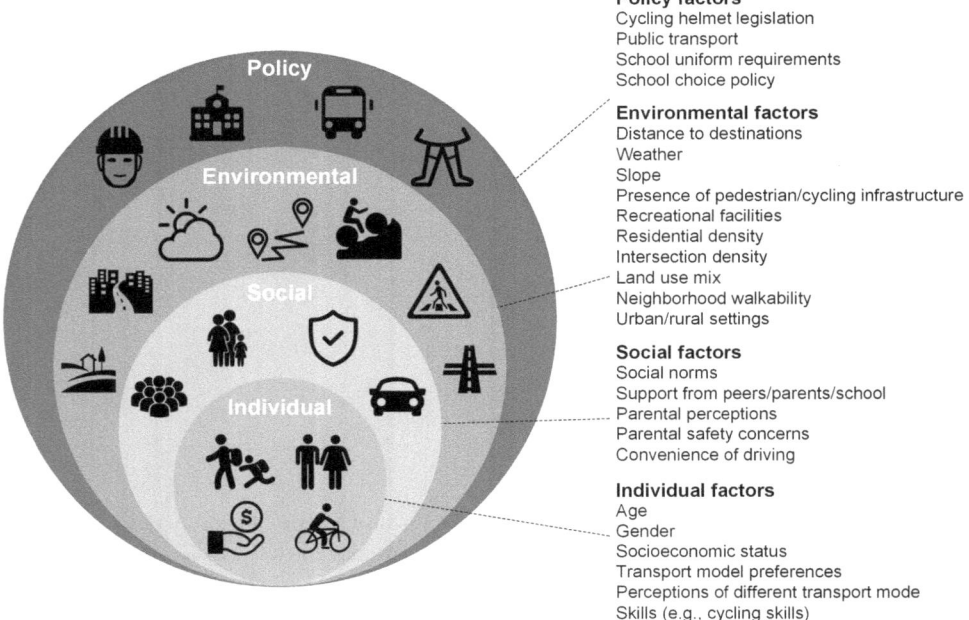

Policy factors
Cycling helmet legislation
Public transport
School uniform requirements
School choice policy

Environmental factors
Distance to destinations
Weather
Slope
Presence of pedestrian/cycling infrastructure
Recreational facilities
Residential density
Intersection density
Land use mix
Neighborhood walkability
Urban/rural settings

Social factors
Social norms
Support from peers/parents/school
Parental perceptions
Parental safety concerns
Convenience of driving

Individual factors
Age
Gender
Socioeconomic status
Transport model preferences
Perceptions of different transport mode
Skills (e.g., cycling skills)

Figure 34.3 Overview of factors influencing active transport in children and youth

to youth has been at least, in part, attributed to increased distance to school when transitioning from primary (elementary) to secondary (high) schools (Duncan et al., 2016; McDonald, 2007). Children from households with fewer vehicles and lower socioeconomic status are more likely to use active transport compared to their counterparts (Pont et al., 2009). Current level and enjoyment of physical activity (Faulkner et al., 2009; Leslie, Kremer, Toumbourou, & Williams, 2010); transport mode preferences, perceptions of different modes of transport, and perceived barriers (e.g., school bag weight (Mandic, Keller, García Bengoechea, Moore, & Coppell, 2018)); skills (such as cycle skills (Hopkins & Mandic, 2017)); and self-efficacy (Trapp et al., 2012) have effects on young people's choice of transport.

Social Factors

Social factors such as social norms and support, parental influences and concerns, and convenience of being driven to places also influence transport behaviors in children and youth. Previous studies emphasized the important role of social support including encouragement from peers, parents, and school (in a case of school transport) in promoting active transport among children and adolescents (Carver, Timperio, Hesketh, & Crawford, 2010; Ikeda, Hinckson et al., 2018; Leslie et al., 2010; Simons et al., 2013; Verhoeven et al., 2016). Children themselves valued social interactions with friends and family members that the school trip affords (Egli et al., 2019). In addition, parental perceptions of safety influence active transport and independent mobility in young people (Foster, Villanueva, Wood, Christian, & Giles-Corti, 2014). Parental concerns related to personal and traffic safety represent key parental barriers to active transport (Broberg & Sarjala, 2015; Buliung et al., 2017; Ikeda, Hinckson et al., 2018; Ikeda et al., 2019), especially for cycling (Mandic, Hopkins et al., 2017) and in adolescent girls (Carver et al., 2005; Esteban-Cornejo et al., 2016). Safety perceptions of active transport in youth are also an important determinant of choosing active versus motorized transport to school (Pocock, Moore, Keall, & Mandic, 2019). Trip-chaining and perceived convenience of being driven to different locations also represent barriers to active transport use among young people (Aibar, Mandic, Generelo Lanaspa, Gallardo, & Zaragoza Casterad, 2018; Gustat et al., 2015; Schlossberg, Greene, Phillips, Johnson, & Parker, 2006). Aibar et al. (2018) reported gender differences in parental perceptions of barriers to active transport to school. Children's extra-curricular activities and lack of children's interest in walking to school were barriers to active transport for mothers but not fathers (Aibar et al., 2018). These findings suggest that future active transport programs and interventions targeting parents may need to be gender-specific. School culture around activity and active transport have been interrelated with local community and the built environment, which all culminated in supporting and discouraging active school transport (Hawley, Witten, Hosking, Mackie, & Smith, 2019).

Environmental Factors

Factors related to the physical (i.e., natural and built) environment also influence transport choices among young people (Davison et al., 2008; Ikeda, Stewart et al., 2018; Panter et al., 2008; Pont et al., 2009; Wong et al., 2011). Distance to destinations has been consistently reported as the strongest negative correlate of active transport in children and youth (Ikeda, Hinckson et al., 2018; Ikeda, Stewart et al., 2018; Rothman et al., 2018). Factors such as weather (Aibar et al., 2015; Gustat et al., 2015; Mandic, Hopkins et al., 2017) and hills (Mandic, Hopkins et al., 2017; Timperio et al., 2006) also influence transport choices. Furthermore, built environment features such as traffic volume and accidents, presence of footpaths and/or cycle lanes, availability of recreational facilities, intersection density, residential density, land use mix, and streetlights are associated with active transport in young people (Dessing et al., 2016; Ikeda, Stewart et al., 2018; Larsen,

Gilliland, & Hess, 2012; Panter et al., 2008; Pont et al., 2009; Wong et al., 2011). Therefore, factors related to both natural and built environments have effects on uptake of active transport in children and youth.

Most previous studies on active transport in children and youth focused on urban settings, whereas few studies have been conducted in youth living in rural areas (Babey et al., 2009; Booth et al., 2007; Dalton et al., 2011; Ikeda, Stewart et al., 2018; McDonald, 2007; Pabayo, Gauvin, & Barnett, 2011). Given that active transport behavior is context-specific, and differences in this behavior between rural and urban contexts can be expected, further research is required particularly in rural settings. Compared to urban areas, rural settings are characterized by greater distances to school (Mandic et al., 2015; Nelson, Foley, O'Gorman, Moyna, & Woods, 2008; Sjolie & Thuen, 2002), different built environment characteristics (Sandercock, Angus, & Barton, 2010), destination accessibilities (Rainham et al., 2012), and greater reliance on transport to access work and leisure activities (Banister, 2009), particularly for children and youth.

Policy Factors

Policy factors such as mandatory helmet use, availability of public transport, and school policies also have important implications on active transport. For example, mandatory helmet use legislation that exists in some countries may represent a barrier for young people to cycle for recreation and/or transportation (Molina-García, Queralt, García Bengoechea, Moore, & Mandic, 2018). Availability and use of public transport may also have implications on active transport use among children and youth (Voss, Winters, Frazer, & McKay, 2015). School uniforms may represent a barrier to active transport to school, particularly for cycling in girls (Hopkins & Mandic, 2017). School policies that do not require adolescents to enroll in a local school increase the distance between home and school (Mandic, Sandretto, Hopkins et al., 2017), and in many cases, private vehicle transport and public transport become the only option for traveling to school (Mandic, Sandretto, García Bengoechea et al., 2017). Other school policies related to active transport such as school start/dismissal times, school drop-off/pick-up, school speed zones, and school siting (Eyler et al., 2008), as well as school transport programs (e.g., Safe Routes to School, School Travel Plans, walking school buses) may play an influential role (Hawley et al., 2019). Hence, school policy and practices may have differential contribution to encouraging and hindering active transport among children and youth.

Active Transport Interventions for Children and Youth

Several interventions have been implemented to promote active transport in children, youth, and/or community internationally (Table 34.1). These interventions mostly integrated multiple components that influence individual, social, environmental, and/or policy factors as identified in the previous section.

Interventions to Promote Walking

Existing evidence regarding active transport interventions for children and youth focused mainly on encouraging walking to school, and more frequently targeted children (under the age of 14) than youth (age 14–18 years) (Chillón, Evenson, Vaughn, & Ward, 2011; Villa-González et al., 2018). For example, *Safe Routes to School* (Boarnet, Anderson, Day, McMillan, & Alfonzo, 2005; Boarnet, Day, Anderson, McMillan, & Alfonzo, 2005; Buckley, Lowry, Brown, & Barton, 2013; Bungum, Clark, & Aguilar, 2014; Hoelscher et al., 2016; McDonald et al., 2014; McDonald, Yang, Abbott, & Bullock, 2013; Staunton, Hubsmith, & Kallins, 2003; Stewart, Moudon, & Claybrooke, 2014),

Table 34.1 Summary of active transport interventions

Intervention (country): Website	Description
Interventions to promote walking	
Safe Routes to School (US): https://www.saferoutesmichigan.org/	Safe Routes to School is a federal program in the US, and aims to make children's school trips safe, convenient, and fun. The Safe Routes to School can be implemented through a combination of infrastructure and non-infrastructure projects and programs (6Es). The 6Es refers to Education, Encouragement, Engineering, Enforcement, Evaluation, and Equity.
School Travel Planning (Canada): https://www.ontarioactiveschooltravel.ca/school-travel-planning/	School Travel Planning is a community-based, school-level action plans that utilize the 5Es (Education, Encouragement, Engineering, Enforcement, and Evaluation) to address road safety issues and increase the number of children using active transport.
Safe School Travel Plans (New Zealand): https://www.at.govt.nz/cycling-walking/travelwise-school-programme/safe-school-travel-plans/	A Safe School Travel Plan is an action plan for road safety and active transport including road safety education, traffic calming, walking school buses, and parking restrictions. The program has been delivered in partnership with the school community, national and regional governments, and other organizations.
Walking School Bus (US): https://www.walkingschoolbus.org/; (New Zealand): https://www.at.govt.nz/cycling-walking/travelwise-school-programme/walking-school-bus/	A walking school bus is a group of children walking to and/or from school along a designated route with one or more adult volunteers.
Interventions to promote cycling	
Ride2School (Australia): https://www.bicyclenetwork.com.au/rides-and-events/ride2school/	The Ride2School is school-based program to promote active transport particularly cycling. The program involves cycling and active transport events including Ride2School Day, Walk and Wheel-a-thon, mapping activities, classroom surveys, infrastructure improvements, as well as customized advice, support, and resources.
Bike Safe (New Zealand): https://www.at.govt.nz/cycling-walking/travelwise-school-programme/bike-safe-training/	The Bike Safe is cycling skills training designed for children in school years 5 and 6 (aged 9–11 years). The program includes a combination of theory and practical components focusing on bike handling, confidence, and safety.
Bikes in Schools (New Zealand): https://www.bikeon.org.nz/bikes-in-schools/	The Bikes in Schools provides cycling program package including bikes, bike helmets, bike storage, and bike skills and safety training to primary (elementary) schools.
Bikeability (UK): https://www.bikeability.org.uk/	The Bikeability is cycling training designed for children in the final years of primary (elementary) school. The goal of the program is to improve children's cycle skills and confidence to cycle safely on the road.

(Continued)

Intervention (country): Website	Description
Interventions to promote walking and cycling	
Te Ara Mua – Future Streets (New Zealand): https://www.futurestreets.org.nz	The "Te Ara Mua – Future Streets" has transformed the streets of an Auckland suburb to improve walking and cycling infrastructure, increase safety, and improve social and health outcomes.
iWay (New Zealand): https://www.iway.org.nz/ Let's Go (New Zealand): https://www.letsgo.org.nz/	The Model Communities program involves two interventions – 'iWay' and 'Let's Go' in which walking and cycling infrastructure changes were implemented to encourage active transport.
Connect2 (UK): https://www.sustransconnect2.org.uk/	The Connect2 program aims to increase physical activity and improve safety of the local community by building a foot or cycle bridge, and creating or retrofitting a pedestrian/cycling path.
Ciclovía Recreativa (17 Latin American countries): https://www.cicloviarecreativa.uniandes.edu.co/english/index.html	The Ciclovía Recreativa programs creates a temporary, safe space for active transport by closing streets to motorized vehicles and opening them for walking and cycling.

School Travel Plans (Buliung, Faulkner, Beesley, & Kennedy, 2011; Hinckson & Badland, 2011; Mammen et al., 2014), and *walking school buses* (Collins & Kearns, 2010; Heelan, Abbey, Donnelly, Mayo, & Welk, 2009; Kong et al., 2009, 2010; Mendoza, Levinger, & Johnston, 2009; Mendoza et al., 2011; Sayers, LeMaster, Thomas, Petroski, & Ge, 2012; Sirard, Alhassan, Spencer, & Robinson, 2008; Zaccari & Dirkis, 2003) have been implemented in some countries to provide safe school trips and promote active transport to and from school for children. The *Safe Routes to School* in the US (Boarnet, Anderson et al., 2005; Boarnet, Day et al., 2005; Buckley et al., 2013; Bungum et al., 2014; Hoelscher et al., 2016; McDonald et al., 2013, 2014; Staunton et al., 2003; Stewart et al., 2014) and the *School Travel Plans* in Canada (Buliung et al., 2011; Mammen et al., 2014) applied the "6Es" and "5Es" approaches which incorporate a combination of infrastructure and non-infrastructure projects and programs, referring to "Education", "Encouragement", "Engineering", "Enforcement", and "Evaluation" (plus "Equity" in the Safe Routes to School). These comprehensive approaches align with the socio-ecological model (Figure 34.3) in which individual, social, environmental and policy factors would be addressed to promote active transport among children and youth. The Safe Routes to School is one of the federal-funded, long-term active transport interventions which was first implemented in 2003 in Marin County, California (Staunton et al., 2003). The Safe Routes to School has provided comprehensive support ranging from extensive resources to funding opportunities for schools and their communities to support active school transport for children.

Similarly, the *Safe School Travel Plans* in New Zealand (Hinckson & Badland, 2011) have been developed to promote active transportation to and from school, reduce school-related traffic congestion, and increase traffic and neighborhood safety. The program consists of six components: engineering, road safety education, enforcement activities, public education, rewards and awards, and policy. It is important that this process involves the engagement of children/youth, parents, caregivers, schools, and the community to translate their voices into practice; however, it is unclear whether or how much their voices have been incorporated into actual plans to date. Given that children/youth and parents/caregivers have different perceptions on school transport behavior (Moran, Rodríguez, & Corburn, 2018; Wilson et al., 2018), listening to and valuing views of both of these groups are critical to change their behavior and develop effective interventions for promoting active transport to school.

A *walking school bus*, in which a group of children walk/cycle to school with one or two adults, has been an internationally recognized program to encourage active transport to school and independent mobility in primary (i.e., elementary) school children (Marzi & Reimers, 2018). Walking school buses can provide social advantages such as catching up with friends and making new friends which lead to enjoyment and motivation of active transport among children (Hinckson, 2016). Children and their parents also felt safe because children walked to school in larger groups (Egli, Ikeda, Stewart, & Smith, 2018; Hinckson, 2016; Tranter & Pawson, 2001). Nevertheless, lack of adult volunteers and inappropriate behaviors of parents (e.g., crossing roads unsafely, parking cars illegally) can be challenging (Hinckson, 2016). Community engagement to increase the availability of adult volunteers, and parent education to improve their behaviors around school should be integrated in future walking school bus interventions.

Interventions to Promote Cycling

Different factors influence walking versus cycling for transport in children and youth (Aarts, Mathijssen, van Oers, & Schuit, 2013; Mandic, Hopkins et al., 2017). Therefore, future interventions for promoting active transport in these groups need to address transport mode-specific barriers. For example, in addition to built environment features and presence or absence of cycling infrastructure, adolescents' choice of cycling for transport is influenced by their cycling skills, parental perceptions of their cycling skills, cycling safety, and previous cycling experiences (including accidents) (Hinckson, 2016; Hopkins & Mandic, 2017; Kerr et al., 2006; Trapp et al., 2011). The *Ride2School* program in Australia (Crawford & Garrard, 2013), the *Bike Safe* program (Auckland Transport, 2018) and the *Bikes in Schools* project in New Zealand (Bike on New Zealand Charitable Trust, 2018), and the *Bikeability* program in the UK (Goodman, van Sluijs, & Ogilvie, 2016) were specifically designed to improve cycle skills in children. The *Ride2School* program incorporated infrastructure improvements (e.g., bicycle storage, pedestrian crossings) and activities (e.g., active transport events, safe school route mapping exercise, online resources, and incentives). The *Bikes in Schools* project has been provided a combination of resources such as bicycles and bicycle storage, as well as cycle skills training (Bike on New Zealand Charitable Trust, 2018). The *Bike Safe* and the *Bikeability* programs focused on safety education and cycle skills training. Cycle skills training improves children's knowledge of road rules, increases their self-efficacy for cycling, and may have positive effects on increasing the rates of cycling to school (Mandic, Flaherty, Pocock et al., 2018). However, existing cycle skills training programs have been designed for children and not for youth. Recent evaluation of cycle skills training for adolescent girls reported improved cycling-related knowledge and increased confidence to cycle on the road (with on-road training component) (Mandic, Flaherty, Ergler et al., 2018). However, the training did not change adolescents' confidence to cycle to school or cycling habits (Mandic, Flaherty, Ergler et al., 2018). Future interventions targeting adolescents are required to promote cycling as a mode of active transport.

Interventions to Promote Walking and Cycling

Wider neighborhood-level infrastructure changes can also influence rates of walking and cycling in children and youth. For example, in New Zealand, *Te Ara Mua – Future Streets* project has implemented community-wide street modifications including cycle lanes and footpath widening to provide greater affordance for walking and cycling in an Auckland suburb (Mackie et al., 2018; Macmillan et al., 2018). Likewise, the *Model Communities* program including *iWay* in Hastings and

Let's Go in New Plymouth were implemented in New Zealand (Keall et al., 2015). The program incorporated walking and cycling infrastructural changes to promote active transport (Keall et al., 2015). Several studies from other countries also focus on improving infrastructure for walking and cycling; however, these studies did not necessarily evaluate the impact of the interventions on walking and cycling in children and youth (Goodman, Sahlqvist, & Ogilvie, 2013; Goodman, Sahlqvist, Ogilvie, & iConnect Consortium, 2014). The *Connect2* project in the UK was a natural experiment to build and improve walking and cycling routes at 79 sites across the country (Goodman et al., 2013, 2014). The *Ciclovía Recreativa* programs in Latin America aim to create a safe and pleasant environment for active transport in the neighborhood (Sarmiento et al., 2017). These programs do not involve infrastructure changes, but a temporary closure of streets (5–55 km) to motorized vehicles and opening exclusively for individuals to walk, jog, skate, or cycle (Sarmiento et al., 2017). Seventeen countries (e.g., Argentina, Brazil, Chile, Colombia, Ecuador, Mexico, Peru) in Latin America have successfully implemented the programs since 2000 (Sarmiento et al., 2017).

Key Issues

Systematic reviews (Chillón et al., 2011; Villa-González et al., 2018) reported that most of the existing interventions did not have strong study designs such as randomized control trials due to the nature of their interventions (e.g., school/community-based approach). Similarly, specific causal relationships between the interventions and the rates of active transport to/from school might be difficult to determine due to a combination of individual, social, environmental, and policy factors that influence active transport to/from school (Benton, Anderson, Hunter, & French, 2016). Objective measures such as GPS may be preferred to accurately examine single- and multi-mode of transport in children and youth; however, subjective measures can capture individuals' perceptions of their usual transport behavior. It is important that existing interventions and studies report what works, what doesn't, and what could be done better to inform the design of future interventions (e.g., Larouche, Mammen, Rowe, & Faulkner, 2018; Witten et al., 2018). Future interventions should also consider a holistic approach posited by a socio-ecological model involving multiple levels of individual, social, environmental, and/or policy supports to change transport behavior (Larouche, Mammen et al., 2018).

Despite the challenges outlined above, the effectiveness of the interventions could improve when increasing the heterogeneity of data (Ikeda, Stewart et al., 2018; Ogilvie, Egan, Hamilton, & Petticrew, 2005). For example, several Safe Route to School programs might collectively and positively impact on the national level of active transport for children and youth in the US. The balance between the consistency of methodologies to make studies comparable and the variance of interventions to effectively change behaviors in each specific setting may be required.

Recommendations for Researchers and Practitioners

In every setting, a combination of individual, social, environmental, and policy factors influences active transport behaviors in children and youth. For instance, countries with strong cycling traditions, such as Belgium (Van Dyck, De Bourdeaudhuij, Cardon, & Deforche, 2010) and Denmark (Cooper et al., 2006), have extensive cycling-friendly infrastructure and a flat landscape which might contribute to high rates of cycling for transportation among all segments of the population, including children and youth. A holistic and context-specific approach (e.g., urban versus rural) is essential for designing effective interventions for increasing rates of active transport among young people. For example, longer distances to school (Mandic et al., 2015) and different built environment features (Sandercock et al., 2010) in rural compared to urban settings need to be taken into account for planning active transport interventions.

Although independent mobility is positively associated with active transport (Buliung et al., 2017; Ikeda et al., 2019; Marzi & Reimers, 2018), few interventions have been implemented to improve independent mobility in children (e.g., 'We go to school alone' program (Prezza, Alparone, Renzi, & Pietrobono, 2009)). Changes in the built environment (e.g., street modifications to increase safety and visibility) and policy (e.g., distinction between independent mobility and inadequate supervision) may provide opportunities for encouraging children's independent mobility (Marzi & Reimers, 2018). Safe and child-friendly environments enabled children to travel around their neighborhood on their own (e.g., playing outside, visiting friends, running small errands), which led to developing their autonomy, sense of community, and social skills (Marzi & Reimers, 2018; Prezza et al., 2009). Given that lower rates of independent mobility have been observed in children versus youth and girls versus boys (Prezza et al., 2009; Shaw et al., 2015), future interventions for encouraging independent mobility should target children and girls.

Improving the availability and accessibility of public transport can also encourage active transport among children and youth (Voss et al., 2015). Young people consider public transport as a place to socialize with friends, and a means to travel to school and other destinations more conveniently and quickly than by car (Hinckson, 2016). In some settings, the availability of public transport may be limited, and public transport fares could be expensive such as in New Zealand and Belgium (Hinckson, 2016; Simons et al., 2013). When young people get driver licenses, it is more likely that driving is perceived as an easy and convenient way to travel around (Hopkins, García Bengoechea, & Mandic, 2019). Increasing the number of young people traveling to school by car poses additional traffic safety issues during the school commuting hours (Kirk & Stamatiadis, 2001), which may risk road safety for children and youth who actively travel to/from school. Likewise, parents chauffeuring their children can create traffic safety issues around schools during drop-off and pick-up times (Carver, Timperio, & Crawford, 2013; Tranter & Pawson, 2001). Designing drop-off/pick-up zones away from a school gate could alleviate these issues, and would encourage active transport between the drop-off/pick-up area and child's school (Vanwolleghem, D'Haese, Van Dyck, De Bourdeaudhuij, & Cardon, 2014). Interventions designed to increase the accessibility and affordability of public transport for children and youth, and traffic regulations in school neighborhoods should be considered as a part of comprehensive efforts to encourage active transport as a part of the school trip. In addition, unique needs and barriers to youth active transport specific to urban and rural areas should be taken into account when planning and designing interventions.

Conclusion

Active transport in children and youth can contribute to higher levels of overall physical activity, help maintain healthy body weight, increase cardiovascular fitness, and contribute to independent mobility. Active transport also contributes to economic benefits and environmental sustainability by reducing traffic congestion and noise, and diminishing transport-related air pollution and global warming. Despite these benefits, the prevalence of active transport in children and youth has been low internationally and declining in recent decades. Multiple individual, social, environmental, and policy factors contribute to the currently low rates of active transport among children and youth globally, and should be considered in future interventions for promoting active transport. Based on existing active transport literature, interventions should be mode-specific and consider a holistic approach to encourage active transport among children and youth. Future interventions for promoting use of public transport targeting youth, and supporting independent mobility, particularly in children and girls, should be considered. Future initiatives should also include the input from children/youth, parents, and community into intervention design and planning.

References

Aarts, M.-J., Mathijssen, J. J. P., van Oers, J. A. M., & Schuit, A. J. (2013). Associations between environmental characteristics and active commuting to school among children: A cross-sectional study. *International Journal of Behavioral Medicine, 20*(4), 538–555. doi:10.1007/s12529-012-9271-0

Adams, M. A., Frank, L. D., Schipperijn, J., Smith, G., Chapman, J., Christiansen, L. B., . . . Sallis, J. F. (2014). International variation in neighborhood walkability, transit, and recreation environments using geographic information systems: The IPEN adult study. *International Journal of Health Geographics, 13*(1), 43. doi:10.1186/1476-072x-13-43

Aibar, A., Bois, J. E., Generelo, E., Bengoechea, E. G., Paillard, T., & Zaragoza, J. (2015). Effect of weather, school transport, and perceived neighborhood characteristics on moderate to vigorous physical activity levels of adolescents from two European cities. *Environment and Behavior, 47*(4), 395–417. doi:10.1177/0013916513510399

Aibar, A., Mandic, S., Generelo Lanaspa, E., Gallardo, L. O., & Zaragoza Casterad, J. (2018). Parental barriers to active commuting to school in children: Does parental gender matter? *Journal of Transport & Health, 9*, 141–149. doi:10.1016/j.jth.2018.03.005

Aubert, S., Barnes, J. D., Abdeta, C., Nader, P. A., Adeniyi, A. F., Aguilar-Farias, N., . . . Tremblay, M. S. (2018). Global Matrix 3.0 physical activity report card grades for children and youth: Results and analysis from 49 countries. *Journal of Physical Activity and Health, 15*(S2), S251–S273. doi:10.1123/jpah.2018-0472

Auckland Transport. (2018). *Bike Safe training* [Internet]. Retrieved from https://at.govt.nz/cycling-walking/travelwise-school-programme/bike-safe-training/

Babey, S. H., Hastert, T. A., Huang, W., & Brown, E. R. (2009). Sociodemographic, family, and environmental factors associated with active commuting to school among US adolescents. *Journal of Public Health Policy, 30*(1), S203–S220. doi:10.1057/jphp.2008.61

Banister, D. (2009). Transport, rural. In R. Kitchin & N. Thrift (Eds.), *International encyclopedia of human geography* (pp. 460–464). Oxford, UK: Elsevier. Retrieved from http://www.sciencedirect.com/science/article/pii/B978008044910400910X, doi:10.1016/B978-008044910-4.00910-X

Benton, J. S., Anderson, J., Hunter, R. F., & French, D. P. (2016). The effect of changing the built environment on physical activity: A quantitative review of the risk of bias in natural experiments. *International Journal of Behavioral Nutrition and Physical Activity, 13*(107), 1–18. doi:10.1186/s12966-016-0433-3

Bike on New Zealand Charitable Trust. (2018). *Bikes in schools.* Retrieved December 14, 2018, from https://bikeon.org.nz/bikes-in-schools/

Boarnet, M. G., Anderson, C. L., Day, K., McMillan, T., & Alfonzo, M. (2005). Evaluation of the California safe routes to school legislation: Urban form changes and children's active transportation to school. *American Journal of Preventive Medicine, 28*(2 Suppl 2), 134–140. doi:10.1016/j.amepre.2004.10.026

Boarnet, M. G., Day, K., Anderson, C. L., McMillan, T., & Alfonzo, M. (2005). California's safe routes to school program: Impacts on walking, bicycling, and pedestrian safety. *Journal of the American Planning Association, 71*(3), 301–317. doi:10.1080/01944360508976700

Booth, M. L., Okely, A. D., Denney-Wilson, E., Hardy, L. L., Dobbins, T., Wen, L. M., & Rissel, C. (2007). Characteristics of travel to and from school among adolescents in NSW, Australia. *Journal of Paediatrics and Child Health, 43*(11), 755–761. doi:10.1111/j.1440-1754.2007.01159.x

Broberg, A., & Sarjala, S. (2015). School travel mode choice and the characteristics of the urban built environment: The case of Helsinki, Finland. *Transport Policy, 37*, 1–10. doi:10.1016/j.tranpol.2014.10.011

Brown, B., Mackett, R., Gong, Y., Kitazawa, K., & Paskins, J. (2008). Gender differences in children's pathways to independent mobility. *Children's Geographies, 6*(4), 385–401. doi:10.1080/14733280802338080

Buckley, A., Lowry, M. B., Brown, H., & Barton, B. (2013). Evaluating safe routes to school events that designate days for walking and bicycling. *Transport Policy, 30*, 294–300. doi:10.1016/j.tranpol.2013.09.021

Buliung, R., Faulkner, G., Beesley, T., & Kennedy, J. (2011). School travel planning: Mobilizing school and community resources to encourage active school transportation. *Journal of School Health, 81*(11), 704–712. doi:10.1111/j.1746-1561.2011.00647.x

Buliung, R., Larsen, K., Faulkner, G., & Ross, T. (2017). Children's independent mobility in the City of Toronto, Canada. *Travel Behaviour and Society, 9*, 58–69. doi:10.1016/j.tbs.2017.06.001

Buliung, R., Mitra, R., & Faulkner, G. (2009). Active school transportation in the Greater Toronto Area, Canada: An exploration of trends in space and time (1986–2006). *Preventive Medicine, 48*(6), 507–512. doi:10.1016/j.ypmed.2009.03.001

Bungum, T. J., Clark, S., & Aguilar, B. (2014). The effect of an active transport to school intervention at a suburban elementary school. *American Journal of Health Education, 45*(4), 205–209. doi:10.1080/19325037.2014.916635

Carver, A., Salmon, J., Campbell, K., Baur, L., Garnett, S., & Crawford, D. (2005). How do perceptions of local neighborhood relate to adolescents' walking and cycling? *American Journal of Health Promotion, 20*(2), 139–147. doi:10.4278/0890-1171-20.2.139

Carver, A., Timperio, A., & Crawford, D. (2013). Parental chauffeurs: What drives their transport choice? *Journal of Transport Geography, 26*, 72–77. doi:10.1016/j.jtrangeo.2012.08.017

Carver, A., Timperio, A., Hesketh, K., & Crawford, D. (2010). Are children and adolescents less active if parents restrict their physical activity and active transport due to perceived risk? *Social Science and Medicine, 70*(11), 1799–1805. doi:10.1016/j.socscimed.2010.02.010

Chillón, P., Evenson, K. R., Vaughn, A., & Ward, D. S. (2011). A systematic review of interventions for promoting active transportation to school. *International Journal of Behavioral Nutrition and Physical Activity, 8*(10), 1–17. doi:10.1186/1479-5868-8-10

Collins, D., & Kearns, R. A. (2010). Walking school buses in the Auckland region: A longitudinal assessment. *Transport Policy, 17*(1), 1–8. doi:10.1016/j.tranpol.2009.06.003

Cooper, A. R., Wedderkopp, N., Wang, H., Andersen, L. B., Froberg, K., & Page, A. S. (2006). Active travel to school and cardiovascular fitness in Danish children and adolescents. *Medicine and Science in Sports and Exercise, 38*(10), 1724–1731. doi:10.1249/01.mss.0000229570.02037.1d

Crawford, S., & Garrard, J. (2013). A combined impact-process evaluation of a program promoting active transport to school: Understanding the factors that shaped program effectiveness. *Journal of Environmental and Public Health, 2013*, 1–14. doi:10.1155/2013/816961

Dalton, M. A., Longacre, M. R., Drake, K. M., Gibson, L., Adachi-Mejia, A. M., Swain, K., . . . Owens, P. M. (2011). Built environment predictors of active travel to school among rural adolescents. *American Journal of Preventive Medicine, 40*(3), 312–319. doi:10.1016/j.amepre.2010.11.008

Davison, K. K., Werder, J. L., & Lawson, C. T. (2008). Children's active commuting to school: Current knowledge and future directions. *Preventing Chronic Disease, 5*(3), 1–11.

Dessing, D., de Vries, S. I., Hegeman, G., Verhagen, E., van Mechelen, W., & Pierik, F. H. (2016). Children's route choice during active transportation to school: Difference between shortest and actual route. *International Journal of Behavioral Nutrition and Physical Activity, 13*(48), 1–11. doi:10.1186/s12966-016-0373-y

D'Haese, S., Vanwolleghem, G., Hinckson, E., De Bourdeaudhuij, I., Deforche, B., Van Dyck, D., & Cardon, G. (2015). Cross-continental comparison of the association between the physical environment and active transportation in children: A systematic review. *International Journal of Behavioral Nutrition and Physical Activity, 12*(145), 1–14. doi:10.1186/s12966-015-0308-z

Duncan, S., White, K., Mavoa, S., Stewart, T., Hinckson, E., & Schofield, G. (2016). Active transport, physical activity, and distance between home and school in children and adolescents. *Journal of Physical Activity and Health, 13*(4), 447–453. doi:10.1123/jpah.2015-0054

Egli, V., Ikeda, E., Stewart, T., & Smith, M. (2018). Interpersonal correlates of active transport to school. In R. Larouche (Ed.), *Children's active transportation* (pp. 115–125). Retrieved from https://www.sciencedirect.com/science/article/pii/B9780128119310000089?via%3Dihub, doi:10.1016/B978-0-12-811931-0.00008-9

Egli, V., Mackay, L., Jelleyman, C., Ikeda, E., Hopkins, S., & Smith, M. (2019). Social relationships, nature, and traffic: Findings from a child-centred approach to measuring active school travel route perceptions. *Children's Geographies*, 1–17. doi:10.1080/14733285.2019.1685074

Esteban-Cornejo, I., Carlson, J. A., Conway, T. L., Cain, K. L., Saelens, B. E., Frank, L. D., . . . Sallis, J. F. (2016). Parental and adolescent perceptions of neighborhood safety related to adolescents' physical activity in their neighborhood. *Research Quarterly for Exercise and Sport, 87*(2), 191–199. doi:10.1080/02701367.2016.1153779

Eyler, A. A., Brownson, R. C., Doescher, M. P., Evenson, K. R., Fesperman, C. E., Litt, J. S., . . . Schmid, T. L. (2008). Policies related to active transport to and from school: A multisite case study. *Health Education Research, 23*(6), 963–975. doi:10.1093/her/cym061

Faulkner, G. E. J., Buliung, R. N., Flora, P. K., & Fusco, C. (2009). Active school transport, physical activity levels and body weight of children and youth: A systematic review. *Preventive Medicine, 48*(1), 3–8. doi:10.1016/j.ypmed.2008.10.017

Foster, S., Villanueva, K., Wood, L., Christian, H., & Giles-Corti, B. (2014). The impact of parents' fear of strangers and perceptions of informal social control on children's independent mobility. *Health & Place, 26*, 60–68. doi:10.1016/j.healthplace.2013.11.006

Fyhri, A., Hjorthol, R., Mackett, R. L., Fotel, T. N., & Kyttä, M. (2011). Children's active travel and independent mobility in four countries: Development, social contributing trends and measures. *Transport Policy, 18*(5), 703–710. doi:10.1016/j.tranpol.2011.01.005

Goodman, A., Sahlqvist, S., & Ogilvie, D. (2013). Who uses new walking and cycling infrastructure and how? Longitudinal results from the UK iConnect study. *Preventive Medicine, 57*(5), 518–524. doi:10.1016/j.ypmed.2013.07.007

Goodman, A., Sahlqvist, S., Ogilvie, D., & iConnect Consortium. (2014). New walking and cycling routes and increased physical activity: One- and 2-year findings from the UK iConnect study. *American Journal of Public Health, 104*(9), e38–e46. doi:10.2105/AJPH.2014.302059

Goodman, A., van Sluijs, E., & Ogilvie, D. (2016). Impact of offering cycle training in schools upon cycling behaviour: A natural experimental study. *International Journal of Behavioral Nutrition and Physical Activity, 13*(34), 1–12. doi:10.1186/s12966-016-0356-z

Grabow, M. L., Spak, S. N., Holloway, T., Stone, B., Mednick, A. C., & Patz, J. A. (2012). Air quality and exercise-related health benefits from reduced car travel in the midwestern United States. *Environmental Health Perspectives, 120*(1), 68–76. doi:10.1289/ehp.1103440

Grize, L., Bringolf-Isler, B., Martin, E., & Braun-Fahrländer, C. (2010). Trend in active transportation to school among Swiss school children and its associated factors: Three cross-sectional surveys 1994, 2000 and 2005. *International Journal of Behavioral Nutrition and Physical Activity, 7*(28), 1–8. doi:10.1186/1479-5868-7-28

Gustat, J., Richards, K., Rice, J., Andersen, L., Parker-Karst, K., & Cole, S. (2015). Youth walking and biking rates vary by environments around 5 Louisiana schools. *Journal of School Health, 85*(1), 36–42. doi:10.1111/josh.12220

Hawley, G., Witten, K., Hosking, J., Mackie, H., & Smith, M. (2019). The journey to learn: Perspectives on active school travel from exemplar schools in New Zealand. *Journal of Transport & Health, 14.* doi:10.1016/j.jth.2019.100600

Heelan, K. A., Abbey, B. M., Donnelly, J. E., Mayo, M. S., & Welk, G. J. (2009). Evaluation of a walking school bus for promoting physical activity in youth. *Journal of Physical Activity and Health, 6*(5), 560–567. doi:10.1123/jpah.6.5.560

Hinckson, E. (2016). Perceived challenges and facilitators of active travel following implementation of the school travel-plan programme in New Zealand children and adolescents. *Journal of Transport & Health, 3*(3), 321–325. doi:10.1016/j.jth.2016.05.126

Hinckson, E., & Badland, H. (2011). School travel plans: Preliminary evidence for changing school-related travel patterns in elementary school children. *American Journal of Health Promotion, 25*(6), 368–371. doi:10.4278/ajhp.090706-ARB-217

Hoelscher, D., Ory, M., Dowdy, D., Miao, J., Atteberry, H., Nichols, D., . . . Wang, S. (2016). Effects of funding allocation for safe routes to school programs on active commuting to school and related behavioral, knowledge, and psychosocial outcomes: Results from the Texas childhood obesity prevention policy evaluation (T-COPPE) study. *Environment and Behavior, 48*(1), 210–229. doi:10.1177/0013916515613541

Hopkins, D., García Bengoechea, E., & Mandic, S. (2019). Adolescents and their aspirations for private car-based transport. *Transportation,* 1–27. doi:10.1007/s11116-019-10044-4

Hopkins, D., & Mandic, S. (2017). Perceptions of cycling among high school students and their parents. *International Journal of Sustainable Transportation, 11*(5), 342–356. doi:10.1080/15568318.2016.1253803

Ikeda, E., Hinckson, E., Witten, K., & Smith, M. (2018). Associations of children's active school travel with perceptions of the physical environment and characteristics of the social environment: A systematic review. *Health & Place, 54,* 118–131. doi:10.1016/j.healthplace.2018.09.009

Ikeda, E., Hinckson, E., Witten, K., & Smith, M. (2019). Assessment of direct and indirect associations between children active school travel and environmental, household and child factors using structural equation modelling. *International Journal of Behavioral Nutrition and Physical Activity, 16*(32), 1–17. doi:10.1186/s12966-019-0794-5

Ikeda, E., Stewart, T., Garrett, N., Egli, V., Mandic, S., Hosking, J., . . . Smith, M. (2018). Built environment associates of active school travel in New Zealand children and youth: A systematic meta-analysis using individual participant data. *Journal of Transport & Health, 9,* 117–131. doi:10.1016/j.jth.2018.04.007

Kalman, M., Inchley, J., Sigmundova, D., Iannotti, R. J., Tynjälä, J. A., Hamrik, Z., . . . Bucksch, J. (2015). Secular trends in moderate-to-vigorous physical activity in 32 countries from 2002 to 2010: A cross-national perspective. *European Journal of Public Health, 25*(Suppl 2), 37–40. doi:10.1093/eurpub/ckv024

Keall, M., Chapman, R., Howden-Chapman, P., Witten, K., Abrahamse, W., & Woodward, A. (2015). Increasing active travel: Results of a quasi-experimental study of an intervention to encourage walking and cycling. *Journal of Epidemiology and Community Health, 69*(12), 1184–1190. doi:10.1136/jech-2015-205466

Kek, C. C., García Bengoechea, E., Spence, J. C., & Mandic, S. (in press). The relationship between transport-to-school habits and physical activity in a sample of New Zealand adolescents. *Journal of Sport and Health Science.* doi:10.1016/j.jshs.2019.02.006

Kerr, J., Rosenberg, D., Sallis, J. F., Saelens, B. E., Frank, L. D., & Conway, T. L. (2006). Active commuting to school: Associations with environment and parental concerns. *Medicine and Science in Sports and Exercise, 38*(4), 787–794. doi:10.1249/01.mss.0000210208.63565.73

Kirk, A., & Stamatiadis, N. (2001). Crash rates and traffic maneuvers of younger drivers. *Transportation Research Record: Journal of the Transportation Research Board*, 1779, 68–74. doi:10.3141/1779-10

Kong, A. S., Burks, N., Conklin, C., Roldan, C., Skipper, B., Scott, S., . . . Leggott, J. (2010). A pilot walking school bus program to prevent obesity in hispanic elementary school children: Role of physician involvement with the school community. *Clinical Pediatrics, 49*(10), 989–991. doi:10.1177/0009922810370364

Kong, A. S., Sussman, A. L., Negrete, S., Patterson, N., Mittleman, R., & Hough, R. (2009). Implementation of a walking school bus: Lessons learned. *Journal of School Health, 79*(7), 319–325. doi:10.1111/j.1746-1561.2009.00416.x

Larouche, R., Mammen, G., Rowe, D. A., & Faulkner, G. (2018). Effectiveness of active school transport interventions: A systematic review and update. *BMC Public Health, 18*(1), 206. doi:10.1186/s12889-017-5005-1

Larouche, R., Sarmiento, O. L., & Stewart, T. (2018). Active transportation – Is the school hiding the forest? In R. Larouche (Ed.), *Children's active transportation* (pp. 243–258). Oxford, UK: Elsevier. Retrieved from http://www.sciencedirect.com/science/article/pii/B978012811931000017X, doi:10.1016/B978-0-12-811931-0.00017-X

Larouche, R., Saunders, T. J., Faulkner, G. E. J., Colley, R., & Tremblay, M. (2014). Associations between active school transport and physical activity, body composition, and cardiovascular fitness: A systematic review of 68 studies. *Journal of Physical Activity and Health, 11*(1), 206–227. doi:10.1123/jpah.2011-0345

Larsen, K., Buliung, R., & Faulkner, G. (2016). School travel route measurement and built environment effects in models of children's school travel behavior. *Journal of Transport and Land Use, 9*(2), 5–23. doi:10.5198/jtlu.2015.782

Larsen, K., Gilliland, J., & Hess, P. M. (2012). Route-based analysis to capture the environmental influences on a child's mode of travel between home and school. *Annals of the Association of American Geographers, 102*(6), 1348–1365. Retrieved from https://www.tandfonline.com/doi/abs/10.1080/00045608.2011.627059, doi:10.1080/00045608.2011.627059

Larsen, K., Gilliland, J., Hess, P. M., Tucker, P., Irwin, J., & He, M. (2009). The influence of the physical environment and sociodemographic characteristics on children's mode of travel to and from school. *American Journal of Public Health, 99*(3), 520–526. doi:10.2105/AJPH.2008.135319

Leslie, E., Kremer, P., Toumbourou, J. W., & Williams, J. W. (2010). Gender differences in personal, social and environmental influences on active travel to and from school for Australian adolescents. *Journal of Science and Medicine in Sport, 13*(6), 597–601. doi:10.1016/j.jsams.2010.04.004

Lindsay, G., Macmillan, A., & Woodward, A. (2011). Moving urban trips from cars to bicycles: Impact on health and emissions. *Australian and New Zealand Journal of Public Health, 35*(1), 54–60. doi:10.1111/j.1753-6405.2010.00621.x

Mackett, R., Brown, B., Gong, Y., Kitazawa, K., & Paskins, J. (2007). Children's independent movement in the local environment. *Built Environment, 33*(4), 454–468.

Mackie, H., Macmillan, A., Witten, K., Baas, P., Field, A., Smith, M., . . . Woodward, A. (2018). Te Ara Mua – Future streets suburban street retrofit: A researcher-community-government co-design process and intervention outcomes. *Journal of Transport & Health, 11*, 209–220. doi:10.1016/j.jth.2018.08.014

Macmillan, A. K., Mackie, H., Hosking, J. E., Witten, K., Smith, M., Field, A., . . . Baas, P. (2018). Controlled before-after intervention study of suburb-wide street changes to increase walking and cycling: Te Ara Mua-future streets study design. *BMC Public Health, 18*(850), 1–13. doi:10.1186/s12889-018-5758-1

Mammen, G., Stone, M. R., Faulkner, G., Ramanathan, S., Buliung, R., O'Brien, C., & Kennedy, J. (2014). Active school travel: An evaluation of the Canadian school travel planning intervention. *Preventive Medicine, 60*, 55–59. doi:10.1016/j.ypmed.2013.12.008

Mandic, S., Flaherty, C., Ergler, C., Kek, C. C., Pocock, T., Lawrie, D., . . . García Bengoechea, E. (2018). Effects of cycle skills training on cycling-related knowledge, confidence and behaviour in adolescent girls. *Journal of Transport & Health, 9*, 253–263. doi:10.1016/j.jth.2018.01.015

Mandic, S., Flaherty, C., Pocock, T., Kek, C. C., McArthur, S., Ergler, C., . . . García Bengoechea, E. (2018). Effects of cycle skills training on children's cycling-related knowledge, confidence and behaviours. *Journal of Transport & Health, 8*, 271–282. doi:10.1016/j.jth.2017.12.010

Mandic, S., Hopkins, D., García Bengoechea, E., Flaherty, C., Williams, J., Sloane, L., . . . Spence, J. C. (2017). Adolescents' perceptions of cycling versus walking to school: Understanding the New Zealand context. *Journal of Transport & Health, 4*, 294–304. doi:10.1016/j.jth.2016.10.007

Mandic, S., Keller, R., García Bengoechea, E., Moore, A., & Coppell, K. (2018). School bag weight as a barrier to active transport to school among New Zealand adolescents. *Children, 5*(129), 1–11. doi:10.3390/children5100129

Mandic, S., Leon de la Barra, S., García Bengoechea, E., Stevens, E., Flaherty, C., Moore, A., . . . Skidmore, P. (2015). Personal, social and environmental correlates of active transport to school among adolescents in Otago, New Zealand. *Journal of Science and Medicine in Sport, 18*(4), 432-437. doi:10.1016/j.jsams.2014.06.012

Mandic, S., Sandretto, S., García Bengoechea, E., Hopkins, D., Moore, A., Rodda, J., & Wilson, G. (2017). Enrolling in the closest school or not? Implications of school choice decisions for active transport to school. *Journal of Transport & Health, 6*(Suppl C), 347–357. doi:10.1016/j.jth.2017.05.006

Mandic, S., Sandretto, S., Hopkins, D., Wilson, G., Moore, A., & García Bengoechea, E. (2017). 'I wanted to go here': Adolescents' perspectives on school choice. *Journal of School Choice, 12*(1), 1–25. doi:10.1080/15582159.2017.1381543

Mandic, S., Williams, J., Moore, A., Hopkins, D., Flaherty, C., Wilson, G., . . . Spence, J. C. (2016). Built environment and active transport to school (BEATS) study: Protocol for a cross-sectional study. *BMJ Open, 6*(5), 1–11. doi:10.1136/bmjopen-2016-011196

Marzi, I., & Reimers, A. (2018). Children's independent mobility: Current knowledge, future directions, and public health implications. *International Journal of Environmental Research and Public Health, 15*(2441), 1–15. doi:10.3390/ijerph15112441

McDonald, N. C. (2007). Active transportation to school: Trends among U.S. school children, 1969–2001. *American Journal of Preventive Medicine, 32*(6), 509–516. doi:10.1016/j.amepre.2007.02.022

McDonald, N. C., Steiner, R. L., Lee, C., Rhoulac Smith, T., Zhu, X., & Yang, Y. (2014). Impact of the safe routes to school program on walking and bicycling. *Journal of the American Planning Association, 80*(2), 153–167. doi:10.1080/01944363.2014.956654

McDonald, N. C., Yang, Y., Abbott, S. M., & Bullock, A. N. (2013). Impact of the safe routes to school program on walking and biking: Eugene, Oregon study. *Transport Policy, 29*, 243–248. doi:10.1016/j.tranpol.2013.06.007

McMillan, T. E. (2005). Urban form and a child's trip to school: The current literature and a framework for future research. *Journal of Planning Literature, 19*(4), 440–456. doi:10.1177/0885412204274173

Mendoza, J. A., Levinger, D. D., & Johnston, B. D. (2009). Pilot evaluation of a walking school bus program in a low-income, urban community. *BMC Public Health, 9*(122), 1–7. doi:10.1186/1471-2458-9-122

Mendoza, J. A., Watson, K., Baranowski, T., Nicklas, T. A., Uscanga, D. K., & Hanfling, M. J. (2011). The walking school bus and children's physical activity: A pilot cluster randomized controlled trial. *Pediatrics, 128*(3), e537–e544. doi:10.1542/peds.2010-3486

Ministry of Health. (2017, May 10). *Updated physical activity guidelines for 5–17 year olds*. Retrieved December 3, 2018, from https://www.health.govt.nz/news-media/news-items/updated-physical-activity-guidelines-5-17-year-olds

Ministry of Transport. (2015). *25 years of New Zealand travel: New Zealand household travel 1989–2014*. Wellington, New Zealand. Retrieved from http://www.transport.govt.nz/assets/Uploads/Research/Documents/25yrs-of-how-NZers-Travel.pdf

Mitchell, H., Kearns, R. A., & Collins, D. C. A. (2007). Nuances of neighbourhood: Children's perceptions of the space between home and school in Auckland, New Zealand. *Geoforum, 38*(4), 614–627. doi:10.1016/j.geoforum.2006.11.012

Mitra, R. (2013). Independent mobility and mode choice for school transportation: A review and framework for future research. *Transport Reviews, 33*(1), 21–43. doi:10.1080/01441647.2012.743490

Molina-García, J., Queralt, A., García Bengoechea, E., Moore, A., & Mandic, S. (2018). Would New Zealand adolescents cycle to school more if allowed to cycle without a helmet? *Journal of Transport & Health, 11*, 64–72. doi:10.1016/j.jth.2018.10.001

Moran, M. R., Rodríguez, D. A., & Corburn, J. (2018). Examining the role of trip destination and neighborhood attributes in shaping environmental influences on children's route choice. *Transportation Research Part D: Transport and Environment, 65*, 63–81. doi:10.1016/j.trd.2018.08.001

Morrow, V. (2003). Improving the neighbourhood for children: Possibilities and limitations of 'social capital' discourses. In P. Christensen & M. O'Brien (Eds.), *Children in the city: Home, neighbourhood and community* (pp. 162–183). London, UK: RoutledgeFalmer.

National Centre for Safe Routes to School. (2011). *How children get to school: School travel patterns from 1969 to 2009*. Retrieved from http://www.safekidsgf.com/Documents/Research%20Reports/NHTS%20School%20Travel%20Report%202011.pdf

National Health Service. (2018, June 25). *Physical activity guidelines for children and young people*. Retrieved December 3, 2018, from https://www.nhs.uk/live-well/exercise/physical-activity-guidelines-children-and-young-people/

Nelson, N. M., Foley, E., O'Gorman, D. J., Moyna, N. M., & Woods, C. B. (2008). Active commuting to school: How far is too far? *International Journal of Behavioral Nutrition and Physical Activity, 5*(1), 1–9. doi:10.1186/1479-5868-5-1

Ogilvie, D., Egan, M., Hamilton, V., & Petticrew, M. (2005). Systematic reviews of health effects of social interventions: 2. Best available evidence: How low should you go? *Journal of Epidemiology and Community Health, 59*(10), 886–892. doi:10.1136/jech.2005.034199

Oliver, M., Parker, K., Witten, K., Mavoa, S., Badland, H. M., Donovan, P., . . . Kearns, R. A. (2016). Children's out-of-school independently mobile tips, active travel, and physical activity: A cross-sectional examination from the kids in the City Study. *Journal of Physical Activity and Health, 13*(3), 318–324. doi:10.1123/jpah.2015-0043

Pabayo, R., Gauvin, L., & Barnett, T. A. (2011). Longitudinal changes in active transportation to school in Canadian youth aged 6 through 16 years. *Pediatrics, 128*(2), e404–e413. doi:10.1542/peds.2010-1612

Panter, J. R., Jones, A. P., & van Sluijs, E. M. F. (2008). Environmental determinants of active travel in youth: A review and framework for future research. *International Journal of Behavioral Nutrition and Physical Activity, 5*(34), 1–14. doi:10.1186/1479-5868-5-34

Piercy, K. L., Troiano, R. P., Ballard, R. M., Carlson, S. A., Fulton, J. E., Galuska, D. A., . . . Olson, R. D. (2018). The physical activity guidelines for Americans. *JAMA, 320*(19), 2020–2028. doi:10.1001/jama.2018.14854

Pocock, T., Moore, A., Keall, M., & Mandic, S. (2019). Physical and spatial assessment of school neighbourhood built environments for active transport to school in adolescents from Dunedin (New Zealand). *Health & Place, 55*, 1–8. doi:10.1016/j.healthplace.2018.10.003

Pont, K., Ziviani, J., Wadley, D., & Abbott, R. (2011). The model of children's active travel (M-CAT): A conceptual framework for examining factors influencing children's active travel. *Australian Occupational Therapy Journal, 58*(3), 138–144. doi:10.1111/j.1440-1630.2010.00865.x

Pont, K., Ziviani, J., Wadley, D., Bennett, S., & Abbott, R. (2009). Environmental correlates of children's active transportation: A systematic literature review. *Health & Place, 15*(3), 849–862. doi:10.1016/j.healthplace.2009.02.002

Prezza, M., Alparone, F. R., Renzi, D., & Pietrobono, A. (2009). Social participation and independent mobility in children: The effects of two implementations of 'we go to school alone'. *Journal of Prevention & Intervention in the Community, 38*(1), 8–25. doi:10.1080/10852350903393392

Rainham, D. G., Bates, C. J., Blanchard, C. M., Dummer, T. J., Kirk, S. F., & Shearer, C. L. (2012). Spatial classification of youth physical activity patterns. *American Journal of Preventive Medicine, 42*(5), e87–e96. doi:10.1016/j.amepre.2012.02.011

Rissel, C., Curac, N., Greenaway, M., & Bauman, A. (2012). Physical activity associated with public transport use – A review and modelling of potential benefits. *International Journal of Environmental Research and Public Health, 9*(7), 2454–2478. doi:10.3390/ijerph9072454

Rissotto, A., & Tonucci, F. (2002). Freedom of movement and environmental knowledge in elementary school children. *Journal of Environmental Psychology, 22*(1), 65–77. doi:10.1006/jevp.2002.0243

Rothman, L., Macpherson, A. K., Ross, T., & Buliung, R. N. (2018). The decline in active school transportation (AST): A systematic review of the factors related to AST and changes in school transport over time in North America. *Preventive Medicine, 111*, 314–322. doi:10.1016/j.ypmed.2017.11.018

Saelens, B. E., Moudon, A. V., Kang, B., Hurvitz, P. M., & Zhou, C. (2014). Relation between higher physical activity and public transit use. *American Journal of Public Health, 104*(5), 854–859. doi:10.2105/ajph.2013.301696

Sallis, J. F., Cervero, R. B., Ascher, W., Henderson, K. A., Kraft, M. K., & Kerr, J. (2006). An ecological approach to creating active living communities. *Annual Review of Public Health, 27*, 297–322. doi:10.1146/annurev.publhealth.27.021405.102100

Sallis, J. F., Owen, N., & Fotheringham, M. J. (2000). Behavioral epidemiology: A systematic framework to classify phases of research on health promotion and disease prevention. *Annals of Behavioral Medicine, 22*(4), 294–298. doi:10.1007/bf02895665

Salmon, J., Timperio, A., Cleland, V., & Venn, A. (2005). Trends in children's physical activity and weight status in high and low socio-economic status areas of Melbourne, Victoria, 1985–2001. *Australian and New Zealand Journal of Public Health, 29*(4), 337–342. doi:10.1111/j.1467-842X.2005.tb00204.x

Sandercock, G., Angus, C., & Barton, J. (2010). Physical activity levels of children living in different built environments. *Preventive Medicine, 50*(4), 193–198. doi:10.1016/j.ypmed.2010.01.005

Sarmiento, O. L., Díaz del Castillo, A., Triana, C. A., Acevedo, M. J., Gonzalez, S. A., & Pratt, M. (2017). Reclaiming the streets for people: Insights from Ciclovías Recreativas in Latin America. *Preventive Medicine, 103*, S34–S40. doi:10.1016/j.ypmed.2016.07.028

Saunders, L. E., Green, J. M., Petticrew, M. P., Steinbach, R., & Roberts, H. (2013). What are the health benefits of active travel? A systematic review of trials and cohort studies. *PloS One, 8*(8). doi:10.1371/journal.pone.0069912

Sayers, S. P., LeMaster, J. W., Thomas, I. M., Petroski, G. F., & Ge, B. (2012). A walking school bus program: Impact on physical activity in elementary school children in Columbia, Missouri. *American Journal of Preventive Medicine, 43*(5 Suppl. 4), S384–S389. doi:10.1016/j.amepre.2012.07.009

Schlossberg, M., Greene, J., Phillips, P. P., Johnson, B., & Parker, B. (2006). School trips: Effects of urban form and distance on travel mode. *Journal of the American Planning Association, 72*(3), 337–346. doi:10.1080/01944360608976755

Schoeppe, S., Duncan, M. J., Badland, H., Oliver, M., & Curtis, C. (2013). Associations of children's independent mobility and active travel with physical activity, sedentary behaviour and weight status: A systematic review. *Journal of Science and Medicine in Sport, 16*(4), 312–319. doi:10.1016/j.jsams.2012.11.001

Shaw, B., Bicket, M., Elliot, B., Fagan-Watson, B., Mocca, E., & Hillman, M. (2015). *Children's independent mobility: An international comparison and recommendations for action.* London, UK: University of Westminster. Retrieved from http://www.psi.org.uk/docs/7350_PSI_Report_CIM_final.pdf

Simons, D., Clarys, P., De Bourdeaudhuij, I., de Geus, B., Vandelanotte, C., & Deforche, B. (2013). Factors influencing mode of transport in older adolescents: A qualitative study. *BMC Public Health, 13*(323), 1–10. doi:10.1186/1471-2458-13-323

Sirard, J. R., Alhassan, S., Spencer, T. R., & Robinson, T. N. (2008). Changes in physical activity from walking to school. *Journal of Nutrition Education and Behavior, 40*(5), 324–326. doi:10.1016/j.jneb.2007.12.002

Sjolie, A. N., & Thuen, F. (2002). School journeys and leisure activities in rural and urban adolescents in Norway. *Health Promotion International, 17*(1), 21–30. doi:10.1093/heapro/17.1.21

Staunton, C. E., Hubsmith, D., & Kallins, W. (2003). Promoting safe walking and biking to school: The Marin County success story. *American Journal of Public Health, 93*(9), 1431–1434. doi:10.2105/ajph.93.9.1431

Stevenson, M., Thompson, J., de Sá, T. H., Ewing, R., Mohan, D., McClure, R., . . . Woodcock, J. (2016). Land use, transport, and population health: Estimating the health benefits of compact cities. *The Lancet, 388*(10062), 2925–2935. doi:10.1016/S0140-6736(16)30067-8

Stewart, O., Moudon, A. V., & Claybrooke, C. (2014). Multistate evaluation of safe routes to school programs. *American Journal of Health Promotion, 28*(3 Suppl), S89–S96. doi:10.4278/ajhp.130430-QUAN-210

Stewart, T., Duncan, S., & Schipperijn, J. (2017). Adolescents who engage in active school transport are also more active in other contexts: A space-time investigation. *Health & Place, 43*, 25–32. doi:10.1016/j.healthplace.2016.11.009

Stewart, T., Schipperijn, J., Snizek, B., & Duncan, S. (2017). Adolescent school travel: Is online mapping a practical alternative to GPS-assessed travel routes? *Journal of Transport & Health, 5*, 113–122. doi:10.1016/j.jth.2016.10.001

Strong, W. B., Malina, R. M., Blimkie, C. J. R., Daniels, S. R., Dishman, R. K., Gutin, B., . . . Trudeau, F. (2005). Evidence based physical activity for school-age youth. *The Journal of Pediatrics, 146*(6), 732–737. doi:10.1016/j.jpeds.2005.01.055

Sun, Y., Liu, Y., & Tao, F.-B. (2015). Associations between active commuting to school, body fat, and mental well-being: Population-based, cross-sectional study in China. *Journal of Adolescent Health, 57*(6), 679–685. doi:10.1016/j.jadohealth.2015.09.002

Timperio, A., Ball, K., Salmon, J., Roberts, R., Giles-Corti, B., Simmons, D., . . . Crawford, D. (2006). Personal, family, social, and environmental correlates of active commuting to school. *American Journal of Preventive Medicine, 30*(1), 45–51. doi:10.1016/j.amepre.2005.08.047

Tranter, P., & Pawson, E. (2001). Children's access to local environments: A case-study of Christchurch, New Zealand. *Local Environment, 6*(1), 27–48. doi:10.1080/13549830120024233

Trapp, G. S. A., Giles-Corti, B., Christian, H. E., Bulsara, M., Timperio, A. F., McCormack, G. R., & Villaneuva, K. P. (2011). On your bike! A cross-sectional study of the individual, social and environmental correlates of cycling to school. *International Journal of Behavioral Nutrition and Physical Activity, 8*(123), 1–10. doi:10.1186/1479-5868-8-123

Trapp, G. S. A., Giles-Corti, B., Christian, H. E., Bulsara, M., Timperio, A. F., McCormack, G. R., & Villaneuva, K. P. (2012). Increasing children's physical activity: Individual, social, and environmental factors associated with walking to and from school. *Health Education and Behavior, 39*(2), 172–182. Retrieved from https://journals.sagepub.com/doi/abs/10.1177/1090198111423272, doi:10.1177/1090198111423272

Tremblay, M. S., Barnes, J. D., González, S. A., Katzmarzyk, P. T., Onywera, V. O., Reilly, J. J., . . . the Global Matrix 2.0 Research Team. (2016). Global Matrix 2.0: Report card grades on the physical activity of children and youth comparing 38 countries. *Journal of Physical Activity and Health, 13*(11 Suppl 2), S343–S366. doi:10.1123/jpah.2016-0594

Tremblay, M. S., Gray, C. E., Akinroye, K., Harrington, D. M., Katzmarzyk, P. T., Lambert, E. V., . . . Tomkinson, G. (2014). Physical activity of children: A Global Matrix of grades comparing 15 countries. *Journal of Physical Activity and Health, 11*(Suppl 1), S113–S125. doi:10.1123/jpah.2014-0177

U.S. Department of Transportation. (1972). *Nationwide personal transportation study: Transportation characteristics of school children.* Retrieved from https://www.fhwa.dot.gov/ohim/1969/q.pdf

Van Dijk, M. L., De Groot, R. H., Van Acker, F., Savelberg, H. H., & Kirschner, P. A. (2014). Active commuting to school, cognitive performance, and academic achievement: An observational study in Dutch adolescents using accelerometers. *BMC Public Health, 14*(1), 799. doi:10.1186/1471-2458-14-799

Van Dyck, D., De Bourdeaudhuij, I., Cardon, G., & Deforche, B. (2010). Criterion distances and correlates of active transportation to school in Belgian older adolescents. *International Journal of Behavioral Nutrition and Physical Activity, 7*(87), 1–9. doi:10.1186/1479-5868-7-87

Vanwolleghem, G., D'Haese, S., Van Dyck, D., De Bourdeaudhuij, I., & Cardon, G. (2014). Feasibility and effectiveness of drop-off spots to promote walking to school. *International Journal of Behavioral Nutrition and Physical Activity, 11*(136), 1–11. doi:10.1186/s12966-014-0136-6

Verhoeven, H., Simons, D., Van Dyck, D., Van Cauwenberg, J., Clarys, P., De Bourdeaudhuij, I., . . . Deforche, B. (2016). Psychosocial and environmental correlates of walking, cycling, public transport and passive transport to various destinations in Flemish older adolescents. *PLoS One, 11*(1), e0147128. doi:10.1371/journal.pone.0147128

Villa-González, E., Barranco-Ruiz, Y., Evenson, K. R., & Chillón, P. (2018). Systematic review of interventions for promoting active school transport. *Preventive Medicine, 111*, 115–134. doi:10.1016/j.ypmed.2018.02.010

Villanueva, K., Giles-Corti, B., & McCormack, G. (2008). Achieving 10,000 steps: A comparison of public transport users and drivers in a university setting. *Preventive Medicine, 47*(3), 338–341. doi:10.1016/j.ypmed.2008.03.005

Voss, C., Winters, M., Frazer, A., & McKay, H. (2015). School-travel by public transit: Rethinking active transportation. *Preventive Medicine Reports, 2*, 65–70. doi:10.1016/j.pmedr.2015.01.004

Wilson, K., Clark, A. F., & Gilliland, J. A. (2018). Understanding child and parent perceptions of barriers influencing children's active school travel. *BMC Public Health, 18*(1053), 1–14. doi:10.1186/s12889-018-5874-y

Witten, K., Carroll, P., Calder-Dawe, O., Smith, M., Field, A., & Hosking, J. (2018). Te Ara Mua – Future streets: Knowledge exchange and the highs and lows of researcher-practitioner collaboration to design active travel infrastructure. *Journal of Transport & Health, 9*, 31–44. doi:10.1016/j.jth.2018.03.001

Wong, B. Y.-M., Faulkner, G. E. J., & Buliung, R. N. (2011). GIS measured environmental correlates of active school transport: A systematic review of 14 studies. *International Journal of Behavioral Nutrition and Physical Activity, 8*(39), 1–22. doi:10.1186/1479-5868-8-39

Woodcock, J., Edwards, P., Tonne, C., Armstrong, B. G., Ashiru, O., Banister, D., . . . Roberts, I. (2009). Public health benefits of strategies to reduce greenhouse-gas emissions: Urban land transport. *The Lancet, 374*(9705), 1930–1943. doi:10.1016/S0140-6736(09)61714-1

Woodward, A., & Lindsay, G. (2010). Changing modes of travel in New Zealand cities. In P. Howden-Chapman, K. Stuart, & R. B. Chapman (Eds.), *Sizing up the city: Urban form and transport in New Zealand.* Wellington, New Zealand: Steele Roberts.

World Health Organization. (2010). *Global recommendations on physical activity for health.* Retrieved from http://apps.who.int/iris/bitstream/10665/44399/1/9789241599979_eng.pdf

World Health Organization. (2018). *Global action plan on physical activity 2018–2030: More active people for a healthier world.* Geneva, Switzerland. Retrieved from http://apps.who.int/iris/bitstream/handle/10665/272722/9789241514187-eng.pdf?ua=1

Zaccari, V., & Dirkis, H. (2003). Walking to school in inner Sydney. *Health Promotion Journal of Australia, 14*(2), 137–140. doi:10.1071/HE03137

Zapata-Diomedi, B., Knibbs, L. D., Ware, R. S., Heesch, K. C., Tainio, M., Woodcock, J., & Veerman, J. L. (2017). A shift from motorised travel to active transport: What are the potential health gains for an Australian city? *PLoS One, 12*(10), e0184799. doi:10.1371/journal.pone.0184799

35

THE ROLE OF TECHNOLOGY IN PROMOTING PHYSICAL ACTIVITY IN YOUTH

Kelly A. Mackintosh, Dale W. Esliger, Andrew P. Kingsnorth,
Adam Loveday, Sam G. M. Crossley, and Melitta A. McNarry

Introduction

Regular participation in physical activity (PA) is beneficial to children's physiological and psychosocial health (Department of Health, 2011), as well as educational attainment (Singh, Uijtdewilligen, Twisk, van Mechelen, & Chinapaw, 2012). Specifically, PA is well accepted to be protective from a number of conditions, including obesity (Jakicic, 2009), diabetes (Jeon, Lokken, Hu, & van Dam, 2007), heart disease (Sofi, Capalbo, Cesari, Abbate, & Gensini, 2008), depression (Teychenne, Ball, & Salmon, 2008), and some cancers (Friedenreich, Neilson, & Lynch, 2010). Despite this, 1 in 3 children do not engage in sufficient sustained PA to accrue such benefits (World Health Organization, 2018b). Moreover, the concomitant high sedentary behaviour (SB), defined as any waking behaviour characterized by an energy expenditure ≤ 1.5 metabolic equivalents (METs), while in a sitting, reclining, or lying posture (Sedentary Behaviour Research Network, 2012), that is typical of many children's daily routines, is independently associated with multiple deleterious health outcomes (Biswas et al., 2015). Indeed, physical inactivity, the absence of sufficient PA to meet current PA recommendations (Tremblay et al., 2017), has been identified as the fourth leading risk factor for mortality globally (World Health Organization, 2009), accounting for approximately 3.2 million deaths per year (World Health Organization, 2018b), contributing to 10% of non-communicable disease (Lim et al., 2012), and costing £54 billion annually worldwide (World Health Organization, 2018b). Consequently, the World Health Organisation (WHO) has set a global target to reduce physical inactivity by 10% and 15% by 2025 and 2030, respectively (World Health Organization, 2018a), which will only be achieved with radical changes in interventional approaches to increasing PA (Das & Horton, 2016). Recent figures from a meta-analysis of 358 population-based studies incorporating 1.9 million people suggest that the 2025 target will not be met unless there are significant efforts to prioritise and scale up policies to increase PA (Guthold, Stevens, Riley, & Bull, 2018).

Traditional interventions to increase PA and decrease SB have been associated with varied degrees of success, but the majority are neither scalable to a public health level nor sustainable beyond intervention cessation (Cobiac, Vos, & Barendregt, 2009; Estabrooks & Gyurcsik, 2003). Technology plays a complicated role in physical inactivity and is often considered a double-edged sword (Sun, Zeng, & Gao, 2017). Specifically, while some technologies have undoubtedly contributed to the physical inactivity epidemic, such as sedentary video games and social media, other technologies have been incorporated into increasingly popular tools to assess and promote PA and health through devices such as personal activity trackers. Indeed, the self-monitoring of PA that these tools enable has been identified as an effective behaviour change technique that has been utilised in numerous behavioural interventions targeting increases in PA levels (Michie et al., 2013). A key challenge in youth populations is ensuring an awareness of their own PA and SB levels and how these translate to the WHO and government guidelines; technology may play a key role in increasing this awareness by allowing personalised, individual feedback and self-monitoring.

Technology is ubiquitous across the developed world, with the introduction of intuitive touch-screen user interfaces on internet-enabled mobile devices, such as smart phones and tablet computers, creating further opportunities for more extensive engagement with technology by youth and at ever younger ages (Straker, Zabatiero, Danby, Thorpe, & Edwards, 2018). For example, in Australia, average weekly screen-time has recently been reported to be 14.2 and 25.9 hours in those less than 2 years (Rhodes, 2017) and 2–5 years (Rideout & Robb, 2017) old, respectively. A central issue in resolving the role of technology as the potential instigator of, or resolution to, this global inactivity epidemic is the conflicting pressures of different agencies (Straker et al., 2018). Specifically, while educators, industries, innovators, and employers promote increased use of digital technology at young ages to enhance, among other aspects, learning, digital skill sets, and engagement in Science, Technology, Engineering and Mathematics (STEM), health agencies advocate limited use of technology due to concerns regarding the associated effects on physical, cognitive, emotional, and social health; well-being; and development. This chapter will consider a range of recent technological advancements and their potential role in the resolution of this conflict, as well as the sustainable promotion of increased PA and decreased SB in youth. Specifically, the ability of these technologies to engender physiological and psychosocial benefits will be explored, highlighting the challenges and issues that remain to be resolved prior to their wide-scale implementation. Finally, key considerations for the development of future technology-focused interventions will be discussed.

Overview of the Literature

Evolution of Technology

Technology is continuously changing and developing, with the nature of this progression and the time taken, varying both between and within technologies, such as between different applications of the same technology. Put simply, a broad conceptualisation is that technological progress can be viewed as evolutionary or revolutionary. While both evolution and revolution describe change, evolution, by its inherent nature, is a more gradual change, whereas revolution is a faster, more dramatic, change on a wider societal scale. As such, revolutionary technologies could arguably include the personal computer (PC), internet, or smart phone (Beaudry, Doms, & Lewis, 2010; Neubeck et al., 2015). Within this context, the current landscape of PA-promoting technology could be considered to reflect an evolution in technology, from the simple pedometer to sophisticated multi-sensor wearables and activity trackers.

Despite the gradual pace of wearable technology evolution, it is still a challenge for researchers to match this pace of iteration in consumer wearables. Indeed, Moore's Law, named after the co-founder of Intel, Gordon Moore, observes that the number of components in an integrated circuit doubles every 18 months to 2 years (Bondyopadhyay, 1998; Schaller, 1997); in short, these advances facilitate a doubling in processing power every 2 years. This is exemplified by current pocket-sized smartphones which have substantially more processing power than the computers used by NASA in the 1960s (Puiu, 2015). Although there is some debate over whether this rate of change may have slowed somewhat (perhaps to every 2.5 years), it serves as a useful illustration for the approximate pace of technological change.

The approximately 2-year pace of technological change stands in stark contrast to the average 17-year pace of translating research findings into clinical practice (Morris, Wooding, & Grant, 2011). With wearable technologies, such as activity trackers, the knowledge translation lag is marked as research papers are published having studied technologies released several years prior (Burton et al., 2018). These studies could therefore be using dated technologies that have been superseded by newer models or, in some cases, using technologies which are no longer commercially available (Orme et al., 2018). That is not to say, however, that studies such as these are devoid of value; commonalities in the features of technologies, and the way they are utilised in interventions, ensure that there will still be important and translatable findings, irrespective of specific brands, models, or designs.

The incongruence between the pace of technological advances and that of academic research has led to some researchers seeking innovative methodologies which are more responsive than traditional ones (Hekler, Michie et al., 2016; Moller et al., 2017). One such example, "Agile Science" (Hekler, Klasnja et al., 2016), is a paradigm from agile software development, which explicitly rejects the notion of a "definitive" scientific trial. This is, at least in part, due to the issues under investigation being complex, and thus, a modular approach is utilised whereby multiple variations of plausibly effective interventions are created for a given population, in a specific place and at a specific time (i.e., a "niche"; Hekler, Klasnja et al., 2016). These specific behaviour change interventions are tested for real-world success against optimisation criteria (i.e., definitions of success and failure). If they are found to be useful, they are then repurposed for different "niches" (i.e., different people, in different places and at different times). The ultimate goal of this approach is to produce interventions that are effective and to determine the context (where, when and for whom), in which a specific intervention should be used. In adults, this contextually tailored approach has shown promising results in initial optimisation trials (Klasnja et al., 2018). Further examples of these innovative methodologies include pragmatic clinical trials, N of 1 studies, and micro-randomised trials (Klasnja et al., 2015; Lillie et al., 2011; Spruijt-Metz et al., 2015). These methodologies, and indeed others, are an important development in harnessing the potential of various technologies as intervention modalities to increase PA and/or reduce SB.

Technologies to Promote PA in Youth

Avatars

An avatar, classified as any human-controlled graphical or textual representation that has the ability to perform actions in real time (Bell, 2008), can provide living metaphor visualisations of feedback. Such visualisations have inspired the design of numerous youth activity trackers and their associated apps. For example, Sqord (2018) is an activity tracker and platform where youths can create their own personal avatar and collect points and rewards for completing PA. Other examples, such as GeoPalz and Zamzee, also utilise an activity tracker and online visual rewards and feedback through personalised avatars. Although these commercially available activity trackers and associated feedback apps have, and continue to have, some degree of success (Miller & Mynatt, 2014), there is a paucity of literature regarding the impact of the living metaphor visualisations to enforce increased engagement in youth PA (Masteller, Sirard, & Freedson, 2017). For example, Masteller et al. (2017) examined 8–9-year-old children's perceptions of the Sqord and Zamzee trackers, as well as their associated visual feedback, to promote PA. The findings revealed that youths liked the 'avatar' feedback represented on the Sqord (75%) and Zamzee (94%) websites as they could change the avatar to depict themselves.

More recent technological developments in the 3D scanning of an individual have enabled researchers to create 'photorealistic' avatars that closely resemble the self (Thompson et al., 2018).

Specifically, Thompson and colleagues (2018) utilised 3D scanning technology to develop an exergame called 'The Nightmare Runner' which involved youth completing physical movements in the real world to control their in-game photorealistic avatar to avoid obstacles and escape the chasing monsters. During the 20-minute gameplay, participants PA levels were measured using an accelerometer, showing that approximately 75% (15.9 minutes), 16% (3.3 minutes), and 10% (1.6 minutes) of gameplay was spent in vigorous, moderate, and light PA, respectively. Interestingly, youth expressed how their photorealistic avatar had a positive impact on their gameplay experience because "it's almost as if [it] was me, like if I were in the videogame I would want to get away from the monster" (p. 5, Thompson et al., 2018). While the findings were based on the short-term effects of photorealistic avatars and the influence of such methods on sustained PA remains to be elucidated, it is suggested that an individual is more likely to be motivated to play the game if the avatar is similar to the self (Jin, 2010; Thin, Brown, & Meenan, 2013). In this way, it could be postulated that exergames that utilise photorealistic avatars would not only get young people to feel more emotionally connected to the game, but may also reap the benefits of enhanced lifestyle behaviors, such as increased PA.

Exergames

Recent statistics demonstrate that 73% of children aged 6–14 years in Great Britain engage in gaming, irrespective of type, format, or device (Interactive Software Federation of Europe, 2018). Despite being slightly lower than their European counterparts (Figure 35.1), game use is by far the highest in youth and peaks at 11–14 years old, prior to declining with age (Interactive Software Federation of Europe, 2018). Games are able to provide an enjoyable and engaging experience for an individual (Deterding, 2014), and have been of considerable interest for health promotion programs for over a decade (Baranowski, Buday, Thompson, & Baranowski, 2008). Technological advances have led to the development of a new generation of video gaming, frequently termed 'exergames', a portmanteau of 'exercise' and 'gaming', that promote physical movements as part of the game (Oh & Yang, 2010). With young people being the largest proportion of society that interact with video games, researchers have sought to capitalise on this medium of entertainment, but with a different public health perspective in mind.

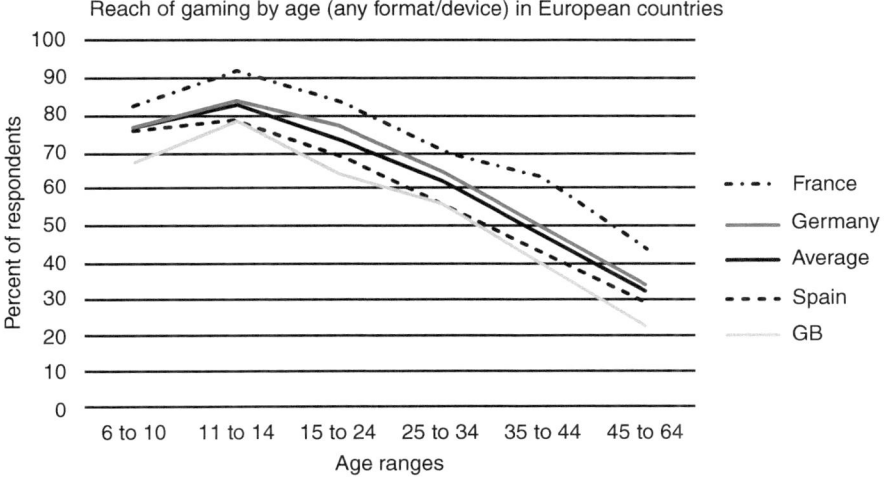

Figure 35.1 Data obtained from the GameTrack Digest Report: Quarter 1 (2018) (Interactive Software Federation of Europe, 2018)

Well-known exergames could be considered to be the Dance Dance Revolution or the Wii generation games that were prevalent during the late 1990s and early 2000s; yet, exergames were developed in the early 1980s, with the Atari Joyboard and Puffer models being some of the earliest exergaming technologies (Finco & Maass, 2014).The terminology to describe these technologies in the literature has been inconsistent, with 'exergaming' historically being most common in non-health-related contexts, while health-related researchers typically opted for terms such as 'active video games' or 'interactive video games' (Oh & Yang, 2010). It has subsequently been suggested that 'exergames' should be used to refer to all video game activities that require physical exertion and also those that include strength, balance and flexibility (Oh & Yang, 2010).

Research has shown that, compared to common sedentary-based games, exergames can acutely increase an individual's energy expenditure (Barnett, Cerin, & Baranowski, 2011; Biddiss & Irwin, 2010; Foley & Maddison, 2010; Guy, Ratzki-Leewing, & Gwadry-Sridhar, 2011; McNarry & Mackintosh, 2016; Peng, Crouse, & Lin, 2013) and have the potential to impact PA behaviours due to their intrinsic appeal (Madden, Lenhart, Duggan, Cortesi, & Gasser, 2013), ease of distribution, and the potential to engage individuals through basic positive motivational processes that have been identified as fundamental drivers to sustained behaviour change (Cole, Yoo, & Knutson, 2012; Koepp et al., 1998). Several systematic reviews have been conducted that have assessed the influence of exergames on health and behavioural outcomes in children and adolescents (Barnett et al., 2011; Biddiss & Irwin, 2010; Campos & del Castillo Fernández, 2016; Guy et al., 2011; Johnson et al., 2016; Pakarinen, Parisod, Smed, & Salantera, 2017; Peng et al., 2013). Overall, the key findings suggest that exergames can elicit positive non-physical effects, such as increasing PA enjoyment (Joronen, Aikasalo, & Suvitie, 2016) and PA (health games) self-efficacy (Pakarinen et al., 2017), as well as reducing sedentary time during the measurement period (i.e., during active video gaming; Norris, Hamer, & Stamatakis, 2016). Moreover, there is strong evidence that in non-typically developing children and adolescents balance can be improved using exergames (Page, Barrington, Edwards, & Barnett, 2017). Additionally, a research study that objectively assessed the activity levels of US children (mean age of 6.89 years) during 20–22-minute exergaming sessions reported that children spent on average 20%, 33%, and 47% in moderate-to-vigorous PA (MVPA), light activity, and SB, respectively (Quan, Pope, & Gao, 2018). In comparison with a traditional PE lesson of similar length, exergames have been reported to be equally effective at promoting children's light PA, MVPA, and energy expenditure, with no negative effects on SB. However, it is pertinent to note the longer duration of typical PE lessons than an exergame, which limits the comparisons that can be drawn to some extent. (Gao, Pope et al., 2017). Similarly, a randomised control trial that used home-based exergaming in overweight/obese children found that exergames of 1-hour per session, three times a week, resulted in a significant, albeit small, decrease in BMI z-score of 0.06 (Staiano et al., 2018). Yet, not all exergaming studies report an increase in PA levels; for example, after 12 weeks of dance exergaming in overweight and obese adolescent girls, there was no change in objectively measured PA but there was an increase in self-efficacy towards PA (Staiano, Beyl, Hsia, Katzmarzyk, & Newton, 2016).

Pokémon Go

A vast majority of exergaming has been focused on the development of interventions during targeted and specific measurable periods of the day; however, the release of Pokémon Go provided a great opportunity to study the effect of exergames in a more free-living setting. Advertised as a 'get up and go' game, it uses a GPS signal from a mobile phone to track a user's location in order to move an avatar on a digitised map (American Heart Association, 2016). The basic premise is that by physically moving, you can interact with many features of the app to gain items or experience points. An early study conducted on this app reported that particularly engaged users increased their steps by an average of 1,473 steps per day compared to their baseline activity levels (Althoff, White, & Horvitz, 2016). Combining gamification (the application of the characteristics and benefits of games to real-world processes/problems), the requirement for PA, and augmented reality, the game encourages its users to walk with the phone active to increase their chances of finding new creatures to collect or to hatch eggs that only complete after a set distance, e.g. 2, 5, or 10 km (LeBlanc & Chaput, 2017).

Visualisations of PA

Tangible Visualisations of PA

As Jansen et al. (2013) advocate, there are many benefits of tangible visualisations over on-screen visualisations. These include (i) allowing for active perception, (ii) leveraging non-visual senses, (iii) integration into the physical world, and (iv) harnessing of the interplay between vision and touch to facilitate cognition. In addition, tangible objects can offer different opportunities for youth interaction when compared to on-screen visualisations, such as being able to trade or display them on a shelf (Ananthanarayan, 2015), which historically aligns with the popularity of art installations and museums (Dragicevic & Jansen, 2012). With the recent rise of the 'maker movement', cost-effective three-dimensional (3D) printers, such as the MakerBot and the Ultimaker, have given rise to health-related researchers utilising their capacities to create tangible visualisations of PA. Specifically, 3D printing is an additive manufacturing process where a tangible object is created by depositing layer by layer of a material (e.g., plastic) onto a print bed. Khot, Hjorth, and Mueller (2014) were the first to encapsulate adult heart rate data into 3D-printed visualisations which took numerical, abstract, and living metaphor forms, such as a physical graph, flower, frog, dice, and ring (Figure 35.2). Findings demonstrated that all the tangible representations of PA allowed participants to relate to their data, showing increased awareness and reflection of their PA

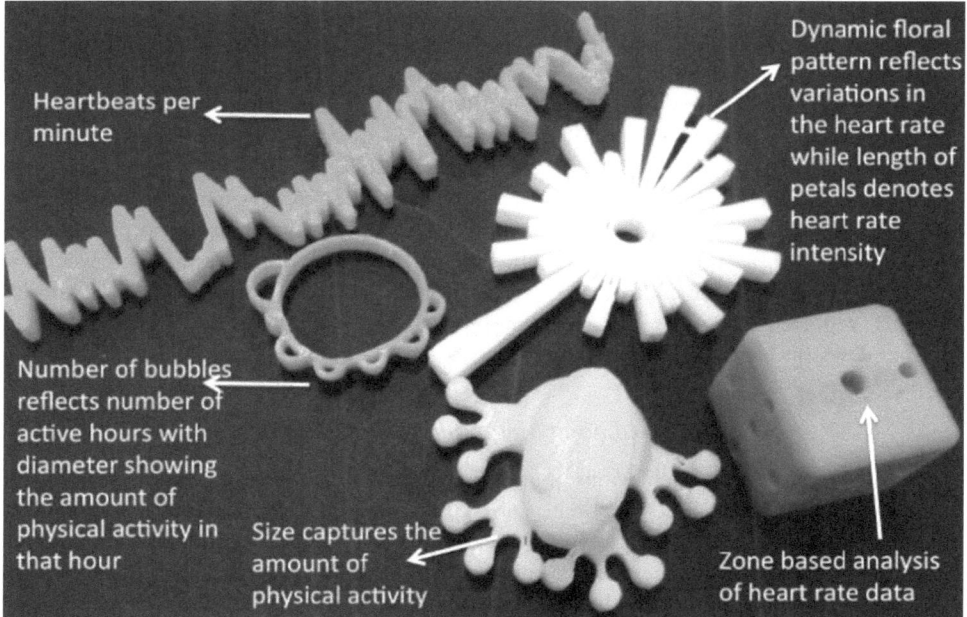

Figure 35.2   3D-printed representations of heart rate. From Khot et al. (2014)

patterns. As described by Khot et al. (2014), this type of 3D-printed data acts as both a reward and a feedback of PA data, which may offer more for youths given that incentive-based interventions have showed some level of promise in promoting PA levels (Christian et al., 2016; Finkelstein et al., 2013; Hardman, Horne, & Fergus Lowe, 2011).

Numerical Visualisations of PA

Visualisations are particularly central to our understanding of data, as "seeing" makes knowledge credible (Bloch, 2008) and a greater visibility of information contributes to an added responsibility to act (Viseu & Suchman, 2010). Moreover, visualisations are known to enable individuals to identify patterns and relationships within their data, leading to the discovery of new concepts and ideas that were previously unknown or only hypothesised (Card, Mackinlay, & Schneiderman, 1999). In the context of PA, visualisations offer individuals awareness of their PA levels, making them actionable and comprehensible in terms of health-related outcomes (Khot, 2016). Over the past decade, there has been an explosion of commercially available activity trackers that incorporate a number of different sensors (e.g., pedometers, heart rate monitors, accelerometers) into one device for self-monitoring PA patterns (Hooke, Gilchrist, Tanner, Hart, & Withycombe, 2016). The multitude of information collected from these devices (e.g., step count, distance travelled, floors climbed, beats per minute, calories burned, sleep patterns, and intensity of PA) can be evaluated through interfaced connections with computers, smartphones, and tablets, which can provide interactive visualisations of feedback. Specifically, these interactive visualisations of data allow an individual to hover over a particular number or graph segment to find a specific numerical value to understand progress towards personal goals (Polzien, Jakicic, Tate, & Otto, 2007).

The increasing number of persuasive technologies has enormous potential for promoting PA (Fogg & Eckles, 2007), with its greatest appeal being in PA interventions, not least due to the large numbers of individuals that can be reached and the ability to communicate large volumes of personalised visual feedback that coincides with health behaviour theory (Ramirez-Marrero, Smith, Sherman, & Kirby, 2005; van Gemert-Pijnen et al., 2011). Indeed, several reviews report that using wearable activity trackers and their visual feedback can increase adult's PA levels (Fanning, Mullen, & McAuley, 2012; Harries et al., 2016; Lewis, Lyons, Jarvis, & Baillargeon, 2015; Li, Dey, & Forlizzi, 2011; Tudor-Locke & Bassett, 2004). However, there is a paucity of evidence to support their use among youth populations (Dean, Voss, De Souza, & Harris, 2016; Gaudet, Gallant, & Bélanger, 2017; Hayes & Van Camp, 2015; Hooke et al., 2016; Jacobsen et al., 2016; Ridgers, McNarry, & Mackintosh, 2016; Schaefer, Ching, Breen, & German, 2016). For example, Hooke et al. (2016) examined the efficacy of the Fitbit One and its feedback to promote youth (6–15 years old) PA in a clinical setting. Specifically, participants wore the Fitbit for 2 weeks, with daily screenshots of the feedback from the associated Fitbit app sent via email to each individual. The findings reported no significant increase in step count; although there were marginal increases in steps per day from weeks 1–2, steps count decreased from weeks 2–3 (Hooke et al., 2016).

Abstract and Living Metaphor Visualisations of PA

Abstract and metaphorical visualisations of feedback allow for data to be communicated in a symbolic way that may have benefits to numerical feedback when data is more difficult or subjective to understand (Khot et al., 2014). Previous research has emphasised the importance of creating more abstract visualisations of feedback to support an individual's positive engagement with data (Consolvo, McDonald et al., 2008). Indeed, abstract visualisations are known to help an individual with the task of impression management, defined as the conscious or subconscious process to influence an individual's perceptions about a behaviour (Goffman, 1959), including the ambiguity to create a 'story' (Aoki & Woodruff, 2005), which enables increased reflection of behaviours (Sunny, David, & James, 2009). Anderson et al. (2007) developed a mobile phone system called 'Shakra' that was designed to represent PA in an abstract form, finding that the visualisations encouraged individuals to reflect on their PA behaviours and motivated them to attain higher PA levels. Congruently, Fan et al. (2012) designed a system called 'Spark' (Figure 35.3), which could represent various abstract and graphical visualisations of PA data (Fan et al., 2012). The findings reported that the abstract displays increased adult's awareness of PA and SB, though data in children remains scarce. Interestingly, some participants preferred the graphical visualisations when looking for specific information or historical patterns of behaviour; however, all participants agreed that abstract visualisations were more appealing and aesthetically pleasing than the graph when "glancing" at their data (Fan et al., 2012). While related to tangible 3D-printed objects, Crossley et al. (2019b) found that adolescents preferred graphical visualisations, whereas younger children preferred more abstract visualisations.

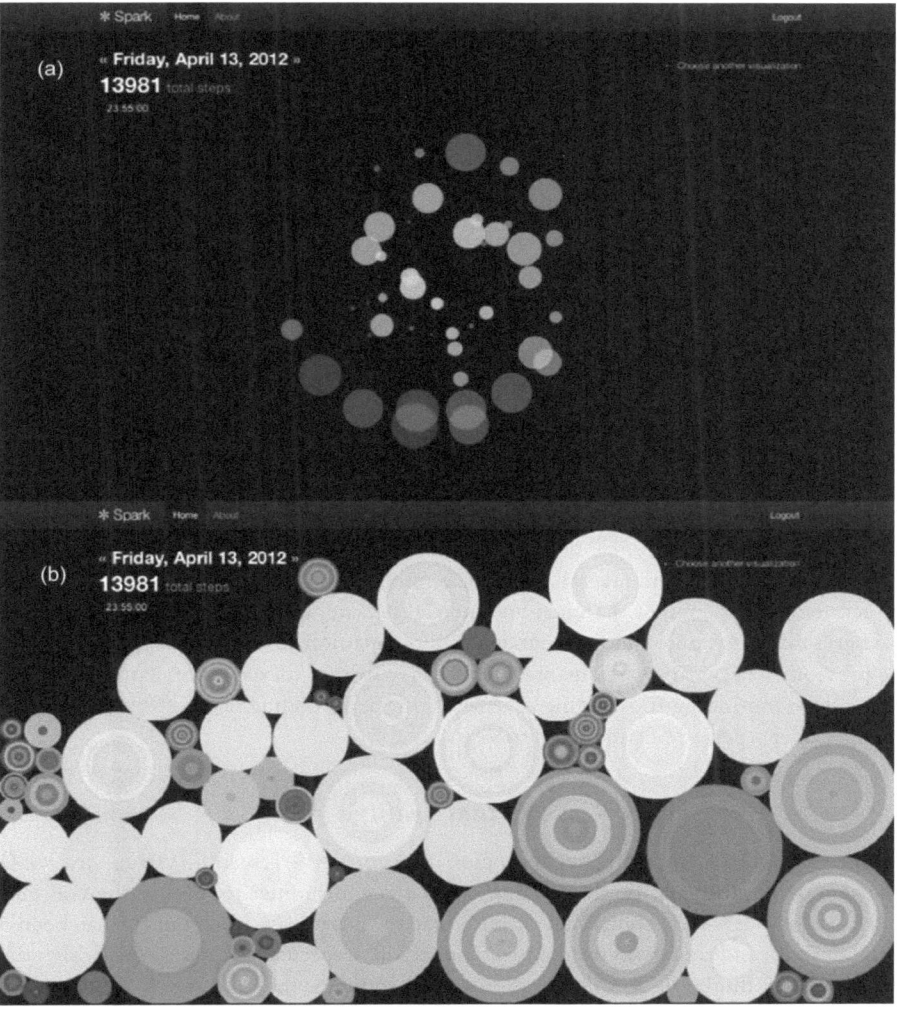

Figure 35.3   Spark abstract visualisations of physical activity: (a) Spiral, (b) Bucket. From Fan et al. (2012)

Similar to abstract visualisations, living metaphors (e.g., flowers, animals) are found to be more engaging, motivating, glanceable, and ambient than graphical and numerical visualisations (Consolvo, Klasnja et al., 2008; Consolvo, McDonald et al., 2008; Fan et al., 2012; Lin, Mamykina, Lindtner, Delajoux, & Strub, 2006). One of the first examples of a living metaphor visualisation was the release of the Nintendo Pocket Pikachu in the late 1990s, which was based on pedometer counts and involved the user increasing or maintaining their step count to keep the virtual Pikachu alive or make them grow (Fogg, 2002). Similarly, Lin et al. (2006) developed a living metaphor through an animated fish that emotional state and size changed to happier and larger, respectively, in response to increased PA, and vice versa. The findings from Lin et al. (2006) did, however, reveal that those individuals who were inactive disengaged with the software as a result of the fish looking unhappy, highlighting that negative framing of data could result in user disengagement. Furthermore, Consolvo, McDonald et al. (2008) designed software called 'Ubifit', which involved users growing a garden with increased levels of PA on their personal mobiles. The findings reported that the garden display helped raise adult's awareness and motivation to maintain their PA levels, though there is no similar data for children. Moreover, users' PA levels did not significantly increase, with concerns expressed over the novelty effect of the system, especially given the study was only a 3-month intervention. Such novelty effects are likely to be more evident in youth.

Wearables and Nearables

Historically, the most commonly used wearable to measure PA in youth was the pedometer, where step count was the only recorded metric presented on a small, digital display (Butcher, Fairclough, Stratton, & Richardson, 2007; Horne, Hardman, Lowe, & Rowlands, 2009; Oliver, Schofield, & McEvoy, 2006; Southard & Southard, 2006). However, in more recent times, there has been a proliferation of commercial wearable technology and activity trackers, with one review identifying 423 devices from 132 companies (Henriksen et al., 2018). Presenting opportunities to increase the user's PA levels, these technologies incorporate behaviour change strategies such as self-monitoring, feedback, and goal-setting (Sanders et al., 2016) which have previously been identified as effective behaviour change techniques for increasing levels of PA (Gardner, Smith, Lorencatto, Hamer, & Biddle, 2016; Michie, Abraham, Whittington, McAteer, & Gupta, 2009; Michie et al., 2013).

These new technologies differ from, for example, traditional pedometers in several key ways:

- They provide feedback on several metrics (i.e., steps, sleep) including proprietary metrics such as "active minutes", rather than just one metric (i.e., steps).
- Data are, normally, automatically synced to a companion smartphone app, thereby reducing the previously necessary participant burden of recording, for example, daily step counts.
- They allow continuous monitoring of metrics through a companion website or app, including tracking over a period of time (days to years).

Virtual Reality

Among the plethora of emerging technologies utilised in PA research, virtual reality (VR) is perhaps the most exciting although, in some ways, it is a misnomer to refer to them as emerging. While the history of VR is somewhat disputed, at the very least, the concept has been around for several decades and there was even a mechanical VR experience in the 1960s which displayed short films while stimulating multiple senses such as sound, smell, and touch (Burdea & Coiffet, 2003; Mazuryk, Gervautz, & Smith, 2013). Indeed, a quick search of the PubMed database for the term "virtual reality" returns papers from as early as 1991. While the concept and application of VR has been around for a long time, modern VR has become more immersive, stimulating, and realistic. Modern VR can therefore be defined as a "real or simulated environment in which a perceiver experiences telepresence" (p. 76; Steuer, 1992). In short, it alters or replaces the real world with a simulated world.

Key Issues

Avatars

Relevance of Avatars

Despite apparent wide-spread success, there is some scepticism regarding on-screen visualisations and their ability to inspire and sustain health behaviours in youth (Wartella, Rideout, Montague, Beaudoin-Ryan, & Lauricella, 2016; WIRED, 2009). For example, a recent study reported that adolescents considered the activity tracker feedback as an "*adult thing*" (Wartella et al., 2016). While this is the case, it can be argued that youths' lack of cohesion with on-screen feedback platforms may be due to current behavioural theories not yet being adapted to leverage their advantages to promote behaviour change (Schembre et al., 2018). Nevertheless, on-screen visualisations of PA are limited to stimulating an individual's visual and auditory senses, which ignore the abundance of other senses including touch (Ullmer & Ishii, 2000). Indeed, a vast body of research in youth educational science (Bara, Gentaz, Colé, & Sprenger-Charolles, 2004; Marshall, 2007; Price, Rogers, Scaife, Stanton, & Neale, 2003; Rogers, Scaife, Gabrielli, Smith, & Harris, 2002) and developmental psychology (Cole & Wertsch, 1996; Fleming & Mills, 1992; Montessori, 1912; Piaget & Cook, 1952; Rita & Dunn, 1979) suggests that manipulation of tangible objects can promote intellectual development, understanding, and enable higher mental functions. More research is therefore required, inclusive of the opinions of the target audience, before avatars can be truly identified as effective behaviour change strategy tools.

Exergaming

Exergames

RELEVANCE AND COMPENSATORY EFFECTS

Despite the aforementioned research suggesting that exergames should be used to increase PA within children, it is important to assess the findings against their relevance or meaningfulness. For instance, Gao et al. (2017) concludes that exergames could be integrated into school-based programs as there was no significant difference between exergames and typical physical education provision. However, it is unclear why a school setting would go through the additional expense if an increase in behaviour was the primary outcome of interest and as other segments of the day, such as the after-school period, could be better utilised to promote children's PA (Gao, Chen, Huang, Stodden, & Xiang, 2017). Additionally, Quan and colleagues (2018) reported that the majority of time spent within an exergaming session (10.34 minutes) was spent sedentary and only provided 4.4 minutes of MVPA, equating to only 7% of the daily US and UK target of 60 minutes of MVPA per day (Department of Health, 2011; Department of Health & Human Services, 2018). The quality of movements and educational experience elicited during exergames should also be questioned; if overall time spent active is similar between exergames and traditional physical education, it could be argued that the latter is likely to promote significantly greater advances in fundamental movement skills and understanding of the importance of these movements for health, which are pivotal for lifelong PA (see Chapter 23).

Further research is required prior to exergaming being advocated for health-related interventions in youth, which should include more rigorous research designs, greater follow-up, and an assessment of compensatory effects (Joronen et al., 2016; Norris et al., 2016; Pakarinen et al., 2017). Indeed, some children have been shown to exhibit something called the 'activitystat' where they compensate for their behaviours (i.e., increased sitting, standing, or stepping on 1 day reduces the same behaviour the next; Ridgers, Timperio, Cerin, & Salmon, 2015). If compensatory effects are not assessed, researchers cannot be sure whether children reduce their PA outside of these sessions in response to the additional PA provided by exergaming (Baranowski, 2017).

Pokémon Go

Novelty

Despite the reported ability to increase PA levels of the app users, one of the drawbacks from this particularly serendipitous behaviour change strategy is that there appears to be a novelty effect, whereby any increase in activity is only short-lived. Indeed, the increased steps as a response to playing Pokémon Go were shown to be attenuated 24 days after download in a study of Hong Kong users (Ma et al., 2018). Corroborated by another study in American users, the number of daily steps recorded by the mobile phone increased by 935 steps, but then declined over 5 weeks until it returned to baseline in the 6th week (Howe et al., 2016). Nevertheless, what sets this mobile game apart from other existing health apps is the ability to reach low activity populations, which have the most to gain by improving their activity levels (Althoff et al., 2016). The popularity of the app has been considerable, with over 800 million people downloading the app by May 2018 (GameRevolution, 2018). Perhaps capitalising on a sense of nostalgia and a fan base from the mid-1990s (American Heart Association, 2016), the game appears to appeal to a wide consumer base and raises important questions regarding why this particular form of game has been so popular and effective at raising PA levels, albeit only in the short term.

Researcher Agility

One of the main aims of health researchers is to develop and evaluate new ways to encourage the population to be more physically active, but success has been equivocal. In contrast, the number of downloads of this app raises the question of whether health researchers are the right people to create games that increase PA levels. It is often reported that it takes, on average, 17 years for research and to put it into practice (Morris et al., 2011), and even if the lag was halved, technology and trends move on rapidly, and therefore, any researcher-developed intervention or games would likely already be replaced by the next craze (Freeman, Chau, & Mihrshahi, 2017). Arguably, the most successful interventions, or utilisation of gamification, would come from health researchers working in collaboration with game developers, whereby researchers can advise and ensure appropriate behaviour change techniques and practices are incorporated within the game, as well as the correct tools to evaluate the games impact through a public health lens (Freeman et al., 2017).

Visualisation of PA

Tangible Visualisations of PA

LACK OF UNDERSTANDING OF TOTAL PA LEVELS

Similar to Khot, Mueller, and Hjorth (2013), Stusak et al. (2014) designed 3D-printed sculptures, in the form of human figures, necklaces, a lamp, and jar that mapped adult running data. However,

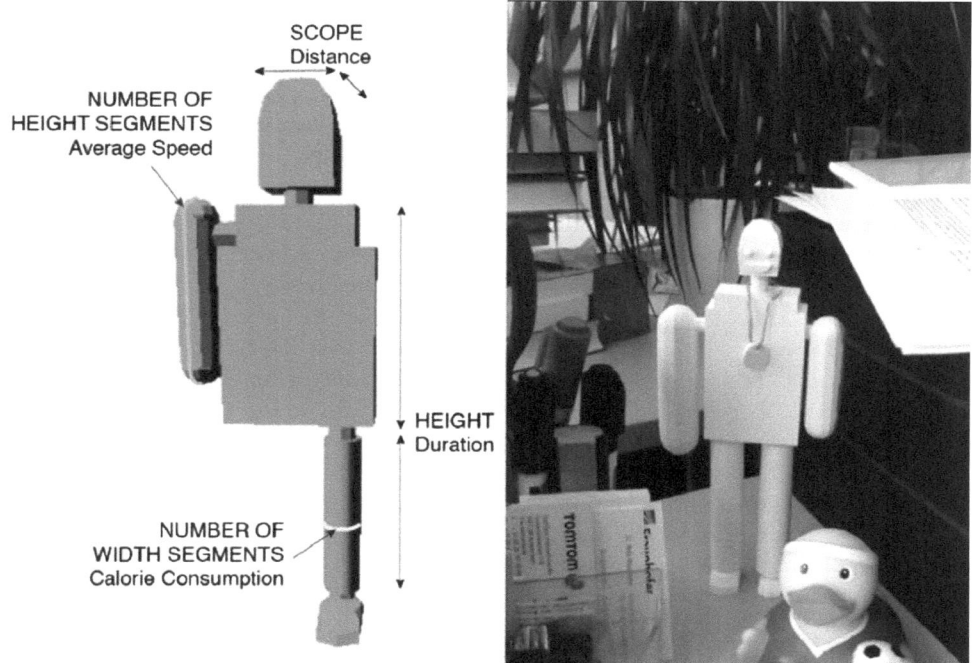

Figure 35.4 Human figure representing running data. From Stusak (2016)

in contrast, Stusak and colleagues' (2014) 3D-printed sculptures were created using a number of variables derived from running data, including the duration, distance, calorie consumption, and elevation gain, which allowed for alternative representations of data to be explored. As shown in Figure 35.4, the 3D-printed human body figure would represent the run duration and the width of the leg would denote the calories burned. The 3D-printed sculptures generated curiosity, discussions, and competition between participants, as well as motivating them to increase their sculptures size following the receipt of previous 3D outputs. Despite this, the 3D-printed sculptures only provided participants with a single bout of exercise data and, therefore, do not provide individuals with feedback on their overall PA levels. Indeed, this is particularly important given that an individual who appears to be active in short bursts of vigorous intensity activity can also be sedentary for prolonged periods within the same day, with very few individuals able to maintain a consistent level of activity (Thompson & Batterham, 2013). Therefore, the 3D-printed sculptures may not provide adequate feedback to raise an individual's awareness and understanding of their true PA levels.

LACK OF RESEARCH ON TANGIBLE FEEDBACK

Using a Fitbit activity tracker to measure PA, Lee et al. (2015) created a 'Patina Engraving System', which engraves a patina-like pattern onto the activity trackers wristband. Over time, the user's wristband would accumulate a visually rich activity pattern that would recognise the individuals' step count, active time, calories, sleep, and walking distance. Although the study focused more on the fashion aspect of the patina patterns for styling activity trackers, it was expressed that participants cherished the activity wristband more due to the personalisation, which led to more spontaneous interactions with other users to discuss their physical efforts. More recently, Sauvé et al.

(2017) developed a system called 'LOOP' which visualises step count data recorded from a Fitbit tracker. The LOOP system is made out of seven inner rings to represent each day of the week, with the smallest and largest rings representing Monday and Sunday, respectively. At the start of a week, each ring starts by facing downwards to represent no steps taken, with the position of the ring designed to mechanically move upwards (updated every hour) depending on the user's step count activity. Converse to previous tangible methods, the LOOP system dynamically changes its shape or position in response to PA. However, the effectiveness of the LOOP system to promote PA is unknown due to a lack of real-world evaluation studies.

To date, there is only a handful of studies that have explored the utility of representing health data through personalised physical visualisations in children (Ananthanarayan, 2015; Ananthanarayan, Siek, & Eisenberg, 2016; Crossley, McNarry, Eslambolchilar, Knowles, & Mackintosh, 2019a; Crossley et al., 2019b; Crossley, McNarry, Rosenberg et al., 2019c). Specifically, Ananthanarayan et al. (2016) invited children to craft their own tangible visualisations using paper and a pre-designed wearable UV tracker, provided by the researchers, to attach to their final design. The UV tracker was designed to send warning alarms, through flashing LED lights and a buzzer, to inform the children they were spending too much time indoors. For example, one participant created an ambient octopus visualisation, with the eyes and tentacles of the octopus illuminating with LED lights in parallel with the sound of a buzzer from the mouth to inform the participant to play outside (Figure 35.5). The study concluded that children's health could benefit from using the personalised health crafting approach. However, it could be argued that feedback through paper visualisations may not provide adequate haptic and proprioceptive experience for youths when compared to 3D-printed PA feedback (Gillet, Sanner, Stoffler, & Olson, 2005). Indeed, research suggests that the manipulation of tangible representations may support a more effective and natural process of learning (Sluis et al., 2004; Terrenghi, Kranz, Holleis, & Schmidt, 2006; Zuckerman, Arida, & Resnick, 2005).

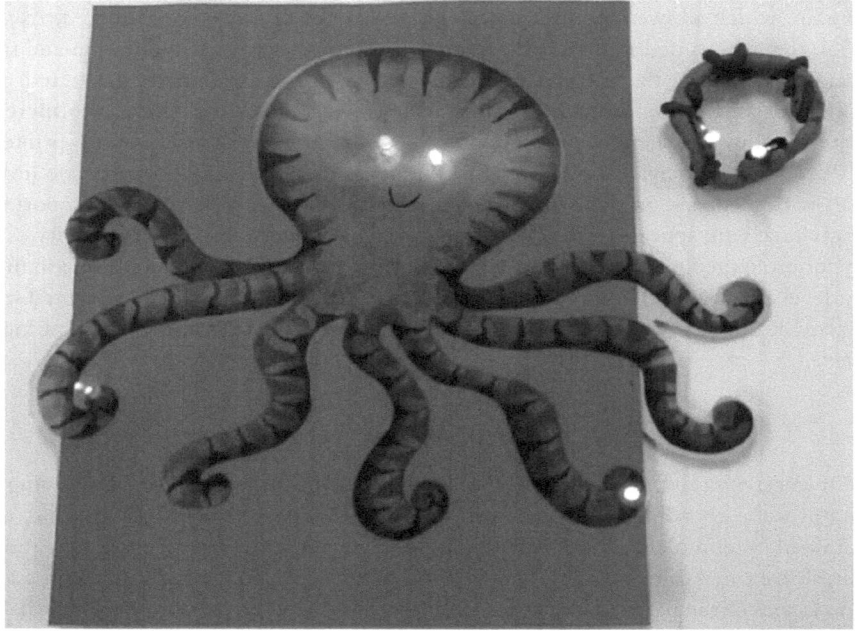

Figure 35.5   Ambient octopus visualisation of activity. From Ananthanarayan (2015)

In accord with Khot et al. (2014), recent formative research has explored youths' perceptions of and designs for 3D-printed visualisations of PA data derived from tri-axial accelerometers. Findings from Crossley et al. (2019b) demonstrated youth's ability to conceptualise 3D-printed models of PA, with 80% of youths expressing that the models would motivate them to engage in more PA. Furthermore, youths expressed a preference for 3D models, represented through abstract and graphical designs, which led to the development of two age-specific 3D-printed models (Figure 35.6), which were further validated in a follow-up study (Crossley, McNarry, Rosenberg et al., 2019c). A 7-week intervention utilising the two age-specific 3D models showed how the models enhanced youths' awareness of their PA levels and provided a motivational tool

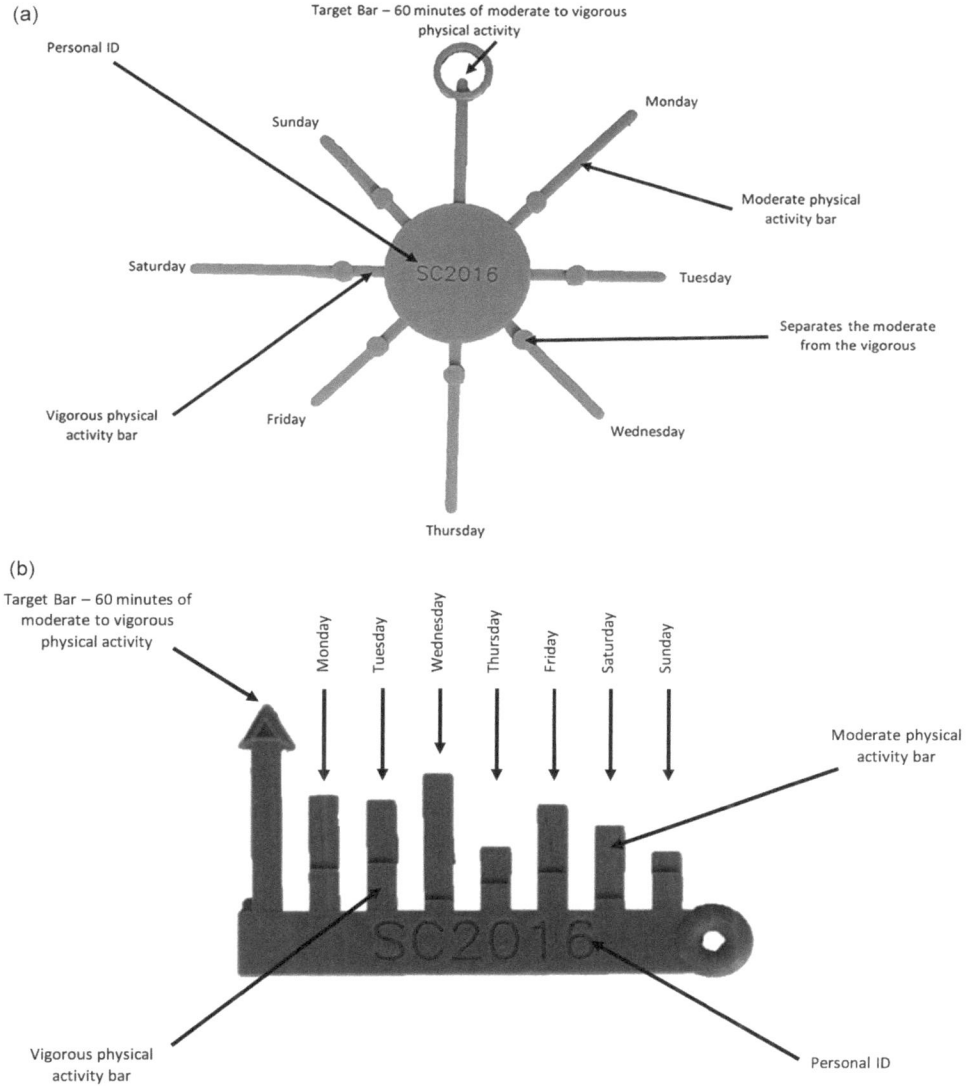

Figure 35.6   Two age-specific 3D models of physical activity: (a) Children's 'sun' 3D model, (b) Adolescents' 'bar chart' 3D model. From Crossley et al. (2019a)

for goal-setting (Crossley, McNarry, Eslambolchilar et al., 2019a). There are, however, concerns regarding the sustainability of such 3D-printed model interventions, as studies to date have only focused on the short-term effects on behaviour change with no long-term follow-up and attention drawn to the costs involved in 3D printing. While 3D printing is conventionally considered to be expensive, the technology is growing rapidly, with experts previously anticipating the rise of more accurate and cheaper 3D printers with time (Anderson, 2010). Indeed, many schools in the UK now own a 3D printer, which makes a 3D model intervention more feasible than has previously been thought (Mercuri & Meredith, 2014).

Numerical Visualisations of PA

COMPLICATIONS

There are many advantages in using activity trackers and their numerical visualisations of feedback, not least in that they only require a small screen (Van Wijk, 2005), with graphs or charts making data easier to understand and glance at to raise an individual's awareness of their PA levels (Yi, ah Kang, & Stasko, 2007). However, research suggests that these numerical or graphical forms of visual feedback are too complicated even for adult users, as they are not skilled at interpreting the statistical data (Ancker & Kaufman, 2007; Galesic & Garcia-Retamero, 2011). As Khot (2016) noted, this could be a result of the visual data being too overwhelming to generate new insights or actionable knowledge. Indeed, this numerical approach to visualising feedback could also be problematic for youths, given that numbers and graphs are associated with Mathematics, which is unlikely to be meaningful and aesthetically pleasing to youth populations (Brian, 2012). As expressed by Hassenzahl, Laschke, and Praest (2016), numbers could make PA feel more like work; there is a need to explore better and richer ways to represent data. In this light, developers and researchers are currently exploring alternative ways of visualising PA data through abstract (Anderson et al., 2007; Fan et al., 2012) and living metaphors (Consolvo, Klasnja et al., 2008; Consolvo, McDonald et al., 2008).

Wearable and Nearables

EQUIVOCAL RESULTS

As well as providing traditional visual feedback (such as step count), wearables also provide automatic feedback, such as vibratory feedback when the wearer has not moved for a defined period of time. Despite the proliferation of these new technologies, there is a relative dearth of scientific evidence on their efficacy as intervention modalities to increase PA in young people. A 2016 review (Ridgers, McNarry & Mackintosh, 2016) identified only five studies consisting of three intervention and two feasibility studies, with just one of these five using a gold standard, randomised controlled trial study design. The included studies were conducted across a wide age range (7–17 years of age), with relatively small sample sizes, and were, with the exception of one study, all conducted in the US. There was some evidence that activity trackers may have a positive effect on young people's PA levels, but differences were largely non-significant with two of the included studies possibly underpowered to detect a statistical difference (Ridgers, McNarry & Mackintosh, 2016). Further studies published since Ridgers et al.'s (2016) review suggests similarly equivocal results. Specifically, Foote and colleagues (2017) found that utilising a wrist-worn activity monitor, coupled with associated feedback, for 3 weeks in 25 10–12-year olds resulted in no significant main effect, and that information alone may not be sufficient to increase young people's PA levels. These conclusions were reminiscent of a study published a decade earlier; although the technology was less advanced, it was noted that feedback from pedometers alone was not sufficient to elicit significant increases in young people's steps. Similarly, Evans et al. (2017) used the Fitbit Zip with 42 participants with an average age of 12 years old in a cluster randomised trial in which participants either received the Fitbit Zip with goals and incentives, only the Fitbit Zip, or were assigned to a control group for 6 weeks. Similar to previous studies, this study found no significant group differences between baseline and follow-up (Evans et al., 2017). In contrast, Gaudet and colleagues (2017) used the Fitbit Charge HR in a group of 23 13–14-year olds for 7 weeks. Although this study did not find an overall effect of wearing the activity tracker, changes in MVPA were related to the stages of behaviour change the participants were in within the transtheoretical model of behaviour change. Participants in the adoption stages showed an increase in MVPA from baseline, whereas those in the pre-adoption phases (i.e., pre-contemplation, contemplation, and preparation) showed no change in daily MVPA levels (Gaudet et al., 2017). This suggests that for adolescents in the adoption phases, simply gaining access to an activity tracker may be sufficient to elicit changes in PA, whereas additional intervention modalities may be necessary for adolescents in pre-adoption phases (Gaudet et al., 2017). Overall, the extant evidence indicates that, while young people generally have a favourable view of activity trackers and their utility (particularly the social aspects), efficacy may be greater in participants in the adoption phases of behaviour change and that these technologies may be more effective as one component within a wider, holistic program to increase PA rather than as the sole intervention modality.

Perception of Wearables

An important mediator in activity tracker efficacy is likely to be the perception of activity trackers among young people themselves. Masteller and colleagues (2017) investigated 16 young people's perceptions of three youth-orientated PA trackers. Of a possible 36 behaviour change techniques, the three trackers back-end website platforms incorporated between 8 and 15 techniques. Interestingly, the participants had a favourable view of the social aspects of these platforms and indicated that they would want to wear the devices more if their friends were also wearing the tracker (Masteller et al., 2017). Similarly, Ridgers et al. (2018) found that adolescents reported the Fitbit Flex to be an easy to use and useful tool, including undertaking challenges with their friends. This highlights the importance of social support in PA interventions.

Virtual Reality

LACK OF RESEARCH

Although VR has developed a solid evidence base in adults, particularly in rehabilitation contexts (Laver, George, Thomas, Deutsch, & Crotty, 2015), there is a paucity of evidence in young people. However, VR has been used both in-school and out-of-school for children's PA promotion. Specifically, VR within a school setting has often been combined with enhancing the learning experience, whereas outside of school its use is more concerned with entertainment, particularly games. Moreover, there remains a paucity of evidence on the effects of VR within physical education, with the evidence base limited by the relatively high cost of implementing VR interventions. Outside of physical education lessons, one area that does show promising results is "virtual field trips".

A feasibility study found that virtual field trips increased light, moderate, and vigorous PA (Norris, Shelton, Dunsmuir, Duke-Williams, & Stamatakis, 2015). Originally developed as sedentary activities, virtual field trips have been modified to incorporate movement in younger age groups (Norris et al., 2015). These virtual field trips allow exploration of virtual maps or

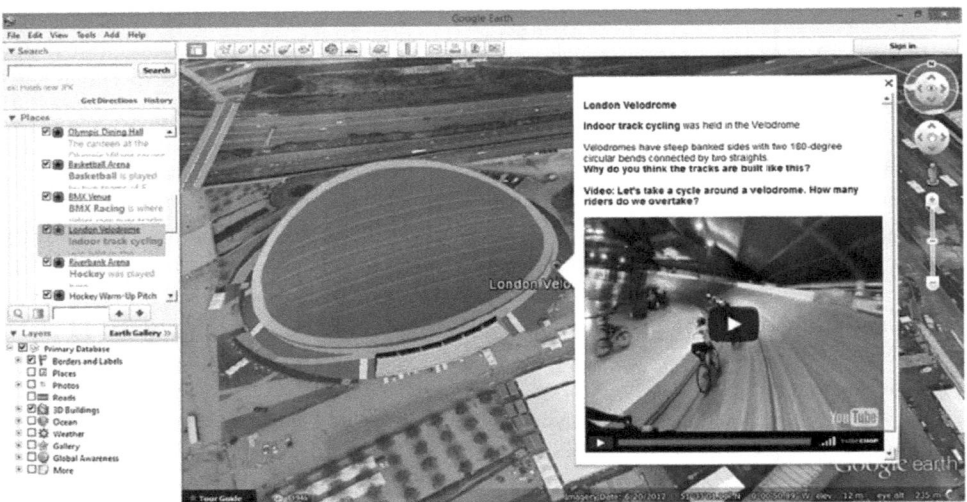

Figure 35.7   Representation of the virtual traveller intervention. Adapted from Norris et al. (2015)

landmarks using, for example, interactive whiteboards with participants standing throughout and simulating movements at, or between, various sites (Norris et al., 2015), as shown in Figure 35.7. These interventions therefore have the important dual benefit of being both educational and, potentially, promoting PA, or at least decreasing SB, in young people.

Importantly, both teachers and students reported that these sessions are, on the whole, feasible and enjoyable (Norris et al., 2015). Indeed, an evaluation using the RE-AIM framework found that the intervention showed potential in primary schools (Norris, Dunsmuir, Duke-Williams, Stamatakis, & Shelton, 2018), although virtual traveller sessions decreased sedentary time and increased MVPA during lessons, it had no effect across overall school or weekend days (Norris et al., 2018). It is also important to note that workload and a resistance to technology were flagged as potential issues by teachers (Norris et al., 2015). Overall, VR shows promise as a PA intervention, but currently has a limited evidence base. There is therefore a need for more and better designed studies to fully elucidate the effects of this "emerging technology".

Emerging Issues

Exergaming

Pokémon Go

SAFETY AND MISUSE CONCERNS

While researchers may consider the mobile gaming format, which is untethered from a console and requires users to roam their environment, as a positive for promoting PA behaviours, it does also pose a few issues. Exergaming, or the use of augmented reality outside the home, provides opportunities for new risks such as increased levels of accidents, abductions, and engagements in risky behaviours and trespassing (Lindqvist, Castelli, Hallberg, & Rutberg, 2018; Serino, Cordrey, McLaughlin, & Milanaik, 2016; Wagner-Greene et al., 2017). Additionally, given the success of Pokémon Go, other companies have utilised the increased usage of such apps as a way to promote other services and even other behaviours that have unhealthy connotations. Indeed, Niantic, the developer behind the game, has stated that they have driven 500 million visitors to sponsored locations such as McDonald's (TechCrunch, 2017). Cashing in on the success of the exergames or augmented reality games was likely inevitable; yet, researchers must be mindful of the potential negatives and ensure they are balanced against potential public health benefits such as increasing PA levels.

Recommendations for Research and Practice

Time-use survey data corroborate the widely held belief that youth today take part in less overall PA, accumulating more time in sedentary pursuits, such as screen-based activities (Mullan, 2019). Further scrutiny of such self-reported data reveals that participation in sports has increased marginally over previous decades, but that unstructured play outside the home decreased to a greater extent. These trends are consistent both with the rising parental concerns of child safety and the increasing importance of education in children's lives, but arguably it is rapid technological development over the past two decades, that is, at least in part, accountable for the erosion of leisure-time PA in youth (Mullan, 2019). However, it is intriguing how sedentary industries, dominated by screens that did not even exist a generation ago, easily seduced and wholly preoccupied the population's leisure time. This success may, in part, be due to the marginal engineering iterations that characterise the **evolutions** in 'active industries' (e.g., sporting goods, gyms, fitness equipment, sports apparel), and the **revolutions** being made at pace in electronic technologies that promote 'sedentary industries' (e.g., PVRs, streaming TV and music, social media, ubiquitous Wi-Fi, computers, gaming consoles, and mobile phones and tablets; Sturm, 2004). However insidious the secular trend towards sedentary time use appears, it does not reflect a market failure. As Sturm (2004) suggests, industry growth reflects demand and market reaction, whether for PA or sedentary pastimes. Nevertheless, there are many aspects of 'sedentary industries' where outcomes are not socially optimal from a public health perspective, even if they appear to yield economic growth.

Many of the commercial technologies discussed in this chapter are being used to promote PA behaviours in millions of youths all over the world. However, many of these technologies will act as a double-edged sword by actually thwarting PA behaviours. Nonetheless, the diverse types of technologies emerging in both the active and sedentary industries, coupled with their accessibility and reach across increasingly representative segments of youth populations, make these novel technologies an attractive intervention platform in their own right, but also allow for the evaluation of PA and/or SB interventions (Department of Health & Human Services, 2018). As the *2018 Physical Activity Guidelines Advisory Committee Scientific Report* from the US suggested, despite this growing interest among the scientific community, the current evidence base remains constrained to less rigorous study designs of short durations and small and often highly selected participant samples that lack heterogeneity, particularly in youth populations. This government advisory committee, a large team of expert scientists, performed a comprehensive review of the evidence from 2011 to 2016 and made two key recommendations, which are in line with the findings of this chapter. The first is to employ additional types of experimental designs and methods that will allow for more rapid testing of technology interventions; given the rapid evolution of the technology interventions discussed in this chapter, traditional 2-arm parallel-arm trial designs may not easily allow researchers to keep up with the emerging technology innovations. Further use of more advanced experimental designs, such as fractional or multi-level factorial designs and just-in-time adaptive interventions, are therefore warranted. The second recommendation is further exploration of methods and pathways for systematically exploiting the vast array of pre-existing, and continuously growing and updating, commercially available PA data and interventions. Specifically, wearable databases have vast potential for accelerating our knowledge concerning the most effective ways of promoting PA among different population groups, yet these remain relatively untouched.

References

Althoff, T., White, R. W., & Horvitz, E. (2016). Influence of Pokemon Go on physical activity: Study and implications. *Journal of Medical Internet Research, 18*(12), e315. doi:10.2196/jmir.6759

American Heart Association. (2016). *Pokémon Go brings video games outside.* Retrieved from https://newsarchive.heart.org/pokemon-go-brings-video-games-outside/

Ananthanarayan, S. (2015). *Health craft: A computational toolkit for motivating health awareness in children* (Computer Science graduate theses & dissertations). University of Colorado, Boulder. Retrieved from https://scholar.colorado.edu/csci_gradetds/107

Ananthanarayan, S., Siek, K., & Eisenberg, M. (2016). *A craft approach to health awareness in children.* Paper presented at the Proceedings of the 2016 ACM Conference on Designing Interactive Systems, Brisbane, Australia.

Ancker, J. S., & Kaufman, D. (2007). Rethinking health numeracy: A multidisciplinary literature review. *Journal of the American Medical Informatics Association, 14*(6), 713–721.

Anderson, C. (2010). In the next industrial revolution, atoms are the new bits. *Wired Magazine*, January 25.

Anderson, I., Maitland, J., Sherwood, S., Barkhuus, L., Chalmers, M., Hall, M., . . . Muller, H. (2007). Shakra: Tracking and sharing daily activity levels with unaugmented mobile phones. *Mobile Networks and Applications, 12*(2), 185–199. doi:10.1007/s11036-007-0011-7

Aoki, P. M., & Woodruff, A. (2005). *Making space for stories: Ambiguity in the design of personal communication systems.* Paper presented at the Proceedings of the SIGCHI Conference on Human Factors in Computing Systems, Portland, OR.

Bara, F., Gentaz, E., Colé, P., & Sprenger-Charolles, L. (2004). The visuo-haptic and haptic exploration of letters increases the kindergarten-children's understanding of the alphabetic principle. *Cognitive Development, 19*(3), 433–449.

Baranowski, T. (2017). Exergaming: Hope for future physical activity? or blight on mankind. *Journal of Sport and Health Science, 6*(1), 44–46.

Baranowski, T., Buday, R., Thompson, D. I., & Baranowski, J. (2008). Playing for real: Video games and stories for health-related behavior change. *American Journal of Preventive Medicine, 34*(1), 74–82.e10. doi:10.1016/j.amepre.2007.09.027

Barnett, A., Cerin, E., & Baranowski, T. (2011). Active video games for youth: A systematic review. *Journal of Physical Activity and Health, 8*(5), 724–737.

Beaudry, P., Doms, M., & Lewis, E. (2010). Should the personal computer be considered a technological revolution? Evidence from US metropolitan areas. *Journal of Political Economy, 118*(5), 988–1036.

Bell, M. W. (2008). Toward a definition of "virtual worlds". *Journal For Virtual Worlds Research, 1*, 1–5.

Biddiss, E., & Irwin, J. (2010). Active video games to promote physical activity in children and youth: A systematic review. *Archives of Pediatrics & Adolescent Medicine, 164*(7), 664–672. doi:10.1001/archpediatrics.2010.104

Biswas, A., Oh, P. I., Faulkner, G. E., Bajaj, R. R., Silver, M. A., Mitchell, M. S., & Alter, D. A. (2015). Sedentary time and its association with risk for disease incidence, mortality, and hospitalization in adults: A systematic review and meta-analysis. *Annals of Internal Medicine, 162*(2), 123–132.

Bloch, M. (2008). Truth and sight: Generalizing without universalizing. *Journal of the Royal Anthropological Institute, 14*(s1), s22–s32.

Bondyopadhyay, P. K. (1998). Moore's law governs the silicon revolution. *Proceedings of the IEEE, 86*(1), 78–81.

Brian, K. (2012). Maths anxiety: The numbers are mounting. *The Guardian*. Retrieved from https://www.theguardian.com/education/2012/apr/30/maths-anxiety-school-support

Burdea, G. C., & Coiffet, P. (2003). *Virtual reality technology.* New York, NY: John Wiley & Sons.

Burton, E., Hill, K. D., Lautenschlager, N. T., Thøgersen-Ntoumani, C., Lewin, G., Boyle, E., & Howie, E. (2018). Reliability and validity of two fitness tracker devices in the laboratory and home environment for older community-dwelling people. *BMC Geriatrics, 18*(1), 103.

Butcher, Z., Fairclough, S., Stratton, G., & Richardson, D. (2007). The effect of feedback and information on children's pedometer step counts at school. *Pediatric Exercise Science, 19*(1), 29–38.

Campos, C. M., & del Castillo Fernández, H. (2016). The benefits of active video games for educational and physical activity approaches: A systematic review. *Journal of New Approaches in Educational Research, 5*(2), 115.

Card, S., Mackinlay, J., & Schneiderman, B. (1999). *Readings in information visualisation.* San Francisco, CA: Kaufmann.

Christian, D., Todd, C., Hill, R., Rance, J., Mackintosh, K., Stratton, G., & Brophy, S. (2016). Active children through incentive vouchers – Evaluation (ACTIVE): A mixed-method feasibility study. *BMC Public Health, 16*(1), 890. doi:10.1186/s12889-016-3381-6

Cobiac, L. J., Vos, T., & Barendregt, J. J. (2009). Cost-effectiveness of interventions to promote physical activity: A modelling study. *PLoS Medicine, 6*(7), e1000110.

Cole, M., & Wertsch, J. V. (1996). Beyond the Individual-social antinomy in discussions of Piaget and Vygotsky. *Human Development, 39*(5), 250–256.

Cole, S. W., Yoo, D. J., & Knutson, B. (2012). Interactivity and reward-related neural activation during a serious videogame. *PLoS One, 7*(3), e33909. doi:10.1371/journal.pone.0033909

Consolvo, S., Klasnja, P., McDonald, D. W., Avrahami, D., Froehlich, J., LeGrand, L., . . . Landay, J. A. (2008). *Flowers or a robot army?: Encouraging awareness & activity with personal, mobile displays.* Paper presented at the Proceedings of the 10th International Conference on Ubiquitous Computing, Seoul, Korea.

Consolvo, S., McDonald, D. W., Toscos, T., Chen, M. Y., Froehlich, J., Harrison, B., . . . Landay, J. A. (2008). *Activity sensing in the wild: A field trial of ubifit garden.* Paper presented at the Proceedings of the SIGCHI Conference on Human Factors in Computing Systems, Florence, Italy.

Crossley, S. G. M., McNarry, M. A., Eslambolchilar, P., Knowles, Z. R., & Mackintosh, K. A. (2019a). The tangibility of personalised 3D printed feedback may enhance youth's physical activity awareness, goal-setting and motivation. *Journal of Medical Internet Research, 21*(6), e12067.

Crossley, S. G. M., McNarry, M. A., Hudson, J., Eslambolchilar, P., Knowles, Z. R., & Mackintosh, K. A. (2019b). Perceptions of visualising physical activity as a 3D printed object: A formative study. *Journal of Medical Internet Research, 21*(1), e12064.

Crossley, S. G. M., McNarry, M. A., Rosenberg, M., Knowles, Z. R., Eslambbolchilar, P., & Mackintosh, K. A. (2019c). Understanding youth's ability to interpret 3D printed physical activity data and identify associated intensity levels. *JMIR mHealth and uHealth, 21*(2), e11253.

Das, P., & Horton, R. (2016). Physical activity-time to take it seriously and regularly. *Lancet, 388*(10051), 1254–1255.

Dean, P., Voss, C., De Souza, A., & Harris, K. (2016). Assessment, assurance, and actuation: The use of activity trackers to monitor physical activity in a pediatric population with congenital heart disease. *Canadian Journal of Cardiology, 32*(10), S130–S131.

Department of Health. (2011). *Start active, stay active: A report on physical activity for health from the four home countries' chief medical officers.* London, UK: Department of Health.

Department of Health & Human Services. (2018). *Physical Activity Guidelines for Americans* (2nd ed.). Washington, DC: Department of Health & Human Services.

Deterding, S. (2014). The ambiguity of games: Histories and discourses of a gameful world. In S. P. Walz & S. Deterding (Eds.), *The gameful world* (pp.23–64). Cambridge: MIT Press.

Dragicevic, P., & Jansen, Y. (2012). *List of physical visualizations.* Retrieved from https://www.dataphys.org/list

Estabrooks, P., & Gyurcsik, N. (2003). Evaluating the impact of behavioral interventions that target physical activity: Issues of generalizability and public health. *Psychology of Sport and Exercise, 4*(1), 41–55.

Evans, E. W., Abrantes, A. M., Chen, E., & Jelalian, E. (2017). Using novel technology within a school-based setting to increase physical activity: A pilot study in school-age children from a low-income, urban community. *BioMed Research International, 2017*, 7.

Fan, C., Forlizzi, J., & Dey, A. K. (2012). *A spark of activity: Exploring informative art as visualization for physical activity.* Paper presented at the Proceedings of the 2012 ACM Conference on Ubiquitous Computing, Pittsburgh, PA.

Fanning, J., Mullen, S. P., & McAuley, E. (2012). Increasing physical activity with mobile devices: A meta-analysis. *Journal of Medical Internet Research, 14*(6), e161.

Finco, M. D., & Maass, R. W. (2014). *The history of exergames: Promotion of exercise and active living through body interaction.* Paper presented at the 2014 IEEE 3rd International Conference on Serious Games and Applications for Health (SeGAH), Rio de Janeiro, Brazil.

Finkelstein, E. A., Tan, Y.-T., Malhotra, R., Lee, C.-F., Goh, S.-S., & Saw, S.-M. (2013). A cluster randomized controlled trial of an incentive-based outdoor physical activity program. *The Journal of Pediatrics, 163*(1), 167–172.e161. doi:10.1016/j.jpeds.2013.01.009

Fleming, N. D., & Mills, C. (1992). Not another inventory, rather a catalyst for reflection. *To Improve the Academy, 11*(1), 137–155.

Fogg, B. (2002). Persuasive technology: using computers to change what we think and do. *Ubiquity, 5*, doi:10/1145/764008.763957

Fogg, B., & Eckles, D. (2007). *The behavior chain for online participation: How successful web services structure persuasion.* Paper presented at the International Conference on Persuasive Technology, Palo Alto, CA.

Foley, L., & Maddison, R. (2010). Use of active video games to increase physical activity in children: A (virtual) reality? *Pediatric Exercise Science, 22*(1), 7–20.

Foote, S. J., Wadsworth, D. D., Brock, S., Hastie, P. H., & Cooper, C. K. (2017). The effect of a wrist worn accelerometer on children's in-school and out-of-school physical activity levels. *Swedish Journal of Scientific Research, 4*(3), 1–6.

Freeman, B., Chau, J., & Mihrshahi, S. (2017). Why the public health sector couldn't create Pokémon Go. *Public health research & practice, 27*(3), 1–3.

Friedenreich, C. M., Neilson, H. K., & Lynch, B. M. (2010). State of the epidemiological evidence on physical activity and cancer prevention. *European Journal of Cancer, 46*(14), 2593–2604.

Galesic, M., & Garcia-Retamero, R. (2011). Graph literacy: A cross-cultural comparison. *Medical Decision Making, 31*(3), 444–457.

GameRevolution. (2018). *Pokemon Go has reached 800 million downloads.* Retrieved November 11, 2018. Retrieved from https://www.gamerevolution.com/news/392129-pokemon-go-has-reached-800-million-downloads

Gao, Z., Chen, S., Huang, C. C., Stodden, D. F., & Xiang, P. (2017). Investigating elementary school children's daily physical activity and sedentary behaviours during weekdays. *Journal of Sports Sciences, 35*(1), 99–104.

Gao, Z., Pope, Z., Lee, J. E., Stodden, D., Roncesvalles, N., Pasco, D., . . . Feng, D. (2017). Impact of exergaming on young children's school day energy expenditure and moderate-to-vigorous physical activity levels. *Journal of Sport and Health Science, 6*(1), 11–16.

Gardner, B., Smith, L., Lorencatto, F., Hamer, M., & Biddle, S. J. (2016). How to reduce sitting time? A review of behaviour change strategies used in sedentary behaviour reduction interventions among adults. *Health Psychology Review, 10*(1), 89–112.

Gaudet, J., Gallant, F., & Bélanger, M. (2017). A bit of fit: Minimalist intervention in adolescents based on a physical activity tracker. *JMIR mHealth and uHealth, 5*(7), e92.

Gillet, A., Sanner, M., Stoffler, D., & Olson, A. (2005). Tangible interfaces for structural molecular biology. *Structure, 13*(3), 483–491. doi:10.1016/j.str.2005.01.009

Goffman, E. (1959). *The presentation of self in everyday life.* London, UK: Penguin Books.

Guthold, R., Stevens, G. A., Riley, L. M., & Bull, F. C. (2018). Worldwide trends in insufficient physical activity from 2001 to 2016: A pooled analysis of 358 population-based surveys with 1·9 million participants. *The Lancet Global Health, 6*(10), e1077–e1086.

Guy, S., Ratzki-Leewing, A., & Gwadry-Sridhar, F. (2011). Moving beyond the stigma: Systematic review of video games and their potential to combat obesity. *International Journal of Hypertension, 2011*, 13. doi:10.4061/2011/179124

Hardman, C. A., Horne, P. J., & Fergus Lowe, C. (2011). Effects of rewards, peer-modelling and pedometer targets on children's physical activity: A school-based intervention study. *Psychology & Health, 26*(1), 3–21. doi:10.1080/08870440903318119

Harries, T., Eslambolchilar, P., Rettie, R., Stride, C., Walton, S., & van Woerden, H. C. (2016). Effectiveness of a smartphone app in increasing physical activity amongst male adults: A randomised controlled trial. *BMC Public Health, 16*(1), 925.

Hassenzahl, M., Laschke, M., & Praest, J. (2016). *On the stories activity trackers tell.* Paper presented at the Proceedings of the 2016 ACM International Joint Conference on Pervasive and Ubiquitous Computing: Adjunct, Heidelberg, Germany.

Hayes, L. B., & Van Camp, C. M. (2015). Increasing physical activity of children during school recess. *Journal of Applied Behavior Analysis, 48*(3), 690–695.

Hekler, E. B., Klasnja, P., Riley, W. T., Buman, M. P., Huberty, J., Rivera, D. E., & Martin, C. A. (2016). Agile science: Creating useful products for behavior change in the real world. *Translational Behavioral Medicine, 6*(2), 317–328.

Hekler, E. B., Michie, S., Pavel, M., Rivera, D. E., Collins, L. M., Jimison, H. B., . . . Spruijt-Metz, D. (2016). Advancing models and theories for digital behavior change interventions. *American Journal of Preventive Medicine, 51*(5), 825–832.

Henriksen, A., Mikalsen, M. H., Woldaregay, A. Z., Muzny, M., Hartvigsen, G., Hopstock, L. A., & Grimsgaard, S. (2018). Using fitness trackers and smartwatches to measure physical activity in research: Analysis of consumer wrist-worn wearables. *Journal of Medical Internet Research, 20*(3), e110.

Hooke, M. C., Gilchrist, L., Tanner, L., Hart, N., & Withycombe, J. S. (2016). Use of a fitness tracker to promote physical activity in children with acute lymphoblastic leukemia. *Pediatric Blood & Cancer, 63*(4), 684–689.

Horne, P., Hardman, C., Lowe, C., & Rowlands, A. (2009). Increasing children's physical activity: A peer modelling, rewards and pedometer-based intervention. *European Journal of Clinical Nutrition, 63*(2), 191.

Howe, K. B., Suharlim, C., Ueda, P., Howe, D., Kawachi, I., & Rimm, E. B. (2016). Gotta catch'em all! Pokémon GO and physical activity among young adults: Difference in differences study. *BMJ, 355*, i6270.

Interactive Software Federation of Europe. (2018). GameTrack Digest: Quarter 1 2018 1.

Jacobsen, R. M., Ginde, S., Mussatto, K., Neubauer, J., Earing, M., & Danduran, M. (2016). Can a home-based cardiac physical activity program improve the physical function quality of life in children with Fontan circulation? *Congenital Heart Disease, 11*(2), 175–182.

Jakicic, J. M. (2009). The effect of physical activity on body weight. *Obesity, 17*(S3), S34–S38.

Jansen, Y., Dragicevic, P., & Fekete, J.-D. (2013). *Evaluating the efficiency of physical visualizations*. Paper presented at the Proceedings of the SIGCHI Conference on Human Factors in Computing Systems, Paris, France.

Jeon, C. Y., Lokken, R. P., Hu, F. B., & van Dam, R. M. (2007). Physical activity of moderate intensity and risk of type 2 diabetes: A systematic review. *Diabetes Care, 30*(3), 744–752. doi:10.2337/dc06-1842

Jin, S.-A. A. (2010). 'I feel more connected to the physically ideal mini me than the mirror-image mini me': Theoretical implications of the 'malleable self' for speculations on the effects of avatar creation on avatar–self connection in Wii. *Cyberpsychology, Behavior, and Social Networking, 13*(5), 567–570.

Johnson, D., Deterding, S., Kuhn, K.-A., Staneva, A., Stoyanov, S., & Hides, L. (2016). Gamification for health and wellbeing: A systematic review of the literature. *Internet Interventions, 6*, 89–106.

Joronen, K., Aikasalo, A., & Suvitie, A. (2016). Nonphysical effects of exergames on child and adolescent well-being: A comprehensive systematic review. *Scandinavian Journal of Caring Sciences, 31*(3), 449–461. doi:10.1111/scs.12393

Khot, R. A. (2016). *Understanding material representations of physical activity*. Melbourne, Australia: RMIT University.

Khot, R. A., Hjorth, L., & Mueller, F. F. (2014). *Understanding physical activity through 3D printed material artifacts*. Paper presented at the Proceedings of the SIGCHI Conference on Human Factors in Computing Systems, Toronto, Canada.

Khot, R. A., Mueller, F. F., & Hjorth, L. (2013). *SweatAtoms: Materializing physical activity*. Paper presented at the Proceedings of the 9th Australasian Conference on Interactive Entertainment: Matters of Life and Death, Melbourne, Australia.

Klasnja, P., Hekler, E. B., Shiffman, S., Boruvka, A., Almirall, D., Tewari, A., & Murphy, S. A. (2015). Microrandomized trials: An experimental design for developing just-in-time adaptive interventions. *Health Psychology: Official Journal of the Division of Health Psychology, American Psychological Association, 34S*, 1220–1228. doi:10.1037/hea0000305

Klasnja, P., Smith, S., Seewald, N. J., Lee, A., Hall, K., Luers, B., . . . Murphy, S. A. (2018). Efficacy of contextually tailored suggestions for physical activity: A micro-randomized optimization trial of heartsteps. *Annals of Behavioral Medicine*. doi:10.1093/abm/kay067

Koepp, M. J., Gunn, R. N., Lawrence, A. D., Cunningham, V. J., Dagher, A., Jones, T., . . . Grasby, P. M. (1998). Evidence for striatal dopamine release during a video game. *Nature, 393*(6682), 266–268. doi:10.1038/30498

Laver, K. E., George, S., Thomas, S., Deutsch, J. E., & Crotty, M. (2015). Virtual reality for stroke rehabilitation. *Cochrane Database Systematic Reviews, 2*, Cd008349. doi:10.1002/14651858.CD008349.pub3

LeBlanc, A. G., & Chaput, J. P. (2017). Pokemon Go: A game changer for the physical inactivity crisis? *Preventive Medicine, 101*, 235–237. doi:10.1016/j.ypmed.2016.11.012

Lee, M.-H., Cha, S., & Nam, T.-J. (2015). *Patina engraver: Visualizing activity logs as patina in fashionable trackers*. Paper presented at the Proceedings of the 33rd Annual ACM Conference on Human Factors in Computing Systems, Seoul, Republic of Korea.

Lewis, Z. H., Lyons, E. J., Jarvis, J. M., & Baillargeon, J. (2015). Using an electronic activity monitor system as an intervention modality: A systematic review. *BMC Public Health, 15*(1), 585.

Li, I., Dey, A. K., & Forlizzi, J. (2011). *Understanding my data, myself: Supporting self-reflection with ubicomp technologies*. Paper presented at the Proceedings of the 13th International Conference on Ubiquitous Computing, Beijing, China.

Lillie, E. O., Patay, B., Diamant, J., Issell, B., Topol, E. J., & Schork, N. J. (2011). The n-of-1 clinical trial: The ultimate strategy for individualizing medicine? *Personalized Medicine, 8*(2), 161-173. doi:10.2217/pme.11.7

Lim, S. S., Vos, T., Flaxman, A. D., Danaei, G., Shibuya, K., Adair-Rohani, H., . . . Memish, Z. A. (2012). A comparative risk assessment of burden of disease and injury attributable to 67 risk factors and risk factor clusters in 21 regions, 1990–2010: A systematic analysis for the global burden of disease study 2010. *Lancet, 380*(9859), 2224–2260. doi:10.1016/s0140-6736(12)61766-8

Lin, J., Mamykina, L., Lindtner, S., Delajoux, G., & Strub, H. (2006). Fish'n'Steps: Encouraging physical activity with an interactive computer game. In P. Dourish & A. Friday (Eds.), *UbiComp 2006: Ubiquitous computing* (Vol. 4206, pp. 261–278): Heidelberg, Germany: Springer.

Lindqvist, A. K., Castelli, D., Hallberg, J., & Rutberg, S. (2018). The praise and price of Pokemon GO: A qualitative study of children's and parents' experiences. *JMIR Serious Games, 6*(1), e1. doi:10.2196/games.8979

Ma, B. D., Ng, S. L., Schwanen, T., Zacharias, J., Zhou, M., Kawachi, I., & Sun, G. (2018). Pokemon GO and physical activity in Asia: Multilevel study. *Journal of Medical Internet Research, 20*(6), e217. doi:10.2196/jmir.9670

Madden, M., Lenhart, A., Duggan, M., Cortesi, S., & Gasser, U. (2013). *Teens and technology 2013.* Washington, DC: Pew Internet & American Life Project.

Marshall, P. (2007). *Do tangible interfaces enhance learning?* Paper presented at the Proceedings of the 1st International Conference on Tangible and Embedded Interaction, Baton Rouge, LO.

Masteller, B., Sirard, J., & Freedson, P. (2017). The physical activity tracker testing in youth (PATTY) study: Content analysis and children's perceptions. *JMIR mHealth and uHealth, 5*(4), e55.

Mazuryk, T., Gervautz, M., & Smith, K. R. (2013). Virtual reality history, applications, technology and future. *Digital Outcasts.* Retrieved from http://citeseerx.ist.psu.edu/viewdoc/download?doi=10.1.1.42.7849&rep=rep1&type=pdf

McNarry, M. A., & Mackintosh, K. A. (2016). Investigating the relative exercise intensity of exergames in prepubertal children. *Games Health Journal, 5*(2), 135–140. doi:10.1089/g4h.2015.0094

Mercuri, R., & Meredith, K. (2014). An educational venture into 3D Printing. In *Integrated STEM Education Conference (ISEC)* (pp. 1–6). IEEE, Princeton, NJ.

Michie, S., Abraham, C., Whittington, C., McAteer, J., & Gupta, S. (2009). Effective techniques in healthy eating and physical activity interventions: A meta-regression. *Health Psychology, 28*(6), 690–701. doi:10.1037/a0016136

Michie, S., Richardson, M., Johnston, M., Abraham, C., Francis, J., Hardeman, W., . . . Wood, C. E. (2013). The behavior change technique taxonomy (v1) of 93 hierarchically clustered techniques: Building an international consensus for the reporting of behavior change interventions. *Annals of Behavioral Medicine, 46*(1), 81–95. doi:10.1007/s12160-013-9486-6

Miller, A. D., & Mynatt, E. D. (2014). *StepStream: A school-based pervasive social fitness system for everyday adolescent health.* Paper presented at the Proceedings of the SIGCHI Conference on Human Factors in Computing Systems, Toronto, Canada.

Moller, A. C., Merchant, G., Conroy, D. E., West, R., Hekler, E., Kugler, K. C., & Michie, S. (2017). Applying and advancing behavior change theories and techniques in the context of a digital health revolution: Proposals for more effectively realizing untapped potential. *Journal of Behavioral Medicine, 40*(1), 85–98. doi:10.1007/s10865-016-9818-7

Montessori, M. (1912). *The Montessori method: Scientific pedagogy as applied to child education in" the children's house", with additions and revisions by the author; Translated from the Italian by Anne E. George; with an Introduction by Professor Henry W. Holmes.* Brooklyn, NY: FA Stokes.

Morris, Z. S., Wooding, S., & Grant, J. (2011). The answer is 17 years, what is the question: Understanding time lags in translational research. *Journal of the Royal Society of Medicine, 104*(12), 510–520. doi:10.1258/jrsm.2011.110180

Mullan, K. (2019). A child's day: Trends in time use in the UK from 1975 to 2015. *The British Journal of Sociology, 70*, 997–1024. doi:10.1111/1468-4446.12369

Neubeck, L., Lowres, N., Benjamin, E. J., Freedman, S. B., Coorey, G., & Redfern, J. (2015). The mobile revolution–using smartphone apps to prevent cardiovascular disease. *Nature Reviews: Cardiology, 12*(6), 350–360. doi:10.1038/nrcardio.2015.34

Norris, E., Dunsmuir, S., Duke-Williams, O., Stamatakis, E., & Shelton, N. (2018). Mixed method evaluation of the virtual traveller physically active lesson intervention: An analysis using the RE-AIM framework. *Evaluation and Program Planning, 70*, 107–114. doi:10.1016/j.evalprogplan.2018.01.007

Norris, E., Hamer, M., & Stamatakis, E. A. (2016). Active video games in schools and effects on physical activity and health: Review. *The Journal of Pediatrics, 172*, 40–46.e5. doi:10.1016/j.jpeds.2016.02.001

Norris, E., Shelton, N., Dunsmuir, S., Duke-Williams, O., & Stamatakis, E. (2015). Virtual field trips as physically active lessons for children: A pilot study. *BMC Public Health, 15*, 366. doi:10.1186/s12889-015-1706-5

Oh, Y. & Yang, S. (2010). *Defining exergames & exergaming.* Paper presented at the Meaningful Play Conference, MI.

Oliver, M., Schofield, G., & McEvoy, E. (2006). An integrated curriculum approach to increasing habitual physical activity in children: A feasibility study. *Journal of School Health, 76*(2), 74–79.

Orme, M. W., Weedon, A. E., Saukko, P. M., Esliger, D. W., Morgan, M. D., Steiner, M. C., . . . Singh, S. J. (2018). Findings of the chronic obstructive pulmonary disease-sitting and exacerbations trial (COPD-SEAT) in reducing sedentary time using wearable and mobile technologies with educational support: Randomized controlled feasibility trial. *Journal of Medical Internet Research* . doi:10.2196/mhealth.9398

Page, Z. E., Barrington, S., Edwards, J., & Barnett, L. M. (2017). Do active video games benefit the motor skill development of non-typically developing children and adolescents: A systematic review. *Journal of Science and Medicine in Sport, 20*(12), 1087–1100. doi:10.1016/j.jsams.2017.05.001

Pakarinen, A., Parisod, H., Smed, J., & Salantera, S. (2017). Health game interventions to enhance physical activity self-efficacy of children: A quantitative systematic review. *Journal of Advanced Nursing, 73*(4), 794–811. doi:10.1111/jan.13160

Peng, W., Crouse, J. C., & Lin, J. H. (2013). Using active video games for physical activity promotion: A systematic review of the current state of research. *Health Education & Behavior, 40*(2), 171–192. doi:10.1177/1090198112444956

Piaget, J., & Cook, M. (1952). *The origins of intelligence in children* (Vol. 8). New York, NY: International Universities Press.

Polzien, K. M., Jakicic, J. M., Tate, D. F., & Otto, A. D. (2007). The efficacy of a technology-based system in a short-term behavioral weight loss intervention. *Obesity, 15*(4), 825–830.

Price, S., Rogers, Y., Scaife, M., Stanton, D., & Neale, H. (2003). Using 'tangibles' to promote novel forms of playful learning. *Interacting with Computers, 15*(2), 169–185. doi:10.1016/S0953-5438(03)00006-7

Puiu, T. (2015). *Your smartphone is millions of times more powerful that all of NASA's combined computing in 1969.* Retrieved from https://www.zmescience.com/research/technology/smartphone-power-compared-to-apollo-432/

Quan, M., Pope, Z., & Gao, Z. (2018). examining young children's physical activity and sedentary behaviors in an exergaming program using accelerometry. *Journal of Clinical Medicine, 7*(10). doi:10.3390/jcm7100302

Ramirez-Marrero, F., Smith, B., Sherman, W., & Kirby, T. (2005). Comparison of methods to estimate physical activity and energy expenditure in African American children. *International Journal of Sports Medicine, 26*(5), 363–371.

Rhodes, A. (2017). *Screen time and kids: What's happening in our homes (detailed report).* Melbourne, Australia: The Royal Childrens Hospital Melbourne.

Rideout, V., & Robb, M. (2017). *The common sense census: Media use by kids age zero to eight.* San Francisco, CA: Common Sense Media.

Ridgers, N. D., McNarry, M. A., & Mackintosh, K. A. (2016). Feasibility and effectiveness of using wearable activity trackers in youth: A systematic review. *JMIR mHealth and uHealth, 4*(4), e129. doi:10.2196/mhealth.6540

Ridgers, N. D., Timperio, A., Brown, H., Ball, K., Macfarlane, S., Lai, S. K., . . . Salmon, J. (2018). Wearable activity tracker use among Australian adolescents: Usability and acceptability study. *JMIR mHealth and uHealth, 6*(4), e86. doi:10.2196/mhealth.9199

Ridgers, N. D., Timperio, A., Cerin, E., & Salmon, J. (2015). Within-and between-day associations between children's sitting and physical activity time. *BMC Public Health, 15*(1), 950. doi:10.1186/s12889-015-2291-3

Rita, D., & Dunn, K. (1979). Learning styles/teaching styles: Should they ... can they ... be matched. *Educational Leadership, 36*(4), 238–244.

Rogers, Y., Scaife, M., Gabrielli, S., Smith, H., & Harris, E. (2002). A conceptual framework for mixed reality environments: Designing novel learning activities for young children. *Presence Teleoperators and Virtual Environments, 11*(6), 677–686. doi:10.1162/105474602321050776

Sanders, J. P., Loveday, A., Pearson, N., Edwardson, C., Yates, T., Biddle, S. J., . . . New, Y. (2016). Devices for self-monitoring sedentary time or physical activity: Review. *Journal of Medical Internet Research, 18*(5), e90. doi:10.2196/jmir.5373

Sauvé, K., Houben, S., Marquardt, N., Bakker, S., Hengeveld, B., Gallacher, S., & Rogers, Y. (2017). *LOOP: A physical artifact to facilitate seamless interaction with personal data in everyday life.* Paper presented at the Proceedings of the 2017 ACM Conference Companion Publication on Designing Interactive Systems, pp. 285–288. doi:10.1145/3064857.3079175

Schaefer, S. E., Ching, C. C., Breen, H., & German, J. B. (2016). Wearing, thinking, and moving: Testing the feasibility of fitness tracking with urban youth. *American Journal of Health Education, 47*(1), 8–16.

Schaller, R. R. (1997). Moore's law: Past, present, and future. *IEEE Spectrum, 34*(6), 52–59.

Schembre, S. M., Liao, Y., Robertson, M. C., Dunton, G. F., Kerr, J., Haffey, M. E., . . . Hicklen, R. S. (2018). Just-in-time feedback in diet and physical activity interventions: Systematic review and practical design framework. *Journal of Medical Internet Research, 20*(3).

Sedentary Behaviour Research Network. (2012). Letter to the editor: Standardized use of the terms 'sedentary' and 'sedentary behaviours'. *Applied Physiology, Nutrition, and Metabolism*, *37*(3), 540–542. doi:10.1139/h2012-024

Serino, M., Cordrey, K., McLaughlin, L., & Milanaik, R. L. (2016). Pokémon Go and augmented virtual reality games: A cautionary commentary for parents and pediatricians. *Current Opinion in Pediatrics*, *28*(5), 673–677. doi:10.1097/MOP.0000000000000409

Singh, A., Uijtdewilligen, L., Twisk, J. W., van Mechelen, W., & Chinapaw, M.J. (2012). Physical activity and performance at school A systematic review of the literature including a methodological quality assessment. *Archives of Pediatrics Adolescent Medicine*, *166*(1), 49–55.

Sluis, R., Weevers, I., Van Schijndel, C., Kolos-Mazuryk, L., Fitrianie, S., & Martens, J. (2004). *Read-it: Five-to-seven-year-old children learn to read in a tabletop environment*. Paper presented at the Proceedings of the 2004 Conference on Interaction Design and Children: Building a Community, MD.

Sofi, F., Capalbo, A., Cesari, F., Abbate, R., & Gensini, G. F. (2008). Physical activity during leisure time and primary prevention of coronary heart disease: An updated meta-analysis of cohort studies. *European Journal of Cardiovascular Prevention Rehabilitation*, *15*(3), 247–257. doi:10.1097/HJR.0b013e3282f232ac

Southard, D. R., & Southard, B. H. (2006). Promoting physical activity in children with MetaKenkoh. *Clinical and Investigative Medicine, 29*(5), 293.

Spruijt-Metz, D., Hekler, E., Saranummi, N., Intille, S., Korhonen, I., Nilsen, W., . . . Pavel, M. (2015). Building new computational models to support health behavior change and maintenance: New opportunities in behavioral research. *Translational Behavioral Medicine*. doi:10.1007/s13142-015-0324-1

Sqord. (2018). *Promote kid fitness and healthy habits*. Retrieved from https://sqord.com

Staiano, A. E., Beyl, R. A., Guan, W., Hendrick, C. A., Hsia, D. S., & Newton, R. L., Jr. (2018). Home-based exergaming among children with overweight and obesity: A randomized clinical trial. *Pediatric Obesity, 13*(11), 724–733. doi:10.1111/ijpo.12438

Staiano, A. E., Beyl, R. A., Hsia, D. S., Katzmarzyk, P. T., & Newton, R. L. (2016). Twelve weeks of dance exergaming in overweight and obese adolescent girls: Transfer effects on physical activity, screen time, and self-efficacy. *Journal of Sport and Health Science, 6*(1), 4–10. doi:10.1016/j.jshs.2016.11.005

Steuer, J. (1992). Defining virtual reality: Dimensions determining telepresence. *Journal of Communication*, 1460–2466 doi:10.1111/j.1460-2466.1992.tb00812.x

Straker, L., Zabatiero, J., Danby, S., Thorpe, K., & Edwards, S. (2018). Conflicting guidelines on young children's screen time and use of digital technology create policy and practice dilemmas. *The Journal of Pediatrics, 202*, 300–303. doi:10.1016/j.jpeds.2018.07.019

Sturm, R. (2004, October 1). The economics of physical activity: Societal trends and rationales for interventions. *American Journal of Preventive Medicine*. doi:10.1016/j.amepre.2004.06.013

Stusak, S. (2016). *Exploring the potential of physical visualizations* (PhD). LMU, München.

Stusak, S., Tabard, A., Sauka, F., Khot, R. A., & Butz, A. (2014). Activity sculptures: Exploring the impact of physical visualizations on running activity. *IEEE Transactions on Visualization and Computer Graphics, 20*(12), 2201–2210. doi:10.1109/TVCG.2014.2352953

Sun, H., Zeng, N., & Gao, Z. (2017). Promoting physical activity and health through emerging technology. In Z. Gao (Ed.), *Technology in physical activity and health promotion* (1st ed., pp. 26–45). London, UK: Routledge.

Sunny, C., David, W. M., & James, A. L. (2009). *Theory-driven design strategies for technologies that support behavior change in everyday life*. Paper presented at the Proceedings of the SIGCHI Conference on Human Factors in Computing Systems, Boston, MA.

TechCrunch. (2017). *Pokémon GO reveals sponsors like McDonald's pay it up to $0.50 per visitor*. Retrieved November from https://techcrunch.com/2017/05/31/pokemon-go-sponsorship-price/?guccounter=1&guce_referrer=aHR0cHM6Ly93d3cuZ29vZ2xlLmNvbS8&guce_referrer_sig=AQAAAFswAHTGHbaQqBkEGIBT1Um1lQ6aQZK9A9lC50TxmxT_1ygXX8B1_7foy2HwJghjSvbOq5mjgRTvOlzjKXsj4TQzLLEZcaYqmOIfxAZKrrSGu946lKm4UgYkYBcM7HaEaaWuaZcRGt-SgeEJ1bT_zgMwQDtektYCNRJ7RqYwJeP2

Terrenghi, L., Kranz, M., Holleis, P., & Schmidt, A. (2006). A cube to learn: A tangible user interface for the design of a learning appliance. *Personal and Ubiquitous Computing, 10*(2–3), 153–158.

Teychenne, M., Ball, K., & Salmon, J. (2008). Physical activity and likelihood of depression in adults: A review. *Preventive Medicine, 46*(5), 397–411. doi:10.1016/j.ypmed.2008.01.009

Thin, A. G., Brown, C., & Meenan, P. (2013). User experiences while playing dance-based exergames and the influence of different body motion sensing technologies. *International Journal of Computer Games Technology, 2013*, 7. doi:10.1155/2013/603604

Thompson, D. I., & Batterham, A. M. (2013). Towards integrated physical activity profiling. *PLoS One, 8*(2), e56427.

Thompson, D. I., Cantu, D., Callender, C., Liu, Y., Rajendran, M., Rajendran, M., . . . Deng, Z. (2018). Photorealistic avatar and teen physical activity: Feasibility and preliminary efficacy. *Games for Health Journal, 7*(2), 143–150.

Tremblay, M. S., Aubert, S., Barnes, J. D., Saunders, T. J., Carson, V., Latimer-Cheung, A. E., . . . on behalf of SBRN Terminology Consensus Project Participants. (2017). Sedentary behavior research network (SBRN) – Terminology consensus project process and outcome. *International Journal of Behavioral Nutrition and Physical Activity, 14*(1), 75. doi:10.1186/s12966-017-0525-8

Tudor-Locke, C., & Bassett, D. R. (2004). How many steps/day are enough? *Sports Medicine, 34*(1), 1–8.

Ullmer, B., & Ishii, H. (2000). Emerging frameworks for tangible user interfaces. *IBM Systems Journal, 39*(3–4), 915–931. doi:10.1147/sj.393.0915

van Gemert-Pijnen, J. E., Nijland, N., van Limburg, M., Ossebaard, H. C., Kelders, S. M., Eysenbach, G., & Seydel, E. R. (2011). A holistic framework to improve the uptake and impact of eHealth technologies. *Journal of Medical Internet Research, 13*(4), e111.

Van Wijk, J. (2005). The value of visualization. In *Proceedings of the IEEE visualisation* (pp. 79–86). Los Alamitos, CA: IEEE Press.

Viseu, A., & Suchman, L. (2010). Wearable augmentations: Imaginaries of the informed body. In J. Edwards, P. Harvey, & P. Wade (Eds.), *Technologized images, technologized bodies* (pp. 161–184). New York, NY: Bergham Books.

Wagner-Greene, V. R., Wotring, A. J., Castor, T., Kruger, J., Mortemore, S., & Dake, J. A. (2017). Pokemon GO: Healthy or harmful? *American Journal of Public Health, 107*(1), 35–36. doi:10.2105/ajph.2016.303548

Wartella, E., Rideout, V., Montague, H., Beaudoin-Ryan, L., & Lauricella, A. (2016). Teens, health and technology: A national survey. *Media Communication, 4*(3), 12.

WIRED. (2009). *Wearables are totally failing the people who need them most.* Retrieved November 11, 2018 from https://www.wired.com/2014/11/where-fitness-trackers-fail

World Health Organization. (2009). *Global health risks: Mortality and burden of disease attributable to selected major risks.* Geneva, Switzerland: World Health Organization.

World Health Organization. (2018a). *Global action plan on physical activity 2018–2030: More active people for a healthier world, 2018–2030.* Geneva, Switzerland: World Health Organization.

World Health Organization. (2018b). *Physical inactivity: A global public health problem.* Retrieved from http://www.who.int/dietphysicalactivity/factsheet_inactivity/en

Yi, J. S., ah Kang, Y., & Stasko, J. (2007). Toward a deeper understanding of the role of interaction in information visualization. *IEEE Transactions on Visualization and Computer Graphics, 13*(6), 1224–1231. doi:10.1109/TVCG.2007.70515

Zuckerman, O., Arida, S., & Resnick, M. (2005). *Extending tangible interfaces for education: Digital montessori-inspired manipulatives.* Paper presented at the Proceedings of the SIGCHI Conference on Human Factors in Computing Systems, Portland, OR.

PART 9

Motor Skill Development, Exercise, and Sport

36

FUNDAMENTAL MOVEMENT SKILL INTERVENTIONS

Lawrence Foweather and James R. Rudd

Introduction

Terminology and Scope

In Chapter 19, which examined the assessment of motor competence, it was noted that there has been a plethora of terms used to describe goal-directed movement within motor development and related disciplines, creating confusion in understanding what constituents of movement are being assessed and what the impact of motor development is on health and wider developmental outcomes. Motor competence, defined as the degree to which an individual can perform goal-directed movements in a coordinated, accurate and relatively error-free manner (Anson, Elliot, & Davids, 2005; Robinson et al., 2015; Rudd et al., 2016), has been proposed as an umbrella term to align research and reduce ambiguity in terminology, and encompasses various terms used interchangeably within past literature (i.e., fundamental movement/motor skills, foundational movement skills, motor proficiency, motor performance, motor coordination, motor creativity and motor ability). Since the turn of the century there has been a large body of research focused on fundamental movement skills (FMS) (also called fundamental motor skills, gross motor skills and fundamental motor patterns; for a review of terminology, see Logan, Ross, Chee, Stodden, & Robinson, 2018), which represent an important element of motor competence. In this chapter, we will begin by defining and examining the importance of FMS before considering the prevalence of skill proficiency among children and adolescents and how these skills develop. The main body of the chapter will focus on literature surrounding interventions to improve the acquisition and mastery of FMS followed by a discussion of key themes emerging from the scientific evidence base. The chapter then concludes with a list of recommendations for FMS interventions in research and practice.

Fundamental Movement Skills

FMS are defined as observable movement patterns involving the combined use of two or more body parts and include stability (e.g., balancing and twisting), locomotor (e.g., running and jumping) and object-control (e.g., catching and throwing) skills (Gallahue, Ozmun, & Goodway, 2012; Logan et al., 2018). FMS are considered the initial building blocks of more advanced, complex movements required to participate in many sports, games and physical activities (Gallahue et al.,

2012; Seefeldt, 1980). For example, advanced forms of kicking transfer to football (soccer), while specialized forms of throwing can be applied in sports such as cricket or baseball. A more detailed understanding of transfer has been proposed by Langendorfer, Roberton, and Stodden (2013), who highlight that the timely coordination among body segments exhibited in more complex coordination and control movement tasks can be learned and enhanced through mastery of foundation skills such as throwing, kicking and striking activities. This is due to enhanced perceptual-motor integration, development of high angular velocities of multiple joints, optimal relative timing of segmental interactions, optimal inter- and intra-muscular coordination and optimal transfer of energy through the kinetic chain. Mastery of a broad repertoire of FMS is therefore considered to enhance opportunities for children and young people to experience success and sustain participation in sports and physical activities (Clark & Metcalfe, 2002; Gallahue et al., 2012; Seefeldt, 1980; Stodden et al., 2008).

Importance of FMS

Developing competence in FMS is important (for more detailed reviews, see Barnett et al., 2016; Bremer & Cairney, 2018; Lubans, Morgan, Cliff, Barnett, & Okely, 2010; Robinson et al., 2015). Strong evidence from cross-sectional and longitudinal studies indicates that relative to those with low FMS competence, children and adolescents with high FMS competence are more likely to participate in physical activity (Figueroa & An, 2017; Foweather et al., 2015; Holfelder & Schott, 2014; Logan, Webster, Getchell, Pfeiffer, & Robinson, 2015; Lubans et al., 2010) and have higher physical fitness (Cattuzzo et al., 2016; Luz, Rodrigues, De Meester, & Cordovil, 2017) and lower prevalence of overweight and obesity (D'Hondt et al., 2014; McWhannell et al., 2018; O'Brien, Belton, & Issartel, 2016b; Rodrigues, Stodden, & Lopes, 2016). Further, children and adolescents with high FMS competence have been found to have higher perceived competence (Babic et al., 2014; Barnett, Morgan, Van Beurden, Ball, & Lubans, 2011; Barnett, Morgan, van Beurden, & Beard, 2008), which is important because youth who feel competent while participating in games, sports and other physical activity contexts are more likely to enjoy involvement and consequently feel intrinsically motivated to continue effort and participation in all forms of physical activity (Harter, 1978). The ability to perform specialized forms of FMS has also been demonstrated to be positively associated with academic achievement and the development of higher order cognitive skills, i.e., executive functions such as working memory, inhibitory control and cognitive flexibility (van der Fels et al., 2015). These functions are critical as they allow children and young people to effectively manage their thoughts, actions and emotions in order to accomplish everyday tasks and also to plan, organize and manage their time. Therefore, poor FMS development has wide-reaching adverse influences on physical, psychological, cognitive, and social and emotional development (Leonard & Hill, 2014), and may provide a barrier to participation in physical activity and sports in later life (Barnett et al., 2009; De Meester et al., 2018; Lloyd, Saunders, Bremer, & Tremblay, 2014; Loprinzi, Davis, & Fu, 2015; Seefeldt, 1980; Stodden et al., 2008).

Despite the above evidence, the premise that mastery over FMS is necessary for participation in physical activity has been critiqued in recent years (Almond, 2014; Pot & van Hilvoorde, 2014). According to Almond (2014), FMS has a weak conceptual base, as not all skills are fundamentally necessary for children to be physically active and to participate in the many sporting opportunities available in modern society. In addition, it is argued that the current list of FMS is not broad enough and that the existing classification of FMS will lead to children participating in only a limited number of sports and activities, and these will, as a result, have limited transfer capability (Afonso, Coutinho, Araújo, Almond, & Pot, 2014; Almond, 2014). The other criticism directed at the conceptual base of FMS is that skills are developed predominantly through experience and do not require explicit teaching (Afonso et al., 2014). However, as noted in a published response by Barnett and other international FMS researchers (2016), the term 'fundamental' represents possessing a base of skill competencies and therefore refers to sets of skills rather than individual skills. More recently, Hulteen, Morgan, Barnett, Stodden, and Lubans (2018) proposed The Life-long Physical Activity Model and replaced the term 'fundamental movement skills' with 'foundational movement skills' to better reflect that these skills represent an underlying base or support. Thus, while developing competency in these skills would support and maximize opportunities for participation in physical activity, failure to master one skill will not necessarily lead to inactivity (Hulteen et al., 2018). Further, the new term 'foundational movement skills' is proposed as inclusive of both traditionally conceptualized FMS (e.g., run, throw and static balance) and skills that support physical activity participation through the life-course, such as cycling, freestyle swimming stroke and bodyweight squatting. The change in terminology to 'foundational' may help dispel the aforementioned critique about FMS not being 'fundamental'. Furthermore, the proposal for a broader classification of movement skills to encapsulate the range of skills that may promote physical activity participation into the elderly years is interesting and should stimulate further debate and research. Though promising, given that research into foundational movement skills is in its infancy, this chapter will focus on traditional FMS, in accordance with the widely used Gallahue et al. (2012) definition.

Prevalence of FMS Proficiency among Children and Young People

The evidence summarized above indicates that FMS are important for positive health and developmental trajectories for children and adolescents. This makes it is imperative to examine and track the prevalence and levels of FMS competence to ensure that children are making sufficient advances in motor skill acquisition to acquire these benefits. Early childhood (2–5 years) is considered a critical phase for FMS, with rapid brain growth and neuromuscular development coinciding with high confidence and fearlessness, which encourages the young child to seek and persist in activities that will develop their skills (Malina, Bouchard, & Bar-Or, 2004; Stodden et al., 2008). In the past decade, several studies have documented levels of FMS competence among preschool children (Brian et al., 2018; Foulkes et al., 2015; Hardy, King, Farrell, Macniven, & Howlett, 2010; Robinson, 2011; Veldman, Jones, Santos, Sousa-Sá, & Okely, 2018). Overall, these studies suggest that, as expected in young children, these skills are at the rudimentary stage of development. With appropriate instruction, encouragement, opportunities and practice, children can master FMS by 7–8 years of age (Gallahue & Donnelly, 2007; Gallahue et al., 2012). It is therefore of concern that low levels of FMS competence have been reported within numerous studies involving primary school-aged children and adolescents living in highly developed western countries such as the United Kingdom (Bryant, Duncan, & Birch, 2014; Duncan, Jones, O'Brien, Barnett, & Eyre, 2018; McWhannell et al., 2018; Morley, Till, Ogilvie, & Turner, 2015), Ireland (Bolger et al., 2018; Farmer, Belton, & O'Brien, 2017; Kelly, O'Connor, Harrison, & Ni Chéilleachair, 2019; Lester et al., 2017; O'Brien, Belton, & Issartel, 2016a; O'Brien et al., 2016b), Italy (Sgrò, Quinto, Messana, Pignato, & Lipoma, 2017), Canada (LeGear et al., 2012), Belgium (Bardid, Rudd, Lenoir, Polman, & Barnett, 2015), Australia (Bardid et al., 2015; Cohen, Morgan, Plotnikoff, Callister, & Lubans, 2014; Hardy, Barnett, Espinel, & Okely, 2013; Rudd et al., 2015), as well as high-income Eastern countries such as Singapore (Mukherjee, Ting Jamie, & Fong, 2017) and middle-income countries such as Brazil in South America (Valentini et al., 2016). Thus, low levels of FMS competence are a global issue, and actions to improve FMS proficiency are required. The following sections of this chapter will therefore explore the factors that influence the development of FMS competence and consider theories and models of FMS development. Following this, we will review the effectiveness of interventions to improve FMS in young children, children and adolescents, and present some examples of good practice.

Theories and Models of FMS Development

Proficient performance of FMS requires the development of motor control, precision and accuracy, which in turn builds movement efficiency and confidence (Gallahue & Donnelly, 2007). Children's motor performance normally improves with age (Branta, Haubenstricker, & Seefeldt, 1984; Ulrich, 2000; Walkley, Holland, Treloar, & Probyn-Smith, 1993), and childhood is a sensitive learning period for reaching proficiency in FMS. In particular, early childhood represents a 'window of opportunity' for FMS development (Gallahue & Donnelly, 2007). However, this process is not automatic; the rate and extent of FMS development is idiosyncratic and non-linear (Gallahue & Donnelly, 2007) and dependent on several factors. Newell (1986) conceptualized the multiple influences on motor development through a triangular model of constraints, proposing that motor development is dynamic and that movement arises from the interaction of constraints associated with a specific task (i.e., the goal of the movement, associated rules and equipment), performed by a learner with structural (i.e., genetics, puberty, maturation and growth, muscular and nervous systems) and functional (i.e., motivation, prior experience, confidence, fear) characteristics, in a precise environmental setting (e.g., surface type, dimensions, gravity or altitude). Children will only develop a rudimentary level of FMS competence through growth and maturation alone. To reach proficiency, children's FMS need to be nurtured through frequent encouragement, access to appropriate equipment and play spaces, high-quality instruction using developmentally appropriate activities, opportunities to practice and refine the skills and a supportive learning environment (Gallahue & Donnelly, 2007; Haywood & Getchell, 2018; Payne & Isaacs, 2017). If such conditions are present, it is possible for children to develop much higher levels of skill than is normally expected for a given age (Wickstrom, 1977). Conversely, if opportunities to develop skill competence are not available, due to factors such as a lack of outdoor space or a highly sedentary lifestyle, FMS development may be delayed. As such, these individual and environmental constraints mean that children can follow very different "developmental trajectories" (Clark & Metcalfe, 2002). Given the dynamic nature of FMS development, it is important to identify any subgroups of children who are likely to be at risk of low FMS competence so that interventions can be targeted accordingly. Furthermore, identifying factors that influence and constrain the development of FMS can also inform the design and effectiveness of interventions and programs to enhance competence at these skills.

Correlates and Determinants of FMS

Barnett, Lai, et al. (2016) conducted a systematic review of individual, socio-cultural and environmental (i.e., socio-ecological) correlates of gross motor competence, including FMS, in children and adolescents. Age (increasing), weight status (healthy), sex (male) and socio-economic background (higher) were each found to be positively correlated with certain aspects of motor competence, suggesting that FMS interventions should perhaps be developed towards younger children, overweight/obese groups, girls and/or children from low socio-economic status backgrounds. Sex differences are evident for object-control skills in particular. While biological differences such as the greater size and power of boys compared to girls may partly explain higher movement performance outcomes for skills such as throwing (i.e., distance, speed), it is also likely that sex differences are due to socio-cultural factors (gender stereotyping, lack of encouragement and support for girls) and a lack of opportunities for girls to engage in sports and activities that enhance these skills at home, in school and in the community (Barnett et al., 2019; Barnett, Lai, et al., 2016). Differences are also formulated in unstructured settings such as school playtime (McWhannell et al., 2018), with boys more likely to participate in ball games and use equipment, whereas girls prefer social and sedentary play, skipping or hopscotch (McWhannell et al., 2018; Ridgers, Fairclough, & Stratton, 2010; Roberts, Fairclough, Ridgers, & Porteous, 2012). The available evidence also indicated that children from higher socio-economic backgrounds possess higher levels of FMS proficiency than those from disadvantaged areas, particularly for locomotor skills (Barnett, Lai, et al., 2016). Children from more affluent areas may have greater access to facilities, be more likely to own sports equipment in the home and have greater parental support and finances to access opportunities to develop these skills.

Childhood obesity was found to be negatively associated with FMS competence, in particular locomotor and stability skills (Barnett, Lai, et al., 2016). Object-control skills tend to be more static and therefore are less difficult to perform for overweight/obese children and adolescents than those locomotor and stability movements that require shifting or controlling a greater body mass (D'Hondt, Deforche, De Bourdeaudhuij, & Lenoir, 2009). Obese children may also demonstrate abnormal gait patterns, which increase the energy cost of locomotion, leading to fatigue and potential biomechanical and musculoskeletal issues in knee and hip joints, which can limit participation in physical activity and time spent practicing locomotor skills (McGraw, McClenaghan, Williams, Dickerson, & Ward, 2000; Stovitz, Pardee, Vazquez, Duval, & Schwimmer, 2008). Overweight and obese children can also suffer from bullying, name-calling and teasing, and may seek to avoid overt victimization by withdrawing from physical activity (Hayden-Wade et al., 2005; Zabinski, Saelens, Stein, Hayden-Wade, & Wilfley, 2003), which, in turn, may limit their opportunities to develop skill competence. As children with more developed FMS are more likely to be active, having poor FMS competence also hinders the perceived competence and motivation of overweight/obese children and adolescents to take part in physical activity (Harter, 1978; Southall, Okely, & Steele, 2004). Thus, low FMS competence leads to low participation in physical activity, and therefore increasing the likelihood of weight gain in what is a vicious cycle with weight gain then impacting further on FMS development and engagement in physical activity (Lima et al., 2017; Stodden et al., 2008).

The review by Barnett, Lai, et al. (2016) also found evidence to support physical activity as a predictor of overall skill competence, though evidence for object-control and locomotor subscales was indeterminate, while few studies examined associations between physical activity and stability skills. Physical activity participation is important to build FMS competence in young children (Stodden et al., 2008). However, while children and adolescents participate in physical activity in many contexts, including sport, play, recess and physical education, little is known about what types, quality and contexts of physical activity better contribute to FMS development. Furthermore, few studies had explored the influence of socio-cultural and environmental factors on FMS development. Evidence from research conducted in the field of physical activity indicates that peer, parental and teacher social influences (e.g., encouragement, support, role modeling) may be important for child and adolescent participation in physical activity, while factors within the physical environment (e.g., available equipment, facilities, outdoor space) at home, in school and in the community can also promote or inhibit opportunities for activity (e.g., see Sterdt, Liersch, & Walter, 2013; Yao & Rhodes, 2015). Further research to explore whether such psychosocial, cultural, environmental and behavioral factors influence FMS competence is therefore necessary to improve our understanding of FMS development.

In summary, the evidence discussed above suggests that to promote FMS development, educators, practitioners and research interventionists should be aware that a child's unique characteristics and the physical, social and environmental conditions of the task affect movement skill proficiency.

Overview of the Literature

Interventions to Improve FMS

The sub-optimal levels of FMS proficiency described earlier in the chapter highlight the need for interventions to enhance skill competence. Over the past decade, a number of systematic reviews have been published on the short- and long-term effects of interventions to improve FMS and related outcomes in children and adolescents. There is some overlap between review studies in terms of included intervention studies, but subtle differences in the foci of reviews, inclusion criteria and populations of interest lead to differences from review to review. In this section, we will summarize systematic reviews of interventions conducted in young/preschool children, children, adolescents and overweight/obese groups in order to explore intervention characteristics and effectiveness.

Young Children (Preschoolers)

Early childhood (2–5 years) is a critical window of opportunity for FMS development. Young children's innate enthusiasm for active play and physical activity can be capitalized upon for FMS development with rich, diverse and quality movement experiences necessary to build competence. As such, the early years should be a key priority for FMS interventions and programs.

Three reviews of interventions to improve FMS in young children were located (Van Capelle, Broderick, van Doorn, Ward, & Parmenter, 2017; Veldman, Jones, & Okely, 2016. Wick et al., 2017). Veldman et al. (2016) updated an earlier systematic review by Riethmuller and colleagues (2009) and reviewed interventions targeting FMS in 0- to 5-year-old typically developing preschool children in studies published between 2007 and January 2015. Veldman et al. reported that six out of seven studies included in the review reported significant intervention effects on FMS, with three studies finding effects for total FMS score and three studies reporting improvements for either locomotor, object-control or individual skills. All interventions took place in early childhood settings (e.g., kindergarten, nursery, childcare centers) and were mostly delivered by setting staff following between one and five sessions of professional development training. Few studies involved parents ($n = 2$). Interventions varied from 2 to 10 months in length and from 2 to 5 sessions per week, and sessions from 15 to 40 minutes in duration. Six interventions included structured FMS programs focused on either implementing one FMS skill per session, focusing on different skills each week, providing circuits of activities, or using structured activities in combination with supervised free play or unstructured activities.

Van Capelle and colleagues (2017) examined preschool-based FMS interventions of at least 4 weeks among children aged 3–5-year. They located 20 studies, including 15 randomized controlled trials and 5 controlled trials involving 4,255 preschoolers, and conducted a meta-analysis to quantify the intervention effects. Overall, participation in the intervention groups was associated with small effects on overall FMS score (Standardized Mean Difference [SMD] = 0.31), moderate effects on locomotor skills (SMD = 0.62) and large effects on object-control skills (SMD = 1.06), though only 23% of studies were rated as being of high methodological quality. Most of the interventions ($n = 13$) were delivered by preschool educators/teachers who had received training and been provided with resources. Some interventions ($n = 6$) were delivered by external professionals such as researchers or specialized sports coaches, while one study exclusively involved provision of education to parents. Interestingly, when the different types of delivery models were examined, there was moderate quality evidence to support teacher-led interventions to improve FMS but limited evidence to support external/specialist delivered approaches (effects were positive, but non-significant). Interventions ranged from 6 to 80 weeks in length, with sessions running for between 2 and 5 days per week and lasting from 15 to 90 minutes in duration. Interventions that reported large effects across different FMS were relatively intensive, delivering sessions lasting at least 30 minutes on 4 or 5 days per week. Intervention components included structured activity sessions/lessons focused on a various aspects of FMS, alongside other intervention components such as parent education, supply of play equipment and the promotion of healthy eating.

Wick et al. (2017) conducted a systematic review and meta-analysis of FMS interventions for 2–6-year-old children conducted in childcare and kindergarten settings. In a search conducted up to August 2015, 30 trials were located (15 randomized controlled trials and 15 controlled trials), involving 6,126 preschoolers. Participation in the interventions was associated with small-to-large effects on overall FMS score (SMD = 0.46), locomotor skills (SMD = 0.94) and object-control skills (SMD = 1.36), though again the overall methodological quality of many of the studies was indicative of high bias. Somewhat in contrast to the findings of the review by Van Capelle et al. (2017), interventions delivered by external experts rather than usual childcare or kindergarten teachers resulted in higher effect sizes. Interventions ranged from 6 weeks to 20 months in length, with sessions lasting from 15 to 65 minutes and occurring from once per week to daily. Interestingly from a dose-response perspective, interventions of 6 months or less were more effective than interventions of a longer duration (i.e., more than 6 months), suggesting that there might be a plateau in FMS development due to the lack of progression within the program, or children may lose interest and motivation. Interventions included either structured activities in lessons/sessions, sometimes combined with additional time for unstructured physical activity, or unstructured physical activity only with increased free play and outdoor play time intended to foster FMS. Eight studies also included a parental component to the intervention.

The findings from these systematic reviews suggest that there is evidence that kindergarten- or nursery- or childcare-based interventions to improve FMS in young children are effective, though more high-quality trials are needed, while the involvement of parents as well as home- and community-based interventions have received relatively little attention. Very few studies included long-term follow-up assessments of FMS, so it is unclear whether the reported positive gains were maintained over time, or whether children in control groups would eventually 'catch-up' with intervention group peers. Each of the reviews highlighted that many intervention programs were not well described, making it difficult to identify the pedagogies or intervention components that best contribute to FMS development.

Children and Adolescents

Childhood and adolescence represent important periods for developing, applying and specializing in FMS. Opportunities for skill development in primary school-aged children include physical education lessons, recess and participation in afterschool program or organized sports. As children mature into youth and transition from primary to middle and high/secondary school, they can participate in a wider variety of games and sports and access more structured competitive sport alongside broader recreational activities that enable them to apply and utilize advanced forms of FMS. The next section provides an overview of systematic review evidence concerning the effectiveness of program to improve FMS among children and adolescents.

One of the earlier systematic reviews in this population, conducted by Dudley and colleagues (Dudley, Okely, Pearson, & Cotton, 2011), focused on physical education or school sport curricular interventions aimed at improving FMS, physical activity and/or enjoyment among 5–18-year-old children and adolescents. Twenty-three studies were located in a search conducted up to June 2010; four studies reported on FMS outcomes, with sample sizes ranging from 311 to 1,131 participants. All four FMS outcome studies reported significant improvements in FMS following participation in the intervention, though only one study was ranked as having high methodological quality. The FMS interventions were all conducted in primary school settings, with three intervention studies delivered by the class teacher or specialist PE teacher following professional development training, and the other delivered by external staff. Three of the FMS interventions were delivered within physical education lessons, with one intervention conducted within the curriculum but in addition to physical education. Interventions ranged from 6 months to 3 years in length. All FMS intervention studies utilized a prescribed FMS curriculum, with three studies implementing direct or explicit teaching strategies, while one study also provided a web-based resource for teachers to access.

In a wider systematic review and meta-analysis published in the same year, Logan and colleagues (Logan, Robinson, Wilson, & Lucas, 2012) located 11 studies that had implemented any type of FMS intervention and assessed FMS outcomes. Studies predominantly targeted children, with FMS interventions reporting significant small positive effects on overall FMS (d [effect size] = 0.39), and similar improvements in object-control (d = 0.41) and locomotor skills (d = 0.45), though methodological quality of the included studies was not appraised. The overall effect size for the control conditions (n = 6 studies) was not significant (d = 0.06), indicating that children who did not receive an intervention did not meaningfully improve skill competence. This lends support to the notion that FMS require encouragement, practice and instruction in order to be attained and highlights the need for FMS programs. Intervention characteristics analyzed within the review were limited. Interventions were between 6 and 15 weeks in length and included between 6 and 24 hours of total session time. However, there was no correlation between intervention dose and effect size, with the authors suggesting that children may plateau in FMS competence after a critical amount of instruction or intervention activities may become tedious and repetitive, leading to disengagement (Logan et al., 2012).

Morgan and colleagues (Morgan et al., 2013) examined school, home and community FMS interventions in typically developing children and adolescents aged 5–18 years. Twenty-two studies were selected for inclusion in the systematic review and meta-analysis, involving sample sizes ranging from 13 to 1,464 participants. Despite there being 19 unique interventions in the review, only one study was targeted at adolescents, with the rest aimed at primary/elementary school-aged children. Four studies were conducted afterschool with the remainder during curricular time. All studies included in the review reported significant intervention effects for at least one FMS, with participation in the intervention compared to control groups associated with very large positive effects for overall FMS (SMD = 1.42), locomotor skills (SMD = 1.42) and object-control skills (SMD = 0.63). However, there was a high risk of bias in many of the included studies (e.g., due to the lack of a power calculation, assessor blinding, poor retention or poor reporting of randomization). Most interventions were delivered by physical education teachers or experienced coaches (n = 16). Interventions ranged from 3 weeks to 3 years, offering between 8 and 195 hours of total instruction time, with both short- (4–8 weeks) and long-term (>6 months) interventions found to be effective. Interventions were predominantly based on direct instruction models of practice and consisted of enhanced physical education curricula focusing on FMS (n = 5), enhanced and extended physical education curricula (n = 8) or simply increased time for physical education (n = 1). Yet, most interventions did not provide sufficient detail about the pedagogical approaches used to underpin the interventions, with half of studies not stating the approach or theory used. Few studies reported involving parents and implementing interventions in community or home settings.

Lai and colleagues (Lai et al., 2014) conducted a systematic review to explore the evidence that FMS, physical activity and/or fitness interventions can maintain and sustain improvements in these outcomes in typically developing children and adolescents. The review included trials that had included a follow-up data collection time point that occurred at least 6 months after post-intervention testing. Fourteen studies, involving baseline samples from 161 to 5,106 participants, were located for the review, though a risk of bias was evident. Only two Australian studies (Barnett et al., 2009; Salmon, Ball, Hume, Booth, & Crawford, 2008) could be located that included long-term follow-up of FMS effects, with both reporting sustained impact on FMS outcomes. The authors concluded that it is probable that FMS is a sustainable outcome in children and adolescents, though more research is required.

Tompsett and colleagues (Tompsett, Sanders, Taylor, & Cobley, 2017) systematically reviewed the effect of FMS interventions on FMS as well as physiological (e.g., strength), behavioral (e.g., physical activity) or psychological (e.g., cognition) outcomes in 5–18-year-old children. The authors located 29 studies, including 14 randomized controlled trials and 10 controlled trials, reporting 24 unique interventions predominantly from Europe and Australia. Sample sizes ranged from 13 to 1,464 participants, with most studies targeting children, except two studies in adolescents. Almost all of the chosen studies (93%) showed significant improvements in FMS as a result of the interventions. Beneficial effects were also observed across a variety of interventions for aerobic fitness, self-perceptions and (predominantly self-reported) physical activity levels, though there was little impact on overweight/obesity indicators, strength or flexibility. Most of the interventions included in the review targeted improvements in specific FMS, though other interventions engaged participants in general sports games and physical activity, active video games, or focused on professional development for teachers. Some studies utilized a multi-component approach, though it is unclear whether this was associated with larger intervention effects. Interventions were primarily conducted in school, though four studies were conducted in afterschool settings. Most interventions were delivered by external specialists ($n = 16$) or by classroom teachers ($n = 4$) or parents ($n = 2$) or a combination ($n = 2$). Interventions lasted from 4 weeks to 11 years, with the number of sessions varying from one in a week to daily, and from 20 to 90 minutes in duration. Variations in the number and duration of sessions per week did not appear to be associated with FMS results. The authors concluded that specialist-led and physical activity-based interventions, taught in conjunction with at home practice and parent involvement, were more efficacious than physical education alone. Furthermore, environments giving students' autonomy were more likely to enhance perceived and actual FMS competence, and best foster physical activity participation.

These systematic reviews provide evidence that school-based interventions utilizing quality instruction and practices aimed at FMS development are effective in improving FMS, though more research is needed in adolescents and out of school settings. Similar to the preschool FMS intervention literature, there is a need for stronger research designs, including long-term follow-up assessments, and better reporting and description of pedagogical approaches and intervention components. Thus, though a minimum of two sessions per week are likely needed to improve FMS competence, the wide range of instructional practices and variation in the dose and duration of interventions again makes it difficult to determine the key ingredients of successful interventions. Likewise, a recent systematic review found that teachers can improve FMS outcomes following professional development, though few studies describe the teacher training offered in sufficient detail (Lander, Eather, Morgan, Salmon, & Barnett, 2017). Therefore, despite professional development being a common component of FMS interventions for children and adolescents, the nature and value of teacher training is poorly understood and replicating effective interventions is challenging. Strategies such as professional development for facilitators are important for adopting FMS programs into practice. However, to date little is known about the sustainability and maintenance of FMS interventions in children and adolescents, and more research is required.

Overweight/Obese Populations

As outlined above, overweight/obese children and adolescents often have low FMS competence, which can lead them to withdraw from participation in physical activity due to low confidence and motivation, therefore increasing the likelihood of weight gain in what is a vicious cycle, with weight gain then impacting further on FMS development and engagement in physical activity (Lima et al., 2017; Stodden et al., 2008). Developing FMS competence in overweight/obese populations could help to break this negative cycle and reduce childhood obesity.

Han et al. (Han, Fu, Cobley, & Sanders, 2018) conducted a systematic review of the effect of physical activity or exercise-based interventions on FMS in overweight/obese children and adolescents. In a search conducted up to May 2015, 17 studies were located including 4 randomized controlled trials and 13 observational studies, involving sample sizes ranging from 13 to 649 children. Of 38 different skill tests examined within the studies, 33 showed increases in FMS following interventions, though results for balance were equivocal. While the average quality of the studies was rated at 64%, only 8 studies investigated FMS with valid and reliable measurement tools, and only 5 out of 17 studies had a long-term follow-up, suggesting some bias is likely present within the reported positive findings. Interventions were all supervised programs, with ten studies including a structured program of activities, six had both structured and unstructured elements, while one was unstructured. Only three of the studies implemented interventions solely focused on FMS improvement, while eight studies included FMS activities alongside other activities considered to impact weight loss such as aerobic training or resistance training. Six studies did not include any FMS activities. As such, the authors' qualitative conclusion was that there is a need for more enjoyable and targeted skill-development interventions aimed at improving FMS in overweight/obese populations.

Key Issues

It is clear from the evidence summarized above that FMS interventions show great promise in improving skill competence. Table 36.1 highlights some examples of successful FMS interventions organized by the type of population studied. These programs were found to be effective following evaluation through cluster-randomized controlled trials that had low risk of bias and included key intervention components such as professional development training of staff and planned FMS activities. Most interventions have been conducted in educational settings in the United States, Australia or Europe. Therefore, there is a need for more evidence in low-and middle-income countries, as well as home and community settings. The reviews also highlighted that there is a need for better quality research evidence, particularly in terms of blinding assessors to intervention conditions, better retention of participants within follow-up assessments, clearer description of randomization procedures and using an intention-to-treat protocol for analysis. Moreover, to move the field on there needs to be more detail reported in study protocols surrounding the theoretical/pedagogical approach used to underpin professional development training and FMS interventions, including how the theoretical components and pedagogical principles were applied in practice (i.e., the teaching strategies, techniques and activities). There is also a need for more process evaluations of FMS interventions to explore their implementation and whether interventions were delivered as intended. This would aid our understanding of how contextual factors influence FMS development and provide information that can be used to support the adoption of FMS interventions into practice. In particular, it is clear that FMS interventions involving researchers can develop FMS for children and adolescents but the sustainability and maintenance of programs once researcher support is removed remains a key challenge that needs to be addressed.

Table 36.1 Examples of successful FMS interventions evaluated through randomized controlled trials

Population study (citation)	Sample	FMS measure	Intervention	Findings
Young Children Munch and Move (Hardy, King, Kelly, Farrell, & Howlett, 2010)	N = 430 Australian 3–5 years	8 Skills TGMD-2	20-week low-intensity preschool-based intervention aimed at promoting healthy eating and physical activity. Intervention included 1-day professional workshop for preschool staff which provided training on physical activity and ideas of incorporating games-based FMS activities into programs and increasing unstructured active play. Intervention also included other strategies to develop related policies, reduce screen time and improve healthy eating. Preschools were also provided with resources (e.g., manual, lanyards with skill components, equipment grant) and contact with health promotion professionals.	Total FMS, locomotor and object-control skills significantly increased following Munch and Move intervention ($p < 0.01$)
Children SCORES (Cohen, Morgan, Plotnikoff, Callister, & Lubans, 2015; Cohen, Morgan, Plotnikoff, Barnett, & Lubans, 2015; Lubans et al., 2012)	N = 460 Australian 7–10 years, in low-SES areas; 54.1% girls	12 Skills TGMD-2	12-month primary school-based intervention focused on physical activity and FMS; guided by socio-ecological framework and including behavior change strategies underpinned by competence motivation theory and self-determination theory. Intervention included student leadership and physical activity promotion tasks; professional development for teachers; parental engagement via newsletters, FMS homework and a parent evening; school policy initiatives to support physical activity/FMS; strategies to improve school-community links (e.g., with local sports organizations). PE lessons included skill development tasks involving skill exploration, guided discovery and application in games.	Overall FMS score significantly increased at post-test ($p = 0.0045$). Changes in overall FMS significantly mediated changes in MVPA. Changes in overall FMS and locomotor skills mediated CRF fitness.

(Continued)

Population study (citation)	Sample	FMS measure	Intervention	Findings
Adolescents Y-PATH (Belton, O'Brien, Meegan, Woods, & Issartel, 2014; McGrane, Belton, Fairclough, Powell, Issartel, 2018)	*N* = 482 Irish 12–13 years; 49% female	15 Skills TGMD-2 Victorian FMS Manual	Multi-component school-based physical activity intervention delivered for 8 months across an academic school year including family component (parent information leaflets and information sessions) and underpinned by Youth Physical Activity Promotion Model. The Y-PATH intervention focused on increasing health-related activity and FMS in PE lessons, and providing students with pathways to access community sports clubs and activities. The intervention was implemented by school PE teachers following a one-day training workshop. In addition, all teaching staff in the school received information leaflets and an information session aimed at improving staff and student physical activity during school time, with a pedometer challenge involving all the school. A website provided resources and information to support intervention delivery.	Total FMS, object-control and locomotor scores significantly increased following Y-PATH intervention at 8-month post-intervention and 3-month retention ($p < 0.0001$), irrespective of gender, weight status or baseline physical activity level.
Overweight/Obese HIKCUPS (Cliff et al., 2011)	*N* = 165 Australian 5.5–9 years; 59% girls; 78% obese	12 Skills TGMD-2	6-month intervention consisting of 10-week face-to-face afterschool program delivered by qualified physical education teachers (phase 1) followed by minimal contact 3-month maintenance phase. Phase 1 included ten 2-hour weekly group sessions (90-minute PA per session) and weekly home PA and skill challenges which encouraged family and friend involvement. PA sessions focused on developing technique in 12 FMS using exploration, discovery, practice and application methods. Phase 2 involved monthly telephone calls to assist parents in behavior change and problem-solving barriers, as well as a single movement skill booster session covering all 12 skills.	Gross motor quotient, locomotor and object-control scores significantly increased after PA intervention ($p < 0.001$), with gains of approximately 13% at 6 months.

Note: FMS: Fundamental movement skills; TGMD-2: Test of Gross Motor Development-2; PA: physical activity; MVPA: moderate-to-vigorous physical activity; CRF: cardiorespiratory fitness; PE: physical education.

Emerging Issues

Pedagogically Informed FMS Interventions

Learning of FMS or learning in any domain is dependent on the pedagogical approaches used by the practitioner or teacher. The evidence reviewed above indicates that while a variety of pedagogical approaches and teaching strategies have been utilized in FMS interventions, it is clear that there is a need for better reporting and description of the theories and pedagogies that are used to underpin interventions. Pedagogy is often placed on a continuum from teacher-centered to learner-centered and includes a number of models of practice such as sport education and teaching games for understanding (Kirk & Haerens, 2014). These models rely on a variety of teaching styles ranging from direct instruction at one end to discovery at the other. Overall, the evidence to date suggests that the most effective strategy to increase children's levels of FMS competency is direct instruction. This finding is consistent with a meta-analysis which suggests that direct instruction teaching strategies have medium effect size on targeted intervention groups in educational settings (Hattie, 2012). However, there is an ongoing debate about which pedagogical approach should be used in the realization of FMS interventions, with the prescriptive and specific nature of direct instruction teaching strategies potentially thwarting the development of wider learning skills and independent learning (Dudley et al., 2011). Rink (2001) suggests that all instructional methodologies are rooted in some form of learning theory and initiating any change process must involve some understanding of the theories that support it and subsequent assumptions about learning. This next section will investigate Information Processing Theory, which is the theory of motor learning that underpins direct instruction models of practice. It also explores a contemporary theory of motor learning – Ecological Dynamics – and considers how this might be enacted within an FMS intervention.

Information Processing Theory – Learning through Direct Instruction

Information Processing Theory postulates that the learning of FMS is a process that unfolds in identifiable linear phases. This approach is hierarchical, suggesting that the human mind is a system that processes information according to a set of logical rules and limitations, similar to those of a computer. Information enters through the sensory system and is encoded and stored in either short-term or long-term memory, depending upon the importance of the information. The central nervous system acts as the 'hardware' whose function is to order, monitor, select and organize the information, which dictates our movement. As such, pedagogically learning from a 'cognitive' Information Processing Theory perspective is considered as a gradual linear process, where the teacher/instructor guides the learner to achieve the correct movement technique. FMS are acquired through repetition of a skill and development of each skill progresses through three identifiable stages of competence (see Fitts & Posner, 1967).

Information Processing Theory underpins teacher-centered pedagogical approaches to learning such as direct instruction. In this model, the lesson is divided into the format of an introductory activity, followed by a skill/drill practice phase focused on developing and improving technique or aspects of technique, finishing with applying the learned skill/technique in a more complex and often-competitive performance context. The main aim of this teacher-centered (*linear*) model is to develop 'technical proficiency', as it emphasizes a skills first orientation where skills are learned in isolation before the introduction of rules and game play. This model of teaching is also characterized by what Light and Kentel (2010) call a 'hard masculinized pedagogy', where the teacher is an authoritative expert passing on objectified knowledge, resulting in a power imbalance between the teacher and the child/learner. This is symptomatic of teacher-led and reproduction teaching styles, such as command and reciprocal (Mosston & Ashworth, 2008). The teaching and learning experience for the child includes both prescriptive (e.g., following technical demonstrations and instructions from the teacher) and repetitive actions (e.g., replication of the optimal technique), where variability is reduced until a performer can execute a skill efficiently and reliably. Feedback is a one-way process: the teacher tells the child what they are doing incorrectly and proposes a different (and better) way of skill development. From a classroom and behavior management perspective, the didactic nature of this linear pedagogy gives the teacher or coach more control over children, enabling focus to be maintained on the learning outcomes of the lesson.

Ecological Dynamics – Discovery-based Learning

A contemporary theory of how we learn FMS is Ecological Dynamics. This theory purports that learning a skill is not simply a matter of processing information and accruing representations, but is the constant active, perceptual engagement of the learner and context (Bailey & Pickard, 2010). This concept is based upon the original insights of Gibson's (1979) direct perception and Bernstein's (1967) dynamical systems theory. Direct perception dictates that there is a constant reciprocal relationship between an individual and their environment, while dynamical systems theory appreciates that each complex system, such as the human body, has many interacting and related parts, and that these interrelating parts constrain movement actions. When combined to form Ecological Dynamics, learners are regarded as complex adaptive systems who are presented with opportunities for action (affordances) from their environment. The concept of affordances highlights the interaction between the environmental features and functional capabilities of the individual child. Furthermore, the Ecological Dynamics approach suggests that goal-directed movements are the product of the interaction between personal, environmental and task constraints. Ecological Dynamics has led to the creation of an alternative learner-centered pedagogy which caters to individual needs and emphasizes an explore–discover–adapt = learning approach called 'Nonlinear Pedagogy' (Chow, Davids, Button, & Renshaw, 2016). Nonlinear Pedagogy outlines five principles: representativeness, constraints manipulation, task simplification, informational constraints and task simplification (for an in-depth discussion of these principles, see Renshaw & Chow, 2018). These are illustrated through the following gymnastics exemplar lesson.

AN EXEMPLAR OF NONLINEAR PEDAGOGY IN ACTION

This section uses an early primary/elementary (5–6-year-old children) gymnastics physical education lesson with a focus on rolling in order to highlight how the theory of Ecological Dynamics can be applied in practice through the principles of Nonlinear Pedagogy.

REPRESENTATIVE LEARNING DESIGN

Perhaps the most important representative learning design for children aged 5–6 years within a physical education setting is that learning is enjoyable and fun (Beni, Fletcher, & Ní Chróinín, 2017; Headrick, Renshaw, Davids, Pinder, & Araújo, 2015). Young children love story-telling, and so this gymnastics lesson is based around a story book called *The Gruffalo* which is commonly read to primary school children in the United Kingdom. This much-loved children's book tells the story of a small mouse who encounters and outwits a host of predators in a deep dark wood. Incorporating *The Gruffalo* into gymnastics lessons captivates the children's imaginations thus creating an abundance of affordances (opportunities for action) that the teacher can exploit. Within the representative learning design of *The Gruffalo*, children are encouraged to adopt the movements of the characters within the book. In a lesson on rolling, the snake is the protagonist and this analogy affords the children to move their bodies close to the floor and over and under equipment.

CONSTRAINTS MANIPULATION

Another exemplar of Nonlinear Pedagogy pertains to the application of constraints coaching. In the rolling gymnastics lesson, as children move around the hall like characters from *The Gruffalo*, the hall and the equipment (e.g., benches, horses, mats) act as the environmental constraints, and the experience and skill levels of the children are the individual constraints. The practitioners make decisions about which task constraints to manipulate based upon their observations of children's interactions within their environment. If the practitioner observes children repeating movement solutions consistently while traveling around the hall, they read further into the book and introduce one of the predators. With a little exaggeration to the story, a game of tag could emerge thus changing the landscape of affordances and taking our 5–6-year-old class back to the edge of chaos, and renew instability within children's movement solutions.

TASK SIMPLIFICATION

A Nonlinear Pedagogy-based lesson encourages learners to practice skills in their entirety rather than being broken down into component parts (i.e., task simplification rather than task decomposition). Movement creates information that we directly perceive, and in turn supports further movement in a cyclical process. At a macro-level, information-movement coupling is maintained within gymnastics lessons by having all large equipment (gym mats, wedges, wall bars) present throughout the duration of each lesson creating the need for children to regulate behavior and self-organize leading to better spatial awareness and being more socially in-tune with their peers over time. At a micro-level, the practitioner does not prescribe the type of motor skill that the child should learn. Instead, they promote creativity and exploration through the use of scenarios and/or mini-games that encourage children to explore and experiment with a broad range of movement skills, meaning movements are learnt in context, and the practitioner does not isolate skills or develop them by separating them into components.

INFORMATIONAL CONSTRAINTS FOCUSING ON MOVEMENT EFFECT

Nonlinear Pedagogy places an emphasis on movement effect, which is considered necessary to support the acquisition of both creative and functional motor skills (Chow, 2013). To develop functional and adaptive movements, practitioners introduce mini-games into the lessons, and utilize and build upon teaching methods such as analogies and questions. As an example within the gymnastics rolling lesson, children take part in a game in which the children play the part of a snake who must move treasure (beanbags) from one side of the water (their mat) to the other. The treasure must not get wet, and each piece bit of treasure must be rolled across the water in different ways to avoid the attention of *The Gruffalo*. These activities create an external attention of focus and at the heart of the activity is problem-solving, which requires functional movement solutions from the child, rather than the teacher/practitioner telling the child exactly what to do.

VARIABILITY IN PRACTICE

If the teacher/practitioner observes a learner who is not progressing, they can act to destabilize the skill performance by altering the task constraints or changing the task goal to create opportunities for the learner (child) to explore and acquire a more functional movement to achieve the task goal. In the example of the snake game played in the gymnastics rolling lesson, the practitioner creates instability in movement by giving children different types of equipment (treasure) to transport (i.e., of different size, shape or weight) across the mat. Changing task constraints will result in new affordances. The practitioner might also create different types of affordances by manipulating other task constraints depending upon how the child is succeeding at the game. In the example of the snake game, these might include space (i.e., putting two mats together), task (i.e., changing the rules of the game) or people (i.e., playing with a partner). These manipulations are made at the practitioner's discretion; however, it is important that it is understood that it is acceptable for children to demonstrate different movement solutions to the same task and also that regression in skill competence is inevitable when altering constraints (such as equipment). The practitioner must also keep in mind that as long as the skill is functional and achieves the outcome of the lesson, then it is to be accepted.

Whichever teaching style one adopts, having a sound theoretical foundation to an FMS intervention such as the ones described above will help guide decisions around intervention design and, more importantly, provide crucial answers to the question concerning why children did or did not improve their FMS. There is, however, a need for more robust evidence from theoretically informed FMS interventions, and in particular the practical application of the theory of Ecological Dynamics warrants further investigation.

Recommendations for Research and Practice

The purpose of this chapter was to identify and provide specific, evidence-based recommendations concerning improving FMS outcomes in children and adolescents. While the number of published FMS intervention studies continues to grow and there is promising evidence of effective programs, we conclude this chapter by proposing recommendations for future research considered necessary to advance the field and provide implications for promoting FMS in practice.

Research Recommendations

- There is a need for more high-quality FMS intervention research study designs. Experimental research should therefore adhere to guidelines such as the "Consolidated Standards of Reporting Trials" (CONSORT: Schulz, Altman, & Moher, 2010), the "Standard Protocol Items: Recommendations for Interventional Trials" (SPIRIT: Chan et al., 2013)" and "Transparent Reporting of Evaluations with NonRandomised Designs" (TREND; Des Jarlais, Lyles, Crepaz, & Group, 2004). In addition, studies should use feasible, valid and reliable assessments of FMS (see Chapter 19) and adjust for potential confounding factors such as socio-economic status and ethnicity within the analysis of intervention effects. Moreover, additional studies are needed that are sufficiently powered to conduct subgroup analysis, for instance, reporting results separately by sex (given the need to increase girls' FMS competence), socio-economic status group or baseline FMS competence level.
- More research is needed on the psychosocial, cultural, environmental and behavioral determinants of FMS competence. Understanding these factors is necessary to ensure that FMS target populations in need of improving the targeting and design of FMS interventions.
- The theoretical and pedagogical approaches utilized within professional development and training of the delivery agents of FMS interventions require further research and should be better described within studies. Furthermore, the characteristics (e.g., qualifications,

experience) of these facilitators should be detailed. This information will help to ensure that future interventions provide delivery agents with comprehensive training that gives them the pedagogic and content knowledge and skills to deliver FMS interventions with confidence.

- Similarly, the theoretical and pedagogical approaches used to underpin FMS interventions aimed at FMS development should receive greater attention. In particular, nonlinear pedagogies such as Ecological Dynamics should be explored. Irrespective of the approach taken, there is a need for better reporting of the pedagogical approaches and teaching and learning activities, as well as the dose, intensity and duration of interventions. Researchers could use the "Template for Intervention Description and Replication" (TIDieR: Hoffmann et al., 2014) to facilitate the better reporting of interventions.

- The pressure on school curricular time highlights the need for broader opportunities for FMS development beyond physical education. Yet to date few FMS interventions have been conducted outside the school setting. More research is therefore needed on home- and community-based FMS interventions, for example, involving parents/carers or community sports clubs. A good example of one such study is the "Multimove for Kids" community intervention, which was delivered to 3–8-year-old Flemish children (Bardid et al., 2017).

- Researchers should include process evaluation methods to explore how contextual and implementation factors influence the effectiveness of FMS interventions. Key aspects of process evaluations that should be examined include *reach* (the proportion and demographics of the target audience who received the intervention), *dose* (the amount of intervention delivered and how the participants responded), *fidelity* (whether the intervention was delivered as intended, including theoretical fidelity) and the *acceptability* of intervention to participants and delivery agents. Future researchers should also seek to gain children's perspectives on the intervention approaches, particularly whether or not they enjoyed the intervention activities and perceived impacts.

- There is much work to be done surrounding translating and up-scaling FMS interventions into practice. Advances in the field of implementation science could provide a framework for future researchers to study factors that encourage the sustained delivery of FMS interventions through existing organizations and settings in collaboration with key stakeholders.

- While there is cross-sectional and longitudinal evidence that proficiency in FMS is important for health and development, more research is needed to understand the causal mechanisms relating to how changes in movement proficiency influence key outcomes such as physical activity behavior, fitness and overweight/obesity, among others. The effect of FMS interventions on these wider physical, cognitive, affective and behavioral outcomes should therefore be further explored and measured. Moreover, given that these outcomes are likely interconnected, more research is needed on the mediating pathways that may affect and explain these relationships.

Practical Implications

Guidelines for improving FMS in young children

- Interventions should include structured high-quality programs including activities specifically aimed at a broad range of FMS, delivered for at least two sessions per week.
- Interventions should be delivered by early years setting staff who have received professional development training around FMS in order to maximize sustainability.
- Interventions should include parent involvement, with setting staff and parents working in partnership to improve FMS.

Guidelines for improving FMS in children and adolescents

- Interventions should include structured high-quality programs including activities specifically aimed at a broad range of FMS, delivered for at least two sessions per week.
- Physical education curricula should include structured and planned learning activities specifically targeting FMS development, particularly in primary school.
- FMS programs should be provided by staff with relevant qualifications and training to design and deliver FMS sessions that are underpinned by an appropriate pedagogy.
- Children and adolescents should also be provided with opportunities to develop FMS beyond the school setting, including home- (e.g., involving parents/carers) and community-based (e.g., afterschool clubs, community sports clubs) intervention strategies.
- Adolescents should be assessed for FMS competence at the start of secondary/high school, with remedial programs offered to those who have low levels of ability.
- Programs should provide girls with additional instruction, practice and opportunities to develop object-control skills.
- Researchers, educators, sports bodies and government should work together to improve the sustainability and adoption of FMS programs into practice.

Practical guidelines for improving FMS in overweight/obese youth

- Assess FMS competence in overweight and obese children to determine if additional support and remedial programs are needed.
- Provide supervised and structured extra-curricular and community programs specifically for overweight/obese children aimed at improving FMS, in particular locomotor and stability skills.
- Programs should seek to build overweight/obese children's perceptions of competence by providing a supportive learning environment with plentiful encouragement, praise and positive feedback.
- Involve parents/carers and family members in programs and encourage them to support their children's skill development.

References

Anson, G., Elliott, D., & Davids, K. (2005). Information processing and constraints-based views of skill acquisition: Divergent or complementary? *Motor control*, *9*(3), 217–241.

Afonso, J., Coutinho, P., Araújo, R., Almond, L., & Pot, N. (2014). Fundamental movement skills: A seriously misguided approach. Retrieved from www.youtube.com/watch?v=sLNppM8UmPg

Almond, L. (2014). Serious flaws in an FMS interpretation of physical literacy. *Science & Sports*, *29*, S60. doi:10.1016/j.scispo.2014.08.121

Babic, M. J., Morgan, P. J., Plotnikoff, R. C., Lonsdale, C., White, R. L., & Lubans, D. R. (2014). Physical activity and physical self-concept in youth: systematic review and meta-analysis. *Sports Medicine*, *44*(11), 1589–1601.

Bailey, R., & Pickard, A. (2010). Body learning: Examining the processes of skill learning in dance. *Sport, Education and Society*, *15*(3), 367–382. doi:10.1080/13573322.2010.493317

Bardid, F., Lenoir, M., Huyben, F., De Martelaer, K., Seghers, J., Goodway, J. D., & Deconinck, F. J. A. (2017). The effectiveness of a community-based fundamental motor skill intervention in children aged 3–8 years: Results of the "Multimove for Kids" project. *Journal of Science and Medicine in Sport*, *20*(2), 184–189.

Bardid, F., Rudd, J. R., Lenoir, M., Polman, R., & Barnett, L. M. (2015). Cross-cultural comparison of motor competence in children from Australia and Belgium. *Frontiers in Psychology*, *6*, 964. doi:10.3389/fpsyg.2015.00964

Barnett, L. M., Lai, S. K., Veldman, S. L. C., Hardy, L. L., Cliff, D. P., Morgan, P. J., . . Ridgers, N. D. (2016). Correlates of gross motor competence in children and adolescents: A systematic review and meta-analysis. *Sports Medicine*, *46*(11), 1663–1688.

Barnett, L. M., Morgan, P. J., Van Beurden, E., Ball, K., & Lubans, D. R. (2011). A reverse pathway? Actual and perceived skill proficiency and physical activity. *Medicine and Science in Sports and Exercise, 43*(5), 898–904. doi:10.1249/MSS.0b013e3181fdfadd

Barnett, L. M., Morgan, P. J., van Beurden, E., & Beard, J. R. (2008). Perceived sports competence mediates the relationship between childhood motor skill proficiency and adolescent physical activity and fitness: A longitudinal assessment. *International Journal of Behavioral Nutrition and Physical Activity, 5*(1), 40.

Barnett, L. M., Stodden, D., Cohen, K. E., Smith, J. J., Lubans, D. R., Lenoir, M., . . . Dudley, D. (2016). Fundamental movement skills: An important focus. *Journal of Teaching in Physical Education, 35*(3), 219–225.

Barnett, L. M., Telford, R. M., Strugnell, C., Rudd, J., Olive, L. S., & Telford, R. D. (2019). Impact of cultural background on fundamental movement skill and its correlates. *Journal of Sports Sciences, 37*(5), 492–499.

Barnett, L. M., van Beurden, E., Morgan, P. J., Brooks, L. O., Zask, A., & Beard, J. R. (2009). Six year follow-up of students who participated in a school-based physical activity intervention: A longitudinal cohort study. *International Journal of Behavioral Nutrition and Physical Activity, 6*(1), 48. doi:10.1186/1479-5868-6-48

Belton, S., O'Brien, W., Meegan, S., Woods, C., & Issartel, J. (2014). Youth-physical activity towards health: Evidence and background to the development of the Y-PATH physical activity intervention for adolescents. *BMC Public Health, 14*(1), 122.

Beni, S., Fletcher, T., & Ní Chróinín, D. (2017). Meaningful experiences in physical education and youth sport: A review of the literature. *Quest, 69*(3), 291–312. doi:10.1080/00336297.2016.1224192

Bernstein, N. A. (1967). *The co-ordination and regulation of movements*. Oxford: Pergamon.

Bolger, L. E., Bolger, L. A., O'Neill, C., Coughlan, E., O'Brien, W., Lacey, S., & Burns, C. (2018). Age and sex differences in fundamental movement skills among a cohort of Irish school children. *Journal of Motor Learning and Development, 6*(1), 81–100.

Branta, C., Haubenstricker, J., & Seefeldt, V. (1984). Age changes in motor skills during childhood and adolescence. *Exercise and Sport Sciences Reviews, 12*, 467–520.

Bremer, E., & Cairney, J. (2018). Fundamental movement skills and health-related outcomes: A narrative review of longitudinal and intervention studies targeting typically developing children. *American Journal of Lifestyle Medicine, 12*(2), 148–159.

Brian, A., Bardid, F., Barnett, L. M., Deconinck, F. J. A., Lenoir, M., & Goodway, J. D. (2018). Actual and perceived motor competence levels of Belgian and United States preschool children. *Journal of Motor Learning and Development, 6*(S2), S320–S336.

Bryant, E. S., Duncan, M. J., & Birch, S. L. (2014). Fundamental movement skills and weight status in British primary school children. *European Journal of Sport Science, 14*(7), 730–736.

Cattuzzo, M. T., dos Santos Henrique, R., Ré, A. H. N., de Oliveira, I. S., Melo, B. M., de Sousa Moura, M., . . . Stodden, D. (2016). Motor competence and health related physical fitness in youth: A systematic review. *Journal of Science and Medicine in Sport, 19*(2), 123–129.

Chan, A.-W., Tetzlaff, J. M., Altman, D. G., Laupacis, A., Gøtzsche, P. C., Krleža-Jerić, K., . . . Berlin, J. A. (2013). SPIRIT 2013 statement: Defining standard protocol items for clinical trials. *Annals of Internal Medicine, 158*(3), 200–207.

Chow, J. Y. (2013). Nonlinear learning underpinning pedagogy: Evidence, challenges, and implications. *Quest, 65*(4), 469–484. doi:10.1080/00336297.2013.807746

Chow, J. Y., Davids, K., Button, C., & Renshaw, I. (2016). *Nonlinear pedagogy in skill acquisition: An introduction*. Abingdon, UK: Routledge.

Clark, J. E., & Metcalfe, J. S. (2002). The mountain of motor development: A metaphor. *Motor Development: Research and Reviews, 2*(163–190), 183–202.

Cliff, D. P., Okely, A. D., Morgan, P. J., Steele, J. R., Jones, R. A., Colyvas, K., & Baur, L. A. (2011). Movement skills and physical activity in obese children: Randomized controlled trial. *Medicine and Science in Sports and Exercise, 43*(1), 90–100. doi:10.1249/MSS.0b013e3181e741e8

Cohen, K. E., Morgan, P. J., Plotnikoff, R. C., Barnett, L. M., & Lubans, D. R. (2015). Improvements in fundamental movement skill competency mediate the effect of the SCORES intervention on physical activity and cardiorespiratory fitness in children. *Journal of Sports Sciences, 33*(18), 1908–1918. doi:10.1080/02640414.2015.1017734

Cohen, K. E., Morgan, P. J., Plotnikoff, R. C., Callister, R., & Lubans, D. R. (2014). Fundamental movement skills and physical activity among children living in low-income communities: A cross-sectional study. *International Journal of Behavioral Nutrition and Physical Activity, 11*(1), 49.

Cohen, K. E., Morgan, P. J., Plotnikoff, R. C., Callister, R., & Lubans, D. R. (2015). Physical activity and skills intervention: SCORES cluster randomized controlled trial. *Medicine and Science in Sports and Exercise, 47*(4), 765–774. doi:10.1249/MSS.0000000000000452

D'Hondt, E., Deforche, B., De Bourdeaudhuij, I., & Lenoir, M. (2009). Relationship between motor skill and body mass index in 5- to 10-year-old children. *Adapted Physical Activity Quarterly, 26*(1), 21–37. doi:10.1123/apaq.26.1.21

D'Hondt, E., Deforche, B., Gentier, I., Verstuyf, J., Vaeyens, R., De Bourdeaudhuij, I., . . . Lenoir, M. (2014). A longitudinal study of gross motor coordination and weight status in children. *Obesity, 22*(6), 1505–1511. doi:10.1002/oby.20723

De Meester, A., Stodden, D., Goodway, J., True, L., Brian, A., Ferkel, R., & Haerens, L. (2018). Identifying a motor proficiency barrier for meeting physical activity guidelines in children. *Journal of Science and Medicine in Sport, 21*(1), 58–62.

Des Jarlais, D. C., Lyles, C., Crepaz, N., & Group, T. (2004). Improving the reporting quality of nonrandomized evaluations of behavioral and public health interventions: The TREND statement. *American Journal of Public Health, 94*(3), 361–366.

Dudley, D., Okely, A., Pearson, P., & Cotton, W. (2011). A systematic review of the effectiveness of physical education and school sport interventions targeting physical activity, movement skills and enjoyment of physical activity. *European Physical Education Review, 17*(3), 353–378.

Duncan, M. J., Jones, V., O'Brien, W., Barnett, L. M., & Eyre, E. L. J. (2018). Self-perceived and actual motor competence in young British children. *Perceptual and Motor Skills, 125*(2), 251–264. doi:10.1177/0031512517752833

Farmer, O., Belton, S., & O'Brien, W. (2017). The relationship between actual fundamental motor skill proficiency, perceived motor skill confidence and competence, and physical activity in 8–12-year-old irish female youth. *Sports, 5*(4), 74.

Figueroa, R., & An, R. (2017). Motor skill competence and physical activity in preschoolers: A review. *Maternal and Child Health Journal, 21*(1), 136–146.

Fitts, P., & Posner, M. (1967). *Human performance*. Oxford, England: Brooks/Cole. Retrieved from http://psycnet.apa.org/record/1967-35040-000

Foulkes, J. D., Knowles, Z., Fairclough, S. J., Stratton, G., O'Dwyer, M., Ridgers, N. D., & Foweather, L. (2015). Fundamental movement skills of preschool children in northwest England. *Perceptual and Motor Skills, 121*(1), 260–283. doi:10.2466/10.25.PMS.121c14x0

Foweather, L., Knowles, Z., Ridgers, N. D., O'Dwyer, M. V, Foulkes, J. D., & Stratton, G. (2015). Fundamental movement skills in relation to weekday and weekend physical activity in preschool children. *Journal of Science and Medicine in Sport, 18*(6), 691–696. doi:10.1016/j.jsams.2014.09.014

Gallahue, D. L., & Donnelly, F. C. (2007). *Developmental physical education for all children*. Champaign, IL: Human Kinetics.

Gallahue, D. L., Ozmun, J. C., & Goodway, J. (2012). *Understanding motor development : Infants, children, adolescents, adults*. McGraw-Hill Humanities, Social Sciences & World Languages. doi:10.1542/peds.2006-0742

Gibson, J. (1979). *The ecological approach to visual perception*. Boston, MA: Houghton Mifflin.

Han, A., Fu, A., Cobley, S., & Sanders, R. H. (2018). Effectiveness of exercise intervention on improving fundamental movement skills and motor coordination in overweight/obese children and adolescents: A systematic review. *Journal of Science and Medicine in Sport, 21*(1), 89–102.

Hardy, L. L., Barnett, L., Espinel, P., & Okely, A. D. (2013). Thirteen-year trends in child and adolescent fundamental movement skills: 1997–2010. *Medicine and Science in Sports and Exercise, 45*(10), 1965–1970. doi:10.1249/MSS.0b013e318295a9fc

Hardy, L. L., King, L., Farrell, L., Macniven, R., & Howlett, S. (2010). Fundamental movement skills among Australian preschool children. *Journal of Science and Medicine in Sport, 13*(5), 503–508.

Hardy, L. L., King, L., Kelly, B., Farrell, L., & Howlett, S. (2010). Munch and move: Evaluation of a preschool healthy eating and movement skill program. *International Journal of Behavioral Nutrition and Physical Activity, 7*(1), 80.

Harter, S. (1978). Effectance motivation recon-sidered: Toward a developmental model. *Human Development, 21*(1), 34–60.

Hattie, J. (2012). *Visible learning for teachers: Maximizing impact on learning*. London: Routledge.

Hayden-Wade, H. A., Stein, R. I., Ghaderi, A., Saelens, B. E., Zabinski, M. F., & Wilfley, D. E. (2005). Prevalence, characteristics, and correlates of teasing experiences among overweight children vs. non-overweight peers. *Obesity Research, 13*(8), 1381–1392. doi:10.1038/oby.2005.167

Haywood, K. M., & Getchell, N. (2018). *Life span motor development*. Champaign, IL: Human Kinetics.

Headrick, J., Renshaw, I., Davids, K., Pinder, R. A., & Araújo, D. (2015). The dynamics of expertise acquisition in sport: The role of affective learning design. *Psychology of Sport and Exercise, 16*, 83–90.

Hoffmann, T. C., Glasziou, P. P., Boutron, I., Milne, R., Perera, R., Moher, D., . . . Johnston, M. (2014). Better reporting of interventions: Template for intervention description and replication (TIDieR) checklist and guide. *BMJ, 348*, g1687.

Holfelder, B., & Schott, N. (2014). Relationship of fundamental movement skills and physical activity in children and adolescents: A systematic review. *Psychology of Sport and Exercise, 15*(4), 382–391. doi:10.1016/j. psychsport.2014.03.005

Hulteen, R. M., Morgan, P. J., Barnett, L. M., Stodden, D. F., & Lubans, D. R. (2018). Development of foundational movement skills: A conceptual model for physical activity across the lifespan. *Sports Medicine, 48*(7), 1533–1540.

Kelly, L., O'Connor, S., Harrison, A., & Ni Chéilleachair, N. J. (2019). Does fundamental movement skill proficiency vary by sex, class group or weight status? Evidence from an Irish primary school setting. *Journal of Sports Sciences, 37*(9), 1055–1063. doi:10.1080/02640414.2018.1543833

Kirk, D., & Haerens, L. (2014). New research programmes in physical education and sport pedagogy. *Sport, Education and Society, 19*(7), 899–911.

Lai, S. K., Costigan, S. A., Morgan, P. J., Lubans, D. R., Stodden, D. F., Salmon, J., & Barnett, L. M. (2014). Do school-based interventions focusing on physical activity, fitness, or fundamental movement skill competency produce a sustained impact in these outcomes in children and adolescents? A systematic review of follow-up studies. *Sports Medicine, 44*(1), 67–79. doi:10.1007/s40279-013-0099-9

Lander, N., Eather, N., Morgan, P. J., Salmon, J., & Barnett, L. M. (2017). Characteristics of teacher training in school-based physical education interventions to improve fundamental movement skills and/or physical activity: A systematic review. *Sports Medicine, 47*(1), 135–161.

Langendorfer, S., Roberton, M. A., & Stodden, D, F. (2013). Biomechanical aspects of the development of object projection skills. In M. De Ste Croix & T. Korff (Eds.), *Peaediatric biomechanics and motor control: theory and application* (pp. 181–201). Oxford, UK: Routledge.

LeGear, M., Greyling, L., Sloan, E., Bell, R. I., Williams, B.-L., Naylor, P.-J., & Temple, V. A. (2012). A window of opportunity? Motor skills and perceptions of competence of children in kindergarten. *International Journal of Behavioral Nutrition and Physical Activity, 9*(1), 29.

Leonard, H. C., & Hill, E. L. (2014). Review: The impact of motor development on typical and atypical social cognition and language: a systematic review. *Child and Adolescent Mental Health, 19*(3), 163–170. doi:10.1111/camh.12055

Lester, D., McGrane, B., Belton, S., Duncan, M., Chambers, F., & O'Brien, W. (2017). The age-related association of movement in Irish adolescent youth. *Sports, 5*(4), 77.

Light, R., & Kentel, J. A. (2010). Soft pedagogy for a hard sport (?) Disrupting hegemonic masculinity in high school rugby through feminist-informed pedagogy. In M. Kehlen & M. Atkinson (Eds.), *Boys' bodies* (pp. 133–152). Oxford, UK: Peter Lang.

Lima, R. A., Pfeiffer, K. A., Bugge, A., Møller, N. C., Andersen, L. B., & Stodden, D. F. (2017). Motor competence and cardiorespiratory fitness have greater influence on body fatness than physical activity across time. *Scandinavian Journal of Medicine & Science in Sports, 27*(12), 1638–1647.

Lloyd, M., Saunders, T. J., Bremer, E., & Tremblay, M. S. (2014). Long-term importance of fundamental motor skills: A 20-year follow-up study. *Adapted Physical Activity Quarterly, 31*(1), 67–78.

Logan, S. W., Webster, K. E., Getchell, N., Pfeiffer, K. A., & Robinson, L. E. (2015). Relationship between fundamental motor skill competence and physical activity during childhood and adolescence: A systematic review. *Kinesiology Review, 4*(4), 416–426. doi:10.1123/kr.2013-0012

Logan, S. W., Robinson, L. E., Wilson, A. E., & Lucas, W. A. (2012). Getting the fundamentals of movement: A meta-analysis of the effectiveness of motor skill interventions in children. *Child: Care, Health and Development, 38*(3), 305–315. doi:10.1111/j.1365-2214.2011.01307.x

Logan, S. W., Ross, S. M., Chee, K., Stodden, D. F., & Robinson, L. E. (2018). Fundamental motor skills: A systematic review of terminology. *Journal of Sports Sciences, 36*(7), 781–796. doi:10.1080/02640414.2017. 1340660

Loprinzi, P. D., Davis, R. E., & Fu, Y.-C. (2015). Early motor skill competence as a mediator of child and adult physical activity. *Preventive Medicine Reports, 2*, 833–838.

Lubans, D. R., Morgan, P. J., Cliff, D. P., Barnett, L. M., & Okely, A. D. (2010). Fundamental movement skills in children and adolescents: Review of associated health benefits. *Sports Medicine, 40*(12), 1019–1035. doi:10.2165/11536850-000000000-00000

Lubans, D. R., Morgan, P. J., Weaver, K., Callister, R., Dewar, D. L., Costigan, S. A., . . . Plotnikoff, R. C. (2012). Rationale and study protocol for the supporting children's outcomes using rewards, exercise and skills (SCORES) group randomized controlled trial: A physical activity and fundamental movement skills intervention for primary schools in low-income communiti. *BMC Public Health, 12*(1), 427.

Luz, C., Rodrigues, L. P., De Meester, A., & Cordovil, R. (2017). The relationship between motor competence and health-related fitness in children and adolescents. *PloS One, 12*(6), e0179993.

Malina, R. M., Bouchard, C., & Bar-Or, O. (2004). *Growth, maturation, and physical activity*. Champaign, IL: Human kinetics.

McGrane, B., Belton, S., Fairclough, S. J., Powell, D., & Issartel, J. (2018). Outcomes of the Y-PATH randomized controlled trial: Can a school-based intervention improve fundamental movement skill proficiency in adolescent youth? *Journal of Physical Activity and Health, 15*(2), 89–98.

McGraw, B., McClenaghan, B. A., Williams, H. G., Dickerson, J., & Ward, D. S. (2000). Gait and postural stability in obese and nonobese prepubertal boys. *Archives of Physical Medicine and Rehabilitation, 81*(4), 484–489. doi:10.1053/mr.2000.3782

McWhannell, N., Foweather, L., Graves, L. E. F., Henaghan, L. J., Ridgers, D. N., & Stratton, G. (2018). From surveillance to intervention: Overview and Baseline Findings for the Active City of Liverpool Active Schools and SportsLinx (A-CLASS) Project. *International Journal of Environmental Research and Public Health.* doi:10.3390/ijerph15040582

Morgan, P. J., Barnett, L. M., Cliff, D. P., Okely, A. D., Scott, H. A., Cohen, K. E., & Lubans, D. R. (2013). Fundamental movement skill interventions in youth: A systematic review and meta-analysis. *Pediatrics, 132*(5), e1361–e1383. doi:10.1542/peds.2013-1167

Morley, D., Till, K., Ogilvie, P., & Turner, G. (2015). Influence of gender and socioeconomic status on the motor proficiency of children in the UK. *Human Movement Science, 44,* 150–156. doi:10.1016/j.humov.2015.08.022

Mosston, M., & Ashworth, S. (2008). Teaching physical education. *Spectrum Institute for Teaching and Learning,* 378. doi:10.17226/18314

Mukherjee, S., Ting Jamie, L. C., & Fong, L. H. (2017). Fundamental motor skill proficiency of 6-to 9-year-old Singaporean children. *Perceptual and Motor Skills, 124*(3), 584–600. doi:10.1177/0031512517703005

Newell, K.. (1986). Constraints in the development of coordination. In M. G. Wade & H. T. Whiting (Eds.), *Motor development in children: Aspects of coordination and control.* Martinus Nijhoff: Dordrecht. doi:10.1007/978-94-009-4460-2_19

O'Brien, W., Belton, S., & Issartel, J. (2016a). Fundamental movement skill proficiency amongst adolescent youth. *Physical Education and Sport Pedagogy, 21*(6), 557–571.

O'Brien, W., Belton, S., & Issartel, J. (2016b). The relationship between adolescents' physical activity, fundamental movement skills and weight status. *Journal of Sports Sciences, 34*(12), 1159–1167.

Payne, V. G., & Isaacs, L. D. (2017). *Human motor development: A lifespan approach.* London, UK: Routledge.

Pot, N., & van Hilvoorde, I. (2014). Fundamental movement skills do not lead necessarily to sport participation. *Science & Sports, 29,* S60–S61. doi:10.1016/j.scispo.2014.08.122

Renshaw, I., & Chow, J.-Y. (2018). A constraint-led approach to sport and physical education pedagogy. *Physical Education and Sport Pedagogy, 24,* 1–14.

Ridgers, N. D., Fairclough, S. J., & Stratton, G. (2010). Variables associated with children's physical activity levels during recess: The A-CLASS project. *The International Journal of Behavioral Nutrition and Physical Activity, 7,* 74. doi:10.1186/1479-5868-7-74

Riethmuller, A. M., Jones, R. A., & Okely, A. D. (2009). Efficacy of interventions to improve motor development in young children: A systematic review. *Pediatrics, 124*(4), e782–e792. doi:10.1542/peds.2009-0333

Rink, J. E. (2001). Investigating the assumptions of pedagogy. *Journal of Teaching in Physical Education, 20*(2), 112–128.

Roberts, S. J., Fairclough, S. J., Ridgers, N. D., & Porteous, C. (2012). An observational assessment of physical activity levels and social behaviour during elementary school recess. *Health Education Journal, 72*(3), 254–262. doi:10.1177/0017896912439126

Robinson, L. E. (2011). The relationship between perceived physical competence and fundamental motor skills in preschool children. *Child: Care, Health and Development, 37*(4), 589–596.

Robinson, L. E., Stodden, D. F., Barnett, L. M., Lopes, V. P., Logan, S. W., Rodrigues, L. P., & D'Hondt, E. (2015). Motor competence and its effect on positive developmental trajectories of health. *Sports Medicine, 45*(9), 1273–1284. doi:10.1007/s40279-015-0351-6

Rodrigues, L. P., Stodden, D. F., & Lopes, V. P. (2016). Developmental pathways of change in fitness and motor competence are related to overweight and obesity status at the end of primary school. *Journal of Science and Medicine in Sport, 19*(1), 87–92.

Rudd, J., Butson, M. L., Barnett, L., Farrow, D., Berry, J., Borkoles, E., & Polman, R. (2016). A holistic measurement model of movement competency in children. *Journal of Sports Sciences, 34*(5), 477–485. doi:10.1080/02640414.2015.1061202

Rudd, J. R., Barnett, L. M., Butson, M. L., Farrow, D., Berry, J., & Polman, R. C. J. (2015). Fundamental movement skills are more than run, throw and catch: The role of stability skills. *PLoS ONE, 10*(10). doi:10.1371/journal.pone.0140224

Salmon, J., Ball, K., Hume, C., Booth, M., & Crawford, D. (2008). Outcomes of a group-randomized trial to prevent excess weight gain, reduce screen behaviours and promote physical activity in 10-year-old children: Switch-play. *International Journal of Obesity, 32*(4), 601.

Schulz, K. F., Altman, D. G., & Moher, D. (2010). CONSORT 2010 statement: Updated guidelines for reporting parallel group randomised trials. *BMC Medicine, 8*(1), 18.

Seefeldt, V. (1980). Developmental motor patterns: Implications for elementary school physical education. In C. Nadeau, W. Holliwell, K. Newell, & G. Roberts (Eds.), *Psychology of motor behavior and sport* (pp. 314–323). Champaign, IL: Human Kinetics.

Sgrò, F., Quinto, A., Messana, L., Pignato, S., & Lipoma, M. (2017). Assessment of gross motor developmental level in Italian primary school children. *Journal of Physical Education and Sport, 17*(3), 1954–1959.

Southall, J. E., Okely, A. D., & Steele, J. R. (2004). Actual and perceived physical competence in overweight and nonoverweight children. *Pediatric Exercise Science, 16*(1), 15–24. doi:10.1123/pes.16.1.15

Sterdt, E., Liersch, S., & Walter, U. (2013). Correlates of physical activity of children and adolescents: A systematic review of reviews. *Health Education Journal, 73*(1), 72–89. doi:10.1177/0017896912469578

Stodden, D. F., Goodway, J. D., Langendorfer, S. J., Roberton, M. A., Rudisill, M. E., Garcia, C., & Garcia, L. E. (2008). A developmental perspective on the role of motor skill competence in physical activity: An emergent relationship. *Quest, 60*(2), 290–306. doi:10.1080/00336297.2008.10483582

Stovitz, S. D., Pardee, P. E., Vazquez, G., Duval, S., & Schwimmer, J. B. (2008). Musculoskeletal pain in obese children and adolescents. *Acta Paediatrica, 97*(4), 489–493. doi:10.1111/j.1651-2227.2008.00724.x

Tompsett, C., Sanders, R., Taylor, C., & Cobley, S. (2017). Pedagogical approaches to and effects of fundamental movement skill interventions on health outcomes: A systematic review. *Sports Medicine, 47*(9), 1795–1819. doi:10.1007/s40279-017-0697-z

Ulrich, D. A. (2000). *Test of gross motor development* (3rd ed.). Austin, TX: Pro-ED.

Valentini, N. C., Logan, S. W., Spessato, B. C., de Souza, M. S., Pereira, K. G., & Rudisill, M. E. (2016). Fundamental motor skills across childhood: Age, sex, and competence outcomes of Brazilian children. *Journal of Motor Learning and Development, 4*(1), 16–36.

Van Capelle, A., Broderick, C. R., van Doorn, N., Ward, R. E., & Parmenter, B. J. (2017). Interventions to improve fundamental motor skills in pre-school aged children: A systematic review and meta-analysis. *Journal of Science and Medicine in Sport, 20*(7), 658–666.

van der Fels, I. M. J., te Wierike, S. C. M., Hartman, E., Elferink-Gemser, M. T., Smith, J., & Visscher, C. (2015). The relationship between motor skills and cognitive skills in 4–16 year old typically developing children: A systematic review. *Journal of Science and Medicine in Sport, 18*(6), 697–703. doi:10.1016/j.jsams.2014.09.007

Veldman, S. L., Jones, R. A., & Okely, A. D. (2016). Efficacy of gross motor skill interventions in young children: An updated systematic review. *BMJ Open Sport & Exercise Medicine, 2*(1), e000067.

Veldman, S. L. C., Jones, R. A., Santos, R., Sousa-Sá, E., & Okely, A. D. (2018). Gross motor skills in toddlers: Prevalence and socio-demographic differences. *Journal of Science and Medicine in Sport, 21*(12), 1226–1231.

Walkley, J., Holland, B., Treloar, R., & Probyn-Smith, H. (1993). Fundamental motor skill proficiency of children. *ACHPER National Journal*, (141), 11–14.

Wick, K., Leeger-Aschmann, C. S., Monn, N. D., Radtke, T., Ott, L. V, Rebholz, C. E., . . . Kriemler, S. (2017). Interventions to promote fundamental movement skills in childcare and kindergarten: A systematic review and meta-analysis. *Sports Medicine (Auckland, N.Z.), 47*(10), 2045–2068. doi:10.1007/s40279-017-0723-1

Wickstrom, R. L. (1977). *Fundamental motor patterns* (3rd ed.). Philadelphia, PA: Lea & Febiger.

Yao, C. A., & Rhodes, R. E. (2015). Parental correlates in child and adolescent physical activity: As meta-analysis. *International Journal of Behavioral Nutrition and Physical Activity, 12*(1), 10. doi:10.1186/s12966-015-0163-y

Zabinski, M. F., Saelens, B. E., Stein, R. I., Hayden-Wade, H. A., & Wilfley, D. E. (2003). Overweight children's barriers to and support for physical activity. *Obesity Research, 11*(2), 238–246. doi:10.1038/oby.2003.37

37

EXERCISE FOR CHILDREN AND ADOLESCENTS

Jordan J. Smith, Nigel Harris, Narelle Eather,
and David R. Lubans

Introduction

Exercise is a subset of physical activity that is planned, structured, repetitive, and done to improve or maintain physical fitness (Caspersen, Powell, & Christenson, 1985). The relative importance of planned exercise increases with age, as habitual physical activity levels decline. Very young children are spontaneously active if provided with opportunities for physical activity and do not require prescribed exercise (Welk, Corbin, & Dale, 2000). However, children's activity levels begin to decline towards the end of elementary school and continue to decrease at a rate of 7% per year during adolescence (Dumith, Gigante, Domingues, & Kohl, 2011). In addition, sport drop-out is common during adolescence (Howie, McVeigh, Smith, & Straker, 2016), resulting in the loss of a structured, regular occurring opportunity for physical activity. As such, late childhood and early adolescence represent an ideal time to introduce young people to structured exercise to ensure they accrue the associated health and performance benefits, and gain the skills, motivation, and confidence to participate in exercise across the lifespan.

It is important to note that children and adolescents are not 'little adults' and exercise programs should recognize the unique characteristics, needs, and interests of this group. The aim of this chapter is to provide an overview of the research literature regarding exercise for children and adolescents. Specifically, this chapter will outline seminal and contemporary research evidence of the benefits of aerobic, resistance, and flexibility training, as well as current recommendations for exercise prescription in this population. To align with the broad focus of this textbook, this chapter will place greater emphasis on exercise delivered in ecologically valid settings such as schools, rather than laboratory-based training studies.

There are different ways of categorizing components of fitness, but a common approach is to distinguish between the two broad categories of 'health-related' and 'skill-related' fitness (Caspersen et al., 1985). Health-related fitness reflects aspects of physical functioning that have been directly linked to health outcomes, while skill-related fitness (also known as performance-related fitness) refers to fitness components necessary for success in sports and other recreational activities (Caspersen et al., 1985). Skill-related fitness components are important for youth to develop, as they will support achievement, enjoyment, and ongoing participation in sport. However, this chapter will focus on the ways in which various forms of exercise can be utilized to improve health-related fitness in young people. Health-related fitness encompasses four distinct dimensions: (i) *cardiorespiratory fitness* (CRF), the capacity of the body to supply oxygen to working muscles for energy production (also known as cardiovascular or aerobic fitness); (ii) *muscular fitness* (MF), the ability to exert force against an external resistance maximally (i.e., maximal strength), or repeatedly under sub-maximal load (i.e., local muscular endurance); (iii) *flexibility*, the site-specific range of motion (ROM) around a joint or group of joints; and (iv) *body composition*, the relative proportion of total body mass composed of fat (i.e., adipose) and fat-free (i.e., muscle and osseous) tissues.

Historically, planned exercise would not have been considered necessary for school-aged youth, who would attain more than enough health-enhancing physical activity through outdoor play, household chores, active transportation, and organized sports. However, much of the incidental activity children once engaged in routinely is a thing of the past (Kyttä, Hirvonen, Rudner, Pirjola, & Laatikainen, 2015; Van der Ploeg, Merom, Corpuz, & Bauman, 2008). Indeed, there have been global declines in CRF (Tomkinson, Lang, & Tremblay, 2017) and MF (Hardy, Merom, Thomas, & Peralta, 2018; Sandercock & Cohen, 2018; Santtila, Pihlainen, Koski, Vasankari, & KyrÖlÄinen, 2018), and increases in overweight/obesity (Abarca-Gómez et al., 2017) over the past four decades. These changes may have serious implications for population health and well-being. Of note, low CRF is among the most strongly predictive risk factors for morbidity and mortality (Sui et al., 2013). For example, low CRF is a stronger predictor of premature mortality than smoking, obesity, and hypertension in adults (Blair, 2009), and even modest improvements in CRF can lead to significant reductions in chronic disease risk. In children and adolescents, physical fitness is also a powerful marker of health (Ortega, Ruiz, Castillo, & Sjostrom, 2008; Smith et al., 2014), and an early indicator of risk for numerous chronic physical and mental health conditions (Henriksson, Henriksson, Tynelius, & Ortega, 2018; Mintjens et al., 2018; Ortega, Silventoinen, Tynelius, & Rasmussen, 2012). For example, elevated cardiovascular risk can be detected in elementary school-aged children, and evidence has shown adequate fitness to be protective at this age (Ekelund et al., 2007; Ruiz et al., 2016). In addition, physical activity and fitness are linked to better mental health, cognitive performance, and academic achievement in school-aged youth (Biddle, Ciaccioni, Thomas, & Vergeer, 2019; Lubans et al., 2016). Given the numerous benefits, planned exercise might be more important than ever for counteracting the adverse health impacts of modern sedentary living.

Exercise is often associated with gyms and fitness centers, and while children and adolescents might engage in exercise in these settings, they are by no means the only places in which to do so. For many youth around the world, gyms and fitness centers can be costly or geographically inaccessible, and/or may enforce minimum age-restrictions precluding access (Parker, 2003). Considering the legitimate barriers to access for many youth, it is important to recognize other places in which exercise can take place. The most obvious and perhaps most ideal of these alternative settings are schools. Indeed, schools have access to the vast majority of youth for a significant portion of their lives, and have trained/qualified personnel, facilities and resources to deliver fitness activities, and a formal curriculum (Physical Education, PE) within which exercise can be offered (Hills, Dengel, & Lubans, 2015). Other important settings include community centers, where out-of-school time programs are routinely delivered (Afterschool Alliance, 2015), as well as summer day camps that are attended by large numbers of young people in certain parts of the world (Afterschool Alliance, 2010). Beyond these structured environments, exercise can also be performed in the family home or in public spaces within the local community (e.g., parks). While these settings pose fewer barriers to access the background knowledge, self-efficacy, and motivation of young people, their parents and peers will likely dictate the degree to which these settings are utilized for exercise.

The ways in which exercise is delivered to children and adolescents should differ to that of adults (Faigenbaum & McFarland, 2016), but there are fundamental training principles common to individuals of all ages that will determine the extent to which exercise improves health-related fitness (Ratamess, 2012). These principles apply to each of the different types of exercise that will be covered in the later sections of this chapter and are as follows: (i) *Overload* refers to providing an appropriate stimulus for attaining a desired level of physical adaptation. Exercise that does not provide a sufficient training stimulus (i.e., insufficient volume and/or intensity) will not result in improvements in fitness; (ii) *Progression* refers to the need for training to change or progress as physiological adaptations take place. The human body has been elegantly shaped by evolution to adapt to the physical demands placed upon it, and over time a given training stimulus will have less of an impact on fitness due to the adaptations that have occurred; (iii) *Specificity* refers to the fact that training adaptations will be specific to the muscle groups, movement patterns, ROM, velocity of movement, and energy systems being trained. As such, the type of exercise performed should correspond with the desired outcomes of training; (iv) *Reversibility* refers to the tendency for fitness gains to be lost following cessation of exercise of sufficient volume and intensity; and (v) *Variety* refers to the regular manipulation of training variables such as intensity, speed of movement, volume, and exercise type to prevent performance plateaus. The body becomes more efficient in response to the same exercise, resulting in gradually diminishing benefits, and variety ensures body systems are continually challenged to adapt. The following sections of this chapter will provide more detail regarding the application of these principles to aerobic, resistance, and flexibility training, and will provide an overview of prior research related to each of these specific forms of exercise conducted with children and adolescents.

Overview of the Literature

Aerobic Training

It's unequivocal that youth of all ages can experience training-induced positive health adaptations from a variety of aerobic exercise modalities (Baquet, van Praagh, & Berthoin, 2003). Biological maturation may be influential for some outcomes, such as VO_{2peak} in that pre-pubertal children experience slightly less improvement compared with youth at later stages of maturation (i.e., post-peak height velocity). Moreover, it has been established that aerobic exercise training can reduce visceral adipose tissue (i.e., the fat tissue found around the organs in the abdominal cavity) (Ismail, Keating, Baker, & Johnson, 2012), which is more strongly linked with cardiovascular and metabolic health risk than subcutaneous adipose tissue (i.e., fat tissue directly under the skin). Aerobic exercise has also been linked to improved metabolic health in young people (García-Hermoso et al., 2017). This section overviews structured aerobic exercise prescription for youth, with particular focus on moderate intensity continuous training (MICT) and high intensity interval training (HIIT).

MICT is commonly associated with structured exercise for CRF improvement, and involves sustained duration, non-stop, physiologically steady-state efforts. A variety of protocols have proven effective with youth, with evidence suggesting 3–4 aerobic exercise sessions per week for 8–12 weeks can increase CRF by 8%–10%, beyond normal increases attributable to age and maturation (Baquet et al., 2003). Some programs are individually prescribed and closely monitored. For example, the Healthy Eating Aerobic and Resistance Training in Youth (HEARTY) randomized controlled trial (Alberga et al., 2016) investigated the effects of 22 weeks MICT versus resistance training (RT), combined training, or a non-exercise control group in a sample of 304 overweight adolescents (14–18 years). All participants received dietary counseling with a maximum daily energy deficit of 250 kcal. The MICT group comprised of 20–45-minute sessions four times weekly at 70%–85% heart rate reserve, utilizing exercise facility equipment and individual supervision for many sessions. The MICT group experienced the greatest improvements in VO_{2peak} (2.7 ml/0_2/kg/min, $p < 0.001$), although the combined group also experienced a significant improvement (1.6 ml/0_2/kg/min, $p < 0.001$). In terms of body composition, the HEARTY trial reported that all three exercise groups experienced small reductions in percent body fat and waist circumference (Sigal et al., 2014).

In contrast, other MICT interventions have been implemented in more real-world settings. For example, the so-termed 'Daily Mile' (Chesham et al., 2018) was a daily 1-mile/15-minute walk or run at a self-selected pace implemented in a Scottish primary school setting (age 4–12 years) during school days. In a quasi-experimental pilot study, improvements were reported for aerobic fitness, body composition, and a range of other outcome measures in the intervention group (approximately 250 participants at 6 months follow-up) compared to a control 'standard practice' schools' group. This study provides provisional evidence, but limitations with the study design and dissemination have been identified (Daly-Smith, Morris, Hobbs, & McKenna, 2019).

Interval training is not a modern phenomenon (Gibala & Hawley, 2017), but over the last two decades, the concept of so-called 'HIIT' has received a great deal of attention in both research and practice. HIIT consists of repeated, effortful work bouts of between a few seconds and several minutes, interspersed with recovery periods. Although previously classified as a form of HIIT, protocols involving supra-maximal efforts (i.e. exercise bouts performed at an intensity greater than maximal aerobic capacity) are now generally referred to as sprint interval training (SIT). Contemporary interest in HIIT was prompted in 1996 when the seminal 'Tabata' research (Tabata et al., 1996) was published. Tabata's protocol involved 8 bouts of 20 seconds at 170% of VO_{2peak} pace on a cycle ergometer, interspersed with 10 seconds rest, and resulted in significantly improved VO_{2max} and anaerobic exercise performance after 6 weeks training. In 2006, Gibala et al. (2006) published results of a protocol involving 4–6 bouts of 30 seconds maximal effort (approximately 700W on a cycle ergometer) interspersed with 4 minutes of active recovery. The training elicited similar improvements in time trial performance and physiological adaptations after 2 weeks compared to a group performing 90–120-minute MICT at 65% VO_{2peak}. That 15-minutes total work period over 2 weeks for the HIIT group induced similar positive adaptations relative to 630 minutes for the MICT group provoked broad interest from researchers, practitioners, and the public alike. Gibala's group later investigated a similar protocol, but reduced to 3 work bouts of 20 seconds all-out effort, and reported similar positive adaptations (Gillen et al., 2016). There has been a substantive body of research on the relative efficacy of a broad range of HIIT protocols in a wide range of settings, compared to the most part to some form of MICT. However, earlier research tended to utilize recreationally trained young adults.

Several recent reviews (Bond, Weston, Williams, & Barker, 2017; Costigan, Eather, Plotnikoff, Taaffe, & Lubans, 2015; Eddolls, McNarry, Stratton, Winn, & Mackintosh, 2017; Garcia-Hermoso et al., 2016; Logan, Harris, Duncan, & Schofield, 2014; Thivel et al., 2018) have provided a summary of the emerging contemporary research on HIIT with youth participants. It is clear that HIIT elicits responses and adaptations in youth analogous to their adult counterparts; hence, HIIT is an efficacious exercise option for youth for a variety of health outcome measures. For example, Dias et al. (2018) demonstrated that 12 weeks of HIIT produced significant increases in CRF compared with MICT (+3.6 ml/kg/min, 95% CI (confidence interval) 1.1 to 6.0) in obese children. Based on the findings from a recent systematic review, it appears that HIIT is superior to MICT in regard to improving CRF (2.6 ml/kg/min, 95% CI 1.8 to 3.3) and body fat percentage (−1.6%, 95% CI −2.9 to −0.5) in young people (Costigan et al., 2015).

Formulation of HIIT prescription parameters involves an interplay of work bout duration and number, prescribed intensity, and the duration of the rest period, but intensity clearly underpins the potency of HIIT, hence defining a minimum threshold is important. Baquet et al. (2003) noted on reviewing 22 studies of a variety of aerobic exercise training programs in youth that significant improvements in VO_{2peak} were produced independent of training frequency and session duration, but that intensity was a key factor, suggesting 80% of maximum heart rate (HR_{max}) was the threshold for significant improvements. No clear consensus exists, partly owing to the variety of methods utilized to quantify effort exerted. The intensity of the most published HIIT protocols ranges from 85% HR_{max} up to 'supramaximal' bouts (i.e., as hard as the individual can perform). The spectrum

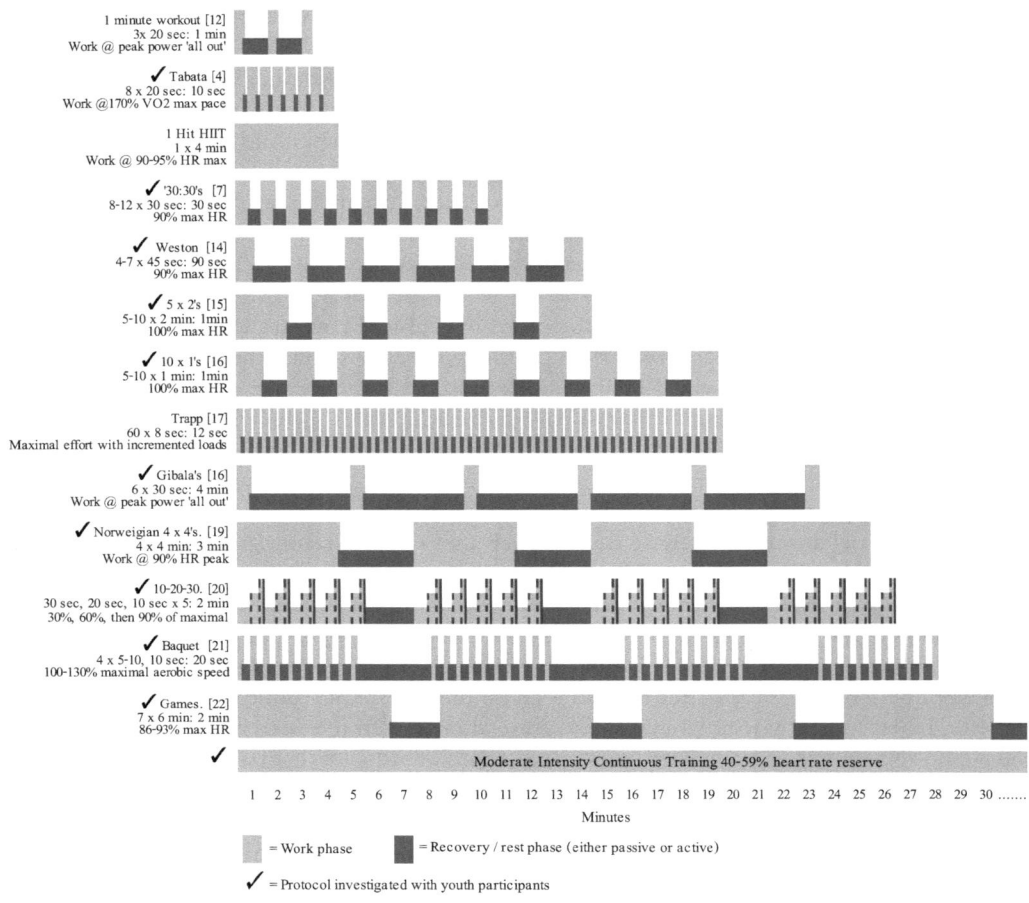

Figure 37.1 A representation of HIIT protocols in order of session duration

of HIIT protocols with some evidence-based efficacy is represented in Figure 37.1, which details the work and rest phases, and total session duration along with intensity prescription parameters. Also indicated is whether the protocol has been investigated with youth participants. Clearly, a broad variety of HIIT formats are efficacious, so it is likely that multiple combinations of HIIT prescription parameters would be potentially effective at least to some extent, facilitating flexible and varied delivery. Structured RT is commonly associated with the intent to elicit specific strength improvements and/or muscular hypertrophy. However, some formats utilizing RT exercises and formats may additionally elicit significant improvements in aerobic capacity, and other health outcomes in youth (Giannaki, Aphamis, Tsouloupas, Ioannou, & Hadjicharalambous, 2016; Mayorga-Vega, Viciana, & Cocca, 2013). The utilization of multi-joint, multi-muscle exercises such as body weight-only squatting induces acute physiological responses in youth indicative of both positive general neuromuscular and cardiovascular chronic adaptations (Harris et al., 2017). So-called 'high intensity functional training' (HIFT) is emergent nomenclature (Feito, Heinrich, Butcher, & Poston, 2018) for formats designed with a variety of consecutive exercises, targeting adaptations to a spectrum of fitness components including cardiorespiratory and muscular. HIFT and HIIT are similar but not synonymous (Feito et al., 2018), in that HIFT may not incorporate passive or low intensity recovery periods, and tends to emphasize more strength-based exercises. Traditional 'circuits', whereby a series of exercises are performed in sequence, either for a set number to completion or a set duration, punctuated by a brief rest periods are also similar to HIFT, with proven efficacy on a range of health outcomes (Mayorga-Vega et al., 2013). Movement competency through progressive instruction is an important foundational aspect if strength-based exercises are to be prescribed with the intention of soliciting repeated strenuous efforts inducing metabolic fatigue.

Recommendations for Children and Adolescents

International physical activity guidelines state that it is important to encourage youth to participate in physical activities that are appropriate for their age and ability, that are enjoyable, and that offer variety. Arguably, ability appropriateness, enjoyment, and variety are exercise recommendations that should not be exclusive to youth, given these aspects are very likely influential on uptake and adherence, irrespective of age.

Training Frequency

Weekly frequency of structured aerobic exercise sessions should be considered in context to accumulated total levels of moderate and vigorous physical activity quantity and quality. The generally considered minimum effective frequency appears to be twice weekly for structured prescription.

Training Intensity

Monitoring intensity for prescribed exercise sessions is important, particularly where a specific intensity threshold is considered a fundamental parameter (e.g., HIIT). There are a several methods utilized to express and measure exercise effort, from simple solicitation of perceptive responses (e.g., Rate of Perceived Exertion scales) to detailed laboratory-based physiological measures such as direct determination of VO_{2peak} via gas analysis, and subsequent prescription of specifically defined workload on ergometry. The relationships between these metrics across a spectrum of intensities have been described, allowing some translation between direct and indirect methods (Riebe, 2018). The detailed laboratory measures and associated prescription parameters are utilized commonly in research settings, but are typically inaccessible to the general population, and also inherently limited in general practical applicability to a range of exercise modalities. Heart rate monitoring provides a reasonably accessible, versatile, and valid intensity metric, normally expressed as a percent of estimated maximum from simple equations, for example: $220 - age$ = estimated HR maximum (Fox, Naughton, & Haskell, 1971) or $207 - 0.7 \times age$ (Tanaka, Monahan, & Seals, 2001) although it is acknowledged that such estimates are subject to inter-individual discrepancy (Mahon, Marjerrison, Lee, Woodruff, & Hanna, 2010). Table 37.1 provides a brief summary of simple heart rate and RPE monitoring metrics from moderate to maximal levels.

Table 37.1 Intensity metrics comparison

Intensity categorization	% Estimated heart rate maximum	Example HR for age 15 years (BPM)	Rating of perceived exertion (on 1–10 scale)	Rating of perceived exertion (on 6–20 scale)
Moderate	64–76	130–155	3–5	12–13
Vigorous	77–95	156–192	6–8	14–17
High intensity interval training	≥85	≥171	≥8	≥17
Sprint interval training	≥96	≥195	≥9	≥18

Heart rate monitoring technology has advanced recently, and a plethora of consumer products are now available. Indirect telemetry remains the most valid portable heart rate monitoring technique, whereby a chest strap transmits heart rate to a receiver unit such as a wristwatch or mobile device. It is important to note that the accuracy of certain devices reliant exclusively on wrist-worn sensor technology (i.e., no chest strap) has questionable validity, particularly at greater exercise intensity. Therefore, caution should be applied to interpretation of HR using this technology at present (Abt, Bray, & Benson, 2018; Evenson, Goto, & Furberg, 2015; Shcherbina et al., 2017; Stahl, An, Dinkel, Noble, & Lee, 2016; Thiebaud et al., 2018; Weiler, Edkins, Cleary, & Saleem, 2017).

The temporal characteristics of HR response to exercise onset or increased intensity should be accommodated in the prescription monitoring for HIIT. That is, HR response is such that it may not represent physiological effort in very brief exercise bouts (such as 20–30 seconds), or until several repeated work bouts have accumulated within a session. Hence, HR targets in HIIT should be utilized towards the completion of work 'sets', rather than as an expected immediate onset response, and also be interpreted with discretion in the early stages of a HIIT session overall. A useful supplementary (or exclusive) approach to intensity prescription and monitoring is the simple Rate of Perceived Exertion (Borg, 1982): an accessible, quick, and valid tool for intensity prescription and monitoring based on the so-termed 'estimation of production paradigm' (Haile, Gallagher, & Robertson, 2014). The commonly utilized 1–10 scale is simply implementable through verbal prompt, although the discretionary use of a pictorial prompt illustrating a character in different stages of physical exertion may be appropriate for youth, for which a variety of age-specific versions exist (Eston & Parfitt, 2007).

Session Duration

The per-session duration of published MICT protocols ranges from 15 minutes upward (including warm-up), sometimes progressed incrementally over a training period. Typically, session duration is between 30 and 60 minutes. For HIIT, Figure 37.1 illustrates that session duration can vary a great deal, given the interplay between prescription parameters. It should be noted that some HIIT sessions occupy similar total time per session to many published MICT protocols (e.g., approximately 30 minutes), so session brevity may not be an exclusive attraction for HIIT for youth, depending on the particular protocol utilized.

Resistance Training

RT is a specialized method of conditioning utilizing a wide range of resistive loads to increase muscle size (i.e., hypertrophy), enhance muscular strength and endurance, improve body composition, and enhance sports performance. A common view of RT involves the use of free (e.g., dumbbells) and machine weights (e.g., chest press) in a gym, but RT also encompasses the use of body weight exercises (e.g., push-up, plank, squat), resistance bands, and other non-traditional forms of resistance (e.g., tractor tires, sand bags, water-filled containers), which can be utilized in a variety of settings. Among adults, RT is considered an integral component of training for many sports, and an appropriate exercise option for those wanting to maintain general health and fitness. However, attitudes towards RT in children and adolescents remain quite negative. For example, a survey of European parents found perceptions of strength activities were far more negative than they were for aerobic activities, with parents citing concerns for injury and impaired physical development, or a belief that RT wasn't necessary if their children were active in other ways (ten Hoor et al., 2015). In addition, RT does not rank highly among popular leisure-time physical activities for children and adolescents around the world (Hulteen et al., 2017).

The claim that RT is particularly risky for children and adolescents has a long history and originates from case reports (Jenkins & Mintowt-Czyz, 1986) and surveillance data (Gould & DeJong, 1994), describing injuries caused by misuse of home weight training equipment, alongside reports of high injury rates in youth powerlifting programs (Brown & Kimball, 1983). However, in a review of experimental studies with pre- and early-pubertal youth, it was concluded that appropriately supervised programs are safe and do not negatively impact physical growth (Malina, 2006). Later investigations corroborated these findings and highlighted that injury rates in youth RT programs were significantly lower than in popular youth sports (Faigenbaum et al., 2009). In addition, the safety and efficacy of RT for children and adolescents has been formally recognized by the American Academy of Pediatrics for some time (Committee on Sports Medicine and Fitness, 2001). Ironically, there is now strong evidence that RT has injury prevention benefits for youth. Indeed, studies have shown that participation in RT is likely to reduce the risk of sports-related injury in young athletes (Faigenbaum & Myer, 2010; Lauersen, Andersen, & Andersen, 2018). Moreover, muscle-strengthening activities often form a key part of return-to-play rehabilitation programs following a sports injury (Moksnes, Engebretsen, & Risberg, 2012).

Beyond concerns for safety, it was once believed that RT simply wasn't useful for pre-pubertal children due to the lack of circulating androgenic hormones considered necessary to stimulate muscle growth (Malina, 2006). While post-pubertal youth do achieve greater gains in muscle strength from RT, evidence has clearly indicated children as young as 5–6 years can also achieve noticeable improvements (Faigenbaum, Westcott, Loud, & Long, 1999). Importantly, it is now understood that increases in lean mass contribute significantly to strength improvements following puberty, whereas strength gains among children are driven primarily by neural adaptations (e.g., enhanced motor unit recruitment and synchronization) (Lloyd, Faigenbaum, & Stone, 2014). Prior experimental studies have demonstrated that programs of at least 8 weeks can result in relative gains in maximal strength of around 30% in untrained children and adolescents (Faigenbaum et al., 2009). RT is beneficial for both males and females (Granacher et al., 2016; Lesinski, Prieske, & Granacher, 2016), and can improve some (but not all) indices of body composition (Collins, Fawkner, Booth, & Duncan, 2018). In addition, prior research has found RT programs improve sports-related motor skills such as jumping, running, and throwing (Granacher et al., 2016; Harries, Lubans, & Callister, 2012; Lesinski et al., 2016), alongside RT-specific movement skills (Kennedy et al., 2017; Lubans, Smith, Plotnikoff, et al., 2016). The mechanisms underpinning the motor skill benefits of RT are not quite clear, and may depend on whether a product (i.e., the distance/speed of the jump, sprint, or throw) or process measure (i.e., the quality of the movement with respect to accepted performance criteria) of motor skill is used. Regardless, it is plausible that RT-induced changes in both MF and neuromuscular coordination may contribute to this effect. Finally, well-designed and thoughtfully delivered RT programs can also have psychosocial benefits, including enhanced physical self-concept (Morgan, Saunders, & Lubans, 2012; Schranz, Tomkinson, Parletta, Petkov, & Olds, 2014; Velez, Golem, & Arent, 2010), greater well-being (Lubans, Smith, Morgan, et al., 2016), and improved RT self-efficacy (Schranz et al., 2014; Smith et al., 2018).

Recommendations for Children and Adolescents

The most complete and up-to-date synthesis of the youth RT literature was published in 2014 by a group of international experts in pediatric exercise science, pediatric medicine, PE, strength and conditioning, and sports medicine (Lloyd et al., 2014). This document echoed the findings of previous reviews and national position statements supporting appropriately designed and supervised RT programs delivered by qualified professionals. Specific recommendations regarding RT exercise prescription for children and adolescents from this international consensus, prior position stands (Behm, Faigenbaum, Falk, & Klentrou, 2008; Faigenbaum et al., 2009; Lloyd et al., 2012; McCambridge & Stricker, 2008) and other recent sources (Faigenbaum, Lloyd, MacDonald, & Myer, 2016; Granacher et al., 2016; Lesinski et al., 2016) are as follows.

Exercise Selection

Prior to commencing RT, instructors must be confident youth have the emotional maturity to listen to and follow instructions, alongside sufficient balance and postural control. Assuming this is the case, there are a range of exercises and equipment that can be used. However, a clear focus on technical competency should be maintained at all times, and 'child sized' equipment (i.e., free weights or machines designed specifically for the grip span and/or body dimensions of children) may be required to facilitate this (Lloyd et al., 2014). Free weights, machine weights, body weight exercises, resistance bands, and medicine balls can all elicit physiological adaptations in youth, but exercise selection should be based primarily on prior training experience (otherwise known as 'training age') and movement competency. Foundational body weight exercises (i.e., squatting, lunging, pressing, and pulling movements) as well as agility and balance training are recommended for novice trainers (Granacher et al., 2016; Lloyd et al., 2014), and progression to more complex RT movements should only occur once technical competency in body weight exercises is demonstrated. Tools such as the Resistance Training Skills Battery (RTSB) (Barnett et al., 2015; Lubans, Smith, Harries, Barnett, & Faigenbaum, 2014) might be useful for determining readiness for progression. Untrained youth have previously demonstrated relatively poor competency in the skills within the RTSB (Smith et al., 2017), but have shown improvements following participation in body weight training (Kennedy et al., 2017; Smith, Morgan, & Plotnikoff, 2014). Importantly, developing quality exercise technique may support improvements in MF (Smith, Morgan, Plotnikoff, Stodden, & Lubans, 2016) as well as reducing injury risk.

When ready, youth should progress to light free weight exercises (i.e., using dumbbells, barbells, or medicine balls) rather than machine weights, as the latter may produce less muscle activation and the former is superior for developing maximal strength (Granacher et al., 2016). Again, the core focus for youth at this stage should be developing appropriate technique, rather than lifting heavy loads. For technically competent youth with sufficient training experience, multi-joint, velocity-specific exercises with free weights of moderate-to-high resistance can be used, assuming the exercises are consistent with the purposes and desired outcomes of training (Lloyd et al., 2014). Finally, exercises should target all of the major muscle groups, should focus on symmetrical muscular development, and should be performed through the full ROM around a joint (McCambridge & Stricker, 2008).

Training Frequency

For most RT programs, 1 week is the standard unit of organization and training frequency is typically expressed as the number of sessions per week. Evidence to date suggests 2–3 sessions per week on non-consecutive days is sufficient to improve MF in youth (Lloyd et al., 2014). However, there are a number of factors that should be considered when prescribing training frequency. For example, children and adolescents often participate in multiple physical activities, including organized sports, active transportation, and general play. Therefore, prescribed training frequency should recognize the cumulative physical activity load, not just that acquired through RT. Training frequency should also be based on training experience (usually related to age), with novice, intermediate, and experienced youth recommended to train on 2 days/week, 2–3 days/week, and 2–4 days/week, respectively (Faigenbaum et al., 2016). Prior evidence has identified a positive association between training frequency and improvements in MF (Behringer, vom Heede, Yue, &

Mester, 2010), but sufficient rest and recovery is essential for achieving training-related adaptations. Moreover, >4 days/week of training does not seem to confer any additional benefit and may increase injury risk (McCambridge & Stricker, 2008).

Training Intensity and Volume

Intensity reflects the resistance to be overcome during a repetition of an exercise, whereas volume refers to the number of repetitions completed in a training session multiplied by the intensity (i.e., reps x kg). Both of these variables are important when prescribing RT for youth, as manipulations in volume and intensity will result in distinct physiological adaptations, and are related to risk of injury and overtraining. Importantly, intensity and volume are inversely related, with increases in intensity (i.e., heavier resistance) necessitating decreases in volume (i.e., fewer repetitions). Typically, prescription of intensity is based on a percentage of an individual's one repetition maximum (1RM), which is the maximum amount of resistance the individual can lift for one repetition. However, for inexperienced and untrained youth 1RM testing is unnecessary and a basic repetition range is much more practical and widely applicable. Beginners should start with low volume training (1–2 sets of 1–3 repetitions) of low-to-moderate intensity (≤60% of 1RM), with concurrent feedback provided to reinforce correct technique (Faigenbaum et al., 2016; Lloyd et al., 2014). When competent, it is generally recommended youth progress to 2–4 sets of 6–12 repetitions of each exercises using an intensity of ≤80% of 1RM. Progression of intensity should be incremental, increasing by approximately 10% at a time (McCambridge & Stricker, 2008). For some youth with an advanced training age and strong technical competency, periodic participation in RT using ≤6 repetitions at ≥85% of 1RM may be appropriate. However, such training should be very closely supervised, and if technique appears suboptimal, the intensity should be reduced.

Rest Intervals

In addition to volume and intensity, rest between sets is another variable that can be manipulated within a youth RT program. Interestingly, children and adolescents have a greater capacity than adults to recover when performing RT (Zaferidis et al., 2005), and it has been suggested that a 1-minute rest period between sets is sufficient for most youth (Lloyd et al., 2014). However, it is difficult to select a single appropriate rest interval, as the suitability of a specified rest period will differ according to the fitness level and training age of the individual, the intensity and complexity of the exercise being performed, and the desired goals of training (often related to sports performance). Consequently, there may be a need to increase rest periods to 2–3 minutes (Lloyd et al., 2014). This is particularly relevant for RT exercises requiring high levels of skill or rapid force production, such as with weightlifting movements or complex plyometric exercises. As noted, promoting technical competency and reducing injury risk are of upmost importance for youth RT programs. Therefore, rest should not be deliberately sacrificed at the expense of proper technique.

Repetition Velocity

Movement velocity, or the speed with which RT movements take place, will vary as a function of the type of exercise, the resistance used, the technical proficiency of the individual, and the desired outcomes of training. For beginners, moderate speed may be required to maintain correct technique and postural control throughout the movement (Lloyd et al., 2014). In addition, even for more advanced youth, a heavy load may mean a moderate speed is all that can realistically be achieved. However, it is generally accepted that the 'intention' to move explosively is important, even if a fast movement velocity is not ultimately realized, as this maximizes neuromuscular adaptations. It is therefore recommended that for the main strength and power exercises within an RT program, individuals with a training history of several months should be exposed to faster movement velocities, assuming appropriate technique can be maintained (Faigenbaum et al., 2016; Lloyd et al., 2014).

Delivery

Although often an afterthought, the quality of session delivery (or pedagogy) is an important consideration for youth RT programs (Morgan, Young, Smith, & Lubans, 2016). While RT is considered a safe, effective, and worthwhile activity for children and adolescents, common sense and a commitment to providing an enjoyable experience are critical for supporting safety, engagement, and adherence. Encouragingly, recommendations for those delivering RT with young people are beginning to recognize the importance of the *qualitative* aspects of the exercise experience (e.g., socialization, fun, autonomy), in addition to the commonly recognized *quantitative* aspects (e.g., volume, frequency, intensity) (Faigenbaum & Bruno, 2017). For example, Faigenbaum and McFarland's (2016) PROCESS framework emphasizes the critical importance of 'psychosocial' features such as creativity (C), enjoyment (E), socialization (S), and supervision (S) within youth RT programs, in addition to the established training principles of progression (P), regularity (R), and overload (O). Practical examples are becoming available in the published literature (Faigenbaum & Bruno, 2017), and should be considered core reading for anyone interested in designing engaging RT programs for children and adolescents.

Flexibility Training

Flexibility is widely accepted as an important component of physical fitness and is defined as the ROM of a joint or a series of joints (Anderson & Burke, 1991). Flexibility is joint specific and affected by a number of factors including sex, age, temperature, physical activity levels, exercise history, and body build (Alter, 2004; Thompson, 2008). Optimal flexibility is believed to facilitate efficient and coordinated movement of the body, provide increased protection against muscle injury, and improve athletic performance (Hedrick, 2000). Stretching can be used to improve or maintain flexibility (McNeal & Sands, 2006). However, acute and chronic training effects of stretching vary for specific populations and for individuals (Sands et al., 2013; Shrier & Gossal, 2000; Stathokostas, Little, Vandervoort, & Paterson, 2012). A summary of popular stretching techniques is presented in Table 37.2. Various forms of dance, gymnastics, and martial arts have endured as popular activities appropriate for developing flexibility (among other physical capacities), especially among young people (Australian Sports Commission, 2016). More recently, less competitive or structured movement forms targeting the development of flexibility have gained popularity among individuals of all ages, including yoga and Pilates (Penman, Cohen, Stevens, & Jackson, 2012), and are readily available in the community through gyms and private providers, and accessible on DVD and smart-phone/computer applications (Thompson, 2008).

Stretching before participation in physical activities, exercise, and sport is common practice for participants at the recreational to competitive levels. In physical activity contexts, stretching is actively promoted as a tool for preventing injury and enhancing performance (Behm & Chaouachi, 2011). However, there is limited evidence indicating that stretching before or after physical activity will prevent injury and muscle soreness, or facilitate improvements in performance (Herbert & Gabriel, 2002; Shrier, 2004; Small, Mc Naughton, & Matthews, 2008; Stodden, Sacko, & Nesbitt, 2017; Thacker, Gilchrist, Stroup, & Kimsey, 2004; Weldon & Hill, 2003). Some evidence suggests that optimal levels of flexibility may exist for some joints with regard to enhancing performance, and that sports performance might be hindered for individuals with poor flexibility (Thacker et al., 2004).

However, optimal flexibility is highly specific to the sport, movement, and individual (Thacker et al., 2004). Researchers have recommended that more rigorous experimental studies be conducted to gain a full understanding of the most effective stretching methods and protocols for individuals and targeted groups (Behm & Chaouachi, 2011; Weerapong, Hume, & Kolt, 2004; Weldon & Hill, 2003).

Traditionally, static stretching has been the most commonly used technique to improve flexibility, and has been shown to be effective for increasing ROM (Weerapong et al., 2004). Studies have reported an increase in short-term static joint flexibility of the knee, hip, trunk, shoulder, and ankle joints (Thacker et al., 2004), and running economy (Shrier, 2004) as a result of acute static stretching. However, static stretching does not affect dynamic flexibility, and a decrease in muscle force and power output is observed when static stretching is conducted immediately prior to exercise (Behm & Chaouachi, 2011; Kay & Blazevich, 2012; Shrier, 2004; Simic, Sarabon, & Markovic, 2013; Weerapong et al., 2004). Based on strong evidence showing impairments in performance when longer duration static stretching (lasting >60 seconds) is performed pre-performance; it is recommended that static stretching for each individual muscle should be less than 30 seconds in total duration – and only used for sport-specific needs (Kay & Blazevich, 2012). Long-term static stretching programs are shown to have benefit for increasing flexibility and musculo-tendinous compliance when used within overall fitness and well-being programs (Kokkonen, Nelson, Eldredge, & Winchester, 2007). However, it is recommended that static stretching be performed independent of other training sessions or competitions to achieve long term or more permanent improvements in flexibility and performance (Behm, Blazevich, Kay, & McHugh, 2015; Behm & Chaouachi, 2011).

Although there are limited high-quality studies, proprioceptive neuromuscular facilitation (PNF) stretching techniques have shown to be effective for improving flexibility and performance. PNF stretching achieves greater improvements in ROM compared to static stretching, particularly when the passive stretching phase of PNF is performed immediately after preisometric contraction (Weerapong et al., 2004). Because PNF is a complicated stretching technique that requires training, experience, and a partner to be performed correctly, the use and rigorous evaluation of PNF stretching is limited, and further investigations are needed to confirm

Table 37.2 Common stretching techniques and movement forms

Type of stretching	Description
Ballistic stretching	Repetitive bouncing movements at the end of joint ROM to force the joint to extend beyond its normal ROM
Dynamic stretching	Involves slow and controlled movement of body parts and a gradual increase in range and/or speed of movement throughout a full ROM
Active stretching	Involves assuming a position and then holding it with no assistance (other than using the strength of the agonist muscles)
Passive (or relaxed) stretching	Involves the individual relaxing the muscle/muscle group and an external force is used to increase ROM (e.g., another person, stretching aide, other body parts)
Static stretching	Involves a passive movement of a muscle to maximum ROM then holding the position for a set period of time (e.g., 15–60 seconds)
Isometric stretching	Involves the resistance of muscle groups through isometric contractions (tensing) of the stretched muscles
Proprioceptive neuromuscular facilitation (PNF)	Techniques generally employ isometric agonist contraction/relaxation where the stretched muscles are isometrically contracted and then relaxed before the stretch is extended further

the benefits of PNF on dynamic muscle properties (e.g. active and passive stiffness), performance, and muscle soreness (Weerapong et al., 2004).

Dynamic stretching, involving controlled movement through the active ROM of a joint, has shown to facilitate improvements in fitness and performance, including flexibility, power output, agility, and sprint and jumping performance (especially when performed for durations longer than 90 seconds) (Behm & Chaouachi, 2011; Herman & Smith, 2008). When dynamic stretching routines combine exercises and calisthenics that simulate the movement patterns necessary for performing an event or sport and increase in intensity, there is opportunity for movement rehearsal, increasing blood flow to the muscles, and nerve-impulse activation (Perrier, Pavol, & Hoffman, 2011). Consequently, the improvements in performance outcomes resulting after a dynamic stretching and warm-up routine have informed guidelines recommending the replacement of static stretches with dynamic stretches in pre-activity preparation (Baechle & Earle, 2008).

Ballistic stretching is considered less desirable and effective than static, dynamic, and PNF stretching given that more tension is created in the muscle and the risk of injury is greater (Smith, 1994). However, if performed correctly, ballistic stretching is more controlled than many athletic or sports-related movements, and is therefore less dangerous than competing or playing sport (Shrier & Gossal, 2000). Additionally, preparation for dynamic sporting performances requires replication of movement patterns encountered during the performance, so often ballistic stretching is the most suitable method (e.g., dance, gymnastics, karate). This said, the lack of experience many youth will have had with this form of stretching means that it should be used judiciously, and in general other forms of stretching will be more appropriate for the majority of children and adolescents.

Yoga and Pilates

A review of comparative studies investigating the impact of yoga on health outcomes supports that in both healthy and diseased populations yoga may be as effective as, or better than, exercise at improving a variety of health-related outcome measures (Raub, 2002; Ross & Thomas, 2010; Sengupta, 2012; Tran, Holly, Lashbrook, & Amsterdam, 2001). Yoga has been shown to have immediate positive effects on physical fitness (such as flexibility, strength, muscular endurance, CRF) (Tran et al., 2001) and psychological health (such as a reducing anxiety levels, increasing feelings of emotional, social, and spiritual well-being), and for improving specific health conditions (such as cardiovascular disease, metabolic conditions, diabetes, and cancer) (Ross & Thomas, 2010; Sengupta, 2012). Recent reviews reporting the impact of yoga on children concur that yoga may be an effective exercise mode for improving physical capacity (fitness and respiration) and mental well-being (anxiety and stress levels) (Galantino, Galbavy, & Quinn, 2008; Hagen & Nayar, 2014; Nanthakumar, 2018). Additionally, targeted school-based yoga programs for children have demonstrated improvements in resilience, mood, and self-regulation skills (Hagen & Nayar, 2014).

Research reporting on the effectiveness of Pilates is limited, despite the fact that Pilates exercises have been used for almost a century. The available research implies that Pilates is effective for improving flexibility, abdominal and lumbo-pelvic stability and endurance, and muscular activity (Kloubec, 2011), and as a rehabilitation tool (particularly for reducing pain and disability) (Byrnes, Wu, & Whillier, 2018; Campos et al., 2016). Evidence suggests participating in Pilates also has other health benefits, such as improved balance, posture and coordination, fitness, prevention and rehabilitation of injuries, and improved mental health, but more rigorous studies are needed to confirm these benefits for varied populations (Cancela, de Oliveira, & Rodríguez-Fuentes, 2014; Cruz-Ferreira, Fernandes, Gomes, et al., 2011; Cruz-Ferreira, Fernandes, Laranjo, Bernardo, & Silva, 2011; Kloubec, 2011). Pilot studies indicate that children enjoy Pilates and that Pilates programs have potential for improving flexibility and for obesity prevention (González-Gálvez, Poyatos, Pardo, Vale, & Feito, 2015; Jago, Jonker, Missaghian, & Baranowski, 2006).

Recommendations for Children and Adolescents

The functioning of the musculoskeletal system affects an individual's overall health status, and is dependent on the system's capacity for enabling muscles to exert force, exert force quickly, resist fatigue, and move freely through a full ROM (S. A. Plowman, 2014). Flexibility becomes increasingly important with age, as high levels of flexibility are associated with improved ability to complete daily tasks, increased functional independence and mobility, and a reduction in falls in older adults (Kell, Bell, & Quinney, 2001; Warburton, Glendhill, & Quinney, 2001). However, high-quality studies investigating and reporting on the link between musculoskeletal performance (assessed using tests of flexibility, strength, and power) and health markers in children and adolescents are scarce (S. A. Plowman, 2014). There is some evidence to support the tracking of musculoskeletal fitness (including flexibility) from childhood to young adulthood in both boys and girls (Beunen et al., 1997; Maia et al., 2001; Malina, 1996; Matton et al., 2007), and the value of fitness levels in adolescents for predicting fitness in adulthood (Mikkelsson et al., 2006). Plowman (2014) questions that lack of evidence linking flexibility and health status, proposing that flexibility may have merely been omitted from quality research studies on a theoretical basis. In fact, there is a call for studies to investigate all aspects of flexibility and health in children and adolescents (Pate, Oria, & Pillsbury, 2012), and to confirm or challenge preliminary evidence regarding flexibility, health, performance, and injury.

The measurement of flexibility within health-related test batteries has been common practice since the 1980s; however, new test batteries do not include the measurement of flexibility (Pate et al., 2012; Ruiz et al., 2011). The exclusion of flexibility in fitness test batteries is of interest, especially given the significant decline in flexibility observed in boys and girls in recent years (Shingo & Takeo, 2002; Tremblay et al., 2010), and the potential impact decreased capacity of the musculoskeletal system may have on a child's ability to develop fundamental movement skills or an adult's quality of life in later years (Tremblay & Lloyd, 2010). Despite this omission, it is still recommended that flexibility assessments be performed in schools within fitness education programs to educate children and adolescents about flexibility as a key component of overall and lifelong musculoskeletal fitness, function, and performance (Pate et al., 2012; Stodden et al., 2017). Furthermore, and despite the inconsistencies, there is evidence supporting the inclusion of stretching within a warm-up routine and within full conditioning programs for improving flexibility, enhancing performance, and preventing injury (Behm et al., 2015; Thacker et al., 2004). Given the recent shift away from static stretching and PNF stretching prior to performance, it is now recommended that a warm-up routine includes submaximal intensity aerobic activity, dynamic stretching, and sport-specific dynamic activities (especially prior to strength, high speed, explosive or reactive activities) (Behm et al., 2015; Behm & Chaouachi, 2011; Small et al., 2008).

Emerging Issues

Physical activity levels decline precipitously during adolescence, and the current generation of children has lower levels of CRF and MF than their parents' generation (Hardy et al., 2018; Sandercock & Cohen, 2018; Santtila et al., 2018; Tomkinson et al., 2017). While there are myriad factors that contribute to the global physical inactivity pandemic, it is clear that structured exercise can form part of the solution. In this chapter, we have highlighted the extensive health and performance benefits that young people can accrue through structured aerobic, resistance, and, to a lesser extent, flexibility training. While children and adolescents will benefit from participating in exercise training programs, it is important they participate in a wide range of enjoyable physical activities (e.g., sport, dance, and other recreational pursuits). As such, exercise should not be promoted as the preferred, ideal, or only physical activity opportunity for young people, but rather one of many options complementing a broad repertoire of movement experiences.

The concept of physical literacy has gained considerable attention in recent years (Edwards, Bryant, Keegan, Morgan, & Jones, 2017; Giblin, Collins, & Button, 2014). Broadly defined as the motivation, confidence, competence, and knowledge to engage in physical activity across the lifespan (Whitehead, 2001), physical literacy is arguably the most important objective of PE. However, much of the early physical literacy research focused on children's fundamental movement skill competency (i.e., ability to run, catch, throw, and kick) (Edwards et al., 2017). These skills are indeed valuable, but not sufficient to support participation in physical activity across the lifespan. Fortunately, there is an emerging recognition that young people need to acquire confidence and competence across the spectrum of movement experiences, including exercise. Hulteen and colleagues (2018) recently published a conceptual model outlining the importance of foundational movement skills for supporting lifelong physical activity participation. In their model, body weight RT skills, such as the squat and the push-up, were conceptualized as foundational movement skills that should be acquired by all young people. Acquisition of such skills requires exposure to exercise training, and even if children and adolescents do not participate in exercise regularly during the schooling years, the skills and knowledge they gain by experiencing exercise may nonetheless have value for later life.

An important but often overlooked factor to consider in the design of exercise programs is delivery. Young people's experiences in physical activity shape their attitudes, motivation, and intentions for future participation. Of concern, many adults vividly recall adverse experiences in PE, such as embarrassment during fitness testing, the use of exercise as punishment, and the displeasure associated with forced exercise (Ladwig, Vazou, & Ekkekakis, 2018; Ruiz-Pérez, Palomo-Nieto, Gómez-Ruano, & Navia-Manzano, 2018). For these reasons, it is important that those responsible for the delivery of exercise programs for children and adolescents utilize evidence-based pedagogical approaches. For example, the SAAFE (Supportive, Active, Autonomous, Fair, and Enjoyable) delivery principles (Lubans et al., 2017) provide instructors with an easy-to-follow framework that can be used to maximize young people's motivation to participate in structured exercise. This may be particularly important for higher intensity activity, which is associated with lower affect and higher rates of drop-out (Ekkekakis, Parfitt, & Petruzzello, 2011). For example, greater enjoyment of physical activity at baseline predicted greater involvement in moderate to vigorous physical activity 8 months later in a cohort of 5–11-year olds (Kruk et al., 2018). It has been conjectured that HIIT is likely to elicit negative responses in non-athletic participants; hence, it may be unsuitable for broader uptake (Biddle & Batterham, 2015; Hardcastle & Costa, 2018). Inherent aspects of HIIT noted as influential on such negative responses include the psychologically aversive nature of high intensity exercise (Decker & Ekkekakis, 2017; Ekkekakis, Hall, & Petruzzello, 2008; Zenko, Ekkekakis, & Ariely, 2016) and subsequent anticipated displeasure, compromising intention to utilize HIIT (Hardcastle & Costa, 2018). However, there is evidence that HIIT is actually perceived as more enjoyable than MICT (Bond et al., 2017; Oliveira, Santos, Kilpatrick, Pires, & Deslandes, 2018; Stork, Gibala, & Martin Ginis, 2018), owing to aspects such as feelings of self-efficacy and reward, and session brevity. There is clearly a need for instructors to consider these factors in the design and delivery of aerobic training sessions to maximize youth engagement and adherence over time.

Recommendations for Researchers/Practitioners

As noted previously, this chapter has a public health focus. Therefore, our research recommendations are focused on the development, implementation, and dissemination of exercise interventions in real-world settings such as schools and community-based youth exercise facilities.

In addition to the abovementioned recommendations for practitioners, the following represent some important areas for further research:

- The majority of HIIT protocols have been developed, assessed, and delivered in laboratory settings, using specialized equipment to facilitate detailed and accurate quantification of workload, often under close supervision by researchers. Determination of longer-term effectiveness in real-world settings needs investigation, although preliminary evidence in settings such as schools is encouraging (Costigan, Eather, Plotnikoff, Hillman, & Lubans, 2016; Costigan et al., 2015; Leahy et al., 2019; Logan et al., 2016; Weston et al., 2016).
- There is a need to better understand young people's perceptive responses to different aerobic exercise formats and modalities in terms of acceptability, enjoyment, and subsequent adherence. Tracking the responses over a duration greater than the typically implemented 12-week training program period would provide worthwhile insights.
- There is a need for more rigorous experimental studies to identify the most effective stretching methods and protocols for individuals and targeted groups. Moreover, experimental studies are needed to determine the health benefits of flexibility for young people.
- The majority of RT studies have been small-scale, short duration, and conducted in controlled settings. As such, there is a need to take RT 'out of the gym'. Training teachers to deliver RT programs in schools with minimal equipment and limited access to facilities is a promising approach that requires further study. For example, encouraging teachers to adopt a 'fitness infusion' approach that embeds resistance-based exercise into regular PE lessons could have substantial public health benefits, and would assist youth to accrue the 3 days/week of muscle-strengthening physical activity recommended within international physical activity guidelines.
- Historically, research on RT has focused on identifying the physiological effects of various training prescriptions (Kraemer et al., 2017), and in youth has focused on establishing evidence of safety and efficacy (Lloyd et al., 2014; Malina, 2006). Although the available data support the benefits of RT for psychological outcomes, this remains a highly understudied area of research in need of further attention. In addition, more research exploring creative ways to engage young people to both adopt and maintain participation in RT would be valuable. Such research may help to shift public perceptions of the appropriateness of RT for children, which despite the research evidence remains negative.

Conclusion

There is growing recognition of the importance of structured exercise programs for children and adolescents, which is reflected in national and international physical activity guidelines. Evidence suggests that high-quality exercise programs can enhance young people's health and performance. To maximize the benefits, exercise programs should be designed and delivered using the recommendations outlined in this chapter.

References

Abarca-Gómez, L., Abdeen, Z. A., Hamid, Z. A., Abu-Rmeileh, N. M., Acosta-Cazares, B., Acuin, C., . . . Aguilar-Salinas, C. A. (2017). Worldwide trends in body-mass index, underweight, overweight, and obesity from 1975 to 2016: A pooled analysis of 2416 population-based measurement studies in 128.9 million children, adolescents, and adults. *The Lancet, 390*(10113), 2627–2642.

Abt, G., Bray, J., & Benson, A. C. (2018). The validity and inter-device variability of the Apple Watch for measuring maximal heart rate. *Journal of Sports Science, 36*(13), 1447–1452. doi:10.1080/02640414.2017. 1397282

Afterschool Alliance. (2010). *Special report on summer: Missed opportunities, unmet demand.* Retrieved from Washington, DC. http://www.afterschoolalliance.org/?gclid=Cj0KCQiAmsrxBRDaARIsANyiD1qE-Z7NyU7f1dIor8cSt5Gfaby6Mcae6gppdeRJlTtJ7dxDDr1dHVPYaAngMEALw_wcB

Afterschool Alliance. (2015). *Kids on the move: Afterschool programs promoting healthy eating and physical activity.* Retrieved from Washington, DC. https://www.afterschoolalliance.org/AA3PM/Kids_on_the_Move.pdf

Alberga, A. S., Prud'homme, D., Sigal, R. J., Goldfield, G. S., Hadjiyannakis, S., Phillips, P., . . . Kenny, G. P. (2016). Effects of aerobic training, resistance training, or both on cardiorespiratory and musculoskeletal fitness in adolescents with obesity: The HEARTY trial. *Applied Physiology, Nutrition, and Metabolism, 41*(3), 255–265. doi:10.1139/apnm-2015-0413

Alter, M. J. (2004). *Science of Flexibility* (3rd ed.). Champaign, IL: Human Kinetics Publishers.

Anderson, B., & Burke, E. R. (1991). Scientific, medical, and practical aspects of stretching. *Clinics in Sports Medicine, 10*(1), 63–86.

Australian Sports Commission. (2016). *AusPlay participation data for the sport sector.* Canberra: Australian Sports Commission. Retrieved from https://www.ausport.gov.au/__data/assets/pdf_file/0007/653875/34648_AusPlay_summary_report_accessible_FINAL_updated_211216.pdf

Baechle, T. R., & Earle, R. W. (2008). *Essentials of strength training and conditioning* (3rd ed.). Champaign, IL: Human Kinetics.

Baquet, G., van Praagh, E., & Berthoin, S. (2003). Endurance training and aerobic fitness in young people. *Sports Medicine, 33*(15), 1127–1143. doi:10.2165/00007256-200333150-00004

Barnett, L., Reynolds, J., Faigenbaum, A. D., Smith, J. J., Harries, S., & Lubans, D. R. (2015). Rater agreement of a test battery designed to assess adolescents' resistance training skill competency. *Journal of Science and Medicine in Sport, 18*(1), 72–76. doi:10.1016/j.jsams.2013.11.012

Behm, D. G., Blazevich, A. J., Kay, A. D., & McHugh, M. (2015). Acute effects of muscle stretching on physical performance, range of motion, and injury incidence in healthy active individuals: A systematic review. *Applied Physiology, Nutrition, and Metabolism, 41*(1), 1–11. doi:10.1139/apnm-2015-0235

Behm, D. G., & Chaouachi, A. (2011). A review of the acute effects of static and dynamic stretching on performance. *European Journal of Applied Physiology, 111*(11), 2633–2651. doi:10.1007/s00421-011-1879-2

Behm, D. G., Faigenbaum, A. D., Falk, B., & Klentrou, P. (2008). Canadian Society for Exercise Physiology position paper: Resistance training in children and adolescents. *Applied Physiology, Nutrition, and Metabolism, 33*(3), 547–561.

Behringer, M., vom Heede, A., Yue, Z., & Mester, J. (2010). Effects of resistance training in children and adolescents: A meta-analysis. *Pediatrics, 126*(5), e1199–e1210.

Beunen, G. P., Malina, R. M., Lefevre, J., Claessens, A. L., Renson, R., Kanden Eynde, B., . . Simons, J. (1997). Skeletal maturation, somatic growth and physical fitness in girls 6–16 years of age. *International Journal of Sports Medicine, 18*(6), 413–419.

Biddle, S. J., & Batterham, A. M. (2015). High-intensity interval exercise training for public health: A big HIT or shall we HIT it on the head? *International Journal of Behavioral Nutrition and Physical Activity, 12*(1), 95.

Biddle, S. J., Ciaccioni, S., Thomas, G., & Vergeer, I. (2019). Physical activity and mental health in children and adolescents: An updated review of reviews and an analysis of causality. *Psychology of Sport and Exercise, 42*, 146–155.

Blair, S. N. (2009). Physical inactivity: The biggest public health problem of the 21st century. *British Journal of Sports Medicine, 43*(1), 1–2.

Bond, B., Weston, K. L., Williams, C. A., & Barker, A. R. (2017). Perspectives on high-intensity interval exercise for health promotion in children and adolescents. *Open Access Journal of Sports Medicine, 8*, 243–265. doi:10.2147/OAJSM.S127395

Borg, G. A. V. (1982). Psychophysical bases of perceived exertion. / Les bases psychophysiques de la perception de l' effort. *Medicine & Science in Sports & Exercise, 14*(5), 377–381.

Brown, E. W., & Kimball, R. G. (1983). Medical history associated with adolescent powerlifting. *Pediatrics, 72*(5), 636–644.

Byrnes, K., Wu, P.-J., & Whillier, S. (2018). Is Pilates an effective rehabilitation tool? A systematic review. *Journal of Bodywork and Movement Therapies, 22*(1), 192–202. doi:10.1016/j.jbmt.2017.04.008

Campos, R. R., Dias, J. M., Pereira, L. M., Obara, K., Barreto, M. S., Silva, M. F., . . . Cardoso, J. R. (2016). Effect of the Pilates method on physical conditioning of healthy subjects: A systematic review and meta-analysis. *A Journal on Sports Medicine, Sports Traumatology and Sports Psychology, 56*(7–8), 864–873.

Cancela, J. M., de Oliveira, I. M., & Rodríguez-Fuentes, G. (2014). Effects of Pilates method in physical fitness on older adults. A systematic review. *European Review of Aging and Physical Activity, 11*(2), 81–94. doi:10.1007/s11556-014-0143-2

Caspersen, C. J., Powell, K. E., & Christenson, G. M. (1985). Physical activity, exercise, and physical fitness: Definitions and distinctions for health-related research. *Public Health Reports, 100*(2), 126–131.

Chesham, R. A., Booth, J. N., Sweeney, E. L., Ryde, G. C., Gorely, T., Brooks, N. E., & Moran, C. N. (2018). The Daily Mile makes primary school children more active, less sedentary and improves their fitness and body composition: A quasi-experimental pilot study. *BMC Medicine, 16*(1), 64.

Collins, H., Fawkner, S., Booth, J. N., & Duncan, A. (2018). The effect of resistance training interventions on weight status in youth: A meta-analysis. *Sports Medicine-Open, 4*(1), 41.

Committee on Sports Medicine and Fitness. (2001). Strength training by children and adolescents. *Pediatrics, 107*(6), 1470–1472.

Costigan, S. A., Eather, N., Plotnikoff, R. C., Hillman, C. H., & Lubans, D. R. (2016). High intensity interval training for cognitive and mental health in adolescents. *Medicine and Science in Sports and Exercise, 48*(10), 1985–1993.

Costigan, S. A., Eather, N., Plotnikoff, R. C., Taaffe, D. R., & Lubans, D. R. (2015). High-intensity interval training for improving health-related fitness in adolescents: A systematic review and meta-analysis. *The British Journal of Sports Medicine, 49*(19), 1253–1261. doi:10.1136/bjsports-2014-094490

Costigan, S. A., Eather, N., Plotnikoff, R. C., Taaffe, D. R., Pollock, E., Kennedy, S. G., & Lubans, D. R. (2015). Preliminary efficacy and feasibility of embedding high intensity interval training into the school day: A pilot randomized controlled trial. *Preventive Medicine Reports, 2*, 973–979. doi:10.1016/j.pmedr.2015.11.001

Cruz-Ferreira, A., Fernandes, J., Gomes, D., Bernardo, L. M., Kirkcaldy, B. D., Barbosa, T. M., & Silva, A. (2011). Effects of Pilates-based exercise on life satisfaction, physical self-concept and health status in adult women. *Women Health, 51*(3), 240–255. doi:10.1080/03630242.2011.563417

Cruz-Ferreira, A., Fernandes, J., Laranjo, L., Bernardo, L. M., & Silva, A. (2011). A systematic review of the effects of Pilates method of exercise in healthy people. *Archives of Physical Medicine and Rehabilitation, 92*(12), 2071–2081. doi:10.1016/j.apmr.2011.06.018

Daly-Smith, A., Morris, J. L., Hobbs, M., & McKenna, J. (2019). Commentary on a recent article on the effects of the 'daily mile'on physical activity, fitness and body composition: Addressing key limitations. *BMC medicine, 17*(1), 96.

Decker, E. S., & Ekkekakis,. P. (2017). More efficient, perhaps, but at what price? Pleasure and enjoyment responses to high-intensity interval exercise in low-active women with obesity. *Psychology of Sport and Exercise.* doi:10.1016/j.psychsport.2016.09.005

Dias, K. A., Ingul, C. B., Tjønna, A. E., Keating, S. E., Gomersall, S. R., Follestad, T.,. . . Haram, M. (2018). Effect of high-intensity interval training on fitness, fat mass and cardiometabolic biomarkers in children with obesity: A randomised controlled trial. *Sports Medicine, 48*(3), 733–746.

Dumith, S. C., Gigante, D. P., Domingues, M. R., & Kohl, H. W. (2011). Physical activity change during adolescence: A systematic review and a pooled analysis. *International Journal of Epidemiology, 40*(3), 685–698.

Eddolls, W. T. B., McNarry, M. A., Stratton, G., Winn, C. O. N., & Mackintosh, K. A. (2017). High-intensity interval training interventions in children and adolescents: A systematic review. *Sports Medicine, 47*(11), 2363–2374. doi:10.1007/s40279-017-0753-8

Edwards, L. C., Bryant, A. S., Keegan, R. J., Morgan, K., & Jones, A. M. (2017). Definitions, foundations and associations of physical literacy: A systematic review. *Sports Medicine, 47*(1), 113–126.

Ekelund, U., Anderssen, S., Froberg, K., Sardinha, L. B., Andersen, L. B., & Brage, S. (2007). Independent associations of physical activity and cardiorespiratory fitness with metabolic risk factors in children: The European Youth Heart Study. *Diabetologia, 50*(9), 1832–1840.

Ekkekakis, P., Hall, E. E., & Petruzzello, S. J. (2008). The relationship between exercise intensity and affective responses demystified: To crack the 40-year-old nut, replace the 40-year-old nutcracker! *Annals of Behavioral Medicine, 35*(2), 136–149. doi:10.1007/s12160-008-9025-z

Ekkekakis, P., Parfitt, G., & Petruzzello, S. J. (2011). The pleasure and displeasure people feel when they exercise at different intensities. *Sports Medicine, 41*(8), 641–671.

Eston, R., & Parfitt, G. (2007). Perceived exertion. In N. Armstrong (Ed.), *Paediatric exercise physiology* (pp. 275–297). Philadelphia, PA: Elsevier.

Evenson, K. R., Goto, M. M., & Furberg, R. D. (2015). Systematic review of the validity and reliability of consumer-wearable activity trackers. *International Journal of Behavioral Nutrition and Physical Activity, 12*, 159. doi:10.1186/s12966-015-0314-1

Faigenbaum, A. D., & Bruno, L. E. (2017). A fundamental approach for treating pediatric dynapenia in kids. *ACSM's Health & Fitness Journal, 21*(4), 18–24.

Faigenbaum, A. D., Kraemer, W. J., Blimkie, C. J., Jeffreys, I., Micheli, L. J., Nitka, M., & Rowland, T. W. (2009). Youth resistance training: Updated position statement paper from the national strength and conditioning association. *The Journal of Strength & Conditioning Research, 23*, S60–S79.

Faigenbaum, A. D., Lloyd, R. S., MacDonald, J., & Myer, G. D. (2016). Citius, Altius, Fortius: Beneficial effects of resistance training for young athletes: Narrative review. *British Journal of Sports Medicine, 50*(1), 3–7.

Faigenbaum, A. D., & McFarland, J. E. (2016). Resistance training for kids: Right from the start. *ACSM's Health & Fitness Journal, 20*(5), 16–22.

Faigenbaum, A. D., & Myer, G. D. (2010). Resistance training among young athletes: Safety, efficacy and injury prevention effects. *British Journal of Sports Medicine, 44*(1), 56–63.

Faigenbaum, A. D., Westcott, W. L., Loud, R. L., & Long, C. (1999). The effects of different resistance training protocols on muscular strength and endurance development in children. *Pediatrics, 104*(1), e5.

Feito, Y., Heinrich, K. M., Butcher, S. J., & Poston, W. S. C. (2018). High-intensity functional training (HIFT): Definition and research implications for improved fitness. *Sports (Basel), 6*(3). doi:10.3390/sports6030076

Fox, S. M., 3rd, Naughton, J. P., & Haskell, W. L. (1971). Physical activity and the prevention of coronary heart disease. *Annals of Clinical Research, 3*(6), 404–432.

Galantino, M. L., Galbavy, R., & Quinn, L. (2008). Therapeutic effects of yoga for children: A systematic review of the literature. *Pediatric Physical Therapy, 20*(1), 66–80.

García-Hermoso, A., Ceballos-Ceballos, R., Poblete-Aro, C., Hackney, A., Mota, J., & Ramírez-Vélez, R. (2017). Exercise, adipokines and pediatric obesity: A meta-analysis of randomized controlled trials. *International Journal of Obesity, 41*(4), 475.

Garcia-Hermoso, A., Cerrillo-Urbina, A. J., Herrera-Valenzuela, T., Cristi-Montero, C., Saavedra, J. M., & Martinez-Vizcaino, V. (2016). Is high-intensity interval training more effective on improving cardiometabolic risk and aerobic capacity than other forms of exercise in overweight and obese youth? A meta-analysis. *Obesity Reviews, 17*(6), 531–540. doi:10.1111/obr.12395

Giannaki, C. D., Aphamis, G., Tsouloupas, C. N., Ioannou, Y., & Hadjicharalambous, M. (2016). An eight week school-based intervention with circuit training improves physical fitness and reduces body fat in male adolescents. *The Journal of Sports Medicine and Physical Fitness, 56*(7–8), 894–900.

Gibala, M. J., & Hawley, J. A. (2017). Sprinting toward fitness. *Cell Metabolism, 25*(5), 988–990. doi:10.1016/j.cmet.2017.04.030

Gibala, M. J., Little, J. P., Van Essen, M., Wilkin, G. P., Burgomaster, K. A., Safdar, A., . . . Tarnopolsky, M. A. (2006). Short-term sprint interval versus traditional endurance training: Similar initial adaptations in human skeletal muscle and exercise performance. *The Journal of Physiology, 575*(3), 901–911.

Giblin, S., Collins, D., & Button, C. (2014). Physical literacy: Importance, assessment and future directions. *Sports Medicine, 44*(9), 1177–1184.

Gillen, J. B., Martin, B. J., MacInnis, M. J., Skelly, L. E., Tarnopolsky, M. A., & Gibala, M. J. (2016). Twelve weeks of sprint interval training improves indices of cardiometabolic health similar to traditional endurance training despite a five-fold lower exercise volume and time commitment. *PLoS One, 11*(4), e0154075. doi:10.1371/journal.pone.0154075

González-Gálvez, N., Poyatos, M. C., Pardo, P. J. M., Vale, R. G. d. S., & Feito, Y. (2015). Effects of a pilates school program on hamstrings flexibility of adolescents. *Revista Brasileira de Medicina do Esporte, 21*, 302–307.

Gould, J. H., & DeJong, A. R. (1994). Injuries to children involving home exercise equipment. *Archives of Pediatrics & Adolescent Medicine, 148*(10), 1107–1109.

Granacher, U., Lesinski, M., Büsch, D., Muehlbauer, T., Prieske, O., Puta, C., . . . Behm, D. G. (2016). Effects of resistance training in youth athletes on muscular fitness and athletic performance: A conceptual model for long-term athlete development. *Frontiers in Physiology, 7*, 164.

Hagen, I., & Nayar, U. S. (2014). Yoga for children and young people's mental health and well-being: Research review and reflections on the mental health potentials of yoga. *Frontiers in Psychiatry, 5*, 35. doi:10.3389/fpsyt.2014.00035

Haile, L., Gallagher, M., & Robertson, J. R. (2014). The estimation–production paradigm for exercise intensity self-regulation. In *Perceived exertion laboratory manual* (pp. 111–129). New York, NY: Springer New York.

Hardcastle, S. J., & Costa, E. C. (2018). Hardcastle takes a hit! Commentary: Why sprint interval training is inappropriate for a largely sedentary population. *Annals of Behavioral Science.* doi:10.21767/2471-7975.100032s

Hardy, L. L., Merom, D., Thomas, M., & Peralta, L. (2018). 30-Year changes in Australian children's standing broad jump: 1985–2015. *Journal of Science and Medicine in Sport, 21*, 1057–1061.

Harries, S. K., Lubans, D. R., & Callister, R. (2012). Resistance training to improve power and sports performance in adolescent athletes: A systematic review and meta-analysis. *Journal of Science and Medicine in Sport, 15*(6), 532–540.

Harris, N. K., Dulson, D. K., Logan, G. R. M., Warbrick, I. B., Merien, F. L. R., & Lubans, D. R. (2017). Acute responses to resistance and high-intensity interval training in early adolescents. *The Journal of Strength & Conditioning Research, 31*(5), 1177–1186. doi:10.1519/jsc.0000000000001590

Hedrick, A. (2000). Dynamic flexibility training. *Strength & Conditioning Journal, 22*(5), 33.

Henriksson, H., Henriksson, P., Tynelius, P., & Ortega, F. B. (2018). Muscular weakness in adolescence is associated with disability 30 years later: A population-based cohort study of 1.2 million men. *British Journal of Sports Medicine*, doi:10.1136/bjsports-2017-098723

Herbert, R. D., & Gabriel, M. (2002). Effects of stretching before and after exercising on muscle soreness and risk of injury: Systematic review. *BMJ, 325*(7362), 468.

Herman, S. L., & Smith, D. T. (2008). Four-week dynamic stretching warm-up intervention elicits longer-term performance benefits. *The Journal of Strength & Conditioning Research, 22*(4), 1286–1297. doi:10.1519/JSC.0b013e318173da50

Hills, A. P., Dengel, D. R., & Lubans, D. R. (2015). Supporting public health priorities: Recommendations for physical education and physical activity promotion in schools. *Progress in Cardiovascular Diseases, 57*(4), 368–374.

Howie, E. K., McVeigh, J. A., Smith, A. J., & Straker, L. M. (2016). Organized sport trajectories from childhood to adolescence and health associations. *Medicine & Science in Sports & Exercise, 48*(7), 1331–1339. doi:10.1249/mss.0000000000000894

Hulteen, R. M., Morgan, P. J., Barnett, L. M., Stodden, D. F., & Lubans, D. R. (2018). Development of foundational movement skills: A conceptual model for physical activity across the lifespan. *Sports Medicine, 48*(7), 1533–1540.

Hulteen, R. M., Smith, J. J., Morgan, P. J., Barnett, L. M., Hallal, P. C., Colyvas, K., & Lubans, D. R. (2017). Global participation in sport and leisure-time physical activities: A systematic review and meta-analysis. *Preventive Medicine, 95*, 14–25. doi:10.1016/j.ypmed.2016.11.027

Ismail, I., Keating, S., Baker, M., & Johnson, N. (2012). A systematic review and meta-analysis of the effect of aerobic vs. resistance exercise training on visceral fat. *Obesity Reviews, 13*(1), 68–91.

Jago, R., Jonker, M. L., Missaghian, M., & Baranowski, T. (2006). Effect of 4 weeks of Pilates on the body composition of young girls. *Preventive Medicine, 42*(3), 177–180. doi:10.1016/j.ypmed.2005.11.010

Jenkins, N., & Mintowt-Czyz, W. (1986). Bilateral fracture-separations of the distal radial epiphyses during weight-lifting. *British Journal of Sports Medicine, 20*(2), 72.

Kay, A. D., & Blazevich, A. J. (2012). Effect of acute static stretch on maximal muscle performance: A systematic review. *Medicine & Science in Sports & Exercise, 44*(1), 154–164. doi:10.1249/MSS.0b013e318225cb27

Kell, R. T., Bell, G., & Quinney, A. (2001). Musculoskeletal fitness, health outcomes and quality of life. *Sports Med, 31*(12), 863–873.

Kennedy, S. G., Smith, J. J., Morgan, P. J., Peralta, L. R., Hilland, T. A., Eather, N., . . . Salmon, J. (2017). Implementing resistance training in secondary schools: A cluster RCT. *Medicine and Science in Sports and Exercise, 50*(1), 62–72.

Kloubec, J. (2011). Pilates: How does it work and who needs it? *Muscles, Ligaments and Tendons Journal, 1*(2), 61–66.

Kokkonen, J., Nelson, A. G., Eldredge, C., & Winchester, J. B. (2007). Chronic static stretching improves exercise performance. *Medicine & Science in Sports & Exercise, 39*(10), 1825–1831. doi:10.1249/mss.0b013e3181238a2b

Kraemer, W. J., Ratamess, N. A., Flanagan, S. D., Shurley, J. P., Todd, J. S., & Todd, T. C. (2017). Understanding the science of resistance training: An evolutionary perspective. *Sports Medicine, 47*(12), 2415–2435.

Kruk, M., Zarychta, K., Horodyska, K., Boberska, M., Scholz, U., Radtke, T., & Luszczynska, A. (2018). From enjoyment to physical activity or from physical activity to enjoyment? Longitudinal associations in parent-child dyads. *Psychology and Health*, 1–15. doi:10.1080/08870446.2018.1489049

Kyttä, M., Hirvonen, J., Rudner, J., Pirjola, I., & Laatikainen, T. (2015). The last free-range children? Children's independent mobility in Finland in the 1990s and 2010s. *Journal of Transport Geography, 47*, 1–12.

Ladwig, M. A., Vazou, S., & Ekkekakis, P. (2018). "My best memory is when I was done with it": PE memories are associated with adult sedentary behavior. *Translational Journal of the American College of Sports Medicine, 3*(16), 119–129.

Lauersen, J. B., Andersen, T. E., & Andersen, L. B. (2018). Strength training as superior, dose-dependent and safe prevention of acute and overuse sports injuries: A systematic review, qualitative analysis and meta-analysis. *British Journal of Sports Medicine*, doi:10.1136/bjsports-2018-099078

Leahy, A. A., Eather, N., Smith, J. J., Hillman, C. H., Morgan, P. J., Plotnikoff, R. C., . . . Lubans, D. R. (2019). Feasibility and preliminary efficacy of a teacher-facilitated high-intensity interval training intervention for older adolescents. *Pediatric Exercise Science, 31*(1), 107–117. doi:10.1123/pes.2018-0039

Lesinski, M., Prieske, O., & Granacher, U. (2016). Effects and dose–response relationships of resistance training on physical performance in youth athletes: A systematic review and meta-analysis. *British Journal of Sports Medicine, 50*(13), 781–795.

Lloyd, R. S., Faigenbaum, A. D., Myer, G., Stone, M., Oliver, J., Jeffreys, I., . . . Pierce, K. (2012). UKSCA position statement: Youth resistance training. *Prof Strength Cond, 26*, 26–39.

Lloyd, R. S., Faigenbaum, A. D., & Stone, M. H. (2014). Position statement on youth resistance training: The 2014 international consensus. *British Journal of Sports Medicine, 48*(7), 498–505. doi:10.1136/bjsports-2013-092952

Logan, G. R., Harris, N., Duncan, S., Plank, L. D., Merien, F., & Schofield, G. (2016). Low-active male adolescents: A dose response to high-intensity interval training. *Medicine & Science in Sports & Exercise, 48*(3), 481–490. doi:10.1249/MSS.0000000000000799

Logan, G. R., Harris, N., Duncan, S., & Schofield, G. (2014). A review of adolescent high-intensity interval training. *Sports Medicine, 44*(8), 1071–1085. doi:10.1007/s40279-014-0187-5

Lubans, D., Richards, J., Hillman, C., Faulkner, G., Beauchamp, M., Nilsson, M., . . . Biddle, S. (2016). Physical activity for cognitive and mental health in youth: A systematic review of mechanisms. *Pediatrics, 138*(3), e20161642. doi:10.1542/peds.2016-1642

Lubans, D. R., Lonsdale, C., Cohen, K., Eather, N., Beauchamp, M. R., Morgan, P. J., . . . Smith, J. J. (2017). Framework for the design and delivery of organized physical activity sessions for children and adolescents: Rationale and description of the 'SAAFE' teaching principles. *International journal of behavioral nutrition and physical activity, 14*(1), 24.

Lubans, D. R., Smith, J. J., Harries, S. K., Barnett, L. M., & Faigenbaum, A. D. (2014). Development, test-retest reliability, and construct validity of the resistance training skills battery. *The Journal of Strength & Conditioning Research, 28*(5), 1373–1380.

Lubans, D. R., Smith, J. J., Morgan, P. J., Beauchamp, M. R., Miller, A., Lonsdale, C., . . . Dally, K. (2016). Mediators of psychological well-being in adolescent boys. *Journal of Adolescent Health, 58*(2), 230–236. doi:10.1016/j.jadohealth.2015.10.010

Lubans, D. R., Smith, J. J., Plotnikoff, R. C., Dally, K. A., Okely, A. D., Salmon, J., & Morgan, P. J. (2016). Assessing the sustained impact of a school-based obesity prevention program for adolescent boys: The ATLAS cluster randomized controlled trial. *International Journal of Behavioral Nutrition and Physical Activity, 13*, 92. doi:10.1186/s12966-016-0420-8

Mahon, A. D., Marjerrison, A. D., Lee, J. D., Woodruff, M. E., & Hanna, L. E. (2010). Evaluating the prediction of maximal heart rate in children and adolescents. *Research Quarterly for Exercise and Sport, 81*(4), 466–471. doi:10.1080/02701367.2010.10599707

Maia, J. A., Lefevre, J., Claessens, A., Renson, R., Vanreusel, B., & Beunen, G. (2001). Tracking of physical fitness during adolescence: A panel study in boys. *Medicine & Science in Sports & Exercise, 33*(5), 765–771.

Malina, R. M. (1996). Tracking of physical activity and physical fitness across the lifespan. *Research Quarterly for Exercise and Sport, 67*, S48–S57.

Malina, R. M. (2006). Weight training in youth-growth, maturation, and safety: An evidence-based review. *Clinical Journal of Sport Medicine, 16*(6), 478–487.

Matton, L., Duvigneaud, N., Wijndaele, K., Philippaerts, R., Duquet, W., Beunen, G., . . . Lefevre, J. (2007). Secular trends in anthropometric characteristics, physical fitness, physical activity, and biological maturation in Flemish adolescents between 1969 and 2005. *American Journal of Human Biology, 19*(3), 345–357.

Mayorga-Vega, D., Viciana, J., & Cocca, A. (2013). Effects of a circuit training program on muscular and cardiovascular endurance and their maintenance in schoolchildren. *Journal of Human Kinetics, 37*, 153–160. doi:10.2478/hukin-2013-0036

McCambridge, T., & Stricker, P. (2008). Strength training by children and adolescents. *Pediatrics, 121*(4), 835–840.

McNeal, J. R., & Sands, W. A. (2006). Stretching for performance enhancement. *Current Sports Medicine Reports, 5*(3), 141–146.

Mikkelsson, L., Kaprio, J., Kautiainen, H., Kujals, U., Mikkelsson, M., & Nupponen, H. (2006). School fitness tests as predictors of adult health- related fitness. *American Journal of Human Biology, 18*, 342–349.

Mintjens, S., Menting, M. D., Daams, J. G., van Poppel, M. N., Roseboom, T. J., & Gemke, R. J. (2018). Cardiorespiratory fitness in childhood and adolescence affects future cardiovascular risk factors: A systematic review of longitudinal studies. *Sports Medicine, 48*(11), 2577–2605.

Moksnes, H., Engebretsen, L., & Risberg, M. A. (2012). Management of anterior cruciate ligament injuries in skeletally immature individuals. *Journal of Orthopaedic & Sports Physical Therapy, 42*(3), 172–183.

Morgan, P., Saunders, K., & Lubans, D. (2012). Improving physical self-perception in adolescent boys from disadvantaged schools: Psychological outcomes from the Physical Activity Leaders randomized controlled trial. *Pediatric Obesity, 7*(3), e27–e32.

Morgan, P. J., Young, M. D., Smith, J. J., & Lubans, D. R. (2016). Targeted health behavior interventions promoting physical activity: A conceptual model. *Exercise and Sport Sciences Reviews, 44*(2), 71–80.

Nanthakumar, C. (2018). The benefits of yoga in children. *Journal of Integrative Medicine-Jim, 16*(1), 14–19. doi:10.1016/j.joim.2017.12.008

Oliveira, B. R. R., Santos, T. M., Kilpatrick, M., Pires, F. O., & Deslandes, A. C. (2018). Affective and enjoyment responses in high intensity interval training and continuous training: A systematic review and meta-analysis. *PLoS One, 13*(6), e0197124. doi:10.1371/journal.pone.0197124

Ortega, F. B., Ruiz, J. R., Castillo, M. J., & Sjostrom, M. (2008). Physical fitness in children and adolescence: A powerful marker of health. *International Journal of Obesity, 32*(1), 1–11.

Ortega, F. B., Silventoinen, K., Tynelius, P., & Rasmussen, F. (2012). Muscular strength in male adolescents and premature death: Cohort study of one million participants. *British Medical Journal 345*, e7279.

Parker, R. J. (2003). *Kids in gyms: Guidelines for running physical activity programs for young people in fitness and leisure centres in NSW.* Sydney, NSW: Department of Tourism, Sport and Recreation.

Pate, R., Oria, M., & Pillsbury, L. (2012). *Fitness measures and health outcomes in youth.* Washington, DC: Institute of Medicine.

Penman, S., Cohen, M., Stevens, P., & Jackson, S. (2012). Yoga in Australia: Results of a national survey. *International Journal of Yoga, 5*(2), 92–101. doi:10.4103/0973-6131.98217

Perrier, E. T., Pavol, M. J., & Hoffman, M. A. (2011). The acute effects of a warm-up including static or dynamic stretching on countermovement jump height, reaction time, and flexibility. *The Journal of Strength & Conditioning Research, 25*(7), 1925–1931. doi:10.1519/JSC.0b013e3181e73959

Plowman, S. A. (2014). Muscular strength, endurance, and flexibility assessments. In S. Plowman & M. D. Meredith (Eds.), *FITNESSGRAM /ACTIVITYGRAM reference guide* (updated 4th ed., pp. 55). Dallas, TX: Cooper Institute.

Plowman, S. A. (2014). Top 10 research questions related to musculoskeletal physical fitness testing in children and adolescents. *Research Quarterly for Exercise and Sport, 85*(2), 174–187.

Ratamess, N. (2012). *ACSM's Foundations of Strength Training and Conditioning.* Philadelphia, PA: Lippincott, Williams and Wilkins.

Raub, J. A. (2002). Psychophysiologic effects of hatha yoga on musculoskeletal and cardiopulmonary function: A literature review. *The Journal of Alternative and Complementary Medicine, 8*(6), 797–812. doi:10.1089/10755530260511810

Riebe, D. (2018). *ACSM's Guidelines for Exercise Testing and Prescription.* Philadelphia, PA: Wolters Kluwer.

Ross, A., & Thomas, S. (2010). The health benefits of yoga and exercise: A review of comparison studies. *The Journal of Alternative and Complementary Medicine, 16*(1), 3–12. doi:10.1089/acm.2009.0044

Ruiz-Pérez, L. M., Palomo-Nieto, M., Gómez-Ruano, M. A., & Navia-Manzano, J. A. (2018). When we were clumsy: Some memories of adults who were low skilled in physical education at school. *Journal of Physical Education, 5*(1), 30–36.

Ruiz, J. R., Cavero-Redondo, I., Ortega, F. B., Welk, G. J., Andersen, L. B., & Martinez-Vizcaino, V. (2016). Cardiorespiratory fitness cut points to avoid cardiovascular disease risk in children and adolescents; what level of fitness should raise a red flag? A systematic review and meta-analysis. *British Journal of Sports Medicine, 50*(23), 1451–1458.

Ruiz, J. R., Espana Romero, V., Castro Pinero, J., Artero, E. G., Ortega, F. B., Cuenca Garcia, M., . . .Castillo, M. J. (2011). ALPHA-fitness test battery: Health-related field-based fitness tests assessment in children and adolescents. *Nutricion Hospitalaria, 26*(6), 1210–1214. doi:10.1590/S0212-16112011000600003

Sandercock, G. R., & Cohen, D. D. (2018). Temporal trends in muscular fitness of English 10-year-olds 1998–2014: An allometric approach. *Journal of Science and Medicine in Sport, 22*, 201–205.

Sands, W. A., McNeal, J. R., Murray, S. R., Ramsey, M. W., Sato, K., Mizuguchi, S., & Stone, M. H. (2013). Stretching and its effects on recovery: A review. *Strength and Conditioning Journal, 35*(5), 30–36.

Santtila, M., Pihlainen, K., Koski, H., Vasankari, T., & KyrÖlÄinen, H. (2018). Physical fitness in young men between 1975 and 2015 with a focus on the years 2005–2015. *Medicine and Science in Sports and Exercise, 50*(2), 292–298.

Schranz, N., Tomkinson, G., Parletta, N., Petkov, J., & Olds, T. (2014). Can resistance training change the strength, body composition and self-concept of overweight and obese adolescent males? A randomised controlled trial. *British Journal of Sports Medicine, 48*(20), 1482–1488.

Sengupta, P. (2012). Health impacts of yoga and pranayama: A state-of-the-art review. *International Journal of Preventive Medicine, 3*(7), 444–458.

Shcherbina, A., Mattsson, C. M., Waggott, D., Salisbury, H., Christle, J. W., Hastie, T., . . . Ashley, E. A. (2017). Accuracy in wrist-worn, sensor-based measurements of heart rate and energy expenditure in a diverse cohort. *Journal of Personalized Medicine, 7*(2). doi:10.3390/jpm7020003

Shingo, N., & Takeo, M. (2002). The educational experiments of school health promotion for the youth in Japan: Analysis of the 'sport test' over the past 34 years. *Health Promotion International, 17*(2), 147–160.

Shrier, I. (2004). Does stretching improve performance?: A systematic and critical review of the literature. *Clinical Journal of Sport Medicine, 14*(5), 267–273.

Shrier, I., & Gossal, K. (2000). Myths and truths of stretching. *The Physician and Sportsmedicine, 28*(8), 57–63. doi:10.3810/psm.2000.08.1159

Sigal, R. J., Alberga, A. S., Goldfield, G. S., Prud'homme, D., Hadjiyannakis, S., Gougeon, R., . . . Doucette, S. (2014). Effects of aerobic training, resistance training, or both on percentage body fat and cardiometabolic risk markers in obese aolescents: The Healthy Eating Aerobic and Resistance Training in Youth randomized clinical trial. *JAMA Pediatrics, 168*(11), 1006–1014.

Simic, L., Sarabon, N., & Markovic, G. (2013). Does pre-exercise static stretching inhibit maximal muscular performance? A meta-analytical review. *Scandinavian Journal of Medicine & Science in Sports, 23*(2), 131–148. doi: 10.1111/j.1600-0838.2012.01444.x

Small, K., Mc Naughton, L., & Matthews, M. (2008). A systematic review into the efficacy of static stretching as part of a warm-up for the prevention of exercise-related injury. *Research in Sports Medicine, 16*(3), 213–231. doi:10.1080/15438620802310784

Smith, C. A. (1994). The warm-up procedure: To stretch or not to stretch. A brief review. *Journal of Orthopaedic & Sports Physical Therapy, 19*(1), 12–17. doi:10.2519/jospt.1994.19.1.12

Smith, J. J., Beauchamp, M. R., Faulkner, G., Morgan, P. J., Kennedy, S. G., & Lubans, D. R. (2018). Intervention effects and mediators of well-being in a school-based physical activity program for adolescents: The 'Resistance Training for Teens' cluster RCT. *Mental Health and Physical Activity, 15*, 88–94.

Smith, J. J., DeMarco, M., Kennedy, S. G., Kelson, M., Barnett, L. M., Faigenbaum, A. D., & Lubans, D. R. (2017). Prevalence and correlates of resistance training skill competence in adolescents. *Journal of Sports Sciences, 36*(11), 1241–1249.

Smith, J. J., Eather, N., Morgan, P. J., Plotnikoff, R. C., Faigenbaum, A., & Lubans, D. R. (2014). The health benefits of muscular fitness for children and adolescents: A systematic review and meta-analysis. *Sports Medicine, 44*(9), 1209–1223. doi:10.1007/s40279-014-0196-4

Smith, J. J., Morgan, P. J., & Plotnikoff, R. C. (2014). Smart-phone obesity prevention trial for adolescent boys in low-income communities: The ATLAS RCT. *Pediatrics, 134*. doi:10.1542/peds.2014-1012

Smith, J. J., Morgan, P. J., Plotnikoff, R. C., Stodden, D. F., & Lubans, D. R. (2016). Mediating effects of resistance training skill competency on health-related fitness and physical activity: The ATLAS cluster randomised controlled trial. *Journal of sports sciences, 34*(8), 772–779. doi:10.1080/02640414.2015.1069383

Stahl, S. E., An, H. S., Dinkel, D. M., Noble, J. M., & Lee, J. M. (2016). How accurate are the wrist-based heart rate monitors during walking and running activities? Are they accurate enough? *BMJ Open Sport & Exercise Medicine, 2*(1), e000106. doi:10.1136/bmjsem-2015-000106

Stathokostas, L., Little, R. M. D., Vandervoort, A. A., & Paterson, D. H. (2012). Flexibility training and functional ability in older adults: A systematic review. *Journal of Aging Research, 2012*, 30. doi:10.1155/2012/306818

Stodden, D., Sacko, R., & Nesbitt, D. (2017). A review of the promotion of fitness measures and health outcomes in youth. *American Journal of Lifestyle Medicine, 11*(3), 232–242. doi:10.1177/1559827615619577

Stork, M. J., Gibala, M. J., & Martin Ginis, K. A. (2018). Psychological and behavioral responses to interval and continuous exercise. *Medicine & Science in Sports & Exercise, 50*(10), 2110–2121. doi:10.1249/MSS.0000000000001671

Sui, X., Li, H., Zhang, J., Chen, L., Zhu, L., & Blair, S. N. (2013). Percentage of deaths attributable to poor cardiovascular health lifestyle factors: Findings from the aerobics center longitudinal study. *Epidemiology Research International, 2013*, 1–9. doi:10.1155/2013/437465

Tabata, I., Nishimura, K., Kouzaki, M., Hirai, Y., Ogita, F., Miyachi, M., & Yamamoto, K. (1996). Effects of moderate-intensity endurance and high-intensity intermittent training on anaerobic capacity and $VO2_{max}$. *Medicine and Science in Sports and Exercise, 28*(10), 1327–1330.

Tanaka, H., Monahan, K. D., & Seals, D. R. (2001). Age-predicted maximal heart rate revisited. *Journal of the American College of Cardiology, 37*(1), 153–156.

ten Hoor, G., Sleddens, E. F., Kremers, S. P., Schols, A. M., Kok, G., & Plasqui, G. (2015). Aerobic and strength exercises for youngsters aged 12 to 15: What do parents think? *BMC Public Health, 15*(1), 1. doi:10.1186/s12889-015-2328-7

Thacker, S. B., Gilchrist, J., Stroup, D. F., & Kimsey, C. D. (2004). The impact of stretching on sports injury risk: A systematic review of the literature. *Medicine and Science in Sports and Exercise, 36*(3), 371–378.

Thiebaud, R. S., Funk, M. D., Patton, J. C., Massey, B. L., Shay, T. E., Schmidt, M. G., & Giovannitti, N. (2018). Validity of wrist-worn consumer products to measure heart rate and energy expenditure. *Digit Health, 4,* 2055207618770322. doi:10.1177/2055207618770322

Thivel, D., Masurier, J., Baquet, G., Timmons, B. W., Pereira, B., Berthoin, S., . . . Aucouturier, J. (2018). High-intensity interval training in overweight and obese children and adolescents: Systematic review and meta-analysis. *The Journal of Sports Medicine and Physical Fitness.* doi:10.23736/S0022-4707.18.08075-1

Thompson, D. L. (2008). Fitness focus copy-and-share: Flexibility. *ACSM's Health & Fitness Journal, 12*(5), 5. doi:10.1249/FIT.0b013e318184516b

Tomkinson, G. R., Lang, J. J., & Tremblay, M. S. (2017). Temporal trends in the cardiorespiratory fitness of children and adolescents representing 19 high-income and upper middle-income countries between 1981 and 2014. *British Journal of Sports Medicine.* doi:10.1136/bjsports-2017-097982

Tran, M. D., Holly, R. G., Lashbrook, J., & Amsterdam, E. A. (2001). Effects of hatha yoga practice on the health-related aspects of physical fitness. *Preventive Cardiology, 4*(4), 165–170.

Tremblay, M., & Lloyd, M. (2010). Physical literacy measurement: The missing piece. *Physical and Health Education Journal, 76*(1), 26–30.

Tremblay, M. S., Shields, M., Laviolette, M., Craig, C. L., Janseen, I., & Gorber, S. C. (2010). Fitness of Canadian children and youth: Results from the 2007–2009 Canadian Health Measures Survey. *Health Reports, 21*(1), Catalogue no. 82-003-x.

Van der Ploeg, H. P., Merom, D., Corpuz, G., & Bauman, A. E. (2008). Trends in Australian children traveling to school 1971–2003: Burning petrol or carbohydrates? *Preventive Medicine, 46*(1), 60–62.

Velez, A., Golem, D. L., & Arent, S. M. (2010). The impact of a 12-week resistance training program on strength, body composition, and self-concept of Hispanic adolescents. *Journal of Strength and Conditioning Research, 24*(4), 1065–1073.

Warburton, D. E., Glendhill, N., & Quinney, A. (2001). The effects of changes in musculoskeletal fitness on health. *Canadian Journal of Applied Physiology, 26*(2), 161–216.

Weerapong, P., Hume, P. A., & Kolt, G. S. (2004). Stretching: Mechanisms and benefits for sport performance and injury prevention. *Physical Therapy Reviews, 9*(4), 189–206. doi:10.1179/108331904225007078

Weiler, D. T., V. S., Edkins, L., Cleary, S., & Saleem, J. J. (2017). *Wearable heart rate monitor technology accuracy in research: A comparative study between PPG and ECG technology.* Paper presented at the Proceedings Human Factors & Ergonomics Society Annual Meeting.

Weldon, S. M., & Hill, R. H. (2003). The efficacy of stretching for prevention of exercise-related injury: A systematic review of the literature. *Manual Therapy, 8*(3), 141–150. doi:10.1016/S1356-689X(03)00010-9

Welk, G. J., Corbin, C. B., & Dale, D. (2000). Measurement issues in the assessment of physical activity in children. *Research quarterly for exercise and sport, 71*(sup2), 59–73.

Weston, K. L., Azevedo, L. B., Bock, S., Weston, M., George, K. P., & Batterham, A. M. (2016). Effect of novel, school-based high-intensity interval training (HIIT) on cardiometabolic health in adolescents: Project FFAB (fun fast activity blasts) – An exploratory controlled before-and-after trial. *PLoS One, 11*(8), e0159116. doi:10.1371/journal.pone.0159116

Whitehead, M. (2001). The concept of physical literacy. *European Journal of Physical Education, 6*(2), 127–138.

Zaferidis, A., Dalamitros, A., Dipla, K., Manou, V., Galanis, N., & Kellis, S. (2005). Recovery during high-intensity intermittent anaerobic exercise in boys, teens, and men. *Medicine & Science in Sports & Exercise, 37*(3), 505–512.

Zenko, Z., Ekkekakis, P., & Ariely, D. (2016). Can you have your vigorous exercise and enjoy it too? Ramping intensity down increases postexercise, remembered, and forecasted pleasure. *Journal of Sport and Exercise Psychology, 38*(2), 149–159. doi:10.1123/jsep.2015-0286

38

IMPORTANCE OF ORGANIZED SPORT PARTICIPATION FOR YOUTH PHYSICAL ACTIVITY

Stewart A. Vella and Matthew J. Schweickle

Introduction

Organized youth sports are one of the most popular leisure-time activities worldwide, and are also one of the most participated-in forms of physical activity among children and young people (Aubert et al., 2018). Globally, over 40% of children and adolescents participate in organized extracurricular sport, with participation rates much greater in high-income countries such as New Zealand, Australia, Canada, and Denmark (Aubert et al., 2018). While definitions of organized sport vary, the core components of these definitions stipulate that organized sports include the following: physical activity (Khan et al., 2012; McPherson, Curtis, & Loy, 1989), which should involve either physical exertion or physical skill (Australian Bureau of Statistics, 2008; Commonwealth of Australia, 2011); a structured or organized setting (Smoll & Smith, 2002); and some level of competition against others (Commonwealth of Australia, 2011; McPherson et al., 1989). Other conditions that are sometimes included in the definition of organized youth sports are the following: formal guidance and supervision provided by adults (Smoll & Smith, 2002); the existence of a formal organization to facilitate participation (Australian Bureau of Statistics, 2008; Commonwealth of Australia, 2011); and a defined goal (Khan et al., 2012). Organized youth sports typically include children and adolescents aged 7–19 years (e.g., Evans et al., 2017), and can be participated in individually or as part of a team (Khan et al., 2012). In this chapter, we refer specifically to extracurricular sports where participation is distinct from schooling and typically occurs in the after-school period and on weekends.

Overview of the Literature

The 2018 Global Matrix of physical activity for children and youth reported on participation in organized sports across 49 countries worldwide. Results showed that the vast majority of countries for which participation data were available reported participation at or above 40% (Aubert et al., 2018). In highly developed countries, participation in organized sports was much higher (often above 70%), and in these countries, sport was the most popular form of physical activity (Aubert et al., 2018). These patterns have been consistent across the last three Global Matrices (Aubert et al., 2018; Tremblay et al., 2014, 2016). Participation in organized sports is positively associated with several sociodemographic indicators, including the Human Development Index (an index measuring the extent to which a nation's population enjoys a long and healthy life, being knowledgeable, and have a decent standard of living), life expectancy at birth, mean years of schooling, growth of national income per capita, public health expenditure as a percentage of gross domestic product, global food security index, improved drinking water coverage, and summer Olympic medal count (Aubert et al., 2018). In contrast, global organized sport participation is negatively correlated with measures of inequality, specifically the Gini index (a measure of wealth distribution) and the gender inequality index (Aubert et al., 2018).

It should be noted that the above prevalence estimates are cross-sectional indicators of organized sport participation. That is, the measure of sport participation that is typically used in national surveillance is the percentage of the population that has engaged in some form of organized sports over the previous 12-month period (e.g., Sport Australia, 2018). While such surveillance, particularly at a national level, is helpful in monitoring participation trends, it tells us very little about secular trends in participation over a number of years. For example, studies using large national samples of Australian youth show that the percentage of individuals that engage in organized sports over a 2-year period is 89% (Vella, Cliff, Magee, & Okely, 2014a, 2014b), compared to 79% in the previous 12 months. This includes 10% of the population who dropped out of sports, and 10% who commenced participation. Thus, while the trend in participation remains at 79% in each year, this statistic obscures the movement of a meaningful number of youths in and out of organized sports over time.

National monitoring (e.g., Sport Australia, 2018) and studies of longitudinal data (e.g., Howie, McVeigh, Smith, & Straker, 2016) both provide evidence that participation in organized sports peaks during early adolescence and then steadily declines thereafter. Although these figures reflect overall participation rates, it should be noted that some dropout is apparent among children and increases with age. In line with global data, national participation data also show that participation in organized sports is positively correlated with indices of socioeconomic advantage and opportunity. In Australia, sports participation is associated with higher socioeconomic status, physically active parents, and residing within a safe neighborhood. Lower rates of sports participation are typically observed among families with lower incomes, and those in rural and remote areas (Sport Australia, 2018; Vella, Cliff, & Okely, 2014). At an individual level, sports participation is higher among children and adolescents who have greater motor coordination, better overall health, better social functioning, better mental health, and fewer injuries, and are more physically active (Vella et al., 2014).

It is notable that measures of health and health behaviors predict participation in organized sports. The vast majority of literature pertaining to the correlates of sports participation hypothesizes that indices of health and health behaviors are the outcomes of participation in organized sports. That is, participation in organized sports leads to better health and greater health behaviors. However, cross-sectional and longitudinal studies do not permit such conclusions (Eime, Young, Harvey, Charity, & Payne, 2013; Lee, Pope, & Gao, 2018; Nelson et al., 2011). For example, when longitudinal data are used to analyze associations over time, the relationship between sports participation and health indices such as mental health may be bidirectional in nature (Vella, Swann, Allen, Schweickle, & Magee, 2017). That is, sports participation is associated with later positive mental health, and positive mental health is associated with later sports participation.

Although establishing directionality and causality is difficult (see below for an extended discussion on this issue), participation in organized sports is associated with a number of health indices and health behaviors. Two systematic reviews (Lee et al., 2018; Nelson et al., 2011) have investigated the associations between participation in organized sports during childhood and adolescence, physical activity, and adiposity. Both reviews found positive associations between sport participation and physical activity. In addition, Lee et al. (2018) demonstrated that this association persists over several years and may even persevere into adulthood. However, given higher levels of physical activity also predict participation in organized sport (Sport Australia, 2018; Vella et al., 2014), it is difficult to assert causality to these findings. In regard to adiposity, both reviews noted an inconsistency in the evidence base. Indeed, Lee et al. (2018) and Nelson et al. (2011) both concluded that there is uncertainty as to whether sports participation helps to prevent or reduce obesity. Directionality may also be important here, as body fat percentage does not predict subsequent time spent in organized sports (Vella & Cliff, 2018). As such, it may be that no association between sports participation and measures of adiposity exist in either direction.

One of the reasons why sports participation may not be associated with measures of adiposity is because it is associated with greater caloric intake. Nelson et al. (2011) demonstrated that young people who participate in organized sports were more likely to consume fruits, vegetables, and milk. However, they were also more likely to eat fast food, drink sugar-sweetened beverages, and consume more calories overall. A study conducted by Vella, Cliff, Okely, Scully, and Morley (2013) provided partial support for this finding. In a large, nationally representative Australian sample, adolescents who participated in organized sports were more likely to meet national fruit and vegetable consumption guidelines. However, no relationship between sport participation and consumption of high fat foods or sugar-sweetened beverages was reported. Furthermore, Vella et al. (2013) reported that organized sports participation was associated with reductions in electronic screen time, supporting previous research reporting this association (Sirard, Pfeiffer, & Pate, 2006). As such, it remains unclear whether sports participation contributes to an overall energy balance.

Consistent associations have been documented between sports participation and various indicators of mental health. A systematic review has shown that youth sports participants report fewer mental health problems, lower depression scores, and fewer anxiety symptoms (Eime et al., 2013). Sports participation is also associated with positive indicators of psychological health such as greater self-esteem, higher psychological resilience, and increased well-being (Eime et al., 2013). Further, sports participation during childhood and adolescence is associated with greater social skills and social functioning (Eime et al., 2013). Evidence from longitudinal studies suggests that early sports participation (i.e., at 4–6 years of age) is associated with positive developmental trajectories of both mental health and quality of life from childhood to adolescence (Vella, Gardner, Swann, & Allen, 2018; Vella, Magee, & Cliff, 2015). However, as previously noted, evidence of bidirectionality in the relationship between sports participation and mental health means that asserting causality is difficult (Vella et al., 2017).

One model capable of explaining the bidirectional nature of relationships between sports participation and a range of health outcomes is the Conceptual Model of Health through Sport (Eime et al., 2013). This model incorporates three distinct components: (1) determinants of sport participation, (2) the nature of sport participation, and (3) the outcomes of sport participation. In conceptualizing the determinants of sport participation, a socioecological approach has been incorporated (Sallis, Owen, & Fotheringham, 2000). Accordingly, the Conceptual Model of Health through Sport posits that there are multiple levels of influence which act together to impact sport participation. These levels include individual (e.g., physical activity levels of the child), interpersonal (e.g., parental physical activity), organizational (e.g., quality of available sporting programs), environmental (e.g., safe neighborhoods), and policy levels (e.g., tax rebates for sporting fees). Subsequently, when young people participate in sport, the nature of that participation falls into one of four broad categories defined by two dimensions: (1) team/individual, and (2) organized/ non-organized. For example, sport participation can be organized team sport, organized individual sport, non-organized team sport, or non-organized individual sport. In turn, the nature of participation leads to a variety of health outcomes across physical, psychological, and social domains. The Conceptual Model of Health through Sport postulates that organized and team sports demonstrate stronger relationships with adaptive psychological and social outcomes than physical health outcomes. In contrast, individual and non-organized sports are supported by stronger relationships with physical health than psychological and social health outcomes. Importantly, the

Conceptual Model of Health through Sport then includes a series of feedback loops, whereby the health outcomes of sport feed back into the socioecological model as intra- and interpersonal determinants of sports participation. In this way, the Conceptual Model of Health through Sport can account for potential bidirectionality in the relationships between sport participation and health among children and adolescents (Eime et al., 2013).

Contribution of Participation in Organized Sports to Overall Physical Activity

Although national organized youth sport participation may be relatively high (see Aubert et al. 2018 for full data from 49 countries) when compared with other forms of physical activity, researchers and policy makers have seen fit to warn that sport participation in isolation is not sufficient for health. For example, the authors of Australia's first ever national physical activity report card, entitled 'Sport is Not Enough' (Schranz et al., 2014), warned Australians against the assumption that sports participation alone provided sufficient physical activity for health benefits. This is consistent with warnings derived from empirical research which show that very few sport participants accumulate enough physical activity during sports practice to meet physical activity guidelines (Leek et al., 2011).

There is relatively little research illuminating exactly how much of one's overall physical activity is derived from participation in organized sports. Wickel and Eisenmann (2007) estimated that organized sports contribute about 23% of daily moderate-to-vigorous physical activity (MVPA) among 6–12-year-old boys. Furthermore, on days when organized sports were not participated in, boys spent more time in sedentary behaviors and less time in both moderate and vigorous intensity physical activities (Wickel & Eisenmann, 2007). Meanwhile, an Australian study derived from time use diaries demonstrated that participation in organized sports contributed 45% of daily MVPA by time, 58% of MVPA by energy expenditure, and a total of 17% of total daily energy expenditure (Olds, Dollman, & Maher, 2009). Notwithstanding that these estimates vary widely (23%–58% of daily MVPA), it appears that a meaningful percentage of total daily MVPA is accumulated among those who participate in organized youth sports.

There is some evidence to suggest that participation in organized sports during childhood and adolescence is associated with higher levels of physical activity during adulthood (e.g., Hirvensalo & Lintunen, 2011). Specifically, sports participation may lead to the acquisition of foundational movement skills. These skills are defined as "goal-directed movement patterns that directly and indirectly impact an individual's capability to be physically active and that can continue to be developed to enhance physical activity participation and promote health across the lifespan" (Hulteen, Morgan, Barnett, Stodden, & Lubans, 2018, p. 2). Foundational movement skills incorporate the traditional movement skills of running, kicking, and throwing, and other skills necessary for lifelong physical activity are riding a bicycle, swimming strokes, and body weight squats. For example, while sports participation is popular during childhood and adolescence, lifelong physical activities such as swimming and walking are more popular during adulthood (Hulteen et al., 2017). Meanwhile, the acquisition of foundational movement skills can also lead to lifelong physical activity through the acquisition of specialized movement skills such as baseball pitching, shooting a basketball, or mountain biking (Hulteen et al., 2018).

Based on the popularity of organized sports, the Global Advocacy for Physical Activity have nominated organized sports as one of the seven best global investments for physical activity (Global Advocacy for Physical Activity (GAPA) the Advocacy Council of the International Society for Physical Activity and Health (ISPAH), 2012). However, a greater evidence base, built from more rigorous evidence, is needed to substantiate such rhetoric. The strength of the above studies is that they are derived from a variety of methodologies, such as accelerometry (e.g., Wickel &

Eisenmann, 2007) and time use diaries (e.g., Olds et al., 2009). However, the extent to which organized sport participation contributes to overall physical activity over an extended period of time (such as a week, month, or year) remains unclear. To generate such knowledge, a combination of extended objective data, such as accelerometry, in combination with detailed subjective data, such as time use diaries, may be needed. Further, rich longitudinal data may be needed to more accurately ascertain the associations between sports participation during childhood and adolescence, and physical activity during adulthood. Ideally, such data would be based on sound theory as to the mechanisms through which sport participation may be associated with lifelong physical activity, facilitating the modeling and testing of causal pathways.

Physical Activity Accumulated during Participation in Organized Sports

When considering the amount of physical activity accumulated during participation in organized sports, it is appropriate to first establish the amount of time young people spend in organized sport practice and competition. Australian data derived from time use diaries found young Australians aged between 9 and 16 years spend, on average, 43 minutes in organized sport participation each day (Olds et al., 2009). This is a total of 5 hours each week. A second study among a larger, nationally representative sample of over 12,000 Australian adolescents aged 12–17 years indicated that adolescents spend on average 7.5 hours in organized sports each week. This was constituted by approximately 8 hours per week for males and 7 hours per week for females (Vella et al., 2013).

One of the most pertinent questions, then, is the amount of physical activity accumulated during participation in organized sports. To our knowledge, three studies have provided evidence on the amount of physical activity accumulated during youth sport practices. Wickel and Eisenmann (2007) found that, among 119 boys aged 6–12 years, just over half (~52%) of all time spent in organized sports was spent in either sedentary or light intensity activities. Approximately 27% of time was spent in moderate intensity activities and 22% in vigorous intensity activities. Leek and Carlson (2011) reported very similar results among 200 7–14-year-old participants in baseball and soccer. Among soccer participants, just over 50% of all time was spent in moderate and vigorous activities, with higher rates among younger participants. Among baseball participants, just over 40% of all time was spent in moderate-to-vigorous intensity activities. These results suggest that there are meaningful differences by sport and potentially differences by age. Lastly, Guagliano, Rosenkranz, and Kolt (2013) found that among 94 girls participating in netball, basketball, and soccer, only one third (33.8%) of practice time was spent in MVPA. However, as opposed to the studies conducted by Wickel and Eisenmann (2007) and Leek and Carlson (2011), which used accelerometry data to measure physical activity, this study used the Systematic Observation for Fitness Instruction Time (SOFIT; McKenzie, Sallis, & Nader, 1992). The SOFIT tool includes observation of instructor behaviors, and it was found that a meaningful amount of time was spent on management (~15%) and knowledge delivery (~18%) behaviors (Guagliano et al., 2013). However, the SOFIT tool has been shown to overestimate physical activity levels when compared with accelerometry (Hollis et al., 2017).

Of the studies investigating physical activity during youth sport participation, only two have examined the amount of physical activity accumulated during *competitive settings*. Guagliano et al. (2013) found that among female athletes participating in competitive netball, basketball, and soccer, less time was spent in MVPA when compared to practice settings. However, the differences were small. The 33.8% of time spent in MVPA during practices was only slightly higher than the 30.6% of time spent in MVPA during competition. This translates to a difference of approximately 2 minutes of extra MVPA for each hour of participation. These estimates are consistent with those of Sacheck, Nelson, Ficker, and Kafka (2011) who reported that children aged 7–10 years spent

33% of time in MVPA during a competitive indoor soccer game. Further, the children spent almost half (49%) of the time in sedentary activities. Thus, despite limited evidence, it does not seem that there is a meaningful difference between the amount of physical activity accumulated during practice and competitive settings.

Organized sports may be a popular mechanism through which to address physical inactivity. However, participation in organized sports alone does not provide sufficient physical activity for children and adolescents to meet physical activity guidelines. There remains scope to improve the structure, content, and environment of organized sports programs to promote physical activity. Guagliano and colleagues followed up their observational study with an intervention to increase girls' physical activity during organized youth basketball (Guagliano, Lonsdale, Kolt, Rosenkranz, & George, 2015). Coaches randomized to an intervention group participated in two coach education sessions designed to help coaches recognize and increase participants' activity levels (Guagliano, Lonsdale, Kolt, & Rosenkranz, 2014). Following coach education, participants in the intervention group increased their MVPA during practice by 15.1%, with a corresponding decrease of 14.2% in sedentary activities (Guagliano et al., 2015). Therefore, it appeared that sedentary activities were replaced by MVPA. In contrast, there was no change in the control group (Guagliano et al., 2015). As such, brief coach education can be successful in helping coaches to facilitate greater levels of physical activity during youth sport practices.

Dropout from Organized Sports and Health Consequences

Organized youth sports are an important source of physical activity for children and adolescents, and the effects of dropout are likely to be numerous. In fact, dropout from organized sport may be considered an important (and negative) public health behavior. Despite this, obtaining an accurate estimate of the dropout rate from organized sport has proved elusive. Based on cross-sectional and longitudinal data, it has been estimated that around 30% of all youth sport participants drop out each year (Balish, McLaren, Rainhaim, & Blanchard, 2014). Given that most countries report national participation rates of between 40% and 80% of all children and adolescents each year (Aubert et al., 2018), this would mean that a total of 12%–24% of all children and adolescents are dropping out of organized sports in each country, each year. Given that organized sports contribute somewhere between 23% and 58% of daily MVPA (Wickel & Eisenmann, 2007; Olds et al., 2009), this rate is alarmingly high.

The health consequences of dropout from organized sport may be detrimental for young people. While it is difficult to establish causality, there are a number of negative health outcomes that are associated with dropout from organized sports. Vella et al. (2014a) indicated that dropout from organized sports is associated with a 10%–20% increase in risk for diagnosis of mental health problem within 3 years, when compared with continued participation. This represents a substantial increase in risk. In a study with the same participants, Vella et al. (2014b) reported that dropout from organized sports is associated with decreases in quality of life when compared to continued participation. Given consistent associations between participation in organized sports and physical activity, dropout from organized sports is likely associated with reductions in physical activity (Lee et al., 2018; Nelson et al., 2011), and in turn the negative health consequences resulting from reduced physical activity (e.g., Janssen & LeBlanc, 2010).

One important way of understanding health behaviors, such as dropout from organized sports, is to examine correlates (Sallis et al., 2000). This sort of descriptive research is useful in identifying the characteristics of people who are most in need of intervention. Importantly, the correlates of dropout may not be the same as the correlates of sport participation. Adopting a socioecological approach, a systematic review conducted by Balish et al. (2014) reported a number of correlates of dropout from organized youth sport, which were reported over multiple levels of influence and supported by high levels of evidence. At a biological level, age is positively associated with dropout. At an intrapersonal level, maladaptive forms of motivation (i.e., amotivation, identified regulation) and intention to dropout are positively associated with dropout. Meanwhile, perceived autonomy, intrinsic motivation for accomplishment, intrinsic motivation for stimulation, perceived competence, and perceived relatedness are all negatively correlated with dropout. At an interpersonal level, a task climate is negatively associated with dropout. Meanwhile, a host of other variables were reported to be associated with dropout, though only had a low level of evidence. These include variables at organizational, community, and policy levels.

A second systematic review provides support for the results presented by Balish et al. (2014). Reviewing studies conducted in over 30 sports, Crane and Temple (2015) reported that intrapersonal and interpersonal constructs were most frequently associated with dropping out of sport. The authors concluded that the reasons for dropout from sports could be integrated into five major areas: (i) lack of enjoyment, (ii) perceptions of competence, (iii) social pressures, (iv) competing priorities, and (v) physical factors (e.g., maturation and injuries). In addition to these five areas, the findings of Balish et al. (2014) indicate that motivation and motivational climate should be added as a sixth group of important correlates, or at least considered in conjunction with enjoyment of sport. Taken together, these reviews highlight the need for systematic investigation into higher levels of influence on dropout from organized sports, including organizational, community, and policy levels. Further, both reviews have identified a great need for higher quality work in this area, including prospective and observational studies (as opposed to cross-sectional studies relying on self-report measures), theory-based research, and simultaneous investigation of correlates at multiple levels of influence (Balish et al., 2014; Crane & Temple, 2015).

According to the Behavioral Epidemiology Framework (Sallis et al., 2000), once correlates of a particular health behavior are identified, the next phase of research should include the testing of interventions to change the behavior. To our knowledge, very few interventions have investigated dropout as an outcome variable. In one study, a Coach Effectiveness Training Program was piloted with eight Little League coaches (Barnett, Smoll, & Smith, 1992). The training program was designed to increase positive coach-player interaction, team cohesion, and a positive view of participation in sport as an opportunity for achievement, rather than a possibility for failure. The program included a 2.5-hour workshop where behavioral guidelines were presented verbally and in written format, in addition to the modeling of both desirable and undesirable coaching behaviors. All coaches also completed a self-monitoring form after every game of the season which prompted reflection on the behavioral guidelines. The program was evaluated against a control group of 10 Little League coaches. The following season, 26% of the athletes from coaches allocated to the control group did not return. In contrast, only 5% of athletes from coaches in the intervention group did not return the following season. This suggests that interventions to prevent dropout from organized sport can be effective, and could be an important public health strategy.

Emerging Issues

What Is a Quality Youth Sport Program?

The outcomes associated with participation in organized youth sports are, in general, positive. Children who participate in organized sports are likely to experience a range of associated psychosocial benefits, including better mental health, increased self-esteem, and greater social functioning (Eime et al., 2013). However, the positive outcomes associated with participation in organized sports are not universal. There are significant negative outcomes that are also associated with sport participation, including pressure, stress, and antisocial behavior (Fraser-Thomas, Côté, &

Deakin, 2005). As such, a focus should be placed on the aspects of youth sport programs that can lead to health benefits. Currently, there are no guidelines on what constitutes a quality youth sport program.

High levels of physical activity are one way of improving the quality of organized sports programs. The use of organized sports programs that are high in MVPA have formed the basis of large-scale health programs (Robinson et al., 2013), and with basic training coaches can meaningfully increase the amount of MVPA during practices. In line with the findings of Balish et al. (2014), high-quality sport programs should also foster adaptive forms of motivation. For example, athletes participating in sport programs that rate highly on a measure of overall program quality perceive significantly greater opportunities for autonomy, relatedness, and choice (Bean, Harlow, Mosher, Fraser-Thomas, & Forneris, 2018). In line with self-determination theory (Ryan & Deci, 2000), the perception of high levels of autonomy, competence, and relatedness will lead to more adaptive forms of motivation (i.e., more self-determined forms of motivation). An alternate, comprehensive framework to encapsulate high-quality sport programs are the Supportive, Active, Autonomous, Fair, and Enjoyable (SAAFE) principles (Lubans et al., 2017). The SAAFE principles represent an evidence-based framework designed to guide the planning, delivery, and evaluation of organized physical activity sessions, including organized community sport programs. However, the SAAFE principles have not yet been tested within organized sports.

The Personal Assets Framework to Sport (Côté, Turnnidge, & Vierimaa, 2016) gives some theory-based guidance as to the variables in sport that account for positive outcomes. First, good quality relationships between the athlete and their coach, parent, and peers are necessary to promote positive outcomes. Further, the structural elements of high-quality sport programs should include the following: (1) a safe environment in which youth develop; (2) an appropriate structure in which youth experience a stable environment; (3) the availability of opportunities for skill building; (4) the integration of family, school, and community efforts; (5) accessibility to different sport contexts; and (6) sport contexts with fewer people, as they increase personal effort and involvement in different roles and positions.

Measuring Participation in Organized Sports

High-quality measures are at the heart of all stages of health behavior research, including surveillance and national monitoring, establishing links with health outcomes, and measuring change within interventions (Sallis et al., 2000). There are several approaches to measuring sports participation. For example, categorical measures are commonly used (Lee et al., 2018; Nelson et al., 2011). These measures can be used to classify children and adolescents into sports participants and non-participants for the purposes of comparing the two groups on health outcomes, or to investigate those variables that predict participation or non-participation. However, one of the drawbacks of this approach is that it is unclear what the minimum threshold should be to constitute 'sport participants'. It has been recommended that a threshold of an average of at least once per week for 3 months (or one school term) is an appropriate starting point (Vella et al., 2016). A second drawback of the categorical approach is that much of the variability in sports participation is lost, including the frequency and duration of participation, which may be important predictors of health outcomes.

One measure capable of capturing the variations in sports participation, including the frequency, duration, and type of sports participation, is the Adolescent Physical Activity Recall Questionnaire (APARQ; Booth, Okely, Chey, & Bauman, 2002). The APARQ has two main components: (1) participation in organized sports and games and (2) participation in non-organized physical activities. As the components are separable, it is possible to administer only the organized sports component of the APARQ. Organized sports and games are described as activities that are usually supervised by adults, and usually involve organized training or practice, and an organized competition. Participants are asked to think about a normal week during summer school terms and a normal week during winter school terms (excluding vacations). Participants are then asked to report separately for each season: each activity they did (up to seven activities could be reported); the frequency with which they participated in that activity in a normal week (including training and competition); and the usual time they spent doing that activity each time they did it (including both training and competition). As such, estimates can be derived for total organized sport participation, participation in training, participation in competitive settings, participation by individual sports, or participation by groups of sports (e.g., individual sports, team sports). However, one of the drawbacks of this approach is that it relies on participant recall, which can be inaccurate.

Recommendations for Researchers/Practitioners

Despite strong rhetoric surrounding the health benefits of participation in organized sport, the field is characterized by very little evidence of causality. That is, few experimental studies have demonstrated that sport participation itself provides health benefits. Evidence to support a relationship between sports participation and indicators of physical, psychological, and social health is entirely cross-sectional and longitudinal in nature (Eime et al., 2013; Lee et al., 2018; Nelson et al., 2011). This means that the direction of relationships and the causal mechanisms which underpin those relationships are unknown. Randomized controlled trials are needed in this regard. Tightly controlled efficacy studies are needed to evaluate the impact of well-implemented sport programs. Such studies may provide evidence that sport participation is causally related to improved health outcomes. Further, effectiveness studies whereby the 'real-life' influence of sports participation can be studied are also needed.

There are, however, clear difficulties in attaining causal evidence regarding the role of sports participation. First, maintaining an adequate control group is difficult. It is foreseeable that participants randomized to any form of control group (i.e., non-sport group) may seek out sports participation elsewhere. Second, researchers would be faced with the task of attempting to measure and account for any school- or community-based organized sports that participants, in either an intervention or control group, may accumulate outside of the study implementation. Researchers would also have to decide how they may account for previous sports participation, if at all. In terms of efficacy studies, genuine questions could be raised as to the generalizability of results to 'real-world' sports participation. In particular, the lack of genuine competitive contexts would be problematic given that competition is inherent in the definition of organized sports. Finally, in terms of effectiveness studies, the genuine allocation of participants to either intervention or control groups may legitimately be impossible.

Despite these limitations, the pursuit of causal evidence should be a priority for the field. Very little research is without any genuine limitations, and limitations should not prevent researchers from attempting to shed light on the causal role (or otherwise) of sports participation on the health and health behaviors of children and adolescents. It is likely that a variety of research designs will be needed, with evidence accumulated and synthesized over time to provide high levels of evidence that can underpin evidence-based program design, implementation, and policy. Until such evidence is forthcoming, it is difficult to provide guidelines to program designers, practitioners, and administrators as to the best way to structure and implement organized sport programs. It is also worth noting that the quality of one's sporting experience is important in enhancing the experience of sport participation, and this is an area that lends itself to robust research designs and high-quality evidence.

Notwithstanding the above, practitioners within organized youth sports would be well advised to (1) maintain high levels of MVPA during practices and competitive settings; (2) facilitate high levels of perceived autonomy, competence, and relatedness on behalf of athletes; (3) encourage engagement with a variety of different sports and roles; (4) facilitate good quality relationships between athletes and their coaches, parents, and peers; and (5) provide a stable and safe environment for participation. These principles are covered in detail in the comprehensive and evidence-based SAAFE principles (Lubans et al., 2017).

References

Aubert, S., Barnes, J. D., Abdeta, C., Nader, P. A., Adeniyi, A. F., Aguilar-Farias, N., . . . Tremblay, M. S. (2018). Global Matrix 3.0 physical activity report card grades for children and youth: Results and analysis from 49 countries. *Journal of Physical Activity and Health, 15*(Suppl 2), S251–S273.

Australian Bureau of Statistics. (2008). *Defining sport and physical activity, a conceptual mode.* Canberra, Australia: Australian Bureau of Statistics.

Balish, S. M., McLaren, C., Rainhaim, D., & Blanchard, C. (2014). Correlates of youth sport attrition: A review and future directions. *Psychology of Sport and Exercise, 15*, 429–439.

Barnett, N. P., Smoll, F. L., & Smith, R. E. (1992). Effects of enhancing coach-athlete relationships on youth sport attrition. *The Sport Psychologist, 6*, 111–127.

Bean, C., Harlow, M., Mosher, A., Fraser-Thomas, J., & Forneris, T. (2018). Assessing differences in athlete-reported outcomes between high and low-quality youth sport programs. *Journal of Applied Sport Psychology, 30*, 456–472.

Booth, M. L., Okely, A. D., Chey, T., & Bauman, A. (2002). The reliability and validity of the adolescent physical activity recall questionnaire. *Medicine and Science in Sports and Exercise, 34*, 1986–1995.

Commonwealth of Australia. (2011). *National sport and active recreation policy framework.* Canberra, Australia: Commonwealth of Australia.

Côté, J., Turnnidge, J., & Vierimaa, M. (2016). A personal assets approach to youth sport. In K. Green & A. Smith (Eds.), *Routledge handbook of youth sport* (pp. 243–256). New York, NY: Routledge.

Crane, J., & Temple, V. (2015). A systematic review of dropout from organized sport among children and youth. *European Physical Education Review, 21*, 114–131.

Eime, R. M., Young, J. A., Harvey, J. T., Charity, M. J., & Payne, W. R. (2013). A systematic review of the psychological and social benefits of participation in sport for children and adolescents: Informing development of a conceptual model of health through sport. *International Journal of Behavioral Nutrition and Physical Activity, 10*, 98.

Evans, M. B., Allan, V., Erickson, K., Martin, L. J., Budziszewski, R., & Côté, J. (2017). Are all sport activities equal? A systematic review of how youth psychosocial experiences vary across differing sport activities. *British Journal of Sports Medicine, 51*, 169–176.

Fraser-Thomas, J. L., Côté, J., & Deakin, J. (2005). Youth sport programs: An avenue to foster positive youth development. *Physical Education and Sport Pedagogy, 10*, 19–40.

Global Advocacy for Physical Activity (GAPA) the Advocacy Council of the International Society for Physical Activity and Health (ISPAH). (2012). NCD prevention: Investments that work for physical activity. *British Journal of Sports Medicine, 46*, 709–712.

Guagliano, J. M., Lonsdale, C., Kolt, G. S., & Rosenkranz, R. R. (2014). Increasing girls' physical activity during an organised youth sport basketball program: A randomised controlled trial protocol. *BMC Public Health, 14*, 383.

Guagliano, J. M., Lonsdale, C., Kolt, G. S., Rosenkranz, R. R., & George, E. S. (2015). Increasing girls' physical activity during a short-term organized youth sport basketball program: A randomized controlled trial. *Journal of Science and Medicine in Sport, 18*, 412–417.

Guagliano, J. M., Rosenkranz, R., & Kolt, G. (2013). Girls' physical activity levels during organised sports in Australia. *Medicine and Science in Sports and Exercise, 45*(1), 116–122.

Hirvensalo, M., & Lintunen, T. (2011). Life-course perspective for physical activity and sports participation. *European Review of Aging and Physical Activity, 8*, 13–22.

Hollis, J. L., Sutherland, R., Williams, A. J., Campbell, L., Nathan, N., Wolfenden, L., . . . Wiggers, J. (2017). A systematic review and meta-analysis of moderate-to-vigorous physical activity levels in secondary school physical education lessons. *International Journal of Behavioral Nutrition and Physical Activity, 14*(52). doi:10.1186/s12966-12017-10504-12960.

Howie, E. K., McVeigh, A. J., Smith, A. J., & Straker, L. M. (2016). Organized sport trajectories from child-hood to adolescence and health associations. *Medicine and Science in Sports and Exercise, 48*, 1331–1339.

Hulteen, R. M., Morgan, P. J., Barnett, L. M., Stodden, D. F., & Lubans, D. R. (2018). Development of foundational movement skills: A conceptual model for physical activity across the lifespan. *Sports Medicine, 48*, 1533–1540.

Hulteen, R. M., Smith, J. J., Morgan, P. J., Barnett, L. M., Hallal, P., Colyvas, K., & Lubans, D. R. (2017). Global participation in sport and leisure-time physical activities: A systematic review and meta-analysis. *Preventive Medicine, 95*, 14–25.

Janssen, I., & LeBlanc, A. G. (2010). Systematic review of the health benefits of physical activity and fitness in school-aged children and youth. *International Journal of Behavioral Nutrition and Physical Activity, 7*, 40.

Khan, K. M., Thompson, A. M., Blair, S. N., Sallis, J. F., Powell, K. E., Bull, F. C., & Bauman, A. E. (2012). Sport and exercise as contributors to the health of nations. *Lancet, 380*, 59–64.

Lee, J. E., Pope, Z., & Gao, Z. (2018). The role of youth sports in promoting children's physical activity and preventing pediatric obesity: A systematic review. *Behavioral Medicine, 44*, 62–76.

Leek, D., Carlson, J. A., Cain, K. L., Henrichon, S., Rosenberg, D., Patrick, K., & Sallis, J. F. (2011). Physical activity during youth sport practices. *Archives of Pediatric and Adolescent Medicine, 165*, 294–299.

Lubans, D. R., Lonsdale, C., Cohen, K., Eather, N., Beauchamp, M., Morgan, P. J., . . . Smith, J. J. (2017). Framework for the design and delivery of organized physical activity sessions for children and adolescents: Rationale and description of the 'SAAFE' teaching principles. *International Journal of Behavioral Nutrition and Physical Activity, 14*(24). doi:10.1186/s12966-12017-10479-x

McKenzie, T. L., Sallis, J. F., & Nader, P. R. (1992). SOFIT: System for observing fitness instruction time. *Journal of Teaching in Physical Education, 11*, 195–205.

McPherson, B. C., Curtis, J. E., & Loy, J. W. (1989). *The social significance of sport: An introduction to the sociology of sport.* Champaign, IL: Human Kinetics.

Nelson, T. F., Stovitz, S. D., Thomas, M., LaVoi, N. M., Bauer, K. W., & Neumark-Sztainer, D. (2011). Do youth sports prevent pediatric obesity? A systematic review and commentary. *Current Sports Medicine Reports, 10*(6), 360–370.

Olds, T. S., Dollman, J., & Maher, C. (2009). Adolescent sport in Australia: Who, when, where and what? *ACPHER Healthy Lifestyles Journal, 56*(1), 11–16.

Robinson, T. N., Matheson, D., Desai, M., Wilson, D. M., Weintraub, D. L., Haskell, W. L., . . . Killen, J. D. (2013). Family, community and clinic collaboration to treat overweight and obese children: Stanford GOALS-A randomized controlled trial of a three-year, multi-component, multi-level, multi-setting intervention. *Contemporary Clinical Trials, 36*(2), 421–435.

Ryan, R. M., & Deci, E. L. (2000). Self-determination theory and the facilitation of intrinsic motivation, social development, and well-being. *American Psychologist, 55*, 68–78.

Sacheck, J. M., Nelson, T., Ficker, L., & Kafka, T. (2011). Physical activity during soccer and its contribution to physical activity recommendations in normal weight and overweight children. *Pediatric Exercise Science, 23*, 281–292.

Sallis, J. F., Owen, N., & Fotheringham, M. J. (2000). Behavioral epidemiology: A systematic framework to classify phases of research on health promotion and disease prevention. *Annals of Behavioral Medicine, 22*, 294–298.

Schranz, N. K., Olds, T. S., Cliff, D. P., Davern, M., Engelen, L., Giles-Corti, B., . . . Tomkinson, G. (2014). Results from Australia's 2014 report card on physical activity for children and youth. *Journal of Physical Activity and Health, 11*(Supp 1), S21–S25.

Sirard, J. R., Pfeiffer, K. A., & Pate, R. R. (2006). Motivational factors associated with sports program participation in middle school students. *Journal of Adolescent Health, 38*, 696–703.

Smoll, F. L., & Smith, R. E. (2002). *Children and youth in sport: A biopsychosocial perspective* (2nd ed.). Dubuque, IA: Kendall/Hunt.

Sport Australia. (2018). *AusPlay focus: Children's participation in organised physical activity outside of school hours.* Canberra, Australia: Sport Australia.

Tremblay, M. S., Barnes, J. D., Gonzalez, S. A., Katzmarzyk, P. T., Onywera, V. O., Reilly, J. J., . . . Global Matrix 2.0 Research Team. (2016). Global Matrix 2.0: Report card grades on the physical activity of children and youth comparing 38 countries. *Journal of Physical Activity and Health, 13*, S343–S366.

Tremblay, M. S., Gray, C. E., Kakinroye, K., Harrington, D. M., Katzmarzyk, P. T., Lambert, E. V., . . . Tomkinson, G. (2014). Physical activity of children: A global matrix of grades comparing 15 countries. *Journal of Physical Activity and Health, 11*(Supp 1), S113–S125.

Vella, S. A., & Cliff, D. P. (2018). Organised sports participation and adiposity among a cohort of adolescents over a two year period. *PLoS One, 13*(12), e0206500.

Vella, S. A., Cliff, D. P., Magee, C. A., & Okely, A. D. (2014a). Associations between sports participation and psychological difficulties during childhood: A two-year follow up. *Journal of Science and Medicine in Sport, 18*, 304–309. doi:10.1016/j.jsams.2014.05.006

Vella, S. A., Cliff, D. P., Magee, C. A., & Okely, A. D. (2014b). Sports participation and parent-reported health-related quality of life in children: Longitudinal associations. *Journal of Pediatrics, 164*(6), 1469–1474.

Vella, S. A., Cliff, D. P., & Okely, A. D. (2014). Socio-ecological predictors of participation and dropout from organised sports during childhood. *International Journal of Behavioral Nutrition and Physical Activity, 11*(1), 62.

Vella, S. A., Cliff, D. P., Okely, A. D., Scully, M., & Morley, B. (2013). Associations between organized sports participation and obesity-related health behaviors in Australian adolescents. *International Journal of Behavioral Nutrition and Physical Activity, 10*, 113.

Vella, S. A., Gardner, L. A., Swann, C., & Allen, M. S. (2018). Trajectories and predictors of risk for mental health problems throughout childhood. *Child and Adolescent Mental Health, 24*(2), 142–148.

Vella, S. A., Magee, C. A., & Cliff, D. P. (2015). Trajectories and predictors of health-related quality of life during childhood. *Journal of Pediatrics, 167*, 422–427.

Vella, S. A., Schranz, N. K., Davern, M., Hardy, L. L., Hills, A. P., Morgan, P. J., . . . Tomkinson, G. (2016). The contribution of organised sports to physical activity in Australia: Results and directions from the active healthy kids Australia 2014 report card on physical activity for children and young people. *Journal of Science and Medicine in Sport, 19*, 407–412.

Vella, S. A., Swann, C., Allen, M. S., Schweickle, M. J., & Magee, C. A. (2017). Bidirectional associations between sport involvement and mental health in adolescence. *Medicine & Science in Sports & Exercise, 49*, 687–694.

Wickel, E. E., & Eisenmann, J. C. (2007). Contribution of youth sport to total daily physical activity among 6- to 12-year old boys. *Medicine and Science in Sports and Exercise, 39*(9), 1493–1500.

INDEX

Note: **Bold** page numbers refer to tables and *italic* page numbers refer to figures.